NUTRITIONAL ASSESSMENT

NUTRITIONAL ASSESSMENT

Third Edition

Robert D. Lee, DrPH, RD
Central Michigan University

David C. Nieman, DrPH, FACSM
Appalachian State University

Boston   Burr Ridge, IL   Dubuque, IA   Madison, WI   New York   San Francisco   St. Louis
Bangkok   Bogotá   Caracas   Kuala Lumpur   Lisbon   London   Madrid   Mexico City
Milan   Montreal   New Delhi   Santiago   Seoul   Singapore   Sydney   Taipei   Toronto

McGraw-Hill Higher Education

*A Division of The **McGraw-Hill** Companies*

NUTRITIONAL ASSESSMENT, THIRD EDITION

Published by McGraw-Hill, a business unit of The McGraw-Hill Companies, Inc., 1221 Avenue of the Americas, New York, NY 10020. Copyright © 2003, 1996, 1993 by The McGraw-Hill Companies, Inc. All rights reserved. No part of this publication may be reproduced or distributed in any form or by any means, or stored in a database or retrieval system, without the prior written consent of The McGraw-Hill Companies, Inc., including, but not limited to, in any network or other electronic storage or transmission, or broadcast for distance learning.

Some ancillaries, including electronic and print components, may not be available to customers outside the United States.

This book is printed on recycled, acid-free paper containing 10% postconsumer waste.

2 3 4 5 6 7 8 9 0 QPD/QPD 0 9 8 7 6 5 4 3 2

ISBN 0–07–292731–3

Publisher: *Colin H. Wheatley*
Senior developmental editor: *Lynne M. Meyers*
Marketing manager: *Tami Petsche*
Senior project manager: *Gloria G. Schiesl*
Senior production supervisor: *Laura Fuller*
Media project manager: *Jodi K. Banowetz*
Senior media technology producer: *Barbara R. Block*
Coordinator of freelance design: *Rick D. Noel*
Cover designer: *Cynthia Crampton*
Cover imagery: *©PhotoDisc*
Lead photo research coordinator: *Carrie K. Burger*
Supplement producer: *Brenda A. Ernzen*
Compositor: *Black Dot Group*
Typeface: *10/12 Times Roman*
Printer: *Quebecor World Dubuque, IA*

Library of Congress Cataloging-in-Publication Data

Lee, Robert D.
  Nutritional assessment / Robert D. Lee, David C. Nieman. — 3rd ed.
    p.   cm.
  Includes bibliographical references and index.
  ISBN 0–07–292731–3
  1. Nutritional—Evaluation. 2. Nutrition surveys. 3. Nutrition disorders—Diagnosis.
I. Nieman, David C., 1950–. II. Title.

RC621 .L43   2003
613.2—dc21   2002067855
                                                           CIP

To Sandra and Cathy

BRIEF CONTENTS

CONTENTS

CHAPTER 4

NATIONAL DIETARY AND NUTRITION SURVEYS   111

CHAPTER 5

COMPUTERIZED DIETARY ANALYSIS SYSTEMS   144

CHAPTER 6

ANTHROPOMETRY   163

CHAPTER 7

ASSESSMENT OF THE HOSPITALIZED PATIENT   *216*

CHAPTER 8

NUTRITIONAL ASSESSMENT IN DISEASE PREVENTION   *251*

PREFACE

The ability to accurately assess nutritional status has become critically important in recent decades, as knowledge of and interest in the relationships between diet and health have increased. Nutrition researchers must be able to measure food and nutrient intake with accuracy and precision before drawing conclusions about how health and risk for disease are influenced by what we eat. Periodic monitoring of the nation's health and nutritional status is necessary to develop effective programs targeting specific health and nutrition concerns, such as high blood cholesterol levels, diabetes, food insecurity and hunger, maternal and infant malnutrition, and overweight. Awareness of these health and nutrition concerns has led the government to establish such programs as the National Cholesterol Education Program; the National Diabetes Education Program; the Food Stamp Program; the Special Supplemental Food Program for Women, Infants, and Children; and Sisters Together: Move More, Eat Better. Periodic nutritional and health monitoring provides data to determine the cost-effectiveness of such programs in attempts to preserve effective programs from changing political agendas and governmental budgetary priorities. Dietitians and physicians rely on objective measures of nutritional status before administering nutritional support to a critically ill patient and to determine that patient's responsiveness to treatment. The public is increasingly interested in the health implications of taking nutritional supplements and of knowing how much of which supplements can actually improve health and prevent disease.

The third edition of *Nutritional Assessment* addresses these and many other topics, including computerized dietary analysis systems, national surveys of dietary intake and nutritional status, assessment techniques and standards for the hospitalized patient, nutritional assessment in the prevention of such diseases as coronary heart disease and diabetes, clinical assessment, and proper counseling techniques. The third edition builds on the strengths of the first two editions and is primarily a textbook for students of dietetics and public health nutrition.

It is also intended to be a valuable reference for health professionals who interact on a regular basis with patients who have diet-related medical problems.

ORGANIZATION

We recommend that study of *Nutritional Assessment* follow the progression of the 11 chapters in the order in which they are presented. Chapter 1 gives a thorough introduction to the topic of nutritional assessment, exploring various definitions and concepts. Chapter 2 reviews the wide assortment of standards for nutrient intake, such as the Dietary Reference Intakes, the Food Exchange System, the *Dietary Guidelines for Americans,* and the Food Guide Pyramid, and it gives practical guidelines for their use.

Methods for measuring diet and the strengths and weaknesses of each technique are outlined in Chapter 3. Results from the Continuing Survey of Food Intakes by Individuals, the National Health and Nutrition Examination Survey, and other diet and nutrition surveys are interpreted in Chapter 4, and statistics on trends in the American diet are summarized. Chapter 5 reviews the use of computerized dietary analysis systems in nutritional assessment and gives guidelines for evaluating the operating features, nutrient databases, and overall strengths and weaknesses of any commercially available program.

Chapters 6 and 7 survey anthropometric techniques for both healthy and ill people, with complete descriptions of how to measure body skinfolds and circumferences and then make appropriate decisions on classification. Nutritional assessment, as it relates to prevention of coronary heart disease, hypertension, osteoporosis, and diabetes, is reviewed in Chapter 8. Seventeen laboratory tests are interpreted, and biochemical methods for assessing protein, iron, calcium, and other nutrient status are discussed in Chapter 9. Chapter 10 gives an overview of the clinical assessment of nutritional status. Chapter 11 reviews the major theories and techniques of both individual and group counseling methods.

NEW TO THIS EDITION

The numerous revisions and additions to the third edition of *Nutritional Assessment* make it the most comprehensive and up-to-date textbook available on the subject. New to this edition is discussion of the American Cancer Society's Guidelines on Nutrition and Physical Activity for Cancer Prevention, detailed information on the Dietary Reference Intakes, a review of the 2000 edition of the Dietary Guidelines for Americans, and a section on food insecurity and hunger in the United States. This edition contains details on the pediatric growth charts recently developed by the Centers for Disease Control and Prevention, new guidelines for the detection, evaluation, and treatment of high blood cholesterol from the National Cholesterol Education Program, and new diagnostic and treatment guidelines from the American Diabetes Association. There are new sections on air displacement plethysmography for assessing body composition, the bicarbonate-urea method for measuring energy expenditure, quantitative ultrasound for assessing risk for osteoporosis, and the Mini Nutritional Assessment questionnaire for assessing the nutritional status of elderly persons. Data and graphics on food and nutrient intake from national surveys have been thoroughly updated, as have the sections on the U.S. Department of Agriculture's nutrient databases and use of computers in nutritional assessment.

NUTRITIONAL ASSESSMENT WEBSITE (www.mhhe.com/leenieman)

This website provides readers with a convenient and authoritative on-line source for additional information and resources on nutritional assessment. Following the organization of the book's chapters, it contains links to private and governmental websites related to nutritional assessment, sources of data from national health and nutrition surveys, and links to suppliers of nutritional assessment equipment. It serves to update readers on new information and developments in the field of nutritional assessment as they become available. It also provides a readily accessible link to the McGraw-Hill Nutrition Website.

FEATURES

Chapter Outline

Each chapter begins with an outline of the contents of the chapter. Reading this before beginning the chapter gives the student an idea of the material to be covered, and it is a useful review tool when the student is studying for exams.

Figures and Tables

There are more than 100 tables in the text, supplemented with 160 graphs, illustations, and photographs. Figures in Chapter 4, for example, illustrate trends in food and nutrient intake based on data from national surveys such as the National Health and Nutrition Examination Survey and the Continuing Survey of Food Intakes by Individuals. Chapters 6 and 7 contain numerous photographs illustrating the exact procedures involved in skinfold measurement and other anthropometric techniques used in assessing nutritional status.

Summaries

A summary at the end of each chapter highlights all important chapter information and will be especially helpful when the student reviews for exams.

References

A complete list of up-to-date references is included at the end of each chapter. This list provides the student and instructor with extensive sources for continued study.

Assessment Activities

Most chapters end with two or three practical assessment activities to help the student better understand the concepts presented in the chapter. For example, activities are given for personal computerized dietary analysis, use of food composition tables, practice of anthropometry and one-on-one counseling, and interpretation of serum lipid and cholesterol results.

Appendixes

Appendixes A and B contain nutrient standards for the United Kingdom and the historically important U.S. Recommended Daily Allowances. Various recording forms and questionnaires used in measuring diet are presented in Appendixes C through J. Appendix K is a nutrient breakdown of more than 2000 foods. The 2001 Behavioral Risk Factor Surveillance System Questionnaire is provided in Appendix L. Appendix M lists suppliers of nutritional assessment equipment. Appendix N gives the recently revised CDC clinical growth charts for children and adolescents. Various anthropometric standards are tabled in Appendixes O through R. Appendix S provides reference data for serum lipid and lipoprotein levels for children, adolescents, and adults. Appendix T contains a form for self-monitoring dietary intake, and Appendix U has a checklist for counseling competencies.

Glossary

Throughout the text, important terms are shown in boldface type. Concise definitions for these nearly 350 terms can be found in the glossary.

ACKNOWLEDGMENTS

We would like to express our sincere gratitude to the editorial and production team at McGraw-Hill. We are particularly indebted to our wives, Sandra and Cathy, for their encouragement, support, and patience. We wish to thank those professors who served as critical reviewers of the third edition. Their suggestions have been helpful, and we are grateful for their contributions. They are

Madge N. Hanson
University of Minnesota
Maren Hegsted
Louisiana State University
Mary B. McDonald
University of Missouri, Emeritus
Phylis B. Moser-Veillon
University of Maryland

Robert D. Lee
David C. Nieman

INTRODUCTION TO NUTRITIONAL ASSESSMENT

INTRODUCTION

Until about the middle of the twentieth century, infectious disease was the leading cause of death in developed countries, and nutritional deficiencies were common. Improved sanitation, vaccine development, improved health care, and increased quality and quantity of food now have virtually eliminated infectious disease as a major killer in developed countries, and nutrient deficiency is much less common.

However, with increased life expectancy, a higher living standard, and an abundance of food has come an epidemic of chronic diseases, many of which are related to excess consumption of high-fat foods and alcoholic beverages and inadequate consumption of foods high in complex carbohydrates and fiber. This situation, along with heightened public and professional interest in the role of nutrition in health and disease, has created an increased need for health professionals proficient in nutritional assessment. The ability to identify persons at nutritional risk and to effectively enhance their health status through improved nutrition has made nutritional assessment an important tool for health professionals concerned about making health care more cost-effective.

GOOD NUTRITION ESSENTIAL FOR HEALTH

Good nutrition is critical for the well-being of any society and to each individual within that society. The variety, quality, and quantity of available food and the patterns of food consumption can profoundly affect health.

Scurvy, for example, was among the first diseases recognized as being caused by a nutritional deficiency. One of the earliest descriptions of scurvy was made in

1250 by French writer Joinville, who observed it among the troops of Louis IX at the siege of Cairo. When Vasco da Gama sailed to the East Indies around the Cape of Good Hope in 1497, more than 60% of his crew died of scurvy.[1] In 1747, James Lind, a British naval surgeon, conducted the first controlled human dietary experiment showing that consumption of citrus fruits cures scurvy.[2]

Deficiency Diseases Once Common

During the nineteenth century and the first half of the twentieth century, scurvy and other **deficiency diseases,** such as **rickets, pellagra, beriberi, xerophthalmia,** and **goiter** (caused by inadequate dietary vitamin D, niacin, thiamin, vitamin A, and iodine, respectively), were commonly seen in the United States and throughout the world and posed a significant threat to human health (Figure 1.1).[3]

Nutritional deficiencies and **infectious disease** remain serious problems in many developing countries and even among certain population groups in the United States and other developed countries.[3] Sanitation measures, improved health care, vaccine development, and mass immunization programs have dramatically reduced the incidence of infectious disease in developed nations. An abundant food supply, **fortification** of some foods with important trace nutrients, **enrichment** to replace certain nutrients lost in food processing, and better methods of determining the nutrient content of foods have made nutrient-deficiency diseases relatively uncommon in developed nations.[3] Among certain groups, however, deficiencies of certain nutrients remain a problem.[4]

Figure 1.1
Poverty in America during the economic depression of the 1930s led to limited food choices and diets lacking essential nutrients. Nutritional deficiency diseases often resulted. Poverty among certain groups in America continues to prevent them from obtaining adequate nutrition and health care.

Chronic Diseases Now Epidemic

Despite the many advances of nutritional science, nutrition-related diseases not only continue to exist but also result in a heavy toll of disease and death. In recent decades, however, they have taken a form different from the nutrient-deficiency diseases common in the early 1900s. Diseases of dietary excess and imbalance now rank among the leading causes of illness and death in America and play a prominent role in the epidemic of chronic disease that Western nations are currently experiencing.[5] In the 1988 *Surgeon General's Report on Nutrition and Health,* 5 of the 10 leading causes of death— **coronary heart disease** (heart attack), certain **cancers, stroke, diabetes mellitus,** and **atherosclerosis**—were linked with diet.[3] Table 1.1 ranks the 15 leading causes of death in 1997. Of these, 5 are linked with diet and 4 (accidents, suicide, homicide, and chronic liver disease and cirrhosis) are linked with excessive alcohol consumption.

The *Surgeon General's Report on Nutrition and Health* points out that, although these diseases are caused by a combination of dietary and nondietary factors and that the exact proportion attributable to diet is uncertain, "it is now clear that diet contributes in substantial ways to the development of these diseases and that modification of diet can contribute to their prevention."[3] The report goes on to say that "for the two out of three adult Americans who do not smoke and do not drink excessively, one personal choice seems to influence long-term health prospects more than any other: what we eat."[3] The report's main conclusion was that "overconsumption of certain dietary components is now a major concern for Americans. While many food factors are involved, chief among them is the disproportionate consumption of foods high in fats, often at the expense of foods high in complex carbohydrates and fiber that may be more conducive to health."[3]

The continuing presence of nutrition-related disease makes it essential that health professionals be able to determine the nutritional status of individuals. Both the American College of Physicians and the U.S. Preventive Services Task Force regard nutritional assessment and counseling as essential components of preventive services offered by physicians and other health professionals.[6] This will help identify persons who might benefit from nutrition intervention to improve their health and which interventions would be appropriate.

NUTRITIONAL SCREENING AND ASSESSMENT

Nutritional screening "is the process of identifying characteristics known to be associated with nutrition problems. Its purpose is to pinpoint individuals who are malnourished or at nutritional risk."[7] If nutritional screening identifies a person at nutritional risk, a more

TABLE 1.1	Estimated Deaths and Percent of Total Deaths for the 15 Leading Causes of Death, United States, 1997

Rank	Cause of Death	Number of Deaths	Percent of Total Deaths
	All causes	2,314,245	100.0
1*	Diseases of the heart	726,974	31.4
2*	Malignant neoplasms	539,577	23.3
3*	Cerebrovascular disease	159,791	6.9
4	Chronic obstructive pulmonary disease	109,029	4.7
5†	Accidents and adverse effects	95,644	4.1
6	Pneumonia and influenza	86,449	3.7
7*	Diabetes mellitus	62,636	2.7
8†	Suicide	30,535	1.3
9	Nephritis, nephrotic syndrome and nephrosis	25,331	1.1
10†	Chronic liver disease and cirrhosis	25,175	1.1
11	Alzheimer's disease	22,475	1.0
12	Septicemia	22,396	1.0
13†	Homicide and legal intervention	19,846	0.9
14	Human immunodeficiency syndrome	16,516	0.7
15*	Atherosclerosis	16,057	0.7
	All other causes	356,394	15.4

Data from the National Center for Health Statistics.

*Causes of death in which diet plays a part.

†Causes of death in which excessive alcohol consumption plays a part.

thorough evaluation of the individual's nutritional status can be performed. Nutritional screening can be done by any member of the health care team such as a dietitian, dietetic technician, dietary manager, nurse, or physician. Nutritional screening and how it fits into the nutritional care process are discussed in greater detail in Chapter 7, and examples of screening instruments are shown there.

Nutritional assessment is an evaluation of the nutritional status of individuals or populations through measurements of food and nutrient intake and evaluation of nutrition-related health indicators. The U.S. Department of Health and Human Services (DHHS) defines nutritional assessment as "the measurement of indicators of dietary status and nutrition-related health status to identify the possible occurrence, nature, and extent of impaired nutritional status," which can range from deficiency to toxicity.[4] The American Dietetic Association defines nutritional assessment as "a comprehensive approach, completed by a registered dietitian, to defining nutrition-

al status that uses medical, nutrition, and medication histories; physical examination; anthropometric measurements; and laboratory data."[7] According to the World Health Organization (WHO), the ultimate purpose of nutritional assessment is to improve human health.[8]

Nutritional Assessment Methods

Four different methods are used to collect data used in assessing a person's nutritional status: anthropometric, biochemical or laboratory, clinical, and dietary (Figure 1.2). The mnemonic "ABCD" can help you remember these different methods.

Anthropometric Methods

Anthropometry is the measurement of the physical dimensions and gross composition of the body. Examples of anthropometry include measurements of height, weight, and head circumference and the use of measurements of **skinfold thickness, body density** (underwater weighing), **air-displacement plethysmography,** and **bioelectrical impedance** to estimate the percentage of fat and lean tissue in the body. These results often are compared with standard values obtained from measurements of large numbers of subjects. Anthropometry will be covered in Chapters 6 and 8. At the end of most chapters are suggested exercises, called assessment activities, that allow you to apply the concepts covered. In the assessment activities of Chapter 6, you will try your hand at skinfold measurements to estimate percent body fat and compare several methods of determining body composition.

Biochemical Methods

In nutritional assessment, biochemical or laboratory methods includes measuring a nutrient or its metabolite in blood, feces, or urine or measuring a variety of other components in blood and other tissues that have a relationship to nutritional status. The quantity of **albumin** and other **serum proteins** frequently is regarded as an indicator of the body's protein status, and **hemoglobin** levels in blood reflect iron status. Blood **cholesterol** levels, which are influenced by diet, reflect coronary heart disease risk.

Biochemical methods are covered in Chapters 7 through 9. An assessment activity in Chapter 8 suggests that you have your blood drawn and tested at a clinical laboratory and compare your results with recommended values. Assessment activities in Chapters 7 and 9 guide you through the application of key concepts as you evaluate biochemical and other data from patient records.

Clinical Methods

The medical history and physical examination are clinical methods used to detect **signs** and **symptoms** of **malnutrition.** Symptoms are disease manifestations that the patient is usually aware of and often complains about. Signs are

Figure 1.2
Examples of the four nutritional assessment methods include (clockwise from upper left) use of a personal computer and nutritional analysis software in diet analysis (dietary methods), skinfold measurements (anthropometric methods), blood tests (biochemical methods), and physical examination (clinical methods).
Source: © Eye Wire.

observations made by a qualified examiner during physical examination. Painful cracks in the angles of the mouth, for example, may be symptomatic of riboflavin or niacin deficiency. Thyroid gland enlargement, sometimes caused by iodine deficiency, is a sign often first discovered by a physician during physical examination. Although the nutrition professional will not often collect this information, it is important to look for it in the medical record and have a keen eye to observe visible clinical signs. Such data may support and reinforce a suspected diagnosis of nutritional deficiency. Clinical signs and symptoms in nutritional assessment will be discussed in Chapter 10.

Dietary Methods

Dietary methods generally involve surveys measuring the quantity of the individual foods consumed during the course of one to several days or assessing the pattern of food use during the previous several months. These can provide data on intake of nutrients or specific classes of foods. Chapters 2 through 4 cover dietary methods. One of the assessment activities in Chapter 3 involves collecting a

24-hour dietary recall from a classmate and analyzing his or her nutrient intake using food composition tables.

Included among dietary methods is the use of the computer to analyze dietary intake. A number of programs for personal computers are available that allow nutritionists and dietitians to quickly analyze the nutrient composition of dietary intake. These programs vary widely in price and certain features, such as the number and types of different foods and nutrients each program contains. Chapter 5 covers selection and use of nutritional analysis software. The assessment activity in Chapter 5 involves computerized analysis of the 24-hour recall and 3-day food record collected as part of the assessment activities in Chapter 3.

Importance of Nutritional Assessment

The use of nutritional assessment to identify diet-related disease has increased in importance in recent years because of our greater knowledge of the relationship between nutrition and health and our expanded ability to alter the nutritional state.[9]

Evidence related to the role of diet in maternal and child health indicates that well-nourished mothers produce healthier children.[10,11] Sufficient intake of energy and nutrients, including appropriate body weight before pregnancy and adequate weight gain during pregnancy, improves infant birth weight and reduces infant **morbidity** and **mortality.** Consequently, nutritional assessment has become an integral part of maternity care at the beginning of pregnancy and periodically throughout pregnancy and lactation.[3,10,11] Nutrition also can have a profound influence on health, affecting growth and development of infants, children, and adolescents; immunity against disease; morbidity and mortality from illness or surgery; and risk of such diseases as cancer, coronary heart disease, and diabetes.[3,12]

Interventions to alter a person's nutritional state can take many forms. In certain situations, nutrient mixes can be delivered into the stomach or small intestine through feeding tubes (**enteral nutrition**) or administered directly into veins (**parenteral nutrition**) to improve nutritional status. Thus, nutritional assessment is important in identifying persons at nutritional risk, in determining what type of nutrition intervention, if any, may be appropriate to alter nutritional status, and in monitoring the effects of nutrition intervention.

OPPORTUNITIES IN NUTRITIONAL ASSESSMENT

Numerous opportunities currently exist for applying nutritional assessment skills. As our understanding of the relationships between nutrition and health increases, these opportunities will also increase. Following are some examples of areas in which nutritional assessment can make a significant contribution to health care.

Meeting the *Healthy People 2010* Objectives

The *Healthy People 2010* objectives outline a comprehensive, nationwide health promotion and disease prevention agenda designed to improve the health of all people in the United States during the first decade of the twenty-first century.[5] Like the preceding *Healthy People 2010* initiative, *Healthy People 2010* is committed to a single, overarching purpose: promoting health and preventing illness, disability, and premature death.[13] The two fundamental goals of the 2010 objectives are to increase quality and years of healthy life and to eliminate disparities in health status indicators and risk factors that are evident in many segments of the population based on gender, age, income, race, and ethnicity.[14] There are a total of 467 objectives organized into 28 focus areas, with each area representing an important public health concern. The 28 focus areas are shown in Box 1.1. Of the 467 objectives, 18 are listed in the nutrition and overweight focus area as shown in Box 1.2. Approximately 40 other nutrition-related objectives are listed under other focus areas, such as cancer, diabetes, food safety, heart disease and stroke, physical activity and fitness, and maternal, infant, and child health.

For example, meeting objective 4 (reduce growth retardation among low-income children under age 5 years) requires health professionals skillful in anthropometry and able to intelligently use various standards for assessing adequate growth. The ability to evaluate dietary intake and interpret laboratory data and physical signs and symptoms reflecting nutritional status would be

---

Box 1.1   *Healthy People 2010* **Focus Areas**

1. Access to quality health care
2. Arthritis, osteoporosis, and chronic back conditions
3. Cancer
4. Chronic kidney disease
5. Diabetes
6. Disability and secondary conditions
7. Educational and community-based programs
8. Environmental health
9. Family planning
10. Food safety
11. Health communication
12. Heart disease and stroke
13. HIV
14. Immunization and infectious diseases
15. Injury and violence prevention
16. Maternal, infant, and child health
17. Medical product safety
18. Mental health and mental disorders
19. Nutrition and overweight
20. Occupational safety and health
21. Oral health
22. Physical activity and fitness
23. Public health infrastructure
24. Respiratory diseases
25. Sexually transmitted diseases
26. Substance abuse
27. Tobacco use
28. Vision and hearing

From U.S. Department of Health and Human Services. 2000. *Healthy People 2010: Objectives for improving health.* Washington, DC: U.S. Government Printing Office.

Box 1.2   *Healthy People 2010* **Objectives for the Nutrition and Overweight Focus Area**

1. Increase the proportion of adults who are at a healthy weight.
2. Reduce the proportion of adults who are obese.
3. Reduce the proportion of children and adolescents who are overweight or obese.
4. Reduce growth retardation among low-income children under age 5 years.
5. Increase the proportion of persons aged 2 years and older who consume at least two daily servings of fruit.
6. Increase the proportion of persons aged 2 years and older who consume at least three daily servings of vegetables, with at least one-third being dark green or deep yellow vegetables.
7. Increase the proportion of persons aged 2 years and older who consume at least six daily servings of grain products, with at least three being whole grains.
8. Increase the proportion of persons aged 2 years and older who consume less than 10% of calories from saturated fat.
9. Increase the proportion of persons aged 2 years and older who consume no more than 30% of calories from fat.
10. Increase the proportion of persons aged 2 years and older who consume 2,400 mg or less of sodium daily.
11. Increase the proportion of persons aged 2 years and older who meet dietary recommendations for calcium.
12. Reduce iron deficiency among young children and females of childbearing age.
13. Reduce anemia among low-income pregnant females in their third trimester.
14. Reduce iron deficiency among pregnant females.
15. Increase the proportion of children and adolescents aged 6 to 19 years whose intake of meals and snacks at schools contributes proportionally to good overall dietary quality.
16. Increase the proportion of worksites that offer nutrition or weight management classes or counseling.
17. Increase the proportion of physician office visits made by patients with a diagnosis of cardiovascular disease, diabetes, or hyperlipidemia that include counseling or education related to diet and nutrition.
18. Increase food security among U.S. households and in so doing reduce hunger.

From U.S. Department of Health and Human Services. 2000. *Healthy People 2010: Objectives for improving health.* Washington, DC: U.S. Government Printing Office.

important in understanding some of the causes of diminished growth and in planning interventions to improve growth. Objective 9 (increase the proportion of persons aged 2 years and older who consume no more than 30% of calories from fat) requires a working knowledge of dietary survey methods to initially assess fat intake and to monitor long-term adherence to the objective.

In Hospitals

Hospitals continue to offer many opportunities for health professionals trained in nutritional assessment. **Protein-energy malnutrition (PEM),** an excessive loss of lean body mass resulting from inadequate consumption of energy and/or protein or resulting from the increased energy and nutrient requirements of certain diseases, is commonly seen in residents of long-term care facilities and patients of acute-care hospitals.[15] Depending on the criteria used, the reported prevalence of PEM in long-term facilities ranges from 19% to 27%, while in acute-care hospitals the prevalence ranges from 33% to 58%.[15] One nutrition researcher characterized this situation by saying, "Malnutrition is the skeleton in the hospital's closet."[16]

Although the relationship between malnutrition and hospital outcome often is obscured by other factors that can affect the outcome of a patient's hospital stay (for example, the nature and severity of the disease process), several researchers have reported that patients with PEM tend to have a longer hospital stay, a higher incidence of complications, and a higher mortality rate.[17–20]

Identifying patients at nutritional risk is a major activity necessary for providing cost-effective medical treatment and helping contain health care costs.[7] Good medical practice and economic considerations make it imperative that hospital patients be nutritionally assessed and that steps be taken, if necessary, to improve their nutritional status. Evaluation of a patient's weight, height, midarm muscle area, and triceps skinfold thickness and values from various laboratory tests can be valuable aids in assessing protein and energy nutriture. Some researchers believe that rapid, nonpurposeful weight loss is the single best predictor of malnutrition currently available.[9] These and other assessment techniques for hospitalized patients will be discussed in detail in Chapter 8.

Diabetes Mellitus

Nutritional assessment has been an important component of managing diabetes in recent decades. However, nutritional assessment plays a major role in the American Diabetes Association's most recent nutrition recommendations and principles for people with diabetes.[21] Goals for the person with diabetes are based on dietary history, nutrient intake, and clinical data. A thorough knowledge of the patient gained through nutritional assessment will assist the dietitian—the primary provider of nutrition therapy—in guiding the patient to a successful treatment outcome. The role of nutritional assessment in managing diabetes is discussed further in Chapter 8.

Weight Management

According to the *Dietary Guidelines for Americans,*[22] a healthy weight range for most adults is defined as a body mass index, or BMI (weight in kilograms divided by height in meters squared), ≥ 18.5 kg/m^2 to < 25 kg/m^2. **Overweight** is defined as a BMI ≥ 25 kg/m^2 to < 30 kg/m^2, while **obesity** is defined as a BMI ≥ 30 kg/m^2. Based on these definitions, 59.4% of U.S. adult males and 49.9% of U.S. adult females are considered either overweight or obese (i.e., they have a BMI ≥ 25 kg/m^2), while 19.9% of U.S. adult males and 25.1% of U.S. adult females are considered obese (i.e., they have a BMI ≥ 30 kg/m^2), as shown in Figure 1.3.[23] Between the years 1976–1994 and 1988–1994, the percentage of U.S. adults considered overweight increased from 46% to 54.6%, respectively. During the same periods, the percentage of U.S. adults considered obese increased from 14.5% to 22.6%.

Using the same definitions, it is estimated that more than half of European adults age 35 to 65 years are either overweight or obese.[24] Throughout North America and Europe, overweight is more common among adult males than adult females while obesity is more common among adult females.

One of the *Healthy People 2010* objectives is to increase the **prevalence** of U.S. adults age 20 years or older who are at a healthy weight from the current proportion of approximately 42% who are at a healthy

weight to the target of 60%.[14] According to the 1996 state-based Behavioral Risk Factor Surveillance System (discussed in Chapter 4), 28.8% and 35.1% of U.S. adult males and females, respectively, reported that they were attempting to lose weight.[25] The 1996 Behavioral Risk Factor Surveillance System also showed that, among those who reported that they were attempting to lose weight, 21.5% of adult males and 19.4% of adult females reported using a combination of eating fewer kilocalories and exercising 150 minutes or more per week. Among adult males attempting to lose weight, the median self-reported weight was 90.4 kg (199 lb) and the goal weight was 81.4 kg (179 lb), with a median difference of 8.6 kg (19 lb), which is 9% of current body weight. Among adult females attempting to lose, the median self-reported weight was 70.3 kg (155 lb) and the goal weight was 59.0 kg (130 lb), with a median difference of 8.9 kg (19.6 lb), which is 13% of current body weight. In addition, data from the survey show that, among U.S. adult females who reported having a BMI in the health range, 28.7% reported trying to lose weight.

National surveys provide important nutritional assessment data, such as prevalence of overweight and obesity in a particular population. Dietary methods can be valuable in initially assessing the quantity and quality of caloric intake and in monitoring dietary intake throughout treatment for obesity. Anthropometry is important in monitoring changes in percent body fat to help ensure that decrements in weight primarily come from body fat stores and that losses of lean body mass (mostly viscera and skeletal muscle) are minimized. Techniques for monitoring changes in percent body fat will be discussed in Chapter 6.

Figure 1.3 Prevalence of overweight American adults, 1960 to 1994.
In the past several decades, the prevalence of overweight among American adults has increased, particularly since the late 1970s. Currently, more than half of all American adults are considered overweight.
Source: Data from the National Center for Health Statistics.

Heart Disease and Cancer

Heart disease and cancer are the first and second leading causes of death in the United States, respectively. Together they accounted for 54.7% of all deaths in 1997. Dietary factors playing a major role in heart disease are high intake of saturated fat, high intake of dietary cholesterol, and an imbalance between energy intake and energy expenditure leading to obesity.

Categories of coronary heart disease (CHD) risk factors are shown in Box 1.3. The "causative risk factors" are the major causal risk factors for CHD. When these are modified, CHD risk is reduced.[26,27] They can account for as much as 90% of the increased CHD risk in persons having these risk factors when compared with nonsmokers who have optimally low levels of blood pressure and total cholesterol, relatively high levels of high-density lipoprotein cholesterol, and no diabetes.[27] The "conditional risk factors" are correlated with CHD risk, but there are insufficient data from large, prospective studies to accurately quantify the extent to which these factors increase CHD risk.

The "predisposing risk factors" contribute to the development of CHD by intensifying or worsening the effects of the causative and conditional risk factors. According to the American Heart Association, two of these, obesity (particularly abdominal obesity) and physical inactivity are considered major risk factors because they are so strongly related to increased risk of CHD. Abdominal obesity is a particularly strong risk factor in postmenopausal women. Here it is defined as a waist circumference > 102 cm (> 40 in.) in males and > 88 cm (> 35 in.) in females. Several of these factors (e.g., elevated blood pressure, diabetes, overweight and obesity, and serum levels of total and LDL-cholesterol, triglycerides, and homocysteine) are related to diet.

Despite a decline of more than 50% in the **age-adjusted death rate** since the 1970s, heart disease remains the leading cause of death in the United States and accounts for 31% of all deaths. Because dietary therapy is the cornerstone of lowering blood cholesterol, nutritional assessment skills are vitally important in its management. Proficiency in measuring diet, for example, would enable a dietitian to assess a client's consumption of saturated fat and cholesterol and suggest appropriate dietary changes. Chapter 3 includes a discussion of a questionnaire for assessing adherence to a cholesterol-lowering diet. Chapter 8 covers nutritional assessment in preventing heart disease.

Cancer is largely a preventable disease and causes nearly 25% of all deaths in North America. In the United States, it is responsible for more than a half-million deaths annually.[28] Roughly two-thirds of all cancer deaths in the United States are linked to tobacco use, obesity, physical inactivity, and certain dietary choices, all of which can be modified by both individual and societal action. The percentage of cancer deaths attributable to dietary factors is estimated to be 35%, with a range of 10% to 70%.[29]

The American Cancer Society guidelines on nutrition and physical activity for cancer prevention are shown in Box 1.4.[30] Methods for assessing dietary levels of fruits, vegetables, cereals, legumes, meats and other animal products, and alcoholic beverages will be necessary in applying these guidelines, as will anthropometric skills.

 Box 1.3   **Categories of Coronary Heart Disease Risk Factors***

Causative Risk Factors

- Cigarette smoking
- Elevated blood pressure
- Elevated serum total cholesterol or elevated serum low-density lipoprotein cholesterol
- Low serum high-density lipoprotein cholesterol
- Diabetes
- Advancing age

Conditional Risk Factors

- Serum triglycerides[†]
- Small low-density lipoprotein particles[†]
- Serum lipoprotein (a)[†]
- Serum homocysteine[†]
- Factors promoting blood coagulation[†]
- Inflammatory markers

Predisposing Risk Factors

- Overweight and obesity[‡]
- Abdominal obesity[‡]
- Physical inactivity[‡]
- Male sex
- Family history of premature coronary heart disease
- Socioeconomic factors
- Behavioral factors (e.g., mental depression)
- Insulin resistance

*A more detailed discussion of this box can be found in Chapter 8.
†These are considered conditional risk factors when serum levels are high.
‡Obesity and physical inactivity are considered major risk factors by the American Heart Association.

Adapted from Smith SC, Greenland P, Grundy SM. 2000. Prevention Conference V: Beyond secondary prevention: Identifying the high-risk patient for primary prevention: Executive summary. *Circulation* 101:111–116.

Box 1.4   **The American Cancer Society Guidelines on Nutrition and Physical Activity for Cancer Prevention**

RECOMMENDATIONS FOR INDIVIDUAL CHOICES

1. Eat a variety of healthful foods, with an emphasis on plant sources.
   - Eat five or more servings of vegetables and fruits each day.
   - Choose whole grains in preference to processed (refined) grains and sugars.
   - Limit consumption of red meats, especially high-fat and processed meats.
   - Choose foods that help maintain a healthful weight.

2. Adopt a physically active lifestyle.
   - Adults: Engage in at least moderate activity for 30 minutes or more on five or more days of the week; 45 minutes or more of moderate-to-vigorous activity on five or more days per week may further enhance reductions in the risk of breast and colon cancer.

- Children and adolescents: Engage in at least 60 minutes per day of moderate-to-vigorous physical activity at least five days per week.

3. Maintain a healthful weight throughout life.
   - Balance caloric intake with physical activity.
   - Lose weight if currently overweight or obese.

4. If you drink alcoholic beverages, limit consumption.

RECOMMENDATION FOR COMMUNITY ACTION

Public, private, and community organizaions should work to create social and physical environments that support the adoption and maintenance of healthful nutrition and physical activity behaviors.

- Increase access to healthful foods in schools, worksites, and communities.
- Provide safe, enjoyable, and accessible environments for physical activity in schools and for transportation and recreation in communities.

From American Cancer Society. 2002. *Cancer prevention and early detection facts and figures—2002*. Atlanta, GA: American Cancer Society.

Nutrition Monitoring

Nutrition monitoring is defined as "those activities necessary to provide timely information about the contributions of food and nutrient consumption and nutritional status to the health of the U.S. population."[31] A milestone in nutrition monitoring in the United States was passage of the National Nutrition Monitoring and Related Research Act of 1990. Key provisions of the act were development of a 10-year comprehensive plan for coordinating the activities of 22 federal agencies involved in nutrition monitoring and assurance of the collaboration and coordination of nutrition monitoring at federal, state, and local levels.[31] This included all data collection and analysis activities associated with health and nutrition status measurements, food composition measurements, dietary knowledge, attitude assessment, and surveillance of the food supply.[4] Considerable nutritional assessment expertise is required for administering such surveys as the National Health and Nutrition Examination Survey and the Continuing Surveys of Food Intakes by Individuals. These will be discussed in Chapter 4.

Nutritional Epidemiology

Practically all nutrition research undertaken by universities, private industry, and government involves some aspect of nutritional assessment. An understanding of the theory behind assessment techniques, an awareness of the strengths and weaknesses of assessment methods, and proficiency in their use are essential skills for anyone currently involved in or contemplating a career in **nutritional epidemiology.**

For example, to arrive at valid conclusions about the relationships between the intake of antioxidant nutrients, such as β-carotene, and risk of cancer or heart disease, nutritional epidemiologists need to know which methods best assess β-carotene nutriture and how to appropriately use those methods. Failing to do so, they would likely arrive at erroneous conclusions and disseminate inaccurate information about diet-health relationships. Methods for measuring diet are discussed in Chapter 3, and measurement of vitamin A status is presented in Chapter 9.

Epidemiologists examining the prevention and treatment of **osteoporosis** must understand, among other things, the strengths and weaknesses of various techniques to assess changes in bone mineralization. Such techniques will be discussed in Chapter 8. Researchers investigating the influence of diet and/or exercise on weight loss and changes in percent body fat use a variety of dietary and anthropometric methods to monitor caloric intake and changes in weight and body composition.

Major limitations of research investigating the relationship between diet and disease are uncertainty in measuring diet and inadequate information on the quantity of certain nutrients and components in food.[32,33] Consequently, there is considerable need for improved methods of measuring diet and assessing the body's vitamin and mineral status, as well as a need for better data on the nutrient composition of foods.

SUMMARY

1. The relationship between nutrition and health has long been recognized. Scientific evidence confirming this relationship began accumulating as early as the mid-eighteenth century, when James Lind showed that consumption of citrus fruits cured scurvy.

2. During the nineteenth and first half of the twentieth centuries, infectious disease was the leading cause of death throughout the world, and nutrient-deficiency diseases were common. Because of sanitation measures, improved health care, vaccine development, mass immunization programs, and an improved food supply, infectious disease is no longer the leading cause of death in developed nations, and nutrient deficiency is relatively uncommon.

3. The current leading causes of death are chronic diseases, such as coronary heart disease, cancer, and stroke. Although a number of factors are responsible, diet contributes in substantial ways to the development of these diseases, and modification of diet can contribute to their prevention. Diet plays a prominent role in 5 of the 15 leading causes of death in America. Excessive alcohol consumption is a factor in at least another 4 of the 15.

4. The main conclusion of the 1988 *Surgeon General's Report on Nutrition and Health* is that "overconsumption of certain dietary components is now a major concern for Americans. While many food factors are involved, chief among them is the disproportionate consumption of foods high in fats, often at the expense of foods high in complex carbohydrates and fiber that may be more conducive to health."

5. The continuing presence of nutrition-related disease makes it important that health professionals be able to assess nutritional status to identify who might benefit from nutrition intervention and which interventions would be appropriate.

6. Nutritional screening allows persons who are at nutritional risk to be identified, so that a more thorough evaluation of the individual's nutritional status can be performed. Nutritional assessment is an attempt to evaluate the nutritional status of individuals or populations through measurements of food and nutrient intake and nutrition-related health. Nutritional assessment techniques can be classified according to four types: anthropometric, biochemical or laboratory, clinical, and dietary. Use of the mnemonic "ABCD" can help in remembering these four types.

7. Our expanded ability to alter the nutritional state of a patient and our increased knowledge of the relationship between nutrition and health has made nutritional assessment an important tool in health care.

8. Objectives related to nutrition and health have a prominent place in the *Healthy People 2010* objectives. Skill in applying nutritional assessment techniques will play a major part in the health professional's efforts to help achieve those objectives.

9. It is estimated that as many as one-quarter of all patients in long-term care facilities and half of all patients in acute-care hospitals suffer from protein-energy malnutrition (PEM). Patients with PEM tend to have longer hospital stays and higher incidence of complications and mortality. Relatively simple techniques often can identify patients at nutritional risk.

10. Nutritional assessment is now a major component of the American Diabetes Association's nutrition recommendations and principles for people with diabetes.

11. Nutritional assessment also plays a significant role in identifying diet-related risk factors for heart disease and cancer and in monitoring efforts to reduce risk.

12. Nutritional assessment is central to current government efforts to monitor and improve the nutritional status of its citizens. It is also a skill essential for nutritional epidemiologists and other nutrition researchers investigating links between diet and health.

REFERENCES

1. Todhunter EN. 1976. Chronology of some events in the development and application of the science of nutrition. *Nutrition Reviews* 34:353–365.

2. Todhunter EN. 1962. Development of knowledge in nutrition. *Journal of the American Dietetic Association* 41:335–340.

3. U.S. Department of Health and Human Services. 1988. *The surgeon general's report on nutrition and health.* Washington, DC: U.S. Government Printing Office.

4. Federation of American Societies for Experimental Biology, Life Sciences Research Office. Prepared for the Interagency Board for Nutrition Monitoring and Related Research. 1995. *Third report on nutrition monitoring in the United*

States. Washington, DC: U.S. Government Printing Office.

5. U.S. Department of Health and Human Services. 2000. *Healthy People 2010: Understanding and improving health.* Washington, DC: U.S. Government Printing Office.

6. U.S. Department of Health and Human Services. 1995. *Guide to clinical preventive services,* 2nd ed. Washington, DC: Office of Public Health and Science, Office of Disease Prevention and Health Promotion.

7. Posthauer ME, Dorse B, Foiles RA, et al. 1994. ADA's definitions for nutrition screening and nutrition assessment. *Journal of the American Dietetic Association* 94:838–839.

8. Beghin I, Cap M, Dujardin B. 1988. *A guide to nutritional assessment.* Geneva, Switzerland: World Health Organization.

9. Starker PM. 1990. Nutritional assessment of the hospitalized patient. *Advances in Nutritional Research* 8:109–118.

10. National Academy of Sciences. 1991. *Nutrition during pregnancy.* Washington, DC: National Academy Press.

11. National Academy of Sciences. 1991. *Nutrition during lactation.* Washington, DC: National Academy Press.

12. Shils ME, Olson JA, Shike M, Ross AC. 1999. *Modern nutrition in health and disease,* 9th ed. Baltimore, MD: Williams & Wilkins.

13. Marwick C. 2000. Healthy People 2010 initiative launched. *Journal of the American Medical Association* 283:989–990.

14. U.S. Department of Health and Human Services. 2000. *Healthy People 2010: Objectives for improving health.* Washington, DC: U.S. Government Printing Office.

15. Dwyer JT. 1991. *Screening older Americans' nutritional health: Current practices and future possibilities.* Washington, DC: Nutrition Screening Initiative.

16. Butterworth CE. 1974. The skeleton in the hospital closet. *Nutrition Today* 9:4–8.

17. Hensrud DD. 1999. Nutrition screening and assessment. *Medical Clinics of North America* 83:1526–1546.

18. Jeejeebhoy KN. 1998. Nutritional assessment. *Gastroenterological Clinics of North America* 27:347–369.

19. Bickford GR, Brugler LJ, Dolsen S, Vickery CE. 1999. Nutrition assessment outcomes: A strategy to improve health care. *Clinical Laboratory Management Review* 13:357–364.

20. Berry JK, Braunschweig CA. 1998. Nutritional assessment of the critically ill patient. *Critical Care Nursing Quarterly* 21:33–46.

21. American Diabetes Association. 2002. Evidence-based nutrition principles and recommendations for the treatment and prevention of diabetes and related complications. *Diabetes Care* 25:S50–S60.

22. U.S. Department of Agriculture/ U.S. Department of Health and Human Services. 2000. *Nutrition and your health: Dietary guidelines for Americans,* 5th ed. Washington, DC: U.S. Government Printing Office.

23. National Center for Health Statistics. 1999. *Health, United States, 1999 with health and aging chartbook.* Washington, DC: U.S. Government Printing Office.

24. Seidell JS, Flegal KM. 1997. Assessing obesity: Classification and epidemiology. *British Medical Bulletin* 53:238–252.

25. Serdula MK, Mokdad AH, Williamson DF, Galuska DA, Mendlein JM, Heath GW. 1999. Prevalence of attempting weight loss and strategies for controlling weight. *Journal of the American Medical Association* 282:1353–1358.

26. Smith SC, Greenland P, Grundy SM. 2000. Prevention Conference V: Beyond secondary prevention: Identifying the high-risk patient for primary prevention: Executive summary. *Circulation* 101: 111–116.

27. Grundy SM, Bazzarre T, Cleeman J, D'Agostino RB, Hill M, Houston-Miller N, et al. 2000. Prevention Conference V: Beyond secondary prevention: Identifying the high-risk patient for primary prevention: Medical office assessment: Writing group I. *Circulation* 101:e3–e11.

28. Greenlee RT, Murray T, Bolden S, Wingo PA. 2000. Cancer statistics, 2000. *CA-A Cancer Journal for Clinicians* 50:7–33.

29. Doll R, Peto R. 1981. The causes of cancer: Quantitative estimates of avoidable risks of cancer in the United States today. *Journal of the National Cancer Institute* 66:1191–1308.

30. American Cancer Society. 2000. *Cancer facts and figures—2000:* Atlanta, GA: American Cancer Society.

31. Kuczmarski MF, Moshfegh A, Briefel R. 1994. Update on nutrition monitoring activities in the United States. *Journal of the American Dietetic Association* 94:753–760.

32. Mertz W, Tsui JC, Judd JT, Reiser S, Hallfrisch J, Morris ER, Steele PD, Lashley E. 1991. What are people really eating? The relation between energy intake derived from estimated diet records and intake determined to maintain body weight. *American Journal of Clinical Nutrition* 54:291–295.

33. National Research Council. 1989. *Diet and health—Implications for reducing chronic disease risk.* Washington, DC: National Academy Press.

2

STANDARDS FOR NUTRIENT INTAKE

INTRODUCTION

This chapter discusses a variety of standards for evaluating the quality of nutrient intake of groups and individuals. Although most of these guidelines originally were designed to serve as standards for nutritional adequacy, to aid in diet planning, or to improve nutritional and health status, they are also useful as standards for evaluating levels and proportions of macronutrients, micronutrients, and various food components in diets.

Prominent among these standards is the Dietary Reference Intakes. You will learn how the Dietary Reference Intakes evolved from early dietary standards, what their intended purposes are, what some of the problems encountered with their application are, and what future plans are for their revision. We will discuss the Reference Daily Intakes and Daily Reference Values developed by the Food and Drug Administration (FDA) for food labeling purposes and briefly consider nutritional labeling of food. You will learn what nutrient density is, how it is calculated, and how it can be used to evaluate dietary intake. This chapter also will discuss how the food exchange system can be used to plan meals and quickly approximate energy and macronutrient intake. Another important standard discussed in this chapter is the report *Healthy People 2000,* which outlines the U.S. health objectives for the year 2000. This chapter's assessment activities will give you the opportunity to develop a greater working knowledge of recommended nutrient intake standards, the index of nutritional quality, and the food exchange system.

Recognition of diet's role in health and disease has led to numerous efforts in the past several decades to formulate dietary guidelines and goals to promote health and prevent disease. A clear consensus has developed among most dietary guidelines and goals: dietary patterns are important factors in several of the leading causes of death, and dietary modifications can, in a number of instances, reduce one's risk of premature disease and death. Nutritional assessment is pivotal to improving dietary intake, thus reducing disease risk and improving health.

EARLY DIETARY STANDARDS AND RECOMMENDATIONS

The earliest formal dietary standard was established in the British Merchant Seaman's Act of 1835. The act made the provision of lemon juice (known as "lime juice") compulsory in the rations of British merchant seamen. This action followed the 1753 treatise by British naval surgeon James Lind stating that citrus fruits cure scurvy and the introduction in 1796 of lemon juice for the British Navy.[1] Throughout the remainder of the nineteenth century, dietary standards for protein, carbohydrates, and fat were proposed by scientists in Europe, the United Kingdom, and North America. These dietary standards had two things in common. First, the catalyst for their development was the occurrence of starvation and the diseases associated with it, resulting from economic dislocation and unemployment.[1,2] Second, they were, for the most part, **observational standards** because they were based on *observed* intakes rather than *measured* needs.[1]

Observational Standards

Carl Voit, a distinguished German physiologist of the late 1800s, made extensive observations of the amounts and kinds of foods eaten by German laborers and soldiers. He concluded that the nutritional needs of a 70-**kilogram (kg)** male of his day doing moderate work would be met by a diet containing 118 g of protein, 500 g of carbohydrate, and 56 g of fat—a total of approximately 3,000 **kilocalories (kcal).**[3] In 1895, W. O. Atwater, a notable American physiologist and nutrition researcher who studied in Germany under Voit, observed the dietary habits of Americans. He recommended that men weighing 70 kg (154 lb) consume 3,400 kcal and 125 g of protein each day.[2,3] For men engaged in more strenuous occupations, Voit and Atwater recommended 145 g and 150 g of protein per day, respectively. Rather than representing the actual physiological needs of the body, these recommendations were based on observations of what people eat when guided by their appetites and financial resources.[3]

One notable exception to the observational nature of dietary standards of the nineteenth century was the work of Edward Smith, a British physician and scientist. Smith conducted a dietary survey of unemployed British workers to determine what kind of diet would maintain health at the lowest cost.[2] His suggested allowances for protein, carbohydrate, and fat were based on actual laboratory measurements of caloric need and nitrogen excretion, as well as clinical observations that included absence of edema and anemia, "firmness of muscle, elasticity of spirits, capability for exertion."[1] Smith recommended approximately 3,000 kcal of energy and 81 g of protein per day and believed that a diet adequate in calories and protein also would provide sufficient quantities of other necessary nutrients.[1,2]

Beginnings of Scientifically Based Dietary Standards

Advances in the early twentieth century in the ability to more accurately estimate actual energy and nutrient needs led to recommendations based on physiologic requirements for protein, carbohydrate, and fat. At the same time, tremendous strides were made in understanding the role of vitamins and minerals in human nutrition.[4] This led to a reassessment and scaling down of protein recommendations in standards established during the 1920s and 1930s by the United Kingdom, America, and the League of Nations. There was also an effort to include recommendations for vitamins and minerals and to make allowances for nutritional needs during pregnancy, lactation, and growth.[2]

Concern about limited resources worldwide and food shortages in European countries during World War I led the British Royal Society to appoint a committee to establish a standard for human energy needs. After reviewing the energy expenditure data of several scientists, the Royal Society Committee accepted the results of calorimetry research conducted by G. Lusk as applicable to the population of the United Kingdom. Lusk recommended 3,000 kcal/day as an average energy requirement for adult males, with an appropriate adjustment for the needs of women and children. This standard also was used in estimating food requirements for the United Kingdom, France, and Italy as a basis for American food exports to these countries during World War I. In addition, the Royal Society Committee recommended that daily protein intake for adult males not fall below 70 g to 80 g, with no less than 25% of calories coming from fat. The committee made no specific recommendation for vitamins and minerals, but it recommended that "processed" foods should not be allowed to constitute a large proportion of the diet and that all diets should include a "certain proportion" of fresh fruits and green vegetables.[1]

The economic depression following the stock market crash in 1929 was the impetus for several dietary standards developed by the United Kingdom, the League of Nations, and the United States. Foremost among these was the standard proposed by Hazel Steibeling of the USDA in 1933. Hers was the first dietary standard to make deliberate recommendations for minerals and vitamins and maintenance of health rather than maintenance of work capacity.[2] In addition to energy and protein, the desirable amounts of calcium, phosphorus, iron, and vitamins A and C were stated. In 1939, these recommendations were expanded to include thiamin and riboflavin.[1]

Beginning in 1935, the League of Nations Technical Commission issued a series of dietary recommendations that were less concerned with defining requirements of food constituents than with outlining desirable allowances of the "protective" foods that had been lacking in so many diets.[1] Consumption of such foods as fruits, leafy vegetables, milk, eggs, fish, and meat was encouraged. These were among what outstanding American biochemist E.V. McCollum termed "protective foods," because of his early observations that they tend to protect against nutritional deficiencies. The recommendations also raised questions about the use of refined sugar, milled grain, and other foods low in vitamins and minerals.[2]

In 1939, the Canadian Council on Nutrition established a Canadian Dietary Standard. Based in part on the recommendations of the League of Nations and on information gathered by the Royal Society Committee, it included recommendations for calories, protein, fat, calcium, iron, iodine, ascorbic acid, and vitamin D.

RECOMMENDED DIETARY ALLOWANCES

In 1940, the U.S. federal government established the Committee of Food and Nutrition under the National

Research Council of the National Academy of Sciences in Washington, DC. In 1941, this committee was established on a permanent basis and renamed the Food and Nutrition Board.[2] The role of the committee was to advise government agencies on problems relating to food and nutrition of the people and on nutrition problems in connection with national defense.[5,6] In 1941, the committee prepared the first Recommended Dietary Allowances (RDAs), as shown in Table 2.1, "to serve as a guide for planning adequate nutrition for the civilian population of the United States."[7] However, it was not until 1943 that the first officially published edition of RDAs appeared.[2] To reflect advances in nutritional science, the RDAs were revised approximately every 5 years until 1989, when the 10th and last edition of *Recommended Dietary Allowances* was released.[8] The 10th edition of the RDAs provided recommendations for energy, protein, 3 electrolytes, 13 vitamins, and 12 minerals.

In essence, the RDAs have served as recommendations for nutrient intakes for 18 life stage and gender groups (life stage considers age and, when appropriate, pregnancy and lactation). The RDAs have accounted for individual differences in nutrient requirements and have included a fairly large margin of safety (i.e., they were set at a level considerably greater than the minimal requirement necessary to prevent deficiency disease).[9] They have been defined as "the levels of intake of essential nutrients that, on the basis of scientific knowledge, are judged by the Food and Nutrition Board to be adequate to meet the known nutrient needs of practically all healthy persons."[8] The first edition of *Recommended Dietary Allowances* was published with the objective of "providing standards to serve as a goal for good nutrition" and to serve as a guide for advising "on nutrition problems in connection with national defense."[8] However, since their inception, the RDAs have been used for a variety of other purposes for which they were not originally intended. These include use in labeling food, evaluating dietary survey data, planning and procuring food supplies for groups, planning food and nutrition information and education programs, and serving as a nutritional benchmark in the Food Stamp Program; the Special Supplemental Food Program for Women, Infants, and Children (WIC); and the School Lunch Program.

For more than 5 decades, the RDAs have served as the premier nutrient standard, not only for the United States but also for many other countries throughout the developed and developing world. However, as our understanding of human nutrition has increased and as nutritional concerns have changed in recent decades, limitations in the RDAs have become apparent. For example, an underlying intent of the RDAs has been to prevent deficiency disease. In recent decades, as chronic degenerative diseases have supplanted infectious and nutrient-deficiency diseases as the leading causes of death, there has been growing interest in the role of diet and nutrition

TABLE 2.1 | The 1941 Recommended Dietary Allowances for Specific Nutrients*

	Kilocalories	Protein (Grams)	Calcium (Grams)	Iron (Milligrams)	Vitamin A† (IU‡)	Thiamin (Milligrams)	Ascorbic Acid (Milligrams)	Riboflavin (Milligrams)	Nicotinic Acid (Milligrams)	Vitamin D (IU)
Man (70 kg)										
Moderately active	3000	70	0.8	12	5000	1.8	75	2.7	18	§
Very active	4500	70	0.8	12	5000	2.3	75	3.3	23	
Sedentary	2500	70	0.8	12	5000	1.5	75	2.2	15	
Woman (56 kg)										
Moderately active	2500	60	0.8	12	5000	1.5	70	2.2	15	§
Very active	3000	60	0.8	12	5000	1.8	70	2.7	18	
Sedentary	2100	60	0.8	12	5000	1.2	70	1.8	12	
Pregnancy (latter half)	2500	85	1.5	15	6000	1.8	100	2.5	18	400–800
Lactation	3000	100	2.0	15	8000	2.3	150	3.0	23	400–800
Children up to 12 Years										
Under 1 year‖	100 per kg	3–4 per kg	1.0	6	1500	0.4	30	0.6	4	400–800
1–3 years¶	1200	40	1.0	7	2000	0.6	35	0.9	6	§
4–6 years	1600	50	1.0	8	2500	0.8	50	1.2	8	
7–9 years	2000	60	1.0	10	3500	1.0	60	1.5	10	
10–12 years	2500	70	1.2	12	4500	1.2	75	1.8	12	
Children over 12 Years										
Girls: 14–15 years	2800	80	1.3	15	5000	1.4	80	2.0	14	§
6–20 years	2400	75	1.0	15	5000	1.2	80	1.8	12	
Boys: 13–15 years	3200	85	1.4	15	5000	1.6	90	2.4	16	§
16–20 years	3800	100	1.4	15	6000	2.0	100	3.0	20	§

*These are tentative allowances toward which to aim in planning practical dietaries. These allowances can be met by a good diet of natural foods that will also provide other minerals and vitamins, the requirements for which are less well known.
†Requirements may be less than the amounts stated if provided as vitamin A and greater if the source is chiefly the pro-vitamin carotene.
‡IU = International Units.
§Vitamin D is undoubtedly necessary for older children and adults. When not available from sunshine, it should be provided probably up to the minimal amounts recommended for infants.
‖Needs of infants increase from month to month. The amounts given are for infants approximately 6 to 18 months of age. The amounts of protein and calcium needed are less if from breast milk.
¶Allowances are based on the middle year for each group (as 2, 5, 8, etc.) and for moderate activity.

in decreasing chronic disease risk, conditions that the RDAs fail to adequately address. For example, the RDAs provide no recommendations for carbohydrate, dietary fibers, total fat, saturated fat, or cholesterol. There are no nutrient recommendations for older persons and no recommendations for food components that are not traditionally defined as nutrients (e.g., phytonutrients, aspartame, caffeine, and alcohol).[10] In addition, the recommended nutrient intake levels of the RDAs are generally limited to amounts obtainable through diet alone, and there is no guidance on the safe and effective use of vitamin, mineral, and other nutrient supplements, despite considerable public interest in use of such supplements.

Consequently, there arose a need for a more comprehensive set of nutritional and dietary standards that adequately address more contemporary nutritional concerns. In response, the Food and Nutrition Board, working in conjunction with scientists from the Canadian Institute of Nutrition and Health Canada, developed a new and expanded set of nutrient intakes known as the Dietary Reference Intakes.[10–12]

DIETARY REFERENCE INTAKES

The Dietary Reference Intakes (DRIs) are defined as "reference values that are quantitative estimates of nutrient intakes to be used for planning and assessing diets for apparently healthy people."[12] As shown in Box 2.1, they include four reference intakes: the Estimated Average Requirement, the Recommended Dietary Allowance, the Adequate Intake, and the Tolerable Upper Intake Level. The DRIs attempt to address the weaknesses of the RDAs and to expand on the original Recommended Dietary Allowances by adding three new reference values.

The initiative to develop the DRIs formally began in June 1993, when the Food and Nutrition Board (FNB) organized a symposium and public hearing entitled "Should the Recommended Dietary Allowances Be Revised?"[9,10] This was followed by several symposia at nutrition-related professional meetings, at which the FNB discussed its tentative plans and invited input from interested nutrition professionals. From these activities arose a clear consensus that a more comprehensive set of nutritional and dietary standards was needed.

During this time period, Health Canada and Canadian scientists were reviewing the need to revise the Recommended Nutrient Intakes.[13] In April 1995, at a symposium cosponsored by the Canadian National Institute of Nutrition and Health Canada, Canadian scientists reached a consensus that the Canadian government should investigate working with the FNB in developing a set of nutrient-based recommendations that will serve, where appropriate, the needs of both countries. In December 1995, the FNB began a close collaboration with the Canadian government and appointed a Standing Committee on the Scientific Evaluation of Dietary Reference Intakes (DRI Committee) composed of scientists from Canada and the United States to conduct and oversee the project. Consequently, the DRIs not only supersede the 10th edition of the *Recommended Dietary Allowances*[8] but also the Canadian Recommended Nutrient Intakes, which were last published in 1990.[13] A liaison from the government of Mexico also serves *ex-officio* on the DRI Committee.

The DRI Committee began its work by grouping the various nutrients and food components into eight or more categories and assigning each nutrient group to a panel of experts on those nutrients. The DRI Committee also formed two subcommittees: a Subcommittee on Upper Reference Levels of Nutrients to assist each panel in the

---

 Box 2.1   **The Dietary Reference Intakes**

Estimated Average Requirement (EAR): This is the daily dietary intake level estimated to meet the nutrient requirement of 50% of healthy individuals in a particular life stage and gender group.

Recommended Dietary Allowance (RDA): This is an average daily dietary intake level sufficient to meet the nutrient requirement of nearly all (97% to 98%) healthy individuals in a particular life stage gender group.

Adequate Intake (AI): This is a recommended daily dietary intake level that is assumed to be adequate

and that is based on experimentally determined approximations of nutrient intake by a group (or groups) of healthy people. The AI is an observational standard used when there are insufficient data available to determine an RDA.

Tolerable Upper Intake Level (UL): This is the highest level of daily nutrient intake that is likely to pose no risk of adverse health effects to almost all apparently healthy individuals in the general population. As intake increases above the UL, the risk of adverse (toxic) effects increases.

Adapted from Standing Committee on the Scientific Evaluation of Dietary Reference Intakes, Food and Nutrition Board, Institute of Medicine. 2000. *Dietary Reference Intakes for vitamin C, vitamin E, selenium, and carotenoids.* Washington, DC: National Academy Press.

development of the Tolerable Upper Intake Levels and a Subcommittee on Interpretation and Uses of Dietary Reference Intakes to determine appropriate examples for using the DRIs.[10–12] The structure of the DRI project and eight of the proposed panels are shown in Figure 2.1. The figure also shows how the Subcommittee on Upper Reference Levels of Nutrients and the Subcommittee on Interpretation and Uses of Dietary Reference Intakes interact with the panels. Box 2.2 shows the tasks of each panel.

The first DRI report, released in August 1997, covered calcium, phosphorus, magnesium, vitamin D, and fluoride. The second DRI report, released in April 1998, included reference intakes for folate and other B vitamins. The third was released in April 2000 and covered vitamins C and E, selenium, and carotenoids. A fourth report was released in January 2001 and covered vitamins A and K and the minerals arsenic, boron, chromium, copper, iodine, iron, manganese, molybdenum, nickel, silicon, vanadium, and zinc.

Table 2.2 shows the Recommended Dietary Allowances (RDAs) and the Adequate Intakes (AIs) for vitamins from these four reports. Table 2.3 shows RDAs and AIs for minerals. The values in bold are RDAs, while those in ordinary type and followed by an asterisk are AIs. The 22 life stage and gender groups included in the DRIs are shown in the column at the extreme left of the table. Table 2.4 shows the Tolerable Upper Intake Levels (ULs) from these four reports. It should be noted that the DRIs use different life stage and gender groups for the ULs than those used for the RDAs and AIs. Updated DRI tables are available on the *Nutritional Assessment* website at www.mhhe.com/hper/nutrition.

Estimated Average Requirement

The Estimated Average Requirement (EAR) is defined as "the daily intake value that is estimated to meet the

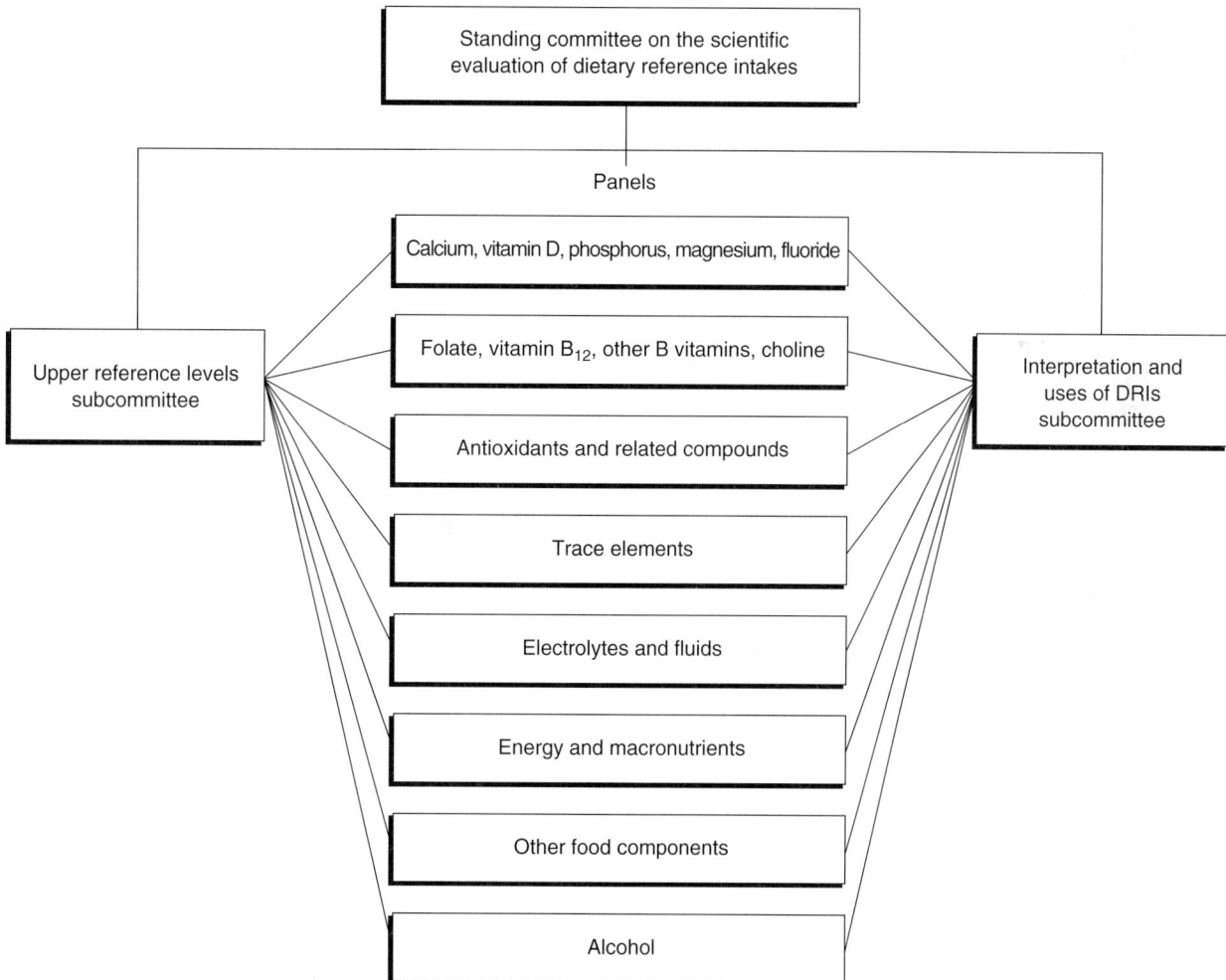

Figure 2.1 **Structure of the DRI project.**
The nutrients and food components are grouped into eight categories, and each is assigned to a panel of experts, who develop the DRIs for each category.

Source: Reprinted from Standing Committee on the Scientific Evaluation of Dietary Reference Intakes, Food and Nutrition Board, Institute of Medicine. 2000. *Dietary Reference Intakes for vitamin C, vitamin E, selenium, and carotenoids.* Washington, DC: National Academy Press. Used with permission.

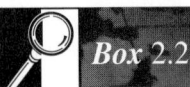

Box 2.2 **Tasks of Each DRI Panel**

- Review the scientific literature for each nutrient or food component under consideration for each of the sex, age, and condition groups
- Consider the roles of each nutrient or food component in decreasing risk of chronic and other diseases and conditions
- Interpret the current nutrient or food component intake data for each of the sex, age, and condition groups in North America
- Develop criteria or indicators of adequacy for each nutrient or food component and provide substantive rationale for each criterion or indicator
- Establish the Estimated Average Requirement (EAR) for each nutrient or food component (assuming that

sufficient data are available) and the Recommended Dietary Allowance (RDA) for each life stage and gender group; if data are insufficient for establishing the EAR/RDA, set the Adequate Intake (AI)
- Participate with the Subcommittee on Upper Reference Levels of Nutrients in estimating the level of nutrient or food component intake above which there is increased risk of toxicity or an adverse reaction—the Tolerable Upper Intake Level (UL)
- Participate with the Subcommittee on Interpretation and Uses of the DRIs in developing practical information and guidance on appropriately using the DRIs

Adapted from Standing Committee on the Scientific Evaluation of Dietary Reference Intakes, Food and Nutrition Board, Institute of Medicine. 1997. *Dietary Reference Intakes for calcium, phosphorus, magnesium, vitamin D, and fluoride.* Washington, DC: National Academy Press.

requirement, as defined by the specified indicator of adequacy, in half of the apparently healthy individuals in a life stage or gender group."[12] The EAR serves as the basis for setting the Recommended Dietary Allowance (RDA). If an EAR cannot be established, then an RDA cannot be set.

Because of individual biological variation in nutrient absorption and metabolism, some individuals have a relatively low (lower than average) requirement for a nutrient, while others have a relatively high (higher than average) requirement. If the requirement of nutrient X in a given life stage and gender group (e.g., 19- to 30-year-old females who are neither pregnant nor lactating) were plotted as shown in Figure 2.2, a normal, or Gaussian, distribution might result, creating a bell-shaped curve. Although it is usually assumed that nutrient requirements are normally distributed, this is not always the case. In some instances, the nutrient requirements of a particular group may not be known because of insufficient data or, in the case of infants, because it would be unethical to perform the types of studies on infants that would be necessary to determine their nutrient requirements.[10–12,14,15] The EARs are sometimes, of necessity, based on scanty data or data drawn from studies with design limitations.[12] As seen in Figure 2.2, some individuals have a requirement for nutrient X that is much less than average, but the proportion of these people in a particular life stage and gender group is small, as indicated by the height of the curve above the horizontal axis. Likewise, the proportion having a requirement much greater than average is also small.

The DRI Committee defines requirement as "the lowest continuing intake level of a nutrient that, for a specified indicator of adequacy, will maintain a defined

level of nutriture in an individual."[10–12] When setting the EAR, a specific criterion (or criteria) of adequacy must first be selected based on a thorough review of the scientific literature.[16] The DRI reports clearly identify the criterion or criteria used in establishing the EAR for each nutrient.[10–12] In some instances, the criterion differs for individuals at different life stages. Criteria used in establishing the EAR include the amount needed to prevent classic deficiency diseases, amounts of the nutrient or its metabolites measured in various tissues during depletion-repletion studies or during induced deficiency states in healthy adult volunteers, and the amount needed to adequately maintain a certain metabolic pathway that is dependent on the nutrient in question. When necessary because of insufficient data on the nutrient requirements of children, adolescents, and pregnant or lactating females, the DRI Committee may choose, when appropriate, to adjust the adult EAR on the basis of differences in reference weights of younger persons or to account for the increased nutrient requirements of the fetus and placenta and for milk production.[10–12] When selecting the criterion to be used, reduction of chronic degenerative disease risk is considered. But despite the intense interest in dietary modification of chronic disease risk, data related to the effects of nutrient intakes on morbidity and mortality from chronic disease in the United States and Canada are limited.

Recommended Dietary Allowance

The Recommended Dietary Allowance (RDA) is defined as "the average daily dietary intake level that is sufficient to meet the nutrient requirement of nearly all (97 to

TABLE 2.2 | **Dietary Reference Intakes: Recommended Intakes for Individuals, Vitamins**

Life Stage Group	Vitamin A (µg/d)[a]	Vitamin C (mg/d)	Vitamin D (µg/d)[b,c]	Vitamin E (mg/d)[d]	Vitamin K (µg/d)	Thiamin (mg/d)	Riboflavin (mg/d)	Niacin (mg/d)[e]	Vitamin B$_6$ (mg/d)	Folate (µg/d)[f]	Vitamin B$_{12}$ (µg/d)	Pantothenic Acid (mg/d)	Biotin (µg/d)	Choline[g] (mg/d)
Infants														
0–6 mo	400*	40*	5*	4*	2.0*	0.2*	0.3*	2*	0.1*	65*	0.4*	1.7*	5*	125*
7–12 mo	500*	50*	5*	5*	2.5*	0.3*	0.4*	4*	0.3*	80*	0.5*	1.8*	6*	150*
Children														
1–3 y	300	15	5*	6	30*	0.5	0.5	6	0.5	150	0.9	2*	8*	200*
4–8 y	400	25	5*	7	55*	0.6	0.6	8	0.6	200	1.2	3*	12*	250*
Males														
9–13 y	600	45	5*	11	60*	0.9	0.9	12	1.0	300	1.8	4*	20*	375*
14–18 y	900	75	5*	15	75*	1.2	1.3	16	1.3	400	2.4	5*	25*	550*
19–30 y	900	90	5*	15	120*	1.2	1.3	16	1.3	400	2.4	5*	30*	550*
31–50 y	900	90	5*	15	120*	1.2	1.3	16	1.3	400	2.4	5*	30*	550*
51–70 y	900	90	10*	15	120*	1.2	1.3	16	1.7	400	2.4[h]	5*	30*	550*
>70 y	900	90	15*	15	120*	1.2	1.3	16	1.7	400	2.4[h]	5*	30*	550*
Females														
9–13 y	600	45	5*	11	60*	0.9	0.9	12	1.0	300	1.8	4*	20*	375*
14–18 y	700	65	5*	15	75*	1.0	1.0	14	1.2	400[i]	2.4	5*	25*	400*
19–30 y	700	75	5*	15	90*	1.1	1.1	14	1.3	400[i]	2.4	5*	30*	425*
31–50 y	700	75	5*	15	90*	1.1	1.1	14	1.3	400[i]	2.4	5*	30*	425*
51–70 y	700	75	10*	15	90*	1.1	1.1	14	1.5	400	2.4[h]	5*	30*	425*
>70 y	700	75	15*	15	90*	1.1	1.1	14	1.5	400	2.4[h]	5*	30*	425*
Pregnancy														
≤18 y	750	80	5*	15	75*	1.4	1.4	18	1.9	600[i]	2.6	6*	30*	450*
10–30 y	770	85	5*	15	90*	1.4	1.4	18	1.9	600[i]	2.6	6*	30*	450*
31–50 y	770	85	5*	15	90*	1.4	1.4	18	1.9	600[i]	2.6	6*	30*	450*
Lactation														
≤18 y	1,200	115	5*	19	75*	1.4	1.6	17	2.0	500	2.8	7*	35*	550*
19–30 y	1,300	120	5*	19	90*	1.4	1.6	17	2.0	500	2.8	7*	35*	550*
31–50 y	1,300	120	5*	19	90*	1.4	1.6	17	2.0	500	2.8	7*	35*	550*

Note: This table (taken from the DRI reports, see www.nap.edu) presents Recommended Dietary Allowances (RDAs) in **bold type** and Adequate Intakes (AIs) in ordinary type followed by an asterisk (*).

aAs retinol activity equivalents (RAEs). 1 RAE = 1 µg retinol, 12 µg β-carotene, 24 µg α-carotene, or 24 µg β-cryptoxanthin in foods. To calculate RAEs from REs of provitamin A carotenoids in foods, divide the REs by 2. For preformed vitamin A in foods or supplements and for provitamin A carotenoids in supplements, 1 RE = 1 RAE.

bCholecalciferol. 1 µg cholecalciferol = 40 IU vitamin D.

cIn the absence of adequate exposure to sunlight.

dAs α-tocopherol.

eAs niacin equivalents (NE). 1 mg of niacin = 60 mg of tryptophan; 0–6 months = preformed niacin (not NE).

fAs dietary folate equivalents (DFE). 1 DFE = 1 µg food folate = 0.6 µg of folic acid from fortified food or as a supplement consumed with food = 0.5 µg of a supplement taken on an empty stomach.

gAlthough AIs have been set for choline, there are few data to assess whether a dietary supply of choline is needed at all stages of the life style, and it may be that the choline requirement can be met by endogenous synthesis at some of these stages.

hBecause 10% to 30% of older people may malabsorb food-bound B$_{12}$, it is advisable for those older than 50 years to meet their RDA mainly by consuming foods fortified with B$_{12}$ or a supplement containing B$_{12}$

iIn view of evidence linking folate intake with neural tube defects in the fetus, it is recommended that all women capable of becoming pregnant consume 400 µg from supplements or fortified foods in addition to intake of food folate from a varied diet.

jIt is assumed that women will continue consuming 400 µg from supplements or fortified food until their pregnancy is confirmed and they enter prenatal care, which ordinarily occurs after the end of the periconceptional period—the critical time for formation of the neural tube.

19

TABLE 2.3	Dietary Reference Intakes: Recommended Intakes for Individuals, Elements											
Life Stage Group	Calcium (mg/d)	Chromium (μg/d)	Copper (μg/d)	Fluoride (mg/d)	Iodine (μg/d)	Iron (mg/d)	Magnesium (mg/d)	Manganese (mg/d)	Molybdenum (μg/d)	Phosphorus (mg/d)	Selenium (μg/d)	Zinc (mg/d)
Infants												
0–6 mo	210*	0.2*	200*	0.01*	110*	0.27*	30*	0.003*	2*	100*	15*	2*
7–12 mo	270*	5.5*	220*	0.5*	130*	11	75*	0.6*	3*	275*	20*	3
Children												
1–3 y	500*	11*	340	0.7*	90	7	80	1.2*	17	460	20	3
4–8 y	800*	15*	440	1*	90	10	130	1.5*	22	500	30	5
Males												
9–13 y	1,300*	25*	700	2*	120	8	240	1.9*	34	1,250	40	8
14–18 y	1,300*	35*	890	3*	150	11	410	2.2*	43	1,250	55	11
19–30 y	1,000*	35*	900	4*	150	8	400	2.3*	45	700	55	11
31–50 y	1,000*	35*	900	4*	150	8	420	2.3*	45	700	55	11
51–70 y	1,200*	30*	900	4*	150	8	420	2.3*	45	700	55	11
>70 y	1,200*	30*	900	4*	150	8	420	2.3*	45	700	55	11
Females												
9–13 y	1,300*	21*	700	2*	120	8	240	1.6*	34	1,250	40	8
14–18 y	1,300*	24*	890	3*	150	15	360	1.6*	43	1,250	55	9
19–30 y	1,000*	25*	900	3*	150	18	310	1.8*	45	700	55	8
31–50 y	1,000*	25*	900	3*	150	18	320	1.8*	45	700	55	8
51–70 y	1,200*	20*	900	3*	150	8	320	1.8*	45	700	55	8
>70 y	1,200*	20*	900	3*	150	8	320	1.8*	45	700	55	8
Pregnancy												
≤18 y	1,300*	29*	1,000	3*	220	27	400	2.0*	50	1,250	60	13
19–30 y	1,000*	30*	1,000	3*	220	27	350	2.0*	50	700	60	11
31–50 y	1,000*	30*	1,000	3*	220	27	360	2.0*	50	700	60	11
Lactation												
≤18 y	1,300*	44*	1,300	3*	290	10	360	2.6*	50	1,250	70	14
19–30 y	1,000*	45*	1,300	3*	290	9	310	2.6*	50	700	70	12
31–50 y	1,000*	45*	1,300	3*	290	9	320	2.6*	50	700	70	12

Sources: Dietary Reference Intakes for Calcium, Phosphorus, Magnesium, Vitamin D, and Fluoride (1997); Dietary Reference Intakes for Thiamin, Riboflavin, Niacin, Vitamin B$_6$, Folate, Vitamin B$_{12}$, Pantothenic Acid, Biotin, and Choline (1998); Dietary Reference Intakes for Vitamin C, Vitamin E, Selenium, and Carotenoids (2000); and Dietary Reference Intakes for Vitamin A, Vitamin K, Arsenic, Boron, Chromium, Copper, Iodine, Iron, Manganese, Molybdenum, Nickel, Silicon, Vanadium, and Zinc (2001). These reports may be accessed via www.nap.edu. Copyright 2001 by The National Academies of Sciences. All rights reserved.

Note: This table presents Recommended Dietary Allowances (RDAs) in **bold type** and Adequate Intakes (AIs) in ordinary type followed by an asterisk (*).

TABLE 2.4 | **Dietary Reference Intakes: Tolerable Upper Intake Levels (UL[a]), Vitamins**

Life Stage Group	Vitamin A (μg/d)[b]	Vitamin C (mg/d)	Vitamin D (μg/d)	Vitamin E (mg/d)[c,d]	Vitamin K	Thiamin	Ribo-flavin	Niacin (mg/d)[d]	Vitamin B$_6$ (mg/d)	Folate (μg/d)[d]	Vitamin B$_{12}$	Pantothenic Acid	Biotin	Choline (g/d)	Carote-noids[e]
Infants															
0–6 mo	600	ND[f]	25	ND	ND	ND	ND	ND	ND	ND	ND	ND	ND	ND	ND
7–12 mo	600	ND	25	ND	ND	ND	ND	ND	ND	ND	ND	ND	ND	ND	ND
Children															
1–3 y	600	400	50	200	ND	ND	ND	10	30	300	ND	ND	ND	1.0	ND
4–8 y	900	650	50	300	ND	ND	ND	15	40	400	ND	ND	ND	1.0	ND
Males, Females															
9–13 y	1,700	1,200	50	600	ND	ND	ND	20	60	600	ND	ND	ND	2.0	ND
14–18 y	2,800	1,800	50	800	ND	ND	ND	30	80	800	ND	ND	ND	3.0	ND
19–70 y	3,000	2,000	50	1,000	ND	ND	ND	35	100	1,000	ND	ND	ND	3.5	ND
>70 y	3,000	2,000	50	1,000	ND	ND	ND	35	100	1,000	ND	ND	ND	3.5	ND
Pregnancy															
≤18 y	2,800	1,800	50	800	ND	ND	ND	30	80	800	ND	ND	ND	3.0	ND
19–50 y	3,000	2,000	50	1,000	ND	ND	ND	35	100	1,000	ND	ND	ND	3.5	ND
Lactation															
≤18 y	2,800	1,800	50	800	ND	ND	ND	30	80	800	ND	ND	ND	3.0	ND
19–50 y	3,000	2,000	50	1,000	ND	ND	ND	35	100	1,000	ND	ND	ND	3.5	ND

(*continued*)

Sources: Dietary Reference Intakes for Calcium, Phosphorus, Magnesium, Vitamin D, and Fluoride (1997); Dietary Reference Intakes for Thiamin, Riboflavin, Niacin, Vitamin B$_6$, Folate, Vitamin B$_{12}$, Pantothenic Acid, Biotin, and Choline (1998); Dietary Reference Intakes for Vitamin C, Vitamin E, Selenium, and Carotenoids (2000); and Dietary Reference Intakes for Vitamin A, Vitamin K, Arsenic, Boron, Chromium, Copper, Iodine, Iron, Manganese, Molybdenum, Nickel, Silicon, Vanadium, and Zinc (2001). These reports may be accessed via www.nap.edu. Copyright 2001 by The National Academies of Sciences. All rights reserved.

[a]UL = The maximum level of daily nutrient intake that is likely to pose no risk of adverse effects. Unless otherwise specified, the UL represents total intake from food, water, and supplements. Due to lack of suitable data, ULs could not be established for vitamin K, thiamin, riboflavin, vitamin B$_{12}$, pantothenic acid, biotin, or carotenoids. In the absence of ULs, extra caution may be warranted in consuming levels above recommended intakes.

[b]As preformed vitamin A only.

[c]As α-tocopherol: applies to any form of supplemental α-tocopherol.

[d]The ULs for vitamin E, niacin, and folate apply to synthetic forms obtained from supplements, fortified foods, or a combination of the two.

[e]β-Carotene supplements are advised only to serve as a provitamin A source for individuals at risk of vitamin A deficiency.

[f]ND = Not determinable due to lack of data of adverse effects in this age group and concern with regard to lack of ability to handle excess amounts. Source of intake should be from food only to prevent high levels of intake.

TABLE 2.4 Dietary Reference Intakes: Tolerable Upper Intake Levels (UL[a]), Elements—*continued*

Life Stage Group	Arsenic[b]	Boron (mg/d)	Calcium (g/d)	Chromium	Copper (µg/d)	Fluoride (mg/d)	Iodine (µg/d)	Iron (mg/d)	Magnesium (mg/d)[c]	Manganese (mg/d)	Molybdenum (µg/d)	Nickel (mg/d)	Phosphorus (g/d)	Selenium (µg/d)	Silicon[d]	Vanadium (mg/d)[e]	Zinc (mg/d)
Infants																	
0–6 mo	ND[f]	ND	ND	ND	ND	0.7	ND	40	ND	ND	ND	ND	ND	45	ND	ND	4
7–12 mo	ND	ND	ND	ND	ND	0.9	ND	40	ND	ND	ND	ND	ND	60	ND	ND	5
Children																	
1–3 y	ND	3	2.5	ND	1,000	1.3	200	40	65	2	300	0.2	3	90	ND	ND	7
4–8 y	ND	6	2.5	ND	3,000	2.2	300	40	110	3	600	0.3	3	150	ND	ND	12
Males, Females																	
9–13 y	ND	11	2.5	ND	5,000	10	600	40	350	6	1,100	0.6	4	280	ND	ND	23
14–18 y	ND	17	2.5	ND	8,000	10	900	45	350	9	1,700	1.0	4	400	ND	ND	34
19–70 y	ND	20	2.5	ND	10,000	10	1,100	45	350	11	2,000	1.0	4	400	ND	1.8	40
> 70 y	ND	20	2.5	ND	10,000	10	1,100	45	350	11	2,000	1.0	3	400	ND	1.8	40
Pregnancy																	
≤ 18 y	ND	17	2.5	ND	8,000	10	900	45	350	9	1,700	1.0	3.5	400	ND	ND	34
19–50 y	ND	20	2.5	ND	10,000	10	1,100	45	350	11	2,000	1.0	3.5	400	ND	ND	40
Lactation																	
≤ 18 y	ND	17	2.5	ND	8,000	10	900	45	350	9	1,700	1.0	4	400	ND	ND	34
19–50 y	ND	20	2.5	ND	10,000	10	1,100	45	350	11	2,000	1.0	4	400	ND	ND	40

aUL = The maximum level of daily nutrient intake that is likely to pose no risk of adverse effects. Unless otherwise specified, the UL represents total intake from food, water, and supplements. Due to lack of suitable data, ULs could not be established for arsenic, chromium, and silicon. In the absence of ULs, extra caution may be warranted in consuming levels above recommended intakes.

bAlthough the UL was not determined for arsenic, there is no justification for adding arsenic to food or supplements.

cThe ULs for magnesium represent intake from a pharmacological agent only and do not include intake from food or water.

dAlthough silicon has not been shown to cause adverse effects in humans, there is no justification for adding silicon to supplements.

eAlthough vanadium in food has not been shown to cause adverse effects in humans, there is no justification for adding vanadium to food, and vanadium supplements should be used with caution. The UL is based on adverse effects in laboratory animals and this data could be used to set a UL for adults but not children and adolescents.

fND = Not determinable due to lack of data of adverse effects in this age group and concern with regard to lack of ability to handle excess amounts. Source of intake should be from food only to prevent high levels of intake.

Figure 2.2 **The distribution of the requirement for nutrient X for a life stage and gender group.**
The Estimated Average Requirement (EAR) and the Recommended Dietary Allowance (RDA) for the group are shown. The nutrient requirement level that is 2 standard deviations greater than the EAR is generally selected for the RDA.

Source: Adapted with permission from Beaton, GH. 1985. Uses and limits of the use of the Recommended Dietary Allowances for evaluating dietary intake data. *American Journal of Clinical Nutrition* 41:155–164.

98 percent) apparently healthy individuals in a particular life stage and gender group."[12] This is essentially the same definition as that used in the 10th edition of the *Recommended Dietary Allowances.*[8] Currently, however, as one of the four DRIs, the only purpose of the RDA is to serve as a goal for dietary intake by healthy individuals.[12] It is not intended to serve as a standard to assess the diets of individuals or groups or to plan diets for groups.[16]

The RDA for a particular nutrient can be set only if the EAR for that nutrient is established. If the requirement for the nutrient among individuals in the life stage and gender group is normally distributed and if data about the variability in requirements are sufficient to calculate the **standard deviation (SD)** of the EAR (SD_{EAR}), the RDA is set at 2 standard deviations above the EAR, as illustrated in Figure 2.2. This is shown mathematically by the following equation:

$$RDA = EAR + 2\ SD_{EAR}$$

Obviously, if the RDA were set at the EAR, the RDA would meet the needs of only half the individuals in a life stage and gender group—those individuals having a requirement equal to or less than the EAR. The requirement for nutrient X for the other half of individuals in the group—those with a requirement greater than the EAR—would not be met. Thus, to meet the needs of nearly all apparently healthy individuals in a particular life stage and gender group, the RDA is set at 2 standard deviations above the EAR. The standard deviation indicates the degree of variation from the mean; in this case, it indicates how different the nutrient requirements of individual group members are from the group mean. At 2 stan-

dard deviations above the mean, the requirement for nutrient X would be met for nearly 98% of individuals in a life stage and gender group.

If data about variability in nutrient requirements are insufficient to calculate a standard deviation, a **coefficient of variation (CV)** for the EAR (CV_{EAR}) of 10% is generally assumed and used in place of the standard deviation.[12,16] The coefficient of variation is the standard deviation divided by the mean, as shown in the following equations:

$$CV_{EAR} = SD_{EAR} \div EAR, or$$
$$SD_{EAR} = CV_{EAR} \times EAR$$

In this situation, the RDA can be calculated as follows:

$$RDA = EAR + 2(CV_{EAR} \times EAR), or$$
$$RDA = EAR + 2(0.1 \times EAR), or$$
$$RDA = 1.2 \times EAR$$

If the nutrient requirement for a particular group is known to be skewed, other approaches can be used to find the intake level sufficient to meet the nutrient requirement of 97% to 98% of healthy persons in a particular life stage and gender group in order to set the RDA.[12,16]

A safety margin also is built into the RDA of a nutrient to compensate for its incomplete use by the body and to account for variations in the levels of the nutrient provided by various food sources. Adjustment also is made in some RDAs to account for the consumption of certain dietary components that are subsequently converted within the body to an essential nutrient. For example, the amino acid tryptophan can be converted to niacin within the body.[11] Examples of RDAs that have been included as part of the DRIs were shown in bold type in Table 2.2. For the current RDAs and other DRIs, visit the *Nutritional Assessment* website at www.mhhe.com/hper/nutrition.

Adequate Intake

If insufficient data are available to calculate an EAR, and thus an RDA cannot be set for a particular nutrient, a separate reference intake, known as Adequate Intake (AI), is used instead of the RDA. Adequate Intake is defined as "a value based on experimentally derived intake levels or approximations of observed mean nutrient intakes by a group (or groups) of healthy people."[10–12] For example, as was shown in Table 2.2, the nutrient intake levels for infants (birth to 12 months of age) are all expressed as AIs instead of RDAs because the types of studies necessary to determine the nutrient requirements of infants (e.g., depletion-repletion studies) cannot ethically be done. The AIs for infants from birth to 6 months of age were calculated based on the mean nutrient intakes of healthy, full-term infants 2 to 6 months of age who were exclusively breast-fed.[10] By weighing these infants before and after breast-feeding, researchers determined that the average volume of milk intake was 780 ml/day. Based on the nutritional composition of human milk, researchers could then determine the average nutritional intake of these infants. For infants 7 to 12 months of age, the AIs are based on the average nutrient intakes of 7- to 12-month-old infants fed a combination of human milk and typical complementary weaning foods used in North America.

As was shown in Table 2.2, the recommended intakes of calcium, fluoride, vitamin D, pantothenic acid, biotin, and choline are expressed as AIs for all life stages and gender groups. This is because there are insufficient data on the requirements of these nutrients, resulting in an inability to establish an EAR and an RDA. As future research provides additional data on the requirements for these nutrients, an EAR and RDA can be set.

It is important to note that the AI is an observational standard—it is based on observed or experimentally derived approximations of average nutrient intake that appear to maintain a defined nutritional state or criterion of adequacy in a group of people.[12,16] Defined nutritional states include normal growth, maintenance of normal circulating nutrient values, and other indicators of nutritional well-being and general health. Because it is set using presumably healthy groups of individuals, the AI is expected to meet or exceed the actual nutrient requirement in practically all healthy members of a specific life stage and gender group. Like the RDA, the AI is intended to serve as a goal for the nutrient intake of healthy individuals. When nutrient requirements are altered due to injury, disease, or some other special health need, the RDA and AI should serve as the basis for an individual's nutrient recommendations, which, depending on the situation, may then need to be adjusted by a registered dietitian or qualified health professional to accommodate the individual's increased or decreased nutrient needs.[16] Unlike the RDA, however, the AI is used when data on nutrient requirements are lacking, and consequently greater uncertainty surrounds the AI.[16] Its use indicates a need for additional research on the requirements for that particular nutrient or food component.

Tolerable Upper Intake Level

The Tolerable Upper Intake Level (UL) is defined as "the highest level of daily nutrient intake that is likely to pose no risk of adverse health effects in almost all individuals in the specified life stage group."[10–12] Examples of these were shown in Table 2.3. The UL is not intended to be a recommended level of nutrient intake but, rather, an indication of the maximum amount of a nutrient that can, with a high degree of probability, be taken on a daily basis without endangering one's health—in

other words, the maximum amount that likely can be *tolerated* by the body when consumed on a daily basis. The term *adverse effect* is defined as "any significant alteration in the structure or function of the human organism" or any "impairment of a physiologically important function that could lead to a health effect that is adverse."[12] To determine the UL, the DRI Committee uses a risk assessment model, which is discussed at length in the DRI reports.[10–12]

The UL was created in response to concerns about the potential for excessive nutrient intakes resulting from recent increases in consumption of nutrient-fortified foods and dietary supplements.[16] Just as inadequate nutrient intake can adversely affect health (e.g., result in nutrient-deficiency disease), so can excessive nutrient intake. As illustrated in Figure 2.3, when a nutrient's level of intake is low, risk of inadequacy increases, as indicated by the curve on the left side of the figure. At a very low intake level, the curve is at its highest point, signifying that risk of inadequacy is 100% (indicated as 1.0 in Figure 2.3). When nutrient intake is very high, there is increased risk of excess nutrient intake (what the DRI Committee calls "risk of adverse effects"), as indicated by the curve on the right side of the figure. An intake level at the UL is unlikely to pose a risk of excessive nutrient intake for most (but not necessarily all) individuals in a specific group. However, as nutrient intake increases above the UL, the risk of adverse health effects increases. When nutrient intake is at the EAR, risk of inadequacy is considered 50% (indicated as 0.5 in Figure 2.3). At the RDA, 97% to 98% of healthy individuals will have their requirement met. Between the RDA and UL is a safe range of intake associated with a very low probability of either inadequate or excessive nutrient intake. However, setting a UL does not suggest that a nutrient intake level greater than the RDA or AI is of any benefit to an individual.

Figure 2.3 does not show the AI because it is an observational standard and set without being able to estimate the requirement. However, the AI is intended to meet or exceed the actual nutrient requirement in practically all healthy members of a specific life stage and gender group and, thus, should be fairly close to the RDA for that nutrient and life stage and gender group, if the RDA is known. Once additional research provides data on the distribution of the requirement for a nutrient and the AI can be replaced with an EAR and RDA, it is likely that the RDA will be slightly less than, if not greater than, the RDA.[16]

Prior to the development of the DRIs, the Recommended Dietary Allowances failed to provide any guidance on the safe use of nutritional supplements and addressed the issue of supplement use only by recommending that the RDAs be met by consuming a diet ". . . composed of a *variety* of foods that are derived from diverse food groups rather than by supplementation or for-

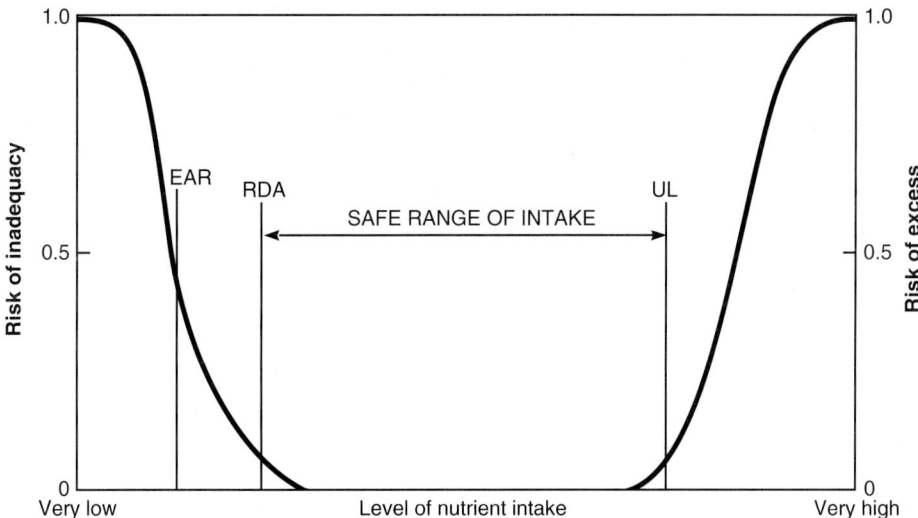

Figure 2.3 **The risk of inadequate or excess intake varies according to the level of nutrient intake. When nutrient intake is very low, the risk of inadequacy is high. When nutrient intake is very high, the risk of excessive intake is high. Between the RDA and UL is a safe range of intake associated with a very low probability of either inadequate or excessive nutrient intake. EAR = Estimated Average Requirement; RDA = Recommended Dietary Allowance; UL = Tolerable Upper Intake Level.**

Sources: Adapted from Health and Welfare, Canada. 1983. *Recommended nutrient intakes for Canadians.* Ottawa: Canadian Publishing Centre; Standing Committee on the Scientific Evaluation of Dietary Reference Intakes, Food and Nutrition Board, Institute of Medicine. 2000. *Dietary Reference Intakes for vitamin C, vitamin E, selenium, and carotenoids.* Washington, DC: National Academy Press.

tification . . . ."[8] It is important to note that this remains an excellent recommendation for a variety of reasons. For example, given the complexity of nutrients and other components in food (some of which we know little, if anything) it is clear that we cannot solely rely on nutritional supplements as a source of these nutrients and other components and must depend primarily on food to obtain them.[17] However, there is need for information on the maximum amounts of supplemental nutrients that can be safely consumed, given the recent proliferation of nutrient-fortified foods in the marketplace, the increased interest in and use of nutritional and dietary supplements by North Americans, and a growing body of scientific evidence demonstrating that in some instances nutrient intakes in excess of the amounts typically obtained solely from diets can reduce chronic disease risk. The ULs help provide this information and fill an important niche.[16] The ULs are not intended to apply to persons receiving nutrient or other dietary supplements under medical supervision.[12]

If adverse effects of excess nutrient consumption are associated with total nutrient intake, the ULs are based on total nutrient intake from food, water, and supplements. If adverse effects are associated only with intakes from supplements or fortified foods, the ULs are based on nutrient intakes from those sources.[12] For many nutrients, there are insufficient data available to set a UL. But the absence of a UL does not imply that a high intake of that nutrient is risk-free. On the contrary, it may suggest

that greater caution is warranted when intakes exceed the RDA or AI.[12]

Uses of the DRIs

The suggested uses of the DRIs fall into two broad categories: assessing nutrient intakes and planning for nutrient intakes. Each of the two categories is further divided into uses pertaining to individuals and uses pertaining to groups. The uses of the DRIs for healthy individuals and groups are outlined in Box 2.3

The DRIs are not intended to serve as the only means of assessing the nutritional adequacy of an individual's diet. An individual's actual nutrient requirement can vary widely from the group average (the EAR), and without various biochemical and physiologic measures it is impossible to determine whether an individual's actual nutrient requirement is close to the group EAR, greater than the EAR, or less than the EAR. In addition, intake of most nutrients varies considerably from one day to the next, requiring many days of measurement to estimate *usual* nutrient intake, as discussed in Chapter 3. Consequently, when assessing the adequacy of an individual's diet, use of multiple nutritional assessment methods— dietary, anthropometric, biochemical, and clinical—must be considered.

If an individual's usual intake of a nutrient is equal to or greater than the RDA or AI, it is unlikely that intake is inadequate. When usual intake is less than the EAR, there

---

Box 2.3   Uses of the Dietary Reference Intakes for Healthy Individuals and Groups

Type of Use	For the Individual	For a Group
Assessment	**EAR**[*]: use to examine the possibility of inadequacy of reported intake	**EAR**[†]: use to estimate the prevalence of inadequate intakes within a group
	AI[*]: intake at this level has a low probability of inadequacy	**AI**[†]: mean intake at this level implies a low prevalence of inadequate intakes
	UL[*]: intake above this level has a risk of adverse effects	**UL**[†]: use to estimate the prevalence of intakes that may be at risk of adverse effects
Planning	**RDA**: aim for this intake	**EAR**: use in conjunction with a measure of variability of the group's intake to set goals for the median intake of a specific population
	AI: aim for this intake	
	UL: use as a guide to limit intake; chronic intake of higher amounts may increase risk of adverse effects	

EAR = Estimated Average Requirement
RDA = Recommended Dietary Allowance
AI = Adequate Intake
UL = Tolerable Upper Intake Level

[*]Requires accurate measure of usual intake. Evaluation of true status requires clinical, biochemical, and anthropometric data.
[†]Requires statistically valid approximation of usual intake.

Reprinted from Standing Committee on the Scientific Evaluation of Dietary Reference Intakes, Food and Nutrition Board, Institute of Medicine. 2000. *Dietary Reference Intakes for vitamin C, vitamin E, selenium, and carotenoids.* Washington, DC: National Academy Press. Copyright 2000 by the National Academy of Sciences. Reprinted courtesy of the National Academy Press, Washington, DC.

---

is a high likelihood that intake is inadequate. However, if usual intake falls between the EAR and RDA, the likelihood of inadequate intake will be difficult to determine, and in such instances use of other assessment techniques is important in determining nutrient adequacy. If an individual's usual intake of a nutrient is less than the UL, there is little risk of excessive intake. Risk of adverse health effects from excessive intake increases when usual intake rises above the UL. When planning a healthy individual's diet, the RDAs and AIs are intended to serve as a goal for average daily nutrient intake over time (over several days to several weeks, depending on the turnover rate of the nutrient in question).

Assessing the adequacy of a group's nutrient intake involves comparing the distribution of usual intakes among group members with the distribution of the requirement for the nutrient. A "cutpoint approach" is typically used to estimate the percentage of group members whose usual intakes are less than the EAR. The RDA is not intended to be used for estimating the prevalence of inadequate intakes in groups.[12] In the absence of an EAR, it may be necessary to use the AI to assess the adequacy of a group's intake, but greater care must be exercised than when using the EAR, given the fact that the AI is an observational standard. The proportion of the population with usual intakes above the UL is likely to be at some

risk of adverse effects due to overconsumption, while the proportion below the UL is likely to be at no risk.

Data from the third National Health and Nutrition Examination Survey (discussed in Chapter 4) indicate that approximately 11% of nonsmoking adult females and 21% of nonsmoking adult males have a usual vitamin C intake (from food and supplements) less than the EAR for vitamin C.[12] Estimating the prevalence of inadequate nutrient intakes in a population requires accurate, quantitative information on usual nutrient intake by the group. Both the U.S. Department of Health and Human Services and the U.S. Department of Agriculture conduct periodic surveys of food and nutrient intake by Americans, which provide these data. The nutritional monitoring activities of these agencies are discussed in Chapter 4.

The EAR is used in planning or making recommendations for the nutrient intake of groups. The group's mean nutrient intake should be high enough so that only a small percentage of group members have an intake less than the EAR but not so high that too many group members have intakes above the UL. If the prevalence of nutrient inadequacy is too high, an appropriate intervention should be undertaken to increase intakes by those at greatest risk of inadequacy while maintaining an acceptably low prevalence of group members with intake above the UL.

NUTRIENT DENSITY

In the nutrient density approach, recommended nutrient intakes and nutritional composition of foods are expressed in terms of *nutrient quantity per 1000 kcal.* The basic concept of nutrient density is that, if the quantity of nutrients per 1000 kcal is great enough, the nutrient needs of a person will be met when his or her energy needs are met.

Nutrient density addresses the issues of overconsumption and the relationships between diet and disease and allows the nutritional qualities of foods and diets to be evaluated and compared easily, quickly, and independently of serving size.

The nutritional value of foods also can be evaluated with respect to their caloric content. This is of particular importance to people consuming low-calorie diets. To achieve nutritional adequacy on a 1000-kcal to 1200-kcal reducing diet (which is roughly half the recommended calorie level for adults), most foods consumed should have a nutrient density approximately double the per 1000-kcal allowance. In other words, the foods selected should be both high in nutrients and low in calories to provide an adequate nutrient intake on a low-calorie diet. Nutrient density is a relatively simple approach to ensuring nutritional adequacy for those on low-calorie diets.

INDICES OF DIET QUALITY

Numerous indices of diet quality have been proposed and reported in the scientific literature.[18] How these indices define diet quality varies considerably, depending on the attributes selected by the creator of the particular index and by the era in which the index was developed. For example, earlier indices tend to define a high-quality diet as one supplying adequate protein and selected micronutrients for a given energy level. More recent indices define diet quality in terms of proportionality (eating more servings of certain food groups and fewer of others), moderation (limiting intake of foods and beverages contributing to excess intake of fat, dietary cholesterol, added sugars, sodium, and alcohol), and variety (thus increasing exposure to a wide range of nutritive and other food components).[18,19] Reflecting the nutritional era in which they were developed, earlier indices tend to focus on prevention of deficiency diseases, while more recent ones tend to address risk of chronic disease.

Diet quality indices are typically based on one of three approaches to assessing diet: comparing intake of certain nutrients and food components to a standard, comparing intake of foods or food groups to a standard, or evaluating both nutrient intake and foods or food groups.[18] The Index of Nutritional Quality compares nutrient and food component intake with such standards as Dietary Reference Intakes, Dietary Guidelines for Americans, and the Daily Values. The Diet Quality Index and the Healthy Eating Index evaluate intake of various nutrients and food components and assess consumption of foods and food groups.

Index of Nutritional Quality

The **Index of Nutritional Quality (INQ)** is a concept related to nutrient density that allows the quantity of a nutrient per 1000 kcal in a food, meal, or diet to be compared with a nutrient standard. The first step in determining the INQ of a food or meal is to calculate a single-value nutrient recommendation for each nutrient from the Dietary Reference Intakes (DRIs) or a similar recommended nutrient intake standard. Unlike the DRIs, which recommend nutrient intakes for 22 *specific groups* of females and males of different ages and physiologic conditions, the INQ generally uses only one recommendation for each nutrient for all people. The method used by scientists at Utah State University, who developed the INQ approach, is to divide the RDAs for each age/sex group by the average kilocalorie recommendation for the group and then multiply by 1000.[20,21] Table 2.5 shows nutrient recommendations per 1000 kcal for persons ages 1 year and older derived from the Recommended Dietary Allowances (RDAs) or the Adequate Intakes (AIs). The single-value recommendations approximate the recommendations for persons whose nutrient-to-calorie needs are the greatest or nearly the greatest. These are usually for persons having the lowest calorie needs (that is, persons in the > 70-year age group).[20] The bottom row of values in Table 2.5 gives the single-value recommendations selected by the authors using the method suggested by R. G. Hansen and others at Utah State University.[20,22]

Table 2.6 shows these single values with the addition of several others (fat, cholesterol, and so on) that are not yet addressed by the DRIs.

The INQ of a food then is calculated using the following formula:[23]

$$INQ = \frac{\text{Amount of nutrient in 1000 kcal of food}}{\text{Allowance of nutrient per 1000 kcal of food}}$$

To calculate the INQ of nonfat or whole milk, for example, determine the amount of nutrients per 1000 kcal in milk from a food composition table or computerized nutritional software (see Chapter 5). Then divide the per 1000-kcal nutrient values by the single-value allowance for each nutrient.

Evaluating Nutrient Content

Figure 2.4 illustrates how the INQ simplifies the evaluation of the nutrient content of foods and allows easy comparison of two or more foods. It compares the INQ of whole milk with that of nonfat milk. When a

TABLE 2.5	Nutrient Recommendations per 1000 Kcal Derived from the Dietary Reference Intakes[*†]

		Water-Soluble Vitamins									
Life Stage and Gender Group	Energy[‡] (kcal)	Vitamin C (mg)	Thiamin (mg)	Riboflavin (mg)	Niacin (mg NE)	Vitamin B$_6$ (mg)	Folate (µg)	Vitamin B$_{12}$ (µg)	Pantothenic Acid (mg)	Biotin (µg)	Choline (mg)
Children											
1–3 years	1300	12	0.4	0.4	4.6	0.4	120	0.7	1.5	6	155
4–8 years	1700	15	0.4	0.4	4.7	0.4	120	0.7	1.8	7	150
Males											
9–13 years	2100	21	0.4	0.4	5.7	0.5	140	0.9	1.9	10	180
14–18 years	2800	27	0.4	0.5	5.7	0.5	140	0.9	1.8	10	200
19–30 years	2600	35	0.5	0.5	6.2	0.5	150	0.9	1.9	12	210
31–50 years	2400	38	0.5	0.5	6.7	0.5	170	1.0	2.1	13	230
51–70 years	2000	45	0.6	0.7	8.0	0.9	200	1.2	2.5	15	275
> 70 years	1700	53	0.7	0.8	9.4	1.0	240	1.4	2.9	18	320
Females											
9–13 years	1700	26	0.5	0.5	7.1	0.6	180	1.1	2.4	12	220
14–18 years	2000	33	0.5	0.5	7.0	0.6	200	1.2	2.5	13	200
19–30 years	2000	38	0.6	0.6	7.0	0.7	200	1.2	2.5	15	210
31–50 years	1800	42	0.6	0.6	7.8	0.7	220	1.3	2.8	17	235
51–70 years	1700	44	0.6	0.6	8.2	0.9	240	1.4	2.9	18	250
> 70 years	1600	47	0.7	0.7	8.8	0.9	250	1.5	3.1	19	265
Single value[§]		50	0.7	0.7	9.0	1.0	250	1.5	30	18	300

[*]Nutrient values calculated by dividing the Recommended Dietary Allowance or Adequate Intake for each life stage and gender group by the energy level for each group and then multiplying by 1000. This results in a recommended nutrient intake level per 1000 kilocalories.

[†]NE = niacin equivalents; RE = retinol equivalents.

[‡]Energy values adapted from median energy intakes from the third National Health and Nutrition Examination Survey (NHANES III).

[§]Single-value recommendations are arrived at by selecting the recommendations for the group having the greatest (or nearly the greatest) nutrient-to-energy needs.

horizontal bar extends to the right of the vertical line labeled "1," a 1000-kcal amount of the food supplies more than the single-value recommendation for that nutrient, as given in Table 2.6. When the horizontal bar reaches the numbers "2" or "3," a 1000-kcal amount of the food supplies two or three times the single-value recommendation, respectively, for that nutrient. For most nutrients, this is desirable. However, in the case of fat (especially saturated fat), cholesterol, and sodium, a relatively low INQ is preferable. Because of the association between consumption of these food components and risk for certain diseases, it is best that they be eaten in relatively low amounts.

Irrespective of the quantity consumed, it is apparent from Figure 2.4 that, on an equal kilocalorie basis, nonfat milk provides significantly less cholesterol and fat and more protein and the vitamins and minerals shown than whole milk. The ease by which the INQ can convey the nutritional content of food is obvious.

A food with an overall INQ substantially greater than "1" is generally considered to be of good quality. It provides important nutrients in excess of calories. On the contrary, a food supplying calories in excess of nutrients would have an INQ less than "1," and a per-

son would have to consume excessive calories to meet his or her recommended intake of nutrients. It is clear that nonfat milk, on a per 1000-kcal basis, is a much better source of nutrients than whole milk. This is mainly because fat (and other components, such as sugar) *dilutes* the nutrient density of food.[22] On a *volume* basis, both foods contain approximately the same amount of calcium, riboflavin, and protein. The extra kilocalories from fat in whole milk, however, significantly reduce its contribution of calcium, riboflavin, and protein on a *per 1000 kcal* basis.

Weaknesses of the Index of Nutritional Quality

The INQ has its weaknesses. Defining the criterion for determining the single-value nutrient recommendation is a major issue of the approach. Dividing an average nutrient requirement plus 2 standard deviations (the RDA, which is sufficient for almost all group members) by an average energy requirement (sufficient for half of the group) is considered by some scientists as convenient but tenuous and lacking a good scientific basis.

		Fat-Soluble Vitamins			Minerals						
Protein (g)	Vitamin A (μg RE)	Vitamin D (μg)	Vitamin E (mg)	Vitamin K (μg)	Calcium (mg)	Fluoride (μg)	Iodine (μg)	Iron (mg)	Phosphorus (mg)	Selenium (μg)	Zinc (mg)
12	310	4	5	12	380	0.5	50	8	350	15	8
15	350	3	4	15	470	0.6	60	6	300	18	6
21	380	3	5	19	620	1.0	60	6	600	19	7
21	360	2	5	23	460	1.0	55	4.5	450	20	5
22	380	2	6	27	380	1.5	60	4	270	21	6
26	400	2	6	33	420	1.7	60	4	300	23	6
32	500	5	8	40	600	2.0	75	5	350	28	7
37	580	9	9	46	710	2.3	90	6	410	32	9
26	470	3	6	24	760	1.2	75	9	740	24	7
22	400	3	8	28	650	1.5	75	8	620	28	6
23	400	3	8	30	500	1.5	75	8	350	28	6
28	440	3	8	36	560	1.7	85	8	390	31	7
29	470	6	9	38	700	1.8	90	6	410	32	7
31	500	9	9	40	750	1.9	90	6	430	34	8
35	550	9	9	45	750	2.0	90	6	700	32	8

Another criticism stems from the fact that nutrient requirements per 1000 kcal of energy expended are higher in sedentary persons compared with physically active persons. Note that the recommendations for several nutrients in Table 2.5 are highest for males and females in the > 70-year age group. This is because, as people age, their energy requirements tend to decrease, while their nutrient requirements, in most instances, remain about the same as those of younger adults. Some scientists object to arbitrarily setting single-value recommendations at an artificially high level to accommodate the needs of persons with a low energy requirement. "Why," they ask, "should the recommendations be so high when the nutrient requirements of more physically active persons can be met with a much lower nutrient quantity per 1000 kcal?"

Expecting a single-value nutrient recommendation to be appropriate for all persons ages 1 year and older is an oversimplification. More than one single-value nutrient recommendation may be necessary—perhaps one for children, one for adolescents and adults, and yet another for pregnant and lactating females. When using nutrient density or INQ in planning meals or evaluating nutrient intake, individual activity levels and energy requirements also should be considered.

Despite their weaknesses, the INQ and nutrient density approach have definite advantages, making them useful tools for meal planning by nutrition professionals, as well as for nutrition education, evaluation of nutrient intake, and food labeling.

Diet Quality Index

The Diet Quality Index (DQI) in an instrument used to assess the overall diet quality of groups and to evaluate risk for chronic disease related to dietary pattern.[19,24] It was originally published in 1994 and was based on 8 dietary recommendations from the National Academy of Sciences publication *Diet and Health: Implications for Reducing Chronic Disease Risk.*[25] It was revised in 1999 to reflect the development of the Food Guide Pyramid, revisions in the Dietary Guidelines for Americans, and the creation of the Dietary Reference Intakes. Table 2.7 shows the recently revised Diet Quality Index (what its creators call the Diet Quality Index Revised). The Diet Quality Index scores diet on the basis of 10 indicators of diet quality. The first 3 indicators reflect macronutrient intake, the next 3 reflect the Food Guide Pyramid's recommendations for fruit, vegetable, and grain consumption, and the 2 recommendations for calcium and iron are based on the Dietary Reference Intakes. The last 2 indicators address the importance of consuming foods from a variety of food groups and having a moderate intake of

TABLE 2.6	Single-Value Nutrient Density Recommendations per 1000 Kilocalories for North Americans Ages 1 Year and Older*

Nutrient or Food Component	Amount†
Vitamin C	50 mg
Thiamin	0.7 mg
Riboflavin	0.7 mg
Niacin	9 mg NE
Vitamin B_6	1 mg
Folate	250 μg
Vitamin B_{12}	1.5 μg
Pantothenic acid	30 mg
Biotin	18 μg
Choline	300 mg
Protein	35 g
Vitamin A	550 μg RE
Vitamin D	9 μg
Vitamin E	9 mg
Vitamin K	45 μg
Calcium	750 mg
Fluoride	2 μg
Iodine	90 μg
Iron	6 mg
Phosphorus	700 mg
Selenium	32 μg
Zinc	8 mg
Carbohydrate (60% kcal)	150 g
Total fat (30% kcal)	33 g
Monounsaturated fat (10% kcal)	11 g
Polyunsaturated fat (10% kcal)	11 g
Saturated fat (10% kcal)	11 g
Cholesterol	150 mg
Dietary fiber	13 g
Sodium	1200 mg

*Recommendations derived from the Dietary Reference Intakes and the Daily Values

†NE = niacin equivalents; RE = retinol equivalents.

sugar, discretionary fat, sodium, and alcoholic beverages.[19] Each of the 10 components contributes a maximum of 10 points to the total DQI score, which has a maximum of 100 points. The higher the score, the higher the diet quality.

One application of the DQI is to assess the diets of groups using data from national nutrition surveys. For example, Haines et al. used the DQI to assess data from the U.S. Department of Agriculture's 1994 Continuing Survey of Food Intakes by Individuals (discussed in Chapter 4). The data were based on two 24-hour recalls (see Chapter 3) obtained from 3202 adults ages 18 and older. The mean DQI score was 63.4 out of a possible

maximum of 100. The DQI scores of survey participants were higher in the areas of dietary cholesterol (66.9% met goal) and iron intakes (59.6% met goal), indicating a greater degree of adherence with those dietary recommendations. Scores were lowest for calcium intakes (16.6% met goal) and the number of servings from the fruit group (19.6% met goal) and the grain group (23.1% met goal).[19]

Healthy Eating Index

The Healthy Eating Index (HEI) is an instrument developed by researchers at the U.S. Department of Agriculture for assessing the quality of the diets of Americans.[26,27] It is a single, summary measure of overall diet quality defined in terms of adequacy, moderation, and variety. The U.S. Department of Agriculture uses the Healthy Eating Index to monitor changes in food consumption patterns, to identify target areas for nutrition education and health promotion programs, and to evaluate those programs.[26] It is the only index issued by the U.S. federal government and computed on a regular basis for gauging the overall diet quality of Americans.

As shown in Figure 2.5, the Healthy Eating Index uses 10 components to determine adherence to the Food Guide Pyramid's serving recommendations for the 5 major food groups (components 1–5), assess intake of total fat and saturated fat as a percent of total energy intake (components 6 and 7), measure intake of dietary cholesterol and sodium (components 8 and 9), and evaluate variety in a person's diet (component 10). As shown by Table 2.8, scores for the 10 components can range from 0 to 10, giving a maximum total score of 100 points.[27] An HEI score greater than 80 points implies a "good" diet; an HEI score between 51 and 80 suggests that the diet "needs improvement"; an HEI score less than 51 points suggests a "poor" diet.

Using data from its Continuing Survey of Food Intakes by Individuals (CSFII), researchers at the U.S. Department of Agriculture calculated HEI scores on the diets of Americans as early as 1989.[26] Trends in the HEI between 1989 and 1994–96 show that the diets of Americans have slightly, but significantly, improved. The overall HEI for 1989 was 61.5, while the overall HEI was 63.8 when applied to data collected by the 1994–96 CSFII. Although this trend is in the desired direction, the diets of most Americans still need improving. In 1996, only 12% of Americans had a diet that could be considered "good," about 18% had "poor" diets, while the diets of most people (approximately 70%) needed improvement.[27] Consistent with the scores from the Diet Quality Index (applied to data collected by the 1994 CSFII), the 1994–96 HEI scores were highest for the cholesterol component and lowest for the components assessing the recommended number of servings from the fruit and milk groups.[27]

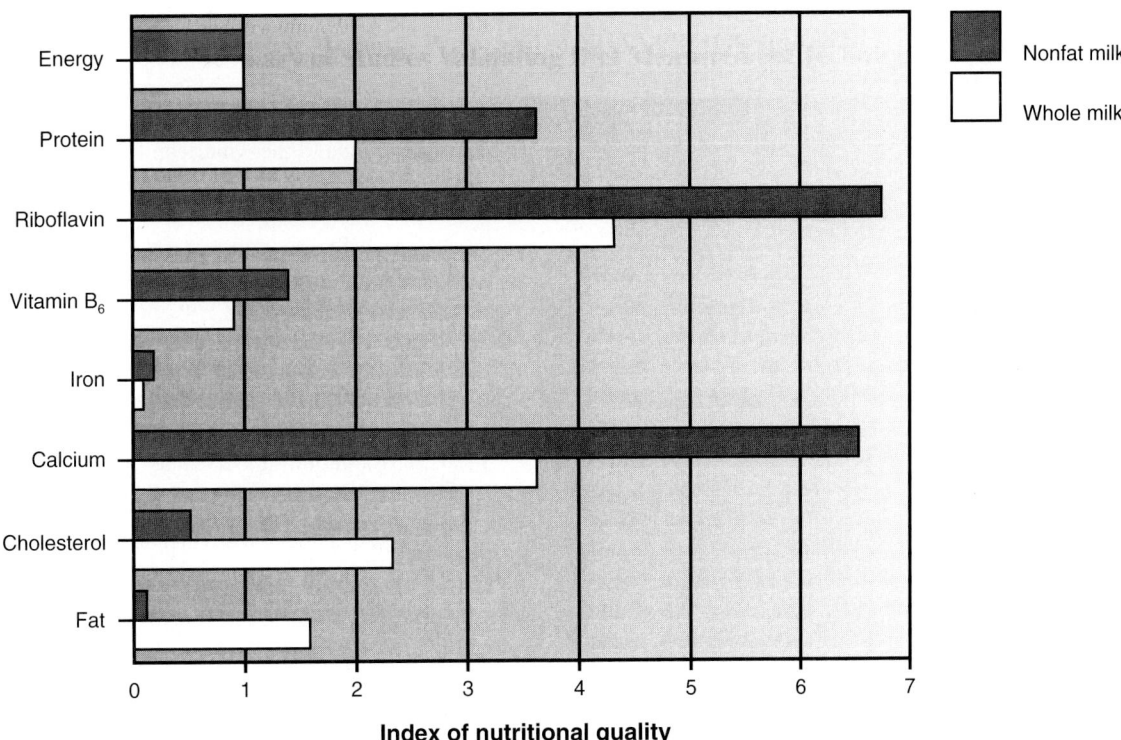

Figure 2.4 Index of nutritional quality of whole milk compared with that of nonfat milk.

DIETARY GUIDELINES

Dietary guidelines or goals can be defined as statements from authoritative scientific bodies translating nutritional recommendations into practical advice to consumers about their eating habits.[28] Rather than merely ensuring adequate nutrient intake, *they are primarily intended to address the more common and pressing nutrition-related health problems, such as heart disease, certain cancers, stroke, hypertension, and diabetes.* They often are expressed as nonquantitative changes from the present average national diet or from people's typical eating habits. Examples of guidelines are "choose a diet that is low in saturated fat and cholesterol and moderate in total fat" and "choose a variety of fruits and vegetables daily." Table 2.9 contrasts the DRIs and dietary guidelines.

Early Dietary Guidelines

Dietary guidelines have existed since time immemorial in the form of cultural practices, taboos, and religious teachings.[28] The first formal set of dietary guidelines of modern times, however, was developed by nutrition professors from Sweden, Finland, Norway, and Denmark and published in 1968.[29,30] Several factors influenced the creation of this set of guidelines for the Nordic countries (Sweden, Finland, Norway, Denmark, and Iceland).[29,30] Dietary surveys showed that the proportion of calories

from fat in the Swedish diet had increased from an average of about 29% at the end of the nineteenth century to 42% by the mid-1960s. There was concern over the high intakes of saturated fat, calories, and refined sugars and low intakes of fruits, vegetables, cereal products, lean meats, and nonfat dairy products. Swedish health authorities were concerned about the association between such dietary practices and obesity, coronary heart disease, hypertension, stroke, and tooth decay.

The Swedish guidelines called for a reduced energy intake (when appropriate) to prevent overweight; decreased consumption of total fat, saturated fat, sugar, and sugar-containing products; increased consumption of vegetables, fruits, potatoes, nonfat milk, fish, lean meat, and cereal products; and regular physical activity, especially for those with sedentary occupations.[29]

These dietary trends were recognized in other Western nations, such as Australia, New Zealand, The Netherlands, the United Kingdom, Germany, and Canada, which, in the early 1970s, issued dietary guidelines of their own.[30]

During this time, a similar situation existed in the United States. Scientists were concerned about trends in the eating habits of Americans. Data from the USDA showed that the distribution of calories from carbohydrate and fat had changed significantly between 1909 and the 1970s. Based on the *disappearance* of food from the marketplace (see Chapter 4), the USDA concluded that

| **TABLE 2.7** | **Diet Quality Index Components and Scoring Guidelines**[*] |

Component	Scoring Criteria	
Total fat ≤ 30% of energy intake	≤ 30%	10 points
	31% to 40%	5 points
	> 40%	0 points
Saturated fat ≤ 10% of energy intake	≤ 10%	10 points
	11% to 13%	5 points
	> 13%	0 points
Dietary cholesterol < 300 mg per day	≤ 300 mg	10 points
	300 to 400 mg	5 points
	> 400 mg	0 points
2–4 servings of fruit per day	10–0 points, proportional to percent of recommended number of servings[*]	
3–5 servings of vegetables per day	10–0 points, proportional to percent of recommended number of servings	
6–11 servings of grains per day	10–0 points, proportional to percent of recommended number of servings	
Calcium intake as a percentage of Adequate Intake for life stage and gender group	10–0 points, proportional to percentage of Adequate Intake for life stage and gender group	
Iron intake as percent of Recommended Dietary Allowance for life stage and gender group	10–0 points, proportional to percentage of Recommended Dietary Allowance for life stage and gender group	
Dietary diversity score	10–0 points, proportional to consumption of foods across 23 food group categories	
Dietary moderation score	10–0 points, based on intake of added sugars, discretionary fat,[†] sodium, and alcohol in excess of recommended levels of intake	

Adapted from Haines PS, Siega-Riz AM, Popkin BM. 1999. The Diet Quality Index Revised: A measurement instrument for populations. *Journal of the American Dietetic Association* 99:697–704.

[*]Serving recommendations based on energy intake according to the Food Guide Pyramid.

[†]Discretionary fat is defined as all excess fat from the five major food groups beyond that which would be consumed if only the lowest fat forms of a given food were eaten. It includes fats added to food in preparation or at the table, including margarine, cheese, oil, meat drippings, and chocolate.

the percent of calories provided by fats had increased from 32% to about 43%, while calories provided by carbohydrate had declined from 57% to 46%. The percent of calories from fats obtained from meat and dairy products had risen sharply, while carbohydrate from fruits, vegetables, and grains had fallen precipitously.[25] At the same time, there was increasingly convincing evidence linking dietary habits to the major causes of death in America: heart disease, cancer, and stroke. Although scientists recognized that heredity, age, and numerous environmental

factors besides diet were involved in the causation of these diseases, diet was one factor over which people had a certain amount of control. This led private agencies, such as the American Medical Association, the American Heart Association, and the American Health Foundation, to publish dietary guidelines.

U.S. Dietary Goals

In February 1977, the report *Dietary Goals for the United States* was issued by the U.S. Senate Select Committee on Nutrition and Human Needs.[31] This was the first of several government reports setting prudent dietary guidelines for Americans.

In its introduction, the Senate Select Committee made this statement:

> The overconsumption of foods high in fat, generally, and saturated fat in particular, as well as cholesterol, refined and processed sugars, salt and/or alcohol has been associated with the development of one or more of six to ten leading causes of death: heart disease, some cancers, stroke and hypertension, diabetes, arteriosclerosis and cirrhosis of the liver.[31]

The committee then submitted seven goals, listed in Box 2.4. The Dietary Goals were to be accomplished through the changes in food selection and preparation listed in Box 2.5.

The reaction to *Dietary Goals for the United States* from U.S. nutrition scientists and professionals was swift, strong, and polarized.[30] *Nutrition Today* published opinions about the goals from some leading nutrition scientists and professionals.[32,33] Some felt the goals were "hastily conceived and based on fragmentary evidence," "premature . . . because the diet has not yet been tested," "blatant sensationalism," "speculation," and "a nutritional debacle." One professional declared that the "Senate Select Committee has perpetrated a hoax." Other scientists believed the goals were "long overdue," "a giant step forward in improving the health of our citizens," "a valid criticism of our current diet," and "a significant achievement" and deserved "the broadest support from all who are concerned with the health and well-being of American citizens." Who was right? Time would tell.

It was immediately clear, however, that, to meet the goals, Americans would need to change the way they ate. Figure 2.6 compares the 1977 U.S. Dietary Goals with the diet of that time and highlights the necessary changes.

The Dietary Guidelines for Americans

In 1980, the U.S. Department of Agriculture and U.S. Department of Health and Human Services jointly published *Nutrition and Your Health: The Dietary Guidelines for Americans*. The Dietary Guidelines provide healthy Americans ages 2 years and older advice about food that promotes health and prevents disease. They also serve as

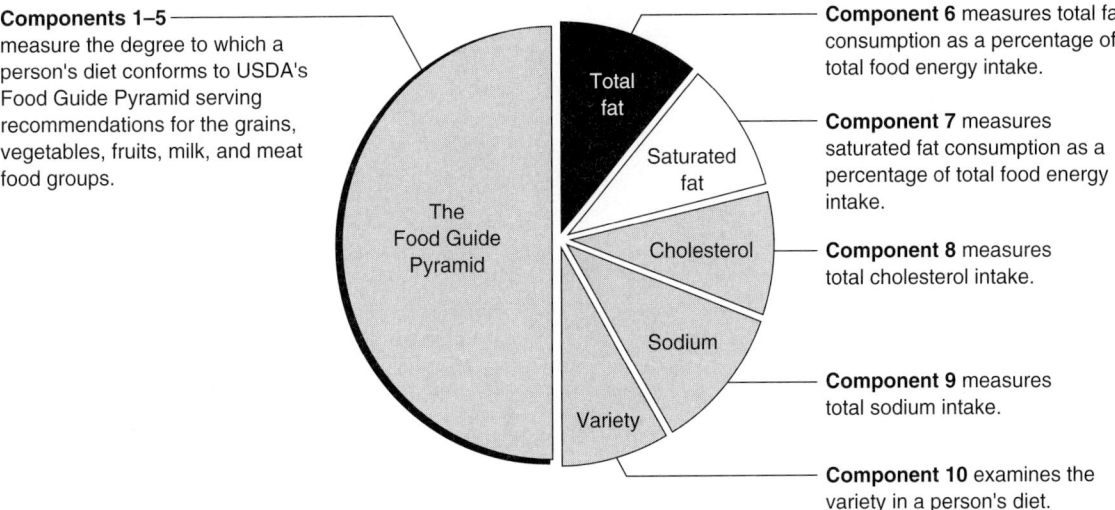

Figure 2.5 Components of the Healthy Eating Index.

Source: Reprinted from Bowman SA, Lino M, Gerrior SA, Basiotis PP. 1998. The Healthy Eating Index, 1994–96. *Family Economics and Nutrition Review* 11(3):2–14.

TABLE 2.8	Components of the Healthy Eating Index and Scoring System		
	Score Ranges[*]	Criteria for Maximum Score of 10	Criteria for Minimum Score of 0
Grain consumption	0 to 10	6–11 servings[†]	0 servings
Vegetable consumption	0 to 10	3–5 servings[†]	0 servings
Fruit consumption	0 to 10	2–4 servings[†]	0 servings
Milk consumption	0 to 10	2–3 servings[†]	0 servings
Meat consumption	0 to 10	2–3 servings[†]	0 servings
Total fat intake	0 to 10	30% or less energy from fat	45% or more energy from fat
Saturated fat intake	0 to 10	Less than 10% energy from saturated fat	15% or more energy from saturated fat
Cholesterol intake	0 to 10	300 mg or less	450 mg or more
Sodium intake	0 to 10	2400 mg or less	4800 mg or more
Food variety	0 to 10	8 or more different items in a day	3 or fewer different items in a day

Reprinted from Bowman SA, Lino M, Gerrior SA, Basiotis PP. 1998. The Healthy Eating Index, 1994–96. *Family Economics and Nutrition Review* 11(3):2–14.

*People with consumption or intakes between the maximum and minimum ranges or amounts were assigned scores proportionately.

†Number of servings depends on the recommended energy intake and are on a per day basis.

TABLE 2.9	The Dietary Reference Intakes (DRIs) and Dietary Guidelines Contrasted
DRIs	**Dietary Guidelines**
Developed earlier	Developed more recently
Only one set per country	Multiple (sometimes incongruent) sets possible in a country
Expressed in quantitative terms as weight of nutrient per day	Often expressed as nonquantitative change from present average national diet
Primarily intended to ensure adequate nutrient intake	Primarily intended to help reduce risk of developing chronic degenerative disease
More firmly established scientifically	More provisional, based more on epidemiologic data
More concerned with micronutrients	Primarily deal with macronutrients but may also address micronutrient intake
Specific recommendations for each life stage and gender group	Generally the same advice for all in the defined target group
Expressed in technical language	Technical language avoided, better understood by the public

Adapted from Truswell AS. 1999. Dietary goals and guidelines: National and international perspectives. In Shils ME, Olson JA, Shike M, Ross AC, eds. *Modern nutrition in health and disease,* 9th ed. Baltimore: Williams & Wilkins.

Box 2.4   1977 Dietary Goals

1. To avoid overweight, consume only as much energy (calories) as is expended; if overweight, decrease energy intake and increase energy expenditure.
2. Increase the consumption of complex carbohydrates and "naturally occurring" sugars from about 28% of energy intake to about 48% of energy intake.
3. Reduce the consumption of refined and processed sugars by about 45% to account for about 10% of total energy intake.
4. Reduce overall fat consumption from approximately 40% to about 30% of energy intake.

5. Reduce saturated fat consumption to account for about 10% of total energy intake and balance that with polyunsaturated and monounsaturated fats, which should account for about 10% of energy intake each.
6. Reduce cholesterol consumption to about 300 milligrams per day.
7. Limit the intake of sodium by reducing the intake of salt to about 5 grams a day.

From Select Committee on Nutrition and Human Needs. 1977. *Dietary goals for the United States.* Washington, DC: U.S. Senate.

Box 2.5   Recommendations from Dietary Goals for the United States

1. Increase consumption of fruits, vegetables, and whole grains.
2. Decrease consumption of refined and other processed sugars and foods high in such sugars.
3. Decrease consumption of foods high in total fat and partially replace saturated fats, whether obtained from animal or vegetable sources, with polyunsaturated fats.
4. Decrease consumption of animal fat and choose meats, poultry, and fish, which will reduce saturated fat intake.

5. Except for young children, substitute low-fat and nonfat milk for whole milk and low-fat dairy products for high-fat dairy products.
6. Decrease consumption of butterfat, eggs, and other high-cholesterol sources. Some consideration should be given to easing the cholesterol goal for premenopausal women, young children, and the elderly to obtain the nutritional benefit of eggs in the diet.
7. Decrease consumption of salt and foods high in salt content.

From Select Committee on Nutrition and Human Needs, 1977. *Dietary goals for the United States.* Washington, DC: U.S. Senate.

the basis for federal nutrition policy and nutrition education activities. The Dietary Guidelines have been revised every 5 years, with editions in 1985, 1990, 1995, and 2000.[34–38] Box 2.6 shows the fifth edition, issued in 2000. Table 2.10 shows the 5 editions of the Dietary Guidelines and how they have evolved over the years.

Originally, the Dietary Guidelines were a modification and reissue of the earlier Dietary Goals for the United States and contained all the essential elements of the Dietary Goals—fewer animal products, more plant products, and less added sugar, salt, and fat. They were also less forceful than the Dietary Goals, more brief, and nonquantitative. For example, the three dietary goals regarding overall fat consumption, saturated/polyunsaturated/monounsaturated fats, and cholesterol were combined into the guideline "Avoid too much fat, saturated fat, and cholesterol," and a guideline regarding alcohol consumption was added.

The 2000 edition contains 10 guidelines grouped in 3 categories. The grouping scheme—"Aim for fitness, Build a healthy base, and Choose sensibly for good health" ("ABCs for good health")—was added to make the guidelines more memorable to consumers, particularly since the number of guidelines in the 2000 edition increased from 7 to 10. As can be seen in Table 2.10, the order of the guidelines was changed to emphasize healthy weight and physical activity, and a separate guideline on activity was included to address concerns about the prevalence of overweight and obesity among Americans. The 1995 guideline "Eat a variety of foods" was replaced with "Let the Pyramid guide your food choices" in order to emphasize the importance of the Food Guide Pyramid in nutrition education and to avoid consumers' misinterpreting the variety message as encouraging overconsumption of energy. The 1995 fruits, vegetables, and grains guideline was divided into two guidelines because of differences in the food groups and to give

Figure 2.6 The 1977 U.S. Dietary Goals (right) compared with the American diet of that time.

expanded emphasis on plant foods as an important foundation of healthful eating. A new guideline on consumer food safety, "Keep food safe to eat," was added in recognition of growing concerns about food-borne illnesses. Minor changes were also made in the guidelines pertaining to fat and cholesterol, added sugars, and salt/sodium.

For links to the complete text of the latest edition of the *Dietary Guidelines for Americans* and for other relevant information, visit the *Nutritional Assessment* website at www.mhhe.com/hper/nutrition.

Toward Healthful Diets

Toward Healthful Diets was a brief report released in 1980 by the Food and Nutrition Board of the National Research Council. It gave dietary recommendations that the Food and Nutrition Board believed would "improve general nutritional status, be beneficial in preventing or delaying the onset of some chronic degenerative diseases, and incur no appreciable risks."[39] The recommendations were more conservative than either the Dietary Goals or Dietary Guidelines, except on the matter of salt.

The report appears to have been a response to concerns about the scientific soundness of the many, and sometimes confusing, dietary recommendations extant during the 1970s.[30,39] In the report's introduction, the Food and Nutrition Board stated its concern about

> the flood of dietary recommendations currently being made to the American public in the hope that a variety of chronic degenerative diseases may be prevented in some persons. These recommendations . . . often lack a sound scientific foundation, and some are contradictory to one another. In an effort to reduce the confusion in the mind of the public that has resulted from these many conflicting recommendations, the Board has prepared the following statement.[39]

The report gave five recommendations (Box 2.7), which were targeted to adults.

The Surgeon General's Report on Nutrition and Health

In 1988, *The Surgeon General's Report on Nutrition and Health* was issued.[40] This was a landmark publication

---

Box 2.6 *Dietary Guidelines for Americans, 2000,* **Fifth Edition**

AIM FOR FITNESS
- Aim for a healthy weight.
- Be physically active every day.

BUILD A HEALTHY BASE
- Let the Pyramid guide your food choices.
- Choose a variety of grains daily, especially whole grains.
- Choose a variety of fruits and vegetables daily.

CHOOSE SENSIBLY
- Choose a diet that is low in saturated fat and cholesterol and moderate in total fat.
- Choose beverages and foods to moderate your intake of sugars.
- Choose and prepare foods with less salt.
- If you drink alcoholic beverages, do so in moderation.

U.S. Department of Agriculture/U.S. Department of Health and Human Services. 1995. *Nutrition and your health: Dietary guidelines for Americans,* 5th ed. Hyattsville, MD: U.S. Department of Agriculture, Center for Nutrition Policy and Promotion.

TABLE 2.10 | Dietary Guidelines for Americans, 1980 to 2000

1980: 7 Guidelines	1985: 7 Guidelines	1990: 7 Guidelines	1995: 7 Guidelines	2000: 10 Guidelines, Clustered into 3 Groups	
Eat a variety of foods.	Eat a variety of foods.	Eat a variety of foods.	Eat a variety of foods.		
Maintain ideal weight.	Maintain desirable weight.	Maintain healthy weight.	Balance the food you eat with physical activity—maintain or improve your weight.	Aim for a healthy weight.	**Aim for Fitness**
				Be physically active each day.	
				Let the Pyramid guide your food choices.	**Build a Healthy Base**
Avoid too much fat, saturated fat, and cholesterol.	Avoid too much fat, saturated fat, and cholesterol.	Choose a diet low in fat, saturated fat, and cholesterol.		Choose a variety of grains daily, especially whole grains.	
Eat foods with adequate starch and fiber.	Eat foods with adequate starch and fiber.	Choose a diet with plenty of vegetables, fruits, and grain products.	Choose a diet with plenty of grain products, vegetables, and fruits.	Choose a variety of fruits and vegetables daily.	
				Keep food safe to eat.	
			Choose a diet low in fat, saturated fat, and cholesterol.	Choose a diet that is low in saturated fat and cholesterol and moderate in total fat.	**Choose Sensibly**
Avoid too much sugar.	Avoid too much sugar.	Use sugars only in moderation.	Choose a diet moderate in sugars.	Choose beverages and foods to moderate your intake of sugars.	
Avoid too much sodium.	Avoid too much sodium.	Use salt and sodium only in moderation.	Choose a diet moderate in salt and sodium.	Choose and prepare foods with less salt.	
If you drink alcohol, do so in moderation.	If you drink alcoholic beverages, do so in moderation.	If you drink alcoholic beverages, do so in moderation.	If you drink alcoholic beverages, do so in moderation.	If you drink alcoholic beverages, do so in moderation.	

Center for Nutrition Policy and Promotion, U.S. Department of Agriculture.

NOTE: Shading indicates how the order in which the guidelines are presented has changed over time.

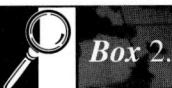

Box 2.7 Recommendations of *Toward Healthful Diets*

1. Select a nutritionally adequate diet from the foods available by consuming appropriate daily servings of dairy products, meats or legumes, vegetables and fruits, and cereal and breads.
2. Select as wide a variety of foods in each of the major food groups as is practicable to ensure a high probability of consuming adequate quantities of all essential nutrients.
3. Adjust dietary energy intake and energy expenditure so as to maintain appropriate weight for height; if

overweight, achieve appropriate weight reduction by decreasing total food and fat intake and by increasing physical activity.
4. If the requirement for energy is low (e.g., reducing diet), reduce consumption of foods such as alcohol, sugars, fats, and oils, which provide calories but few other essential nutrients.
5. Use salt in moderation; adequate but safe intakes are considered to range between 3 and 8 g of sodium chloride daily.

From Food and Nutrition Board, National Research Council. 1980. *Toward healthful diets.* Washington, DC: National Academy Press.

Box 2.8 Recommendations of *The Surgeon General's Report on Nutrition and Health*

ISSUES FOR MOST PEOPLE

- *Fats and cholesterol:* Reduce consumption of fat (especially saturated fat) and cholesterol. Choose foods relatively low in these substances, such as vegetables, fruits, whole-grain foods, fish, poultry, lean meats, and low-fat dairy products. Use food preparation methods that add little or no fat.
- *Energy and weight control:* Achieve and maintain a desirable body weight. To do so, choose a dietary pattern in which energy (caloric) intake is consistent with energy expenditure. To reduce energy intake, limit consumption of foods relatively high in calories, fats, and sugars and minimize alcohol consumption. Increase energy expenditure through regular and sustained physical activity.
- *Complex carbohydrates and fiber:* Increase consumption of whole-grain foods and cereal products, vegetables (including dried beans and peas), and fruits.
- *Sodium:* Reduce intake of sodium by choosing foods relatively low in sodium and limiting the amount of salt added in food preparation and at the table.
- *Alcohol:* To reduce the risk for chronic disease, take alcohol only in moderation (no more than two drinks a day), if at all. Avoid drinking any alcohol before or

while driving, operating machinery, taking medications, or engaging in any other activity requiring judgment. Avoid drinking alcohol while pregnant.

OTHER ISSUES FOR SOME PEOPLE

- *Fluoride:* Community water systems should contain fluoride at optimal levels for prevention of tooth decay. If such water is not available, use other appropriate sources of fluoride.
- *Sugars:* Those who are particularly vulnerable to dental caries (cavities), especially children, should limit their consumption and frequency of use of foods high in sugars.
- *Calcium:* Adolescent girls and adult women should increase consumption of foods high in calcium, including low-fat dairy products.
- *Iron:* Children, adolescents, and women of childbearing age should be sure to consume foods that are good sources of iron, such as lean meats, fish, certain beans, and iron-enriched cereals and whole-grain products. This issue is of special concern for low-income families.

From U.S. Department of Health and Human Services. 1988. *The Surgeon General's report on nutrition and health.* Washington, DC: U.S. Government Printing Office.

summarizing the scientific evidence linking specific dietary factors to health maintenance and disease prevention and presenting recommendations for dietary change to improve the health of the American people.[41] The report recognized that what we eat can affect our risk for several of the leading causes of death and identified, as of primary

importance, the need to reduce consumption of fat, especially saturated fat. It served as an authoritative source of information on which to base nutrition policy decisions and distinguished recommendations appropriate for the general public from those for special populations.[42] The report's recommendations are given in Box 2.8.

Diet and Health

In 1989, the book *Diet and Health: Implications for Reducing Chronic Disease Risk* was published by the Committee on Diet and Health of the National Research Council.[25] It represented the view that dietary recommendations should go beyond the prevention of nutrient deficiencies to the prevention of chronic disease. From their extensive review of the scientific literature, the committee members concluded that, in addition to genetic and environmental factors, "dietary patterns are important factors in the **etiology** of several major chronic diseases and that dietary modifications can reduce such risks." The influence of diet is "very strong" for coronary heart disease and hypertension and "highly suggestive" for certain cancers (esophagus, stomach, large bowel, breast, lung, and prostate). The committee stated that dietary habits also play a role in dental caries, chronic liver disease, and obesity, which increases the risk of **type 2 diabetes mellitus.** Of particular concern was the need for Americans to reduce consumption of fats, saturated fats, and cholesterol and increase intake of fruits, vegetables, legumes, and whole-grain cereals. The committee's dietary recommendations are summarized in Box 2.9.

In 1991, the Food and Nutrition Board published *Improving America's Diet and Health,* which proposed detailed strategies and options for the implementation of the dietary guidelines presented in *Diet and Health.*[43] In 1992, the Food and Nutrition Board published *Eat for Life,* a book intended to help translate the dietary guidelines in *Diet and Health* into practical guidelines for individuals and families.[44]

Other Dietary Guidelines

Since the U.S. Dietary Goals were issued in 1977, numerous scientific organizations and professional groups have studied the impact of American dietary practices on health and disease and have issued their own dietary guidelines. Only those considered most important have been discussed here. Some of the more important ones are summarized in Table 2.11.

Although the various dietary recommendations shown in Table 2.11 span more than 2 decades, there is a remarkable degree of similarity in their major tenets. After reviewing the scientific basis for these recommendations, the Nutrition Committee of the American Heart Association concluded that there is substantial evidence showing that following them will reduce risk of developing heart disease, cancer, diabetes, and obesity—the major causes of morbidity and mortality in North America.[45] Although some of the recommendations require special emphasis because of the unique needs of minorities, children, women, and the elderly, the available evidence suggests that all the major recommendations (summarized in Table 2.12) apply across population groups. To achieve the recommendations in Table 2.12, the Nutrition

---

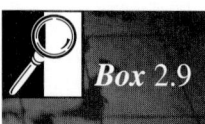

Box 2.9   Summary of Dietary Recommendations from *Diet and Health: Implications for Reducing Chronic Disease Risk*

1. Reduce total fat intake to 30% or less of calories. Reduce saturated fatty acid intake to less than 10% of calories and the intake of cholesterol to less than 300 mg daily. The intake of fat and cholesterol can be reduced by substituting fish, poultry without skin, lean meats, and low-fat or nonfat dairy products for fatty meats and whole-milk dairy products; by choosing more vegetables, fruits, cereals, and legumes; and by limiting oils, fats, egg yolks, and fried and other fatty foods.

2. Eat five or more servings every day of a combination of vegetables and fruits, especially green and yellow vegetables and citrus fruits. Also, increase intake of starches and other complex carbohydrates by eating six or more daily servings of a combination of breads, cereals, and legumes. (An average serving is equal to a half cup for most fresh or cooked vegetables, fruits, dry or cooked cereals and legumes, one medium piece of fresh fruit, one slice of bread, or one roll or muffin.)

3. Maintain protein intake at moderate levels.

4. Balance food intake and physical activity to maintain appropriate body weight.

5. The committee does not recommend alcohol consumption. For those who drink alcoholic beverages, the committee recommends limiting consumption to the equivalent of less than 1 oz of pure alcohol in a single day. This is the equivalent of two cans of beer, two small glasses of wine, or two average cocktails. Pregnant women should avoid alcoholic beverages.

6. Limit total daily intake of salt (sodium chloride) to 6 g or less. Limit the use of salt in cooking and avoid adding it to food at the table. Salty, highly processed salty, salt-preserved, and salt-pickled foods should be consumed sparingly.

7. Maintain adequate calcium intake.

8. Avoid taking dietary supplements in excess of the Recommended Dietary Allowance in any one day.

9. Maintain an optimal intake of fluoride, particularly during the years of primary and secondary tooth formation and growth.

From National Research Council: Food and Nutrition Board. 1989. *Diet and health: Implications for reducing chronic disease risk.* Washington, DC: National Academy Press.

TABLE 2.11 | **Summary of Major Dietary Recommendations**

Nutrient or Food Component	U.S. Dietary Goals, 1977	Surgeon General's Report on Nutrition and Health, 1988	Diet and Health, NRC,* 1989	ACS* Guidelines on Diet, Nutrition, and Cancer Prevention, 1998	Dietary Guidelines for Americans, USDA/USDHHS,* 2000	Dietary Guidelines for Healthy American Adults, AHA,* 1996	American Diabetes Association, 2000†
Total fat (% of kcal)	≤ 30%	Reduce intake	≤ 30%	Limit intake of high-fat foods, particularly from animal sources	≤ 30%	≤ 30%	Must be individualized
Saturated fatty acids (% of kcal)	≤ 10%	Reduce intake	< 10%		< 10%	< 10%	< 10%
Polyunsaturated fatty acids (% of kcal)	≤ 10%	NS	≤ 10%	NC	NS	≤ 10%	≤ 10%
Monounsaturated fatty acids (% of kcal)	≤ 10%	NS	NS	NC	NS	10% to 15%	10% to 15%
Trans fatty acids	NC	NC	NS	NC	Limit intake	Limit intake	NC
Dietary cholesterol (mg/day)	250–300 mg/day	Reduce intake	< 300 mg/day	NC	< 300 mg/day	< 300 mg/day	≤ 300 mg/day
Added sugars	Limit	Limit intake	Consume in moderation	NC	Consume in moderation	Consume in moderation	Priority given to total carbohydrate intake
Carbohydrate (% of kcal)	> 55%	Increase consumption	≥ 55%	Choose most foods from plant sources	Emphasizes unrefined grain products as the foundation of diet	55% to 60%	Must be individualized
Dietary fiber	Increase	Increase consumption	NS	NC	Emphasizes unrefined grains, fruits, vegetables	25–30 g/day	20–35 g/day
Sodium (mg/day)	≤ 2000 mg/day	Reduce intake	≤ 2400 m g/day	NC	≤ 2400 mg/day	≤ 2400 mg/day	≤ 2400 mg/day
Moderate alcohol consumption, if any	Yes	Yes	Yes	Yes	Yes	Yes	Yes, may cause hypoglycemia
Maintain healthy weight, be physically active	Yes	Yes	Yes	Yes	Yes	Yes	Yes
Other	Reduce additives and processed foods	Foods rich in calcium and iron, fluoridated water for some people	Adequate fluoride and calcium intake, moderate protein intake, avoid excess supplement use	NS	Emphasizes following the Food Guide Pyramid and food safety	Children need adequate energy and nutrients for normal growth and development	Chromium and magnesium supplementation only when medically indicated

*NRC = National Research Council; ACS = American Cancer Society; AHA = American Heart Association; USDA = U.S. Department of Agriculture; USDHHS = U.S. Department of Health and Human Services.

†Many of these recommendations must be individualized to suit the personal lifestyle and treatment goals of the individual with diabetes. See Chapter 8 for additional details.

NC = No comment; NS = Not specified.

TABLE 2.12	**Common Recommendations of Dietary Guidelines**

- Saturated fat $< 10\%$ of kcal
- Total fat $\leq 30\%$ of kcal
- Polyunsaturated fat $\leq 10\%$ of kcal
- Monounsaturated fat $\leq 15\%$ of kcal
- Dietary cholesterol ≤ 300 mg/day
- Carbohydrates $\geq 55\%$ of kcal
- Energy intake to achieve and maintain healthy weight
- Sodium intake < 2400 mg/day

Adapted from Deckelbaum RJ, Fisher EA, Winston M, et al. 1999. Summary of a scientific conference on preventive nutrition: Pediatrics to geriatrics. *Circulation* 100:450–456.

Committee of the American Heart Association suggests following the Food Guide Pyramid and the Dietary Guidelines for Americans.[45]

NUTRITION LABELING OF FOOD

Nutrition labeling of food in the United States began in 1973, when the U.S. Food and Drug Administration (FDA) established labeling regulations. These included creating the U.S. Recommended Daily Allowances and instituting specific guidelines for food labeling.

U.S. Recommended Daily Allowances

In 1973, the FDA issued regulations requiring the nutrition labeling of any food containing one or more added nutrients or whose label or advertising included claims about the food's nutritional properties or its usefulness in the daily diet. Nutrition labeling was voluntary for almost all other foods. The *U.S. Recommended Daily Allowances (U.S. RDAs)* were nutrient standards developed by the FDA at that time for use in regulating the nutrition labeling of food. They replaced the Minimum Daily Requirement, which had been in use since 1940 for labeling vitamin and mineral supplements, breakfast cereals, and some special foods.

The U.S. RDAs (shown in Appendix B) included 19 nutrients and recommendations for 4 categories of people. Three sets of nutrient standards (those for infants, children under 4 years of age, and pregnant and lactating females) were used for labeling specialty foods and supplements marketed specifically to infants, children, and pregnant or lactating women. The fourth and most familiar set was for males and nonpregnant, nonlactating females 4 or more years of age; this was the standard seen on most food labels in the United States. It was developed by selecting the highest value for each nutrient given in the 1968 RDA table for males and nonpregnant,

nonlactating females 4 or more years of age, except for calcium and phosphorus, which were set at the midpoint of the RDA values for males and females.

The Nutrition Labeling and Education Act

Between 1973 and 1993, there was growing awareness that the major nutritional problem facing North Americans was overconsumption of foods rich in total fat, saturated fat, and cholesterol and low in complex carbohydrates. There were also major breakthroughs in our knowledge of essential nutrient requirements (for example, the RDAs had been revised three times). Despite these advances, the U.S. RDAs had not been updated, and food labeling regulations remained virtually unchanged. During the same period, the public and various professional and consumer interest groups called for food labels that were easily understood, that were truthful, and that reflected awareness of the relationship between diet and health. In 1990, the FDA's **Nutrition Labeling and Education Act (NLEA)** was passed, mandating nutrition labeling for almost all processed foods regulated by the FDA and authorizing appropriate health claims on the labels of such products. It brought about the most extensive food labeling reform in U.S. history. The NLEA also called for activities to educate consumers about nutrition information on the label and the importance of using that information in maintaining healthful dietary practices. The NLEA's final regulations were published in the 6 January 1993 *Federal Register.* 8 August 1994 was the final deadline for manufacturers to comply. The USDA's Food Safety and Inspection Service, responsible for the inspection of meat and poultry, issued parallel regulations that governed the labeling of meat and poultry.

The NLEA requires virtually all processed foods to carry nutrition information on the label (Figure 2.7). Foods exempted from the regulations include plain coffee and tea, some spices and flavorings, and other foods having insignificant nutritional value; ready-to-eat food prepared primarily on-site, such as deli and bakery items; foods in very small packages; restaurant food; bulk food that is not resold; and foods produced by businesses with food sales of less than $50,000 per year or total sales less than $500,000 per year unless the food item contains a nutrition claim. Nutrition labeling is voluntary for most raw foods. The 20 most frequently eaten raw fruits, vegetables, and fish are included in the FDA's voluntary point-of-purchase nutrition information program. The 45 major cuts of meat and poultry are covered under the USDA's voluntary point-of-purchase program.

The nutrients and food components required on the label were selected because of their relationship to current health concerns, and the order in which they are list-

More consistent serving sizes, in both household and metric units, replace those that used to be set by manufacturers.

This mandatory component helps consumers meet dietary guidelines recommending no more than 30% of energy from fat.

Nutrients required on nutrition panel are those most important to today's consumers, most of whom need to reduce intake of certain items (fat, cholesterol, etc.) and increase intake of other items (dietary fiber, etc.).

Percent of Daily Value for mandatory dietary components shows how the food fits into the overall diet. If a food is fortified or enriched with any of the optional dietary components, or if a claim is made about any of them, the pertinent nutrition information then becomes mandatory.

These vitamins and minerals of current concern are still mandatory.

Daily Reference Values help consumers learn good diet basics. They can be adjusted, depending on a person's energy needs.

Conversion guide helps consumers learn caloric value of the energy-yielding nutrients.

Figure 2.7 **Key aspects of the Nutrition Facts label.**

ed reflects their public health significance. Box 2.10 shows the mandatory and voluntary nutrients and dietary components in the order they must appear on food labels. The mandatory nutrients and dietary components are required on all food labels. Listing of the voluntary ones is optional. If a food is fortified or enriched with any of the voluntary nutrients or dietary components, or if a health or nutrient content claim is made about any of them, the pertinent nutrition information then becomes mandatory. Total calories, total fat, total carbohydrate,

protein, sodium, vitamins A and C, calcium, and iron were carryovers from the previous label. Saturated fat, cholesterol, sugars, dietary fiber, and calories from fat were added by the new regulations. Niacin, thiamin, and riboflavin are now voluntary nutrients.

Serving sizes listed on the label are specified by the FDA, are uniform across all product lines so consumers can more easily compare brands, and are closer to the amounts people actually eat. Using data from USDA food consumption surveys, the FDA determined the

Box 2.10   **Mandatory (in Italics) and Voluntary Nutrients and Dietary Components in the Order They Must Appear on the Nutrition Facts Label**

- *Total calories*
- *Calories from fat*
- Calories from saturated fat
- *Total fat*
- *Saturated fat*
- Stearic acid (on meat and poultry products only)
- Polyunsaturated fat
- Monounsaturated fat
- *Cholesterol*
- *Sodium*
- Potassium
- *Total carbohydrate*
- *Dietary fiber*

- Soluble fiber
- Insoluble fiber
- *Sugars*
- *Sugar alcohols*
- Other carbohydrates
- *Protein*
- *Vitamin A*
- Percent of vitamin A as beta-carotene
- *Vitamin C*
- *Calcium*
- *Iron*
- Other essential vitamins and minerals

amounts of various foods that people customarily consume per eating occasion. These are called **reference amounts** and are expressed in metric units. The serving size listed on food labels is the amount in common household measures closest to the reference amount. It is important to note that serving sizes as defined by the FDA do not always agree with the serving sizes recommended in such dietary guidelines as the Food Guide Pyramid or the exchange system.

A list of all ingredients must appear on all processed and packaged foods. When appropriate, ingredient lists must include any FDA-certified color additives, the sources of any protein hydrolysates, a declaration that caseinate is a milk derivative when caseinate is found in foods claiming to be nondairy, and a declaration of the total percentage of juice in any beverage claiming to contain juice.

An important feature of the NLEA is that it regulates nutrient content claims and health claims on food labels or other labeling of food, such as advertisements. Nutrient content claims are those describing the amount of nutrients in foods, such as "cholesterol free," "low fat," "light," or "lean." Examples of these are shown in Table 2.13. In addition to the nutrient claims shown in Table 2.13 are those using the word *reduced* or *less*. A food making the claim "reduced or less sodium" has to contain at least 25% less sodium per serving than an appropriate food used for comparison purposes. For example, potato chips labeled "low sodium" must contain at least 25% less sodium than comparable potato chips (the "reference food").

The FDA defines a health claim as any claim on the package label or other labeling of a food that characterizes the relationship of any nutrient or other substance in the food to a disease or health-related condition. Accord-

ing to FDA regulations, health claims are allowed only under certain circumstances and must be scientifically based and standardized. Allowable health claims are shown in Box 2.11. The NLEA stipulates that foods bearing health claims must not contain any nutrient or substance in an amount that increases the risk of a disease or a health condition. Foods bearing health claims must contain 20% or less of the Daily Value of fat, saturated fat, cholesterol, and sodium per serving. For example, whole milk (which is high in calcium) may not bear a calcium-osteoporosis claim because its fat content exceeds 20% of the Daily Value for fat. Skim and 1% fat milk easily qualify for the calcium-osteoporosis claim. According to FDA regulation, claims that a substance will prevent a disease are drug claims. Health claims on food labels are limited to saying that a food "may" or "might" reduce the risk of a disease or health condition.

As shown in Figure 2.8, the Nutrition Facts label of foods for children under age 2 years (except infant formula, which has special labeling rules under the Infant Formula Act of 1980) may not carry information about saturated fat, polyunsaturated fat, monounsaturated fat, cholesterol, calories from fat, or calories from saturated fat. This is to prevent parents from wrongly assuming that infants and toddlers should restrict their fat intake, when, in fact, they should not. Fat is important during these years to ensure adequate growth and development. The labels of foods for children under age 4 years may not include the Percent of Daily Values for total fat, saturated fat, cholesterol, sodium, potassium, total carbohydrate, and dietary fiber because the FDA has not established Daily Values for these nutrients in this age category. However, the label may carry the Percent of Daily Values for protein, vitamins, and minerals, which the FDA has established.

TABLE 2.13	Examples and Meanings of Some Allowable Nutrient Content Claims

Example of Nutrient Content Claim	Meaning of Nutrient Content Claim
Sugar free	Less than 0.5 g sugars per serving
Calorie free	Less than 5 kcal per serving
Low calorie	40 kcal or less per serving
Fat free	Less than 0.5 g fat per serving
Saturated fat free	Less than 0.5 g saturated fat and less than 0.5 g *trans* fat per serving
Low fat	3 g or less per serving
Low saturated fat	1 g or less of saturated fat and less than 0.5 g *trans* fat per serving*
Trans fat free	Less than 0.5 g *trans* fat and less than 0.5 g saturated fat per serving*
Cholesterol free	Less than 2 mg of cholesterol and 2 g or less of both saturated fat and *trans* fat*
Low cholesterol	20 mg or less of cholesterol and 2 g or less of both saturated fat and *trans* fat*
Sodium free	Less than 5 mg sodium per serving
Low sodium	140 mg or less per serving
Very low sodium	35 mg or less per serving
Lean meat or poultry	Less than 10 g total fat, less than 4.5 g of saturated and *trans* fat combined, and less than 95 mg cholesterol per serving and per 100 g for individual foods*
Extra lean meat or poultry	Less than 5 g total fat, less than 2 g saturated and *trans* fat combined, and less than 95 mg cholesterol per serving and per 100 g for individual foods*
High, rich in	20% or more of Daily Value to describe protein, vitamins, minerals, dietary fiber, or potassium per serving
Good source of	10% to 19% or more of Daily Value per serving
More, added	Contains a nutrient that is at least 10% percent of Daily Value more than the reference food, regardless of whether the food is altered (fortified or enriched)
Light, lite	One-third fewer calories or half the fat of the reference food; if the food derives 50% or more of its calories from fat, the reduction must be 50% of the fat; can also mean that sodium content has been reduced by at least 50%

Source: U.S. Food and Drug Administration, Center for Food Safety and Applied Nutrition.

*The language used reflects new rules for *trans* fatty acids proposed by the FDA in November 1999.

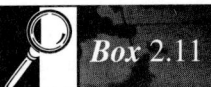

Box 2.11 | **Health Claims Allowed on the Nutrition Facts Label**

- Calcium and reduced risk for osteoporosis
- Sodium and increased risk for hypertension
- Dietary saturated fat and cholesterol and increased risk for coronary heart disease
- Dietary fat and increased risk for cancer
- Fiber-containing grain products, fruits, and vegetables and reduced risk for cancer
- Fruits, vegetables, and grain products that contain fiber, particularly soluble fiber, and reduced risk for coronary heart disease

- Fruits and vegetables and reduced risk for cancer
- Folic acid and reduced risk for neural tube defects
- Sugar alcohols and reduced risk for dental caries
- Soluble fiber and reduced risk for coronary heart disease
- Soy protein and reduced risk for coronary heart disease

Daily Values

The **Daily Values** are dietary reference values intended to help consumers use food label information to plan healthy diets. They serve as the basis for quantifying the amounts of various nutrients and food components on food labels. They are to be used for regulatory purposes only and are not intended to serve as recommended intakes. The basis for calculating the Daily Values are

two separate sets of nutrient reference values: the **Daily Reference Values (DRVs)** and the **Reference Daily Intakes (RDIs).**

Daily Reference Values

The DRVs are reference values for nutrients and food components for which no set of standards (e.g., the RDAs or U.S. RDAs) previously existed. Table 2.14 shows the DRVs

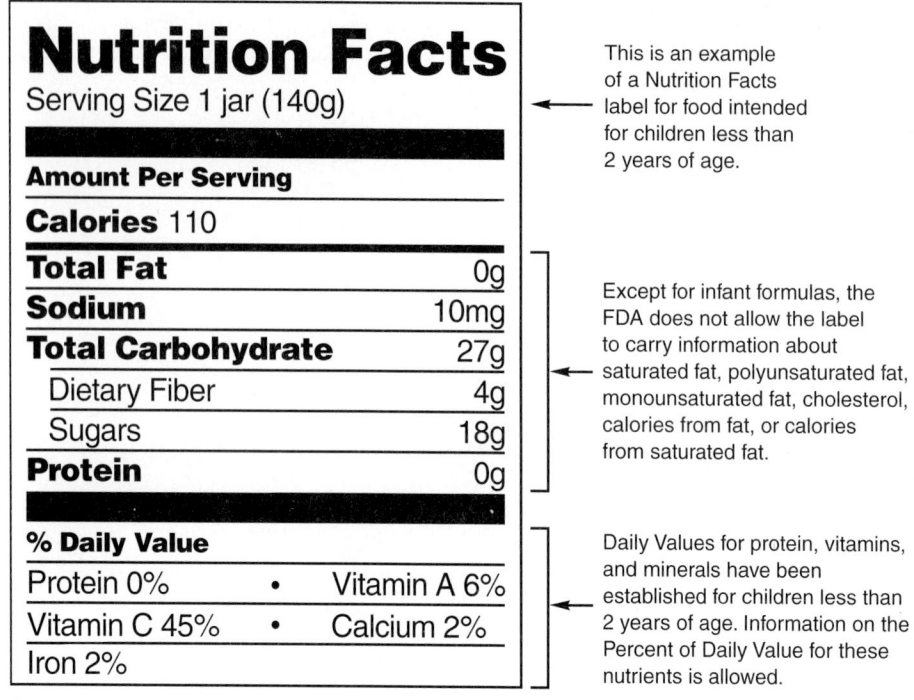

This is an example of a Nutrition Facts label for food intended for children less than 2 years of age.

Except for infant formulas, the FDA does not allow the label to carry information about saturated fat, polyunsaturated fat, monounsaturated fat, cholesterol, calories from fat, or calories from saturated fat.

Daily Values for protein, vitamins, and minerals have been established for children less than 2 years of age. Information on the Percent of Daily Value for these nutrients is allowed.

A

This is an example of a Nutrition Facts label for a food intended for children less than 4 years of age.

The label may not include the Percent of Daily Value for total fat, saturated fat, cholesterol, sodium, potassium, total carbohydrate, and dietary fiber.

Daily Values for protein, vitamins, and minerals have been established for this age group and information on the Percent of Daily Value for these nutrients is allowed.

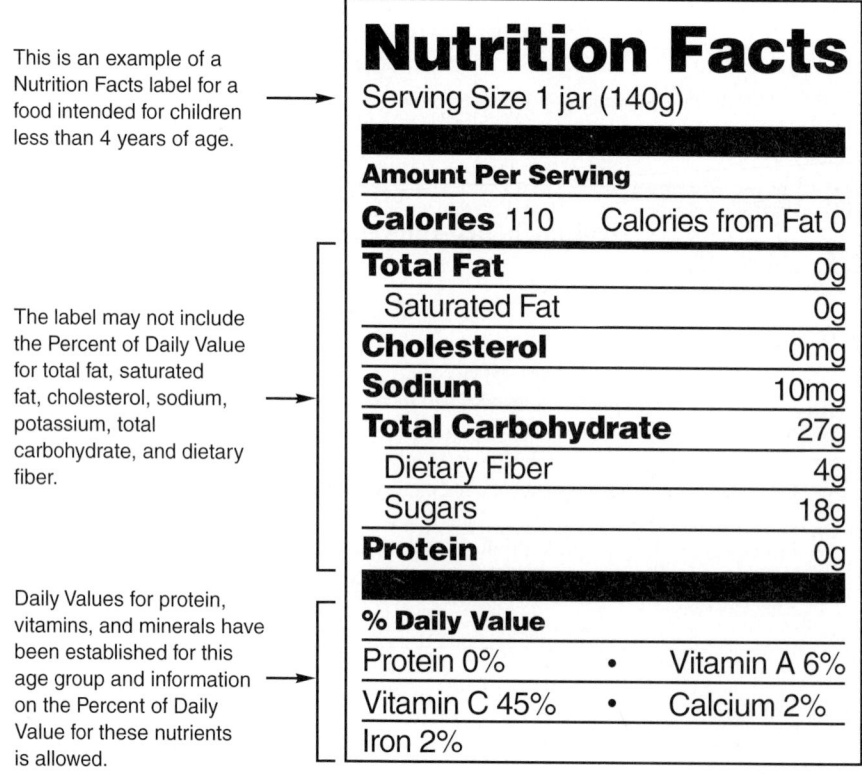

B

Figure 2.8 Examples of mandatory differences in the Nutrition Facts labels for foods designed for children less than 2 years of age (A) and for foods intended for children less than 4 years of age (B).

Source: U.S. Food and Drug Administration, Center for Food Safety and Applied Nutrition.

TABLE 2.14	The Food and Drug Administration's Daily Reference Values (DRVs) for 2000-kcal and 2500-kcal diets

	Daily Reference Value	
Food Component	**2000 kcal**	**2500 kcal**
Fat	< 65 g	< 80 g
Saturated fatty acids	< 20 g	< 25 g
Cholesterol	< 300 mg	< 300 mg
Total carbohydrate	300 g	375 g
Fiber	25 g	30 g
Sodium mg	< 2400 mg	< 2400
Potassium	3500 mg	3500 mg
Protein*	50 g	63 g

*The DRV for protein applies only to children older than 4 years and adults. The RDIs for protein for infants, children 1 to 4 years, pregnant females, and nursing females are 14 g, 16 g, 60 g, and 65 g, respectively.

TABLE 2.15	The Food and Drug Administration's Reference Daily Intakes (RDIs)*

Nutrient	Amount
Vitamin A	5000 IU[†]
Vitamin C	60 mg
Thiamin	1.5 mg
Riboflavin	1.7 mg
Niacin	20 mg
Calcium	1000 mg
Iron	18 mg
Vitamin D	400 IU
Vitamin E	30 IU
Vitamin B_6	2.0 mg
Folic acid	400 μg
Vitamin B_{12}	6 μg
Phosphorus	1000 mg
Iodine	150 μg
Magnesium	400 mg
Zinc	15 mg
Copper	2 mg
Biotin	300 μg
Pantothenic acid	10 mg

*Based on the National Academy of Sciences' 1986 Recommended Dietary Allowances.
[†]IU = international units.

for 2000-kcal and 2500-kcal diets. For labeling purposes, 2000 kcal is the reference for calculating Percent of Daily Values, although some labels may also include DRVs for a higher energy intake, such as 2500 kcal. The DRVs include values for total fat, saturated fatty acids, cholesterol, total carbohydrate, dietary fiber, sodium, potassium, and protein. Some of the DRVs are based on recommendations to increase or maintain intake of the particular food component (carbohydrate, dietary fiber, and potassium), whereas other DRVs reflect levels that are limitations on intake (total fat, saturated fat, cholesterol, and sodium).

Four of the seven food components for which DRVs have been established require a specific energy intake to quantify reference values. Those for total fat, saturated fat, and carbohydrate are based on intake levels of approximately 30%, 10%, and 60% of total energy, respectively. The DRV for protein is based on 10% of energy from protein for adults and children 4 years of age and older. The reference value for dietary fiber is based on an intake of approximately 11.5 g per 1000 kcal. The DRV for cholesterol is based on recommendations that individuals, regardless of energy intake, limit their consumption to less than 300 mg/day. The value for sodium resulted from recommendations that all persons limit their *salt* intake to less than 6 g/day, which is a sodium intake of less than 2.4 g/day. The DRV for potassium is 3500 mg, a level associated with decreased risk of hypertension.

Reference Daily Intakes

The RDIs serve as reference values for vitamins and minerals and are the U.S. RDAs (discussed in the section "U.S. Recommended Daily Allowances" and shown in Appendix B), with a new name. The RDIs are shown in Table 2.15. In 1990, the FDA proposed updating the U.S. RDAs but was temporarily prevented from doing so by Congress. Part of the rationale for changing the name of the U.S. RDAs to RDIs was to decrease confusion over the terms "RDA" and "U.S. RDA." The FDA plans to update the RDIs in the near future, so that they will be more representative of our contemporary understanding of nutrient requirements.

FOOD GUIDES

A food guide is a nutrition education tool translating scientific knowledge and dietary standards and recommendations into an understandable and practical form for use by those who have little or no training in nutrition.[29,45] Food guides are problem oriented and address specific nutritional problems identified within the targeted population. Typically, foods are classified into basic groups according to similarity of nutrient content or some other criteria. If a certain number of servings from each group is consumed, a balanced and adequate diet is thought likely to result.

The USDA has been at the forefront of food guide development in the United States. The major food guides developed by the USDA are outlined in Table 2.16. The USDA's first food guides are credited to Caroline Hunt, a nutrition specialist in USDA's Bureau of Home Economics.[46] In 1916, she developed *Food for Young Children*, followed in 1917 by *How to Select Foods*. In these, foods

TABLE 2.16   Major USDA Food Guides (1916–1995), Showing Food Groups and Numbers of Servings*

Food Guide	Number of Food Groups	Protein-Rich Foods — Milk	Protein-Rich Foods — Meat	Breads	Vegetables	Fruits	Other — Fats	Other — Sugars
Caroline Hunt buying guides (1916)	5	Meats and other protein-rich foods 10% of energy from milk 10% of energy from other foods 1 c milk + 2–3 svgs of other foods based on 3-oz svg		Cereals and other starchy foods 20% of energy 9 svgs based on 1 oz or ¾ c dry cereal	Vegetables and fruits 30% of energy 5 svgs based on average 8-oz svg		Fatty foods 20% of energy 9 svgs based on 1-Tbsp svg	Sugars 10% of energy 10 svgs based on 1-Tbsp svg
H. K. Stiebeling buying guide (1930s)	12	Milk 2c Lean meat, poultry, fish 9–10 svgs/wk	Dry, mature beans, peas, nuts 1 svg/wk Eggs 1	Flours, cereals as desired	Leafy green, yellow 11–12 svgs per wk Potato, sweet potato 1 svg Other vegetables and fruit 3 svgs	Tomato and citrus 1 svg	Butter Other fats	Sugars
Basic Seven foundation diet (1940s)	7	Milk and milk products 2 or more svgs svg = 1 c	Meat, poultry, fish, eggs, dried beans, peas, nuts 1–2 svgs	Breads, flour, and cereals every day	Leafy green, yellow 1 or more svgs Potato and other fruits and vegetables 2 or more svgs	Citrus, tomato, cabbage, salad greens 1 or more svgs	Butter, fortified margarine some daily	
Basic Four foundation diet (1956–1970s)	4	Milk group 2 or more svgs	Meat group 2 or more svgs 2–3 oz svgs	Bread, cereal 4 or more svgs 1 oz dry, 1 slice ½–¾ c cooked	Vegetable-fruit group 4 svgs include dark green/yellow vegetables frequently ½ c or typical portion			
Hassle-Free foundation diet (1979)	5	Milk-cheese group 2 svgs 1 c, 1½ oz cheese	Meat, poultry, fish, and bean group 2 svgs 2- to 3-oz svg	Bread-cereal group 4 or more svgs 1 oz dry, 1 slice ½–¾ c cooked	Vegetable-fruit group 4 svgs include vitamin C source daily and dark-green/yellow vegetables frequently ½ c or typical portion		Fats, sweets, alcohol group use dependent on calorie needs	
Food Guide Pyramid total diet (1984)	6	Milk, yogurt, cheese 2–3 svgs 1 c, 1½ oz cheese	Meat, poultry, fish eggs, dry beans, nuts 2–3 svgs 5–7 oz total/day	Breads, cereals rice pasta 6–11 svgs whole-grain and enriched 1 slice, ½ c cooked	Vegetable 3–5 svgs dark green deep yellow starchy/legumes other ½ c raw ½ c cooked	Fruit 2–4 svgs citrus other ½ c or average	Fats, oils, sweets total fat not to exceed 30% of energy sweets vary according to energy need	

Source: U.S. Department of Agriculture, Center for Nutrition Policy and Promotion.

*Number of servings are daily unless noted otherwise; svg 5 serving.

were categorized into five groups—milk and meat; cereals; vegetables and fruits; fats and fat foods; and sugars and sugary foods. These "buying guides" were designed to ensure adequate energy intake from fat, carbohydrate, and protein while encouraging sufficient variety for minerals and some of the newly discovered body-regulating substances we now know as vitamins. The financial constraints imposed by the economic depression of the early 1930s led to the development of food guides providing advice to families for purchasing foods at various cost levels. Hazel Stiebeling, a food economist in USDA's Bureau of Home Economics, led in the development of these buying guides. She emphasized a balance between high-energy foods (e.g., fats and sweets) and "protective" or nutrient-dense foods supplying essential nutrients. Among the protective foods are milk, which supplies calcium, and fruits and vegetables, which supply vitamins A and C.[46]

Hunt's and Stiebeling's buying guides gave way to food guides promoting "foundation diets." These food guides recommended a minimum number of servings from different food groups, which provided a foundation diet supplying a major portion of the RDAs. It was assumed that, to meet their energy needs, most people would consume more food than the guide specified. This extra food would provide not only necessary energy but additional nutrients as well. It was further assumed that such a diet would meet requirements for all essential nutrients, not just those included in the RDAs.[45,46] During the mid-1940s, the USDA developed the "Basic Seven," which was widely used for many years. Its complexity and lack of specific serving sizes led to the development of the "Basic Four" in 1956.[45,46] The assumption underlying development of the Four Food Groups was that eating the specified numbers of servings from the different food groups would supply approximately 1200 kcal, approximately 100% of the RDAs for vitamins A and C and calcium, and at least 80% of the RDAs for the remaining five nutrients of the 1953 revision of the RDAs.[45] Vitamins A and C and calcium were given priority status because they were shown to be **shortfall nutrients** (nutrients whose intakes were below recommended levels among a significant part of the population).[45]

In 1979, the USDA issued the Hassle-Free Guide to a Better Diet. This was a revision of the Four Food Groups that gave more attention to micronutrients in food groups and included a fifth food group: fats, sweets, and alcohol. The purpose of including this fifth group was to help consumers recognize fats, sweets, and alcohol as empty calories and to draw attention to the need for considering them in meal planning, since no servings from this group were recommended. The Hassle-Free guide highlighted the need to use fat, sugars, and alcohol moderately and gave special attention to calories and dietary fiber.[46]

Publication of the *Dietary Goals for the United States* in 1977 (review Figure 2.6 and Box 2.4) was a turning point for dietary guidance and food guides. Following this landmark event, the USDA and USDHHS published the *Dietary Guidelines for Americans* in 1980, with revisions following every 5 years. In 1980, the USDA began working on a new food guide to replace the Basic Four. This led to development of the food guide shown in Table 2.17. Three key messages of this guide were variety (eating a selection of foods of various types that together meet nutritional needs); proportionality (eating appropriate amounts of various types of foods to meet nutritional needs); and moderation (avoiding too much of food components in the total diet that have been linked to diseases).[46] Despite dissemination of the food guide in several publications developed by the USDA and other groups (including the 1990 edition of *Dietary Guidelines for Americans*), the perception remained among the public and professionals that the USDA was still using the Basic Four developed in the 1950s.[46,47] This led the USDA to develop a separate publication explaining the food guide and containing an appealing illustration conveying the key messages of the guide.

Food Guide Pyramid

In 1988, the USDA contracted with a private market research firm to develop and extensively test a publication and graphics to communicate its new food guide. Of the various graphic alternatives tested, a pyramid proved to be the most effective visual approach for communicating the messages of variety, proportionality, and moderation.[46,47] The pyramid underwent extensive peer review by nutrition educators and was enthusiastically received by these groups. The pyramid was the centerpiece of a colorful nutrition education brochure developed by the USDA and USDHHS that better reflected the current

TABLE 2.17	Daily Food Guide Developed by the USDA to Replace the Basic Four*
Food Group	**Suggested Servings**
Vegetables	3–5
Fruits	2–4
Breads, cereals, rice, and pasta	6–11
Milk, yogurt, and cheese	2–3
Meats, poultry, fish, dry beans and peas, eggs, and nuts	2–3

From USDA/USDHHS. 1990. *Nutrition and your health: Dietary guidelines for Americans,* 3rd ed. Washington, DC: U.S. Government Printing Office.

*Eat a variety of foods daily, choosing different foods from each group. Most people should have at least the lower number of servings suggested from each food group. Some people may need more because of their body size and activity levels. Young children should have a variety of foods but may need small servings.

state of nutritional knowledge. On the day that printing of the brochure was to be completed, then Secretary of Agriculture Edward Madigan canceled the project. According to a former top USDA official, Secretary Madigan canceled the project 10 days after meeting with members of the National Cattlemen's Association, who were reportedly "incensed" over the pyramid graphic. The National Milk Producers Federation also voiced complaints about the graphic.[48,49] Both groups contended that the placement of their products within the graphic would lead to decreased consumption of their products. It was alleged that cancellation was to allow further testing of the pyramid graphic. However, the media widely reported that the project was killed because of meat and dairy industry objections to the pyramid.[50–53] After a year of additional testing at a cost of $855,000, the USDA finally released the Food Guide Pyramid in 1992 (see Figure 2.9).

The Food Guide Pyramid graphically suggests the number of servings of foods from five major groups in an easily understandable way. Recommendations are made for cereals/grains, vegetables, fruits, dairy products, and protein-rich foods. At the pyramid's bottom is the bread, cereal, rice, and pasta group; these should compose the largest portion of the diet, about 6 to 11 servings per day. At the very top of the pyramid are fats, oils, and sweets; placement there indicates caution to use these sparingly.

The pyramid shows a range of food servings for each food group. The number of servings a person should eat depends on the number of kilocalories needed, which in turn depends on that person's age, sex, size, and physical activity. As shown in Table 2.18, the low number of servings from each group provides approximately 1600 kcal per day, while the high number of servings from each group provides approximately 2800 kcal per day. Examples of serving sizes are shown in Table 2.19.

Alternative Food Guides

The Food Guide Pyramid has been criticized by some as representing "a mix of well-supported findings, educated guesses, and political compromises with powerful economic interests such as the dairy and meat industries."[54] Some feel that the recommended number of servings of meat (two to three per day) may be unhealthy and that the Food Guide Pyramid ignores important differences in types of fat, such as saturated and *trans* fatty acids, as opposed to monounsaturated fatty acids.[54] Others object

Figure 2.9 **The U.S. Department of Agriculture's Food Guide Pyramid.**
Source: USDA.

TABLE 2.18	Sample Diets for a Day at Three Energy Levels		
Food Group	Lower, About 1600 kcal	Moderate, About 2200 kcal	Higher, About 2800 kcal
Bread group servings	6	9	11
Vegetable group servings	3	4	5
Fruit group servings	2	3	4
Milk group servings*	2–3	2–3	2–3
Meat group servings† (ounces)	5	6	7
Total fat (grams)	53	73	93
Total added sugars (teaspoons)	6	12	18

*Women who are pregnant or breast-feeding, teenagers, and young adults to age 24 years need 3 servings.

†Meat group amounts are in total ounces.

TABLE 2.19	Examples of Serving Sizes Used in the Food Guide Pyramid
Bread, cereal, rice, and pasta group	1 slice bread 1 oz ready-to-eat cereal ½ c cooked cereal, rice, or pasta
Vegetable group	1 c raw leafy vegetables ½ c other vegetables, cooked, chopped, or raw ¾ c vegetable juice
Fruit group	1 medium apple, banana, or orange ½ c chopped, cooked, or canned fruit ¾ c fruit juice
Milk, yogurt, and cheese group	1 c milk or yogurt 1½ oz natural cheese 2 oz processed cheese
Meat, poultry, fish, dry beans, eggs, and nuts group	2–3 oz cooked lean meat, poultry, or fish or ½ c cooked dry beans, 1 egg, or 2 Tbsp. peanut butter count as 1 oz of lean meat

to the USDA's approach to grouping foods—for example, grouping nonfat dairy products (skim milk or nonfat yogurt, for example) with higher-fat dairy products, such as ice cream and many cheeses, or grouping legumes with meat, many of which are high in fat. The USDA's failure to emphasize sources of calcium other than dairy products is regarded by some as insensitive to individuals of African, Asian, or Hispanic descent, who are more likely to experience lactose malabsorption than are those of Northern European descent. In response to these and other concerns, alternative pyramids have been developed. Among these are the Mediterranean Pyramid and the Vegetarian Pyramid.

Mediterranean Pyramid

The Mediterranean Pyramid (Figure 2.10) was based on the dietary patterns typically followed by persons living in Greece and southern Italy in the 1960s. (Recently, however, diets in these countries have become more similar to those eaten in North America.) Persons in these countries had very low death rates from coronary heart disease and long life expectancies.[54] The Mediterranean Pyramid has several things in common with the USDA's pyramid. Both emphasize grain products as the basis of the diet and liberal daily intake of fruits and vegetables; however, the Mediterranean Pyramid places greater emphasis on whole-grain foods than does the USDA's pyramid. The Mediterranean Pyramid recommends consuming only small amounts of dairy products each day; eating poultry, sweets, and eggs only a few times a week; and eating lean red meats only a few times a month. It also identifies olive oil as the preferred type of fat. In addition to daily exercise, it suggests the controversial option of one glass of wine per day for women and up to two glasses per day for men, with the warning that drinking should be avoided when doing so would put the drinker or others at risk. Despite evidence suggesting that moderate alcohol consumption raises HDL cholesterol, lowers risk of coronary heart disease, and lowers overall mortality, alcohol consumption is a major factor in motor vehicle accidents, homicide, suicide, and domestic violence. There is considerable evidence that even one or two drinks per day can increase risk for breast cancer in females.

Vegetarian Pyramid

The New York Medical College's Vegetarian Pyramid (Figure 2.11) was developed for use by nutritionists and dietitians in counseling their vegetarian clients. In many respects, is it similar to the Food Guide Pyramid. There are some differences, however. Included with the bread, cereal, rice, and pasta group are starchy vegetables, such as potatoes, green peas, and corn. Starchy vegetables are excluded from the vegetable group, and no limit is set on vegetable consumption. The milk and milk substitutes group includes fortified soy milk to provide vegans and ovo-vegetarians with nutrients they might otherwise be lacking. One cup of fortified soy milk contains 200 mg of calcium and 1000 IU of vitamin D, roughly 20% of an adult's RDAs. This explains the upper limit of four servings from this group for those not consuming dairy products. The meat/fish substitutes group recommends such foods as beans, protein-rich seeds, peanut butter, and tofu. A cupful of cooked dry beans is considered a serving, and two or three servings per day are suggested. At the top of the pyramid is the "vegans must consume daily" group.

THE TRADITIONAL HEALTHY MEDITERRANEAN DIET PYRAMID

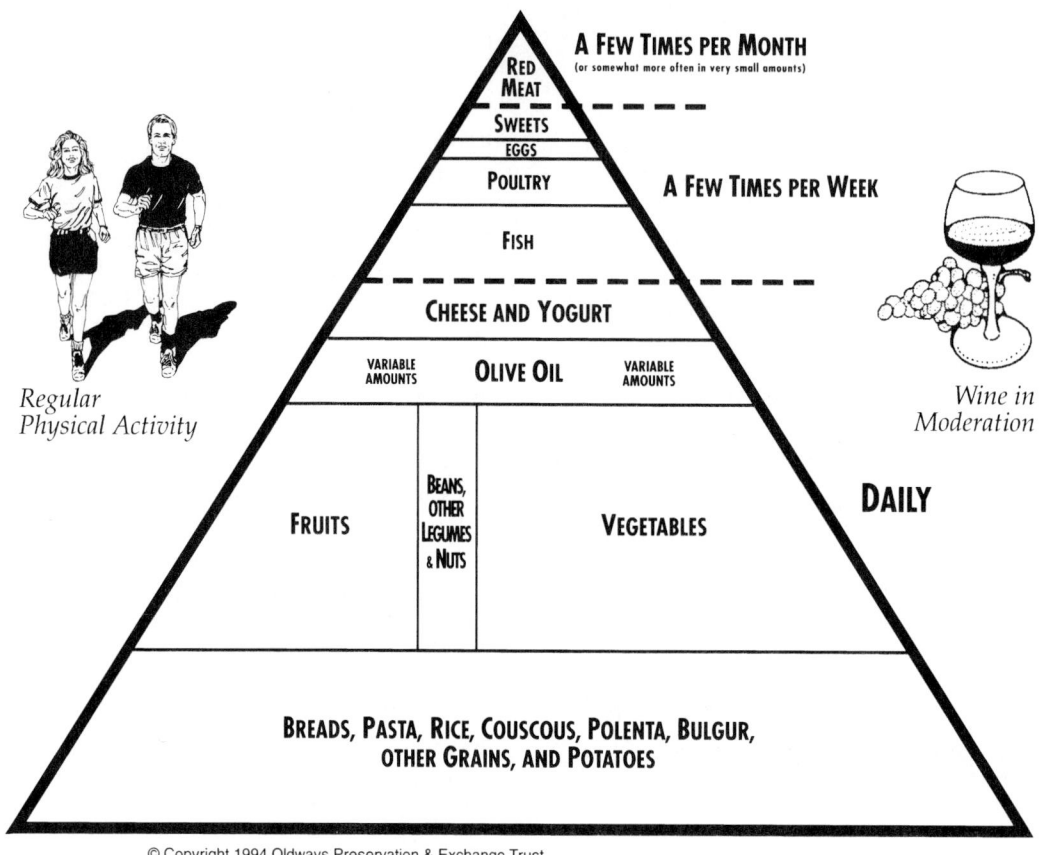

A FEW TIMES PER MONTH (or somewhat more often in very small amounts)

RED MEAT

SWEETS

EGGS

POULTRY

A FEW TIMES PER WEEK

FISH

CHEESE AND YOGURT

VARIABLE AMOUNTS   **OLIVE OIL**   VARIABLE AMOUNTS

Regular Physical Activity

Wine in Moderation

FRUITS

BEANS, OTHER LEGUMES & NUTS

VEGETABLES

DAILY

BREADS, PASTA, RICE, COUSCOUS, POLENTA, BULGUR, OTHER GRAINS, AND POTATOES

Figure 2.10 The Mediterranean Diet Pyramid.
Source: Oldways Preservation and Exchange Trust.

This includes a tablespoon each per day of blackstrap molasses (supplies iron and calcium) and brewer's yeast (supplies riboflavin and B₁₂). The three to five teaspoons of vegetable oil serve as a source of added energy.

FOOD EXCHANGE SYSTEM

The **food exchange system** is a method of planning meals that simplifies controlling energy consumption (particularly from carbohydrate), helps ensure adequate nutrient intake, and allows considerable variety in food selection. Also, once a person becomes familiar with the system, he or she can use it to quickly approximate kilocalorie and macronutrient levels in individual foods or an entire meal.

The food exchange system and accompanying exchange lists originally were developed in 1950 by the American Dietetic Association and the American Dia-

betes Association in cooperation with the U.S. Public Health Service for use in planning diabetic diets.[55] Before then, no standardized method for planning diabetic diets existed, and many health professionals and people with diabetes complained that meal planning often was laborious and difficult to adapt to individual food preferences.

The system categorizes foods into three main groups—the carbohydrate group, the meat and meat substitutes group, and the fat group. The carbohydrate group lists foods that supply most of their energy in the form of carbohydrate: starches, fruits, dairy products, vegetables, and other carbohydrates. The meat and meat substitutes group includes foods that serve as good protein sources, supply variable amounts of fat, and generally provide little, if any, carbohydrate. Foods in this group are listed on the basis of the amount of fat they supply: very lean, lean, medium-fat, and high-fat. Foods in the fat group provide fat and little, if any, pro-

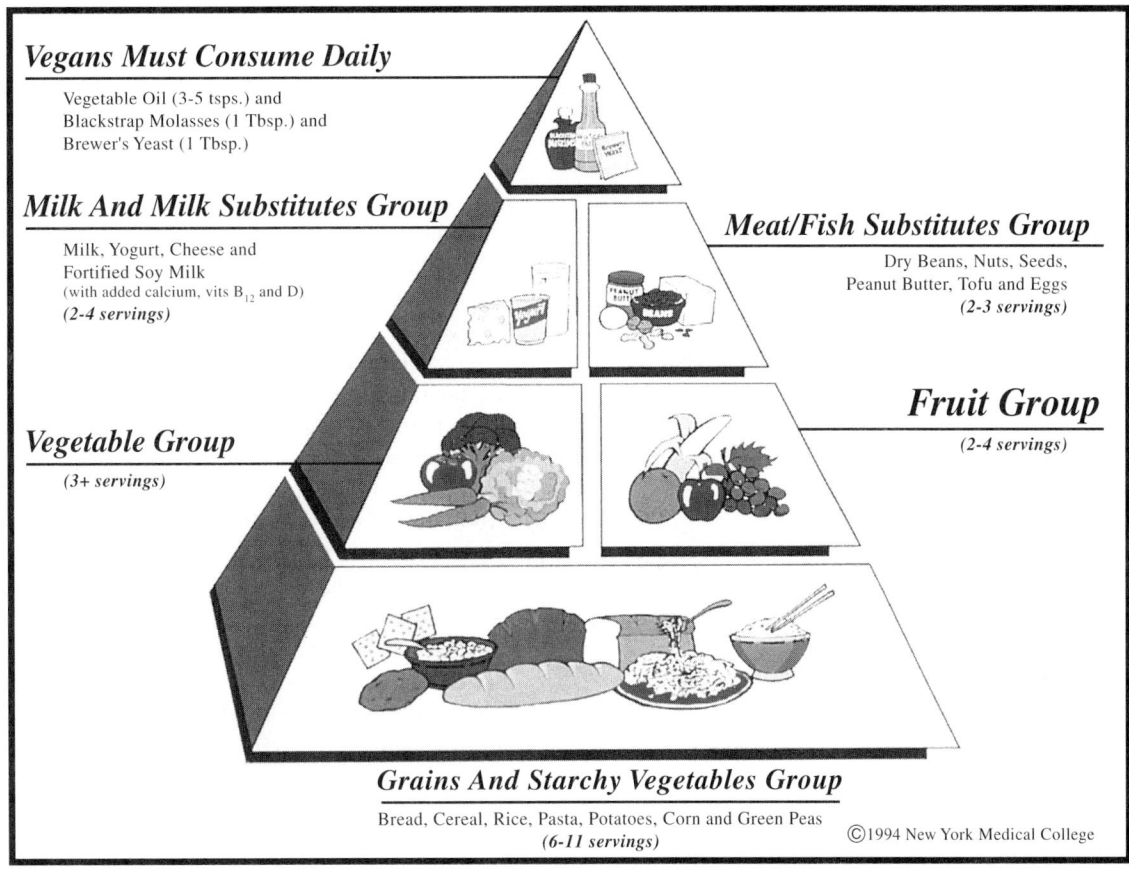

Figure 2.11 The New York Medical College Vegetarian Pyramid.
Source: New York Medical College.

tein and carbohydrate. The fats are divided among three lists on the basis of the major fatty acid they supply: monounsaturated, polyunsaturated, and saturated. There is also a "free foods list" and a list of combination foods and fast foods.

These lists are referred to as "exchange lists" because foods on the same list provide, on average, a similar number of kilocalories and grams of carbohydrate, protein, and fat, as shown in Table 2.20. When planning a meal, foods on the same list can be "exchanged," or traded, for any other on the list without changing the approximate amount of carbohydrate, protein, fat, and energy supplied by the meal. At breakfast, for example, a person could exchange a slice of bread for ¾ cup of unsweetened, ready-to-eat cereal. Each of these foods equals one choice from the starch exchange list and, consequently, has an equal amount of macronutrient and energy content. A detailed listing of foods within the exchange lists and their serving sizes are given in Table 2.21. Unless otherwise indicated, portion sizes are for cooked foods. Note in Table 2.21 that serving sizes differ among the various foods within one exchange list. For example, ⅓ cup of grape juice and 1¼ cup of

cubed watermelon are both considered a fruit exchange. Each provides approximately 15 g of carbohydrate and 60 kcal. However, because grape juice is a more concentrated source of energy compared with watermelon, its serving size is smaller.

Note that foods are not always where you might expect them to be. This is because foods are categorized primarily according to their carbohydrate, protein, and fat content. Olives and peanuts are considered monounsaturated fat exchanges. Corn is in the starchy vegetable exchange list because of its high carbohydrate content. The same is true of green peas, potatoes, and winter squash.

The American Dietetic Association and the American Diabetes Association have developed exchange lists for foods commonly eaten by a number of ethnic and regional groups. Included among these are Alaska native, Jewish, Mexican, Chinese, Navajo, Hmong, Filipino, Indian and Pakistani, Cajun and Creole, soul, and traditional Southern. An exchange list for foods commonly eaten by vegetarians has also been developed.

Sample meal plans using the exchange lists and providing 1500, 2000, and 2500 kcal/day are given in

TABLE 2.20	Average Kilocalorie and Macronutrient Contents of the Exchange Lists*			
Group/List	Carbohydrate (g)	Protein (g)	Fat (g)	Calories
Carbohydrate Group				
Starch	15	3	1 or less	80
Fruit	15	—	—	60
Milk				
Skim	12	8	0–3	90
Low-fat	12	8	5	120
Whole	12	8	8	150
Other carborhydrates	15	Varies	Varies	Varies
Vegetables	5	2	—	25
Meat and Meat Substitutes Group				
Very lean	—	7	0–1	35
Lean	—	7	3	55
Medium-fat	—	7	5	75
High-fat	—	7	8	100
Fat Group	—	—	5	45

From the American Diabetes Association, Inc., and the American Dietetic Association, 1995.

*The exchange lists are based on material in the Exchange Lists for Meal Planning prepared by committees of the American Diabetes Association, Inc., and the American Dietetic Association in cooperation with the National Institute of Arthritis, Metabolism, and Digestive Diseases and the National Heart, Lung, and Blood Institute, Public Health Service, U.S. Department of Health and Human Services.

Table 2.22. A person following the 2000-kcal/day plan, for example, would eat eight servings from the starch/bread exchange list, seven from the meat list, three from the vegetable list, six from the fruit list, three from the milk list, and three from the fat list.

Ideally, when diabetes is diagnosed in a patient, a dietitian works with the patient to design a meal plan individualized to the patient's dietary preferences, daily schedule, medications, body weight, serum lipid levels, and exercise habits. This meal plan can be expressed in terms of the number of foods from each of the six exchange lists. Many weight management programs and meal plans for people with diabetes are based on the exchange system because it simplifies the task of counting calories. An outstanding feature of the exchange system is that, rather than specifying a particular food, it gives a person an almost unlimited variety of foods from which to choose in planning meals. A person following one of the meal patterns in Table 2.22 can select a number of different foods from the starch list to get his or her exchanges from that list. The same is true for the protein, fruit, milk, and fat selections. The important thing is to select the specified *number* of exchanges and the correct *serving size* from each exchange list.

TABLE 2.21	The Exchange Lists for Meal Planning

Starch List

One starch exchange equals 15 g carbohydrate, 3 g protein, 0 to 1 g fat, and 80 calories. Cereals, grains, pasta, breads, crackers, snacks, starchy vegetables, cooked dried beans, peas, and lentils are starches. In general, one starch is

- 1/2 cup of cereal, grain, pasta, or starchy vegetable
- 1 ounce of a bread product, such as 1 slice of bread
- 3/4 to 1 ounce of most snack foods (some snack foods may also have added fat)

Nutrition Tips

1. Most starch choices are good sources of B vitamins.
2. Foods made from whole grains are good sources of fiber.
3. Dried beans and peas are a good source of protein and fiber.

Selection Tips

1. Choose starches made with little fat as often as you can.
2. Starchy vegetables prepared with fat count as one starch and one fat.
3. Bagels and muffins can be 2, 3, or 4 ounces in size and can, therefore, count as 2, 3, or 4 starch choices. Check the size you eat.
4. Dried beans, peas, and lentils are also found on the meat and meat substitutes list.
5. Regular potato chips and tortilla chips are found on the other carbohydrates list.
6. Most of the serving sizes are measured after cooking.
7. Always check Nutrition Facts on the food label.

Bread

Bagel	1/2 (1 oz)
Bread, reduced-calorie	2 slices (1½ oz)

TABLE 2.21 | **The Exchange Lists for Meal Planning—*continued***

Bread (continued)

Bread, white, whole-wheat, pumpernickel, rye	1 slice (1 oz)
Bread sticks, crisp, 4 in. long × 1/2 in.	2 (2/3 oz)
English muffin	1/2
Hot dog or hamburger bun	1/2 (1 oz)
Pita, 6 in. across	1/2
Roll, plain, small	1 (1 oz)
Raisin bread, unfrosted	1 slice (1 oz)
Tortilla, corn, 6 in. across	1
Tortilla, flour, 6 in. across	1
Waffle, 4½ in. square, reduced-fat	1

Cereals and Grains

Bran cereals	1/2 cup
Bulgur	1/2 cup
Cereals	1/2 cup
Cereals, unsweetened, ready-to-eat	3/4 cup
Cornmeal (dry)	3 Tbsp.
Couscous	1/3 cup
Flour (dry)	3 Tbsp.
Granola, low-fat	1/4 cup
Grape-Nuts	1/4 cup
Grits	1/2 cup
Kasha	1/2 cup
Millet	1/4 cup
Muesli	1/4 cup
Oats	1/2 cup
Pasta	1/2 cup
Puffed cereal	1½ cups
Rice milk	1/2 cup
Rice, white or brown	1/3 cup
Shredded Wheat	1/2 cup
Sugar-frosted cereal	1/2 cup
Wheat germ	3 Tbsp.

Starchy Vegetables

Baked beans	1/3 cup
Corn	1/2 cup
Corn on cob, medium	1 (5 oz)
Mixed vegetables with corn, peas, or pasta	1 cup
Peas, green	1/2 cup
Plantain	1/2 cup
Potato, baked or boiled	1 small (3 oz)
Potato, mashed	1/2 cup
Squash, winter (acorn, butternut, pumpkin)	1 cup
Yam, sweet potato, plain	1/2 cup

Crackers and Snacks

Animal crackers	8
Graham crackers, 2½ in. square	3
Matzoh	3/4 oz
Melba toast	4 slices
Oyster crackers	24
Popcorn (popped, no fat added or low-fat microwave)	3 cups
Pretzels	3/4 oz
Rice cakes, 4 in. across	2

continued

TABLE 2.21 | The Exchange Lists for Meal Planning—*continued*

Crackers and Snacks (continued)

Saltine-type crackers	6
Snack chips, fat-free (tortilla, potato)	15–20 (3/4 oz)
Whole-wheat crackers, no fat added	2–5 (3/4 oz)

Dried Beans, Peas, Lentils (Count as 1 Starch Exchange plus 1 Very Lean Meat Exchange)

Beans and peas (garbanzo, pinto, kidney, white, split, black-eyed)	1/2 cup
Lima beans	2/3 cup
Lentils	1/2 cup
Miso*	3 Tbsp.

Starchy Foods Prepared with Fat (Count as 1 Starch Exchange, plus 1 Fat Exchange)

Biscuit, 2½ in. across	1
Chow mein noodles	1/2 cup
Corn bread, 2 in. cube	1 (2 oz)
Crackers, round butter type	6
Croutons	1 cup
French-fried potatoes	16–25 (3 oz)
Granola	1/4 cup
Muffin, small	1 (1½ oz)
Pancake, 4 in. across	2
Popcorn, microwave	3 cups
Sandwich crackers, cheese or peanut butter filling	3
Stuffing, bread (prepared)	1/3 cup
Taco shell, 6 in. across	2
Waffle, 4½ in. square	1
Whole-wheat crackers, fat added	4–6 (1 oz)

Starches often swell in cooking, so a small amount of uncooked starch will become a much larger amount of cooked food. The following table shows some of the changes.

Food (Starch Group)	Uncooked	Cooked
Oatmeal	3 Tbsp.	1/2 cup
Cream of Wheat	2 Tbsp.	1/2 cup
Grits	3 Tbsp.	1/2 cup
Rice	2 Tbsp.	1/3 cup
Spaghetti	1/4 cup	1/2 cup
Noodles	1/3 cup	1/2 cup
Macaroni	1/4 cup	1/2 cup
Dried beans	1/4 cup	1/2 cup
Dried peas	1/4 cup	1/2 cup
Lentils	3 Tbsp.	1/2 cup

Fruit List

One fruit exchange equals 15 g carbohydrate and 60 calories. The weight includes skin, core, seeds, and rinds. Fresh, frozen, canned, and dried fruits and fruit juices are on this list. In general, one fruit exchange is

- 1 small to medium fresh fruit
- 1/2 cup of canned or fresh fruit or fruit juice
- 1/4 cup of dried fruit

Nutrition Tips

1. Fresh, frozen, and dried fruits have about 2 g of fiber per choice. Fruit juices contain very little fiber.
2. Citrus fruits, berries, and melons are good sources of vitamin C.

Selection Tips

1. Count 1/2 cup cranberries or rhubarb sweetened with sugar substitutes as free foods.
2. Read the Nutrition Facts on the food label. If one serving has more than 15 g of carbohydrate, you will need to adjust the size of the serving you eat or drink.

*400 mg or more of sodium per serving.

TABLE 2.21 | **The Exchange Lists for Meal Planning—*continued***

Selection Tips (continued)

3. Portion sizes for canned fruits are for the fruit and a small amount of juice.
4. Whole fruit is more filling than fruit juice and may be a better choice.
5. Food labels for fruits may contain the words "no sugar added" or "unsweetened." This means that no sucrose (table sugar) has been added.
6. Generally, fruit canned in extra light syrup has the same amount of carbohydrate per serving as the "no sugar added" or the juice pack. All canned fruits on the fruit list are based on one of these three types of pack.

Fruit

Apple, unpeeled, small	1 (4 oz)
Applesauce, unsweetened	1/2 cup
Apples, dried	4 rings
Apricots, fresh	4 whole (5½ oz)
Apricots, dried	8 halves
Apricots, canned	1/2 cup
Banana, small	1 (4 oz)
Blackberries	3/4 cup
Blueberries	3/4 cup
Cantaloupe, small	1/3 melon (11 oz) or 1 cup cubes
Cherries, sweet, fresh	12 (3 oz)
Cherries, sweet, canned	1/2 cup
Dates	3
Figs, fresh	1½ large or 2 medium (3½ oz)
Figs, dried	1½
Fruit cocktail	1/2 cup
Grapefruit, large	1/2 (11 oz)
Grapefruit sections, canned	3/4 cup
Grapes, small	17 (3 oz)
Honeydew melon	1 slice (10 oz) or 1 cup cubes
Kiwi	1 (3½ oz)
Mandarin oranges, canned	3/4 cup
Mango, small	1/2 fruit (5½ oz) or 1/2 cup
Nectarine, small	1 (5 oz)
Orange, small	1 (6½ oz)
Papaya	1/2 fruit (8 oz) or 1 cup cubes
Peach, medium, fresh	1 (6 oz)
Peaches, canned	1/2 cup
Pear, large, fresh	1/2 (4 oz)
Pears, canned	1/2 cup
Pineapple, fresh	3/4 cup
Pineapple, canned	1/2 cup
Plums, small	2 (5 oz)
Plums, canned	1/2 cup
Prunes, dried	3
Raisins	2 Tbsp.
Raspberries	1 cup
Strawberries	1¼ cup whole berries
Tangerines, small	2 (8 oz)
Watermelon	1 slice (13½ oz) or 1¼ cup cubes

Fruit Juice

Apple juice/cider	1/2 cup
Cranberry juice cocktail	1/3 cup
Cranberry juice cocktail, reduced-calorie	1 cup
Fruit juice blends, 100% juice	1/3 cup
Grape juice	1/3 cup
Grapefruit juice	1/2 cup

continued

TABLE 2.21 | **The Exchange Lists for Meal Planning—*continued***

Fruit Juice (continued)

Orange juice	1/2 cup
Pineapple juice	1/2 cup
Prune juice	1/3 cup

Milk List

One milk exchange equals 12 g carbohydrate and 8 g protein. Different types of milk and milk products are on this list. Cheeses are on the meat list, and cream and other dairy fats are on the fat list. Based on the amount of fat they contain, milks are divided into fat-free/low-fat milk, reduced-fat milk, and whole milk. One choice of these includes

	Carbohydrate (g)	Protein (g)	Fat (g)	Calories
Fat-free/low-fat	12	8	0–3	90
Reduced-fat	12	8	5	120
Whole	12	8	8	150

Nutrition Tips

1. Milk and yogurt are good sources of calcium and protein. Check the food label.
2. The higher the fat content of milk and yogurt, the greater the amount of saturated fat and cholesterol. Choose lower-fat varieties.
3. Those who are lactose intolerant should look for lactose-reduced or lactose-free varieties of milk.

Selection Tips

1. One cup equals 8 fluid ounces or 1/2 pint.
2. Look for chocolate milk, frozen yogurt, and ice cream on the other carbohydrates list.
3. Nondairy creamers are on the free foods list.
4. Look for rice milk on the starch list.
5. Look for soy milk on the medium-fat meat list.

Fat-Free and Low-Fat Milk (0–3 g Fat per Serving)

Fat-free milk	1 cup
1/2% milk	1 cup
1% milk	1 cup
Fat-free or low-fat buttermilk	1 cup
Evaporated fat-free milk	1/2 cup
Fat-free dry milk	1/3 cup dry
Plain nonfat yogurt	3/4 cup
Nonfat or low-fat fruit-flavored yogurt sweetened with aspartame or with a nonnutritive sweetener	1 cup

Reduced-Fat (5 g Fat per Serving)

2% milk	1 cup
Plain low-fat yogurt	3/4 cup
Sweet acidophilus milk	1 cup

Whole Milk (8 g Fat per Serving)

Whole milk	1 cup
Evaporated whole milk	1/2 cup
Goat's milk	1 cup
Kefir	1 cup

Other Carbohydrates List

One exchange equals 15 g carbohydrate, or 1 starch, or 1 fruit, or 1 milk. You can substitute food choices from this list for a starch, fruit, or milk choice on your meal plan. Some choices will also count as one or more fat choices.

Nutrition Tips

1. These foods can be substituted in your meal plan, even though they contain added sugars or fat. However, they do not contain as many important vitamins and minerals as the choices on the starch, fruit, or milk list.
2. When planning to include these foods in your meal, be sure to include foods from all the lists to eat a balanced meal.

TABLE 2.21 │ **The Exchange Lists for Meal Planning—*continued***

Selection Tips

1. Because many of these foods are concentrated sources of carbohydrate and fat, the portion sizes are often very small.
2. Always check Nutrition Facts on the food label. It will be your most accurate source of information.
3. Many fat-free or reduced-fat products made with fat replacers contain carbohydrate. When eaten in large amounts, they may need to be counted. Talk with your dietitian to determine how to count these in your meal plan.
4. Look for fat-free salad dressings in smaller amounts on the free foods list.

Food	Serving Size	Exchanges per Serving[*]
Angel food cake, unfrosted	1/12 cake	2 C
Brownie, small, unfrosted	2 in. square	1 C, 1 F
Cake, unfrosted	2 in. square	1 C, 1 F
Cake, frosted	2 in. square	2 C, 1 F
Cookie, fat-free	2 small	1 C
Cookie or sandwich cookie with creme filling	2 small	1 C, 1 F
Cranberry sauce, jellied	1/4 cup	2 C
Cupcake, frosted	1 small	2 C, 1 F
Doughnut, plain cake	1 medium (1½ oz)	1½ C, 2 F
Doughnut, glazed	3¾ in. across (2 oz)	2 C, 2 F
Fruit juice bars, frozen, 100% juice	1 bar (3 oz)	1 C
Fruit snacks, chewy (pureed fruit concentrate)	1 roll (3/4 oz)	1 C
Fruit spreads, 100% fruit	1 Tbsp.	1 C
Gelatin, regular	1/2 cup	1 C
Gingersnaps	3	1 C
Granola bar	1 bar	1 C, 1 F
Granola bar, fat-free	1 bar	2 C
Honey	1 Tbsp.	1 C
Hummus	1/3 cup	1 C, 1 F
Ice cream	1/2 cup	1 C, 2 F
Ice cream, light	1/2 cup	1 C, 1 F
Ice cream, fat-free, no sugar added	1/2 cup	1 C
Jam or jelly, regular	1 Tbsp.	1 C
Milk, chocolate, whole	1 cup	2 C, 1 F
Pie, fruit, 2 crusts	1/6 pie	3 C, 2 F
Pie, pumpkin or custard	1/8 pie	2 C, 2 F
Potato chips	12–18 (1 oz)	1 C, 2 F
Pudding, regular (made with low-fat milk)	1/2 cup	2 C
Pudding, sugar-free (made with low-fat milk)	1/2 cup	1 C
Salad dressing, fat-free[†]	1/4 cup	1 C
Sherbert, sorbet	1/2 cup	2 C
Spaghetti or pasta sauce, canned[†]	1/2 cup	1 C, 1 F
Sugar	1 Tbsp.	1 C
Sweet roll or Danish	1 (2½ oz)	2½ C, 2 F
Syrup, light	2 Tbsp	1 C
Syrup, regular	1 Tbsp	1 C
Syrup, regular	1/4 cup	4 C
Tortilla chips	6–12 (1 oz)	1 C, 2 F
Vanilla wafers	5	1 C, 1 F
Yogurt, frozen, low-fat, fat-free	1/3 cup	1 C, 0–1 F
Yogurt, frozen, fat-free, no sugar added	1/2 cup	1 C
Yogurt, low-fat with fruit	1 cup	3 C, 0–1 F

[*]C = carbohydrate exchange; F = fat exchange.

[†]400 mg or more of sodium per serving.

continued

| **TABLE 2.21** | **The Exchange Lists for Meal Planning—*continued*** |

Vegetable List

One vegetable exchange equals 5 g carbohydrate, 2 g protein, 0 g fat, and 25 calories. Vegetables that contain small amounts of carbohydrates and calories are on this list. Vegetables contain important nutrients. Try to eat at least 2 to 3 vegetable choices each day. In general, one vegetable exchange is

- 1/2 cup of cooked vegetables or vegetable juice
- 1 cup of raw vegetables

If you eat 1 or 2 vegetable choices at a meal or snack, you do not have to count the calories or carbohydrates because they contain small amounts of these nutrients.

Nutrition Tips

1. Fresh and frozen vegetables have less added salt than canned vegetables. Drain and rinse canned vegetables if you want to remove some salt.
2. Choose more dark green and dark yellow vegetables, such as spinach, broccoli, romaine, carrots, chilies, and peppers.
3. Broccoli, brussels sprouts, cauliflower, greens, peppers, spinach, and tomatoes are good sources of vitamin C.
4. Vegetables contain 1 to 4 grams of fiber per serving.

Selection Tips

1. A 1-cup portion of broccoli is a portion about the size of a light bulb.
2. Tomato sauce is different from spaghetti sauce, which is on the other carbohydrates list.
3. Canned vegetables and juices are available without added salt.
4. If you eat 3 cups or more of raw vegetables or 1½ cups of cooked vegetables at one meal, count them as 1 carbohydrate choice.
5. Starchy vegetables, such as corn, peas, winter squash, and potatoes, which contain larger amounts of calories and carbohydrates are on the starch list.

Artichoke	Okra
Artichoke hearts	Onions
Asparagus	Pea pods
Beans (green, wax, Italian)	Peppers (all varieties)
Bean sprouts	Radishes
Beets	Salad greens (endive, escarole, lettuce, romaine, spinach)
Broccoli	Sauerkraut*
Brussels sprouts	Spinach
Cabbage	Summer squash
Carrots	Tomato
Cauliflower	Tomatoes, canned
Celery	Tomato sauce*
Cucumber	Tomato/vegetable juice*
Eggplant	Turnips
Green onions or scallions	Water chestnuts
Greens (collard, kale, mustard, turnip)	Watercress
Kohlrabi	Zucchini
Leeks	
Mixed vegetables (without corn, peas, or pasta)	
Mushrooms	

*400 mg or more of sodium per exchange.

Meat and Meat Substitutes List

Meat and meat substitutes that contain both protein and fat are on this list. In general, one meat exchange is

- 1 oz of meat, fish, poultry, or cheese
- 1/2 cup beans, peas, or lentils

Based on the amount of fat they contain, meats are divided into very lean, lean, medium-fat, and high-fat lists. This is done so you can see which ones contain the least amount of fat. One ounce (one exchange) of each of these includes

	Carbohydrate (g)	**Protein (g)**	**Fat (g)**	**Calories**
Very lean	0	7	0–1	35
Lean	0	7	3	55
Medium-fat	0	7	5	75
High-fat	0	7	8	100

TABLE 2.21 | **The Exchange Lists for Meal Planning—*continued***

Nutrition Tips

1. Choose very lean and lean meat choices whenever possible. Items from the high-fat group are high in saturated fat, cholesterol, and calories and can raise blood cholesterol levels.
2. Meats do not have any fiber.
3. Dried beans, peas, and lentils are good sources of fiber.
4. Some processed meats, seafood, and soy products may contain carbohydrate when consumed in large amounts. Check the Nutrition Facts on the label to see if the amount is close to 15 g. If so, count it as a carbohydrate choice as well as a meat choice.

Selection Tips

1. Weigh meat after cooking and removing bones and fat. Four ounces of raw meat is equal to 3 ounces of cooked meat. Some examples of meat portions are
   - 1 ounce cheese = 1 meat choice and is about the size of a 1-inch cube
   - 2 ounces meat = 2 meat choices, such as 1 small chicken leg or thigh and 1/2 cup cottage cheese or tuna
   - 3 ounces meat = 3 meat choices and is about the size of a deck of cards, such as 1 medium pork chop, 1 small hamburger, 1/2 of a whole chicken breast, or 1 unbreaded fish fillet
2. Limit your choices from the high-fat group to three times per week or less.
3. Most grocery stores stock Select and Choice grades of meat. Select grades of meat are the leanest meats. Choice grades contain a moderate amount of fat, and Prime cuts of meat have the highest amount of fat.
4. "Hamburger" may contain added seasoning and fat, but ground beef does not.
5. Read labels to find products that are low in fat and cholesterol (5 g or less of fat per serving).
6. Dried beans, peas, and lentils are also found on the starch list.
7. Peanut butter, in smaller amounts, is also found on the fat list.
8. Bacon, in smaller amounts, is also found on the fat list.

Meal Planning Tips

1. Bake, roast, broil, grill, poach, steam, or boil these foods rather than fry.
2. Place meat on a rack, so that fat will drain off during cooking.
3. Use nonstick spray and a nonstick pan to brown or fry foods.
4. Trim off visible fat before or after cooking.
5. If you add flour, bread crumbs, coating mixes, fat, or marinades when cooking, ask your dietitian how to count them in your meal plan.

Very Lean Meat and Substitutes List

One exchange equals 0 g carbohydrate, 7 g protein, 0–1 g fat, and 35 calories. One very lean meat exchange is equal to any one of the following items:

Poultry:	Chicken or turkey (white meat, no skin), Cornish hen (no skin)	1 oz
Fish:	Fresh or frozen cod, flounder, haddock, halibut, trout, tuna (fresh or canned in water)	1 oz
Shellfish:	Clams, crab, lobster, scallops, shrimp, imitation shellfish	1 oz
Game:	Duck or pheasant (no skin), venison, buffalo, ostrich	1 oz
Cheese (1 g or less fat per ounce):	Nonfat or low-fat cottage cheese	1/4 cup
	Fat-free cheese	1 oz
Other:	Processed sandwich meats with 1 g or less fat per ounce, such as deli thin, shaved meats; chipped beef;* turkey ham	1 oz
	Egg whites	2
	Egg substitutes, plain	1/4 cup
	Hot dogs with 1 g or less fat per ounce	1 oz
	Kidney (high in cholesterol)	1 oz
	Sausage with 1 g or less fat per ounce	1 oz
Count as one very lean meat and one starch exchange:	Dried beans, peas, lentils (cooked)	1/2 cup

*400 mg or more sodium per exchange.

Lean Meat and Substitutes List

One exchange equals 0 g carbohydrate, 7 g protein, 3 g fat, and 55 calories.
One lean meat exchange is equal to any one of the following items:

Beef:	USDA Select or Choice grades of lean beef trimmed of fat, such as round, sirloin, and flank steak; tenderloin; roast (rib, chuck, rump); steak (T-bone, porterhouse, cubed), ground round	1 oz
Pork:	Lean pork, such as fresh ham; canned, cured, or boiled ham; Canadian bacon,* tenderloin, center loin chop	1 oz
Lamb:	Roast, chop, leg	1 oz

continued

TABLE 2.21 | **The Exchange Lists for Meal Planning**—*continued*

Lean Meat and Substitutes List (continued)

Veal:	Lean chop, roast	1 oz
Poultry:	Chicken, turkey (dark meat, no skin), chicken white meat (with skin), domestic duck or goose (well-drained of fat, no skin)	1 oz
Fish:	Herring (uncreamed or smoked)	1 oz
	Oysters	6 medium
	Salmon (fresh or canned), catfish	1 oz
	Sardines (canned)	2 medium
	Tuna (canned in oil, drained)	1 oz
Game:	Goose (no skin), rabbit	1 oz
Cheese:	4.5%-fat cottage cheese	1/4 cup
	Grated parmesan	2 Tbsp.
	Cheeses with 3 g or less fat per ounce	1 oz
Other:	Hot dogs with 3 g or less fat per ounce[*]	1½ oz
	Processed sandwich meat with 3 g or less fat per ounce, such as turkey, pastrami, or kielbasa	1 oz
	Liver, heart (high in cholesterol)	1 oz

[*]400 mg or more sodium per exchange.

Medium-Fat Meat and Substitutes List

One exchange equals 0 g carbohydrate, 7 g protein, 5 g fat, and 75 calories. One medium-fat meat exchange is equal to any one of the following items:

Beef:	Most beef products (ground beef, meat loaf; corned beef; short ribs; Prime grades of meat trimmed of fat, such as prime rib)	1 oz
Pork:	Top loin, chop, Boston butt, cutlet	1 oz
Lamb:	Rib roast, ground	1 oz
Veal:	Cutlet (ground or cubed, unbreaded)	1 oz
Poultry:	Chicken dark meat (with skin), ground turkey or ground chicken, fried chicken (with skin)	1 oz
Fish:	Any fried fish product	1 oz
Cheese (5 g or less per ounce):	Feta	1 oz
	Mozzarella	1 oz
	Ricotta	1/4 cup (2 oz)
Other:	Egg (high in cholesterol, limit to 3 per week)	1
	Sausage with 5 g or less fat per ounce	1 oz
	Soy milk	1 cup
	Tempeh	1/4 cup
	Tofu	4 oz or 1/2 cup

High-Fat Meat and Substitutes List

One exchange equals 0 g carbohydrate, 7 g protein, 8 g fat, and 100 calories. Remember, these items are high in saturated fat, cholesterol, and calories and may raise blood cholesterol level if eaten on a regular basis. One high-fat meat exchange is equal to any one of the following items:

Pork:	Spareribs, ground pork, pork sausage	1 oz
Cheese:	All regular cheeses, such as American,[*] cheddar, Monterey Jack, Swiss	1 oz
Other:	Processed sandwich meats with 8 g or less fat per ounce, such as bologna, pimento loaf, salami	1 oz
	Sausage such as bratwurst, Italian, knockwurst, Polish, smoked	1 oz
	Hot dog (turkey or chicken)	1 (10/lb)
	Bacon	3 slices (20 slices/lb)

Count as one high-fat meat plus one fat exchange:

Hot dog (beef, pork, or combination)[*]	1 (10/lb)
Peanut butter (contains unsaturated fat)	2 Tbsp.

[*]400 mg or more sodium per exchange.

TABLE 2.21 | The Exchange Lists for Meal Planning—*continued*

Fat List

Fats are divided into three groups based on the main type of fatty acids they contain: monounsaturated, polyunsaturated, and saturated. Small amounts of monounsaturated and polyunsaturated fats in the foods we eat are linked with good health benefits. Saturated fats are linked with heart disease and cancer. In general, one fat exchange is

- 1 teaspoon of regular margarine or vegetable oil
- 1 tablespoon of regular salad dressing

Nutrition Tips

1. All fats are high in calories. Limit serving sizes for good nutrition and health.
2. Nuts and seeds contain small amounts of fiber, protein, and magnesium.
3. If blood pressure is a concern, choose fats in the unsalted form, such as unsalted peanuts, to help lower sodium intake.

Selection Tips

1. Check the Nutrition Facts on food labels for serving sizes. One fat exchange is based on a serving size containing 5 g of fat.
2. When selecting regular margarine, choose one with liquid vegetable oil as the first ingredient. Soft margarine is not as saturated as stick margarine. Soft margarines are healthier choices. Avoid those listing hydrogenated or partially hydrogenated fat as the first ingredient.
3. When selecting low-fat margarines, look for liquid vegetable oil as the second ingredient. Water is usually the first ingredient.
4. When used in smaller amounts, bacon and peanut butter are counted as fat choices. When used in larger amounts, they are counted as high-fat meat choices.
5. Fat-free salad dressings are on the other carbohydrates list and the free foods list.
6. See the free foods list for nondairy coffee creamers, whipped topping, and fat-free products, such as margarines, salad dressings, mayonnaise, sour cream, cream cheese, and nonstick cooking spray.

Monounsaturated Fats List (One Fat Exchange Equals 5 g Fat and 45 Calories)

Avocado, medium	1/8 (1 oz)
Oil (canola, olive, peanut)	1 tsp
Olives	
ripe (black)	8 large
green, stuffed*	10 large
Nuts	
almonds, cashews	6 nuts
mixed (50% peanuts)	6 nuts
peanuts	10 nuts
pecans	4 halves
Peanut butter, smooth or crunchy	2 tsp.
Sesame seeds	1 Tbsp.
Tahini paste	2 tsp.

*400 mg or more sodium per exchange.

Polyunsaturated Fats List (One Fat Exchange Equals 5 g Fat and 45 Calories)

Margarine	
stick, tub, or squeeze	1 tsp.
lower-fat (30% to 50% vegetable oil)	1 Tbsp.
Mayonnaise	
regular	1 tsp.
reduced-fat	1 Tbsp.
Miracle Whip Salad Dressing®	
regular	2 tsp.
reduced-fat	1 Tbsp.
Nuts, walnuts, English	4 halves
Oil (corn, safflower, soybean)	1 tsp.
Salad dressing:	
regular*	1 Tbsp.
reduced-fat	2 Tbsp.
Seeds (pumpkin, sunflower)	1 Tbsp.

*400 mg or more sodium per exchange.

continued

| TABLE 2.21 | The Exchange Lists for Meal Planning—*continued* |

Saturated Fats List (One Fat Exchange Equals 5 g Fat and 45 Calories)

Bacon, cooked	1 slice
	(20 slices/lb)
Bacon, grease	1 tsp.
Butter	
stick	1 tsp.
whipped	2 tsp.
reduced-fat	1 Tbsp.
Chitterlings, boiled	2 Tbsp. (1/2 oz)
Coconut, sweetened, shredded	2 Tbsp.
Cream, half and half	2 Tbsp.
Cream cheese	
regular	1 Tbsp. (1/2 oz)
reduced-fat	2 Tbsp. (1 oz)
Fatback or salt pork†	
Shortening or lard	1 tsp.
Sour cream	
regular	2 Tbsp.
reduced-fat	3 Tbsp.

*Saturated fats can raise blood cholesterol levels.

†Use a piece 1 in. × 1 in. × 1/4 in. if you plan to eat the fatback cooked with vegetables. Use a piece 2 in. × 1 in. × 1/2 in. when eating only the vegetables with the fatback removed.

Free Foods List

A *free food* is any food or drink that contains less than 20 calories or less than 5 g of carbohydrate per serving. Foods with a serving size listed should be limited to 3 servings per day. Be sure to spread them out throughout the day. If you eat all 3 servings at one time, it could affect your blood glucose level. Foods listed without a serving size can be eaten as often as you like.

Fat-Free or Reduced-Fat Foods

Cream cheese, fat-free	1 Tbsp.
Creamers, nondairy, liquid	1 Tbsp.
Creamers, nondairy, powdered	2 tsp.
Mayonnaise, fat-free	1 Tbsp.
Mayonnaise, reduced-fat	1 tsp.
Margarine, fat-free	4 Tbsp.
Margarine, reduced-fat	1 tsp.
Miracle Whip®, nonfat	1 Tbsp.
Miracle Whip®, reduced-fat	1 tsp.
Nonstick cooking spray	
Salad dressing, fat-free	1 Tbsp.
Salad dressing, fat-free, Italian	2 Tbsp.
Salsa	1/4 cup
Sour cream, fat-free, reduced-fat	1 Tbsp.
Whipped topping, regular or light	2 Tbsp.

Sugar-Free or Low-Sugar Foods

Candy, hard, sugar-free	1 candy
Gelatin dessert, sugar-free	
Gelatin, unflavored	

TABLE 2.21 | **The Exchange Lists for Meal Planning—***continued*

Sugar-Free or Low-Sugar Foods (continued)

Gum, sugar-free

Jam or jelly, low-sugar or light   2 tsp.

Sugar substitutes*

Syrup, sugar-free   2 Tbsp.

*Sugar substitutes, alternatives, or replacements that are approved by the Food and Drug Administration are safe to use. Common brand names include

   Equal® (aspartame)

   Splenda® (sucralose)

   Sprinkle Sweet® (saccharin)

   Sweet One® (acesulfame K)

   Sweet-10® (saccharin)

   Sugar Twin® (saccharin)

   Sweet 'n Low® (saccharin)

Drinks

Bouillon, broth, consomme*

Bouillon or broth, low-sodium

Carbonated or mineral water

Cocoa powder, unsweetened   1 Tbsp.

Coffee

Club soda

Diet soft drinks, sugar-free

Drink mixes, sugar-free

Tea

Tonic water, sugar-free

Condiments

Catsup   1 Tbsp.

Horseradish

Lemon juice

Lime juice

Mustard

Pickles, dill*   1½ large

Soy sauce, regular or light*

Taco sauce   1 Tbsp.

Vinegar

*400 mg or more of sodium per choice.

Seasonings

Be careful with seasonings that contain sodium or are salts, such as garlic or celery salt and lemon pepper.

Flavoring extracts

Garlic

Herbs, fresh or dried

Pimento

Spices

Tabasco® or other hot pepper sauce

Wine, used in cooking

Worcestershire sauce

Combination Foods List

Many of the foods we eat are mixed together in various combinations. These combination foods do not fit into any one exchange list. Often it is hard to tell what is in a casserole dish or prepared food item. This is a list of exchanges for some typical combination foods. This list will help you fit these foods into your meal plan. Ask your dietitian for information about any other combination foods you would like to eat.

continued

TABLE 2.21 | **The Exchange Lists for Meal Planning**—*continued*

Food	Serving Size	Exchanges per Serving[*]
Entrees		
Tuna noodle casserole, lasagna, spaghetti with meatballs, chili with beans, macaroni and cheese[†]	1 cup (8 oz)	2 C, 2 MFM
Chow mein (without noodles or rice)	2 cups (16 oz)	1 C, 2 LM
Pizza, cheese, thin crust[†]	1/4 of 10 in. (5 oz)	2 C, 2 MFM, 1 F
Pizza, meat topping, thin crust[†]	1/4 of 10 in. (5 oz)	2 C, 2 MFM, 2 F
Pot pie[†]	1 (7 oz)	2 C, 1 MFM, 4 F
Frozen Entrees		
Salisbury steak with gravy, mashed potato	1 (11 oz)	2 C, 3 MFM, 3–4 F
Turkey with gravy, mashed potato, dressing	1 (11 oz)	2 C, 2 MFM, 2 F
Entree with less than 300 calories	1 (8 oz)	2 C, 3 LM
Soups		
Bean[†]	1 cup	1 C, 1 VLM
Cream (made with water)[†]	1 cup (8 oz)	1 C, 1 F
Split pea (made with water)[†]	1/2 cup (4 oz)	1 C
Tomato (made with water)[†]	1 cup (8 oz)	1 C
Vegetable beef, chicken noodle, or other broth-type	1 cup (8 oz)	1 C

[*]C = carbohydrate exchange; VLM = very lean meat exchange; LM = lean meat exchange; MFM = medium-fat meat exchange; F = fat exchange.
[†]400 mg or more sodium per exchange.

Fast Foods[*]	Serving Size	Exchanges per Serving[*]
Burritos with beef[‡]	2	4 C, 2 MFM, 2 F
Chicken nuggets[‡]	6	1 C, 2 MFM, 1 F
Chicken breast and wing, breaded and fried	1 each	1 C, 4 MFM, 2 F
Fish sandwich/tartar sauce[‡]	1	3 C, 1 MFM, 3 F
French fries, thin	20–25	2 C, 2 F
Hamburger, regular	1	2 C, 2 MFM
Hamburger, large[‡]	1	2 C, 3 MFM, 1 F
Hot dog with bun[‡]	1	1 C, 1 HFM, 1 F
Individual pan pizza[‡]	1	5 C, 3 MFM, 3 F
Soft-serve cone	1 medium	2 C, 1 F
Submarine sandwich[‡]	1 sub (6 in.)	3 C, 1 V, 2 MFM, 1 F
Taco, hard shell[‡]	1 (6 oz)	2 C, 2 MFM, 2 F
Taco, soft shell[‡]	1 (3 oz)	1 C, 1 MFM, 1 F

[*]Ask at your fast-food restaurant for nutrition information about your favorite fast foods.
[†]C = carbohydrate exchange; MFM = medium-fat meat exchange; HFM = high-fat meat exchange; F = fat exchange; V = vegetable exchange.
[‡]400 mg or more sodium per serving.

The Exchange Lists are the basis of a meal planning system designed by a committee of the American Diabetes Association and the American Dietetic Association. While designed primarily for people with diabetes and others who must follow special diets, the Exchange Lists are based on principles of good nutrition that apply to everyone. © 1995 American Diabetes Association, Inc., The American Dietetic Association.

TABLE 2.22 | Sample Meal Patterns Using the Exchange Lists for Meal Planning

1500-Kilocalorie Diet with Two Snacks

	Breakfast	Lunch	Snack	Dinner	Snack
Starch	2	2	½	2	½
Meat, medium-fat	1	2	1	2	
Vegetable		1		1	
Fruit	1	1		1	
Milk, skim	½	½			½
Fat	1	1		1	

	Kcal	Carbohydrate	Protein	Fat
Total	1510	178 g	79 g	45 g
Percent of energy		50%	22%	28%

2000-Kilocalorie Diet with Two Snacks

	Breakfast	Lunch	Snack	Dinner	Snack
Starch	2	2	½	3	½
Meat, medium-fat	1	2	1	2	1
Vegetable		1		2	
Fruit	2	2		2	
Milk, skim	1	1		1	
Fat	1	1		1	

	Kcal	Carbohydrate	Protein	Fat
Total	2005	261 g	103 g	50 g
Percent of energy		55%	22%	23%

2500-Kilocalorie Diet with Two Snacks

	Breakfast	Lunch	Snack	Dinner	Snack
Starch	3	3	1	4	1
Meat, medium-fat	1	3	1	3	1
Vegetable		2		2	
Fruit	2	2		2	
Milk, skim	1	1		1	
Fat	1	1		1	

	Kcal	Carbohydrate	Protein	Fat
Total	2500	326 g	131 g	60 g
Percent of energy		55%	22%	23%

SUMMARY

1. A number of tools and methods are available for nutrition professionals to use in evaluating dietary intakes of individuals and groups. Included among these are standards of recommended nutrient intake, measurements of nutrient density, dietary guidelines or goals, and food guides.

2. With a few exceptions, dietary standards up until the twentieth century were observational and lacked a firm scientific base. Advances in metabolic, vitamin, and mineral research during the early twentieth century led to the establishment of scientifically based estimates of human nutrient requirements by the League of Nations and several European countries, Canada, and the United States.

3. One of the earliest and most familiar of the dietary standards is the Recommended Dietary Allowance (RDA), developed by the Food and Nutrition Board of the National Research Council. The RDAs provided specific nutrient recommendations for healthy persons in each life stage and gender group. They were originally developed in 1941 and revised about every 5 years. Their primary focus was prevention of micronutrient deficiency. The last edition of the RDAs was published in 1989.

4. Limitations in the RDAs became apparent as nutritional science advanced and as the primary nutrition concern of North America changed from nutrient deficiency to food and nutrient overconsumption, with an attendant increase in chronic disease risk. In addition, the RDAs had no recommendations for carbohydrate, fiber, fat, cholesterol, and food components not traditionally regarded as nutrients (e.g., phytonutrients). They failed to address the role of nutrition in reducing chronic disease risk and gave no guidance on use of nutritional supplements.

5. In response to the RDAs' limitations, scientists from the Food and Nutrition Board, the Canadian Institute of Nutrition, and Health Canada developed a new set of nutrient reference values, known as the Dietary Reference Intakes (DRIs). The DRIs include four reference values: Estimated Average Requirement (EAR), Adequate Intake (AI), Tolerable Upper Intake Level (UL), and Recommended Dietary Allowance (RDA).

6. EAR is the daily dietary intake level estimated to meet the nutrient requirement of 50% of healthy individuals in a particular life stage and gender group. The EAR is the basis for establishing the RDA, which, as traditionally defined, is an intake level sufficient to meet the nutrient requirement of nearly all healthy individuals in a particular life stage and gender group.

7. If there are insufficient data to establish an EAR, then the AI is used instead of the RDA. The AI is actually an observational standard and is defined as a recommended intake level that is assumed to be adequate and that is based on experimentally determined approximations of nutrient intake by a group (or groups) of healthy people. The UL is the highest level of daily nutrient intake that is likely to pose no risk of adverse health affects to almost all apparently healthy individuals in the general population.

8. The suggested uses of the DRIs are clearly delineated and fall into two broad categories: assessing nutrient intakes of individuals and groups and planning for nutrient intakes of individuals and groups. The DRIs address health promotion and the prevention of both chronic and deficiency disease. They also provide guidance on using nutritional supplements. They are intended to be used in conjunction with other nutritional assessment approaches, rather than as the only means of assessing nutrient adequacy.

9. The arduous task of developing the DRIs formally began in 1993. The first DRI report was released in 1997 and covered calcium, fluoride, magnesium, phosphorus, and vitamin D. The second, published in 1998, covered folate and the other B vitamins. The third was published in 2000, covering vitamins C and E, selenium, and carotenoids.

10. In nutrient density, recommended nutrient intakes and nutritional composition of foods are expressed in terms of nutrient quantity per 1000 kcal. It allows the nutritional qualities of foods and diets to be evaluated and compared easily, facilitates meal planning, addresses the issue of overconsumption, and allows the nutritive value of foods to be evaluated with respect to their caloric content.

11. The index of nutritional quality (INQ) of a food equals the amount of a nutrient in 1000 kcal of that food divided by the recommended allowance of that nutrient per 1000 kcal. A food with an overall INQ substantially greater than "1" has a high nutrient density and provides important nutrients in excess of calories.

12. Dietary guidelines, or goals, are dietary standards primarily intended to address the more common and pressing nutrition-related health problems of chronic disease. They often are expressed as

nonquantitative change from the present average national diet or from people's typical eating habits.

13. Since the late 1960s, numerous dietary guidelines have been issued by Western governments and various health organizations. Overall, they have consistently called for maintenance of healthy body weight, decreased consumption of fat (especially saturated fat), increased consumption of complex carbohydrates, and use of alcoholic beverages in moderation, if at all.

14. Nutrition labeling in the United States began in 1973, when the Food and Drug Administration established the U.S. Recommended Daily Allowances (U.S. RDAs). In 1990, Congress passed the Nutrition Labeling and Education Act, which made sweeping changes in nutrition labeling regulations, replaced the U.S. RDAs with the Reference Daily Intakes (RDIs), and established the Daily Reference Values (DRVs). The RDIs and DRVs are collectively referred to as the Daily Values.

15. Food guides are nutrition education tools that translate dietary standards and recommendations into understandable and practical forms for use by those who have little or no training in nutrition. Generally, foods are classified into groups according to their similarity in nutrient content. If a certain number of servings from each group is consumed, a balanced and adequate diet is thought likely to result.

16. The food exchange system simplifies meal planning for persons limiting energy consumption and helps ensure adequate nutrient intake. Originally developed to facilitate meal planning for persons with diabetes, it is easily adapted to personal food preferences and is useful for quickly approximating kilocalorie and macronutrient levels in foods. The specified serving sizes of foods within each exchange list are approximately equal in their contribution of energy and macronutrients.

17. With the help of a dietitian, people can develop an easily followed meal plan to control energy intake in which the number of servings to be selected from the various exchange lists for each meal is outlined. Meal planning simply involves selecting the correct number of servings from each list and observing the specified serving size.

REFERENCES

1. Leitch I. 1942. The evolution of dietary standards. *Nutrition Abstracts and Reviews* 11:509–521.

2. Harper AE. 1985. Origin of recommended dietary allowances—An historic overview. *American Journal of Clinical Nutrition* 41:140–148.

3. McCollum EV. 1957. *A history of nutrition.* Boston: Houghton Mifflin.

4. Todhunter EN. 1976. Chronology of some events in the development and application of the science of nutrition. *Nutrition Reviews* 34:353–365.

5. Roberts LJ. 1958. Beginnings of the Recommended Dietary Allowances. *Journal of the American Dietetic Association* 34:903–908.

6. Miller DF, Voris L. 1969. Chronologic changes in the Recommended Dietary Allowances. *Journal of the American Dietetic Association* 54:109–117.

7. Committee on Food and Nutrition, National Research Council. 1941. Recommended allowances for the various dietary essentials. *Journal of the American Dietetic Association* 17:565–567.

8. Food and Nutrition Board, National Research Council. 1989. *Recommended Dietary Allowances,* 10th ed. Washington, DC: National Academy Press.

9. Food and Nutrition Board, Institute of Medicine. 1994. *How should the Recommended Dietary Allowances be revised?* Washington, DC: National Academy Press.

10. Standing Committee on the Scientific Evaluation of Dietary Reference Intakes, Food and Nutrition Board, Institute of Medicine. 1997. *Dietary Reference Intakes for Calcium, Phosphorus, Magnesium, Vitamin D, and Fluoride.* Washington, DC: National Academy Press.

11. Standing Committee on the Scientific Evaluation of Dietary Reference Intakes, Food and Nutrition Board, Institute of Medicine. 1998. *Dietary Reference Intakes for Thiamin, Riboflavin, Niacin, Vitamin B$_6$, Folate, Vitamin B$_{12}$, Pantothenic Acid, Biotin, and Choline.* Washington, DC: National Academy Press.

12. Standing Committee on the Scientific Evaluation of Dietary Reference Intakes, Food and Nutrition Board, Institute of Medicine. 2000. *Dietary Reference Intakes for Vitamin C, Vitamin E, Selenium, and Carotenoids.* Washington, DC: National Academy Press.

13. Health and Welfare Canada. 1990. *Nutrition Recommendations.* Ottawa: Canadian Government Publishing Centre.

14. National Research Council. 1986. *Nutrient adequacy: Assessment using food consumption surveys.* Washington, DC: National Academy Press.

15. Beaton GH. 1985. Uses and limits of the use of the Recommended Dietary Allowances for evaluating dietary intake data. *American Journal of Clinical Nutrition* 41:155–164.

16. Yates AA, Schlicker SA, Suitor CW. 1998. Dietary Reference Intakes: The new basis for recommendations for calcium and related nutrients, B vitamins, and choline. *Journal of the American Dietetic Association* 98:699–706.

17. Monsen ER. 2000. Dietary Reference Intakes for the antioxidant nutrients: Vitamin C, vitamin E, and carotenoids. *Journal of the American Dietetic Association* 100:637–640.

18. Kant AK. 1996. Indexes of overall diet quality: A review. *Journal of the American Dietetic Association* 96:785–791.

19. Haines PS, Siega-Riz AM, Popkin BM. 1999. The Diet Quality Index Revised: A measurement instrument for populations. *Journal of the American Dietetic Association* 99:697–704.

20. Hansen RG, Wyse BW. 1980. Expression of nutrient allowances per 1,000 kilocalories. *Journal of the American Dietetic Association* 76:223–227.

21. Hansen RG, Windham CT, Wyse BW. 1985. Nutrient density and food labeling. *Clinical Nutrition* 4:164–170.

22. Wyse BW, Windham CT, Hansen RG. 1985. Nutrition intervention: Panacea or Pandora's box? *Journal of the American Dietetic Association* 85:1084–1090.

23. Windham CT, Wyse BW, Hansen RG. 1983. Nutrient density of diets in the USDA Nationwide Food Consumption Survey, 1977–1978. II. Adequacy of nutrient density consumption practices. *Journal of the American Dietetic Association* 82:34–43.

24. Patterson RE, Haines PS, Popkin BM. 1994. Diet Quality Index: Capturing a multidimensional behavior. *Journal of the American Dietetic Association* 94:57–64.

25. Food and Nutrition Board, National Research Council. 1989. *Diet and health: Implications for reducing chronic disease risk.* Washington, DC: National Academy Press.

26. Kennedy ET, Ohls J, Carlson S, Fleming K. 1995. The Healthy Eating Index: Design and applications. *Journal of the American Dietetic Association* 95:1103–1108.

27. Bowman SA, Lino M, Gerrior SA, Basiotis PP. 1998. The Healthy Eating Index, 1994–96. *Family Economics and Nutrition Review* 11(3):2–14.

28. Berger S. 1987. The implementation of dietary guidelines—Ways and difficulties. *American Journal of Clinical Nutrition* 45:1383–1389.

29. Truswell AS. 1999. *Dietary goals and guidelines: National and international perspectives.* In Shils ME, Olson JA, Shike M, Ross AC, eds. *Modern Nutrition in Health and Disease,* 9th ed. Baltimore: Williams & Wilkins.

30. Truswell AS. 1987. Evolution of dietary recommendations, goals, and guidelines. *American Journal of Clinical Nutrition* 45:1060–1072.

31. Select Committee on Nutrition and Human Needs, U.S. Senate. 1977. *Dietary Goals for the United States.* Washington, DC: U.S. Government Printing Office.

32. Twenty commentaries. 1977. *Nutrition Today* 12(6):10–27.

33. Additional commentaries. 1978. *Nutrition Today* 13(1):30–32.

34. U.S. Department of Agriculture/ U.S. Department of Health and Human Services. 1980. *Nutrition and your health: Dietary Guidelines for Americans.* Washington, DC: U.S. Government Printing Office.

35. U.S. Department of Agriculture/U.S. Department of Health and Human Services. 1985. *Nutrition and your health: Dietary Guidelines for Americans,* 2nd ed. Washington, DC: U.S. Government Printing Office.

36. U.S. Department of Agriculture/U.S. Department of Health and Human Services. 1990. *Nutrition and your health: Dietary Guidelines for Americans,* 3rd ed. Washington, DC: U.S. Government Printing Office.

37. U.S. Department of Agriculture/ U.S. Department of Health and Human Services. 1995. *Nutrition and Your Health: Dietary Guidelines for Americans,* 4th ed. Hyattsville, MD: U.S. Department of Agriculture, Human Nutrition Information Service.

38. U.S. Department of Agriculture/ U.S. Department of Health and Human Services. 2000. *Nutrition and Your Health: Dietary Guidelines for Americans,* 5th ed. Hyattsville, MD: U.S. Department of Agriculture, Center for Nutrition Policy and Promotion.

39. Food and Nutrition Board, National Research Council. 1980. *Toward healthful diets.* Washington, DC: National Academy Press.

40. U.S. Department of Health and Human Services. 1988. *The surgeon general's report on nutrition and health.* Washington, DC: U.S. Government Printing Office.

41. Nestle M. 1988. The surgeon general's report on nutrition and health: New federal dietary guidance policy. *Journal of Nutrition Education* 20:252–254.

42. McGinnis JM, Nestle M. 1989. The surgeon general's report on nutrition and health: Policy implications and implementation strategies. *American Journal of Clinical Nutrition* 49:23–28.

43. Food and Nutrition Board. 1991. *Improving America's diet and health: From recommendations to action.* Washington, DC: National Academy Press.

44. Food and Nutrition Board. 1992. *Eat for life: The Food and Nutrition Board's guide to reducing your risk of chronic disease.* Washington, DC: National Academy Press.

45. Deckelbaum RJ, Fisher EA, Winston M, et al. 1999. Summary of a scientific conference on preventive nutrition: Pediatrics to geriatrics. *Circulation* 100:450–456.

46. Welsh SO, Davis C, Shaw A. 1993. USDA's food guide: Background and development. Hyattsville, MD: U.S. Department of Agriculture, Human Nutrition Information Service.

47. Welsh S, Davis C, Shaw A. 1992. A brief history of food guides in the United States. *Nutrition Today* 27(6):6–11.

48. Combs GF. 1991. What's happening at USDA. *American Institute of Nutrition Notes* 27(3):6.

49. Anonymous. 1991. Official blows whistle on pyramid cancellation. *Community Nutrition Institute Nutrition Week* 21(46):6–7.

50. Nestle M. 1994. The politics of dietary guidance—A new opportunity. *American Journal of Public Health* 84: 713–715.

51. Nestle M. 1993. Food lobbies, the food pyramid, and U.S. nutrition policy. *International Journal of Health Services* 23:483–496.

52. Burros M. 1991. U.S. delays issuing nutrition chart. *New York Times,* 27 April, p. A9.

53. Toufexis A. 1991. Playing politics with our food. *Time* 138(2):57–58.

54. Willett WC. 1994. Diet and health: What should we eat? *Science* 264:532–537.

55. Caso EK. 1950. Calculation of diabetic diets. *Journal of the American Dietetic Association* 26:575–583.

ASSESSMENT ACTIVITY 2.1

Using Standards to Evaluate Nutrient Intake

Nutrient standards are indispensable in establishing a benchmark from which to assess adequacy of nutrient intake. This assessment activity will help you become familiar with the reference nutrient intakes from the United Kingdom (RNIs) and the dietary reference intakes (DRIs) as you assess a defined diet and compare results from these two standards.

Table 2.23 shows mean intakes for five nutrients and energy by women age 20 to 29 years from the third National Health and Nutrition Examination Survey (NHANES III) (see Chapter 4). The data were averaged from 24-hour dietary recalls.

1. Locate the recommended intakes of the five nutrients and energy for females from the recommended nutrient intake tables for the United States (19–30 years old, Tables 2.2 and 2.4) and the United Kingdom (19–50 years old, Appendix A). Record these in Table 2.23 in the appropriate

"Standard" columns. (Note that values present in one table may not be found in another; enter "N/A" for any missing values.)

2. Calculate how intakes compare with each standard by using the following formula. Enter the percent of standard value in the appropriate "Percent of Standard" columns in Table 2.23.

$$\text{Percent of standard} = \frac{\text{Intake of certain nutrient}}{\text{Recommended level of intake for that nutrient}}$$

3. Which of the average nutrient intakes are greater than recommended? Which are lower than recommended?

4. Note that recommended nutrient levels vary among countries. The intake of calcium, for example, may exceed the recommended intake level of one country but not that of another.

TABLE 2.23   **Mean Intakes of Selected Nutrients and Energy of U.S. Females 20–29 Years Old and How They Compare With United Kingdom and U.S. Nutrient Intake Standards**

Nutrient	Mean Intake[*]	United Kingdom Standard	United Kingdom Percent of Standard	United States Standard	United States Percent of Standard
Energy	1957 kcal				
Protein	69 g				
Vitamin C	87 mg				
Folate	230 μg				
Calcium	778 mg				
Iron	12.4 mg				

*From U.S. Department of Health and Human Services.

ASSESSMENT ACTIVITY 2.2

Index of Nutritional Quality (INQ)

This assessment activity will familiarize you with calculating the INQ and using it to compare different foods or meals. Table 2.24 provides values for energy and selected nutrients found in two meals:

TABLE 2.24	**Values for Energy and Selected Nutrients Found in Two Meals**	
Nutrient	**Meal 1**	**Meal 2**
Energy (kcal)	837	814
Protein (g)	24	42
Carbohydrate (g)	87	96
Total fat (g)	44	30
Saturated fat (g)	19	9
Calcium (mg)	230	523
Iron (mg)	5	7
Folate (μg)	72	139

Meal 1

1 cheeseburger with lettuce, tomato, pickle, and mayonnaise
2 servings of French fries
24-ounce diet cola

Meal 2

1 broiled chicken breast sandwich with mayonnaise
1 baked potato topped with ¼ cup nonfat yogurt
1 small tossed salad
1 tablespoon of low-calorie dressing
8 fluid ounces of nonfat milk

Table 2.25 provides the nutrient values per 1000 kcal (rounded to the nearest whole number) and the INQs (rounded to the nearest tenth) for meal 1. The table also provides blank spaces for entering the nutrient values per 1000 kcal and the INQs for meal 2. Your task is to calculate the nutrient values per 1000 kcal and the INQs for meal 2 and record them in the blank spaces of the table.

1. The first step in converting nutrient levels for meal 2 to a *per 1000 kcal* basis is to divide 1000 by the number of kilocalories provided by meal 2.

$$1000 \div 814 = 1.23$$

Store this number in your calculator's memory and multiply it by each of the nutrient values for meal 2 provided in Table 2.24. For example, the grams of protein *per 1000 kcal* provided by meal 2 is 52.

$$1.23 \times 42 \text{ g of protein} = 52 \text{ g of protein per } 1000 \text{ kcal}$$

Perform the same calculations for each of the other nutrient values given for meal 2 and record these in Table 2.25 in the "Per 1000 Kcal" column.

2. Use the following formula to calculate the INQs of meal 2. Nutrient allowances per 1000 kcal are given in Table 2.6.

$$\text{INQ} = \frac{\text{Amount of nutrients in 1000 kcal of food}}{\text{Allowance of nutrients per 1000 kcal}}$$

The INQ of protein in meal 2, for example, is 1.9. This value was reached by dividing the amount of protein per 1000 kcal in meal 2 (52 g) by the single-value protein recommendation per 1000 kcal (35 g) found in Table 2.6. Calculate the remaining INQs for meal 2 and record these in the "INQ" column.

3. Now compare the two meals on the basis of nutrient density (nutrients provided per 1000 kcal) and the INQ. Which of the two meals has an overall higher nutrient density? Which has an overall higher INQ?

4. What do you think is the primary difference between the two meals? Although they supply roughly the same number of kilocalories, the cheeseburger and French fries in meal 1 give it a significantly greater fat content. Fats and refined sugars are common *nutrient diluents* of the Western diet. Foods high in fat (such as French fries or potato chips) tend to have higher INQs for fat than do low-fat foods (such as baked or boiled potatoes with little or no added fat). Remember that, although it is desirable to have a *high* INQ for most nutrients, it is preferable to have *low* INQs for fats (especially saturated fats), cholesterol, and sodium. Which of the meals has the lower INQs for total and saturated fats?

TABLE 2.25	Nutrient and Energy Values per 1000 Kcal and Index of Nutritional Quality (INQ) for Two Meals				

	Meal 1		Meal 2	
Nutrient	**Per 1000 Kcal**	**INQ**	**Per 1000 Kcal**	**INQ**
Energy (kcal)	1000	1	1000	1
Protein (g)	29	0.9	52	1.5
Carbohydrate (g)	104	0.7	———	———
Total fat (g)	53	1.6	———	———
Saturated fat (g)	23	2.1	———	———
Calcium (mg)	275	0.4	———	———
Iron (mg)	6	1.0	———	———
Folate (μg)	86	0.3	———	———

ASSESSMENT ACTIVITY 2.3

Food Exchange System

Using the food exchange system to plan meals and assess macronutrient intake is quite easy once you become accustomed to the technique and familiar with the exchange lists. Let's begin this assessment activity by planning an evening meal and snack for two days using the meal pattern in the far left column of Table 2.26. To manage energy intake and promote dental health, it is probably best for most people to limit eating to meal times and avoid snacking. However, persons taking insulin often need midafternoon and late-evening snacks to maintain adequate blood sugar levels.

1. In the spaces provided under "Meal Plan 1" and "Meal Plan 2," write foods from the exchange lists (see Table 2.21) and their serving sizes that would match the meal pattern. An example of three

exchanges from the starch list is a small baked potato, ½ cup of green peas, and a small, plain roll. One strength of the exchange system is that it allows almost unlimited variety and can be easily adapted to personal or cultural eating practices.

2. Once you become familiar with the exchange lists, you can use them to rapidly approximate energy and macronutrient levels in individual foods or entire meals. The far left column of Table 2.27 lists a typical American breakfast. Using Table 2.20 (which gives the average kilocalorie and macronutrient content of the six exchanges) and Table 2.21 (which details the food exchange lists), enter in the appropriate columns the quantities of energy, carbohydrate, protein, and fat for each food and then total them.

TABLE 2.26	Planning Meals and Snacks Using an Exchange List Meal Pattern	
Meal Pattern	**Meal Plan 1**	**Meal Plan 2**
Evening Meal		
Starch—3 exchanges	_____	_____
	_____	_____
	_____	_____
Lean meat and substitutes—2 exchanges	_____	_____
	_____	_____
Vegetables—2 exchanges	_____	_____
	_____	_____
Fruit—1 exchange	_____	_____
Fat—2 exchanges	_____	_____
	_____	_____
Evening Snack		
Starch—1/2 exchange	_____	_____
Low-fat milk—1/2 exchange	_____	_____

TABLE 2.27	Estimating Energy and Macronutrient Levels in Foods Using the Exchange Lists			
Food	**Energy (kcal)**	**Carbohydrate (g)**	**Protein (g)**	**Fat (g)**
Bran Chex, 1½ cup	_____	_____	_____	_____
Milk, 2% fat, 1 cup	_____	_____	_____	_____
Banana, 1/2	_____	_____	_____	_____
Orange, 1 medium	_____	_____	_____	_____
Bagel, 1/2	_____	_____	_____	_____
Cream cheese, 1 Tbsp.	_____	_____	_____	_____
Totals	_____	_____	_____	_____

MEASURING DIET

INTRODUCTION

Measurement of nutrient intake is probably the most widely used indirect indicator of nutritional status. It is used routinely in national nutrition monitoring surveys, epidemiologic studies, nutrition studies of free-living participants (those living outside a controlled setting), and various federal and state health and nutrition program evaluations. To the uninitiated, measurement of nutrient intake may appear to be straightforward and fairly easy. However, estimating an individual's usual dietary and nutrient intake is difficult. The task is complicated by weaknesses of data-gathering techniques, human behavior, the natural tendency of an individual's nutrient intake to vary considerably from day to day, and the limitations of nutrient composition tables and databases. Despite these weaknesses, nutrient intake data are valuable in assessing nutritional status when used in conjunction with anthropometric, biochemical, and clinical data.

This chapter discusses the reasons for measuring diet and different ways of approaching the topic. Techniques for measuring diet are described along with their strengths and weaknesses. The issues of accuracy and validity are examined, and the number of days of individual dietary intake required to characterize the usual nutrient intake of groups and individuals is discussed.

In some instances, data on the kinds and amounts of food eaten by groups or individuals are important because they allow the estimation of nutrient intake. However, conversion of dietary intake data to nutrient intake data requires information on the nutrient content of foods. This is provided by food composition tables and nutrient databases, which are subject to certain limitations and potential sources of error.

REASONS FOR MEASURING DIET

Assessing dietary status includes considering the types and amounts of foods consumed and the intake of the nutrients and other components contained in foods. When food consumption data are combined with information on the nutrient composition of food, the intake of particular nutrients and other food components can be estimated.[1]

Why measure diet? The ultimate reason is to improve human health.[2–4] Nutritional problems are at the root of the leading causes of death, particularly in developed nations. Food and nutrient intake data are critical for investigating the relationships between diet and these diseases, identifying groups at risk for nutrient deficiency or excess, and formulating food and nutrition policies for disease reduction and health promotion.[5] In general, however, there are four major uses of dietary intake data: assessing and monitoring food and nutrient intake, formulating and evaluating government health and agricultural policy, conducting epidemiologic research, and using the data for commercial purposes.[6] These are outlined in Box 3.1.

Planning national and international food and nutrition programs depends on estimates of per capita (per person) food, energy, and nutrient consumption. Although per capita consumption cannot easily be measured directly, estimates of food disappearance (or availability) (discussed in detail in Chapter 4) are frequently used indirect indicators of consumption. Food consumption data are used in formulating public and private agricultural policies for the production, distribution, and consumption of food.

Repeated surveys estimating food disappearance, such as those conducted by the U.S. Department of Agriculture (USDA), suggest important trends in overall patterns of food consumption over time. Among these are changes in the American diet since the early 1900s in sources of energy, composition of foods, consumption of specific food groups, and eating patterns (such as snacking and eating away from home), all of which can have profound health, social, and economic implications. Dietary assessment is used in determining the extent of malnutrition in a population, developing nutrition intervention and consumer education programs, constructing food guides, devising low-cost food plans, and providing a basis for food and nutrition legislation. Comparisons of dietary practices and nutritional intake with the distribution of disease have demonstrated important links between diet and disease and have shown how dietary changes can modulate disease risk and enhance health.

APPROACHES TO MEASURING DIET

Various methods for collecting food consumption data are available. It is important to note, however, that no single best method exists, and diet measurement will always be accompanied by some degree of error.[7] Each method has its own advantages and disadvantages. Despite these disadvantages and the inevitability of error, properly collected and analyzed, dietary intake data have considerable value, as summarized in Box 3.1. Being informed about the strengths and weaknesses of the methods available will better enable you to scrutinize nutrition research and to draw your own conclusions about a study's results. It will also allow researchers to choose the approach best suited for the task and enable them to use the methods in ways that improve data quality. Selecting the appropriate measurement method, correctly applying it, and using proper data analysis techniques can make the difference between data showing a diet-disease relationship and data showing no relationship where one may actually exist. Choosing the appropriate method for measuring diet depends on such considerations as the research design, characteristics of the study participants, and available resources.

Research Design Considerations

Let's consider four types of research designs: correlational; survey, or cross-sectional; case-control; and longitudinal, or cohort. **Correlational studies** compare the level of some factor (e.g., saturated fat intake) with the level of another factor (e.g., coronary heart disease mortality) in the same population. They are considered most useful for generating hypotheses regarding the associations between suspected risk factors and disease risk. The data used in correlational studies often are only a rough estimate of dietary intake derived from food disappearance studies (discussed in Chapter 4) and are not based on actual dietary intake measurements obtained by the methods discussed in this chapter. Much of these data are readily available from national and international

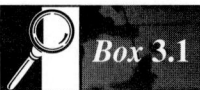

Box 3.1   Reasons for Measuring Diet

Assessing and Monitoring Food and Nutrient Intake

Ensuring adequacy of the food supply	Data from national surveys and food disappearance indicate the adequacy of food, energy, and nutrient supply.
Estimating the adequacy of dietary intakes of individuals and groups	Individual nutrient intake data combined with anthropometric, biochemical, and clinical measures allow assessment of nutritional status.
	The proportion of group members having adequate or inadequate intake of a particular nutrient can be determined when the average group intake and the distribution of that intake are known.
Monitoring trends in food and nutrient consumption	Trends in percent of energy from fat, carbohydrate, and protein per person can be derived from dietary surveys and food disappearance data.
Estimating exposure to food additives and contaminants	The FDA's Total Diet Study monitors average intakes of pesticides, toxins, industrial chemicals, and radioactive substances to determine whether they constitute a health risk.

Formulating and Evaluating Government Health and Agricultural Policy

Planning food production and distribution	Data indicating a marginal or an inadequate supply of energy and/or nutrients can provide direction for planning food production, regulating food imports and exports, and setting priorities for food aid.
	Food consumption data allow certain groups or income levels to be targeted for food assistance programs, such as WIC, food stamps, and the school lunch program.
Establishing food and nutrition regulations	National and individual consumption data allow identification of potential problems to be addressed by food regulations (e.g., labeling) and programs for food enrichment or fortification.
Establishing programs for nutrition education and disease risk reduction	The National Cholesterol Education Program is in part a response to dietary studies indicating that many Americans consume too much total fat, saturated fat, and cholesterol.
	National survey data showing increasing average body weights for Americans indicate the need for a national strategy for weight management.
Evaluating the success and cost-effectiveness of nutrition education and disease risk reduction programs	The decline in the average serum total cholesterol of Americans suggests that cholesterol-lowering campaigns have been successful.

Conducting Epidemiologic Research

Studying the relationships between diet and health	The purpose of many studies is to investigate the relationship between dietary and nutritional intake and health and disease—for example, the relationships between diet and coronary heart disease, cancer, hypertension, and anemia.
Identifying groups at risk of developing diseases because of their diet and/or nutrient intake	Nutrient consumption data show that women of childbearing age often have low folate intake, which increases the risk of their children being born with neural tube defects.
Commercial Purposes	Data from national nutrition surveys are used by food manufacturers to develop advertising campaigns or new food products.

From Sabry JH. 1988. Purposes of food consumption surveys. In *Manual on methodology for food consumption studies,* Cameron ME, Van Staveren WA, eds. New York: Oxford University Press. (See also references 5 and 6.)

agencies. Using such data, early researchers into the causes of coronary heart disease (CHD) showed that saturated fat consumption is positively correlated with risk of CHD. This association led to more definitive studies that demonstrated a cause-and-effect relationship between high saturated fat intake and increased risk of CHD.

Surveys, or **cross-sectional studies,** provide a "snapshot" of the health of a population at a specific point in time. Various health and dietary measurements are performed on a relatively small group of people that is representative of the larger general population. The much smaller "sample" is selected from the "population" using statistical sampling techniques to ensure that it is representative of the larger population. Analysis of the data collected from the sample allow conclusions to be drawn about the health and dietary habits of the population from which the sample has been taken. Examples of surveys include the National Health and Nutrition Examination Survey, the National Health Interview Survey, the Continuing Survey of Food Intakes by Individuals, and the Diet and Health Knowledge Survey, all of which are discussed in Chapter 4. The goal is to collect information on the current diet or dietary habits in the immediate past. The 24-hour recall is the most common method used in surveys, although food records (or food diaries) and food frequency questionnaires are sometimes used.

Case-control studies compare levels of *past exposure* to some factor of interest (e.g., some nutrient or dietary component) in two groups of study participants (cases and controls) to determine how the past exposure relates to a currently existing disease. *Cases* are those people in whom the disease is already diagnosed (e.g., coronary heart disease, cancer, or osteoporosis). *Controls* do not have the disease but share certain characteristics with the cases. The investigators then look *retrospectively* (backward in time) to assess each group's level of exposure to the factor to determine if the disease was preceded by the exposure. Thus, case-control studies require methods that measure dietary intake in the recent past (e.g., the year before diagnosis) or in the distant past (e.g., 10 years ago or in childhood). Methods that focus on current behavior, such as the 24-hour recall and food records, are not suitable. The only good choices for case-control studies are food frequency questionnaires and diet history, which assess diet in the past.

Numerous case-control studies have compared fruit and vegetable intake with risk of cancer at various sites. Past intake of fruits and vegetables among persons diagnosed with cancer (cases) has been compared with that of persons apparently free of cancer (controls). In these studies, increased fruit and vegetable consumption is consistently linked with reduced risk of cancer of the lung and stomach.[9]

Longitudinal, or **cohort, studies** compare *future exposure* to various factors in a group or *cohort* of study participants in an attempt to determine how exposure to the factors relates to diseases that may develop. These are also known as *prospective* studies. Thus, longitudinal studies require methods that measure current diet or dietary habits in the immediate past, such as 24-hour recalls, food records, and food frequency questionnaires.[8,10]

The Framingham Heart Study is an example of a longitudinal study. Initiated in 1949, the cohort consisted of more than 5000 30- to 62-year-old residents of Framingham, Massachusetts. Since joining the study, the participants have undergone regular examinations and dietary assessments in an attempt to identify factors contributing to the subsequent development of coronary heart disease and high blood pressure. Only 2% of the study participants have been lost to follow-up, and approximately one-half of the original participants are still alive. This and other prospective studies have shown that reducing fat intake, controlling body weight and blood pressure, avoiding smoking, and exercising regularly can reduce risk for coronary heart disease and stroke.

Sometimes the goal of dietary assessment is to quickly screen a group of people for probable dietary risk. In these instances, a brief questionnaire identifying people with a high intake of fat, cholesterol, or sodium or a low intake of dietary fiber, fruits, or vegetables can be administered. Two such instruments—the "fat screener," developed by researchers at the National Cancer Institute, and the MEDFICTS questionnaire—are discussed in the section on food frequency questionnaires. The food frequency questionnaire and the 24-hour recall are also suitable for this purpose.[10]

Time and budgetary constraints are major factors influencing the choice of a dietary measurement method. Analyzing the nutrient content of foods recorded in 24-hour recalls and food records can be labor intensive and costly. These methods also require research staff time in checking them over and reviewing them with study participants for completeness and accuracy (Figure 3.1).[5,6] Self-administered food frequency questionnaires, on the other hand, can save considerable time and expense. They can be mailed to study participants, who can complete them on their own and then mail them back to the researchers for data entry and processing. Some food frequency questionnaires are designed to be optically scanned, thus resulting in further saving of staff time and expense.

Characteristics of Study Participants

Factors influencing the selection of a dietary measurement technique include literacy, memory, commitment,

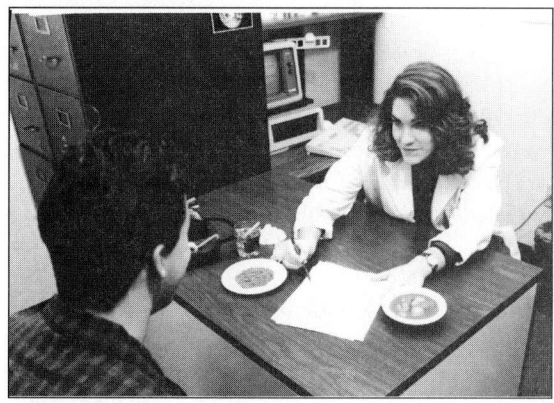

Figure 3.1
Studies of dietary practices and nutritional intake have shown the important role that diet plays in health and disease.

age, ability to communicate, and culture of the participants. If some study participants are likely to be unable to read and/or write, the best methods are the 24-hour recall and the food frequency questionnaire administered by a member of the research team. The food record or self-administered food frequency questionnaire is not recommended. The 24-hour recall and food frequency questionnaire require the ability to remember past eating habits. Food records and self-administered food frequency questionnaires require the training and active participation of the study participants. The level of effort required can also lead participants to change their dietary patterns during the recording period. Consequently, there is concern about response rates, the comparability of recording skills among participants, and the quality of dietary intake results.[8]

The ability to communicate may be limited in study participants who are very young, elderly, developmentally disabled, victims of stroke or Alzheimer's disease, or deceased. In these instances, dietary intake data may have to be collected from another person familiar with the study participant, such as a parent, spouse, child, or sibling. This other person is known as a **surrogate source.** Surrogate sources are discussed later in this chapter in the section "Surrogate Sources." A food inventory method can be useful for older persons living at home. Direct observation of eating habits of persons in institutional care facilities can also be done.[10] The eating habits of children have been assessed using the 24-hour recall, food records, and food frequency questionnaires. Assessing the diets of younger children may require information from surrogates or use of the "consensus recall method," in which the child and both parents give combined responses on a 24-hour recall. This approach has been shown to give more accurate information than a recall from either parent alone.[10]

Assessing the diets of ethnic populations requires modification of existing methods. If participants are interviewed, it is preferable that these be done by persons of the same ethnic or cultural background, so that dietary information can be gathered more effectively. Nutrient analyses of ethnic foods and dishes will likely require changes in food composition databases. Food frequency questionnaires will have to be modified to include food common to the ethnic group being studied.[10]

Available Resources

Some methods for measuring diet are more expensive and labor intensive to administer than others. Before a study begins, the budget must be carefully considered, so that the costs entailed will match the available resources. The 24-hour recall, for example, must be administered by a trained interviewer. If the food record is used, study participants should be trained to properly record their diets. Considerable labor is required to enter data from 24-hour recalls and food records into a computer for analysis. Food frequency questionnaires can be self-administered, and responses can be marked on a form, which is then optically scanned. Data can then be downloaded into a computer for analysis, thus saving considerable time, effort, and expense. Food records and 24-hour recalls tend to be more feasible methods to use in research with smaller numbers of participants. Food frequency questionnaires, on the other hand, are often preferred by researchers studying large numbers of people.

TECHNIQUES IN MEASURING DIET

Measurement of dietary intake usually is conducted for one of three purposes: to compare average nutrient intakes of different groups, to rank individuals within a group, and to estimate an individual's usual intake. Dietary measurement techniques can be categorized as daily food consumption methods (food record and 24-hour recall) and recalled "usual" or average food consumption methods (diet history and food frequency questionnaire).[6] These techniques have also been categorized as meal-based (food record and 24-hour recall) and list-based (food frequency questionnaire).[5]

24-Hour Recall

In the dietary recall method, a trained interviewer asks the respondent to recall in detail all the food and drink consumed during a period of time in the recent past. The interviewer then records this information for later coding and analysis. (In coding, a number is assigned to each kind of food, allowing it to be identified easily for computer analysis.) In most instances, the time period is the previous 24 hours. Thus, the method is most commonly known as the **24-hour recall.**[11] Occasionally, however, the time period is the previous 48 hours, the past 7 days, or, in rare instances, even the preceding month.[12] However, memories of intake may fade rather quickly beyond the most recent day or two, so that loss in accuracy may exceed gain in representativeness.[13,14]

In addition to recording responses, the interviewer helps the respondent remember all that was consumed during the period in question and assists the respondent in estimating portion sizes of foods consumed. (See Appendix C for an example of the 1998 Continuing Survey of Food Intakes by Individuals 24-hour recall form.) A common technique of the 24-hour recall is to begin by asking what the respondent first ate or drank on last awakening. The recall proceeds from the morning of the present day to the current moment. The interviewer then begins at the point exactly 24 hours in the past and works forward to the time of awakening. Some researchers ask respondents to recall their diet from midnight to midnight of the previous day. Asking the respondent about his or her activities during the day and inquiring how they might have been associated with eating or drinking can help in recalling food intake. An inquiry about the previous evening's activities, for example, will stimulate the respondent's memory and may help him or her recall the snack eaten while watching a favorite television program.

After the interview, the recall is checked for omissions and/or mistakes. A respondent may have to be contacted later by telephone or mail to clarify an entry or to obtain information such as brand names, preparation methods, and serving sizes. The recall can then be analyzed using a computerized diet analysis program. Most programs allow research staff to enter the name of the food into the computer and then select the appropriate method of preparation, serving size, and number of servings from a list of choices displayed on the computer screen. In some instances, however, each food may have to be coded using a unique number or food code that identifies each food. For the food "green beans," there may be separate code numbers for cooked frozen green beans, canned green beans, cooked fresh green beans, and so on. This code then is entered into the analysis software (to identify the food) along with the serving size and number of servings to calculate the nutrients of that food.

The 24-hour recall has several strengths. It is inexpensive, it is quick to administer (20 minutes or less), and it can provide detailed information on specific foods, especially if brand names can be recalled.[11,15] It requires only short-term memory. It is well accepted by respondents because they are not asked to keep records, and their expenditure of time and effort is relatively low. Thus, probability sampling within populations and individuals is possible. The method is considered by some to be more objective than the dietary history and food frequency questionnaire, and its administration does not alter the usual diet.[16,17] The 24-hour recall was selected as the primary instrument for measuring dietary intake in the third National Health and Nutrition Examination Survey (NHANES III).[6] Recalls were collected using an automated interview system known as the Dietary Data Collection System.[18] This system is discussed in greater detail in Chapter 4.

Recalls have several limitations. Respondents may withhold or alter information about what they ate because of poor memory or embarrassment or to please or impress the interviewer and researchers. Respondents tend to underreport binge eating, consumption of alcoholic beverages, and consumption of foods perceived as unhealthful. Respondents also tend to overreport consumption of name-brand foods, expensive cuts of meat, and foods considered healthful.[15] Foods eaten but not reported are known as **missing foods,** while foods not eaten but reported are known as **phantom foods.**[19] Several researchers report that, when respondents' actual food consumption is low, they have a tendency to overestimate the amount recalled, and, when their actual consumption is high, they underestimate the amount recalled. Some researchers call this phenomenon the "flat-slope syndrome."[20,21] Energy intake often is underestimated if drinks, sauces, and dressings are not reported.

Underreporting can be limited by using a *multiple-pass 24-hour recall method,* in which the interviewer and respondent review the previous day's eating episodes several times to obtain detailed and accurate information about food intake.[20,21] In one version of the method, a *quick list* of foods eaten in the previous 24 hours is initially compiled. In the second pass, a *detailed description* of foods on the quick list is obtained. The respondent is asked to clarify the description and preparation methods of foods on the quick list. For example, if a respondent reports eating breakfast cereal, the interviewer will ask whether milk was used on the cereal and, if so, what kind of milk and how much was used. In the third pass, called the *review,* the interviewer reviews the data collected, probes for additional eating occasions, and clarifies food portion sizes using household dishes and measures (e.g., cups, bowls, glasses, spoons), geometric shapes (e.g., circles, triangles, rectangles), and food labels.

A five-step, multiple-pass 24-hour recall method was developed for the 1999–2000 National Health and Nutritional Examination Survey (discussed in Chapter 4). In the first pass, a quick list of foods is obtained. In the second pass, information about the meal, time, and place where foods are eaten is recorded. Information about foods that may have been forgotten is collected in the third pass. Additional food details are collected and a final review is completed in the fourth and fifth passes.[21] Use of the multiple-pass method, thorough training and retention of interviewers, and use of other quality-control measures should assure collection of accurate data from this national survey.[22]

The primary limitation of the method is that data on a *single day's diet,* no matter how accurate, are a very poor descriptor of an individual's *usual* nutrient intake because of day-to-day or **intraindividual variability.**[15,23] Even if several 24-hour recalls are collected from one person, it may be impossible to measure intake of infrequently eaten foods, such as liver.[8] However, a sufficiently large number of 24-hour recalls may provide a reasonable estimate of the mean nutrient intake of a group.[11,12,15] Depending on the purpose for which data are used, multiple 24-hour recalls performed on an individual and spaced over various seasons may provide a reasonable estimate of that person's usual nutrient intake.[1,11,24] For example, approximately 3500 participants in NHANES III who were 50 years of age or older completed two additional and unscheduled 24-hour recalls, which were collected by telephone interviews approximately 8 and 16 months after their initial 24-hour recall.[18] This was part of the Supplemental Nutrition Survey of Older Americans, a study collecting data on the diets of older Americans.

The necessary number of days of data collection depends on several factors: whether estimates of usual intake are for individuals or groups, the nutrients of interest, sample size, and degree of intraindividual and interindividual variability.[1,25,26] Twenty-four-hour recalls can provide reasonably accurate data about the preceding day's dietary intake, but reports of diet for the preceding week or month do not accurately characterize dietary intake during those periods.[27] Box 3.2 summarizes the strengths and limitations of the 24-hour recall method.

Food Record, or Diary

In this method, the respondent records, at the time of consumption, the identity and amounts of all foods and beverages consumed for a period of time, usually ranging from 1 to 7 days. An example of a food record form is given in Appendix D. Food and beverage consumption can be quantified by estimating portion sizes, using household measures, or weighing the food or beverage on scales. In many instances, household measures such as cups, tablespoons, and teaspoons or measurements made with a ruler are used to quantify portion size. Certain items, such as eggs, apples, or 12-oz cans of soft drinks, may be thought of as units and simply counted. This method is sometimes referred to as the **estimated food record** because portion sizes are estimated (that is, in terms of coffee cups, dippers, bowls, glasses, and so on), or household measures are used. When food is weighed, the record may be referred to as a **weighed food record.** Box 3.3 compares these two methods. The use of food scales is preferred by European nutrition researchers, who consider it more accurate than using household measures, as is typically done by North American researchers. The degree of accuracy from household measures appears acceptable for most research purposes, especially when considering whether respondents will adhere to the program if they must weigh everything they eat.

The food record does not depend on memory because the respondent ideally records food and beverage consumption (including snacks) at the time of eating. In addition, it can provide detailed food intake data and important information about eating habits (for example, when, where, and with whom meals are eaten and the respondent's mood when choosing certain foods). Data from a multiple-day food record also is more representative

 Box 3.2 **Strengths and Limitations of the 24-Hour Recall**

Strengths

Requires less than 20 minutes to administer

Inexpensive

Easy to administer

Can provide detailed information on types of food consumed

Low respondent burden

Probability sampling possible

Can be used to estimate nutrient intake of groups

Multiple recalls can be used to estimate nutrient intake of individuals.

More objective than dietary history

Does not alter usual diet

Useful in clinical settings

Limitations

One recall is seldom representative of a person's usual intake.

Underreporting/overreporting occurs.

Relies on memory.

Omissions of dressings, sauces, and beverages can lead to low estimates of energy intake.

May be a tendency to overreport intake at low levels and overreport intake at high levels of consumption.

Data entry can be very labor intensive.

Box 3.3   **Comparison of the Estimated Food Record and the Weighed Food Record**

Estimated Food Record

Amounts of food and leftovers are measured in household measures (cups, tablespoons, teaspoons) or estimated using such measures as coffee cups, bowls, glasses, and dippers. The researchers then quantify these measures by volume and weight.

Considered less accurate than the weighed food record

Considered an acceptable method for collecting group intake data

Puts less burden on the respondent than the weighed food record and thus cooperation rates are likely to be higher, especially over long recording periods

As effective in ranking subjects into thirds and fifths as weighed records

Weighed Food Record

Food and leftovers are weighed using scales or computerized techniques supplied by researchers.

Considered more accurate than the estimated food record

Preferred by some researchers for gathering data on individuals

Requires a greater degree of subject cooperation than the estimated food record and thus is likely to have a greater impact on eating habits than the estimated food record

Cost of scales may be prohibitive in some instances

From Bingham SA, Nelson M, Paul AA, et al. 1988. Methods for data collection at an individual level. In Cameron ME and Van Staveren WA (eds.). *Manual on methodology for food consumption studies.* New York: Oxford University Press.

of usual intake than are single-day data from either a 24-hour recall or a 1-day food record. However, multiple food records from nonconsecutive, random days (including weekends) covering different seasons are necessary to arrive at useful estimates of usual intake.[11,28,29]

Food records have several limitations. They require a literate and cooperative respondent who is able and willing to expend the time and effort necessary to record dietary intake. However, such a respondent may not be representative of the general population.[21] The act of recording food intake after several days can lead even motivated respondents to reduce the number of foods and snacks eaten and to decrease the complexity of their diets to simplify the recording process.[28] When asked directly about recording their food intake, 30% to 50% of respondents have

reported changing their eating habits while keeping a food record.[29,30] Thus, the food record may significantly underreport energy and nutrient intakes.[31] Box 3.4 summarizes the strengths and limitations of the food record.

Food Frequency Questionnaires

Food frequency questionnaires assess energy and/or nutrient intake by determining how frequently a person consumes a limited number of foods that are major sources of nutrients or of a particular dietary component in question. The questionnaires consist of a list of approximately 150 or fewer individual foods or food groups that are important contributors to the population's intake of energy and nutrients. Respondents indicate how many

Box 3.4   **Strengths and Limitations of the Food Record**

Strengths

Does not depend on memory

Can provide detailed intake data

Can provide data about eating habits

Multiple-day data more representative of usual intake

Reasonably valid up to 5 days

Limitations

Requires high degree of cooperation

Response burden can result in low response rates when used in large national surveys

Subject must be literate

Takes more time to obtain data

Act of recording may alter diet

Analysis is labor intensive and expensive

times a day, week, month, or year that they usually consume the foods.[11,15,23,24] In some food frequency questionnaires, a choice of portion size is not given. These generally use "standard" portion sizes (the amounts customarily eaten per serving for various age/sex groups) drawn from large-population data.[11,12,23,24] An example of this format is given in Figure 3.2A. It simply asks how many times a year, month, week, or day a person eats dark bread or ice cream. This is sometimes referred to as a **simple,** or **nonquantitative food frequency questionnaire** format. The **semiquantitative food frequency questionnaire,** shown in Figure 3.2B, gives respondents an idea of portion size. It asks how many times a year, month, week, or day a person eats a slice of dark bread or a ½ cup serving of ice cream. In addition to asking the frequency of consumption, the **quantitative food frequency questionnaire,** shown in Figure 3.2C asks the respondent to describe the size of his or her usual serving as small, medium, or large relative to a standard serving.[15] The portion numbers and sizes then are entered into a computer database, which multiplies these by the nutrients contained in each food or food group and arrives at an estimated nutrient intake.[23,24,32] An alternative to this is for respondents to mark their answers on an answer sheet,

which can then be optically scanned, so that their responses can be directly downloaded into a computer for analysis, thus saving the researchers considerable time and money. This feature makes food frequency questionnaires a cost-effective approach for measuring diet in large epidemiologic studies.

Some questionnaires, known as "screeners," have been designed to assess intake of individual nutrients or food components, such as vitamin A, fat, or calcium, for studies investigating the relationships between diet and such conditions as cancer and cardiovascular disease.[12,33–37] Others have been developed to assess a wide spectrum of macronutrients and micronutrients.[23] Figure 3.3 shows several questions from a nonquantitative food frequency questionnaire used in NHANES III. NHANES and other national surveys are discussed in detail in Chapter 4. The entire diet portion of the NHANES III questionnaire for respondents age 17 years and older is shown in Appendix E.

Figure 3.4 shows a 13-item questionnaire developed by researchers at the U.S. National Cancer Institute for identifying groups whose mean percent fat intake is high (or low).[33] The database and age- and sex-specific portion sizes for food items necessary to score the questionnaire

A

Food Item	Average Use During Past Year					
	< 1 month	1–3 month	1–4 week	5–7 week	2–4 day	5+ day
coffee						
dark bread						
ice cream						

B

Food Item	Average Use During Past Year								
	< 1 month	1–3 month	1 week	2–4 week	5–6 week	1 day	2–3 day	4–5 day	6+ day
coffee (1 cup)									
dark bread (1 slice)									
ice cream (1/2 cup)									

C

Food Item	Medium Serving	Your Serving Size			How Often?				
		S	M	L	Day	Week	Month	Year	Never
coffee	(1 cup)								
dark bread	(1 slice)								
ice cream	(1/2 cup)								

Figure 3.2 **Examples of three food frequency questionnaire formats: (A) the simple, or nonquantitative, format; (B) the semiquantitative format; (C) the quantitative format.**

Source: Adapted from Bingham SA, Cummings JH. 1985. Urine nitrogen as an independent validatory measure of dietary intake: A study of nitrogen balance in individuals consuming their normal diet. *American Journal of Clinical Nutrition* 42:1276–1289.

N3. Fruit and Fruit Juices	
Next are fruit juices and fruit. Include all forms — fresh, frozen, canned, and dried.	
a. How often did you have orange juice, grapefruit juice, and tangerine juice?	____ per 1☐D 2☐W 3☐M or 4☐N 9☐DK
b. Other fruit juices such as grape juice, apple juice, cranberry juice, and fruit nectars	____ per 1☐D 2☐W 3☐M or 4☐N 9☐DK
c. Citrus fruits including oranges, grapefruits, and tangerines	____ per 1☐D 2☐W 3☐M or 4☐N 9☐DK
d. Melons including cantaloupe, honeydew, and watermelon	____ per 1☐D 2☐W 3☐M or 4☐N 9☐DK
e. Peaches, nectarines, apricots, guava, mango, and papaya	____ per 1☐D 2☐W 3☐M or 4☐N 9☐DK
f. How often did you have any other fruits such as apples, bananas, pears, berries, cherries, grapes, plums, and strawberries? (include plantains)	____ per 1☐D 2☐W 3☐M or 4☐N 9☐DK

Figure 3.3 Several questions from a food frequency questionnaire used in the third National Health and Nutrition Examination Survey (note that portion size is not assessed).

Source: From National Center for Health Statistics.

are given in Appendix F. The screening tool, which can be administered either by the respondent or by an interviewer, is intended to identify those who might be further studied for the health consequences of their high- or low-fat diet, who may need further dietary assessment, or who might benefit from dietary intervention. It takes about 4 minutes to administer and does essentially as well as three 4-day food records in ranking respondents in terms of their intake in grams of total fat and saturated, oleic, and linoleic fatty acids.[33]

A questionnaire developed to quickly estimate how frequently foods high in total fat, saturated fatty acids, and cholesterol are eaten is shown in Appendix G. It is called the MEDFICTS Dietary Assessment Questionnaire (**M**eats, **E**ggs, **D**airy, **F**ried foods, **I**n baked goods, **C**onvenience foods, **T**able fats, **S**nacks) and is recommended by the National Cholesterol Education Program as a simple approach to assess a person's intake of total fat, saturated fat, and dietary cholesterol.[38]

	Medium Serving	Your Serving Size			How Often?					Office Use
		S	M	L	Day	Week	Month	Year	Rarely/Never	
EXAMPLE: Hamburgers, cheeseburgers, meat loaf	1 medium									
Hamburger, cheeseburgers, meat loaf	1 medium									11 __ __ __ __
Beef steaks, roasts	4 oz.									15 __ __ __ __
Pork, including chops, roast	2 chops or 4 oz.									19 __ __ __ __
Hot dogs	2 dogs									23 __ __ __ __
Ham, lunch meats	2 slices									27 __ __ __ __
Whole milk not incl. on cereal	8 oz. glass									31 __ __ __ __
Cheese, excluding cottage	2 slices or 2 oz.									35 __ __ __ __
Doughnuts, cookies, cake, pastries	1 pc. or 3 cookies									39 __ __ __ __
Eggs	1 egg = small, 2 eggs = medium									43 __ __ __ __
White bread, rolls, bagels, etc., incl. on sandwiches	2 slices, 3 crackers									47 __ __ __ __
Margarine or butter	2 pats									51 __ __ __ __
Salad dressing or mayonnaise (incl. on sandwiches)	2 Tblsp.									55 __ __ __ __
French fries, fried potatoes	3/4 cup									59 __ __ __ __
Do you eat the following foods every day?										
Breakfast cereal ☐ Yes ☐ No										63 __
Dark bread such as whole wheat, rye, or pumpernickel? ☐ Yes ☐ No										64 __

Figure 3.4 A 13-item screening questionnaire for fat intake (see Appendix F for information on coding and scoring).

Source: Courtesy of Dr. Gladys Block.

MEDFICTS focuses on foods that are major contributors of total fat, saturated fat, and cholesterol commonly eaten by North Americans. Within each of the questionnaire's eight categories, foods are placed into either a high-fat, high-cholesterol group (Group 1) or a low-fat, low-cholesterol group (Group 2). Group 1 foods are major contributors of dietary fat and cholesterol, and to the right of these groups is a series of boxes with numbers representing points under each box. Group 2 foods are minor contributors of fat and cholesterol. No points are given for Group 2 foods except if a respondent indicates a large portion size for Group 2 meats, in which case six points are given. In completing the questionnaire, the respondent simply checks the boxes representing his or her frequency of weekly consumption and typical serving size for each food group. The points for weekly consumption (shown below each box) are multiplied by the points for serving size and totaled in the score column. The points from each side of the questionnaire are totaled and compared with the key. A total score or 70 or more indicates a need for dietary change to reduce intake of total fat, saturated fat, and dietary cholesterol. A score between 40 and 69 suggests that the respondent is following a "heart-healthy diet" as defined by the National Cholesterol Education Program.[38] A score less than 40 suggests adherence to the National Cholesterol Education Program's therapeutic lifestyle changes diet, which is discussed in Chapter 8 and outlined in the *Third Report of the Expert Panel on Detection, Evaluation, and Treatment of High Blood Cholesterol in Adults*.[38] Studies suggest that the MEDFICTS does a good job of estimating intake of total fat, saturated fat, and cholesterol, compared with intake estimates based on 3-day and 7-day food records.[39,40]

Numerous food frequency questionnaires have been developed and tested. Three of the more common ones used in nutritional epidemiology research are those developed by Willett and coworkers at Harvard University School of Public Health, Block and coworkers at the National Cancer Institute, and Subar and Thompson at the National Cancer Institute.

Willett Questionnaire

Beginning in 1979, a team of Harvard University nutritionists and epidemiologists headed by Walter C. Willett developed a series of self-administered semiquantitative food frequency questionnaires to conduct epidemiologic research on the relationships between nutrient and food intake and risk of chronic disease. Over the years, their original 61-item questionnaire was modified several times.[15,41–43] A more recently developed 131-item questionnaire (shown in Appendix H) was designed to classify individuals according to levels of average daily intake of nutrients and certain foods and food components during the past year.[44] Its format is similar to that shown in Figure 3.2b. It is self-administered and machine readable, thus making it convenient for use in large epidemiologic studies. Foods included in the questionnaire are those that are major sources of the nutrients, foods, and food components of interest to the researchers. Open-ended questions are also included to identify specific brands of margarine, ready-to-eat cereals, cooking oils, vitamin/mineral supplements, and other foods eaten at least once per week.[44] For each item on the questionnaire, respondents are given nine choices ranging from less than once per month to six or more times per day. Nutrient values are calculated by multiplying nutrient content of each item by frequency of use.

The Willett questionnaire has been designed to be self-administered by nurses and other health professionals in such epidemiologic studies as the Nurses' Health Study and the Health Professionals Follow-up Study with populations of more than 120,000 female nurses and nearly 50,000 male health professionals, respectively.[45,46] However, the similar food frequency questionnaire has been used successfully in a group of socioeconomically diverse group of older women living in Iowa.[47] Among the diet-disease relationships reported in studies using these food frequency questionnaires are the following: significant reductions in coronary heart disease risk in males and females using vitamin E supplements; a lack of association between dietary fat intake and breast cancer; increased risk for colon cancer in females consuming diets high in animal fat; increased risk for coronary heart disease in men consuming alcoholic beverages; and an association between intake of vitamin A, niacin, and zinc and progression of human immunodeficiency virus (HIV) infection to acquired immune deficiency syndrome (AIDS) in HIV-positive homosexual and bisexual males.[45,46,48–50]

Researchers at Harvard University Medical School and Brigham and Women's Hospital in Boston have adapted the Willett food frequency questionnaire for assessing the diets of children and adolescents ages 9 to 18. Known as the Youth/Adolescent Questionnaire (YAQ), it is self-administered and includes a list of 151 foods. According to reproducibility studies, it has a reasonable ability to assess the eating habits of children and adolescents. It is shown in Appendix I.

Block Questionnaire

Another food frequency questionnaire, known as the Health Habits and History Questionnaire (HHHQ), was developed by Gladys Block and coworkers at the National Cancer Institute to collect data on diet and well-established risk factors for cancer and total mortality. Although the questionnaire originally was designed to supplement data from more specific questionnaires collecting data on the relationships between disease and potential causative factors, it has proven useful in assessing total dietary intake.[23,32] The questionnaire was developed using data from the 24-hour recalls of a statistically representative sample of nearly 12,000 American adults who participated in the second National Health and Nutrition Examination Survey (NHANES II), conducted from 1976 to 1980.[23] The 2244 different food codes recorded in these 24-hour recalls were grouped into 147 conceptually similar food items based on several criteria, including similarity in nutrient content per usual serving (for example, 11 different codes for green beans were consolidated into 1 food item labeled "string beans, green beans"). The decision of whether an item should be included on the food list was based on its energy and nutrient content, the frequency of its consumption by the population, and the typical serving size. Foods that were important contributors of energy and nutrients in the NHANES II database were included in the questionnaire. Items included in the food list represent 94% of all food items reported in the NHANES II data and more than 90% of the nation's total energy and nutrient intake.

Diet History Questionnaire

The Diet History Questionnaire (DHQ) is a self-administered, scannable food frequency questionnaire developed by Amy Subar and Frances Thompson at the National Cancer Institute. The DHQ is based on research that led to the development of the Block Health Habits and History Questionnaire (HHHQ). However, its designers consider it an improvement on the HHHQ in two ways.[51] First, the design of the DHQ incorporates results from extensive cognitive testing and addresses commonly encountered problems in food frequency questionnaires related to comprehension, order of food items, intake of seasonal foods, intake averages from multiple food items, and format. Second, the DHQ uses an improved method to convert information about frequency of food intake and portion sizes into daily nutrient intake estimates. The DHQ is currently in use in several epidemiologic studies sponsored by the National Cancer Institute, such as the Prostate, Lung, Colorectal, and Ovarian Screening Study and the Agricultural Health Study.[51] The DHQ's food list and range of portion sizes are based on food intake data from the U.S. Department of Agriculture's 1994–1996 Continuing Survey of Food Intakes by Individuals. The DHQ's food list contains a large number of low-fat foods introduced into the food supply in recent years.[51]

Researchers at the National Cancer Institute have compared the DHQ with the Block and Willett food frequency questionnaires. In a validation study conducted by Subar and fellow researchers at the National Cancer Institute, nutrient intake estimates were obtained from 1,300 subjects, who completed four telephone 24-hour recalls. The subjects were then asked to complete both the DHQ and the HHHQ, or both the DHQ and the Willett questionnaire. Compared with the 24-hour recalls, the DHQ did the best job of estimating absolute intakes of energy and more than 27 nutrients. After the data were adjusted for energy, all three food frequency questionnaires performed similarly.

The DHQ and its analysis software are available for downloading at no charge from the website of the National Cancer Institute. A link to this website is provided on the *Nutritional Assessment* website at www.mhhe.com/hper/nutrition. Several pages of the DHQ are shown in Appendix J. The DHQ software provides quantitative data on the intake of more than 50 nutrients, fatty acids, carotenoids, and other food components, as indicated in Table 3.1. Data on Food Guide Pyramid servings are also available. New foods and nutrients can be added to the database, and other modifications can be made in the DHQ software with relative ease. The current version of the questionnaire is for self-administration or for administration by an interviewer. A computer-assisted personal interview version of the instrument is planned in the near future.

Strengths and Limitations

Food frequency questionnaires have several strengths. They place a modest demand on the time and energy of

TABLE 3.1	**Nutrients and Food Components Analyzed by the Diet History Questionnaire**

Energy	Theobromine
Protein	Phosphorus
Total fat	Magnesium
Saturated fat	Iron
Monounsaturated fat	Zinc
Polyunsaturated fat	Copper
Cholesterol	Sodium
Carbohydrate	Potassium
Dietary fiber	Fatty acid 4:0
Alcohol	Fatty acid 6:0
Vitamin A	Fatty acid 8:0
Carotene	Fatty acid 10:0
Alpha-carotene	Fatty acid 12:0
Beta-carotene	Fatty acid 14:0
Beta-cryptoxanthin	Fatty acid 16:0
Lutein and zeaxanthin	Fatty acid 18:0
Lycopene	Fatty acid 16:1
Vitamin E	Fatty acid 18:1
Vitamin C	Fatty acid 20:1
Thiamin	Fatty acid 22:1
Riboflavin	Fatty acid 18:2
Niacin	Fatty acid 18:3
Vitamin B_6	Fatty acid 18:4
Folate	Fatty acid 20:4
Vitamin B_{12}	Fatty acid 20:5
Calcium	Fatty acid 22:5
Selenium	Fatty acid 22:6
Caffeine	

Data from the National Cancer Institute, National Institutes of Health.

respondents and generate estimates of food and nutrient intake that may be more representative of usual intake than a few days of diet records. They are relatively quick to administer. Approximately 30 minutes are required to complete the diet section of the Health Habits and History Questionnaire, and another 12 to 15 minutes are needed for the nondiet section.[32] They can be self-administered and machine readable and thus are relatively economical to use in large-scale studies.[11,43,52,53] However, data quality may be better when the questionnaire is administered by a trained interviewer. Estimates of nutrient and food intake from repeat administrations of food frequency questionnaires generally compare favorably, showing reasonable reproducibility (see the section "Reproducibility" later in this chapter).[15,41–44,53]

There are questions about how well food frequency questionnaires estimate the actual average nutrient intakes of individuals and groups—what is called validity. Studies comparing nutrient or food intake estimates obtained from food frequency questionnaires with estimates obtained from "criterion methods," such as multiple food records or 24-hour recalls, suggest that food frequency questionnaires are appropriate for estimating mean intakes of energy and some nutrients for groups and for ranking persons as having a low, average, or high consumption of energy and certain nutrients.[41,42,44,47,54,55] Some investigators, however, challenge these conclusions.[56,57] Food frequency questionnaires do not appear appropriate for estimating the nutrient intake of groups (see the section "Validity" later in this chapter).

Food frequency questionnaires have definite limitations. Because the food list is limited to approximately 100 to 150 foods and food groups, these must be representative of the most common foods consumed by respondents in the sample. Short questionnaires are faster and easier to administer but lack comprehensiveness. Long questionnaires may do a better job of assessing nutrient intake but also require respondents to make an almost overwhelming number of decisions. Longer food frequency questionnaires have the disadvantage of being tedious to complete. Individual foods listed on the questionnaire are more likely to be remembered than foods grouped under such headings as "any other fruit" or "any other vegetable" unless a trained interviewer carefully probes the respondent.[52] Grouping foods under broad categories precludes the ability to collect information about specific food items.[56] For example, the Block questionnaire groups doughnuts, cookies, cakes, and pastry within a single group. Portion sizes allow limited choices as well, and they must be the most typical of what is usually eaten. Questionnaires lacking portion size selections or having poorly chosen ones may identify only individuals at the extremes of the nutrient-intake distribution. However, the usefulness of such portion size information is questioned by research suggesting that defined portion

sizes may not be meaningful to some respondents.[27] However, frequency is a more important determinant of nutrient intake than portion size.[58] Another limitation is reliance on the ability of the respondent to describe his or her diet.[13,52,59]

It is important that food frequency questionnaires be culturally sensitive. The Block questionnaire, for example, is best suited for white, middle-class people, who composed the majority of the NHANES II population. Failure to include foods commonly eaten by various groups may result in underestimates of nutrient intake, particularly if the foods are major sources of certain nutrients or food components. The Block and Willett questionnaires address this shortcoming by providing space for respondents to write in foods that they at least occasionally eat but that are not included in the food list. Food lists also must be periodically updated to keep pace with the thousands of new food products entering the marketplace each year.

Despite these limitations, the food frequency questionnaire was used in NHANES III to collect information on water and alcohol consumption, the intake of selected foods and food groups, food sources of calcium and vitamins A and C, and milk intake, although the 24-hour recall was the primary approach for measuring diet.[6] The food frequency questionnaire is considered by some as the method of choice for research on diet-disease relationships on both the macronutrient and micronutrient levels.[11,58]

Box 3.5 summarizes the strengths and limitations of food frequency questionnaires.

Diet History

Diet history is used to assess an individual's usual dietary intake over an extended period of time, such as the past month or year.[11,60,61] Traditionally, the diet history approach has been associated with the method of assessing a respondent's usual diet developed by B. S. Burke during the 1940s.[62]

Burke's original method involved four steps: (1) collect general information about the respondent's health habits, (2) question the respondent about his or her usual eating pattern, (3) perform a cross-check on the data given in step 2, and (4) have the respondent complete a 3-day food record.[62]

A trained nutritionist begins the interview by asking questions about the number of meals eaten per day; appetite; food dislikes; presence or absence of nausea and vomiting; use of nutritional supplements; cigarette smoking; habits related to sleep, rest, work, and exercise; and so on. This allows the interviewer to become acquainted with the respondent in ways that may be helpful in obtaining further information. This is followed by a 24-hour recall, in which the interviewer also inquires about the respondent's usual pattern of eating during and

Box 3.5   Strengths and Limitations of Food Frequency Questionnaires

Strengths

Can be self-administered

Machine readable

Modest demand on respondents

Relatively inexpensive for large sample sizes

May be more representative of usual intake than a few days of diet records

Design can be based on large population data.

Considered by some as the method of choice for research on diet-disease relationships

Limitations

May not represent usual foods or portion sizes chosen by respondents

Intake data can be compromised when multiple foods are grouped within single listings.

Depend on ability of subject to describe diet

Not appropriate for determining absolute nutrient intake in large surveys, such as NHANES III

between meals, beginning with the first food or drink of the day. The interviewer records the respondent's description of his or her usual food intake, including types of food eaten, serving sizes, frequency and timing, and significant seasonal variations.

With the respondent's stated usual dietary practices recorded, the interviewer then cross-checks the data by asking specific questions about the respondent's dietary preferences and habits. For example, the respondent may have said that he or she drinks an 8-oz glass of milk every morning. The interviewer then should inquire about the participant's milk-drinking habits to clarify and verify the information given about the respondent's milk intake. Finally, the participant is asked to complete a 3-day food record, which serves as an additional means of checking the usual intake. Burke admits that this is the least helpful part of the method, and it generally is omitted by the few researchers who currently use this method.

The strengths of the diet history approach are that it assesses the respondent's usual nutrient intake, including seasonal changes, and data on all nutrients can be obtained.[11] The method is one of the preferred methods for obtaining estimates of usual nutrient intake.[11,60] Estimates

of protein intake by the method correlate well with measures of nitrogen excretion. If what is needed for research purposes is a list of items that is typical of an individual's diet rather than a specific list of items eaten during a certain period of time, the diet history appears adequate to determine the typical diet. Most people are able to report what they typically eat, even if they cannot report exactly what they ate during a specific period of time.[27]

Among the method's limitations are that 1 to 2 hours are required to conduct the interview, highly trained interviewers are needed, coding is difficult and expensive, and nutrient intake tends to be overestimated.[11,61,62] The method also requires a cooperative respondent with the ability to recall his or her usual diet.

Box 3.6 summarizes the strengths and limitations of the diet history method.

Duplicate Food Collections

Collection of food consumption data generally is not an end in itself but, rather, a means of eventually arriving at an estimate of nutrient intake. The limitations of using food consumption data to arrive at nutrient intake are the

Box 3.6   Strengths and Limitations of the Diet History Method

Strengths

Assesses usual nutrient intake

Can detect seasonal changes

Data on all nutrients can be obtained.

Can correlate well with biochemical measures

Limitations

Lengthy interview process

Requires highly trained interviewers

Difficult and expensive to code

May tend to overestimate nutrient intake

Requires cooperative respondent with ability to recall usual diet incompleteness of food composition tables, mistakes in coding and entering data, and nutrient losses during food storage and preparation that may not be accounted for in food composition tables.[4] A more direct method of calculating nutrient intake that avoids these particular problems is **duplicate food collections.**

When performing duplicate food collections, participants place in collection containers identical portions of all foods and beverages consumed during a specified period.[63] This then is chemically analyzed at a laboratory for nutrient content. To prevent bacterial decomposition of the duplicate samples, they should be kept refrigerated and delivered to the laboratory daily.

This method has the strength of potentially providing a more accurate determination of actual nutrient intake, compared with calculations based on food composition data. Values in composition tables may not be representative of nutrient levels in the particular foods that respondents consume because of seasonal or regional differences, agricultural practices, and losses during marketing and preparation. A participant may have eaten a food that was introduced recently into the marketplace that is not listed in a food composition table or database. Among the method's limitations are the necessity of preparing the additional amount of food to be collected and the work involved in measuring or weighing exactly duplicate portions of food and beverage. In a 1-year dietary intake study conducted by researchers at the USDA Human Nutrition Research Center in Beltsville, Maryland, respondents kept daily food records throughout the 1-year period and provided duplicate food collections for 1 week during each of the four seasons of the year.[63,64] The participants' mean calculated nutrient intake was 12.9% less during the 4 weeks when duplicate food collections were done. Reductions were greatest for foods rich in fat and protein—often the most expensive foods. The respondents may have felt guilty about "wasting" food that went into the collection jar or were concerned about the food's expense, despite receiving payment for their participation in the study. Thus, intakes during food collection periods may not be representative of habitual nutrient intake.

Box 3.7 summarizes the strengths and limitations of the duplicate food collection method.

Food Accounts

Food accounts are used to measure dietary intake within households and institutions where congregate feeding is practiced, such as penal institutions, nursing homes, military bases, and boarding schools.[65] The method accounts for all food on hand in the home or institution at the beginning of the survey period, all that is purchased or grown throughout the period, and all that remains by the end of the survey. Inventories establish amounts of food on hand at the beginning and ending of the survey period, and invoices or other accounting methods provide records of food purchased or obtained from a farm or garden. Trained personnel make site visits at the beginning and ending of the survey period and as necessary throughout the period to assist in recordkeeping.

The daily mean consumption per person is calculated for each food item from the total amount of food consumed during the survey period and the number of people in the household or institution.[65] This method was used in the Finnish Mental Hospital Study, which showed that, when soft margarine and skim milk with added soy oil replaced butter and whole milk in the diets of institutionalized persons, serum cholesterol levels and heart disease mortality dropped, in contrast to a similar institution where no such dietary changes were made.[66,67]

When used to measure household food consumption, the usual survey period is 2 to 4 weeks. To capture seasonal variations, some researchers may record consumption over different seasons for shorter periods. In addition to the amounts of different foods consumed by family members, it is necessary to account for the number of people present at each meal, the number of meals eaten away from home, and the number served to visitors.[65]

The strengths of the method are that the survey can include a large sample size, food consumption can be monitored for a relatively long period of time, and data on the annual mean consumption and general food patterns and habits of the population can be obtained. The likelihood that the method will alter the diet is less than with the food record method. The method is also relatively economical because personnel need only make periodic visits for supervising and controlling the recording.[65]

Included among the limitations of the method are its inability to account for food that is given to animals,

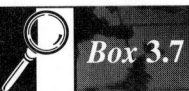
Box 3.7   **Strengths and Limitations of the Duplicate Food Collection Method**

Strengths

Can provide more accurate measurements of actual nutrient intake than calculations based on food composition tables

Limitations

Expense and effort of preparing more food

Effort and time to collect duplicate samples

May underestimate usual intake

thrown away due to spoilage, or discarded as plate waste or for other reasons. Because respondent literacy and cooperation are necessary, families or institutions willing to keep food accounts may not be representative of the population of interest. Accuracy may suffer due to forgetfulness or lack of faithfulness in maintaining food accounts. The method provides information only on the mean daily consumption of the whole family; it does not indicate how food is distributed among the various family members. Thus, it is only appropriate for measuring food consumption of groups.[65]

Box 3.8 summarizes the strengths and limitations of the food account method.

Food Balance Sheets

The **food balance sheet** is a method of indirectly estimating the amounts of food consumed by a country's population at a certain time. It provides data on food *disappearance* (sometimes referred to as *food availability*) rather than actual food consumption. It is calculated using beginning and ending inventories, figures on food production, imports and exports, and adjustments for nonhuman food consumption (for example, cattle feed, pet food, seed, and industrial use). Food disappearance can be thought of as the amount of food that "disappears" from the food distribution system. Much of this is purchased by consumers at supermarkets; however, a considerable amount is lost due to spoilage.

Mean per capita annual amounts are calculated by dividing total disappearance of food by the country's population.[65] This method has been valuable for detecting trends in the amount of food that disappears from the food distribution system within a country over time and thus has been used to roughly indicate likely trends in consumption as well. It is useful for promoting agricultural production in various parts of the world and for encouraging a more even distribution of food among different countries.[65] Because these data are collected in a roughly similar manner in countries around the world, they are useful in epidemiologic research across coun-

tries.[9] We will discuss food disappearance data in greater detail in Chapter 4 in connection with national surveys.

The strengths of the method are that it can give a total view of the food supplies of a country, can be used in drawing conclusions about general food habits and dietary trends within a country, and is valuable in planning international nutrition policy and formulating food programs.[65] In some instances, information on food disappearance may be the only accessible data representing a country's food consumption practices.

The method has a number of limitations. The accuracy of data depends on available statistics, the quality of which can vary greatly, depending on a country's level of development. The data represent only the total amount of food that reportedly leaves the food distribution system, apparently for consumption. Note that it is not an estimate of what was actually consumed. It also does not show how food was distributed among individuals or groups within a particular country. The method also does not account for food that is wasted or fed to animals (for example, pets).[65]

Box 3.9 summarizes the strengths and limitations of the food balance sheet.

Telephone Interviews

Telephone interviewing has, in recent years, become an accepted and widely used method for collecting dietary intake data. Investigators have used the technique to administer 24-hour recalls and food frequency questionnaires, particularly to follow up on face-to-face interviews. This approach was used in NHANES III as part of a study of the eating habits of Americans age 50 years and older. After a face-to-face 24-hour recall, a series of two additional 24-hour recalls were collected by telephone from a subset of older respondents.[6,10,18] In the 1985–1986 Continuing Survey of Food Intakes by Individuals (CSFII), the U.S. Department of Agriculture (USDA) collected some of its 24-hour recalls by telephone interviews after the initial household contact and first 24-hour recall was conducted in person.[10] Telephone

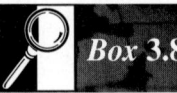 *Box* **3.8**   **Strengths and Limitations of the Food Account Method**

Strengths

Suitable for use with large sample sizes

Can be used over relatively long periods

Gives data on dietary patterns and habits of families and other groups

Less likely to lead to alterations in diet than some other methods

Relatively economical

Limitations

Does not account for food losses

Respondent literacy and cooperation necessary

Not appropriate for measuring individual food consumption

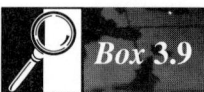

Box 3.9   **Strengths and Limitations of the Food Balance Sheet**

Strengths	Limitations
Can give a total view of a country's food supplies	Accuracy of data may be questionable
Indicates food habits and dietary trends	Only represents food available for consumption
Used to plan international nutrition policies and food programs	Does not represent food actually consumed
May be the only data available on a country's food consumption practices	Does not indicate how food was distributed
	Does not account for wasted food

interviews are now the USDA's principal method of collecting dietary intake data.[68,69] Preadolescent children were shown to be able to provide 24-hour recall data during telephone interviews that compared favorably with written records of their intake unobtrusively collected by parents.[70] Recalls obtained by telephone interview showed good agreement with the observed intake of both college students and elderly participants.[71] Telephone reporting has been shown to be an acceptable method of collecting food record data, whether the data are reported directly to an individual or left on a recording device, such as a telephone answering machine.

Telephone interviews have several strengths. Cost of the method has been reported to be approximately one-fourth to one-half that of comparable personal interviews.[72,73] They also have the potential of easing the time, logistical, and personnel constraints associated with nutrition surveys.[68,74] Telephone surveys have higher response rates than mail surveys.[10] The respondent burden may be somewhat lower with this method, compared with personal interviews. In an era of pervasive suspicion of strangers resulting from rising crime rates, some respondents may find this method more conducive to personal safety than interviews within their homes.[75]

Twenty-four-hour recall or food frequency data collected over the telephone is subject to the same limitations as that collected in personal interviews. The problem of estimating portion sizes can be addressed by providing respondents with measuring cups, spoons, and two-dimensional food models.[42] The tendency of 24-hour recalls to underestimate energy and nutrient intake can be ameliorated by using the multiple-pass 24-hour recall method.[68,69,76] Although 97% of the U.S. population has a telephone, there is lower telephone coverage among blacks, Hispanics (except for Cuban Americans), unemployed persons, and the poor. Households in the South are twice as likely to be without telephones than those in other areas of the United States.[73]

Box 3.10 summarizes the strengths and limitations of telephone interviews.

Photographic and Video Records

Several investigators have developed photographic and video methods to record dietary intake in an attempt to reduce respondent burden and increase validity of dietary intake data.[77–80] In one approach, respondents were provided with an easily operated camera with a built-in electronic flash.[77] Participants photographed all their food before eating it (on plates, in bowls, and so on) and what was left over after eating. In a manual, they recorded descriptions of their food and preparation methods, especially those that would not be apparent in the photographs. The exposed slide film was returned to the investigators for development and evaluation. The slides were projected onto a screen, and estimates were made of each

Box 3.10   **Strengths and Limitations of Telephone Interviews**

Strengths	Limitations
One-quarter to one-half the cost of a comparable personal interview	Subject to many of the same disadvantages of collecting 24-hour recall and food record data
Fewer time, logistical, and personnel constraints	Estimating portion sizes in recalls may be difficult unless steps are taken to address the problem.
Lower respondent burden	
Gives respondent more personal security	

food. Using a second projector, slides of known food portions could be projected beside the respondent's slides to help in estimating portion sizes.

When compared with results of weighed food records, the photographic method was reported to provide very similar results, with no significant difference in nutrient calculations between the two methods.[78] In another validation study, conducted in a cafeteria setting, on-site observers recorded the identity of foods selected by participants. This record compared favorably with the identification of foods from slides.[79]

More recently, the validity and reproducibility of video recordings to assess dietary intake were tested.[80] Video recordings of test trays containing foods of known volume or weight were evaluated independently by two trained observers. Food amounts estimated from the videos were closely correlated with measured amounts, indicating that this method has good validity. Results obtained independently by the two observers who identified food items on the same set of videotaped meals then were compared. These were shown to agree favorably, indicating that the method has good reproducibility.

The validity of the photographic and video methods appears to be good, as does the reproducibility of video records.[78–80] The actual time to record food intake using the methods is less than that for 24-hour recalls, food records, or weighed-food records. Respondent burden also is considerably less with the two methods, and the practice of photographing food within the home has been acceptable to participants. These advantages may lead to fewer of the alterations in diet that inevitably result from the recording process. The methods appear useful for evaluation of food selection in institutional settings, such as retirement facilities, nursing homes, or cafeterias. They may be especially well suited for assessing intake of groups with cognitive, visual, or verbal impairment.[80]

Considerable initial expense is involved in both methods. Aside from the cost of video equipment or cameras, a greater amount of labor and expense is required in developing comparison photographs or slides of standard foods of known portion size. However, these costs may be offset by the greater efficiency and reduced long-term costs of the methods. Considerable skill is needed to interpret the slide or video records, and the coding procedure and time needed for clerical work remains the same as for traditional methods.[53] The methods are not suited for distinguishing between visually similar foods (for example, skim milk versus whole milk or premium ice cream versus ice milk). Some form of written or verbal records will continue to be necessary to document preparation methods and identify visually similar foods.[78,79] The likelihood of technical problems' spoiling the data will increase as the sophistication of recording devices increases.

Box 3.11 summarizes the strengths and limitations of the photographic and video methods.

Computerized Techniques

To reduce respondent burden and increase validity of dietary intake data and the cost-effectiveness of collecting such data, computerized techniques to record dietary intake have been developed. Researchers at the USDA's Western Human Nutrition Research Center have developed what they call a Nutrition Evaluation Scale System.[81–84] Also, computer-assisted self-interviewing has been studied by researchers at the University of North Carolina at Chapel Hill.[86,87]

Nutrition Evaluation Scale System

The Nutrition Evaluation Scale System (NESSy) (Figure 3.5) is an electronic scale interfaced with a laptop computer with a built-in modem.[81–84] The user enters the identity of foods into the system by typing a brief description of each food into the computer prior to eating. The user then matches this description with the appropriate food item within the laptop's database. The

---

 Box 3.11   Strengths and Limitations of Photographic and Video Methods

Strengths

Photographic method has good validity.

Video method has good validity and reproducibility.

Recording food intake takes less time than 24-hour recalls or food records.

Respondent burden is less.

Methods appear to be acceptable to subjects.

Eating habits may be less affected by recording.

Well suited for institutional settings and for disabled persons

Limitations

Large initial expense is involved, but this may be offset by lower long-term costs.

Periodic revalidations are recommended.

Unable to distinguish visually similar foods or document preparation methods

Subject to technical problems caused by sophisticated equipment

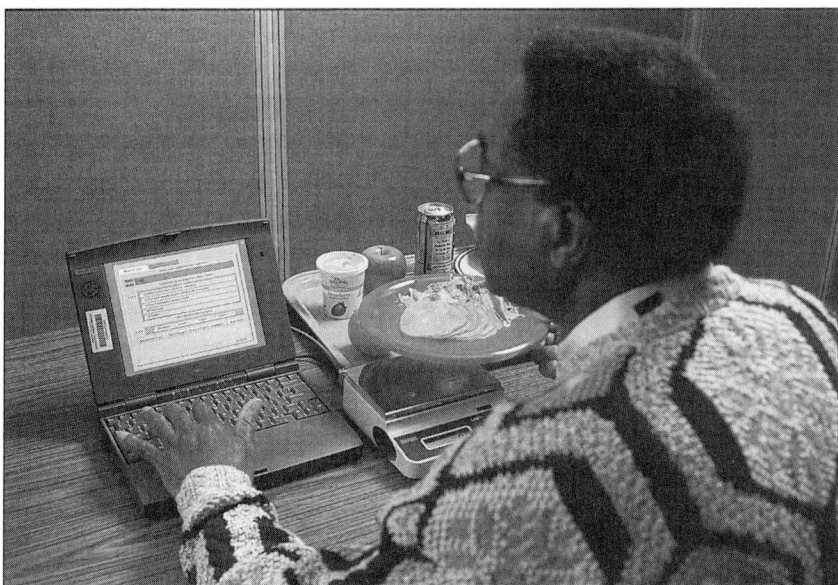

Figure 3.5
The Nutrition Evaluation Scale System is an innovative approach to simplifying the collection of dietary intake data.
Source: Photo courtesy of Dr. MJ Kretsch, USDA, ARS, San Francisco.

computer then directs the user through the weighing of foods, containers, and leftovers. Users do not need to know how to operate the scale or computer, only how to respond to visual and audio instructions from the computer. The software is user-friendly, using icons, sounds, and on-screen prompts to guide users through the process of entering data. The identity and weights of foods consumed are saved in the computer's memory. These data then can be transferred via modem or disk to another computer for review by a dietitian and eventual analysis using a food composition database.

In a validation study, nine participants used the NESSy to record their food intake during a 16-day period. These data were compared with those obtained from weighed-food records kept at the same time by research staff. There were no significant differences in group means between the two methods for energy or any nutrient.[84] When the two methods were compared on the basis of time required to weigh and record food, the NESSy provided savings in time and labor of about 80%.[82] Research has shown the instrument to be a reliable and valid method of measuring dietary intake by persons of both sexes and by free-living teenagers, adults, and older persons having no more than about 12 years of formal education.[83] The NESSy shows considerable promise as a method of providing precise quantitative data of an individual's dietary intake while significantly reducing the labor, time, and costs associated with collecting such data. The developers of NESSy are working with a private technology firm to transform the system into a portable, wireless dietary assessment and intervention tool.[85]

Computer-Assisted Self-interviewing

Using computers to administer an interactive, multimedia dietary intake interview has the potential of offering the flexibility of a personal interview without the cost imposed by a trained interviewer.[86] This potentially promising application of computer technology in dietary measurement has been called computer-assisted self-interviewing (CASI). Researchers at the University of North Carolina at Chapel Hill have developed a computerized, multimedia diet history instrument that conducts an automated, personalized, in-depth interview to obtain a meal-by-meal assessment of one's usual diet.[87] The software is designed to standardize data collection with appropriate levels of probing, to automate the entry of food intake data, to make certain all responses are complete, and to encourage subjects to review and correct any inconsistent data entries. The prototype's interactive and multimedia design improves participation and motivates subjects. Technical expertise is not required, and respondents set their own pace. Hundreds of realistic, lively, and colorful images help the respondent remember foods, preparation methods, and serving sizes, thus facilitating recall to a much greater extent than more traditional instruments. Using text, sound, and colorful video and still images makes the system suitable for the hearing-impaired and for those with a low literacy level.

Surrogate Sources

There are times when a respondent may not be able to provide the dietary intake data that investigators desire. In some instances, a respondent may have a problem with hearing, speech, or memory due to disease, trauma, or advanced age. This is especially a problem with elderly respondents participating in case-control studies. In such instances, obtaining information from **surrogate sources** may improve information quality and provide data otherwise unavailable from deceased or incompetent participants. Potential surrogate respondents include the respondent's spouse or partner, children, other close relatives, and friends.[10,88]

Several investigators have studied the use of surrogate sources of dietary intake. A review of these studies demonstrates that "surrogate respondents can provide dietary information, but that incomplete responses must be anticipated."[88] In some cases, surrogate respondents provide more valid data than the respondents themselves. Surrogate sources often can provide good information on specific foods or nutrients. The availability of data from surrogate respondents varies with the surrogate's relationship to the participant, the surrogate's sex (e.g., females provide more accurate data about the eating habits of males than males do about the eating habits of females), and the number of shared meals. There may be considerable difference in the quality of surrogate data between spouses or partners of deceased participants and spouses or partners of living participants.[10]

Surrogate sources are good in studies in which there is rapid mortality of study participants, in which there is concern about biased recall from participants, or in which participants have problems with memory impairment or difficulty communicating because of such causes as stroke or Alzheimer's disease. In some instances, data from surrogates are good enough for ranking persons in quintiles (one of five levels) in terms of their nutrient intake (i.e., as having an intake that is very low, low, average, high, or very high). In any event, surrogate sources must be carefully selected and data closely scrutinized because misclassification of dietary intake can occur easily when relying on surrogate sources alone.[10,88]

CONSIDERATIONS FOR CERTAIN GROUPS

Adaptations in dietary measurement can be made for certain groups, such as young persons, the reading-impaired, individuals having problems recalling their diet, persons who are visually or hearing-impaired, and the obese. These considerations, summarized in Box 3.12, facilitate collection of intake data from persons who otherwise might have difficulty participating in surveys.

ISSUES IN DIETARY MEASUREMENT

Validity

Validity is the ability of an instrument to actually measure what it is intended to measure.[31,97,98] In most instances, investigators are interested in knowing what a respondent's

usual intake is or has been. Thus, validating an instrument involves comparing estimates of intake obtained by that instrument with a respondent's usual intake. Because it is difficult if not impossible to know a person's true usual intake, investigators must turn to *relative,* or *criterion, validity.* Relative, or criterion, validity is defined as the comparison of a new instrument with another instrument (a so-called gold standard), which has a greater degree of *demonstrated,* or *face, validity.*[31,98] However, if the two instruments fail to compare favorably, the question must be asked, "Which instrument (if any) gives the best estimate of usual intake?" The failure of one instrument to compare favorably with another may not lie in the instrument's being validated; it actually may have given the best estimate of usual intake. The fault may lie in the criterion instrument.

The validity of food frequency questionnaires has been examined by comparing estimates of food and nutrient intake obtained from food frequency questionnaires with estimates obtained from multiple food records or 24-hour recalls, which are thought to give a more detailed and quantitative estimate of dietary intake over an extended period.[41,42,98-100] Researchers at Harvard University, for example, collected four 1-week weighed-diet records over the course of a year from 173 participants.[41] These served as an estimate of usual intake during the 1-year period and the criterion against which intake data from the food frequency questionnaire were compared. Results of the study showed that a simple self-administered food frequency questionnaire can provide useful information about individual nutrient intakes over a 1-year period. To study the questionnaire's ability to assess diet in the recent past, the researchers administered it to the same group of participants 3 to 4 years after the weighed-food records were collected, and they concluded that the questionnaire was useful in estimating nutrient intake 4 years in the past.[42] A number of other validation studies have been done as well.[44,47,54,55] Nutrient estimates derived from food frequency questionnaires compared favorably with those derived from criterion methods, suggesting that food frequency questionnaires can be appropriate to use in epidemiologic research. Overall, these studies support the use of food frequency questionnaires for estimating a group's average intake for energy and some nutrients. They also suggest that the method is appropriate for ranking individuals in terms of nutrient intake (e.g., categorizing individuals as having a low, average, or high intake of some nutrient).[41,99] Other investigators, however, question the use of food frequency questionnaires in epidemiologic research.[56,57]

The validity of a food frequency questionnaire depends in large part on items included in the food list and assumptions about portion size and nutrient content of the various groups.[24] Another important consideration in validation studies is the appropriateness of the criterion instrument. Given the weaknesses of food records and

Box 3.12   Considerations When Measuring Diet in Certain Groups

Group	Considerations
Young persons	Dietary intake data on children under 8 years of age are best obtained from the person responsible for meals. For information on food eaten away from home, interview the child in the presence of the parent or guardian. Data on meals eaten at school, kindergarten, or day care center can be obtained from those responsible for their meals.
	Reliable data on intake in the previous 24 hours can be obtained from children 8 years of age and older.
Persons with recall problems	There appears to be no firm evidence that memory of past diet is impaired during aging despite popular belief to the contrary. The ability to recall past diet may be more a function of how much attention is paid to what is eaten.[30]
	Diet recall can be helped through the use of checklists and visual aids, such as food models and photographs.[30] Information obtained from surrogates (spouse, sibling, or caregiver) can improve the quality of data.[88] Reproducibility of recall of diet many years in the past by older persons has been shown to be good but is reduced by older age, cognitive impairment, and male sex.[89]
Persons with impaired vision or hearing	Intake measurement instructions can be communicated to the visually impaired through large-print materials, tape recordings, radio, telephone, personal interview, and Braille. Some visually impaired persons have video equipment that will enlarge print to a readable size. Data can be collected through personal interview, by telephone or tape recorder, or over specially equipped computer systems.
	Communication of instructions to and collection of data from hearing-impaired persons is easily done with self-explanatory and well-prepared printed materials. Use of an interpreter of sign language and visual aids, such as food models or photographs, can be helpful. Verbal responses to an interviewer can facilitate collection of data.
Persons who cannot read well	Personal interviews, tape recorders, and telephone contacts can all be used in collecting dietary intake data from the reading-impaired. Persons with limited reading ability may be able to use printed materials having an appropriate vocabulary. Food models and photographs are especially helpful. Printed forms relying heavily on pictures may be appropriate for collecting data.
The obese	Several studies have questioned the validity of reported energy intake in obese persons, indicating a tendency to underreport energy intake using the dietary history[90] and food records.[90-94] Other studies indicate this is a problem seen in both obese and normal-weight populations.[95,96]

From Cameron ME, Van Staveren WA. 1988. *Manual on methodology for food consumption studies.* New York: Oxford University Press, and other indicated sources.

24-hour recalls in characterizing usual intake, how appropriate are they to use as a truth measure against which to judge another instrument, such as the food frequency questionnaire? If, in a validation study, data from food frequency questionnaires compare unfavorably to data from a criterion method, is it necessarily the fault of the food frequency questionnaire? A proposal for circumventing this dilemma is to include a biological marker as a *third* criterion method in the validation process.[58] Biological markers are discussed in the section "Use of Biological Markers."

Some investigators have compared estimates of dietary intake using various methods with respondents' *actual* intake, which the investigators observed surreptitiously.[20–22,52] Usually, the respondents ate all or at least most of their meals in a cafeteria or residential metabolic research facility where their food intake could be observed. Different assessment methods then could be used to measure respondents' intake during the period when their diet was observed. Among these were the 24-hour recall,[21,22,69,101,102] food records,[21,52] and food frequency questionnaires.[52] However, such comparisons over relatively short periods of time in monitored or controlled situations fail to adequately validate a method intended to assess the usual, self-selected diets of free-living persons.[98] Validation studies of the various diet measurement techniques are summarized in Box 3.13.

Use of Biological Markers

Another approach to validating dietary measurement methods is to compare intake data with certain biological markers associated with dietary intake.[10,58,110–113] Biological markers offer the advantages of being easily accessible (urine, feces, blood, tissue samples) and providing a validity check of dietary intake independent of respondents' accuracy and truthfulness. A major problem, however, is that many factors other than dietary intake can affect nutrient concentrations in tissues, even in well-fed persons.[10] Although many biological markers have potential for use, only a limited number have been investigated. Among these are nitrogen and sodium in urine, fatty acids in adipose tissue, and assessment of energy expenditure and body weight.[58,110–115]

Analysis of nitrogen in multiple 24-hour urine samples, the most well-known biological marker, has been used to verify protein intake in dietary surveys.[110,112,115] If acceptable agreement exists between urinary nitrogen excretion and estimated protein intake, it can be assumed that intake of other nutrients is fairly well represented. Use of this method depends on several assumptions: that respondents are in nitrogen balance (there is no accumulation of protein for growth or repair or unusual losses due to starvation or injury); that estimates of extrarenal nitrogen excretion sufficiently cover losses through the feces, hair, skin, and other routes; and that all urine has been collected over the course of the collection period.[110,112] Researchers have attempted to use urinary levels of 3-methylhistidine, an amino acid released during muscle catabolism and excreted unchanged in the urine, in assessing meat consumption. Unfortunately, correlations between meat intake and 3-methylhistidine excretion have been low, apparently because of wide variability in 24-hour baseline excretion among individuals even when

not consuming meat.[110] The presence of creatinine in meat makes 24-hour urine creatinine measurements ill suited for validating dietary estimates.[112]

Urinary sodium is a useful measure of dietary sodium intake, especially because amounts used at the table and in cooking are difficult to assess. Fecal sodium losses are minimal, and in temperate climates it is assumed that amounts in sweat are negligible. Differences in urinary sodium and estimated dietary intakes have been shown to be as low as 5%.[110] Because fecal losses of potassium are greater and more variable than with sodium, urinary potassium has not proven as suitable for validating dietary potassium intake.

A potential problem with measurements of nitrogen and sodium in 24-hour urine samples is the necessity of obtaining a *complete* 24-hour urine sample—a requirement some participants have difficulty adhering to. One approach to checking on the completeness of 24-hour urine samples is use of the para-amino-benzoic acid (PABA) marker. Participants take one PABA tablet three times a day with their meals. The PABA is excreted in the urine. A 24-hour urine collection containing less than 85% of the PABA marker is considered unsatisfactory, either because the participant did not take all the PABA tablets or one or more urine specimens was omitted from the collection.[112]

Measurement of the urine osmolality (the number of dissolved particles per kilogram of urine) has been suggested as a method of assessing accuracy of reported dietary intake.[111] Urine osmolality is determined largely by nitrogen-containing substances and sodium and potassium salts in urine. It is measured using a 24-hour urine sample. It also can be predicted from dietary intake data obtained from food records and 24-hour dietary recalls. A measured osmolality significantly less than the predicted value indicates a lower food intake than that reported by the participant. A measured osmolality significantly greater than predicted indicates a greater food intake than that reported by the participant. As with urine nitrogen and sodium, the usefulness of this method depends on participants' obtaining complete 24-hour urine specimens.

Linoleic acid in adipose tissue can be used as an index of dietary intake of linoleic acid over the past 2 to 3 years, whereas the linoleic acid content of erythrocytes (red blood cells) can be an index of dietary linoleic acid during the past 6 to 8 weeks.[116] A small piece of adipose tissue can be easily removed from beneath the skin and measured for linoleic acid. This can be an independent way of estimating dietary fat intake. Such measurements have been shown to compare favorably with estimates of usual intake based on 2 weeks of weighed-food records and a food frequency questionnaire.[113] Another study showed that concentrations of monounsaturated and polyunsaturated fatty acids in adipose tissue compared closely with the type of fatty acids consumed by groups as assessed by 2-day food records.[110]

Box 3.13 | **Summary of Studies Validating Diet Measurement Techniques**

Measurement Technique

24-hour recall

Food record or diary

Food frequency questionnaire (FFQ)

Results of Validation Studies

The 24-hour recall can be validated directly by comparing with actual intake observed surreptitiously, as in a cafeteria,[69] congregate meal site,[21,22] summer camp,[101] school lunch program,[102] or hospital.

Comparisons with 7-day food record[27] or diet history[73] may not be appropriate, since these methods measure diet over a different time frame than 24-hour recall.

For most groups, validity of the 24-hour recall is good for average group intakes of energy and certain nutrients.[103,104] Some researchers report overestimates of average group intakes in children[101] and the elderly.[22,105] Other researchers report the validity of 24-hour recalls for estimating group means when used in conjunction with food records.[106]

In a direct validation study (actual weighed intake of noon meals over 7 days was compared with records of those meals), food records underestimated actual intake of energy and thiamin, while no significant differences were seen for other nutrients studied.[21]

Attempts to validate food records with periodic duplicate food collections have proved unsuccessful because of a decrease in energy and nutrient intake when duplicate food portions are collected.[97,98]

Over a 7-day period, diet records for first 2 days were more valid than those for last 3 days. Education and motivation of respondents will affect validity of the last several days of diet records kept over a 7-day period.[21]

This method has been compared against actual intake observed over 28 days in a cafeteria[59] and during 2 weeks in a metabolic unit.[52] The former study showed that a large percentage of college students could accurately estimate their intake with the FFQ, while others had difficulty. In the latter study, the FFQ underestimated energy and nutrient intake. In comparison against food records, people report frequency of food consumption with reasonable accuracy.[27]

Intake data from a semiquantitative FFQ compared favorably with that obtained from four 1-week weighed-food records collected over a 12-month period.[41] A follow-up study using the FFQ to assess diet 3 to 4 years in the past showed the FFQ to be useful in assessing past diet.[42] In a similar study, correlations between an FFQ and diet records were lowest for selenium and vitamin A and highest for dietary fiber and polyunsaturated fats.[99]

Comparisons with the diet history method show good correlations in terms of group averages but not for individuals.[61]

When compared with reference methods, correlations tend to be low for highly variable nutrients, such as vitamin A. However, the fault may not lie entirely with FFQs, as the reference data may not reflect usual intake.[98]

continued

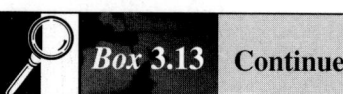
Box 3.13   Continued

Measurement Technique (*continued*)

Diet history

In the few validation studies done, diet histories tend to overestimate group mean intakes compared with the reference method, which is generally 7-day estimated or weighed records.[61]

As noted with FFQs, when compared with reference methods, correlations tend to be low for highly variable nutrients, such as vitamin A. Again, the fault may not lie entirely with the diet history method, since reference data may not be representative of usual intake.[98]

Researchers attempting to measure past dietary intake using the diet history have noted that current diet can influence perceptions of past diet.[107–109]

From Gibson RS. 1990. *Principles of nutritional assessment.* New York: Oxford University Press, and other indicated sources.

Energy Expenditure and Weight Maintenance

Another approach to validating dietary measurement methods is to compare reported energy intake with body weight and energy expenditure calculated from an equation or measured using the doubly labeled water method. Self-reported energy intake has been compared with energy expenditure determined through use of the doubly labeled water method (discussed in greater detail in Chapter 8). Briefly, participants drink a known amount of water labeled with deuterium (^{2}H) and oxygen-18 (^{2}H$_2$^{18}O).[117] They provide periodic samples of urine or saliva over the next 2 weeks or so, which allows monitoring of the body's elimination of deuterium and oxygen-18. Knowledge of the rates at which these isotopes are eliminated allows researchers to calculate energy expenditure in free-living participants with considerable accuracy and precision, despite certain limitations discussed in Chapter 8.

During a 10-day field exercise in the Canadian Arctic, the self-reported energy intake of 20 infantry soldiers was 39% less than their actual energy expenditure measured by doubly labeled water.[118] Researchers from the Ontario Cancer Institute and the University of British Columbia studied the accuracy of reported energy intakes from 7 consecutive days of food records obtained from a subset of 29 women participating in the Canadian Diet and Breast Cancer Prevention Trial. The mean body mass index (BMI, weight in kilograms divided by height in meters squared, or kg/m^2) of the subjects was 23.1 ±2.5 (mean ± standard deviation) and thus essentially within what is considered a healthy range for BMI. Reported energy intakes averaged 20% less than mean total energy expenditure determined by doubly labeled water.[119] Researchers from Maastricht University compared total energy expenditure measured by doubly labeled water with reported energy estimates from 7-day food records completed by

30 adult males. The subjects had a mean BMI (kg/m^2) of 34 ±4 (mean ± standard deviation) and thus were considered obese. Reported energy intakes averaged 37% less than mean total energy expenditure. The researchers estimated that, during the week that subjects kept food records, their energy consumption averaged 26% less than the previous week, when subjects were not recording their intake. These results suggest that, not only do subjects underreport energy intake, but they also are likely to eat less food during the recording period.[120]

Researchers from the University of Vermont compared total energy expenditure measured by doubly labeled water with estimates of energy intake based on four multiple-pass 24-hour recalls obtained over a 2-week period in a group of 35 low-income adult females. Underreporting of energy intake averaged 17%. However, underreporting was greater in subjects who were obese and in those who had lower literacy (difficulty reading and spelling), compared with nonobese subjects and those who had a higher degree of literacy.[121] In another study, energy intake was measured in 118 fourth- and fifth-graders who kept 8-day food records with the help of parents and nutritionists. Average daily energy intake was found to range from 17% to 33% less than total energy expenditure measured by doubly labeled water.[122]

Researchers at the USDA Beltsville Human Nutrition Research Center compared self-reported energy intakes with the amount of energy the participants actually required to maintain their body weight to within ±0.9 kg. The data, collected from 266 research participants over a 14-year period, showed that only 11% of self-reported energy intakes were accurate to within ±100 kcal and that 81% of participants underreported their energy intake by 700 kcal ±379 kcal (mean ± standard deviation).[123]

Another approach to check for underreporting is to compare reported usual energy intake with **resting energy expenditure** (REE), calculated using various equations, such as those shown in Table 3.2. If a subject's reported usual energy intake is < 1.2 times his or her calculated REE, underreporting of energy, and therefore nutrient, intake is highly likely.[94,124] Using data from the third National Health and Nutrition Examination Survey, researchers at the National Center for Health Statistics compared reported energy intakes of nearly 8,000 adult survey participants with their calculated resting energy expenditure.[125] About 18% of males and 28% of females were classified as underreporters. Underreporting was highest in females and in persons who were older, overweight, or trying to lose weight. Researchers at the USDA Western Human Nutrition Research Center compared reported energy intakes from 7-day food records with energy intake necessary to maintain a stable body weight in 22 adult females of widely varying body weight.[126] The subjects completed a variety of behavioral questionnaires that measured hunger, restrained eating, emotional eating (excessive eating in response to anger, fear, or anxiety), anxiety, and depression. Cognitive performance tests were also administered to the subjects. These assessed mental acuity, the ability to sustain or focus attention, short-term memory, and manual dexterity. Underreporting of energy by nonobese females (mean BMI 21.3 kg/m^2) was estimated at 10%, while that of obese subjects (mean BMI 34.2 kg/m^2) was nearly 20%. In the obese group, the presence of emotional factors related to depression were linked to greater likelihood of underreporting.

The observation that underreporting of food intake is common led researchers at the Beltsville Human Nutrition Research Center to propose the hypothesis of the "uncertainty principle of food-intake measurements: the degree of deviation of reported from real intake is proportional to the degree of attention focused on the intake."[123] Although the task of maintaining food records resulted in an 18% underestimate of energy intake, collection of duplicate food portions resulted in a decline of an additional 13%.[63,123] Thus, although the collection of dietary data is critical to our understanding of nutrition, *dietary intake data must be interpreted with considerable caution,* whether self-reported or obtained by observers of whose presence respondents are aware.[123,127] These findings led another research team to recommend that, "ideally, all dietary studies should include independent measures of validity."[94]

Despite the difficulty of accurately measuring usual dietary intake, our ability to quantify the degree of misreporting and to identify some of the characteristics of subjects related to misreporting represents progress toward the goal of accurately measuring diet. The potential now exists for "targeting specific areas of dietary assessment techniques to prevent or at least to minimize the effect of each factor on collection of valid data."[128]

Factors Affecting Validity

Several factors can affect the validity of an instrument. Among these are differences between usual diet and that measured in the study, inherent limitations or weaknesses of assessment methods, respondent characteristics, and observer characteristics. Examples of these are shown in Box 3.14. Sources of error in the different methods of measuring food intake are summarized in Table 3.3.

Reproducibility

Reproducibility, or **reliability,** can be defined as the ability of a method to produce the same estimate on two or more occasions, assuming that nothing has changed in the interim.[98] Reproducibility is concerned only with whether a method is capable of providing the *same or similar answer* two or more times and does not necessarily indicate whether the answer is *correct.* Reproducibility studies can partially answer the validity question; a method cannot give a correct answer every time unless it gives approximately the same answer each time.[98] Problems in instrument design, respondent instructions, or quality control also can be uncovered by reproducibility studies.

How Many Days?

In studies comparing dietary and nutrient intakes with measures of health and disease, it is important to know how long dietary intake must be measured before a sufficiently

TABLE 3.2	Equations for Calculating Resting Energy Expenditure*

World Health Organization

Females	3–9 years old	22.5 W + 499
	10–17 years old	12.2 W + 746
	18–29 years old	14.7 W + 496
	30–60 years old	8.7 W + 829
	> 60 years old	10.5 W + 596
Males	3–9 years old	22.7 W + 495
	10–17 years old	17.5 W + 651
	18–29 years old	15.3 W + 679
	30–60 years old	11.6 W + 879
	> 60 years old	13.5 W + 487

Harris-Benedict (Values Rounded for Simplicity)

Females	REE = 655 + 9.6W + 1.9S − 4.7A
Males	REE = 66 + 13.8W + 5S − 6.8A

*REE = resting energy expenditure; W = body weight in kg; S = stature in cm; A = age in years.

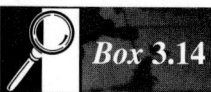

Box 3.14   Sources of Variation Between Actual Dietary Intake and That Measured by Various Methods

Causes of Variation	Examples
Differences between usual diet and that measured in the study	Study group is unrepresentative of the general population.
	Individual's diet is unrepresentative of usual diet because sampling method fails to capture the type of variability that is present (e.g., weekday versus weekends, season to season, spells of illness, periodic episodes of weight reduction diets, binges among bulimics, eating at home versus at business, travel, alternating day and night shifts).
	Number of observations made is inadequate.
Assessment method	Retrospective methods involve forgetting, which may be selective or nonuniform from food to food and may be influenced by frequency of consumption (seldom-eaten items remembered poorly), "telescoping," or including two weekends in one week.
	Prospective methods may lead to unconscious alteration of usual diets during reporting periods, especially in the first few days.
	Errors are present in food composition tables or nutrient database.
Respondent	Underreporting is common among
	• Those who are nonadherent to therapeutic diets • Obese persons (especially early in reporting period for snacks, sweets, desserts) • Heavy drinkers and alcoholics (for alcohol)
	Overreporting is common among
	• Recipients of food or meal program benefits • Anorectics and parents of infants with nonorganic failure to thrive • Those embarrassed about meager intakes
	Alterations of a selective type
	• Respondents report their preconceived notions of ideal or desirable intakes. • Respondents report what they think interviewers wish them to eat, especially respondents who have high needs for social approval or who fear loss of benefits or chastisement from those in power.
Observer	It is difficult to collect data about
	• Very old or very young persons (infants and children) • Ill, retarded, or confused persons (the mentally ill, alcoholics, drug addicts) • Non-English-speaking persons or persons who cannot read • Subjects who lack interest or motivation • Subjects who desire to conceal true intake • Subjects who have chaotic and/or unstructured food intakes

Table by Dwyer JT, used with permission from Stallones RA. 1982. Comments on the assessment of nutritional status in epidemiological studies and surveys of populations. *American Journal of Clinical Nutrition* 35:1290–1291.

reliable estimate of *usual intake* is obtained.[10,25,26,129] A few days of dietary observations, whether by 24-hour recall or food records, are not sufficient to adequately estimate an individual's usual intake. Because eating patterns vary between weekdays and weekends and across seasons, it is important to capture eating behavior in all parts of the week and in all seasons of the year.[10]

Investigators have tested approaches for calculating the number of days that dietary intake data must be collected.[25,26,129] Although a detailed discussion of these calculations is beyond the scope of this text, it should be noted that the number of days that data must be collected before usual intake can be estimated is related to an individual's day-to-day variation in nutrient intake (intraindividual variation) and the degree to which various individuals differ from one another in their nutrient intake (interindividual variation).[130,131] Estimation of usual dietary intake is facilitated when intraindividual variation is small in relation to interindividual variation. When the opposite condition exists (intraindividual variation is large relative to interindividual variation), characterization of usual intake requires a greater number of days.[130,131]

Other factors affecting the number of days of data collection include the purpose of the study, the sex and age of the group surveyed, and the nutrient(s) of interest. For most nutrients, fewer days are required to characterize the usual intake of persons 4 years old or younger (who typically consume a less varied diet) than for older children, adolescents, and adults (who generally consume a more varied diet).[26] The largest number of days is

required for such nutrients as copper, vitamin A, vitamin B$_{12}$, and polyunsaturated fats.[25,26]

Table 3.4 illustrates the problem of trying to estimate usual intake with a single 24-hour recall.[98] The precision of a single 24-hour recall in estimating kilocalorie intake for a typical male would be ±51%. In other words, if a 24-hour recall estimated energy intake at 2300 kcal, the true long-term intake could be 51% greater or less than that estimate and thus could range from 1150 to 3450 kcal. Estimates for vitamin A have a precision of only ±293% for males and ±224% for females.

Data from the Beltsville 1-year dietary intake study have been used to calculate the number of days of food records needed to estimate an individual's true usual intake.[129,132] In the Beltsville study, 29 individuals kept food records for 365 consecutive days while consuming their customary diets. The ranges and averages for males and females, shown in Table 3.5, indicate the number of days of food records required for estimates of nutrient intake to be within ±10% of true usual intake 95% of the time (that is, to have a *confidence index [CI] of 95%*).

It is apparent from Table 3.5 that the number of days needed to estimate usual intake of individuals varies among different participants and for different nutrients. Energy requires the least number of records, whereas vitamin A requires the greatest number. A minimum of 14 days of records was required for capturing usual intake of energy of the 29 participants, but 1 male required 84 days of records and 1 female

Sources of Error	Duplicate Portion	Weighed Record	Estimated Record	24-hour Recall	Dietary History
TABLE 3.3	**Sources of Error in Methods Estimating Food Consumption***				
Response errors					
Omitting foods	−	±	±	+	+
Adding foods	−	−	−	+	+
Estimating weight of foods	−	−	+	+	+
Estimating frequency of consumption of foods	−	−	−	−	+
Day-to-day variation	+	+	+	+	−
Changes in diet	+	+	±	−	−
Coding errors	−	+	+	+	+
Errors in conversion of nutrients					
Food composition tables	−	+	+	+	+
Sampling errors	+	−	−	−	−
Direct analysis	+	−	−	−	−

From Bingham SA, Nelson M, Paul AA, Haraldsdottir J, Loken EB, Van Staveren WA. 1988. Methods for data collection at an individual level. In Cameron ME, Van Staveren WA (eds.). *Manual on methodology for food consumption studies.* New York: Oxford University Press. Reprinted by permission of Oxford University Press.

*− indicates error is unlikely; + indicates error is likely; ± indicates variable effect on error.

TABLE 3.4	Precision of Estimates from One 24-Hour Recall

Dietary Component	Males (%)	Females (%)
Kilocalories	±51	±63
Protein	±71	±62
Carbohydrate	±59	±72
Total fat	±62	±79
Polyunsaturated fat	±100	±150
Cholesterol	±105	±109
Vitamin C	±134	±130
Vitamin A	±293	±224

Adapted from Block GS, Hartman AM. 1989. Issues in reproducibility and validity of dietary studies. *American Journal of Clinical Nutrition* 50:1133–1138.

required 60 days.[129] These differences among different individuals, sexes, and nutrients reflect intraindividual variability in nutrient intake. Nutrient intake over several days tends to vary less in some persons than in oth-

ers. Among all persons, day-to-day fluctuations in energy intake are much less than for nutrients such as vitamin C or vitamin A.

In contrast with estimating the usual intake of individuals, fewer days of data collection are necessary if the study's purpose is to estimate usual intake of groups or to rank the nutrient intake of individuals.[129,131] Data from the Beltsville study (Table 3.6) indicate the number of days of food records needed to estimate true average intake for groups of individuals with a precision of ±10% and a CI of 95%.[129]

ESTIMATING PORTION SIZE

A variety of approaches can be used to help participants estimate portion sizes. Among the simplest and least costly are "food models" composed of various geometric shapes cut out of poster board, as shown in Figure 3.6. Circles of various diameters can be used to help estimate the diameter of round foods, such as apples, oranges, tomato slices, hamburger patties, hamburger buns, and

TABLE 3.5	Ranges and Averages of Number of Days Required to Estimate True Average Intake for an Individual with Given Statistical Confidence*

	Range and Average Number of Days Required					
	Males (*n* = 13)			Females (*n* = 16)		
Component	Minimum	Average	Maximum	Minimum	Average	Maximum
Food energy	14	27	84	14	35	60
Iron	18	68	130	28	66	142
Vitamin A	115	390	1,724	152	474	1,372
Protein	23	36	72	23	48	70
Fat	34	57	131	32	71	114
Saturated fat	30	71	156	42	87	149
Oleic acid	35	68	163	31	85	145
Linoleic acid	77	145	225	82	166	237
Cholesterol	85	139	195	104	200	443
Carbohydrate	10	37	177	16	41	77
Crude fiber	43	82	146	51	86	138
Calcium	30	74	140	35	88	168
Phosphorus	18	32	62	19	41	62
Potassium	17	34	67	25	48	83
Sodium	27	58	140	36	73	116
Thiamin	46	138	405	41	198	728
Riboflavin	13	57	135	31	90	231
Niacin	27	53	89	48	78	126
Vitamin C	90	249	900	83	222	328

From Basiotis PP, Welsh SO, Cronin FJ, Kelsay JL, Mertz W. Number of days of food intake records required to estimate individual and group nutrient intakes with defined confidence. *Journal of Nutrition* 117:1638–1641.

*Estimated using intake data from 1-year dietary intake study by the U.S. Department of Agriculture's Beltsville Human Nutrition Research Center.

TABLE 3.6	Number of Days Required to Estimate True Average Intake for Groups of Individuals with Given Statistical Confidence*

Estimated Number of Days Required for Each Group

Component	Males (*n* = 13)	Females (*n* = 16)
Food energy	3	3
Iron	7	6
Vitamin A	39	44
Protein	4	4
Fat	6	6
Saturated fat	8	7
Oleic acid	6	7
Linoleic acid	13	12
Cholesterol	13	15
Carbohydrate	5	4
Crude fiber	9	9
Calcium	10	7
Phosphorus	4	5
Potassium	4	5
Sodium	6	6
Thiamin	13	16
Riboflavin	7	7
Niacin	5	6
Vitamin C	33	19

From Basiotis PP, Welsh SO, Cronin FJ, Kelsay JL, Mertz W. 1987. Number of days of food intake records required to estimate individual and group nutrient intakes with defined confidence. *Journal of Nutrition* 117:1638–1641.

*Estimated using intake data from 1-year dietary intake study by the U.S. Department of Agriculture's Beltsville Human Nutrition Research Center.

cookies. Square and rectangular pieces are useful in estimating the length and width of bread, cake, some cuts of meat, and cheese. Pie-shaped pieces of various radii can be used in estimating portion sizes of pie, round cake, watermelon, and pizza. Two-dimensional food models have been shown to be as effective as three-dimensional models for estimating portion size in nutritional research.[133]

Pieces of polyurethane foam 3 to 4 inches square and of varying thicknesses can be used to help respondents estimate the thickness of foods. Individual pieces can be used, or several can be stacked to achieve the desired thickness. An alternate approach is to have a number of pieces of cardboard cut 3 to 4 inches square, which can then be stacked to aid in estimating the thickness of food. Polystyrene balls of various diameters are useful in estimating sizes of round food objects. Bowls, plates, measuring cups and spoons, and drinking cups of various sizes also can be used to help respondents estimate serving sizes of soup, breakfast cereal, salad, beverages, sugar, and margarine.

Some investigators use photographs to facilitate portion size estimation.[134] The photographs, similar to the one shown in Figure 3.7, illustrate each food in the three most frequent serving sizes. The plate used in the photograph is available to provide a sense of scale.

When, during an interview, identification of particular brand names of foods consumed is important, a notebook containing photographs of various foods, pictures cut from magazine advertisements, or actual food labels can be used. A photograph of a supermarket dairy case, for example, can help respondents identify the brand of margarine used at home. During the course of a 24-hour recall, for example, a child is likely to remember the brand of potato or corn chips he or she ate but perhaps not the particular bag size. Including in the notebook an assortment of snack food wrappers (for candy, chips, and chewing gum of various brands and sizes) can be helpful in collecting accurate intake data. Lifelike food models, such as those shown in Figure 3.8, also can be used to help respondents estimate food portion sizes. Research suggests that memory of food portion sizes is not long-lasting and that food models are useful only for collecting very crude portion size information.

Figure 3.6
Simple geometric shapes representing foods are sometimes used to help survey participants estimate food portion size. Each piece has a known dimension (surface area or thickness) and is made from poster board or other materials.

Figure 3.7
Some investigators use photographs to help respondents more accurately estimate food portion size.

Figure 3.8
Lifelike food models can be used to improve accuracy in estimating food portion sizes.

SUMMARY

1. The ultimate reason for measuring diet is to improve human health. Other reasons include assessing and monitoring food and nutrient intake, formulating and evaluating government health and agricultural policy, conducting epidemiologic research, and using the data for commercial purposes.

2. No single best method exists for measuring dietary intake. Each method possesses certain advantages and disadvantages. The method used depends on research design considerations, characteristics of the study participants, available resources, and whether the intent is to estimate average group intake, rank individuals within a group, or estimate an individual's usual intake.

3. In the 24-hour recall method, a trained interviewer asks the respondent to remember all foods and beverages consumed during the past 24 hours. The 24-hour recall is quickly administered, has a low respondent burden, but does not give data representative of an individual's usual intake.

4. When keeping a food record, or diary, the respondent records, at the time of consumption, the identity and amounts of all foods and beverages consumed during a 1- to 7-day period. Foods can be either quantified using household measures or weighed, in which case the method is called weighed-food recording. This method does not rely on memory, can provide detailed intake data, requires a high degree of respondent cooperation, and may result in alterations of diet.

5. A food frequency questionnaire assesses nutrient intake by determining the frequency of consumption of a limited number of foods known to be major sources of the dietary components of interest. Respondents indicate how many times a day, week, month, or year the foods usually are consumed.

Relatively high-quality data can be gathered on large groups of respondents; data may be more representative of usual intake than a few days of diet records; respondents must be able to describe their diets; and foods and portion sizes included in questionnaires must be carefully chosen.

6. Collection of duplicate food portions is a more direct method of assessing nutrient intake that avoids some of the problems associated with coding and entering data and the limitations of food composition tables, such as nutrient losses during food storage and preparation. Respondents collect identical portions of all foods and beverages consumed during a specified period, which are then analyzed for nutrient content. Respondent concern about the expense of duplicate portions can alter eating habits, resulting in underestimates of nutrient intake.

7. Food accounts estimate dietary intake within households and institutions where congregate feeding is practiced. The food inventory at the end of the survey period is subtracted from the sum of the beginning inventory and food obtained during the study period. Daily mean consumption per person is calculated by dividing total food consumed by number of meals served. This is a relatively economical method of assessing dietary intake of large groups. It does not account for food losses or meals eaten outside the group and cannot provide estimates of individual food intake.

8. The food balance sheet provides data on food disappearance (or availability) rather than actual food consumption. Mean per capita annual amounts are calculated by dividing total food disappearance by the country's population. It detects trends in food

availability within a country over time and generates data that are useful in epidemiologic research across countries. The data represent only food that disappeared from the food distribution system and may be of questionable accuracy.

9. The high cost of research has led to innovations in the collection of dietary intake data. Included among these are telephone interviewing, photographic and video records, and computers interfaced with electronic scales for recording the identities and weights of foods consumed. Some of these methods have the potential for reducing respondent burden and increasing the validity of dietary intake data and the cost-effectiveness of collecting such data.

10. Surrogate sources are necessary when intake data are needed from persons unwilling or unable to provide them. Potential surrogate respondents include the spouse, partner, children, other close relatives, and friends of the respondent.

11. Validity is the ability of an instrument to measure what it is intended to measure. Validating a method involves comparing measurements of intake obtained by that method with estimates obtained using another method that is thought to have a greater degree of demonstrated, or face, validity.

Some biological markers can provide a validity check of dietary intake independent of respondents' accuracy and truthfulness.

12. Reproducibility, or reliability, is the ability of a method to produce the same estimate on two or more occasions, assuming that nothing has changed in the interim. Reproducibility studies are important in partially answering the validity question; a method cannot give a correct answer every time unless it gives approximately the same answer each time.

13. To estimate usual nutrient intake, diet must be measured for multiple days, for different days of the week (weekdays vs. weekends), and throughout the seasons of the year. The number of days required largely depends on the nutrient of interest, whether individuals or groups are studied, the degree of interindividual variation in nutrient intake, and the desired degree of precision.

14. Estimates of portion sizes can be sources of error in measuring dietary intake. A number of tools have been developed to assist respondents in accurately reporting amounts of foods consumed. These include photographs of food, geometric shapes of various sizes, measuring devices, and lifelike plastic food models.

REFERENCES

1. Federation of American Societies for Experimental Biology, Life Sciences Research Office. Prepared for the Interagency Board for Nutrition Monitoring and Related Research. 1995. *Third report on nutrition monitoring in the United States.* Washington, DC: U.S. Government Printing Office.

2. Begin I, Cap M, Dujardin B. 1988. *A guide to nutritional assessment.* Geneva, Switzerland: World Health Organization.

3. Stamler J. 1994. Assessing diets to improve world health: Nutritional research on disease causation in populations. *American Journal of Clinical Nutrition* 59(suppl):146S–156S.

4. Sabry JH. 1988. Purposes of food consumption surveys. In Cameron ME, Van Staveren WA (eds.). *Manual on methodology for food consumption studies.* New York: Oxford University Press.

5. Buzzard IM. 1994. Rationale for an international conference series on dietary assessment methods.

American Journal of Clinical Nutrition 59(suppl):143S–145S.

6. Sempos CT, Briefel RR, Johnson C, Woteki CE. 1992. Process and rationale for selecting dietary methods for NHANES III. In National Center for Health Statistics. *Dietary methodology workshop for the Third National Health and Nutrition Examination Survey.* Hyattsville, MD: U.S. Department of Health and Human Services, Public Health Service, Centers for Disease Control.

7. Beaton GH. 1994. Approaches to analysis of dietary data: Relationship between planned analyses and choice of methodology. *American Journal of Clinical Nutrition* 59(suppl):253S–261S.

8. Liu K. 1992. Statistical issues related to the design of dietary survey methodology for NHANES III. In National Center for Health Statistics. *Dietary methodology workshop for the Third National Health and Nutrition Examination Survey.*

Hyattsville, MD. U.S. Department of Health and Human Services, Public Health Service Centers for Disease Control.

9. Willett WC. 1999. Goals for nutrition in the year 2000. *CA—A Cancer Journal for Clinicians* 49:331–352.

10. Thompson FE, Byers T. 1994. Dietary assessment resource manual. *Journal of Nutrition* 124(suppl):2245S–2317S.

11. Block G. 1989. Human dietary assessment: Methods and issues. *Preventive Medicine* 18:653–660.

12. Lee Han H, McGuire V, Boyd NF. 1989. A review of the methods used by studies of dietary measurement. *Journal of Clinical Epidemiology* 42:269–279.

13. Block G. 1982. A review of validations of dietary assessment methods. *American Journal of Epidemiology* 115:492–505.

14. Dwyer JT, Krall EA, Coleman KA. 1987. The problem of memory in nutritional epidemiology research.

Journal of the American Dietetic Association 87:1509–1512.

15. Feskanich D, Willett WC. 1993. The use and validity of food frequency questionnaires in epidemiologic research and clinical practice. *Medicine, Exercise, Nutrition, and Health* 2:143–154.

16. Briefel RR. 1994. Assessment of the U.S. diet in national nutrition surveys: National collaborative efforts and NHANES. *American Journal of Clinical Nutrition* 59(suppl):164S–167S.

17. Guenther PM. 1994. Research needs for dietary assessment and monitoring in the United States. *American Journal of Clinical Nutrition* 59(suppl):168S–170S.

18. National Center for Health Statistics. 1994. *Plan and operation of the Third National Health and Examination Survey, 1988–94.* Hyattsville, MD: U.S. Department of Health and Human Services, Public Health Service, Centers for Disease Control.

19. Crawford PB, Obarzanek E, Morrison J, Sabry ZI. 1994. Comparative advantage of 3-day food records over 24-hour recall and 5-day food frequency validated by observation of 9- and 10-year-old girls. *Journal of the American Dietetic Association* 94:626–630.

20. Johnson RK, Driscoll P, Goran MI. 1996. Comparison of multiple-pass 24-hour recall estimates of energy intake with total energy expenditure determined by the doubly labeled water method in young children. *Journal of the American Dietetic Association* 96:1140–1144.

21. McNutt S, Hall J, Cranston B, Soto P, Hults S. 2000. The 24-hour dietary recall data collection and coding methodology implemented for the 1999–2000 National Health and Nutrition Examination Survey. *FASEB Journal* 14:A759.

22. McNutt S, Hall J, Cranston B, Soto P, Hults S. 2000. Quality control procedures implemented for the dietary assessment component of the 1999–2000 National Health and Nutrition Examination Survey. *FASEB Journal* 14:A759.

23. Block G, Hartman AM, Dresser CM, Carroll MD, Gannon J, Gardner L. 1986. A data-based approach to diet questionnaire design and testing. *American Journal of Epidemiology* 124:453–469.

24. Block G. 1992. Dietary assessment issues related to cancer for NHANES III. In National Center for Health Statistics. *Dietary methodology workshop for the Third National Health and Nutrition Examination Survey.* Hyattsville, MD: U.S. Department of Health and Human Services, Public Health Service, Centers for Disease Control.

25. Beaton GH, Milner J, McGuire V, Feather TE, Little JA. 1983. Source of variance in 24-hour dietary recall data: Implications for nutrition study design and interpretation. Carbohydrate sources, vitamins, and minerals. *American Journal of Clinical Nutrition* 37:986–995.

26. Nelson M, Black AE, Morris JA, Cole TJ. 1989. Between- and within-subject variation in nutrient intake from infancy to old age: Estimating the number of days required to rank dietary intakes with desired precision. *American Journal of Clinical Nutrition* 50:155–167.

27. Smith AF. 1991. Cognitive processes in long-term dietary recall. *Vital and Health Statistics 6(4).* Hyattsville, MD: National Center for Health Statistics.

28. Rebro SM, Patterson RE, Kristal AR, Cheney CL. 1998. The effect of keeping food records on eating patterns. *Journal of the American Dietetic Association* 98:1163–1165.

29. Macdiarmid JI, Blundell JE. 1997. Dietary underreporting: What people say about recording their food intake. *European Journal of Clinical Nutrition* 51:199–200.

30. Forster JL, Jeffrey RW, VanNatta M, Pirie P. 1990. Hypertension prevention trial: Do 24-hr food records capture usual eating behavior in a dietary change study? *American Journal of Clinical Nutrition* 51:253–257.

31. Sawaya AL, Tucker K, Tsay R, Willett W, Saltzman E, Dallal GE, Roberts SB. 1996. Evaluation of four methods for determining energy intake in young and older women: Comparison with doubly labeled water measurements of total energy expenditure. *American Journal of Clinical Nutrition* 63:491–499.

32. Smucker R, Block G, Coyle L, Harvin R, Kessler L. 1989. A dietary and risk factor questionnaire and analysis system for personal computers. *American Journal of Epidemiology* 129:445–449.

33. Block G, Clifford C, Naughton MD, Henderson M, McAdams M. 1989. A brief dietary screen for high fat intake. *Journal of Nutrition Education* 21:199–207.

34. Yaroch AL, Resnicow K, Khan LK. 2000. Validity and reliability of qualitative dietary fat index questionnaires: A review. *Journal of the American Dietetic Association* 100:240–244.

35. Samet JM, Humble CG, Skipper BE. 1984. Alternatives in the collection and analysis of food frequency interview data. *American Journal of Epidemiology* 120:572–581.

36. Thompson FE, Kipnis V, Subar AF, Krebs-Smith SM, et al. 2000. Evaluation of 2 brief instruments and a food frequency questionnaire to estimate number of servings of fruit and vegetables. *American Journal of Clinical Nutrition* 71:1503–1510.

37. Brown JL, Griebler R. 1993. Reliability of a short and long version of the Block food frequency form for assessing changes in calcium intake. *Journal of the American Dietetic Association* 93:784–789.

38. National Institutes of Health. 2001. *Third report of the Expert Panel on Detection, Evaluation, and Treatment of High Blood Cholesterol in Adults.* Washington, DC: National Institutes of Health, National Heart, Lung, and Blood Institute.

39. Srinath U, Shacklock F, Shannon BM, Mitchell DC, Kris-Etherton PM, Scott L, Jaax S, Pearson TA.

1993. MEDFICTS—A dietary assessment instrument for evaluating fat, saturated fat, and cholesterol intake. *Circulation* 88(no. 4, part 2):I–634.

40. Srinath U, Shacklock F, Scott LW, Jaax S, Kris-Etherton PM. 1993. Development of MEDFICTS—A dietary assessment instrument for evaluating fat, saturated fat, and cholesterol intake. *Journal of the American Dietetic Association* 93:A–105.

41. Willett WC, Sampson L, Stampfer MJ, Rosner B, Bain C, Witschi J, Hennekens CH, Speizer FE. 1985. Reproducibility and validity of a semiquantitative food frequency questionnaire. *American Journal of Epidemiology* 122:51–65.

42. Feskanich D, Rimm EB, Giovannucci EL, Colditz GA, Stampfer MJ, Litin LB, Willett WC. 1993. Reproducibility and validity of food intake measurements from a semiquantitative food frequency questionnaire. *Journal of the American Dietetic Association* 93:790–796.

43. Willett WC. 1998. *Nutritional epidemiology,* 2nd ed. New York: Oxford University Press.

44. Rimm EB, Giovannucci EL, Stampfer MJ, Colditz GA, Litin LB, Willett WC. 1992. Reproducibility and validity of an expanded self-administered semiquantitative food frequency questionnaire among male health professionals. *American Journal of Epidemiology* 135:1114–1126.

45. Liu S, Manson JE, Stampfer MJ, Rexrode KM, Hu FB, Rimm EB, Willett WC. 2000. Whole grain consumption and risk of ischemic strike in women. *Journal of the American Medical Association* 284:1534–1540.

46. Hu FB, Rimm EB, Stampfer MJ, Ascherio A, Spiegelman D, Willett WC. 2000. Prospective study of major dietary patterns and risk of coronary heart disease in men. *American Journal of Clinical Nutrition* 72:912–921.

47. Munger RG, Folsom AR, Kushi LH, Kaye SA, Sellers TA. 1992. Dietary assessment of older Iowa women with a food frequency questionnaire: Nutrient intake, reproducibility, and comparison with 24-hour dietary recall interviews. *American Journal of Epidemiology* 136:192–200.

48. Willett WC, Hunter DJ, Stampfer MJ, et al. 1992. Dietary fat and fiber in relation to risk of breast cancer: An 8-year follow-up. *Journal of the American Medical Association* 268:2037–2044.

49. Willett WC, Stampfer MJ, Colditz GA, Rosner BA, Speizer FE. 1990. Relation of meat, fat, and fiber intake to the risk of colon cancer in a prospective study among women. *New England Journal of Medicine* 323:1664–1672.

50. Tang AM, Graham NMH, Kirby AJ, McCall D, Willett WC, Saah AJ. 1993. Dietary micronutrient intake and risk of progression to acquired immunodeficiency syndrome (AIDS) in human immunodeficiency virus type 1 (HIV-1)-infected homosexual men. *American Journal of Epidemiology* 138:937–951.

51. Subar AF. Personal communication, 14 November 2000.

52. Krall EA, Dwyer JT. 1987. Validity of a food frequency questionnaire and a food diary in a short-term recall situation. *Journal of the American Dietetic Association* 87:1374–1377.

53. Zulkifli SN, Yu SM. 1992. The food frequency method for dietary assessment. *Journal of the American Dietetic Association* 92:681–685.

54. Hu FB, Rimm E, Smith-Warner SA, Feskanich D, Stampfer MJ, Ascherio A, Sampson L, Willett WC. 1999. Reproducibility and validity of dietary patterns assessed with a food-frequency questionnaire. *American Journal of Clinical Nutrition* 69:243–249.

55. Block G, Woods M, Potosky A, Clifford C. 1990. Validation of a self-administered diet history questionnaire using multiple diet records. *Journal of Clinical Epidemiology* 43:1327–1335.

56. Briefel RR, Flegal KM, Winn DM, Loria CM, Johnson CL, Sempos CT. 1992. Assessing the nation's diet: Limitations of the food frequency questionnaire. *Journal of the American Dietetic Association* 92:959–962.

57. Schaefer EJ, Augustin JL, Schaefer MM, Rasmussen H, Ordovas JM, Dallal GE, Dwyer JT. 2000. Lack of efficacy of a food-frequency questionnaire in assessing dietary macronutrient intakes in subjects consuming diets of known composition. *American Journal of Clinical Nutrition* 71:746–751.

58. Willett WC. 1994. Future directions in the development of food-frequency questionnaires. *American Journal of Clinical Nutrition* 59(suppl):171S–174S.

59. Mullen BJ, Krantzler NJ, Grivetti LE, Schutz HG, Meiselman HL. 1984. Validity of a food frequency questionnaire for the determination of individual food intake. *American Journal of Clinical Nutrition* 39:136–143.

60. Van Staveren WA, de Boer JO, Burema J. 1985. Validity and reproducibility of a dietary history method estimating the usual food intake during one month. *American Journal of Clinical Nutrition* 42:554–559.

61. Jain M. 1989. Diet history: Questionnaire and interview techniques used in some retrospective studies of cancer. *Journal of the American Dietetic Association* 89:1647–1652.

62. Burke BS. 1947. The dietary history as a tool in research. *Journal of the American Dietetic Association* 23:1041–1046.

63. Kim WW, Mertz W, Judd JT, Marshall MW, Kelsay JL, Prather ES. 1984. Effect of making duplicate food collections on nutrient intakes calculated from diet records. *American Journal of Clinical Nutrition* 40:1333–1337.

64. Mertz W. 1992. Food intake measurements: Is there a "gold standard"? *Journal of the American Dietetic Association* 82:1463–1465.

65. Pekkarinen M. 1970. Methodology in the collection of food consumption data. *World Review of Nutrition and Dietetics* 12:145–171.

66. Turpeinen O, Karvonen MJ, Pekkarinen M, Miettinen M,

Elosuo R, Paavilainen E. 1979. Dietary prevention of coronary heart disease: The Finnish Mental Hospital Study. *International Journal of Epidemiology* 8:99–118.

67. Turpeinen O, Miettinen M, Karvonen MJ, Roine P, Pekkarinen M, Lehtosuo EJ, Alivirta P. 1968. Dietary prevention of coronary heart disease: Long-term experiment. *American Journal of Clinical Nutrition* 21:255–276.

68. Casey PH, Goolsby SLP, Lensig SY, Perloff BP, Bogle ML. 1999. The use of telephone interview methodology to obtain 24-hour dietary recalls. *Journal of the American Dietetic Association* 99:1406–1411.

69. Tran KM, Johnson RK, Soultanakis RP, Matthews DE. 2000. In-person vs telephone-administered multiple-pass 24-hour recalls in women: Validation with doubly labeled water. *Journal of the American Dietetic Association* 100:777–780, 783.

70. Van Horn LV, Gernhofer N, Moag-Stahlberg A, Ferris R, Hartmuller G, Lasser VI, Stumbo P, Craddick S, Ballew C. 1990. Dietary assessment in children using electronic methods: Telephones and tape recorders. *Journal of the American Dietetic Association* 90:412–416.

71. Dubois S, Boivin JF. 1990. Accuracy of telephone dietary recalls in elderly subjects. *Journal of the American Dietetic Association* 90:1680–1687.

72. Morgan KJ, Johnson SR, Rizek RL, Reese R, Stampley GL. 1987. Collection of food intake data: An evaluation of methods. *Journal of the American Dietetic Association* 87:888–896.

73. Fox TA, Heimendinger J, Block G. 1992. Telephone surveys as a method for obtaining dietary information: A review. *Journal of the American Dietetic Association* 92:729–732.

74. Posner BM, Borman CL, Morgan JL, Borden WS, Ohls JC. 1982. The validity of a telephone-administered 24-hour dietary recall methodology. *American Journal of Clinical Nutrition* 36:546–553.

75. Medlin C, Skinner JD. 1988. Individual dietary intake methodology: A 50-year review of progress. *Journal of the American Dietetic Association* 88:1250–1257.

76. Jonnalagadda SS, Mitchell DC, Smiciklas-Wright H, Meaker KB, Van Heel N, Karmally W, Ershow AG, Kris-Etherton PM. 2000. Accuracy of energy intake data estimated by a multiple-pass, 24-hour dietary recall technique. *Journal of the American Dietetic Association* 100:303–308, 311.

77. Elwood PC, Bird G. 1983. A photographic method of diet evaluation. *Human Nutrition: Applied Nutrition* 37A:474–477.

78. Bird G, Elwood PC. 1983. The dietary intakes of subjects estimated from photographs compared with a weighed record. *Human Nutrition: Applied Nutrition* 37A:470–473.

79. Weiss EH, Kien CL, Clark G. 1988. Validation of a photographic method for recording the selection of foods by individuals. *Journal of the American Dietetic Association* 88:599–600.

80. Brown J, Tharp TM, Dahlberg-Luby EM, Snowdon DA, Ostwald SK, Buzzard IM, Rysavy DM, Wieser MA. 1990. Videotape dietary assessment: Validity, reliability, and comparison of results with 24-hour dietary recalls from elderly women in a retirement home. *Journal of the American Dietetic Association* 90:1675–1679.

81. Kretsch MJ. 1989. New computerized techniques for assessing food intake. In Livingston GE (ed.). *Nutritional status assessment of the individual.* Trumbull, CT: Food & Nutrition Press.

82. Fong AKH, Kretsch MJ. 1990. Nutrition evaluation scale system reduces time and labor in recording quantitative dietary intake. *Journal of the American Dietetic Association* 90:664–670.

83. Kretsch MJ, Fong AKH. 1993. Validity and reproducibility of a new computerized dietary assessment method. Effects of gender and educational level. *Nutrition Research* 13:133–146.

84. Kretsch MJ, Fong AKH. 1990. Validation of a new computerized technique for quantitating individual dietary intake: The Nutrition Evaluation Scale System (NESSy) vs the weighed food record. *American Journal of Clinical Nutrition* 51:477–484.

85. Kretsch MJ. Personal communication, 7 November 2000.

86. Kohlmeier L. 1995. Future of dietary exposure assessment. *American Journal of Clinical Nutrition* 61(suppl):702S–709S.

87. Kohlmeier L, Mendez M, McDuffie J, Miller M. 1997. Computer-assisted self-interviewing: A multimedia approach to dietary assessment. *American Journal of Clinical Nutrition* 65(suppl):1275S–1281S.

88. Samet JM. 1989. Surrogate measures of dietary intake. *American Journal of Clinical Nutrition* 50:1139–1144.

89. Cumming RG, Klineberg RJ. 1994. A study of the reproducibility of long-term recall in the elderly. *Epidemiology* 5:116–119.

90. Andersson I, Rössner S. 1989. Energy intake of obese women. *International Journal of Obesity* 13:247–253.

91. Bandini LG, Schoeller DA, Cyr HN, Dietz WH. 1990. Validity of reported energy intake in obese and nonobese adolescents. *American Journal of Clinical Nutrition* 52:421–425.

92. Lansky D, Brownell KD. 1982. Estimates of food quantity and calories: Errors in self-report among obese patients. *American Journal of Clinical Nutrition* 35:727–732.

93. Lichtman SW, Pisarska K, Berman ER, Pestone M, Dowling H, Offenbacher E, Weisel H, Heshka S, Matthews DE, Heymsfield SB. 1992. Discrepancy between self-reported and actual caloric intake and exercise in obese subjects. *New England Journal of Medicine* 327:1893–1898.

94. Black AE, Prentice AM, Goldberg GR, Jebb SA, Bingham SA, Livingstone MBE, Coward WA. 1993. Measurements of total energy expenditure provide insights into the validity of dietary measurements of energy intake. *Journal of the American Dietetic Association* 93:572–579.

95. Blake AJ, Guthrie HA, Smiciklas-Wright H. 1989. Accuracy of food portion estimation by overweight and normal-weight subjects. *Journal of the American Dietetic Association* 89:962–964.

96. Myers RJ, Klesges RC, Eck LH, Hanson CL, Klem ML. 1988. Accuracy of self-reports of food intake in obese and normal-weight individuals: Effects of obesity on self-reports of dietary intake in adult females. *American Journal of Clinical Nutrition* 48:1248–1251.

97. Cameron ME, Van Staveren WA. 1988. *Manual on methodology for food consumption studies.* New York: Oxford University Press.

98. Block G, Hartman AM. 1989. Issues in reproducibility and validity of dietary studies. *American Journal of Clinical Nutrition* 50:1133–1138.

99. Pietinen P, Hartman AM, Haapa E, Räsänen L, Haapakoski J, Palmgren J, Albanes D, Virtamo J, Huttunen JK. 1988. Reproducibility and validity of dietary assessment instruments. I. A self-administered food use questionnaire with a portion size picture booklet. *American Journal of Epidemiology* 128:655–666.

100. Pietinen P, Hartman AM, Haapa E, Räsänen L, Haapakoski J, Palmgren J, Albanes D, Virtamo J, Huttunen JK. 1988. Reproducibility and validity of dietary assessment instruments. II. A qualitative food frequency questionnaire. *American Journal of Epidemiology* 128:667–676.

101. Carter RL, Sharbaugh CO, Stapell CA. 1981. Reliability and validity of the 24-hour recall. *Journal of the American Dietetic Association* 79:542–547.

102. Emmons L, Hayes M. 1973. Accuracy of 24-hour recalls of young children. *Journal of the American Dietetic Association* 62:409–415.

103. Stunkard AJ, Waxman M. 1981. Accuracy of self-reports of food intake. *Journal of the American Dietetic Association* 79:547–551.

104. Greger JL, Entyre GM. 1978. Validity of 24-hour recalls by adolescent females. *American Journal of Public Health* 68:70–72.

105. Campbell VA, Dodds ML. 1967. Collecting dietary information from groups of older people. *Journal of the American Dietetic Association* 51:29–33.

106. Lytle LA, Nichaman MZ, Obarzanek E, Glovsky E, Montgomery D, Nicklas T, Zive M, Feldman H. 1993. Validation of 24-hour recalls assisted by food records in third-grade children. *Journal of the American Dietetic Association* 93:1431–1436.

107. Van Staveren WA, West CE, Hoffmans MDAF, Bos P, Kardinaal AFM, Poppel GAFG, Schipper HJA, Hautvast JGJA, Hayes RB. 1986. Comparison of contemporaneous and retrospective estimates of food consumption made by a dietary history method. *American Journal of Epidemiology* 123:884–893.

108. Jain MG, Howe GR, Johnson KC, Miller AB. 1980. Evaluation of a diet history questionnaire for epidemiologic studies. *American Journal of Epidemiology* 111:212–219.

109. Hebert JR, Miller DR. 1988. Methodologic considerations for investigating the diet-cancer link. *American Journal of Clinical Nutrition* 47:1068–1077.

110. Bingham SA. 1987. The dietary assessment of individuals: Methods, accuracy, new techniques and recommendations. *Nutrition Abstracts and Reviews* 57:705–743.

111. Roberts SB, Ferland S, Young VR, Morrow F, Heyman MB, Melanson KJ, Gullans SR, Dallal GE. 1991. Objective verification of dietary intake by measurement of urine osmolality. *American Journal of Clinical Nutrition* 54:774–782.

112. Bingham SA. 1994. The use of 24-h urine samples and energy expenditure to validate dietary assessments. *American Journal of Clinical Nutrition* 59(suppl):227S–231S.

113. Hunter DJ, Rimm EB, Sacks FM, Stampfer MJ, Colditz GA, Litin LB, Willett WC. 1992. Comparison of measures of fatty acid intake by subcutaneous fat aspirate, food frequency questionnaire, and diet records in a free-living population of U.S. men. *American Journal of Epidemiology* 135:418–427.

114. Roberts SB, Morrow FD, Evans WJ, Shepard DC, Dallal GE, Meredith CN, Young VR. 1990. Use of *p*-aminobenzoic acid to monitor compliance with prescribed dietary regimens during metabolic balance studies in man. *American Journal of Clinical Nutrition* 51:485–488.

115. Bingham SA, Cummings JH. 1985. Urine nitrogen as an independent validatory measure of dietary intake: A study of nitrogen balance in individuals consuming their normal diet. *American Journal of Clinical Nutrition* 42:1276–1289.

116. Feunekes GIJ, Van Staveren WA, De Vries JHM, Burema J, Hautvast JGAJ. 1993. Relative and biomarker-based validity of a food-frequency questionnaire estimating intake of fats and cholesterol. *American Journal of Clinical Nutrition* 58:489–496.

117. Speakman JR. 1998. The history and theory of doubly labeled water technique. *American Journal of Clinical Nutrition* 68(suppl):932S–938S.

118. Jones PJH, Jacobs I, Morris A, Duchmarme MB. 1993. Adequacy of food rations in soldiers during an Arctic exercise measured by doubly labeled water. *Journal of Applied Physiology* 75:1790–1797.

119. Martin LJ, Su W, Jones PJ, Lockwood GA, Tritchler DL, Boyd NF. 1996. Comparison of energy intakes determined by food records and doubly labeled water in women participating in a dietary-intervention trial. *American Journal of Clinical Nutrition* 63:483–490.

120. Goris AHC, Westerterp-Plantenga MS, Westerterp KR. 2000. Undereating and underrecording of habitual food intake in obese men: Selective underreporting of fat intake. *American Journal of Clinical Nutrition* 71:130–134.

121. Johnson RK, Soultanakis RP, Matthews DE. 1998. Literacy and body fatness are associated with underreporting of energy intake in US low-income women using the multiple-pass 24-hour recall: A doubly labeled water study. *Journal of the American Dietetic Association* 98:1136–1140.

122. Champagne CM, Baker NB, DeLany JP, Harsha DW, Bray

GA. 1998. Assessment of energy intake underreporting by doubly labeled water and observations on reported energy intake in children. *Journal of the American Dietetic Association* 98:426–430, 433.

123. Mertz W, Tsui JC, Judd JT, Reiser S, Hallfirsch J, Morris ER, Steele PD, Lashley E. 1991. What are people really eating? The relation between energy intake derived from estimated diet records and intake determined to maintain body weight. *American Journal of Clinical Nutrition* 54:291–295.

124. Goldberg GR, Black AE, Jebb SA, Cole TJ, Murgatroyd PR, Coward WA, Prentice AM. 1991. Critical evaluation of energy intake data using fundamental principles of energy physiology. I. Derivation of cut-off limits to identify underrecording. *European Journal of Clinical Nutrition* 45:569–581.

125. Briefel RR, Sempos CT, McDowell MA, Chien S, Alaimo K. 1997. Dietary methods research in the third National Health and Nutrition Examination Survey: Underreporting of energy intake.

American Journal of Clinical Nutrition 65(suppl):1203S–1209S.

126. Kretsch MJ, Fong AKH, Green MW. 1999. Behavioral and body size correlates of energy intake underreporting by obese and normal-weight women. *Journal of the American Dietetic Association* 99:300–306.

127. Schoeller DA. 1999. Recent advances from application of doubly labeled water to measurement of human energy expenditure. *Journal of Nutrition* 129:1765–1768.

128. Kubena KS. 2000. Accuracy in dietary assessment: On the road to good science. *Journal of the American Dietetic Association* 100:775–776.

129. Basiotis PP, Welsh SO, Cronin J, Kelsay JL, Mertz W. 1987. Number of days of food intake records required to estimate individual and group nutrient intakes with defined confidence. *Journal of Nutrition* 117:1638–1641.

130. Beaton GH, Milner J, McGuire V, Feather TE, Little JA. 1979. Sources of variance in 24-hour

dietary recall data: Implications for nutrition study design and interpretation. *American Journal of Clinical Nutrition* 32:2456–2459.

131. Liu K, Stamler J, Dyer A, McKeever J, McKeever P. 1978. Statistical methods to assess and minimize the role of intra-individual variability in obscuring the relationship between dietary lipids and serum cholesterol. *Journal of Chronic Diseases* 31:399–418.

132. Mertz W, Kelsay JL. 1984. Rationale of the Beltsville one-year dietary intake study. *American Journal of Clinical Nutrition* 40:1323–1326.

133. Posner BM, Smigelski C, Duggal A, Morgan JL, Cobb J, Cupples A. 1992. Validation of two-dimensional models for estimating portion size in nutrition research. *Journal of the American Dietetic Association* 92:738–741.

134. Hankin JH. 1986. 23rd Lenna Frances Cooper Memorial Lecture: A diet history method for research, clinical, and community use. *Journal of the American Dietetic Association* 86:868–875.

ASSESSMENT ACTIVITY 3.1

Collecting a 24-Hour Recall

The 24-hour recall is probably the most commonly used technique for measuring diet. Consequently, it is important that health professionals involved in nutritional assessment understand, practice, and master this technique. In this assessment activity, you will collect a 24-hour recall from a classmate and calculate that person's intake of kilocalories, protein, carbohydrate, total fat, calcium, and iron from a food composition table. Be sure to have a classmate collect a 24-hour recall from you, too. This will provide you with additional experience with recalls. You also will need your own 24-hour recall for an assessment activity in Chapter 5.

This assessment activity also will help you become more familiar with using food composition tables. Experience in using food composition tables is valuable. Sometimes it is faster and easier to refer to a food composition table for a nutrient value than to use a computer. Familiarity with food composition tables will also make that task easier.

1. For this assessment activity, we suggest you use a photocopy of the form provided on page 109. It not only provides space for recording the names and

quantities of foods and beverages consumed, but it also allows you to easily record values for energy and nutrients for reported foods.

2. Familiarize yourself with the form *before* beginning your interview. Enter the name of the person being interviewed and the day and date.

3. After completing the recall form, manually calculate the intakes of kilocalories, protein, carbohydrate, total fat, calcium, and iron, using the food composition table in Appendix K. If you cannot find a particular food or beverage in the food composition table, use a similar food or beverage or refer to another food composition table.

4. As you do this assignment, think about the following questions:
   How representative of your respondent's usual dietary intake is this one day of intake data?
   Did you have any difficulty finding any foods in the food composition table?
   If you had to substitute one food for another, how do you think that substitution affected the total nutrient values?

24-Hour Recording Form for Assessment Activity 3.1

Name of person interviewed _____ **Date** _____ **Day of week** _____

Food/Drink	Type/How Prepared	Quantity	Kilocalories	Protein	Carbohydrate	Total Fat	Calcium	Iron
Total								

ASSESSMENT ACTIVITY 3.2

Completing a 3-Day Food Record

Obtaining dietary intake data that is representative of the usual intake of *individuals* requires data from multiple days. According to the research reported in Table 3.5, estimating usual intake of energy (kilocalories) requires an average of approximately 30 days of intake data. Vitamin A requires approximately 400 days of data. Fewer days of data are required when characterizing the average intake of groups, as shown in Table 3.6.

Although this assessment activity will not even come close to giving you the data necessary to estimate your usual nutrient intake, it will give you an idea of what is involved in collecting multiple-day intake data. In this assignment, you will complete a 3-day food record on yourself using the food diary recording form in Appendix D or one provided by your professor. You may want to analyze your food record using the diet analysis software available from the publisher or at your school's computer lab.

1. Familiarize yourself with the form in Appendix D and accompanying instructions *before* beginning your diary.

2. Record your food and beverage intake for two weekdays (Monday through Friday) and one weekend day (Saturday or Sunday). Because most people eat differently on weekend days than on weekdays, this will make your record more representative of your usual intake throughout the entire week.

3. Do not alter your normal diet during the recording period. Provide responses that are as accurate as possible. Record your food and beverage intake as soon after eating as possible.

4. You may save your completed food record for later analysis using diet analysis software.

ASSESSMENT ACTIVITY 3.3

Diet History Questionnaire

Compared with other techniques for measuring diet, food frequency questionnaires are a recent development. There is considerable interest in food frequency questionnaires as a relatively simple and inexpensive approach to characterizing the usual food and nutrient intake of individuals. A food frequency questionnaire developed by researchers at the U.S. National Cancer Institute (NCI) and used in several epidemiologic studies sponsored by the NCI is the Diet History Questionnaire (DHQ). The DHQ is explained in greater detail in this chapter. Several pages of the DHQ are shown in Appendix J, and the entire questionnaire can be downloaded from the website of the NCI. A link to this website is available at the *Nutritional Assessment* website at www.mhhe.com/hper/nutrition. The software for analyzing the DHQ, along with supporting documentation, are also available from the NCI's website, which can be accessed using a link available through the *Nutritional Assessment* website.

Instructors may wish to administer the DHQ to students and use the software to process the questionnaires to develop nutrient intake data for discussion purposes. These data could be compared with national averages. Output from multiple groups of students from different disciplines could be compared to see if significant differences in food and nutrient intake exist among groups of students.

NATIONAL DIETARY AND NUTRITION SURVEYS

INTRODUCTION

Nutritional monitoring is an important activity for any government serious about promoting its citizens' health. The principle goal of nutritional monitoring is to accurately measure the dietary and nutritional status of a population and the quality, quantity, and safety of the food it consumes.[1] Data on the nutritional and health status of a population that are generated by nutritional monitoring are used for many purposes. They can identify nutritional problems of the country as a whole (e.g., excessive fat and cholesterol consumption) and groups at nutritional risk (e.g., low calcium intake by adolescent females). These data are used to justify changes in government policy and the spending of billions of dollars for planning and implementing programs related to food, nutrition, and health promotion, such as the Special Supplemental Nutrition Program for Women, Infants, and Children (WIC) and the National Cholesterol Education Program. They are important in evaluating the cost-effectiveness of such programs, particularly when voters and legislators express concern about reducing budget deficits, controlling the high cost of government, cutting taxes, or limiting government involvement in issues related to diet and health. These data are also critical to research into the relationships between nutrition and health. This chapter discusses nutritional monitoring in the United States and the most important surveys comprising the federal government's nutrition and health surveillance activities. It also discusses the major findings of these surveys.

IMPORTANCE OF NATIONAL DIETARY AND NUTRITION SURVEYS

National dietary and nutrition surveys have a number of important functions and can provide much valuable information. They can show how food supplies are distributed according to such demographic factors as region, income, sex, race, and ethnicity. Survey data are important in monitoring nutritional status of a country's popu-

lation. By observing trends in the health and dietary practices of a population, relationships between diet and health can be elucidated. They identify groups that are at nutritional risk and that may benefit from food assistance programs. They are important for developing the Thrifty Food Plan, which forms the basis for determining benefit levels for participants of the Food Stamp Program. They are also used for evaluating the effectiveness of various USDA food assistance programs. For example, a before-and-after comparison of food consumption practices by Food Stamp Program participants revealed that the program allowed families to purchase more nutritious foods and increased the market for surplus agricultural products. After analyzing nutritional and health survey data, the U.S. General Accounting Office (GAO) reported that women participating in the WIC program had a 25% reduction in low birth weight births (under 2500 g, or 5.5 lb) and a 44% reduction in very low birth weight births (under 1500 g, or 3.3 lb) compared with similar women not participating in the WIC program.[2] The GAO estimated that, for each tax dollar invested in WIC benefits, nearly $3.00 were saved within the first year by federal, state, and local governments and private insurance companies in reduced health care costs and xspecial education. These and other uses of data from nutrition and health surveys are summarized in Box 4.1.

Box 4.1   **Uses of Data from Nutrition and Health Surveys**

PUBLIC POLICY

Monitoring Surveillance

- Identify high-risk groups and geographic areas with nutrition-related problems to facilitate implementation of public health intervention programs and food assistance programs
- Evaluate changes in agricultural policy that may affect the nutritional quality and healthfulness of the U.S. food supply
- Assess progress toward achieving the nutrition objectives in *Healthy People 2010*
- Evaluate the effectiveness of nutritional initiatives of military feeding systems
- Report health and nutrition data from state-based programs to comply with federal administrative program requirements
- Monitor food production and marketing

Nutrition-Related Programs

- Nutrition education and dietary guidance *(Dietary Guidelines for Americans)*
- Food assistance programs

- Nutrition intervention programs
- Public health programs

Regulatory

- Food labeling
- Food fortification
- Food safety

SCIENTIFIC RESEARCH

- Nutrient requirements (Dietary Reference Intakes)
- Diet-health relationships
- Knowledge and attitudes and their relationship to dietary and health behavior
- Nutritional monitoring research—national and international
- Food composition analysis
- Economic aspects of food consumption
- Nutrition education research

From various surveys conducted by the U.S. Department of Health and Human Services and the U.S. Department of Agriculture.

Data from dietary surveys can be used to track food consumption trends over time, examine current dietary practices of specific groups of people, and monitor average intakes of pesticides, toxic substances, radioactive substances, and industrial chemicals. Studies of nutritional status allow monitoring of the general health of a population through health and medical histories, dietary interviews, physical examinations, and laboratory measurements.[3]

Dietary and nutrition surveys are important to government agencies that supervise their country's agriculture and food industries. Data from surveys provide a sound basis for developing policies and programs related to agricultural production, marketing agricultural products, projecting supply and demand, and determining the adequacy of the available food supply.[4] These data provide early warning of impending food shortages and can indicate how such crises may be prevented or alleviated.[5] They have been used to develop the *Dietary Guidelines for Americans* and the nutrition and related health objectives included in *Healthy People 2010.*

Using food balance sheets (see Chapter 3), a government can estimate the "disappearance" of food from its food distribution system and thus arrive at an indirect and rough estimate of food consumption by its citizens. Data on food disappearance or "availability" do not measure actual food consumption, only what enters and leaves the food distribution system. However, these data allow comparisons among different countries and the creation of a world food picture. These comparisons, in turn, can serve as the basis for the formulation of international policies designed to improve the world food and nutrition situation and prevent imbalances in dietary standards among countries.[6]

NUTRITIONAL MONITORING IN THE UNITED STATES

Nutritional monitoring can be defined as "the assessment of dietary or nutritional status at intermittent times with the aim of detecting changes in the dietary or nutritional status of a population."[7] It involves data collection and data analysis in five general areas:

- Nutritional and health status measurements
- Food consumption measurements
- Food composition measurement and nutrient data banks
- Dietary knowledge, behavior, and attitude assessments
- Food supply and demand determinations[1]

Since about the middle of the twentieth century, the U.S. government has sought to obtain objective data on which to base decisions regarding nutrition-related public policies. This was done by the U.S. Department of Agriculture (USDA), which collected food disappear-

ance data and began conducting national household food consumption surveys.

More recently, the federal government has evaluated the food intake of individual Americans through the USDA's Continuing Survey of Food Intakes by Individuals and has assessed the nutritional and health status of the public through the U.S. Department of Health and Human Service's (DHHS) National Health and Nutrition Examination Survey.[8] Some nutritional monitoring activities are conducted at the state level, providing state-specific data on nutritional and health status that may not be available from national surveys. Many of these state activities are supported and coordinated by federal agencies, such as the USDA and DHHS.

NATIONAL NUTRITIONAL MONITORING AND RELATED RESEARCH PROGRAM

As early as 1971, Congress, the nutrition community, various private groups, and expert panels expressed concern about problems with the federal government's nutritional monitoring program and the lack of coordination between the USDA and DHHS. Issues were raised about the frequency and costs of data collected by the two agencies, delays in reporting data, the low response rates seen in some surveys, and, in certain instances, the poor quality of data.[1,8–10] Problems in the two agencies' nutritional monitoring activities were addressed by a number of reports by the National Research Council, the Federation of American Societies for Experimental Biology, and the General Accounting Office (a research arm of Congress that audits government programs and highlights areas of waste and fraud). These reports called for the agencies to develop better methods for collecting dietary intake data, to use standardized data collection techniques that allow data to be compared across the different surveys, and to improve coverage of groups at nutritional risk, such as pregnant and lactating women, infants, preschool children, adolescents, and older persons.[1]

Recognition of the need to improve nutrition monitoring led to passage of the National Nutrition Monitoring and Related Research Act of 1990 (PL 101–445). This legislation required the secretaries of the USDA and DHHS to prepare and implement a comprehensive 10-year plan for integrating the nutritional monitoring activities of the two agencies. This 10-year coordinated effort was called the National Nutrition Monitoring and Related Research Program (NNMRRP).[1,11] The legislation also calls for the creation of an Interagency Board for Nutrition Monitoring and Related Research and a National Nutrition Monitoring Advisory Council.

The NNMRRP coordinates the nutrition monitoring activities of 22 federal agencies under the joint direction of the USDA and DHHS. The program encompasses a group of more than 50 surveys and surveillance activities assessing the health and nutritional status of the U.S. population.[12] The program's goal is to "establish a comprehensive nutrition monitoring and related research program for the federal government by collecting quality data that are continuous, coordinated, timely, and reliable; using comparable methods for data collection and reporting of results; and efficiently and effectively disseminating and exchanging information with data users."[11] Critical to the success of reaching this goal are three overall national objectives and three objectives addressing state and local nutrition monitoring efforts. The three national objectives are (1) to achieve continuous and coordinated data collection, (2) to improve the comparability and quality of data collected by the USDA and DHHS, and (3) to improve the research base for nutrition monitoring. The three state and local objectives are (1) to develop and strengthen state and local capacities for continuous and coordinated data collection; (2) to improve methodologies to enhance comparability of NNMRRP data across federal, state, and local levels; and (3) to improve the quality of state and local nutrition monitoring data.[1,11] The NNMRRP also addresses the need for better nutrition monitoring information about selected population subgroups, more efficient and effective data dissemination to users, and better ways to meet the needs of data users.

The National Nutrition Monitoring and Related Research Act of 1990 placed responsibility for coordinating the NNMRRP with the USDA and DHHS. The Interagency Board for Nutrition Monitoring and Related Research assists in implementing the NNMRRP. The board's members come from approximately 20 other federal agencies (e.g., the Departments of Labor, Commerce, Defense, and Veterans Affairs, as well as the Environmental Protection Agency) and are responsible for representing their agencies in all areas of nutrition monitoring. The board's activities include preparing an annual budget report on nutrition monitoring, preparing biennial reports on the progress of the coordinated program, and preparing periodic scientific reports on the nutritional and related health status of the population.[11]

The act also requires the establishment of the National Nutrition Monitoring Advisory Council. The council is composed of the secretaries of the USDA and DHHS and nine voting members with expertise in the areas of public health, nutrition monitoring research, and food production and distribution. Five of these voting members are appointed by the president and the other four by Congress. The council provides scientific and technical input to the board, evaluates the scientific and technical quality of the comprehensive plan and the effectiveness of the coordinated program, and recommends areas for improvement.[11] The organizational structure of the NNMRRP and members of the Interagency Board are shown in Figure 4.1.

To facilitate data dissemination, the National Nutrition Monitoring and Related Research Act of 1990 requires periodic publication of reports on the dietary, nutritional, and health-related status of the U.S. population. For example, every year the National Center for Health Statistics publishes *Health: United States.* This outstanding publication highlights and updates nutrition monitoring data, information, and research in a user-friendly format, using colorful graphics, extensive data tables, and brief narratives. To improve communication among data users, *The Directory of Federal and State Nutrition Monitoring and Related Research Activities* is periodically published by the Interagency Board for Nutrition Monitoring and Related Research. The directory contains information about federal and state nutrition monitoring activities, the sponsoring agency, contact persons, and the survey's purpose, date, target population, and design.[13] Both of these publications can be downloaded from the website of the National Center for Health Statistics (www.cdc.gov/nchs).

Data collected through surveys are made available in a variety of forms, such as journal articles, government publications, magnetic tapes, CD-ROMs, computer diskettes, and electronic files available for download from various government websites, such as those of the USDA's Food Surveys Research Group and the DHHS's National Center for Health Statistics. Links to these and other websites related to nutrition monitoring can be found at the *Nutritional Assessment* website at www.mhhe.com/hper/nutrition.

ROLE OF THE U.S. DEPARTMENT OF AGRICULTURE

The earliest efforts at nutritional monitoring in the United States were carried out by the USDA.[1,4,14] In the late 1800s and early 1900s, USDA researchers used the food inventory method to collect data on the amounts and costs of food consumed by a relatively small, nonrepresentative group of households. Between 1935 and 1948, the USDA conducted three nationwide, nonrepresentative surveys of food consumption at the household level. Beginning in 1955, the USDA began a series of four nationally representative surveys of food consumption at the household level. The first of these was the 1955 Household Food Consumption Survey (HFCS). This was followed by the 1965–66 HFCS, the 1977–78 Nationwide Food Consumption Survey (NFCS), and the 1987–88 NFCS; these three surveys also measured food intake by individual household members. Following the 1987–88 NFCS, the USDA discontinued efforts to measure household food consumption and focused entirely on assessing individual food intake through the Continuing Survey of Food Intakes by Individuals (CSFII) and the

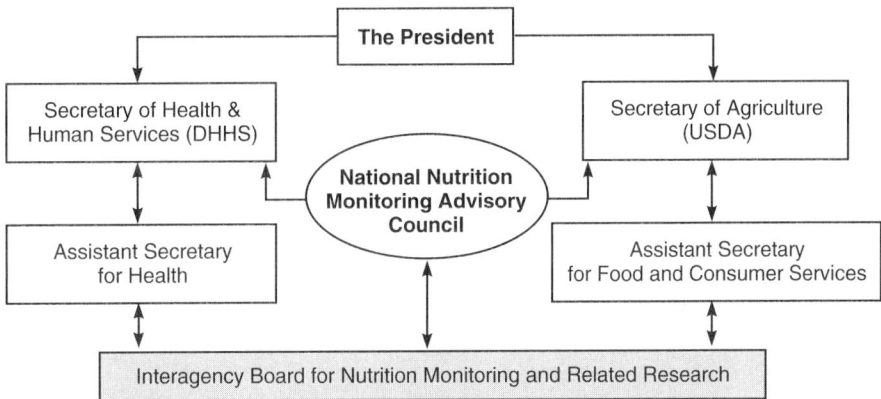

Members:
- Agency for International Development
- Agricultural Research Service, USDA
- Bureau of the Census, DOC
- Bureau of Labor Statistics, DOL
- Cooperative State Research Service, USDA
- Department of Defense
- Department of Education
- Department of Veterans Affairs
- Economic Research Service, USDA
- Environmental Protection Agency
- Extension Service, USDA
- Food and Drug Administration, DHHS
- Food and Nutrition Service, USDA
- Food Safety and Inspection Service, USDA
- Health Resources and Services Administration, DHHS
- Human Nutrition Information Service, USDA
- Indian Health Service, DHHS
- National Center for Chronic Disease Prevention and Health Promotion, CDC, DHHS
- National Center for Health Statistics, CDC, DHHS
- National Institutes of Health, DHHS
- National Marine Fisheries Service, NOAA, DOC
- Substance Abuse and Mental Health Services Administration, DHHS

Figure 4.1

Organizational structure of the National Nutrition Monitoring and Related Research Program and members of the Interagency Board.

Source: U.S. Department of Health and Human Services, U.S. Department of Agriculture. 1994. Ten-year comprehensive plan for the National Nutrition Monitoring and Related Research Program; notice. *Federal Register* 58(111):32751–32806.

dietary knowledge and attitudes of CSFII respondents through the Diet and Health Knowledge Survey. In 1998, the USDA initiated the Supplemental Children's Survey to the CSFII to provide a sample of sufficient size in order to adequately estimate exposure to pesticide residues in the diets of children. The USDA also collects data on the amounts of food passing through the wholesale and retail food distribution system (called food disappearance data) and evaluates food insecurity and hunger in America. Recent, current, and planned nutritional monitoring activities of the USDA and DHHS are described in Table 4.1.

Food Disappearance

Since about the middle of the twentieth century, the USDA has been developing annual estimates of the amount of food that has "disappeared" from the U.S. food distribution system. Known as *food disappearance,* these estimates are also referred to as food available for consumption by the public, or *per capita food availability.*[15,16] These are not direct measures of actual food consumption but, rather, estimates of food that has left the wholesale and retail food distribution system. These estimates, also known as the U.S. Food Supply Series, were the outgrowth of several factors: the need to track food surpluses during World War I, legislation in the early 1930s to ensure an adequate food supply for domestic consumption, and concerns about potential food shortages during the droughts of 1934 and 1936. Estimates of food disappearance for approximately 300 foods were first summarized by the USDA in 1941 to assess food requirements and supplies during World War II. In 1949, food disappearance data from as far back as 1909—the first year for which reliable data were available—were compiled and published.[4]

TABLE 4.1 | **Recent, Current, and Planned Nutritional Monitoring Activities of the USDA and DHHS**

Date	Dept.	Agency	Survey	Target U.S. Population
Nutrition and Related Health Measurements				
Annual	DHHS	CDC/NCHS	National Health Interview Survey (NHIS)	Civilian, noninstitutionalized individuals
Annual	DHHS	CDC/NCHS	National Hospital Discharge Survey	Discharges from nonfederal general and short-stay specialty hospitals
Continuous	DHHS	CDC/NCHS	Vital Statistics Program	Total U.S. population
Continuous	DHHS	CDC/NCCDPHP	Pregnancy Nutrition Surveillance System	Low-income, high-risk pregnant women
Continuous	DHHS	CDC/NCCDPHP	Pediatric Nutrition Surveillance System	Low-income, high-risk children, ages birth to 17 years
Annual	DHHS	CDC/NCHS	National Ambulatory Medical Care Survey	Office visits to nonfederal, office-based physicians
1992—continuous	DHHS	CDC/NCHS	NHANES II Mortality Follow-up Survey	Individuals examined in NHANES II, ages 35–75 years at baseline
1992—continuous	DHHS	CDC/NCHS	Hispanic HANES (HHANES) Mortality Follow-up Survey	Individuals interviewed in HHANES, ages 20–74 years of baseline
1992—annual	DHHS	CDC/NCHS	National Hospital Ambulatory Medical Care Survey	Visits to hospital emergency and outpatients departments of nonfederal, short-stay, general, and specialty hospitals
1992—continuous	DHHS	CDC/NCHS	NHANES III Longitudinal Follow-up Survey	Individuals interviewed and examined in NHANES III, ages 20+ years at baseline
1992—continuous	DHHS	CDC/NCHS	Research on statistical methods: Model-based estimates of NHIS items for states	NA
1994—continuous	DHHS	CDC/NCCDPHP	Adult Nutrition Surveillance System	Adults, ages 18+ years participating in local public health programs
(1997+)	DHHS	CDC/NCHS	National Health and Nutrition Examination Survey (NHANES '97+)	U.S. noninstitutionalized population
Continuous	USDA	ARS	Determination of Nutrient Requirements	U.S. population
Continuous	USDA	ARS	Methods of Assessing Nutritional Status	NA
Continuous	DHHS	CDC/NCEH	Methods of Assessing Nutritional Status	NA or varies
Continuous	USDA	CSRS	Nutrition Research in Support of Nutrition Monitoring	NA or varies
Continuous	DHHS	NIH	Nutrition Research in Support of Nutrition Monitoring	NA or varies
Periodic	DHHS, USDA	TBA	User conferences	NA
Food and Nutrient Consumption				
1994–96—annual	USDA	HNIS	Continuing Survey of Food Intakes by Individuals (CSFII)	Individuals of all ages residing in eligible households nationwide, oversampling of individuals in low-income households
1996	USDA	HNIS	Household Food Consumption Survey	Civilian households, oversampling of low-income households
(1997+)	DHHS	CDC/NCHS	NHANES '97+	See preceding NHANES listing
Annual	DHHS	FDA	Total Diet Study	Representative diets of specific age-sex groups
Continuous	DOD	USARIEM	Nutritional Evaluation of Military Feeding Systems and Military Populations	Enlisted personnel of the Army, Navy, Marine Corps, and Air Force
Continuous	DOL	BLS	Consumer Expenditure Survey	Civilian, noninstitutionalized population and a portion of the institutionalized population in the United States

Frequency	Dept.	Survey/Activity	Agency	Population
Continuous	DOC	Survey of Income and Program Participation	Census	Civilian, noninstitutionalized population of the United States
Continuous	USDA	Research Program on Food Demand	ERS	NA
Periodic	DHHS, USDA	User conferences	TBA	NA

Knowledge, Attitudes, and Behavior Assessments

Frequency	Dept.	Survey/Activity	Agency	Population
Biennial	DHHS	Youth Risk Behavior Survey	CDC/NCCDPHP	Civilian, noninstitutionalized adolescents, ages 12–18 years
1994–96	USDA	Diet and Health Knowledge Survey	HNIS	Selected adults, ages 20+ years in households and noninstitutionalized group quarters participating in the CSFII
Continuous	DHHS	Behavioral Risk Factor Surveillance System	CDC/NCCDPHP	Individuals, ages 18+ years, residing in participating states in households with telephones
Biennial	DHHS	Health and Diet Survey	FDA	Civilian, noninstitutionalized individuals in households with telephones, ages 18+ years
Periodic	DHHS, USDA	User conference	TBA	NA

Food Composition and Nutrient Databases

Frequency	Dept.	Survey/Activity	Agency	Population
Annual	DHHS	Total Diet Study	FDA	NA
Biennial	DHHS	Food Label and Package Survey	FDA	NA
Continuous	USDA	National Nutrient Data Bank	HNIS	NA
Continuous	USDA	Survey Nutrient Data Base	HNIS	NA
Continuous	USDA	Nutrient Composition Laboratory	ARS	NA
Continuous	DHHS	Measurement of Nutrients in Foods	NIH	NA
Periodic	USDA	User conferences	TBA	NA

Food Supply Determinations

Frequency	Dept.	Survey/Activity	Agency	Population
Annual	DOC	Fisheries of the United States	NOAA/NMFS	NA
Annual	USDA	U.S. Food and Nutrition Supply Series	ERS	NA
	USDA	Estimate of Food Available	HNIS	
		Estimate of Nutrients		
Periodic	USDA	User conferences	TBA	NA

Data from the U.S. Department of Health and Human Services and the U.S. Department of Agriculture.

ARS = Agricultural Research Service (USDA); CDC = Centers for Disease Control and Prevention (DHHS); CSRS = Cooperative State Research Service (USDA); (Date) = tentative date; DHHS = U.S. Department of Health and Human Service; DOC = Department of Commerce; DOD = Department of Defense; DOL = Department of Labor; FDA = Food and Drug Administration (DHHS); HHANES = Hispanic Health and Nutrition Examination Survey; HNIS = Human Nutrition Information Service (USDA); NA = not applicable; NCCDPHP = National Center for Chronic Disease Prevention and Health Promotion (DHHS); NCEH = National Center for Environmental Health (DHHS); NCHS = National Center for Health Statistics (DHHS); NHANES = National Health and Nutrition Examination Survey; NIH = National Institutes of Health (DHHS); NMFS = National Marine Fisheries Service (DOC/NOAA); NOAA = National Oceanic and Atmospheric Administration; TBA = to be announced; USARIEM = United States Army Research Institute of Environmental Medicine (DOD); USDA = U.S. Department of Agriculture

Food disappearance data are derived using the **balance sheet approach.** Annual data on food exports, food not meant for human consumption (for example, livestock feed, seed, and food used for industrial purposes), military procurements, and year-end inventories are subtracted from data on beginning-year inventories, total food production, and imports to arrive at an estimate of food available for domestic consumption.[3,4] This estimate then is divided by the U.S. population count to derive per person disappearance (or per capita availability) of food. Per capita availability of energy and a number of nutrients are then calculated using food composition tables.[3,4]

This approach has several drawbacks. It depends almost entirely on data collected for other purposes. The data can vary considerably in adequacy, accuracy, and accessibility. These estimates fail to account for food fed to pets and food losses due to spoilage, disposal of inedible parts, and trimming by the consumer. It does not provide information relating to food consumption on a regional, household, or individual basis. Consequently, these data must be interpreted with care.[4]

Despite these weaknesses, however, the data reflect changes in overall patterns of food disappearance over time and have been the only source of information on food and nutrient trends since the beginning of the twentieth century.[3,7,14] When used in conjunction with similar data developed in other countries, epidemiologists have been able to study the relationships between diet and disease. For example, scientists have investigated how different levels of dietary fat and cholesterol intake across countries relate to coronary heart disease death rates in those countries.[3] Food disappearance data also serve as a rough check on the reasonableness of results from household food consumption surveys.[4] Trends in the per capita availability of energy and nutrients in the U.S. food supply are summarized in the "Dietary Trends" section of this chapter.

Continuing Survey of Food Intakes by Individuals

In 1985, the USDA began a national survey of individual dietary intake known as the *Continuing Survey of Food Intakes by Individuals (CSFII).* The CSFII was initially designed to be conducted annually, except for those years when data were being collected for the NFCS.[7,14] However, it has only been conducted during 1985–86, 1989–91, and 1994–96. The CSFII replaced the NFCS as the USDA's primary survey for estimating individual food and nutrient intake.[1,14] The CSFII provides timely information on U.S. diets; allows further study of the dietary habits of certain population groups thought to be at nutritional risk (e.g., low-income people); provides data on "usual" diets by measuring several days of data

collected over the course of a year; and demonstrates how diets vary over time for individuals and groups of people.

In the 1985–86 CSFII, dietary intake data were collected using 24-hour recalls. In the surveys of women and children, basic household information was obtained, and six 24-hour recalls were collected at approximately 2-month intervals. This not only provided data somewhat more representative of usual dietary intake but also diminished seasonal influence on dietary intake because data were collected throughout the year.

All information in the 1985–86 CSFII was collected by trained interviewers employed by a private contracting agency. Basic household information and the first of the six 24-hour recalls on all age-eligible participants were obtained from the female head of the household or the main meal planner/preparer.[7] An attempt was made to obtain subsequent 24-hour recalls by telephone interview. In the 1985–86 CSFII, about 90% of subsequent 24-hour recalls were obtained by telephone. In households not having a telephone or where the respondent requested to be interviewed in person, succeeding 24-hour recalls were collected by personal interview.[4,7]

In the 1989–91 CSFII, data were collected using one 24-hour recall and a 2-day food diary. In the 1994–96 CSFII, popularly known as the "What We Eat in America" survey, data were collected using two multiple-pass 24-hour recalls administered in the home by trained interviewers. The recalls were conducted on 2 nonconsecutive days, 3 to 10 days apart. In addition to dietary intake data, socioeconomic and health-related information was also collected from respondents.[7,14]

The 1994–96 CSFII was conducted by Westat, Incorporated, a private research firm under contract to the USDA's Agricultural Research Service. A nationally representative sample of approximately 16,000 individuals of all ages from all 50 states participated in the survey. It sampled a disproportionately larger number of low-income people, young children, and older persons to better ascertain their dietary practices. This is known as "oversampling." The response rate was impressive, with 80% of respondents providing at least 1 day of dietary intake data and 76% of respondents providing 2 days of dietary intake data. In addition to providing data on food and nutrient intake in gram and milligram quantities, the 1994–96 CSFII provided data on number of servings of food consumed. This allowed easy comparison of CSFII data with Food Guide Pyramid recommendations. Figure 4.2 compares the average American diet as measured by the 1994–96 CFSII, with recommendations from the Food Guide Pyramid. The figure shows that the average American diet barely meets the minimum recommended number of servings from the grain and vegetable groups, while average consumption from the fruit, dairy, and meat groups falls below the minimum recommended by the pyramid. In contrast, consumption of energy from

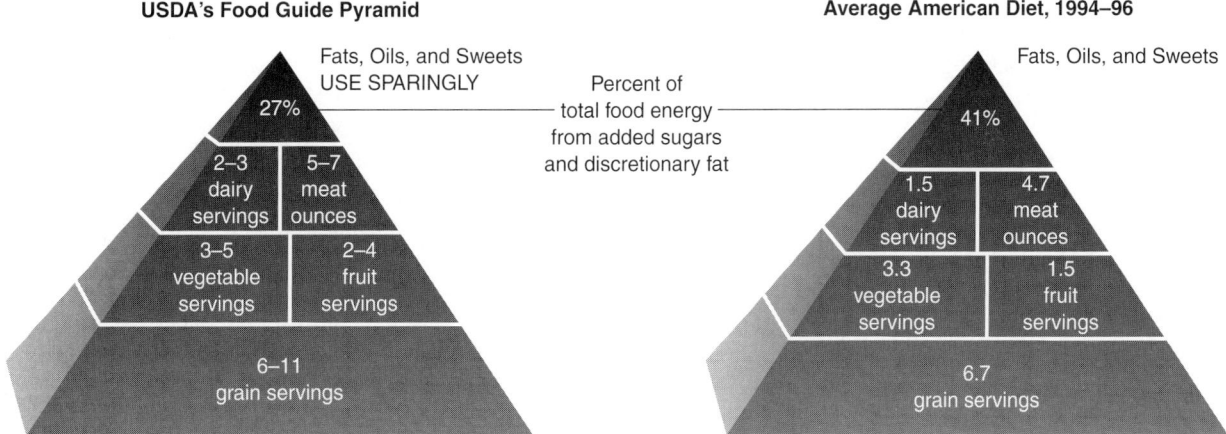

Figure 4.2 The recommendations of the Food Guide Pyramid (on the left) in contrast to the average American diet (all individuals age 2 years and older) as measured by the 1994–96 CFSII (on the right).
Source: Data are from the Food Surveys Research Group, Agricultural Research Service, USDA.

fats, oils, and sweets is much higher (averaging 41% of daily energy intake) than recommended by the pyramid (averaging about 27% of daily energy intake).

Diet and Health Knowledge Survey

During the 1989–91 CSFII, the Diet and Health Knowledge Survey (DHKS) was initiated. The purpose of the DHKS is to measure the attitudes and knowledge of Americans about diet and health. The DHKS provides information about Americans' perceptions about the adequacy of their own food and nutrient intakes, the personal importance they place on dietary guidance messages, their self-appraised weight status, the importance they place on factors related to buying food, and the beliefs they hold that may influence dietary behavior.[14] For example, 56% of respondents in the 1994–96 CSFII/ DHKS reported that they thought their diet was "about right" in calcium. However, nearly two-thirds of these persons had a mean calcium intake less than the 1989 RDA for calcium. Among those adults reporting that their weight was "about right," 45% of adult males and 17% of adult females had a body mass index that placed them in the "overweight" or "obese" category, based on self-reported height and weight.

The DHKS is conducted after the CSFII is completed. For example, approximately 2 weeks after the second 24-hour recall was collected in the 1994–96 CSFII, a group of nearly 6000 persons ages 20 years and older were randomly selected by a computerized process from among all adults who had provided 2 days of dietary intake data. These persons were then contacted by telephone and asked to answer a series of questions on knowledge and attitudes about dietary guidance and health. Administering the DHKS shortly after the completion of the CSFII allows individuals' attitudes and

knowledge about healthy eating to be linked with their food choices and nutrient intakes.

In addition to providing detailed benchmark data on the food and nutrient intakes and eating patterns of the general and low-income populations, the USDA uses data from the CSFII/DHKS to assess the nutritional impact of its food assistance programs, to monitor food security and hunger, and to estimate demand for agricultural products.[14] The USDA and DHHS use these data to evaluate the American diet relative to the *Dietary Guidelines for Americans,* the Food Guide Pyramid, and the *Healthy People 2010* objectives. The Food and Drug Administration uses these data to develop its policies on food enrichment and fortification and food labeling. The data are also used by the National Academy of Sciences in developing the Dietary Reference Intakes and by the Environmental Protection Agency in assessing exposure to pesticide residues, food additives, and contaminants.

Supplemental Children's Survey

The purpose of the Supplemental Children's Survey was to collect dietary intake data from a representative group of children of sufficient size in order to estimate exposure to pesticide residues in the diets of American children. Between December 1997 and November 1998, two 24-hour recalls were collected from roughly 5000 children up to age 9 years. The recalls were obtained through in-person interviews on 2 nonconsecutive days. For infants and children under 6 years of age, a parent or knowledgeable caregiver was asked to provide the data. For children 6 to 9 years of age, the child was interviewed with adult assistance. In addition to the in-home 24-hour recall, interviewers contacted schools, baby-sitters, and day-care providers for information about food eaten away from home.

The Supplemental Children's Survey was a response to concerns about pesticide residues in the diets of infants and children and the lack of good data to accurately assess youngsters' exposure to pesticide residues in the foods they were eating. Concerns about children's exposure to pesticides were heightened by a 1993 report of the National Academy of Sciences entitled "Pesticides in the Diets of Infants and Children." This report was instrumental in passage of the Food Quality Protection Act of 1996, which required the USDA to provide the Environmental Protection Agency with statistically valid information on the food consumption patterns of American infants and children, so that children's exposure to pesticide residues could be estimated with reasonable accuracy.

Food Insecurity and Hunger

The terms *food security, food insecurity,* and *hunger* are defined in Box 4.2. Although hunger in North America (so-called first-world hunger) does not compare in severity to that experienced by many in developing countries (so-called third-world hunger), it is a problem nevertheless. Hunger in North America has been a long-term concern of public health nutritionists on the continent and among some of the more enlightened legislators and policy makers. However, it was only in the 1990s that the U.S. government actually developed a comprehensive national measure of the severity of food insecurity and hunger in the United States.[17] One of the mandates of the National Nutrition Monitoring and Related Research Program (NNMRRP) was that the USDA's Food and Nutrition Service and the DHHS's National Center for Health Statistics jointly develop "a standardized mechanism and instrument(s) for defining and obtaining data on

the prevalence of 'food insecurity' or 'food insufficiency' in the U.S. and methodologies that can be used across the NNMRRP and at state and local levels." In response to this mandate, the USDA led a several-year collaborative effort to draft, pilot-test, and refine an instrument to measure the prevalence and severity of food insecurity and hunger in America, building on the prior work of several nongovernmental organizations. Most notable among these organizations were Cornell University's Division of Nutritional Sciences and the Community Childhood Hunger Identification Project, sponsored by the advocacy organization Food Research and Action Center.[17] Since 1995, the U.S. Bureau of the Census has administered this instrument as part of its annual Current Population Survey, thus providing statistically valid, nationally representative data on the prevalence and severity of food insecurity and hunger in America.[17,18]

The USDA estimates that, in the 12-month period ending in April 1999, nearly 90% of American households were food secure, 7% of American households experienced food insecurity at some time during the year, and 3% experienced food insecurity with hunger at some time during the year, as shown in Figure 4.3 and Table 4.2. Figure 4.4 shows the prevalence for children in U.S. households. It should be noted in Table 4.2 that the prevalence of food insecurity with and without hunger in U.S. children (13.1% and 3.8%, respectively) is greater than that for U.S. adults (7.0% and 2.5%, respectively). Also, the prevalence of food insecurity among black non-Hispanic and Hispanic households is three times greater than in white non-Hispanic households.[19]

The USDA measures food insecurity and hunger using responses to 18 questions about conditions and behaviors known to characterize households having diffi-

---

 Box 4.2   **Definitions of Food Security, Food Insecurity, and Hunger**

FOOD SECURITY

Access by all people at all times to enough food for an active, healthy life. Food security includes at a minimum: (1) the ready availability of nutritionally adequate and safe foods, and (2) an assured ability to acquire acceptable foods in socially acceptable ways (e.g., without resorting to emergency food supplies, scavenging, stealing, or other coping strategies).

FOOD INSECURITY

Limited or uncertain availability of nutritionally adequate and safe food or limited or uncertain ability to acquire acceptable foods in socially acceptable ways.

HUNGER

The uneasy or painful sensation caused by a lack of food. The recurrent and involuntary lack of access to food. Hunger may produce malnutrition over time. It is a potential, although not necessary, consequence of food insecurity.

Source: Andrews M, Nord M, Bickel G, Carlson S. 1999. Household food security in the United States, 1999. *Food Assistance and Nutrition Research Report No. 8.* Food and Rural Economics Division, Economic Research Service, U.S. Department of Agriculture.

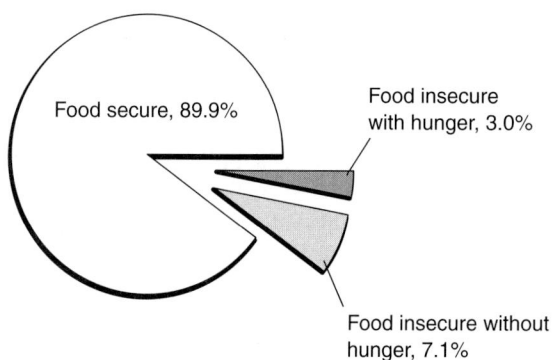

Figure 4.3 **Prevalence of food security, food insecurity, and hunger, U.S. households, 1999.**
Just over 10% of U.S. households experience food insecurity, which continues to be a problem facing millions of Americans. These percentages are for the 12-month period ending in April 1999.
Source: Data from the Economic Research Center, USDA.

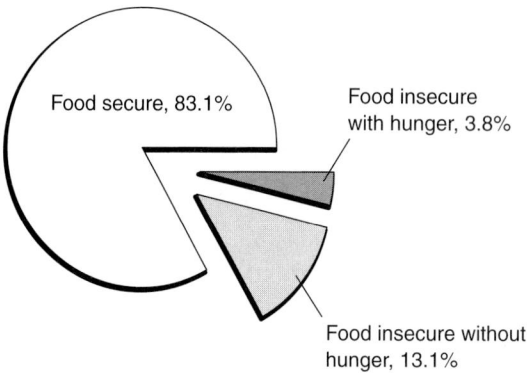

Figure 4.4 **Prevalence of food security, food insecurity, and hunger, U.S. children, 1999.**
Nearly 17% of U.S. children experience food insecurity. More than any other demographic group, children are particularly susceptible to food insecurity and hunger due to their dependence on adults and the nutrient requirements of rapid growth and development. These percentages are for the 12-month period ending in April 1999.
Source: Data from the Economic Research Center, USDA.

culty meeting basic food needs. Each question asks whether the condition or behavior occurred during the previous 12 months and whether the reason for the condition or behavior was a lack of money or other resources to obtain food.[19,20] For example, an interviewer would read the following statement: "We worried whether our food would run out before we got money to buy more." The interviewer would then ask whether, in the past 12 months, this was often, sometimes, or never true in the household. Or the interviewer would ask the following question: "In the past 12 months were you ever hungry, but didn't eat, because you couldn't afford enough food?"

Nationwide Food Consumption Surveys

The Nationwide Food Consumption Surveys were conducted in 1977–78 and 1987–88. Populations targeted by the two surveys included private households in the 48 contiguous states and persons residing in those house-

holds. The surveys included two samples: a basic sample of all households and a low-income sample of households with incomes at or below 130% of the poverty level—a level consistent with eligibility for the Food Stamp Program. The USDA no longer conducts the NFCS, using instead the CSFII.

ROLE OF THE U.S. DEPARTMENT OF HEALTH AND HUMAN SERVICES

The U.S. Department of Health and Human Services (DHHS) has been involved in nutritional and health-related monitoring since the late 1950s, at which time it was known as the Department of Health, Education, and Welfare. Its current name was adopted in 1979. The DHHS's

TABLE 4.2	Prevalence of Food Security, Food Insecurity, and Hunger in the United States by Selected Characteristics, by Percent, 1999 (Percentages Are for the 12-Month Period Ending April 1999)			
		Food Insecure		
Category	**Food Secure**	**All**	**Without Hunger**	**With Hunger**
All households	89.9	10.1	7.1	3.0
All persons in households	88.5	11.5	8.6	2.9
Adults in households	90.5	9.5	7.0	2.5
Children in households	83.1	16.9	13.1	3.8
White non-Hispanic households	93.0	7.0	4.9	2.1
Black non-Hispanic households	78.8	21.2	14.8	6.4
Hispanic households	79.2	20.8	15.3	5.5

Source: Andrews M, Nord M, Bickel G, Carlson S. 1999. Household food security in the United States, 1999. *Food Assistance and Nutrition Research Report No. 8.* Food and Rural Economics Division, Economic Research Service, U.S. Department of Agriculture.

involvement in nutritional monitoring began in response to the National Health Survey Act of 1956, which mandated a continuing survey of the U.S. population for statistical data on amount, distribution, and effects of illness and disability in the United States. To comply with the 1956 act, DHHS conducted a series of three National Health Examination Surveys. These were followed by the landmark Ten-State Nutrition Survey and then the National Health and Nutrition Examination Surveys, including the Hispanic Health and Nutrition Examination Survey. In addition to these, the DHHS is responsible for a number of other surveys related to diet and nutrition, health, knowledge and attitudes, and food labeling. Included among these are the Adult Nutrition Surveillance System, the National Health Interview Survey, the Pediatric Nutrition Surveillance System, the Total Diet Study, the Health and Diet Study, the Behavioral Risk Factor Surveillance System, and the Food Label and Package Survey. These and other surveys related to nutritional monitoring were outlined in Table 4.1.

National Health Examination Surveys

The National Health Examination Surveys (NHES) were a series of three health surveys conducted by the National Center for Health Statistics of the DHHS. NHES I was conducted from 1960 to 1962 and examined the prevalence of selected chronic diseases and health conditions in nearly 7000 Americans 18 to 79 years of age.[21] Using a variety of physical and physiologic measurements, such as blood pressure, serum cholesterol, skinfold measurements, height and weight, and electrocardiography, NHES I was able to focus on such conditions as coronary heart disease, arthritis, rheumatism, and diabetes.[21]

NHES II was conducted from 1963 to 1965 and sampled more than 7000 children 6 to 11 years old. From 1966 to 1970, NHES III studied nearly 7000 persons 12 to 17 years old. A primary task of NHES I and NHES II was to measure growth and development in American children and adolescents. This provided much of the data used by the National Center for Health Statistics in formulating its original growth charts, which have been updated using data from NHANES III (described in Chapter 6 and shown in Appendix N).

Ten-State Nutrition Survey

The Ten-State Nutrition Survey was the nation's first comprehensive survey to assess the nutritional status of a large segment of the U.S. population.[8] During the 1960s, concerns about hunger and malnutrition in America escalated, leading legislators, health professionals, and private citizens to investigate the problem. Their reports revealed "chronic hunger and malnutrition in every part of the United States"[22] and described the situation as "shocking" and having reached "emergency propor-

tions."[8] Congress responded by mandating the Department of Health, Education, and Welfare to conduct a "comprehensive survey of the incidence and location of serious hunger and malnutrition and health problems incident thereto in the United States."[8]

The Ten-State Nutrition Survey targeted geographic areas having high proportions of low-income persons, inner-city residents, and migrant workers. Between 1968 and 1970, data were collected in the following 10 states: California, Kentucky, Louisiana, Massachusetts, Michigan, New York (including New York City), South Carolina, Texas, Washington, and West Virginia.[8]

Although the survey helped reveal the extent and severity of hunger and malnutrition in America, groups surveyed were not representative of the general U.S. population, and consequently its findings could not be extrapolated to the overall population. The survey also demonstrated the difficulty and complexity of assessing nutritional status and recognized the need for additional data on the nutritional status of the U.S. population and the need for a continuing program of national nutritional surveillance. This led to the addition of a nutritional assessment component to the National Health Examination Survey and the beginning of the National Health and Nutrition Examination Survey.[8,23]

National Health and Nutrition Examination Survey

The **National Health and Nutrition Examination Survey (NHANES)** is conducted by the National Center for Health Statistics (NCHS), an agency of the DHHS. Its purpose is to monitor the overall nutritional status of the U.S. population through detailed interviews and comprehensive examinations. Interviews include dietary, demographic, socioeconomic, and health-related questions. Examinations consist of a medical and dental examination, physiologic measurements, and laboratory tests.[12,23,24]

First National Health and Nutrition Examination Survey (NHANES I)

NHANES I, conducted from 1971 to 1975, was designed to assess general health status, with particular emphasis on nutritional status and health of the teeth, skin, and eyes. Its target population was a representative sample of approximately 29,000 noninstitutionalized civilian Americans ages 1 to 74 years. The nutrition component of NHANES I consisted of four major parts: dietary intake based on a 24-hour recall and food frequency questionnaire; biochemical levels of various nutrients based on assays of whole blood, serum, and urine samples; clinical signs of nutrient-deficiency disease; and anthropometric measurements. Although NHANES I originally was designed to provide data on the population's health and nutritional status at the time of the survey (in other words, a **cross-sectional survey**), the

NHANES I Epidemiologic Follow-up Study, conducted in 1982–84, allowed subjects to be reexamined to assess the influence of nutritional status on development of disease and death.

Second National Health and Nutrition Examination Survey (NHANES II)

NHANES II was conducted from 1976 to 1980. It targeted nearly 28,000 noninstitutionalized civilian Americans 6 months to 74 years of age, of which more than 25,000 (91%) were interviewed and more than 20,000 (73%) were examined. Examination components included dietary interviews, anthropometric measurements, a variety of biochemical assays on whole blood, serum, and urine, glucose tolerance tests, blood pressure measurement, electrocardiography, and radiography of the chest and cervical and lumbar spine.[7]

Hispanic Health and Nutrition Examination Survey (HHANES)

HHANES was the largest and most comprehensive Hispanic health survey ever conducted in the United States. Planning for the survey began in 1979, and the actual data were collected from 1982 to 1984 under the direction of the NCHS.[25] The survey collected health and nutritional data on the three largest subgroups of Hispanics living in the 48 contiguous states: nearly 9500 Mexican Americans residing in five southwestern states (Arizona, California, Colorado, New Mexico, and Texas); more than 2000 Cuban Americans living in Dade County, Florida; and more than 3500 Puerto Ricans residing in the New York City metropolitan area (selected countries in New York, New Jersey, and Connecticut).[25,26] Response rates ranged from 79% to 89% for interviews and from 61% to 75% for physical examinations. Because HHANES was not designed as a national Hispanic survey, its results do not necessarily apply to all Hispanics living in the United States. However, the sampled population included about 76% of the Hispanic-origin population of the United States as of 1980.[25]

Rather than providing a comprehensive picture of the health status or total health care needs of Hispanics,

HHANES was designed to obtain basic data on certain chronic conditions and baseline health and nutritional information. As in NHANES, HHANES used five data-collecting techniques: interviews, physical examinations, diagnostic testing, anthropometrics, and laboratory tests.[25,27,28] Interviews were conducted at the homes of survey participants, followed by examinations at a mobile examination center, which consisted of three connected semitrailers, which were specially designed and equipped for testing.[27] The nutritional component included an evaluation of iron status and anemia, serum vitamin A levels, and food consumption as related to diabetes, digestive diseases, overweight, dental health, and alcohol consumption.[25]

Third National Health and Nutrition Examination Survey (NHANES III)

Data collection for NHANES III began October 1988 and ended October 1994.[12,24,29] The survey was conducted in two phases of equal length and sample size. A total of approximately 40,000 noninstitutionalized Americans ages 2 months and older were asked to complete an extensive examination and interview. The response rates for the interview and examination were 86% and 78%, respectively.[12] Four population groups were specially targeted for examination: children ages 2 months to 5 years, persons 60 years of age and older, black Americans, and Mexican Americans.[24] A disproportionately large number of persons in these four groups were examined to appropriately assess their nutritional and health status. The five primary goals of NHANES III are shown in Box 4.3.

In planning for the survey in 1985, the NCHS intended it to provide several types of data: prevalence estimates of compromised nutritional status and trends in nutrition-related risk factors; data on the relationships among diet, nutritional status, and health; prevalence estimates of overweight and obesity in the U.S. population; and anthropometric data on children and adolescents, allowing revision of the original NCHS growth charts (see Chapter 6 and Appendix N), which were based on

---

 Box **4.3**   **Goals of NHANES**

1. To estimate the number and percent of persons in the U.S. population and designated subgroups with selected diseases and risk factors
2. To monitor trends in the prevalence, awareness, treatment, and control of selected diseases
3. To monitor trends in risk behaviors and environmental exposures

4. To analyze risk factors for selected diseases
5. To study the relationship among diet, nutrition, and health
6. To explore emerging public health issues and new technologies
7. To establish a national probability sample of genetic material for future genetic testing

Source: National Center for Health Statistics.

data collected before 1976.[30,31] Four areas received special emphasis: child health, health of older Americans, occupational health, and environmental health.

The Food and Drug Administration (FDA) is using data from NHANES III to evaluate the need to change fortification regulations for the nation's food supply. NHANES III data have been used in evaluating public education efforts, such as the National Cholesterol Education Program. Many of the health objectives for the year 2010, including several in the nutrition priority area, rely on data from NHANES III. The National Institute of Occupational Safety and Health is comparing certain data (for example, pulmonary and central nervous system functioning) with those obtained in smaller studies of workers' health in various occupational settings.[23]

Examination and interviews were conducted in specially equipped and designed mobile examination centers (MEC), which traveled to survey locations throughout the country. Each MEC consisted of four trailers, approximately 48 feet long by 8 feet wide, providing about 1570 square feet of space. Several days before a survey was to begin at a particular location, the trailers were transported to the survey site, aligned, and leveled (as shown in Figure 4.5), and

Figure 4.5 **The mobile examination center used in the third National Health and Nutrition Examination Survey.**

all connections of the passageways, electricity, water, and sewer were made. Each MEC contained a laboratory; examination rooms for physical, dental, and X-ray examinations; a computer room; and other rooms for conducting interviews and collecting specimens.[24] The floor plan of the MEC is shown in Figure 4.6. There were three MECs and

Figure 4.6 **The floor plan of the mobile examination centers used in the third National Health and Nutrition Examination Survey.**

Source: Adapted from the National Center for Health Statistics. 1994. *Plan and operation of the Third National Health and Examination Survey, 1988–1994.* Hyattsville, MD: U.S. Department of Health and Human Services, Public Health Service, Centers for Disease Control and Prevention.

two separate examination teams. Therefore, a set of trailers could always be moved from one survey site to another, parked, set up, and made ready by the time an examination team arrived. A link to the National Center for Health Statistics' "virtual tour" of the MEC is available at the *Nutritional Assessment* website at www.mhhe.com/hper/nutrition.

In NHANES III, the 24-hour recall served as the primary dietary assessment method. Recalls were collected in the MEC (unless participants were unable to leave home). Most of the food frequency questionnaires were completed at home at the same time a detailed health questionnaire was completed by each participant. Recalls were completed using an automated, interactive, micro-computer-based interview procedure called the NHANES III Dietary Data Collection (DDC) system. The DDC was developed by the University of Minnesota's Nutrition Coordinating Center and includes a standardized interview format and automated probes to obtain detailed information about foods, including brand names, food preparation methods, and ingredients used in food preparation, particularly ingredients that contribute fat and sodium.[32] Information recorded in the 24-hour recalls included the time foods were consumed, food names, type of meal or snack, and where the foods were consumed.

Approximately 3500 participants in NHANES III who were 50 years of age or older completed two additional and unscheduled 24-hour recalls, which were collected by telephone interviews approximately 8 and 16 months after the initial 24-hour recall.[24] This was part of the Supplemental Nutrition Survey of Older Americans, a special study collecting data on the diets of older Americans.

NHANES III also used a food frequency questionnaire to provide supplemental information on food and food group consumption; intake of alcohol, calcium, and caffeine; and vitamin and mineral supplement use. The questionnaire was designed to provide qualitative data for ranking respondents by intake of specific foods and food groups. It was not intended to collect quantitative data on the actual amounts of nutrients consumed. It used a 1-month reference period and did not collect information on portion sizes. Researchers were particularly interested in foods containing nutrients related to risk for cancer, cardiovascular disease, and osteoporosis. As part of data collected to study osteoporosis, adults were asked to report their milk consumption during five age periods: 5–12 years, 13–17 years, 18–35 years, 36–65 years, and 65 years of age and older. Responses were recorded as "more than once per day," "once per day," "less than once per day, but more than once per week," "once per week," "less than once per week," or "never." Additional questions were asked about water intake, use of vitamin and mineral supplements, meal and snack patterns, infant feeding practices, and alcohol intake.

NHANES III also studied the impact of food insecurity on dietary intake, nutritional status, and health. At the family level, questions were asked about the number of days per month on which there was no food or money to buy food and the reasons for the problem. Individuals were asked the frequency of and reasons for skipping meals and going without food. Table 4.3 summarizes the nutrition-related information collected in NHANES III by respondent age and information type.

Each of the two examination teams consisted of a group of 16 persons, who worked and traveled together. They included two dietary interviewers, a physician, a dentist, an ultrasonographer, four X-ray technicians, a phlebotomist, three medical technologists, a health interviewer, a home examiner, and a coordinator. Two locally hired staff supplemented the team at each site. Most of the staff, especially the interviewers, were fluent in both Spanish and English. Although the interviewing staff were not required to have academic credentials, most were experienced interviewers who represented a cross section of society. A large staff of interviewers conducted the household interviews. In each location, local health and government officials were notified of the upcoming survey. Households in the survey received an advance letter and booklet to introduce the survey.

TABLE 4.3	Nutrition-Related Information Collected in NHANES III by Respondent Age and Information Type
Information	**Age**
24-hour dietary recall	2 months and over
Food security*	2 months and over
Food program participation*	2 months and over
Drinking water source* and quantity	2 months and over
Vitamin and mineral supplement usage	2 months and over
Salt use frequency and type	2 months and over
Instant food frequency	2 to 11 months
Breakfast practices	1 year and over
Dietary changes for health reasons	1 year and over
Infant feeding practices, including breast-feeding	2 months to 5 years
Food frequency	12 years and over
Alcohol use	12 years and over
Antacids use	17 years and over
Lifetime milk frequency	20 years and over
Self- (or proxy-) reported height and weight	2 months and over
Self- (or proxy-) assessed weight status	2 months and over
Birth weight	2 months to 11 years
Weight loss practices and reasons	1 year and over
Desired weight	12 years and over
Weight history	25 years and over

From National Center for Health Statistics. 1994. *Plan and operation of the Third National Health and Examination Survey, 1988–1994.* Hyattsville, MD: U.S. Department of Health and Human Services, Public Health Services Centers for Disease Control and Prevention.

*Also collected at the household (family) level.

Participants were provided with transportation to and from the MEC. Participants received $30 cash for completing the 4-hour examination and an additional $20 if they arrived at the MEC on time and, if requested, were fasting. As shown in Table 4.4, all participants received a physical examination, various anthropometric measures, hearing tests, and a dietary interview. Depending on the participant's age, additional examination components were performed. In general, the older the participant, the more extensive the examination. Those unable to go to the MEC were given a less extensive examination in their homes.

NHANES III included several diagnostic procedures not used in previous NHANES studies, including bioelectrical impedance (see Chapter 6) and bone densitometry measurements using dual-energy X-ray absorptiometry (see Chapter 9). A variety of measures were used to assess nutritional status in NHANES III (see Figure 4.7). In addition to numerous biochemical tests, a variety of anthropometric measures were performed on participants, as shown in Table 4.5.

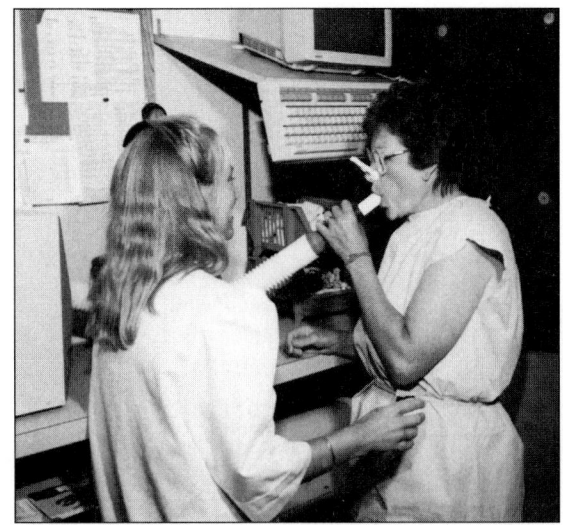

Figure 4.7 A pulmonary function test is an example of the many types of diagnostic procedures performed as part of the third National Health and Nutrition Examination Survey.

TABLE **4.4**	**Examination Components of NHANES III by Age Group**				
2 Months to 5 Years	**6 to 19 Years**	**20 to 39 Years**	**40 to 59 Years**	**60 to 74 Years**	**75 Years and Over**
Physician's examination	Physician's examination	Physician's examination	Physician's examination	Physician's examination	Physician's examination
Dental examination*	Dental examination	Dental examination	Dental examination	Dental examination	Dental examination
Body measurements†	Body measurements	Body measurements†	Body measurements†	Body measurements†	Body measurements†
Venipuncture*	Venipuncture	Venipuncture†	Venipuncture†	Venipuncture†	Venipuncture†
Dietary interview	Dietary interview	Dietary interview	Dietary interview	Dietary interview	Dietary interview
Health interview	Health interview	Health interview	Health interview	Health interview	Health interview
	Urine collection	Urine collection	Urine collection	Urine collection	Urine collection
	Spirometry‡	Spirometry†	Spirometry†	Spirometry†	Spirometry†
	Bioelectric impedance§	Bioelectric impedance	Bioelectric impedance	Bioelectric impedance	Bioelectric impedance
	Allergy test	Allergy test‖	Allergy test‖	———	———
	Audiometry	———	———	———	———
	Tympanometry	———	———	———	———
	Cognitive test¶	———	———	Cognitive test†	Cognitive test†
		Bone density examination	Bone density examination	Bone density examination	Bone density examination
		Ultrasound examination	Ultrasound examination	Ultrasound examination	———
		CNS test‖	CNS test‖	———	———
		Fundus photography	Fundus photography	Fundus photography	
		Electrocardiography	Electrocardiography	Electrocardiography	
				Performance test†	Performance test†
				Hand/knee X rays	Hand/knee X rays

From National Center for Health Statistics. 1994. *Plan and operation of the Third National Health and Examination Survey, 1988–1994.* Hyattsville, MD: U.S. Department of Health and Human Services, Public Health Service, Centers for Disease Control and Prevention.

*1 year of age and over.   §12 years of age and over.

†Also included in the home examination.   ‖Half-sample only. (CNS is central nervous system.)

‡8 years of age and over.   ¶6–16 years of age.

TABLE 4.5	Anthropometric Measures Performed in NHANES III by Age Group[*]					
	2 to 23 Months	24 to 47 Months	4 to 7 Years	8 to 19 Years	20 to 59 Years	60+ Years
Standing height		X	X	X	X	X
Recumbent length	X	X				
Sitting height		X	X	X	X	X
Knee height						X
Upper-leg length		X	X	X	X	X
Upper-arm length	X	X	X	X	X	X
Head circumference	X	X	X			
Midthigh circumference		X	X	X	X	
Calf circumference		X	X	X	X	X
Waist circumference		X	X	X	X	X
Buttocks circumference		X	X	X	X	X
Midupper-arm circumference	X	X	X	X	X	X
Subscapular skinfold	X	X	X	X	X	X
Suprailiac skinfold		X	X	X	X	X
Midthigh skinfold		X	X	X	X	
Triceps skinfold	X	X	X	X	X	X
Biiliac breadth		X	X	X	X	X
Elbow breadth		X	X	X	X	X
Wrist breadth		X	X	X	X	X
Biacromial breadth		(36–47 months)[†]	X	X	X	X
Weight	X	X	X	X	X	X
Bioelectrical impedance				(12+ years)	X	X

From Woteki CE, Briefel RR, Kuczmarski R. 1988. Contributions of the National Center for Health Statistics. *American Journal of Clinical Nutrition* 47:320–328.

[*]NHANES III = third National Health and Examination Survey.

[†]Numbers in parentheses indicate ages of participants who received certain examinations. For example, (36–47 months) indicates that a particular test within the age group only was conducted on participants ages 36 to 47 months.

The Future of NHANES

A number of important changes have been made in the National Health and Nutrition Examination Survey in response to the recommendations of the National Nutrition Monitoring and Related Research Act of 1990. For example, NHANES is now a continuous, annual survey that is better integrated with other nutritional monitoring activities of the U.S. federal government, such as the CSFII and the National Health Interview Survey. Every year, data are collected from a representative sample of the U.S. population, from newborns to older persons, whereas previously it took as long as 6 years before a representative population sample was assessed. This change permits results to be reported in a more timely manner, whereas before this change researchers sometimes had to wait as long as 10 years before gaining access to data that were representative of the entire U.S. population. In addition, the DHHS and USDA have decided to merge NHANES and the CSFII and to call the integrated survey the National Food and Nutrition Survey. By working cooperatively and combining the expertise of their respective staffs, the two agencies can provide more comprehensive and more accurate infor-

mation on the health and nutrition characteristics of the U.S. population in a cost-effective and timely manner.

Other DHHS Surveys

Other surveys providing important data on health and food and nutrient intake include the Total Diet Study, the Navajo Health and Nutrition Survey, the Pregnancy Nutrition Surveillance System, the Pediatric Nutrition Surveillance System, the Health and Diet Survey, and the Behavioral Risk Factor Surveillance System.

The Total Diet Study is conducted annually by the Food and Drug Administration. It provides national estimates of average dietary intakes for 11 nutritional elements, four toxic metals, and various pesticide residues, industrial chemicals, additives, and radionuclides for 14 age-sex groups. Four or more times a year, the FDA purchases foods in grocery stores in selected cities in four geographic areas of the United States. These foods are among a group of approximately 265 "core" foods in the U.S. diet (i.e., foods that are among the most commonly eaten by Americans). These foods are then analyzed for nutrients, toxic metals, and pesticides, among other things. Data from these analyses are then combined with food consumption data from the CSFII and NHANES to arrive at estimates of daily intakes of these substances. The Total Diet Study allows the FDA to monitor the exposure of Americans to these substances, some of which are harmful if consumed in excess. If necessary, the FDA can take action to limit the use of pesticides, additives, and industrial chemicals in agriculture and food processing to maintain the public's exposure to these substances within desirable ranges.[11]

The Navajo Health and Nutrition Survey was planned by the Indian Health Service to establish prevalence data on nutrition-related chronic diseases and to generate a valid description of nutritional status and dietary behaviors of the Navajo people in general and for selected subgroups within that population. The sample size goal was 1700, and data collection took place over a 5-month period during 1991–92. Information was collected on dietary intake, food frequency, anthropometric measurements, lipid profiles, blood pressure, and full blood chemistries, including glucose tolerance tests.[11]

The Pregnancy Nutrition Surveillance System, conducted by the Centers for Disease Control and Prevention (CDC), is designed to monitor the prevalence of nutrition-related problems and behavioral risk factors that are related to infant mortality and low birth weight among high-risk prenatal populations. These include overweight,

underweight, smoking, and alcohol consumption. The system also is studying the relationship of nutritional status to weight gain during pregnancy and birth outcome. Data are collected from health, nutrition, and food assistance programs for pregnant women, such as WIC and prenatal clinics funded by Maternal and Child Health Block Grant and state monies.[11]

The Pediatric Nutrition Surveillance System, conducted by the CDC, is designed to continuously monitor the prevalence of major nutritional problems among high-risk, low-income infants and children from birth to 17 years of age. The system is based on information routinely collected by health, nutrition, and food assistance programs, such as WIC; Early and Periodic Screening, Diagnosis, and Treatment (EPSDT); Head Start; and child health clinics operating under the Maternal and Child Health Block Grant. The Pediatric Nutrition Surveillance System was designed to improve the management of state child health programs and to allow states to develop and monitor state-based nutrition objectives. Program managers use this information to target high-risk subgroups of the population for interventions and to evaluate the effectiveness of interventions designed to reduce nutrition problems in infants and children.[11] An example of data collected by the Pediatric Nutrition Surveillance System is shown in Figure 4.8. This figure shows that, between 1980 and

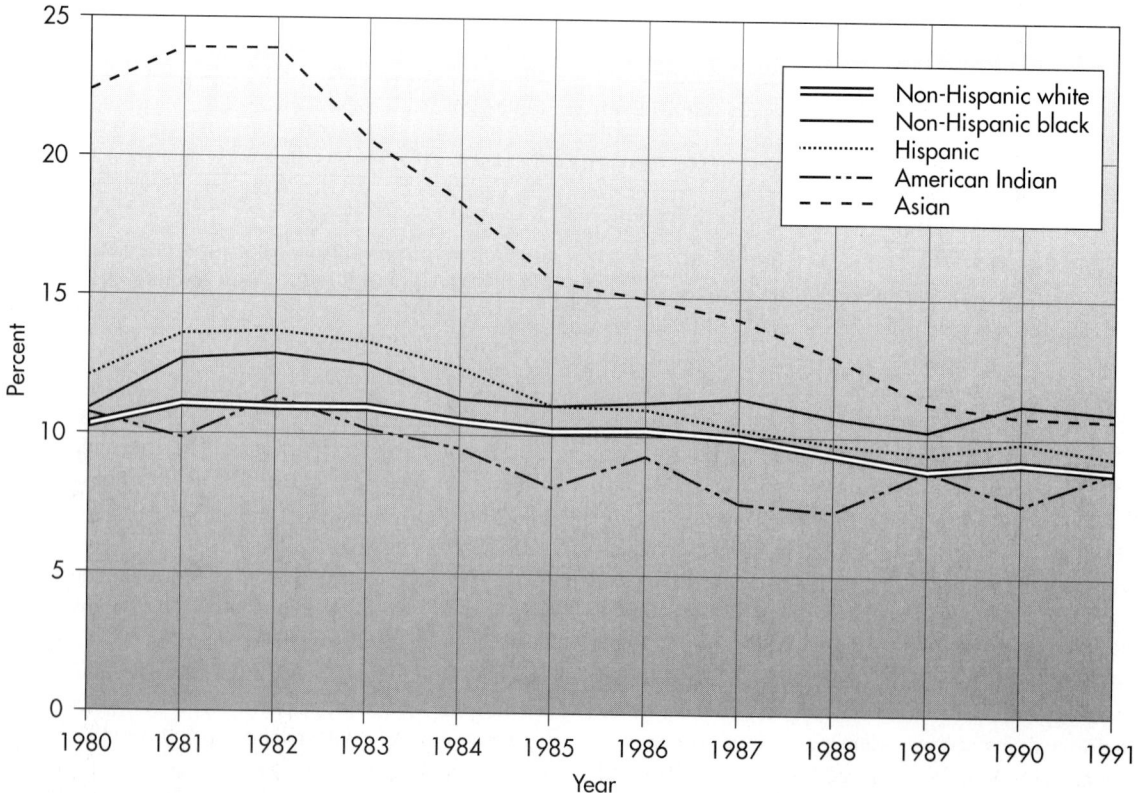

Figure 4.8 **Percent of children 2 to 5 years of age with height-for-age less than the 5th percentile, by race and ethnicity, 1980–1991.**

This is an example of data collected by the Pediatric Nutrition Surveillance System.

Source: Data from the Centers for Disease Control and Prevention, National Center for Chronic Disease Prevention and Health Promotion, Division of Nutrition, Pediatric Nutrition Surveillance System.

1991, the prevalence of short stature for low-income Asian children 2 to 5 years of age (represented by a height-for-age less than the 5th percentile) declined. This indicates that the nutritional status of this group (predominantly Southeast Asian refugees) improved markedly. During the same time, growth status remained stable for the other groups represented in the figure.[33]

The Health and Diet Survey is a telephone survey of a nationally representative sample of American households conducted biennially (every 2 years) by the FDA. Participants are asked a core set of questions relating to health and nutrition that are included in each survey and additional questions that provide timely information on current health and diet issues or special topics. Topics covered by the survey include knowledge and perceptions about sodium, cholesterol, fats, and food labels; self-reported health-related behaviors, such as dieting, sodium avoidance, and efforts to lower blood pressure and blood cholesterol levels; and beliefs about the relationships between diet and cancer, high blood pressure, and heart disease. Survey data have been used to evaluate the effectiveness of public education initiatives of various federal agencies, such as the National Cholesterol Education Program.[11]

The Behavioral Risk Factor Surveillance System (BRFSS) was established in 1984 by the Centers for Disease Control and Prevention and is one of the world's largest ongoing health surveillance systems.[34,35] It is a state-based telephone survey of the civilian, non-institutionalized adult population intended to provide state-based data on the prevalence of personal health practices identified as risk factors for 1 or more of the 10 leading causes of death. In contrast, NHANES and other national surveys do not provide data that are specific to a particular state or region within a state. Data from the BRFSS are used by state and local health departments to plan, initiate, and guide health promotion and disease prevention programs, as well as to monitor the success of such programs over time. The BRFSS is administered by state health departments each month in all 50 states, the District of Columbia, and Puerto Rico. The questionnaire used in the BRFSS includes a core set of questions asked of respondents in all states, an "optional module" of questions developed by the CDC that states can elect to use if they wish, and "state-added questions" developed by individual states. In addition to demographic questions (e.g., sex, age, race, marital status, income, county of residence), the questionnaire asks about health status, health care access, exercise, weight control, diabetes, oral health, tobacco use, alcohol consumption, fruit and vegetable intake, awareness of hypertension and cholesterol, and the like. Several pages from a recent BRFSS questionnaire are shown in Appendix L.

Figure 4.9 shows the prevalence of obesity in 1991 and 1998, based on data collected by the BRFSS.

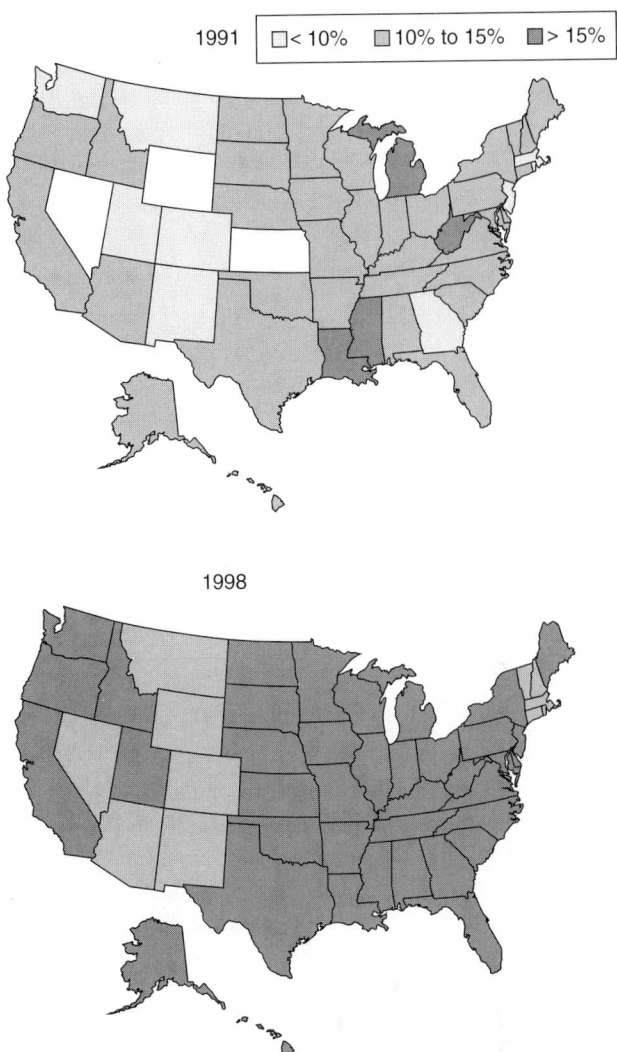

Figure 4.9

This is an example of data collected by the Behavioral Risk Factor Surveillance System, showing the prevalence of obesity (defined as BMI $\geq$ 30 kg/m^2) in American adults in 1991 and 1998, by state. In this figure, BMI is calculated from self-reported height and weight. States are white in 1991 because height and weight data were not collected.

Source: Data from the National Center for Chronic Disease Prevention and Health Promotion, Centers for Disease Control and Prevention.

In Figure 4.9, obesity is defined as a body mass index (BMI) $\geq$ 30 kg/m^2, which is calculated using self-reported height and weight data collected by a telephone interview. Given the fact that overweight participants in self-reported studies tend to underestimate their weight and all participants tend to overestimate their height, it is reasonable to assume that these data underestimate the true prevalence of obesity.[36,37] Despite the problems associated with self-reported data, the BRFSS is the most important source of state-based data on nutrition and health.

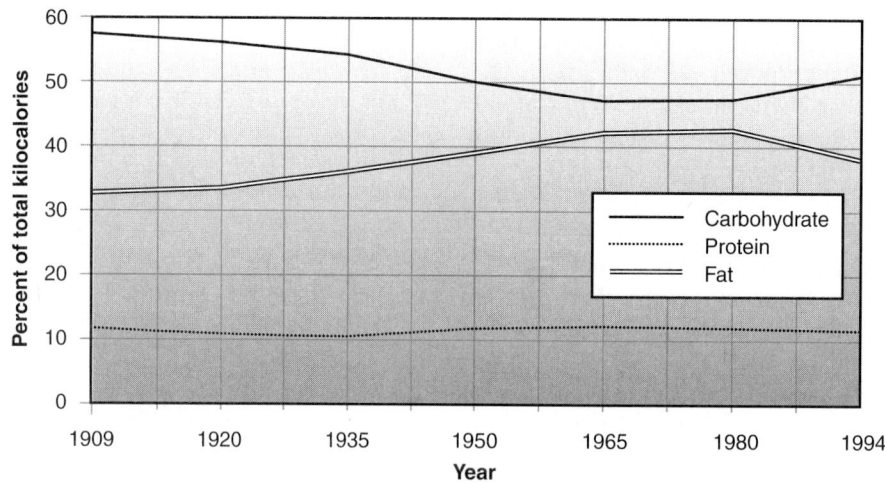

Figure 4.10 Percent of food energy (percent of total kilocalories) contributed by carbohydrate, protein, and fat from 1909 to 1994, based on U.S. Department of Agriculture data.

DIETARY TRENDS

Data on food disappearance and consumption at the individual level have revealed a number of significant changes in the American diet.[3] These include changes in the sources of food energy; average amounts of energy consumed by Americans; use of specific food groups, including alcoholic and nonalcoholic beverages, and changes in eating patterns; such as snacking and eating away from home. In the following sections, some of the data presented are based on food disappearance (or availability), whereas other data are derived from surveys that measured actual food consumption (or at least attempted to). Food disappearance data fail to consider food lost from spoilage, cooking, removal of inedible parts of food, or food fed to animals.

Sources of Food Energy

The distribution of food energy from carbohydrate, fat, and protein has changed since the USDA's Economic Research Service first began compiling food disappearance data. This is shown in Figure 4.10. From 1909 to 1994, energy available from protein remained essentially unchanged at 11% to 12% of total kilocalories. Percentage of kilocalories available from carbohydrate declined from 57% in 1909 to 46% in the 1970s and then increased modestly to about 51% in 1994. Fat availability ranged from a low of about 33% in 1909 to a high of about 43% in the 1970s. In more recent years, fat availability appears to have declined slightly to about 38% of total kilocalories in 1994.

Data from NHANES III for percent of kilocalories from carbohydrate, fat, protein, and alcohol are shown in Figure 4.11. Values for persons ages 2 months to 19 years are shown in part **A,** while values for persons ages 20 years and over are shown in part **B.** Mean percentages of kilocalories from carbohydrate, fat, protein, and alcohol for both males and females ages 20 years and older, as measured by the 1994–96

A   B

Figure 4.11 Percent of kilocalories from carbohydrate, fat, protein, and alcohol, based on data from NHANES III. Values for persons ages 2 months to 19 years are shown in **A.** Values for persons ages 20 years and over are shown in **B.** Numbers may not add up to 100 due to rounding.

Source: Data from McDowell MA, Briefel RR, Alaimo K, Bischof AM, Caughman CR, Carroll MD, Loria CM, Johnson CL. 1994. Energy and macronutrient intakes of persons ages 2 months and over in the United States: Third National Health and Nutrition Examination Survey, Phase 1, 1988–1991. *Advance Data from Vital and Health Statistics.* No. 255. Hyattsville, MD: National Center for Health Statistics.

CSFII, are shown in Figure 4.12. According to surveys conducted between 1965 and 1996 that measured actual food and nutrient intake, the percentage of kilocalories from fat has ranged from a high of 42.1% to a low of 32.8%, as shown in Figure 4.13. Although the percentages in Figure 4.13 seem somewhat inconsistent from one survey to the next, the figure does suggest that the mean percent of kilocalories from fat in the diets of American adults has gradually declined in recent years but is still higher than the recommended upper limit of 30%.

It is important to note that factors other than changes in food consumption practices over time influence the reported percentages of kilocalories from fat in the various surveys represented in Figure 4.13. Among these are differences in how surveys collect dietary intake data, changes in the public's perceptions regarding certain "sensitive food items," ways in which foods are coded, and changes in nutrient content databases. Not all of the surveys represented in Figure 4.13 used the same methods to collect dietary intake data. Research on food intake methodology and advances in technology have led to considerable change and improvement in the way dietary intake data are collected. For example, compared with NHANES II, there was a greater percentage of 24-hour recalls collected for weekend days in NHANES III. In NHANES II, the 24-hour recalls were collected on paper forms and manually coded by dietary interviewers, whereas NHANES III used the Dietary Data Collection system. In addition, the interviewers systematically probed for detailed information about all foods consumed and items added at the table. There were also differences between NHANES II and NHANES III in food coding and the nutrient composition databases used. An important change in the CSFII 1994–96 was use of the multiple-pass approach to collecting 24-hour recalls (discussed in Chapter 3), which likely improved the quality of data collected in that survey, compared with the data collected by the survey of previous years.

As mentioned in Chapter 3, underreporting of food intake by as much as 25% frequently occurs, particularly in females, overweight persons, and those who are weight conscious. In NHANES III, this was addressed by comparing a participant's reported energy intake

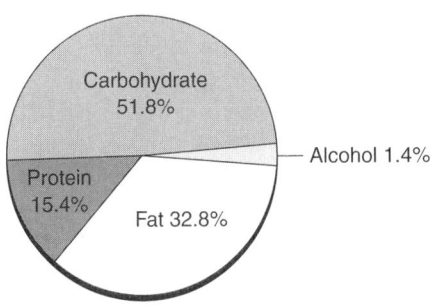

Figure 4.12 **Mean percent of kilocalories from carbohydrate, fat, protein, and alcohol for both males and females ages 20 years and older, from the 1994–96 CSFII.**

Source: Data from USDA, Food Survey Research Group.

Figure 4.13 **Percent of kilocalories from fat in the diets of American adults for selected years, 1965–96.**
Although these percentages seem somewhat inconsistent from one survey to the next, the data suggest that mean percentage of kilocalories from fat has gradually declined in recent years. This is particularly evident in the figure's last three surveys, which have benefited from improvements in food intake data collection methodology.

Source: Data from the USDHHS National Center for Health Statistics and the USDA Foods Survey Research Group.

with his or her calculated resting energy expenditure. If the reported usual energy intake was < 1.2 times the participant's calculated resting energy expenditure, underreporting of energy intake, and therefore, nutrient intake, was probable. The stigma or status attached to consuming certain foods and beverages (so-called sensitive items) can result in either underreporting or overreporting of these foods. For example, changes in public attitudes toward moderate alcohol consumption can influence a respondent's honesty in reporting his or her alcoholic beverage consumption. Given the efforts made to ensure the collection of high-quality data, the estimates of food and nutrient intake from NHANES III and the CSFII 1994–96 are probably among the best available to date.

Major dietary surveys of the past several decades indicate that the percent of kilocalories from carbohydrate in the American diet is increasing. According to data from the CSFII 1994–96 and NHANES III, percent of kilocalories from carbohydrate (excluding alcoholic beverages) for all persons averaged 51.8% and 49%, respectively. Percentage of energy from carbohydrate for males and females ages 20 years and over and for all persons of both sexes are shown in Figure 4.14. Females tend to have a greater carbohydrate intake than males, as do children and adolescents compared with older persons. In contrast, the percent of kilocalories from protein has changed little over the past several decades. Average protein intake for adults was 15.4% kilocalories, according to the CSFII 1994–96.

Based on data from NHANES III, protein provided 16% of kilocalories. Sources of protein in the U.S. diet based on data collected by NHANES III are shown in Figure 4.15.

Trends in Carbohydrates

Availability of total carbohydrates declined from about 488 g/day during 1909 to a low of about 370 g/day between 1963 and 1965. This decline was primarily due to decreased use of starches from grain products (flour and cereals), as shown in Figure 4.16. Since the mid-1960s, availability of carbohydrates increased to about 491 g/day in 1994. Figure 4.17 shows that, between the NFCS 1977–78 and the CSFII 1994–96, there were noticeable increases in the consumption of soft drinks, fruit drinks and ades, beer, all beverages, bananas, and mixed dishes containing red meat, poultry, and fish. During the same time, consumption of all milk and whole milk decreased.[38]

Based on NHANES III data, mean dietary fiber intake for males and females of all ages is 17.0 g/day and 12.8 g/day, respectively.[39] Mean dietary fiber intakes from CSFII 1994–96 were 18.6 g and 13.9 g for males and females ages 20 and older, respectively. These values remain below the 20 to 35 g/day recommended by the Life Sciences Research Office's Expert Panel on Dietary Fiber. According to NHANES III data, females consume more dietary fiber per 1000 kcal (7.36 g/1000 kcal) than males (6.86 g/1000 kcal).

Figure 4.14   Percent of kilocalories from carbohydrate for males and females ages 20 years and over and for both sexes of all ages, based on data collected by the National Health and Nutrition Examination Survey III and the Continuing Survey of Food Intakes by Individuals 1994–96.
Source: Data from the USDHHS National Center for Health Statistics and the USDA Foods Survey Research Group.

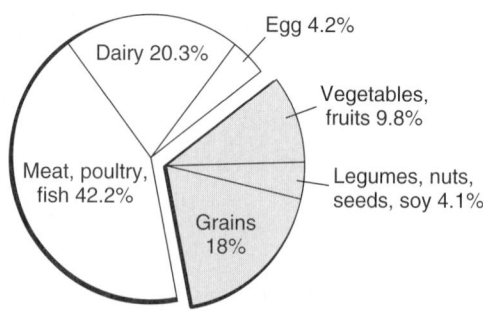

Figure 4.15
On average, Americans obtain approximately two-thirds of their protein from foods of animal origin (meat, poultry, fish, dairy foods, and eggs) and roughly one-third from plant foods (grains, vegetables, fruits, legumes, nuts, seeds, and soy). These data are from phase 1 of NHANES III, which was conducted between 1988 and 1991. The percentages do not add up to 100% due to rounding of the values.
Source: Data from Smit E, Nieto J, Crespo CJ, Mitchell P. 1999. Estimates of animal and plant protein intake in US adults: Results from the Third National Health and Nutrition Examination Survey, 1988–1991. *Journal of the American Dietetic Association* 99:813–820.

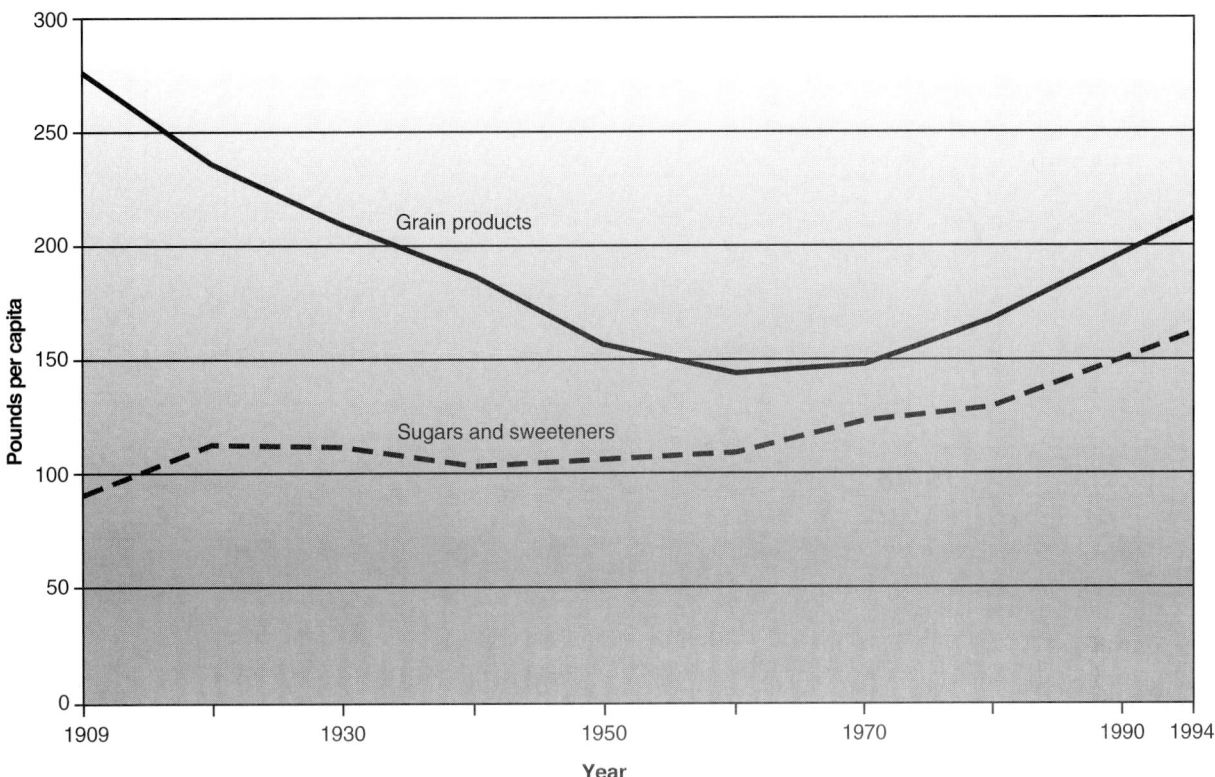

Figure 4.16   **Annual per capita availability of grain products and sugars and sweeteners from the U.S. Food Supply from 1909 to 1994.**

Source: Data from the USDA Economic Research Service.

*MPF mixtures = mixtures containing red meat, poultry, and fish.

Figure 4.17

Between the NFCS 1977–78 and the CSFII 1994–96, there were noticeable increases in the consumption of soft drinks, fruit drinks and ades, beer, all beverages, bananas, and mixed dishes containing red meat, poultry, and fish. During the same time, consumption of all milk (fluid milk) and whole milk decreased.

Source: Data from Enns CW, et al. 1997. Trends in food and nutrient intakes by adults: NFCS 1977, CSFII 1989–91, and CSFII 1994–95. *Family Economics and Nutrition Review* 10(4):2–15.

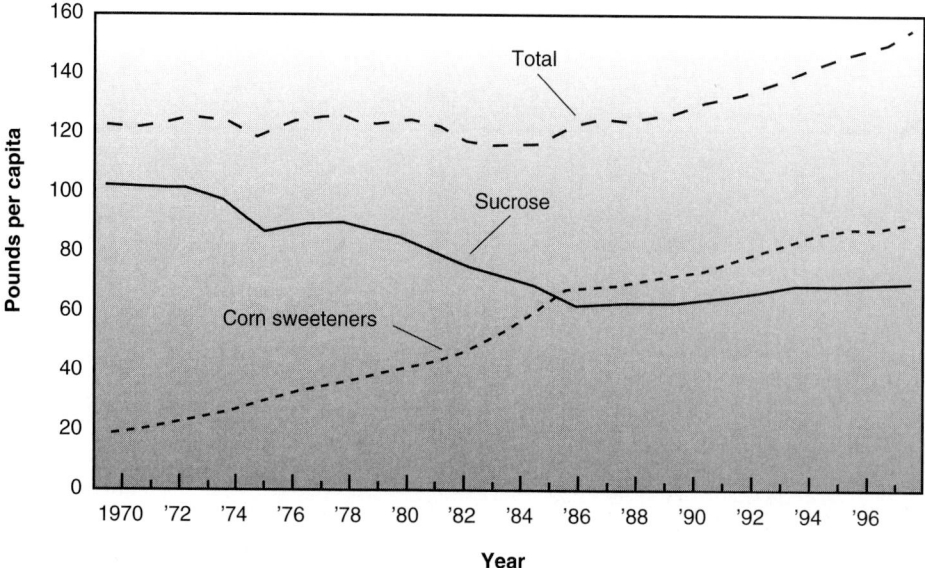

Figure 4.18

Corn sweeteners have surpassed sucrose as the most common caloric sweetener in the diets of Americans. Based on availability data, Americans consume more than 190 g of caloric sweeteners per day.

Source: Data from the USDA Economic Research Service.

Trends in Sugars

Estimates of sugar consumption come from two sources: food availability and food consumption data. Based on food disappearance data, the annual per capita availability of total sugars held relatively steady during the 1970s at about 125 lb but increased gradually to about 154 lb by 1997, as shown in Figure 4.18. These figures are sometimes reported as the average per capita amount of sugars *consumed* in America. What may not be apparent, however, is that these estimates are based on *disappearance* data, not *consumption* data. Estimates of actual consumption are considerably less. According to the CSFII 1994–96, estimated average consumption of all added sweeteners for Americans ages 2 years and older is 82 g/day, or about 66 lb/year.[40] This accounts for 16% of total energy intake. Figure 4.19 shows the percentage of total intake of added sweeteners by food category for persons 2 years of age and older, based on CSFII 1994–96 data. Regular soft drinks are the major contributor of added sweeteners in the diets of Americans ages 2 years and older.[40]

How much sugar and sweeteners do Americans, on the average, actually consume each year? The value of 154 lb is an overestimation. Based on availability, or disappearance, data, it fails to account for waste, spoilage, and nonfood uses of sugars (for example, in the production of alcoholic beverages). Estimates of sugar availability are based on shipments of sweeteners by refiners and importers to buyers such as food industries, wholesalers, and retailers. They are valuable for indicating trends in total sweetener use and use of specific sweeteners in the food supply. The 66 lb estimate based on consumption data from the CSFII 1994–96 is

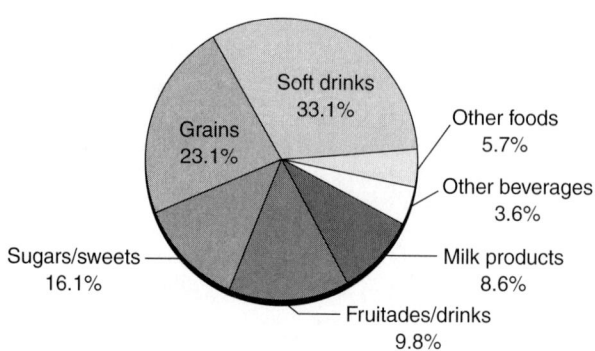

Figure 4.19 **The percentage of total intake of added sweeteners by food category for persons 2 years of age and older, based on CSFII 1994–96 data.**

Source: Data from Guthrie JF, Morton JF. 2000. Food sources of added sweeteners in the diets of Americans. *Journal of the American Dietetic Association* 100:43–48, 51.

probably an underestimate. People tend to underreport their food consumption.[41-44] Actual per capita sugar consumption is somewhere between these two values. However, given the difficulties of measuring diet, the exact value may never be known.

Trends in Dietary Fats

Because of its relation to coronary heart disease, cancer, and obesity, fat consumption is of considerable public health significance. Intake of specific fatty acids also is related to coronary heart disease, as discussed in Chapter 9. Between 1909 and 1994, total fat disappearance increased from 124 to 159 g per capita per day. This increase was primarily due to an increase in the disappearance of polyunsaturated and monounsaturated fatty acids. Although disappearance data indicate a shift away from animal fats to vegetable fats, monounsaturated and saturated fatty acids remain the predominate types of fat in the American diet.

Changes in the sources of fats and oils in the U.S. food supply in 1970 and 1994 are shown in Figure 4.20.

Between 1970 and 1994, the contribution of the meat, poultry, and fish group to total fat disappearance declined 10% to 25%. This was largely due to increased trimming of fat from meat at the processor and retail levels, changes in animal breeding practices resulting in lower–fat flesh, and increasing substitution of poultry and fish for red meat.

Trends in Dairy Products

Americans have made substantial changes in the types of milk they are consuming. Disappearance of whole milk has decreased, while that of low-fat and skim milk has increased markedly. Between 1955 and 1990, for example, disappearance of whole milk fell from 123 to 61 quarts per person per year. During the same period, disappearance of low-fat and skim (nonfat) milk rose from 3 to 41 quarts per person per year. The gains in low-fat and skim milk have not offset the decline in whole milk, and overall, total milk disappearance is down. Changes in the disappearance of milk are

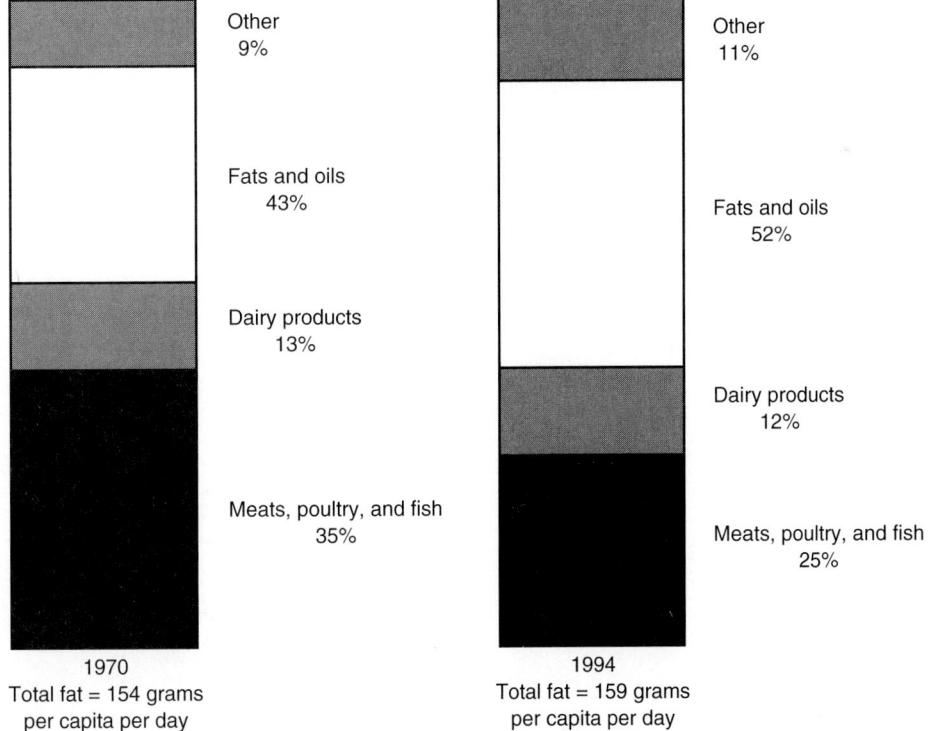

Figure 4.20

Although per capita disappearance of fats and oils increased a modest 5% between 1970 and 1994, 10% less total fat was contributed by meat, poultry, and fish.

Source: Data from the USDA Economic Research Service and Center for Nutrition Policy and Promotion.

summarized in Figure 4.21. According to food disappear-ance data, per capita egg usage has declined steadily since the end of World War II. Between 1970 and 1991, total annual per capita egg use decreased from 309 to 231 eggs, while annual per capita use of eggs in the form of egg products rose from 33 to 51 eggs. Figure 4.22 shows trends in the disappearance of eggs between 1970 and 1998. Some experts believe that the primary reason for these changes is concern about consuming too much cholesterol and saturated fat. Others point out that Americans are eating more meals away from home and are eating fewer cooked breakfasts at home.

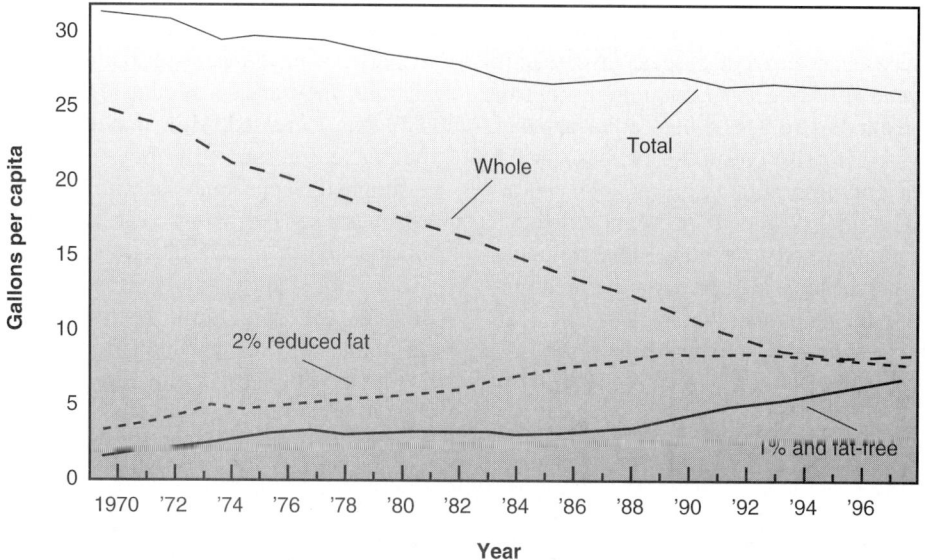

Figure 4.21

Between 1970 and 1997, per capita disappearance of whole milk declined sharply, while disappearance of lower-fat milks increased modestly. Overall, annual per capita disappearance of all milk combined ("total") declined from 31 gallons to 24 gallons.

Source: Data from the USDA Economic Research Service.

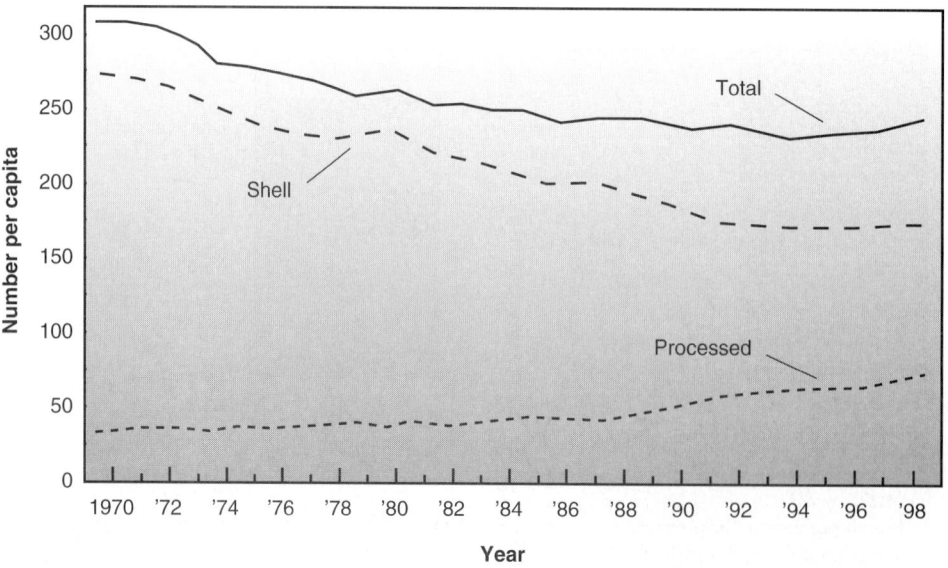

Figure 4.22

Between 1970 and 1989, per capita disappearance of total eggs declined but remained fairly constant during the 1990s. While disappearance of eggs purchased in cartons in the grocery store (shell eggs) declined steadily, disappearance of processed eggs has increased in recent years.

Source: Data from the USDA Economic Research Service.

Trends in Beverages

Another factor in milk's drop in popularity is competition from other beverages, especially soft drinks, which are now America's favorite type of beverage. Milk is the second most popular beverage, followed by coffee, beer, fruit juices, fruit drinks, tea, and wine. However, as a group, alcoholic beverages—beer, wine, and distilled spirits, combined—surpass milk in per capita

consumption. Promotion and advertising of these beverages and greater preference for soft drinks while eating out also have contributed to declining milk consumption. Figure 4.23 shows the per capita disappearance of beverages in the United States in gallons for 1997. Figure 4.24 shows the change in per capita disappearance of carbonated soft drinks and milk between 1945 and 1997.

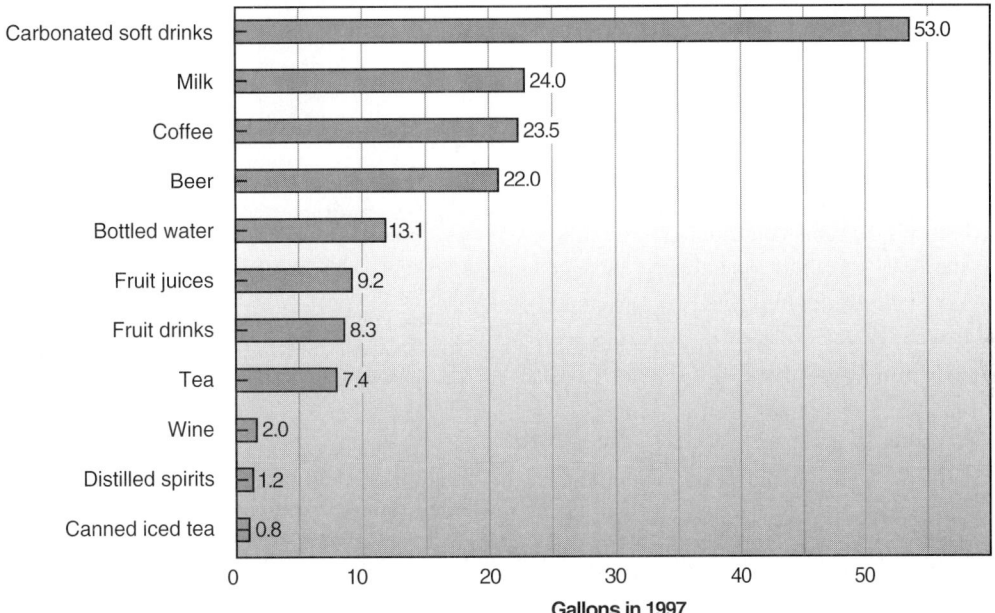

Figure 4.23 **Per capita disappearance of beverages in the United States in gallons for 1997.**
By a wide margin, carbonated soft drinks are the most popular beverage in the United States. When all alcoholic beverages are combined in one group, they become the second most popular beverage in the United States.
Source: Data from the USDA Economic Research Service.

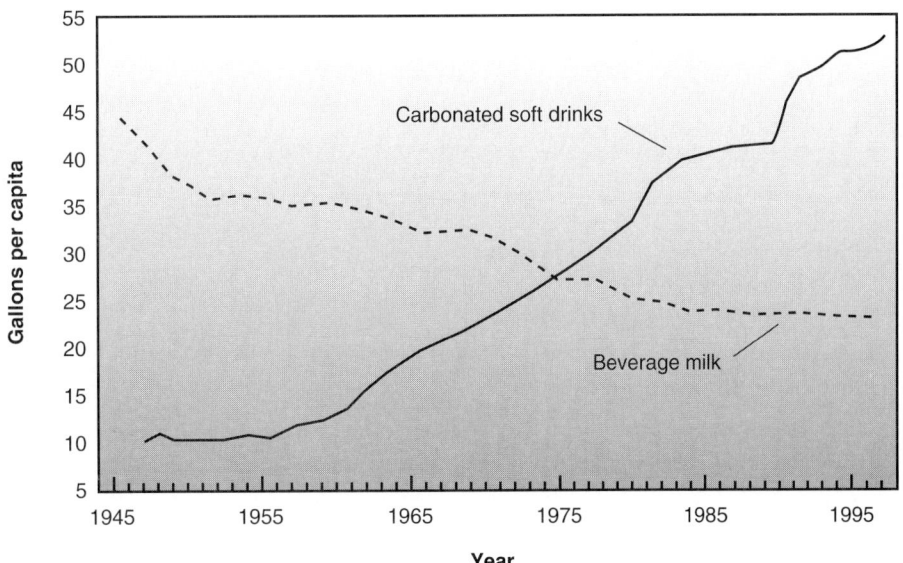

Figure 4.24 **Changes in the per capita disappearance of carbonated soft drinks and beverage milk between 1945 and 1997.**
Disappearance data for soft drinks begin in 1947, the first year for which soft drink data are available.
Source: Data from the USDA Economic Research Service.

Trends in Red Meat, Poultry, and Fish

Based on food disappearance data from the USDA, annual total per capita meat consumption was 19 lb greater in 1998 than in 1970. Although per capita disappearance of red meat (beef, pork, lamb, veal) has declined since 1970, the large increase in the disappearance of chicken has more than offset the decline in red meat. Figure 4.25 shows trends in the disappearance of beef, pork, chicken, and turkey between 1970 and 1998. The primary reasons for these changes seem to be lower prices for poultry due to technological advances and production efficiencies and aggressive marketing by the poultry industry. Concerns about red meat consumption and risk of coronary heart disease may also play a role in these changes.

Data from the CSFII 1994–96 show that Americans are eating more meat and grain mixtures, such as hamburgers on a bun, pizzas, and meat and rice mixtures. Fewer steaks and roasts are being eaten separately and not in a mixture with grains.

Trends in Fruits and Vegetables

As shown in Figure 4.26, total per capita disappearance of fruits and vegetables increased 24% between 1970 and 1997. Factors contributing to this increase include better quality, increased variety, and year-round availability of fresh produce. Public awareness of the health benefits of fruit and vegetable consumption may also be a factor.

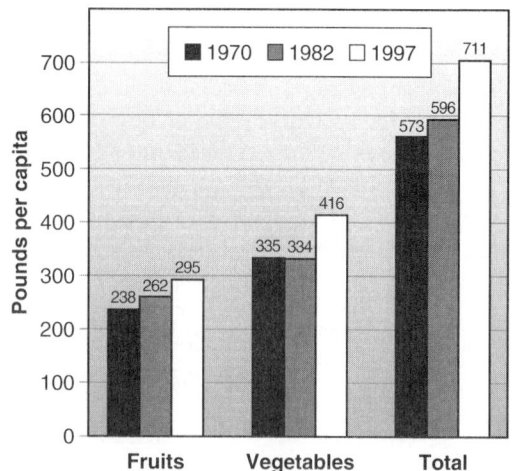

Figure 4.26

Total annual per capita disappearance of fruits and vegetables increased 24% between 1970 and 1997. Eighty percent of this increase occurred since 1982, when the U.S. National Academy of Sciences published its landmark report "Diet, Nutrition, and Cancer," which encouraged greater fruit and vegetable consumption to reduce cancer risk.

Source: Data from the USDA Economic Research Service

Eighty percent of this increase occurred since 1982, when the U.S. National Academy of Sciences published its landmark report "Diet, Nutrition, and Cancer," which emphasized the importance of increased fruit and

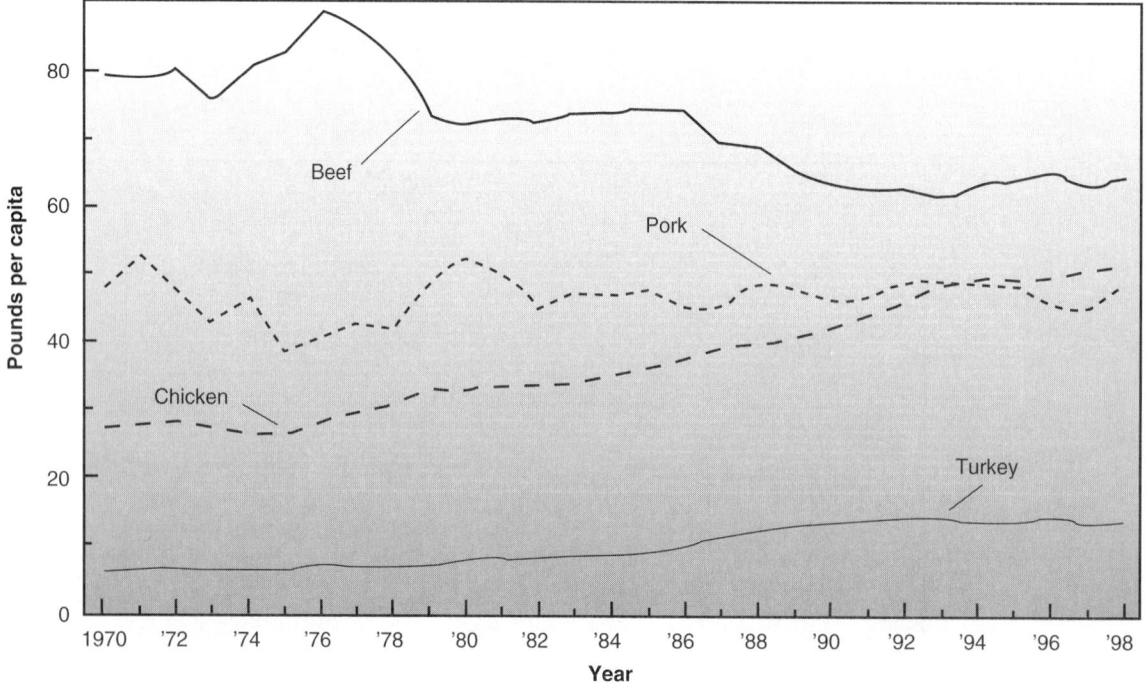

Figure 4.25

Trends in the disappearance of beef, pork, chicken, and turkey between 1970 and 1998 show that disappearance of red meats declined, while that of chicken and turkey increased. The decline in the disappearance of red meat was offset by increased disappearance of chicken and turkey.

Source: Data from the USDA Economic Research Service.

vegetable consumption as part of a comprehensive program to reduce cancer risk.

This increased disappearance has been tempered by the fact that the price of fruits and vegetables has increased more than any other food item, as shown in Figure 4.27. Between 1982 and 1997, the rise in the price of fresh fruits and vegetables was more than double that of processed fruits and vegetables. Despite these increases, the percentage of disposable income Ameri-

cans spend on food has steadily declined since 1960, as shown in Figure 4.28.

Disappearance data also indicate changes in the kinds of fruits and vegetables Americans are purchasing. For example, in recent years per capita disappearance of iceberg lettuce has declined, while that of romaine and leaf lettuces has increased. Specialty lettuces not tracked by the USDA, such as radicchio, frisee, and arugula, have also gained in popularity.

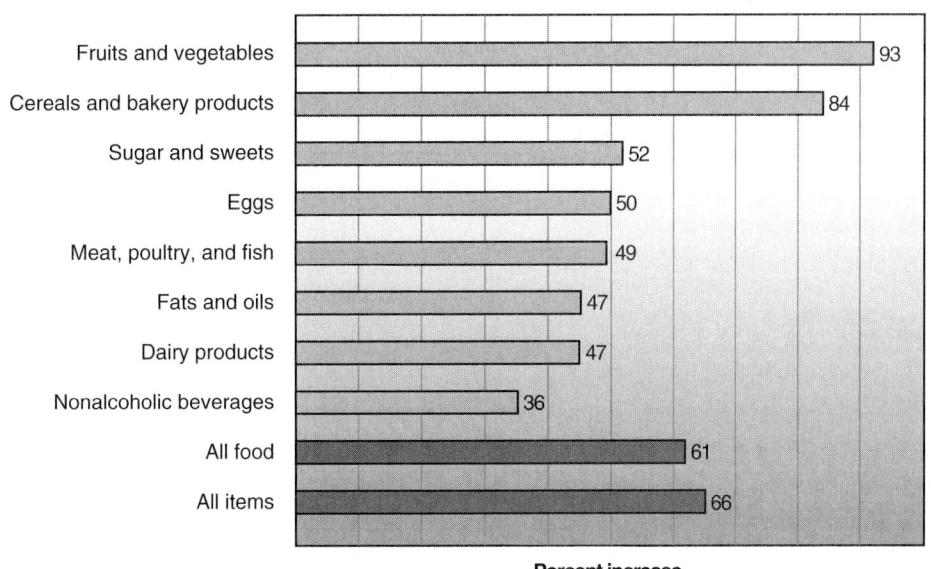

Figure 4.27

Between 1982 and 1997, the percent increase in the price of fruits and vegetables surpassed that of any other food item.

Source: Data from the USDA Economic Research Service.

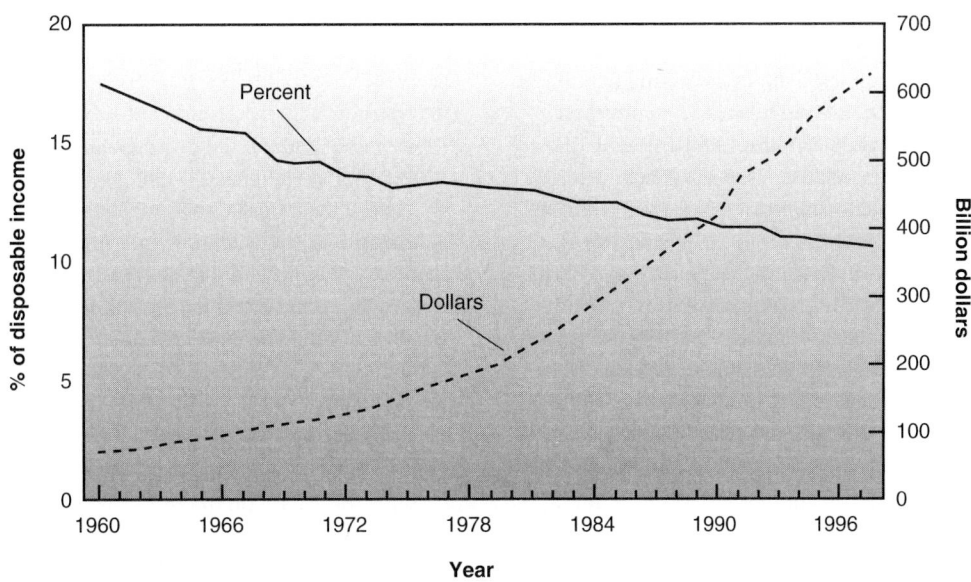

Figure 4.28

Despite the sharp rise in the price of fruits and vegetables, Americans actually spend a smaller percentage of their disposable income for food now than they did in 1960.

Source: Data from the USDA Economic Research Service.

SUMMARY

1. National dietary and nutrition survey data are important in monitoring the nutritional status of a country's population, revealing the relationships between diet and health, identifying groups at nutritional risk and those who may benefit from food assistance programs, and evaluating the cost-effectiveness of food assistance and health education programs. These data are used to track food consumption trends and to monitor intakes of pesticides and other toxic substances.

2. Survey data provide a sound basis for agricultural policy and program development. They provide an early warning of impending food shortages and indicate how such crises may be prevented or alleviated. Food balance sheets estimate the disappearance of food from the food distribution system and provide an indirect estimate of food consumption.

3. Nutritional monitoring is the assessment of dietary or nutritional status at intermittent times to detect changes in the dietary or nutritional status of a population. In the United States, this has been conducted by two federal agencies: the U.S. Department of Agriculture (USDA) and the U.S. Department of Health and Human Services (DHHS).

4. Passage of the National Nutrition Monitoring and Related Research Act of 1990 required the USDA and DHHS to coordinate the nutritional monitoring activities of 22 federal agencies, which encompassed more than 50 surveys and surveillance activities assessing the health and nutritional status of the U.S. population.

5. The USDA has been involved in collecting data on food disappearance, individual food consumption, and household food consumption. Since 1909, the USDA has used the balance sheet approach to determine per capita disappearance of food from the food distribution system. Disappearance (or food availability) is not an actual measure of food consumption. It fails to account for losses resulting from spoilage, disposal of inedible parts, trimming by the consumer, and cooking. It is useful for examining food trends, making international comparisons, and studying the relationships between diet and disease.

6. The USDA began assessing individual food intake with the Household Food Consumption Survey, which had both an individual and a household component. This was later renamed the Nationwide Food Consumption Survey (NFCS) and was conducted during 1977–78 and 1987–88.

The Continuing Survey of Food Intakes by Individuals replaced the NFCS. It provides timely information on U.S. diets, studies the dietary habits of persons at nutritional risk, provides data on "usual" diets by collecting several days of data over the course of a year, and demonstrates how diets vary over time.

7. Other nutritional monitoring activities of the USDA include development of food composition and nutrient databases, reporting of food and nutrient disappearance data, the Diet and Health Knowledge Survey (DHKS), and the Supplemental Children's Survey. The DHKS studies how attitudes and knowledge about healthy eating affect actual dietary practices. The Supplemental Children's Survey measures children's food consumption, so that pesticide residue exposure in children can be calculated.

8. Surveys conducted by the DHHS include the National Health and Nutrition Examination Survey (NHANES), Hispanic Health and Nutrition Examination Survey (HHANES), Total Diet Study, Navajo Health and Nutrition Survey, Pregnancy Nutrition Surveillance System, Pediatric Nutrition Surveillance System, the Health and Diet Survey, and the Behavioral Risk Factor Surveillance System.

9. The NHANES monitors overall nutritional status of the U.S. population through detailed interviews (using dietary, demographic, socioeconomic, and health-related questions) and comprehensive physical examinations, including medical and dental examinations, anthropometric measurements, and diagnostic and laboratory tests.

10. NHANES III was conducted from 1988 to 1994. It provided data on the prevalence of compromised nutritional status and trends in nutrition-related risk factors; data on the relationships among diet, nutritional status, and health; prevalence estimates of overweight and obesity in the U.S. population; and anthropometric data on children and adolescents, allowing revision of the National Center for Health Statistics growth charts.

11. The HHANES was the largest and most comprehensive Hispanic health survey ever carried out in the United States. It collected health and nutritional data on the three largest subgroups of Hispanics living in the 48 continental states: Mexican Americans residing in five southwestern states, Cuban Americans living in Dade County, Florida, and Puerto Ricans residing in the New York City metropolitan area.

12. Food availability data show that the percent of kilocalories from protein has held fairly steady at 11% to 12% since 1909 to the present. During the same period, the percent of kilocalories available from carbohydrate has decreased, while the percent of energy available from fat has increased.

13. Data from NHANES III indicate that adult Americans obtain about 16%, 49%, and 34% of their total energy from protein, carbohydrate, and fat, respectively. Data from the CSFII 1994–96 indicate that American adults obtain 15.4%, 51.8%, and 32.8% of their total energy from protein, carbohydrate, and fat, respectively.

14. Consumption of carbohydrate has declined because Americans now eat fewer grain and flour products and potatoes. Sugar consumption has increased, and estimated annual per capita sugar intake based on food consumption data is about 66 lb. Estimates based on food disappearance are considerably higher. Based on data from NHANES III, dietary fiber intake is estimated to average about 13 and 17 g/day for females and males, respectively. Data from the CSFII 1994–96 indicate 13.9 g and 18.6 g for females and males, respectively.

15. The availability of kilocalories from fat has increased since the early 1900s because of increased consumption of polyunsaturated and monounsaturated fats. The percent of kilocalories from saturated fat remained relatively constant throughout the twentieth century.

16. Overall, Americans are drinking less milk and more soft drinks. Reasons for this include the popularity of soft drinks in restaurants and fast-food outlets, more meals eaten away from home, concern about saturated fat intake in dairy products, and the heavy advertising of soft drinks. When Americans do drink milk, they are now more likely to drink low-fat or skim milk than whole milk.

17. The disappearance of red meat, poultry, and fish has increased steadily since 1909 to the present. In recent years, however, Americans have shown an increased preference for poultry because of its lower price.

18. Annual per capita disappearance of fruits and vegetables has increased 24% since 1970, even though the percentage price increase of fruits and vegetables has exceeded that of other food items. Despite the rising cost of food, the percent of disposable income Americans spend on food has gradually declined since 1960.

REFERENCES

1. U.S. General Accounting Office. 1994. *Nutrition monitoring: Progress in developing a coordinated program.* Washington, DC: United States General Accounting Office. GAO/PEMD-94-23.

2. U.S. General Accounting Office. 1992. *Early intervention: Federal investments like WIC can produce savings.* Washington, DC: United States General Accounting Office. GAO/HRD-92-18.

3. National Research Council. 1989. *Diet and health: Implications for reducing chronic disease risk.* Washington, DC: National Academy Press.

4. Pao EM, Sykes KE, Cypel YS. 1989. *USDA methodological research for large-scale dietary intake surveys, 1975–88.* Washington, DC: U.S. Department of Agriculture, Human Nutrition Information Service.

5. Mason JB, Habicht JP, Tabatabai H, Valverde V. 1984. *Nutritional surveillance.* Geneva, Switzerland: World Health Organization.

6. Food and Agriculture Organization. 1990. *Bibliography of food consumption surveys.* Rome, Italy: Food and Agriculture Organization of the United Nations.

7. Life Science Research Office, Federation of American Societies for Experimental Biology. 1989. *Nutrition monitoring in the United States: An update report on nutrition monitoring.* Washington, DC: U.S. Government Printing Office.

8. Ostenso GL. 1984. National nutrition monitoring system: A historical perspective. *Journal of the American Dietetic Association* 84:1181–1185.

9. Brown GE. 1984. National nutrition monitoring system: A congressional perspective. *Journal of the American Dietetic Association* 84:1185–1189.

10. Brown GE. 1988. Remarks. *American Journal of Clinical Nutrition* 47:333–335.

11. U.S. Department of Health and Human Services, U.S. Department of Agriculture. 1993. Ten-year comprehensive plan for the national nutrition monitoring and related research program; notice. *Federal Register* 58(111):32751–32806.

12. Briefel RR. 1994. Assessment of the U.S. diet in national nutrition surveys: National collaborative efforts and NHANES. *American Journal of Clinical Nutrition* 59(suppl):164S–167S.

13. Interagency Board for Nutrition Monitoring and Related Research. Bialostosky K, ed. 2000. *Nutrition monitoring in the United States: The directory of federal and state nutrition monitoring and related research activities.* Hyattsville, MD: National Center for Health Statistics.

14. Tippett KS, Enns CW, Moshfegh AJ. 1999. Food consumption surveys in the United States Department of Agriculture. *Nutrition Today* 34:33–46.

15. Nesheim RO. 1982. Measurement of food consumption—Past, present, and future. *American Journal of Clinical Nutrition* 35:1292–1296.

16. Welsh SO, Martson RM. 1982. Review of trends in food use in the United States, 1909–1980. *Journal of the American Dietetic Association* 81:120–125.

17. Carlson SJ, Andrews MS, Bickel GW. 1999. Measuring food insecurity and hunger in the United States: Development of a national benchmark measure and prevalence estimates. *Journal of Nutrition* 129:510S–516S.

18. Frongillo EA. 1999. Validation of measures of food insecurity and hunger. *Journal of Nutrition* 129 (suppl):506S–509S.

19. Andrews M, Nord M, Bickel G, Carlson. 1999. Household food security in the United States, 1999. *Food Assistance and Nutrition Research Report No. 8.* Food and Rural Economics Division, Economic Research Service, U.S. Department of Agriculture.

20. Nord M, Jemison K, Bickel G. 1999. Prevalence of food insecurity and hunger, by state, 1996–1998. *Food Assistance and Nutrition Research Report No. 2.* Food and Rural Economics Division, Economic Research Service, U.S. Department of Agriculture.

21. Yetley E, Johnson C. 1987. Nutritional applications of the health and nutrition examination surveys (HANES). *Annual Review of Nutrition* 7:441–463.

22. Citizens Board of Inquiry into Hunger and Malnutrition. 1968. *Hunger—USA.* Washington, DC: New Community Press.

23. Woteki CE, Hitchcock DC, Briefel RR, Winn DM. 1988. National health and nutrition examination survey—NHANES. *Nutrition Today* 23(1):25–27.

24. National Center for Health Statistics. 1994. *Plan and operation of the Third National Health and Examination Survey, 1988–94.* Hyattsville, MD: U.S. Department of Health and Human Services, Public Health Service, Centers for Disease Control and Prevention.

25. Delgado JL, Johnson CL, Roy I, Treviño FM. 1990. Hispanic Health and Nutrition Examination Survey: Methodological considerations. *American Journal of Public Health* 80(suppl):65–105.

26. Woteki CE. 1990. The Hispanic Health and Nutrition Examination Survey (HHANES 1982–1984): Background and introduction. *American Journal of Clinical Nutrition* 51(suppl):897S–901S.

27. Chumlea WC, Guo S, Kuczmarski RJ, Johnson CL, Leahy CK. 1990. Reliability for anthropometric measurements in the Hispanic Health and Nutrition Examination Survey (HHANES 1982–1984). *American Journal of Clinical Nutrition* 51(suppl):902S–907S.

28. Roche AF, Guo S, Baumgartner RN, Chumlea WC, Ryan AS, Kuczmarski RJ. 1990. Reference data for weight, stature, and weight/stature in Mexican Americans from the Hispanic Health and Nutrition Examination Survey (HHANES 1982–1984). *American Journal of Clinical Nutrition* 51(suppl):917S–924S.

29. Woteki CE, Briefel R, Hitchcock D, Ezzati T, Maurer K. 1990. Selection of nutrition status indicators for field surveys: The NHANES III design. *Journal of Nutrition* 120:1440–1445.

30. Woteki CE, Briefel RR, Kuczmarski R. 1988. Contributions of the National Center for Health Statistics. *American Journal of Clinical Nutrition* 47:320–328.

31. Kuczmarski RJ, Ogden CL, Grummer-Strawn LM, Flegal KM, Guo SS, et al. 2000. *CDC growth charts: United States. Advance data from vital and health statistics; no. 314.* Hyattsville, MD: National Center for Health Statistics.

32. McDowell MA, Briefel RR, Alaimo K, Bischof AM, Caughman CR, Carroll MD, Loria CM, Johnson CL. 1994. Energy and macronutrient intakes of persons ages 2 months and over in the United States: Third National Health and Nutrition Examination Survey, phase 1, 1988–91. *Advance Data from Vital and Health Statistics.* No. 255. Hyattsville, MD: National Center for Health Statistics.

33. Interagency Board for Nutrition Monitoring and Related Research. 1993. *Nutrition monitoring in the United States, chartbook 1: Selected findings from the National Nutrition Monitoring and Related Research Program.* Hyattsville, MD: Public Health Service.

34. Bloom Y, Figgs LW, Baker EA, Dugbatey K, Stanwyck CA, Brownson RC. 2000. Data uses, benefits, and barriers for the Behavioral Risk Factor Surveillance System: A qualitative study of users. *Journal of Public Health Management Practice* 6:78–86.

35. Bolen JC, Rhodes L, Powell-Griner EE, Bland SD, Holtzman D. 2000. State-specific prevalence of selected health behaviors, by race and ethnicity: Behavioral Risk Factor Surveillance System, 1997. *Morbidity and Mortality Weekly Report* 49:1–60.

36. Rowland ML. 1990. Self-reported weight and height. *American Journal of Clinical Nutrition* 52:1125–1133.

37. Palta M, Prineas RJ, Berman R, Hannan P. 1982. Comparison of self-reported and measured height and weight. *American Journal of Epidemiology* 115:223–230.

38. Enns CW, Goldman JD, Cook A. 1997. Trends in food and nutrient intakes by adults: NFCS 1977, CSFII 1989–91, and CSFII 1994–95. *Family Economics and Nutrition Review* 10(4):2–15.

39. Alaimo K, McDowell MA, Briefel RR, Bischof AM, Caughman CR, Loria CM, Johnson CL. 1994. Dietary intake of vitamins, minerals, and fiber of persons ages 2 months and over in the United States: Third National Health and

Nutrition Examination Survey, phase 1, 1988–91. *Advance Data from Vital and Health Statistics.* No. 258. Hyattsville, MD: National Center for Health Statistics.

40. Guthrie JF, Morton JF. 2000. Food sources of added sweeteners in the diets of Americans. *Journal of the American Dietetic Association* 100:43–48, 51.

41. Mertz W, Tsui JC, Judd JT, Reiser S, Hallfrisch J, Morris ER, Steele PD, Lashley E. 1991. What are people really eating? The relation between energy intake derived from estimated diet records and intake determined to maintain body weight. *American Journal of Clinical Nutrition* 54:291–295.

42. Mertz W, Kelsay JL. 1984. Rationale and design of the Beltsville one year diet study. *American Journal of Clinical Nutrition* 40(suppl):1323S–1326S.

43. Hallfrisch J, Steele P, Cohen L. 1982. Comparison of seven-day diet records with measured food intake of twenty-four subjects. *Nutrition Research* 2:263–273.

44. Schoeller DA. 1990. How accurate is self-reported dietary energy intake? *Nutrition Reviews* 48:373–379.

5

COMPUTERIZED DIETARY ANALYSIS SYSTEMS

INTRODUCTION: USING COMPUTERS IN NUTRITIONAL ASSESSMENT

Prior to the development of computers and diet analysis software, the manual nutritional analysis of diets was difficult and time consuming. Consider, for example, the steps you would take to manually calculate intake of energy, protein, carbohydrate, total fat, calcium, iron, vitamin C, and other nutrients from a 24-hour recall using nutrient data from a published table. Your first step would be to find the appropriate food in the table and then compare the amount you actually ate with the portion size listed for the food. If these differed, you would have to mathematically adjust all of the nutrient values before listing them on a spreadsheet table. After doing this for each food in your 24-hour recall, you would have to add all of the values for each nutrient to calculate your final 24-hour intake. Next you would have to compare intake to a dietary standard, such as the RDA/DRI, and express this as a percentage. And you can imagine how much more difficult this process would be if you were analyzing a 7-day food record in which nutrient intake would have to be expressed as a daily average.

Clearly, computers are perfectly suited to this task of nutrient analysis, which is nothing more than number crunching, saving time, labor, and expense while reducing error (Figure 5.1).[1-5] Hundreds of software programs have been developed since the mid-1980s for all sorts of nutrition-related tasks, including analysis of food records and food frequency questionnaires, menu planning and forecasting, analysis of recipes, food service and food management tasks, nutrition education, patient interviews and counseling, and research.

The purpose of this chapter is to delineate important characteristics of computerized dietary analysis systems to aid you in selecting an appropriate software package for the analysis of food records, food frequency questionnaires, and recipes. A growing number of dietary analysis systems are now available on the Internet, and the strengths and weaknesses of these systems will be described.

Figure 5.1

Computers are well suited to the task of nutrient analysis.

Source: © Eye Wire.

Descriptions of computer applications in nutrition and dietetics first appeared in the literature in the late 1950s. Computer hardware cost is no longer the prohibitive factor it once used to be, and most hospitals, clinics, businesses, and educational facilities provide personal computer work stations for their employees. Computerized dietary intake analysis is an important skill for dietitians and nutritionists to master.

FACTORS TO CONSIDER IN SELECTING A COMPUTERIZED DIETARY ANALYSIS SYSTEM

Hundreds of dietary analysis software packages are available, ranging from simplified programs designed for elementary school students to comprehensive programs designed for researchers. In selecting a dietary analysis program, the first step is to establish the major needs for obtaining the software, with specific tasks defined. Once this has been accomplished, choose a dietary analysis system that is suitable to these needs and tasks. For example, a research professor in a university nutrition department will probably need a completely different type of computerized dietary analysis system than a public health nutritionist working with pregnant women at nutritional risk in a county health department.

In comparing software programs, dietitians and other health professionals should consider aspects of the database, program operation, and system output.[6–9] The *Journal of the American Dietetic Association* provides regular reviews of computerized dietary analysis systems.

Nutrient Database

The most important consideration to make when selecting a computerized diet analysis system is its nutrient database.[1,2,7] The database must be accurate, well documented, and large enough to meet all intended tasks. Software vendors begin development of their databases with data from the U.S. Department of Agriculture (USDA). The USDA began publishing food composition values in 1896 and has continually revised and expanded its food composition tables ever since.[10] The USDA has also contributed to the development of food composition tables for other countries for many years and has participated in the International Network of Food Data Systems (INFOODS), organized first in 1983. INFOODS is a comprehensive effort, under the United Nations University Food and Nutrition Program and cosponsored by the Food and Agriculture Organization (FAO) of the United Nations, to improve data on the nutrient composition of foods from all parts of the world. See www.fao.org/infoods/ for more information on INFOODS. A link to this and other websites related to computers in nutritional assessment are available on the *Nutritional Assessment* website at www.mhhe.com/hper/nutrition.

USDA Nutrient Data Laboratory

The Nutrient Data Laboratory (NDL) of the USDA is one of seven units in the Beltsville Human Nutrition Research Center (BHNRC) of the Agricultural Research Service (ARS). NDL has an interdisciplinary staff comprised of nutritionists, food technologists, and computer specialists. The mission of the NDL is to develop authoritative food composition databases and state-of-the-art methods to acquire, evaluate, compile, and disseminate composition data on foods available in the United States. As part of its mission, the NDL operates the National Nutrient Databank, a computerized information system for storing and summarizing data on the composition of foods. See Box 5.1 for a glossary of terms and acronyms used by the NDL.

The USDA NDL develops and maintains a number of databases, including the USDA Nutrient Database for Standard Reference (SR) and the Primary Data Set for USDA Nationwide Food Surveys (PDS). SR and PDS nutrient data serve as the core for most commercial and

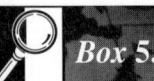

Box 5.1 **Glossary of Terms and Acronyms**

T he following is a list of terms and acronyms with definitions used in this chapter and by the Nutrient Data Laboratory (NDL).

Analytical	Data from laboratory analysis of one or more food samples
AOAC	Association of Official Analytical Chemists, independent scientific organization which published a reference of methods used in analyzing the composition of foods
ARS	Agricultural Research Service, USDA
Atwater System	System developed by W. O. Atwater to calculate the energy contributed by protein, fat, and carbohydrates to foods
BHNRC	Beltsville Human Nutrition Research Center
Calculated	Nutrient values computed or estimated by mathematical adjustment; normalizing nutrients to an average moisture or fat value, use of retention factors, and substitution of similar ingredients in a formulation or recipe are examples of calculated values
CN	Child Nutrition Database
CNPP	Center for Nutrition Policy and Promotion, USDA; produces the Dietary Analysis Program, Food Guide Pyramid, and Healthy Eating Index
FDA	Food and Drug Administration, U.S. Department of Health and Human Services
FNIC	Food and Nutrition Information Center; one of National Agricultural Library (NAL's) information centers.
FNS	Food and Nutrition Service, USDA
Food group	NDL categorizes foods into similar groups and assigns a food group code, such as cereal grains and pasta, beverages, and vegetables.
Food group code	Two-digit numeric code identifying individual food groups; food groups are further classified by subcodes, to produce a four-digit numeric code; for example, fresh pork is 1010, while cured pork is 1020; food group codes are independent of NDB numbers
Food survey	USDA Nationwide Food Surveys
Formulation	The estimated proportion by weight of ingredients in a multi-ingredient commercial food item when other characteristics of the food item are known or can be set; characteristics that may be known or can be set include order of predominance of ingredients, retention codes, target moisture level of individual ingredients and final product, and lower and upper bounds on the proportion of any individual ingredient; as a minimum, to derive a formulation, some nutrient values must be known and flagged for matching
FSRG	Food Surveys Research Group, ARS, BHNRC, USDA; responsible for conducting USDA's food surveys, including the Continuing Survey of Food Intakes by Individuals (CSFII), the Diet Health and Knowledge Survey (DHKS), and the Nationwide Food Consumption Survey (NFCS)
Handbook 8 (AH-8)	USDA *Agriculture Handbook No. 8, Composition of Foods*
HG-72	*Home and Garden Bulletin No. 72, Nutritive Value of Foods*
Household measure	Standard weight (sometimes with dimensions) or portion of individual food; sometimes called serving size
Imputed	Nutrient values developed when analytical values are unavailable; nutrient values from another form of the same food or another species of the same genus are examples of imputed values
INFOODS	International Network of Food Data Systems
Item	Individual food or food product
Key foods	Identification of foods most highly consumed and best sources of nutrients deemed

continued

Box 5.1   Continued

	important to national dietary health; key foods are identified as those foods contributing up to 75% of any one nutrient; key foods are used by NDL to set priorities for nutrient analysis contracts		ingredient food item; amounts of ingredients may be expressed in household volume measure units, such as cups and tablespoons, or may be expressed as gram weights. The term *recipe* is generally applied to a food item prepared from component ingredients in a household or an institutional setting; the term may also apply to a commercial multi-ingredient food item for which the amounts of ingredients are set, rather than estimated (e.g., by Standards of Identity)
Label	Data printed on a food label, as supplied by its manufacturer; the values are primarily company analytical or imputed; however, the values have been rounded and/or adjusted to provide uniform serving size weights		
NAL	National Agricultural Library, part of the U.S. Department of Agriculture (USDA) and the Agricultural Research Service (ARS)	Refuse	Portion of food removed before consumption (meat bones, fruit pits, etc.)
NHANES	National Health and Nutrition Examination Survey; conducted by the National Center for Health Statistics, U.S. Department of Health and Human Services	RM	Reference Material used for evaluating the reliability of analytical methods
		Source code	One-character numeric code to document source of nutrient data
NDB No.	Identification number for food item in USDA Nutrient Database	SRM	Standard Reference Material from NTIS used for evaluating the reliability of analytical methods
NDBS	Nutrient Databank System		
NIH	National Institutes of Health	Standard Reference	USDA Nutrient Database for Standard Reference (SR)
NLEA	National Labeling and Education Act of 1990; refers to food labeling regulations promulgated by the FDA	Tagname	INFOODS tagnames identify individual nutrients for international interchange of nutrient data.
NNDB	USDA National Nutrient Databank	UPC	Universal Product Code; a unique product identification number found on most product labels; represented by bar and number codes
NTIS	National Technical Information Service, U.S. Department of Commerce		
PDS	Primary Data Set for USDA Nationwide Food Surveys	USDA	U.S. Department of Agriculture
Recipe	The known weight or measure of ingredients in a multi-	USDHHS	U.S. Department of Health and Human Services

many foreign databases and are the numerical foundation of essentially all public and private work in the field of human nutrition.

USDA Nutrient Databases

The Nutrient Databank System (NDBS) is a repository for information on up to 113 nutrients and food components found in more than 7300 foods. Until recently, most of this information was published in the form of

Agriculture Handbook 8 (AH-8). However, AH-8 is no longer available in printed form. To facilitate dissemination, the information contained in AH-8 is now provided in the SR at the website of the USDA NDL (www.nal.usda.gov/fnic/foodcomp/). The SR includes the 21 sections and 4 supplements of AH-8. The SR is expanding its inclusion of brand name food items and has begun adding items under a new food group: meals, entrees, and sidedishes.

As information is updated, new versions of the SR database are released. Release 14 (SR14) was published in July 2001 and contained data on 6039 food items and up to 113 nutrients and food components. Table 5.1 lists the 23 food groups included in SR14. It replaced SR13, issued in February 2000, and added new nutrient values (e.g. starch, individual sugars, individual tocopherols, individual phytosterols, and several additional fatty acids) for a limited number of foods.

Data for SR14 were compiled from published and unpublished sources. Published sources included the scientific and technical literature. Unpublished data were from the food industry, other government agencies, and research conducted under contracts initiated by the Agricultural Research Service (ARS). Values in the database may be based on the results of laboratory analyses or calculated by the use of appropriate factors or recipes, and this is indicated by the source code in the Nutrient Data File.

The USDA Table of Nutrient Retention Factors is the major source of nutrient retention data for SR14. Food composition data are needed for the uncooked and cooked forms of foods. However, nutrient data are frequently lacking for cooked foods. The nutrient composition of a cooked food may be calculated from the uncooked food by applying nutrient retention factors. Most public and private sector databases use these retention factors to calculate nutrient values when analytical data for cooked foods are unavailable. The resulting values quantify the nutrient content retained in a food after nutrient losses due to heating or other food preparations.

Every food item may not contain a complete nutrient profile. Thus, blanks in the SR14 database are regarded as "missing data" or an indication of lack of reliable data. Table 5.2 summarizes the number of foods in the SR14 database containing selected nutrients.

Nutrient values per 100 grams and in edible portions of common measures (e.g., cup, tablespoon, or teaspoon) are contained in SR14. Other data are listed to further describe the mean value including the standard error, number of data points upon which the mean is based, and the source code. The source code field indicates how the data value was determined (for example, analytical, calculated, or assumed zero). Several support files that accompany SR14 provide more specific information on the source code, descriptive information about the food items, and descriptions of inedible material (for example, seeds, bone, skin). SR14 is the first release from NDL's new Nutrient Databank System (NDBS). The NDBS contains several important new features for individuals seeking detailed information on statistical attributes that describe the mean (most of which are available in support files):

- Number of studies—the number of analytical studies used to general mean values.
- Minimum value—the smallest observed value in a range of values.
- Maximum value—the largest observed value in a range of values.
- Lower and upper error bounds—represent a range of values the mean is expected to fall within a 95% confidence level.
- Derivation code—a code giving more information about how a value was calculated or imputed.

Table 5.3 gives an example of the data that are available for each food in SR14. Analytical values represent the total amount of the nutrient present in the edible portion of the food, including any nutrients added in processing. The values do not necessarily represent the nutrient amounts available to the body.

The Primary Data Set for USDA Nationwide Food Surveys (PDS) is used to develop the Survey Nutrient Database for the USDA Continuing Survey of Food Intakes by Individuals (CFSII) and for calculating nutrients in the food supply (see Chapter 4). PDS food composition data are also used as the basis of data used in the USDHHS National Health and Nutrition Examination Survey (NHANES). The PDS contains nutrient values for

TABLE 5.1	USDA Nutrient Database for Standard Reference, Release 14

Food Group

01	Dairy and Egg Products
02	Spices and Herbs
03	Baby Foods
04	Fats and Oils
05	Poultry Products
06	Soups, Sauces, and Gravies
07	Sausages and Luncheon Meats
08	Breakfast Cereals
09	Fruits and Fruit Juices
10	Pork Products
11	Vegetables and Vegetable Products
12	Nut and Seed Products
13	Beef Products
14	Beverages
15	Finfish and Shellfish Products
16	Legumes and Legume Products
17	Lamb, Veal, and Game Products
18	Baked Products
19	Sweets
20	Cereal Grains and Pasta
21	Fast Foods
22	Meals, Entrees, and Sidedishes
25	Snacks

Source: U.S. Department of Agriculture, Agricultural Research Service. 2001. USDA Nutrient Database for Standard Reference, Release 14. Nutrient Data Laboratory Home Page, www.nal.usda.gov/fnic/foodcomp. (Release numbers change as new versions are released.)

NOTE: Separate PDF files are available for each food group at the USDA Internet site, www.nal.usda.gov/fnic/foodcomp. The SR databases are also available on CD-ROM and may be purchased from the Government Printing Office. Printed copies of AH-8, *Composition of Foods,* are no longer available.

TABLE 5.2	Number of Foods in SR14 Database (n=6,039) Containing Selected Nutrients		
Nutrient	**Number of Foods**	**Nutrient**	**Number of Foods**
Protein	6039	Vitamin D	157
Total lipid (fat)	6039	Vitamin E, ATE	3301
Water	6039	Alpha-tocopherol	386
Carbohydrate, by difference	6039	Beta-tocopherol	21
Total dietary fiber	5362	Gamma-tocopherol	28
Starch	21	Delta-tocopherol	22
Total sugar	722	Ascorbic acid	5805
Sucrose	63	Thiamin	5656
Glucose	79	Riboflavin	5664
Fructose	79	Niacin	5657
Lactose	58	Pantothenic acid	5284
Galactose	6	Vitamin B_6	5510
Ash	6016	Folate, total	5481
Calcium	5923	Folic acid	5282
Iron	5940	Food folate	5282
Magnesium	5628	Folate, DFE	5282
Phosphorus	5677	Vitamin B_{12}	5539
Potassium	5765	Cholesterol	5931
Sodium	6034	Total saturated fatty acids	5849
Zinc	5608	Total monounsaturated fatty acids	5644
Copper	5536	Total polyunsaturated fatty acids	5651
Manganese	5049	Phytosterols	610
Selenium	4988	Sitosterol	30
Vitamin A (IU)	5868	Stigmasterol	30
Vitamin A (RE)	5404	Campesterol	29

Source: www.nal.usda.gov/fnic/foodcomp/

more than 3150 food items, including all ingredients used in USDA survey recipe calculations.

The Child Nutrition (CN) Database serves the National School Lunch and School Breakfast programs as part of the School Meals Initiative for Healthy Children, which is coordinated by USDA's Food and Nutrition Service (FNS). Data for the CN are collected for 15 nutrients using data from SR. Other datasets developed by NDL include retention tables and tables of special interest on nutrients such as carotenoids, *trans* fatty acids, selenium, vitamin D, and vitamin K. (See Box 5.2.) The USDA sponsors a yearly conference, the "National Nutrient Databank Conference," to facilitate cooperation among the USDA, university researchers, food companies, and others interested in nutrient data. (See www.nal.usda.gov/fnic/foodcomp/conf/ for more details.)

Criteria for Developing High-Quality Databases

Developers of commercial computerized dietary analysis systems are faced with several challenges in formulating high-quality databases.[6–9] Box 5.3 summarizes a checklist of criteria in choosing a good nutrient database.

The first challenge is to decide on how many foods and nutrients to include in the software program. Even though the USDA SR provides values on more than 100

nutrients and food components for more than 6000 foods, relatively few recipes and name brand foods are included. And, as emphasized in Table 5.2, a surprising number of foods also have missing values for some nutrients, such as manganese, selenium, vitamin E, and newly introduced nutrients such as individual sugars and tocopherols.

Although the USDA releases substantial amounts of new or updated information each year, the typical supermarket contains more than 20,000 brand name food products, while more than 10,000 new food items are introduced to consumers each year.[11] The best software vendors attempt to provide their customers with database updates at least once a year, they use non-USDA sources to give information on brand name and ethnic foods, and they fill in missing data.

The total number of food items included in a database is important to ensure that substitution (choosing a similar food when the specific food is not in the database) is kept at a minimum. For example, if a patient in a cardiac rehabilitation program provides a 3-day food record that includes several low-fat items not found in the database, some less than ideal substitutions with other similar foods will have to be made. However, more is not necessarily better. As the database size increases, the

TABLE 5.3	An Example of the Nutrient Data Available for Each Food in SR14

NDB No. 09003
Apples, raw, with skin
Malus sylvestris

Refuse: 8% Core and stem

		Amount in 100 Grams of Edible Portion				Amount in Edible Portion of Common Measures of Food		
Nutrients and Units		**Mean**	**Std. Error**	**Number of Data Points**	**Source Code**	**Measure 1**	**Measure 2**	**Measure 3**
Proximates:								
Water	g	83.93	0.189	126	1	104.91	92.32	177.93
Energy	kcal	59		0	4	74	65	125
Energy	kj	247			4	309	272	523
Protein (N × 6.25)	g	0.19	0.003	119	1	0.24	0.21	0.40
Total lipid (fat)	g	0.36	0.039	35	1	0.45	0.40	0.76
Ash	g	0.26	0.005	116	1	0.33	0.29	0.55
Carbohydrate, by difference	g	15.25		0	4	19.06	16.78	32.33
Fiber, total dietary	g	2.7		0	1	3.4	3.0	5.7
Sugars, total	g							
Starch	g							
Minerals:								
Calcium, Ca	mg	7	0.519	34	1	9	8	15
Iron, Fe	mg	0.18	0.019	119	1	0.23	0.20	0.38
Magnesium, Mg	mg	5	0.100	114	1	6	6	11
Phosphorus, P	mg	7	0.232	114	1	9	8	15
Potassium, K	mg	115	2.561	74	1	144	127	244
Sodium, Na	mg	0	0.064	47	1	0	0	0
Zinc, Zn	mg	0.04	0.007	15	1	0.05	0.04	0.08
Copper, Cu	mg	0.041	0.002	119	1	0.051	0.045	0.087
Manganese, Mn	mg	0.045	0.003	119	1	0.056	0.050	0.095
Selenium, Se	mcg	0.3	0.076	7	1	0.4	0.3	0.6
Vitamins:								
Vitamin C, total ascorbic acid	mg	5.7	0.766	25	1	7.1	6.3	12.1
Thiamin	mg	0.017	0.000	6	1	0.021	0.019	0.036
Riboflavin	mg	0.014	0.001	6	1	0.018	0.015	0.030
Niacin	mg	0.077	0.028	6	1	0.096	0.085	0.163
Pantothenic acid	mg	0.061	0.004	6	1	0.076	0.067	0.129
Vitamin B-6	mg	0.048	0.004	7	1	0.060	0.053	0.102
Folate, total	mcg	3	0.611	23	1	4	3	6
Folic acid	mcg	0		0	7	0	0	0
Folate, food	mcg	3	0.611	23	1	4	3	6
Folate, DFE	mcg_DFE	3		0	4	4	3	6
Vitamin B-12	mcg	0.00		0	7	0.00	0.00	0.00
Vitamin A, IU	IU	53	11.878	6	1	66	58	112
Vitamin A, RE	mcg_RE	5	1.188	6	1	6	6	11
Vitamin E	mg_ATE	0.320		0	1	0.400	0.352	0.678
Tocopherol, alpha	mg	0.32		0	1	0.40	0.35	0.68
Tocopherol, beta	mg							
Tocopherol, gamma	mg							
Tocopherol, delta	mg							

continued

TABLE **5.3**	An Example of the Nutrient Data Available for Each Food in SR14—*continued*

NDB No. 09003
Apples, raw, with skin
Malus sylvestris

Refuse: 8% Core and stem

Nutrients and Units		Amount in 100 Grams of Edible Portion				Amount in Edible Portion of Common Measures of Food		
		Mean	Std. Error	Number of Data Points	Source Code	Measure 1	Measure 2	Measure 3
Tocotrienol, alpha	mg							
Tocotrienol, beta	mg							
Tocotrienol, gamma	mg							
Tocotrienol, delta	mg							
Vitamin D	IU							
Lipids:								
Fatty acids, total saturated	g	0.058		0	1	0.073	0.064	0.123
4:0	g	0.000		0	1	0.000	0.000	0.000
6:0	g	0.000		0	1	0.000	0.000	0.000
8:0	g	0.000		0	1	0.000	0.000	0.000
10:0	g	0.000		0	1	0.000	0.000	0.000
11:0	g							
12:0	g	0.001		1	1	0.001	0.001	0.002
13:0	g							
14:0	g	0.002		1	1	0.003	0.002	0.004
15:0	g							
16:0	g	0.048		4	1	0.060	0.053	0.102
17:0	g							
18:0	g	0.007		4	1	0.009	0.008	0.015
19:0	g							
20:0	g							
22:0	g							
24:0	g							
Fatty acids, total monounsaturated	g	0.015		0	1	0.019	0.017	0.032
14:1	g							
15:1	g							
16:1 undifferentiated	g	0.001		1	1	0.001	0.001	0.002
17:1	g							
18:1 undifferentiated	g	0.014		4	1	0.018	0.015	0.030
20:1	g	0.000		0	1	0.000	0.000	0.000
22:1 undifferentiated	g	0.000		0	1	0.000	0.000	0.000
24:1 c	g							
Fatty acids, total polyunsaturated	g	0.105		0	1	0.131	0.116	0.223
18:2 undifferentiated	g	0.087		4	1	0.109	0.096	0.184
18:3 undifferentiated	g	0.018		4	1	0.023	0.020	0.038
18:4	g	0.000		0	1	0.000	0.000	0.000
20:2 n-6 c,c	g							
20:3 undifferentiated	g							
20:4 undifferentiated	g	0.000		0	1	0.000	0.000	0.000
20:5 n-3	g	0.000		0	1	0.000	0.000	0.000
22:2	g							
22:5 n-3	g	0.000		0	1	0.000	0.000	0.000
22:6 n-3	g	0.000		0	1	0.000	0.000	0.000

continued

TABLE 5.3	An Example of the Nutrient Data Available for Each Food in SR14—*continued*

NDB No. 09003
Apples, raw, with skin
Malus sylvestris

Refuse: 8% Core and stem

Nutrients and Units		Amount in 100 Grams of Edible Portion				Amount in Edible Portion of Common Measures of Food		
		Mean	Std. Error	Number of Data Points	Source Code	Measure 1	Measure 2	Measure 3
Fatty acids, total trans	g							
Cholesterol	mg	0		0	7	0	0	0
Phytosterols	mg	12		0	1	15	13	25
Amino Acids:								
Tryptophan	g	0.002		1	1	0.003	0.002	0.004
Threonine	g	0.007		2	1	0.009	0.008	0.015
Isoleucine	g	0.008		2	1	0.010	0.009	0.017
Leucine	g	0.012		2	1	0.015	0.013	0.025
Lysine	g	0.012		2	1	0.015	0.013	0.025
Methionine	g	0.002		2	1	0.003	0.002	0.004
Cystine	g	0.003		1	1	0.004	0.003	0.006
Phenylalanine	g	0.005		2	1	0.006	0.006	0.011
Tyrosine	g	0.004		2	1	0.005	0.004	0.008
Valine	g	0.009		2	1	0.011	0.010	0.019
Arginine	g	0.006		2	1	0.008	0.007	0.013
Histidine	g	0.003		2	1	0.004	0.003	0.006
Alanine	g	0.007		2	1	0.009	0.008	0.015
Aspartic acid	g	0.034		2	1	0.043	0.037	0.072
Glutamic acid	g	0.020		2	1	0.025	0.022	0.042
Glycine	g	0.008		2	1	0.010	0.009	0.017
Proline	g	0.007		2	1	0.009	0.008	0.015
Serine	g	0.008		2	1	0.010	0.009	0.017
Hydroxyproline	g							
Others:								
Alcohol, ethyl	g	0.0		0	7	0.0	0.0	0.0
Caffeine	mg	0		0	7	0	0	0
Theobromine	mg	0		0	7	0	0	0

NOTE: Blanks in the Mean column indicate lack of reliable data. The Number of Data Points column is the number of analyses upon which the mean is based. A sample of zero indicates the mean was estimated, usually from a recipe, another form of the same food, or similar food.

Common Measures:

Measure 1 = 125.000g: 1 cup, quartered or chopped

Measure 2 = 110.000g: 1 cup slices

Measure 3 = 212.000g: 1 large (3-1/4″ dia) (approx 2 per lb)

Source: USDA Nutrient Database for Standard Reference, Release 14 (2001).

Calories Factors:

Protein 3.36

Fat 8.37

Carbohydrate 3.6

Food Group:

09 Fruits and Fruit Juices

difficulty in finding the right food and the processing time can increase.

Some software packages report having more than 100 nutrients and food components in their databases, while others contain fewer than 30. Again, more is not necessarily better, because values for certain trace minerals (e.g., chromium, selenium, molybdenum, manganese), amino acids, some fatty acids, and some vitamins (e.g., alpha-tocopherol, total tocopherol, vitamin D, vitamin K, biotin) are unknown for many foods. Thus, with an increasing number of food components, the software package developer has to cope with an expanding

Box 5.2   Databases Available from the USDA, Agricultural Research Service, Nutrient Data Laboratory (www.nal.usda.gov/fnic/foodcomp/)

1. *USDA Nutrient Database for Standard Reference, Release 14.* The USDA Nutrient Database for Standard Reference, Release 14 (2001), contains data on 6,039 foods for up to 113 nutrients. It replaces SR13, issued in February 2000. You can search the database online, display reports of all the foods in the database, and download the database for use on your computer. Updated databases will be posted at this Internet site when released. The USDA Nutrient Database for Standard Reference, Release 14, and other special interest tables produced by NDL are also available on CD-ROM from the Government Printing Office.

2. *USDA—Iowa State University Database on the Isoflavone Content of Foods—2000.* This site contains data on daidzein, genistein, glycitein, and total isoflavone content for 128 foods.

3. *USDA Table of Nutrient Retention Factors, Release 4 (1998).* Release 4, of this dataset, replaces the previous release, Release 3, issued in 1986. The dataset contains the factors for calculating retention of 16 vitamins and minerals and alcohol during food preparation. Factors for the 16 vitamins and minerals are the same as those in Release 3. Factors for alcohol retention have been added to this release.

4. *USDA–NCC Carotenoid Database for U.S. Foods—1998.* This site contains new and revised data on five carotenoids (alpha-carotene, beta-carotene, beta-cryptoxanthin, lycopene, and lutein+zeaxanthin) in 215 food items.

5. *Selected Foods Containing Trans Fatty Acids.* This site provides analytical data on the trans fatty acid content of 214 foods obtained under USDA contract.

6. *Vitamin K.* This file contains data from "Provisional Table on the Vitamin K Content of Foods, Revised 1994."

7. *Key foods.* Key foods are identified as those foods contributing up to 75% of any one nutrient. When total nutrient contributions of these key foods are aggregated, they account for approximately 90% of the nutrient content of the U.S. diet for nutrients examined. The key foods list is used to set priorities for NDL's nutrient analysis contracts.

8. *Primary Nutrient Dataset for USDA Nationwide Food Surveys.* The Primary Nutrient Datasets (PDS) for the 1987 NFCS and the 1989–91 CSFII were prepared by NDL and used to generate the Survey Nutrient Database. Links to the later versions are also available.

bank of missing values. If missing data are entered as zero and not flagged (indicated by the software as missing), nutrient totals will appear lower than they actually are. During counseling sessions with patients or clients, some confusion can develop because, for many of these nutrients, low values represent a "database deficiency," not a deficiency in the diet of the patient. The best software packages will give information on how many missing values are present for each nutrient or will warn the dietitian or user about the issue.

One way to judge the quality of a computerized diet analysis system is to determine how the developer met the challenge of missing data in the management of its database.[7–9] Some developers go to unusual lengths to ensure that missing values are substituted with either non-USDA data or imputed values. Many food companies provide information on the nutrient content of their products on request, but usually only for a small number of nutrients. Data on the composition of foods are frequently published in the scientific literature, with several journals (e.g., *Journal of Food Science* and *Journal of Food Composition*) specializing in reporting food composition data. Following established NDL criteria, the nutrient content of mixed dishes and recipes can be estimated. Calculations are also frequently used to impute values using data for another form of food or for a similar food.[2,12,13] (See Table 5.4 for procedures to impute nutrient values.) Replacing missing values with imputed values is not an easy process, and it is

especially difficult when only limited information exists for a certain nutrient (e.g., trace minerals). The process requires nutritionists with expertise in data evaluation, and it is a technique that is still evolving.

The computerized dietary analysis system should at a minimum include the 33 basic nutrients and nutrient factors available from the USDA SR (review Box 5.3):

- Twelve basic components: energy, total fat, total carbohydrate, total protein, alcohol, water, cholesterol, total dietary fiber, caffeine, total saturated fatty acids, total monounsaturated fatty acids, and total polyunsaturated fatty acids
- Eleven vitamins (total vitamin A activity in retinol equivalents, total vitamin E activity in alpha-tocopherol equivalents, vitamin D, vitamin C, thiamin, riboflavin, niacin, pantothenic acid, vitamin B_6, folate, and vitamin B_{12}).
- Ten minerals (calcium, iron, magnesium, phosphorus, potassium, sodium, zinc, copper, manganese, and selenium)

Ensure that calculated nutrient factors, such as percent of calories as fat, saturated fat, carbohydrate, protein, and alcohol, are included. Decide if you need the large number of individual fatty acids ($n = 25$) and amino acids ($n = 18$) provided by the USDA SR and some software programs. Look for special features, such as *trans* fatty acids, animal and vegetable protein,

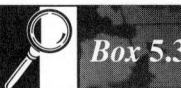

Box 5.3 Basic Checklist for Computerized Dietary Analysis Systems

1. The Nutrient Database

- How many food items are in the database? Aim for more than 15,000 to minimize food substitution decisions during data entry.
- Does the database contain a significant number of brand name items, fast foods, baby foods, and ethnic foods? If the database contains only the 6210 foods found in the USDA SR, few brand name foods will be available, and considerable food substitution decisions will have to be made.
- How many nutrients and nutrient factors does the software program analyze for? It should at a minimum include 33: the 12 basic components (energy sources, water, cholesterol, lipids, dietary fiber, and caffeine), 11 vitamins, and 10 minerals available from the USDA SR. Ensure that calculated nutrient factors such as percent of calories as fat, saturated fat, carbohydrate, protein, and alcohol are included. Decide if you need the large number of individual fatty acids (25) and amino acids (18) provided by the USDA SR and some software programs. Look for special features, such as *trans* fatty acids, animal and vegetable protein, carbohydrate components (fructose, sucrose, starch, etc.), soluble and insoluble dietary fiber, and unique nutrients, such as beta-carotene equivalents, vitamin K, tocopherol components, lycopene, and aspartame. Also review the software for its ability to provide nutrient ratios, such as the polyunsaturated to saturated fat ratio, cholesterol to saturated fatty acid index, calcium to phosphorus ratio, and potassium to sodium ratio.
- How many missing values are in the database? The best software companies go well beyond the USDA SR to scientific journals, food composition tables from other countries, and food manufacturers to not only add additional foods but also ensure that blanks in the nutrient database are filled in with an appropriate value.
- Can you add new food items to the database?
- How often are database updates provided? Aim for one update every 1 to 2 years.

2. Program Operation

- What is the cost of the software package? Most of the high-quality professional computerized dietary analysis systems cost more than $500.
- What type of computer is needed to run the program? Make sure that you have the hardware to run the software.
- How easy is it to search for foods in the database? The best programs allow you to type in any variation of the food name and still ensure that the food will be listed during the search.

- Can the portion size or volume and weight measure be easily adapted to conform to those listed in your food record?
- Can you view the nutrients for a food item during data entry? Access to this information makes food substitution decisions easier.
- How easy is it to edit the food list during entry? You are bound to make mistakes during data entry, and the best programs make it easy to correct your errors.
- Can you easily average multiple days of dietary input to derive a daily nutrient intake average?
- Does the software package allow you to compare dietary intake with a wide variety of standards, such as the RDA/DRI, Canadian RNI, and USDA Dietary Guidelines for Americans?
- How fast is the overall process of entering foods, analyzing and comparing with nutrient standards, and printing results? Some programs are slow and cumbersome to use.
- Is the program so complex that it is difficult to learn and use? The best programs are user-friendly, with a small learning curve and a good help screen system.

3. System Output

- Does the software provide nutrient information in the form of tables and graphs, and does it allow you to adapt the reports as desired? The best programs provide a diversity of attractive reports, which can be adapted and shared with a variety of clients and patients. Some programs allow you to add comments via a word processor.
- Can you print out food exchanges or a Food Guide Pyramid that compares food group intake with USDA standards? Food Guide Pyramid values are often among the most important data to provide clients and patients during counseling.
- Can the nutrient report be printed out as a Nutrition Facts food label? This feature can enhance communication during counseling.
- Can you rank or sort foods in a food record from high to low for any nutrient in the database? Nutrient sorting enhances your ability to personalize comments made to clients and patients during counseling.
- Can you export nutrient output data to a spreadsheet for additional analyses? This is an important feature for investigators and administrators.
- Does the program give an indication of the number of missing values when calculating nutrient intake? This feature can improve the decisions made during the preparation of reports to the client or patient.

---

carbohydrate components (e.g., fructose, sucrose, starch), soluble and insoluble dietary fiber, and unique nutrients, such as beta-carotene equivalents, vitamin K, tocopherol components, lycopene, and aspartame. Also review the

software for its ability to provide nutrient ratios, such as the polyunsaturated-to-saturated fat ratio, cholesterol-to-saturated fatty acid index, calcium-to-phosphorus ratio, and potassium-to-sodium ratio.

TABLE 5.4	Summary of Procedures to Impute Nutrient Values

1. Substitute one or more values from a similar or representative food (e.g., impute dietary fiber for pine nuts based on value for hickory nuts, which are similar in total carbohydrate content).

2. Calculate values from a different form of the same food based on moisture contents and/or retention factors (e.g., impute calcium for cooked horsemeat based on calcium in raw horsemeat, using a retention factor [from the USDA] for calcium in roasted beef).

3. Calculate values for commercial products based on

   a. A single major ingredient source of the missing nutrient(s) (e.g., impute fatty acids in split-pea soup based on the fatty acid profile of butter, which is the major type of fat in split-pea soup)

   b. An estimation of ingredient amounts from product ingredient lists and nutrient profiles provided by manufacturers (e.g., missing nutrients in taco seasoning mix based on estimated amounts of each ingredient)

   c. A representative published recipe or product formula (e.g., missing nutrients in egg bagels calculated from a formula published in the scientific literature)

Source: Schakel SF, Sievert YA, Buzzard IM. Sources of data for developing and maintaining a nutrient database. 1988. *Journal of the American Dietetic Association* 88:1268–1271.

Other important measures for judging a vendor's ability to provide a high-quality database are the strength of its service policy, the number of years the vendor and the software have been in business, the frequency with which the nutrient database is updated, the credentials of the database developers, and the cost of upgrades and technical support.

In summary, the content quality of nutrient databases from different software vendors may vary widely, depending on the number of food items and nutrients included, whether the most recent USDA releases have been incorporated, and the degree to which non-USDA sources (e.g., food industry, scientific literature) or estimating calculations are used to fill in the missing values. Three questions to ask when evaluating a nutrient database for personal or professional use are

- Does the database contain all of the foods and nutrients of interest?
- Is the database complete for the nutrients of interest (i.e., few missing values)?
- Is the nutrient database kept up-to-date with the changing marketplace and the availability of new nutrient data?[2]

Program Operation

General operating features of the computerized diet analysis system are extremely important, determining whether a software package is easy to use while generating the desired information.[6-9] (Review Box 5.3 for a checklist of features to look for in the program operation of computerized dietary analysis systems.)

Important operating features include computer hardware requirements, cost of the software package, quality of help screens and user's manual, methods of searching for and entering foods to be analyzed (e.g., food codes, food names, and/or food groups), ability to preview single food nutrients while entering foods, ability to assign a variety of volume or weight measures for each food item, ease of editing the food list, food entry number limit, ease of averaging multiple days of dietary input, ability to compare results with a variety of dietary standards, and quality and variety of printed reports. The ability to modify the database (e.g., adding new foods, deleting old ones, or altering the nutrient values) is another important concern.

Most of the modern computerized diet analysis systems have been developed for IBM or compatible personal computers, although several vendors also offer Macintosh versions. The amount of conventional RAM (random access memory), required hard disk space, type of central process unit (CPU), and Windows operating system version vary widely among software systems, and the user must carefully compare software requirements with hardware capabilities. Computer novices should seek the help of a local computer specialist before buying a diet analysis software program. Software package prices are typically more than $500 for high-quality programs used by nutrition professionals and researchers. However, some research-based systems can cost much more than this.

Several of the best computerized diet analysis systems come with help screens, which users can "pop up" during any segment of program operation (in other words, "context sensitive"). All software packages come with user's manuals, although the quality of these can vary widely. While many of the early computerized diet analysis systems were rather difficult to use, more recent versions tend to be user-friendly. A user-friendly software package can usually be operated without use of the manual because the various menus and help screens are simple to use and self-explanatory.

The method for searching and entering foods to be analyzed by the microcomputer is one of the most important program operation features. Most software programs allow users to search and enter foods by full name, partial name, or code numbers. However, diet analysis systems have different ways of accomplishing this task, with some requiring more effort and keystrokes than others. For example, some programs require the user to choose a food group prior to selecting the specific food, a step that can slow down the food entry process. Users tend to prefer searching for the appropriate foods using food names rather than code numbers (which requires use of a food code manual) or food groups. Most of the best programs have nearly instantaneous listing of foods after the user enters the food name. Some programs have a search capability, which allows the user to find the food quickly and directly using only a few appropriate keystrokes (e.g., the first few letters of each word of the food description in any order).

While searching the database for the appropriate food from a patient or client diet record, substitutions (using a food that is as similar as possible) often have to be made, even with databases containing more than 6000 food items. Finding appropriate substitutes is much easier when the user is allowed to preview the nutrient breakdown of a certain food. Most of the top-quality programs provide a pop-up window during food search and entry, summarizing the nutrient components for the specific amount of the food chosen.

Once the appropriate food has been located in the database, the user must assign a volume or weight measure for each food item. In comparison with earlier software programs, many current diet analysis programs allow users to assign a wide variety of such measures in an easy and accurate manner.

Often there is the need to edit the food list either during or following food search and entry. Ease of editing the food list is an important feature to evaluate when deciding on a software program. The best programs allow users to easily delete or insert foods or allow the volume or weight measure to be changed with little additional effort.

Some of the earlier computerized diet analysis systems set low limits on the number of foods the user could enter prior to analysis. Although this wasn't a problem if only a 1-day food record was being analyzed, multiple-day food record analysis proved to be quite cumbersome, requiring multiple savings as separate meals and/or days prior to averaging. Many systems allow users to enter 200 or more food items, making it much easier to analyze multiple-day food records. For example, a typical 7-day food record may have 150 food items. All of these items can be entered into one list (without having to save each day separately), with nutrient values automatically divided by 7 after designating this number as the divisor.

Software packages often include a wide variety of dietary standards against which individual nutrient intake can be compared. These dietary standards typically include the Dietary Reference Intakes (DRIs), the Canadian Recommended Nutrient Intakes (RNIs), and the Food Guide Pyramid (see Chapter 2). Additionally, most programs compare basic food component intake (e.g., total fat, saturated fat, cholesterol, dietary fiber) with the USDA Dietary Guidelines for Americans. This comparison allows the tables and graphs to look complete and professional.

Food composition data are continually being updated. Users need to ensure that they are using the most current data available. There are times when a user may want to add foods, delete old ones, or add nutrients to the database. Nearly all dietary analysis systems allow users to modify the database in this fashion.

System Output

Once the data have been entered into the computerized dietary analysis system, two important features are the software program's ability to print out a variety of reports and its ability to export data to electronic files for further analysis. (Review Box 5.3.)

Most software packages allow users to preview the output in both tabular and graphic form on the monitor prior to storage on a disk and/or printing. A variety of output formats are desirable to present the nutrient analysis data, including graphic and tabular comparisons with the DRI, RNI, or other nutrient standards, and a spreadsheet table that outlines the nutrient values for each food in the analysis. While some software programs print a spreadsheet table with all of the nutrients for each food after one or two keystrokes, others will print only two to five nutrients for each food at a time, requiring the user to print out a series of repeated reports.

A few computerized dietary analysis systems have unique features that greatly improve the value of printed information. Few nutrient databases have no missing values. To aid in the interpretation of results, some software programs list missing nutrient values. For example, if a nutritionist is analyzing a 3-day food record with 70 foods, the number of missing values for zinc, vitamin E, copper, and so on are listed separately beside each nutrient. Some software packages allow users to sort and print the analyzed diet for nutrients that may be of concern. For example, if a patient's diet is low in iron, the iron values for each food within the diet can be printed in descending order, allowing the nutritionist to make individualized recommendations. A few software packages also allow personal messages from the nutritionist to the client or patient to be included with each printed report through use of a text editor. Another feature that is extremely useful is the automatic calculation of food exchanges or Food Guide Pyramid food groups contained within the analyzed diet. This allows the nutritionist to counsel the client or patient about potential deficiencies from a food group perspective. The scope, content, and presentation of the information generated vary greatly from one program to another, and users should ensure that printouts are appropriate, meaningful, and useful for specific needs.

Another system output feature that is useful to some nutritionists and most researchers is the ability of the software package to export the nutrient data to electronic files in a format that is useful for further statistical analysis. For example, if a researcher is analyzing the 7-day food records of 100 cancer patients, being able to electronically transport the nutrient summaries of each individual patient to a spreadsheet software program prior to statistical analysis can save a tremendous amount of effort.

Computerized Dietary Analysis Systems

Although several nutrition periodicals and journals regularly review general features of microcomputer dietary analysis systems (e.g., *Nutrition Today, Journal of Nutrition Education, Food and Nutrition News,* and *Journal of the American Dietetic Association*), very few comparative analyses have been published within the past 10 years.[6–8] In general, the few reports in the literature demonstrate that use of different computerized dietary analysis systems may yield widely discrepant results.

Box 5.4 lists general information on five computerized dietary analysis systems that meet most of the criteria listed in Box 5.3. ESHA Research (P.O. Box 13028, Salem, OR 97309) released the first version of Food Processor in 1984, and this was followed soon thereafter by Nutritionist I (at that time from N-squared Computing, and now from First DataBank Inc., 1111 Bayhill Drive, San Bruno, CA 94066). Multiple versions have been released since then, and these two programs are the most popular and critically acclaimed computerized dietary analysis systems among dietitians, nutritionists, nutrition professors, and allied health personnel.

In 1988, the Nutrition Coordinating Center (NCC) at the University of Minnesota released the Nutrition Data System, a microcomputer-based version of the mainframe computer system that had been developed beginning in 1974 in collaboration with the National Heart, Lung and Blood Institute (NHLBI) and outside experts in nutrition, statistics, computer science, and education. In 1998, NCC released the Nutrition Data System for Research (NDS-R), a Windows-based software package incorporating an up-to-date interface with its highly accurate database. The strength of the NDS-R is its extensive database, which contains more than 16,000 foods, 7600 brand name products, and many ethnic foods, with values for up to 117 nutrients and nutrient ratios, with virtually no missing nutrient values. There is a price, however, for this comprehensive database ($8500), and most users include medical and nutrition researchers, epidemiologists, and food and restaurant industries.

CyberSoft, Inc., entered the high-end dietary analysis software industry during the mid-1990s, with its Clinical NutriBase system (3851 E. Thunderhill Place, Phoenix, AZ 85044-6679). The NutriBase software package is an extremely sophisticated program, which contains a high number of food items and an amazing number of unique program operating features. Some may find this package too difficult to use, however, because it is complex, with a high learning curve. CyberSoft, Inc., maintains an excellent Internet site (www.nutribase. com), which provides an involved comparison of its products with those from ESHA Research and First DataBank. This website also provides the most complete list of computerized dietary analysis systems, with information on more than 50 companies.

FoodWorks from The Nutrition Company features a large database and numerous attractive reports at a moderate price. Analysis results can be exported for use with word processors, and spreadsheet and presentation software. FoodWorks uses four dietary standards: RDA/DRI, Daily Values, Canadian RNI, and FAO/WHO. Users can estimate daily energy expenditure using an extensive list of physical activities. Foods can be searched by name, content of a selected nutrient, or by nutrient density. FoodWise by McGraw-Hill is a smaller version of FoodWorks, and is available for users of this textbook and other students. FoodWise has over 8000 foods in its

---

Box 5.4   General Information for Selected Computerized Dietary Analysis Systems That Meet Most of the Criteria Listed in Box 5.3

Feature	Food Processor	Nutritionist V	NutriBase 2001 Clinical	Nutrition Data System for Research	FoodWorks
Company name	ESHA Research	First DataBank	CyberSoft, Inc.	Nutrition Coordinating Center	The Nutrition Company
Telephone number	800-659-3742	800-633-3453	800-959-4849	612-626-9450	888-659-6757
Internet site http://www.	www. esharesearch.com	www. firstdatabank.com	www. nutribase.com	www. ncc.umn.edu	www. nutritionco.com
2001 list price	$599	$595	$495	$8500	$200
Number of foods database	22,000+	16,000+	40,000+	16,000+	15,000+
Number of nutrients/ food components	114	80	111	117	84

database and provides analysis and three different types of reports for 30 nutrients and food components. Food-Wise features a weight management option that allows students to calculate energy expenditure, energy intake, and personal weight goals.

DIETARY ANALYSIS ON THE INTERNET

Use of the Internet through work and home personal computers became widespread during the late 1990s and commonplace early in the twenty-first century. Thousands of websites provide nutrition-based information, and the quality of this information ranges from excellent to very poor. Box 5.5 lists a few websites providing sound nutrition information. The Tufts University Nutrition Navigator is especially useful for rating the accuracy of nutrition content and usability of nutrition websites. A link to this and other websites related to computers in nutritional assessment are available on the *Nutritional Assessment* website at www.mhhe.com/hper/ nutrition.

Free dietary analysis on the Internet first became available during the mid-1990s. Box 5.6 summarizes five of the best Internet sites for dietary assessment. The Diet Analysis Web Page was the first online dietary analysis site, and it currently provides a table and graph of 16 nutrients from a 1-day food record. The top-rated online dietary assessment tool is the Interactive Healthy Eating

Index (IHEI) by the USDA's Center for Nutrition Policy and Promotion. Users at this site can enter food intake from 1 day and receive a score on the overall quality of their diet, nutrient intake data compared with the RDA for 24 nutrients, and a graphic comparison with the Food Guide Pyramid. The IHEI program is based on the Healthy Eating Index, which measures how well the American diet complies with the recommendations of the Dietary Guidelines for Americans and the Food Guide Pyramid (see Chapter 2).

Online dietary assessment tools will become increasingly valuable to nutrition professionals and will more than likely supplant dietary analysis software programs for the PC as Internet access becomes more widespread, faster, and more sophisticated. The Food and Nutrition Information Center (FNIC) maintains an up-to-date listing of online dietary assessment tools (www.nal.usda. gov/fnic).

Currently, online dietary assessment programs fall far short of dietary analysis software programs in several ways (although it is just a matter of time until these are resolved):

- Are slower and more cumbersome to use, and editing is more difficult
- Do not generally allow nutrient analysis of food intake from multiple days
- Have databases with fewer foods and nutrients

Box 5.5   Internet Sources for Sound Nutrition Information

- Tufts University Nutrition Navigator
  navigator.tufts.edu
  Provides a rating of the accuracy of nutrition content and usability of nutrition websites
- Mayo Health Oasis
  www.mayohealth.org
  Provides consumers with good nutrition information in a fun, user-friendly format
- Consumer Information Center
  www.pueblo.gsa.gov
  Provides access to hundreds of educational materials
- FDA Center for Food Safety and Applied Nutrition
  vm.cfsan.fda.gov/list.html
  Provides government updates on food and nutrition issues and basic nutrition guidelines
- Meals for You (My Menus)
  www.MealsForYou.com
  Provides thousands of recipes with menu plans, shopping lists, and nutritional analysis
- USDA Food and Nutrition Information Center
  www.nal.usda.gov/fnic
  Connects readers to the vast nutrition-related resources of the National Agricultural Library

- Healthfinder
  www.healthfinder.gov
  Organizes the health and nutrition information from federal and state agencies
- Vegetarian Resource Group
  www.vrg.org
  Provides nutrition information and recipes for those interested in the vegetarian diet
- American Dietetic Association
  www.eatright.org
  Provides nutrition information for both consumers and dietitians
- International Food Information Council
  ificinfo.health.org
  Provides guidelines on nutrition and food safety for consumers and professionals
- Cyberdiet
  www.cyberdiet.com
  Gives information on foods, recipes, vitamins and minerals, and food planning

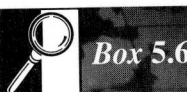

Box 5.6 Dietary Assessment on the Internet

Interactive Healthy Eating Index (http://147.208.9.133)

This online dietary assessment tool is based on the Healthy Eating Index developed by the U.S. Department of Agriculture's Center for Nutrition Policy and Promotion. The Healthy Eating Index measures how well your diet complies with the recommendations of the Dietary Guidelines for Americans and the Food Guide Pyramid. Enter a day's worth of diet intake, and you will receive a score on the overall quality of your diet for that day, nutrient intake data compared with the RDA for 24 nutrients, and a graphic comparison with the Food Guide Pyramid.

Diet Analysis Web Page (http//dawp.anet.com/)

This online dietary analysis provides a tabular and graphic report for 16 nutrients from a 1-day food record. The program uses the USDA Nutrient Database for Standard Reference, Release 13. It was developed by Chris Roberts.

Nutrition Analysis Tool (NAT) (www.nat.uiuc.edu/)

NAT is provided as an Internet public service by the Food Science and Human Nutrition Department at the University of Illinois. The database used by NAT is composed of the *USDA Handbook #8* and information from food companies. The tabular report compares intake from a 1-day food record with the RDA for 19 nutrients. NAT provides a strong help function, and users can save food intake data to a diskette.

DietSite Diet and Recipe Analysis
(www.dietsite.com/main.htm)

This Internet diet analysis program was developed by a dietitian to aid consumers in analyzing their diets. Users can enter a 1-day food record and receive tabular information on 27 nutrients in comparison with the RDA. The database includes 5600 foods from the USDA's *Handbook 8.*

Agricultural Research Service Nutrient Data Laboratory (www.nal.usda.gov/fnic/cgi-bin/nut_search.pl)

This Internet page provides access to Release 13 of the *USDA Nutrient Database for Standard Reference.* You can either view the data or download the data files and documentation in several different formats for use later on your computer. A search tool is also provided, so you can look up the nutrient content (more than 28 nutrients and a complete breakdown of fatty acids and amino acids) of more than 6200 foods directly from this page. Users can view the nutrient content for one food at a time but cannot enter a 1-day food record for analysis.

NOTE: A link to these and other websites related to computers in nutritional assessment are available on the *Nutritional Assessment* website at www.mhhe.com/hper/nutrition.

- Do not have as many special features (for example, nutrient sorting and database editing), and reports often limited to simple tables and graphs
- Often lack an adequate help function

As discussed in Chapter 3, there are both strengths and limitations in assessing dietary intake using 24-hour recalls, food records or food diaries, and food frequency questionnaires. An important feature that is being included with some computerized dietary analysis systems is the option to enter foods either by the standard diet record approach (specific quantities of foods unique to each patient) or from a food frequency list. In the latter option, the number of specified portions of listed foods is entered according to frequency of use (per day, week, or month).

The National Cancer Institute (NCI) has developed dietary analysis software for the analysis of food frequency questionnaires. The Block-NCI Health Habits and History Questionnaires (HHHQ) are food frequency questionnaires developed by Dr. Gladys Block and her colleagues at the NCI and have been repeatedly validated and used in epidemiologic studies.[14,15] Dr. Block is now associated with the University of California at Berkeley. The DietSys software was originally developed in the early 1980s as an analysis tool for the first Block-NCI HHHQ and then updated in 1987 and 1992 as the HHHQ was adapted. (See www.nutritionquest. com/ for more information.) This software program is cumbersome and difficult to use, and it is primarily recommended for research purposes, especially the study of diet-disease relationships. The DietSys software program estimates intake of 33 nutrients and up to 20 user-defined food groups from the HHHQ. The NCI does not support the use of the 1992 HHHQ unless it is modified to keep up with recent changes in the food supply, particularly the increased number of low-fat and nonfat foods available in the marketplace and changes in the fat content of meat.

NCI investigators have developed a self-administered, scannable food frequency questionnaire, the Diet History Questionnaire (DHQ). Validity and calibration studies indicate that the DHQ performs better than the Block-NCI HHHQ in several ways, and it captures changes in the food supply since the 1990s. The DHQ and its analysis software can be downloaded from the NCI Internet site: appliedresearch.cancer.gov/. The DHQ is recommended by the NCI for epidemiologic research and for nutrition professionals who prefer food frequency questionnaires over food records for estimation of nutrient intake.

SUMMARY

1. Computers are perfectly suited to the task of nutrient analysis, which is one of the most widespread applications of computer technology in dietetics. Computerized nutrient analysis tasks include clinical, educational, administrative, epidemiologic, and metabolic/experimental applications.

2. There are many factors to consider in selecting computerized dietary analysis systems. The first step is to establish the major needs for obtaining the software, with specific tasks defined. Once this has been accomplished, the next step is to choose a dietary analysis system that is suitable to these needs and tasks. There are three characteristics of software programs that dietitians and other health professionals can use to compare programs: (a) aspects of the database, (b) software program operation, and (c) system output.

3. The most important consideration to make when selecting a computerized diet analysis system is the nutrient database. The database must be accurate, verified, and large enough to meet all intended tasks.

4. The USDA Nutrient Data Laboratory develops and maintains a number of databases, including the USDA Nutrient Database for Standard Reference (SR) and the Primary Data Set for USDA Nationwide Food Surveys (PDS). SR and PDS nutrient data serve as the core for most commercial and many foreign databases and are the numerical foundation of essentially all public and private work on the field of human nutrition. These USDA nutrient databases can be downloaded from the Internet.

5. Developers of commercial computerized dietary analysis systems are faced with several challenges in formulating a high-quality database. These include deciding on how many foods and nutrients to include in the software program and use of non-USDA sources to give information on certain brand name foods and to fill in the missing data. The contents of nutrient databases from different software vendors may vary widely, depending on the number of food items and nutrients included, whether or not the most recent USDA releases have been incorporated, and the degree to which non-USDA sources (e.g., food industry, scientific literature) or estimating calculations are used to fill in the missing values.

6. The general operating features of the computerized diet analysis system are extremely important, determining whether a software package is easy to use while generating the desired information. These features include everything from search and entry of food items to the comparison of results with a variety of dietary standards.

7. Once the data have been entered into the computerized dietary analysis system, two important features are the software program's ability to print out a variety of printed reports, and export the data to a variety of electronic files for further analysis.

8. Use of the Internet through work and home personal computers became widespread during the late 1990s and commonplace early in the twenty-first century. Free dietary analysis on the Internet first became available during the mid-1990s. Online dietary assessment tools will become increasingly valuable to nutrition professionals and more than likely will supplant dietary analysis software programs for the PC as Internet access becomes more widespread, faster, and more sophisticated. Currently, online dietary assessment programs fall far short of dietary analysis software programs.

REFERENCES

1. Thompson FE. 1994. Dietary assessment resource manual. *Journal of Nutrition* 124(11 suppl):2245S–2317S.

2. Buzzard IM, Price KS, Warren RA. 1991. Considerations for selecting nutrient-calculation software: Evaluation of the nutrient database. *American Journal of Clinical Nutrition* 54:7–9.

3. Block G, Miller M, Harnack L, Kayman S, Mandel S, Cristofar S. 2000. An interactive CD-ROM for nutrition screening and counseling. *American Journal of Public Health* 90:781–785.

4. Kohlmeier L, Mendez M, McDuffie J, Miller M. 1997. Computer-assisted self-interviewing: A multimedia approach to dietary assessment. *American Journal of Clinical Nutrition* 65(4 suppl):1275S–1281S.

5. Jonnalagadda SS, Mitchell DC, Smiciklas-Wright H, Meaker KB, Van Heel N, Karmally W, Ershow AG, Kris-Etherton PM. 2000. Accuracy of energy intake data estimated by a multiple-pass, 24-hour dietary recall technique. *Journal of the American Dietetic Association* 100:303–308.

6. McCullough ML, Karanja NM, Lin PH, Obarzanek E, Phillips KM, Laws RL, Vollmer WM, O'Connor EA, Champagne CM, Windhauser MM. 1999. Comparison of 4 nutrient databases with chemical

composition data from the Dietary Approaches to Stop Hypertension trial. *Journal of the American Dietetic Association* 99(suppl):S45–S53.

7. Lee RD, Nieman DC, Rainwater M. 1995. Comparison of eight microcomputer dietary analysis programs with the USDA Nutrient Data Base for Standard Reference. *Journal of the American Dietetic Association* 95:858–867.

8. Nieman DC, Butterworth DE, Nieman CN, Lee KE, Lee RD. 1992. Comparison of six microcomputer dietary analysis systems with the USDA Nutrient Database for Standard Reference. *Journal of the American Dietetic Association* 92:48–56.

9. Nieman DC, Nieman CN. 1987. A comparative study of two microcomputer nutrient databases with the USDA Nutrient Database for Standard Reference. *Journal of the American Dietetic Association* 87:930–932.

10. Pao EM, Sykes KE, Cypel YS. 1990. Dietary intake—Large scale survey methods. *Nutrition Today* 25(6):11–17.

11. Stillings BR. 1994. Trends in foods. *Nutrition Today* 29(5):6–13.

12. Schakel SF, Sievert YA, Buzzard IM. 1988. Sources of data for developing and maintaining a nutrient database. *Journal of the American Dietetic Association* 88:1268–1271.

13. Schakel SF, Buzzard IM, Gebhardt SE. 1997. Procedures for estimating nutrient values in food composition databases. *Journal of Food Composition Analysis* 10:102–114.

14. Potischman N, Carroll RJ, Iturria SJ, Mittl B, Curtin J, Thompson FE, Brinton LA. 1999. Comparison of the 60- and 100-item NCI-Block questionnaires with validation data. *Nutrition and Cancer* 34:70–75.

15. Velie E, Kulldorff M, Schairer C, Block G, Albanes D, Schatzkin A. 2000. Dietary fat, fat subtypes, and breast cancer in postmenopausal women: A prospective cohort study. *Journal of the National Cancer Institute* 92:833–839.

ASSESSMENT ACTIVITY 5.1

Analysis of Your 24-Hour Recall on the Internet

Fill out a 24-hour recall (see Chapter 3) and analyze your nutrient intake using the Interactive Healthy Eating Index (IHEI) as described in Box 5.6 (http://147.208.9.133). Also, analyze your 24-hour recall using one other Internet dietary assessment tool listed in Box 5.6. Print out results from each program, and compare them in the following table. Then answer the questions that follow the table.

Nutrient	IHEI	Other Internet Program
Energy (kcal)		
Protein (gm)		
Carbohydrate (gm)		
Dietary fiber (gm)		
Total fat (gm)		
Cholesterol (mg)		
Vitamin A (RE)		
Vitamin C (mg)		
Calcium (mg)		
Iron (mg)		
Zinc (mg)		
Sodium (mg)		

1. Did you find that some nutrient intake estimates from the two Internet programs varied more than 10%? List the nutrients that varied 10% or more.

2. What reasons can you list to explain the differences listed in question #1? Consider issues such as differences in databases, food substitution, program operation features, and program output.

Assessment Activity 5.2

Comparison of Computerized Dietary Analysis Systems

Box 5.3 contained a checklist to evaluate computerized dietary analysis systems. Copy this checklist three times, and then go to the CyberSoft, Inc., website at www.nutribase.com. Click on Visit Our Competitors, review some of the listed dietary analysis systems, choose three systems that seem interesting to you, and answer as many of the questions in the Box 5.3 checklist as you can from the information provided by each company. Take this comparison to class and compare notes with other students.

Assessment Activity 5.3

Internet Sources for Sound Nutrition Information

Box 5.5 summarized 11 Internet sites that provide sound nutrition information. A link to this and other websites related to computers in nutritional assessment are available on the Nutritional Assessment website at www.mhhe.com/hper/ nutrition. One of these sites, the Tufts University Nutrition Navigator (navigator.tufts.edu), provides a rating of the accuracy of nutrition content and usability of nutrition websites. Go to the Tufts University Nutrition Navigator site and list three sites that include dietary analysis and have received high ratings.

Three Internet sites that contain some aspect of dietary analysis and are highly rated:

1. Name of Internet site: _____

Basic description: _____

_____

_____

2. Name of Internet site: _____

Basic description: _____

_____

_____

3. Name of Internet site: _____

Basic description: _____

_____

_____

_____

_____

INTRODUCTION

Anthropometry is of considerable interest to scientists and the public. It is a valuable adjunct in assessing nutritional status. Concerns about the social and health implications of overweight and obesity have led many people to question the appropriateness of their weight, body composition, and body image. This has resulted in debate and confusion about which methods and standards should be used in assessing body weight and composition. Unfortunately, in some people it has led to such a preoccupation with body weight that their eating habits and body image have become disordered.

The effect of nutrition on human growth and development has made accurate measurement of the body's dimensions and weight indispensable to the practice of nutritional assessment. Properly assessing growth and development requires that standardized methods be followed for measuring the body. Assessment of the body's protein and muscle stores is fundamental to the diagnosis and treatment of malnutrition and to the evaluation of a patient's response to nutrition and other therapy. Nutritional research often depends on methods of accurately assessing changes in body growth and composition.

This chapter describes the available techniques for measuring the body's dimensions and composition. Some of these techniques will be used daily by practitioners, and others will be limited to nutritional research. This chapter establishes an essential foundation for applying the principles for assessing growth and development, nutritional status, and response to nutrition and other therapy.

Mastering and intelligently applying the techniques and information in this chapter will provide you with skills that will be invaluable to your work in the field of nutrition.

WHAT IS ANTHROPOMETRY?

Anthropometry is the measurement of body size, weight, and proportions.[1–3] Measures obtained from anthropometry can be sensitive indicators of health,

development, and growth in infants and children.[2] Anthropometric measures can be used to evaluate nutritional status, whether it be obesity caused by overnutrition or emaciation resulting from protein-energy malnutrition. They are valuable in monitoring the effects of nutritional intervention for disease, trauma, surgery, or malnutrition.[1,4] Anthropometry also is considered the method of choice for estimating body composition in a clinical setting.[5]

MEASURING LENGTH, STATURE, AND HEAD CIRCUMFERENCE

Measurements of length, stature (or height), weight, and head circumference are among the most fundamental and easily obtained anthropometric measurements. Among infants and children, these measurements are the most sensitive and commonly used indicators of health. A child's growth and development can be assessed by comparing stature for age, weight for age, weight for stature, and BMI for age with standards obtained from studies of large numbers of healthy, normal children. The measurement of stature is important for calculating certain indices such as weight for stature, weight divided by stature, and the creatinine height index and for estimating basal energy expenditure.[6]

In measurements of length and stature, reference will be made to positioning the head in the **Frankfort horizontal plane.** As shown in Figure 6.1, this plane is represented by a line between the lowest point on the margin of the orbit (the bony socket of the eye) and the *tragion* (the notch above the tragus, the cartilaginous projection just anterior to the external opening of the ear). With the head in line with the spine, this plane should be horizontal.[7]

Figure 6.1
Length and stature are measured with the head in the Frankfort horizontal plane. This plane is represented by a line between the lowest point on the margin of the orbit (the bony socket of the eye) and the tragion (the notch above the tragus, the cartilaginous projection just anterior to the external opening of the ear).

In all anthropometric measurements, consistency in technique and units of measurement (feet/inches, centimeter/millimeter, and so on) will help eliminate potential sources of error.[1,2]

Length

Length (also referred to as recumbent length) is obtained with the subject lying down and generally is reserved for children less than 24 months of age or for children between 24 and 36 months of age who cannot stand erectly without assistance.[2,7] The growth charts used for persons birth to 36 months of age are based on recumbent length, whereas the growth charts for those age 2 to 18 years are based on stature.[8] Measurement of recumbent length requires a special measuring device (Figure 6.2) with a stationary headboard and moveable footboard that are perpendicular to the backboard. The device's measuring scale (in millimeters or inches) should have its zero end at the edge of the headboard and allow the child's length to be read from the footboard.[2]

Two persons are required to measure recumbent length, as shown in Figure 6.2. With the child in the supine position (lying on his or her back), one person holds the child's head against the backboard, with the crown securely against the headboard and with the Frankfort plane perpendicular to the backboard. This person also keeps the long axis of the child's body aligned with the center line of the backboard, the child's shoulders and buttocks securely touching the backboard, and the shoulders and hips at right angles to the long axis of the body. The other person keeps the child's legs straight and against the backboard, slides the footboard against the bottom of the feet (without shoes or socks) with the toes pointing upward, and reads the measurement. The footboard should be pressed firmly enough to compress the soft tissues of the soles but without diminishing the vertebral column length. Length should be recorded to the nearest 0.1 cm or ⅛ in., using a consistent unit over re-

peated measurements.[2,7] Gentle restraint is often required to keep a squirming infant properly positioned during measuring. When this is not possible, the best estimate should be recorded with a notation of the circumstances.[2]

Stature

Stature, or standing height, can be measured for subjects 2 to 3 years of age and older who are cooperative and able to stand without assistance.[2,7] Stature can be measured in several ways. The simplest is to fasten a measuring stick or nonstretchable tape measure to a flat, vertical surface (for example, a wall) and use a right-angle headboard for reading the measurement. If a wall is used, it should not have a thick baseboard, and the subject should not stand on carpet, which could affect the accuracy of measurements.[7] Using the moveable rod on a platform scale is not recommended because it often lacks rigidity, the headboard is not always correctly aligned, there is no rigid surface against which to position the body, and the platform height will vary depending on the subject's weight.[9]

Another approach is to use a **stadiometer,** such as the Harpenden stadiometer or one manufactured by Seca Corporation or Measurement Concepts. A list of suppliers of nutritional assessment equipment can be found in Appendix M or at the *Nutritional Assessment* website at www.mhhe.com/hper/nutrition. When being measured with the stadiometer, the subject should be barefoot and wear minimal clothing to facilitate correct positioning of the body. The subject should stand with heels together, arms to the side, legs straight, shoulders relaxed, and head in the Frankfort horizontal plane ("look straight ahead"). Heels, buttocks, scapulae (shoulder blades), and back of the head should, if possible, be against the vertical surface of the stadiometer, as shown in Figure 6.3. Some people may not be able to touch all four points against the stadiometer because of obesity, protruding buttocks, or curvature of the spine. Rather than creating an embarrassing situation by trying to force a subject into

Head placed in Frankfort plane, with crown of head touching headboard

Heels against footboard

Shoulders and buttocks touching backboard

Long axis of body in line with center of backboard

Figure 6.2 Special device for measuring the length of children who cannot stand erectly without assistance; the device has a stationary headboard and a moveable footboard.

Source: Drawing by William Gagnon, Jr.

Figure 6.3 Body position when measuring stature.

Measurer's eyes level with headboard.

Headboard flat against the wall and resting on crown of head. Head in the Frankfort plane.

Head, shoulder blades, and buttocks against the wall.

Shoulders relaxed, arms at sides.

Feet bare, flat on floor. Heels close together and against the wall.

a physically impossible position, have the subject touch two or three of the four points to the vertical surface of the stadiometer or estimate height from knee height, as is discussed in Chapter 7.

Just before the measurement is taken, the subject should inhale deeply, hold the breath, and maintain an erect posture ("stand up tall") while the headboard is lowered on the highest point of the head with enough pressure to compress the hair.[1,2,7] The measurement should be read to the nearest 0.1 cm or ⅛ in. and with the eye level with the headboard to avoid errors caused by **parallax,** which is a difference in the apparent reading of a measurement scale or a skinfold caliper's needle when these are viewed from various points not in a straight line with the eye.[1,2,7] Hair ornamentation may have to be removed if this interferes with the measurement.

Nonambulatory Persons

In nonambulatory persons (those unable to walk) or those who have such severe spinal curvature that measurement of height would be inaccurate, stature can be estimated from knee height.[1,6] This and other recumbent measures and their application in nutritional assessment of older persons are discussed in Chapter 7.

Head Circumference

Head circumference measurement is an important screening procedure to detect abnormalities of head and brain growth, especially in the first year of life. Although these conditions may or may not be related to nutritional factors, discussion of head circumference measurement is included here for convenience.[2,9] Head circumference

increases rapidly during the first 12 months of life but, by 36 months, growth is much slower.[10] Therefore, it is recommended that head circumference be measured routinely on infants and young children up to age 36 months.[2]

Head circumference is most easily measured when the infant or child is sitting on the lap of the caregiver, although older children can be measured when they are standing.[2,7] A flexible, nonstretchable measuring tape is required. Objects such as pins should be removed from the hair. As shown in Figure 6.4, the lower edge of the

Just above the supraorbital ridges

Over part of occiput

Head in Frankfort plane

Figure 6.4
When measuring head circumference, the lower edge of the tape should be just above the eyebrows and ears, around the occipital prominence of the head, tight enough to compress the hair.

tape should be positioned just above the eyebrows, above (not over) the ears, and around the back of the head, so that the maximum circumference is measured. The tape should be in the same plane on both sides of the head and pulled snug to compress the hair. The measurement is read to the nearest 0.1 cm or ⅛ in. and written in the infant's file. Reliability of the measurement should be verified with a second reading.[2,7]

MEASURING WEIGHT

One of the most important measurements in nutritional assessment is body weight. Weight is an important variable in equations predicting caloric expenditure and in indices of body composition.[11]

Body weights should be obtained using an electronic scale or a balance-beam scale with nondetachable weights, as shown in Figure 6.5. Compared with balance beam scales, electronic scales tend to be lighter in weight, somewhat more portable, and faster and easier to use. They provide easy-to-read digital output in either metric or English units and, when properly calibrated, are highly accurate. Errors are commonly made in reading scale, dials, and rulers. The large, easily read digital output from electronic scales can help reduce this error. Digital scales can record a subject's weight quickly. This can be an advantage in weighing infants, who tend to resist lying still for very long.

Scales should be placed on a flat, hard surface that will allow them to sit securely without rocking or tipping. The zero weight on the scale's horizontal beam should be checked periodically and after the scale has been

Figure 6.5
Balance beam scales (platform on the left and pan type on the right) are used in weighing subjects. The zero weight on the horizontal beam of the scale should be checked periodically and after the scale has been moved.

moved.[1,2] On balance beam scales this can be done by sliding the main and fractional weights to their respective zero positions and adjusting the zeroing weight until the beam balances at zero. Two or three times a year the accuracy of the scales should be further assured by using standard weights or by a professional dealer. Because spring-type bathroom scales may not provide the required accuracy after repeated use, they are not recommended.[1,2,7] Balance-beam scales with wheels that are moved from one location to another are not recommended either because scales must be recalibrated every time they are moved.

Infants

Infants should be weighed on a pan-type pediatric electronic or balance-beam scale that is accurate to within 10 g (0.01 kg) or ½ oz, as shown in Figure 6.5.[2,7] Any cushion (for example, either a towel or diaper) used in the pan should be in place when the zero adjustments are made on the scale or its weight should be subtracted from the infant's weight. Whatever practice is used, it must be uniformly followed and noted in the infant's file. Infants can be weighed nude, or the weight of the infant's diaper can be subtracted from the infant's weight. The infant should be set lying down in the middle of the pan. The average of two or three weighings is recorded numerically in the infant's file to the nearest 10 g (0.01 kg) or ½ oz and then is plotted on the growth chart in the presence of the subject's caregiver. If, on comparison with previous data, the current values appear unusual, the measurements should be repeated.[2,7]

Excessive infant movement can make it difficult to obtain an accurate weight, in which case the weighing can be deferred until later in the examination. When too active to weigh on a baby scale, an infant can be weighed on a platform scale while being held by an adult with the weight derived by difference. Because this weight will be less accurate than desired (but still better than no weight), the method should be noted in the infant's chart.

Children and Adults

Children and adults who can stand without assistance are weighed on a platform electronic or balance-beam scale that is accurate to 100 g (0.1 kg) or ¼ lb, as shown in Figure 6.5.[1,2,7] The subject should stand still in the middle of the scale's platform without touching anything and with the body weight equally distributed on both feet. The weight should be read to the nearest 100 g (0.1 kg) or ¼ lb and recorded. Two measurements taken in immediate succession should agree to within 100 g (0.1 kg) or ¼ lb.[1] The weight of children then can be plotted on their growth charts. As with infants, if there seems to be any discrepancy between the current and past values, the measurement should be repeated for verification. Diurnal variations (cyclical changes occurring throughout the day) in weight of about 1 kg in children and 2 kg in adults are known to occur.[7,11] For this reason, it is a good practice to also record the time weight was measured.

Ideally, children and adults should be weighed after voiding and dressed in an examination gown of known weight or in light underclothing with the scales placed where adequate privacy is provided.[1,2,7] Should the weight of clothing be subtracted from the subject's weight? It depends on the purpose for which measurements are obtained and how accurate they need to be. In settings requiring a high degree of accuracy, subjects can be clothed in an examination gown of known weight for which consideration can be easily made. In situations having somewhat less stringent requirements, a reasonable estimate of clothing weight can be subtracted from a subject's weight.[1,7]

Nonambulatory Persons

Persons who cannot stand unassisted on a scale can be weighed in a bed scale or chair scale.[1,7] The subject to be weighed in the bed scale (shown in Figure 6.6) is comfortably positioned in the weighing sling, which then is gently raised until the subject is suspended off the bed. In a chair scale, the subject sits upright in the center of the chair while leaning against the backrest. Using either method, once the subject is still, weight can be read and recorded to the nearest 100 g (0.1 kg) or ¼ lb. Reliability of the measurement can be verified with a second reading, which should agree to within 100 g or ¼ lb.[1]

Body weight also can be computed from knee height, calf circumference, midarm circumference, and subscapular skinfold thickness.[1,10] Descriptions of these anthropometric measurements and computational formulas for computing body weight are given in Chapter 7.

Figure 6.6
A bed scale can be used to weigh bedridden patients.

CDC Growth Charts

Growth charts are a fundamental screening tool for assessing the nutritional status and general well-being of infants, children, and adolescents.[8] They allow a child's physical development (size and growth) to be compared with that of other healthy children of the same sex and age. Many countries have developed growth charts based on large-scale cross-sectional surveys, which have collected data on the length, stature, weight, and head circumference of a nationally representative sample of apparently healthy and well-nourished infants and children. An excellent example of pediatric growth charts are those developed for the United States by the U.S. Centers for Disease Control and Prevention (CDC).[8] The CDC growth charts are a revision of growth charts originally developed by the U.S. National Center for Health Statistics (NCHS) in the 1970s (what are referred to as the "1977 NCHS charts"). Work on the current CDC growth charts began in 1985 and they were published in 2000. Figure 6.7 shows a CDC growth chart developed for assessing length-for-age and weight-for-age in females from birth to 36 months of age.

The CDC has developed growth charts for females and males for two age intervals: birth to 36 months and 2 to 20 years. The charts for the age interval birth to 36 months give percentile curves for weight-for-age, length-for-age, weight-for-length, and head circumference-for-age. For the age interval 2 to 20 years, the charts give percentile curves for stature-for-age, weight-for-age, body mass index-for-age, and weight-for-stature. Figure 6.8 shows the body mass index-for-age chart for males ages 2 to 20 years. The charts also come in two separate sets that differ in the outer limits of their percentile curves. The first set has curves at the 5th, 10th, 25th, 50th, 75th, 90th, and 95th percentiles, with the outer limits of the curves at the 5th and 95th percentiles. It is expected that this set of charts (included in Appendix N) will be used for the majority of routine clinical assessments. The second set has curves at the 3rd, 10th, 25th, 50th, 75th, 90th, and 97th percentiles, with the outer limits of the curves at the 3rd and 97th percentiles. This set would be used relatively infrequently to assess children whose growth is at the extremes of the distribution. Both sets can be downloaded from the website of the National Center for Health Statistics (www.cdc.gov/nchs/). A link to this website and others relating to growth charts can be found on the *Nutritional Assessment* website at www.mhhe.com/ hper/nutrition.

When using the birth-to-36-month charts, length is measured in the recumbent position (lying down). When using the charts for persons 2 to 20 years old, stature (height) should be measured with the child standing. The median difference between length and stature at 2 to 3 years of age is about 0.2 in., or 0.5 cm.[12] Head circumference, a variable included in the birth-to-36-month age charts, is omitted in the charts for 2- to 20-year-olds.

Birth to 36 months: Girls
Length-for-age and weight-for-age percentiles

NAME _____

RECORD # _____

AGE (MONTHS)

Mother's Stature _____
Father's Stature _____

Gestational
Age: _____ Weeks

Comment

Date	Age	Weight	Length	Head Circ.	
Birth					

SOURCE: Developed by the National Center for Health Statistics in collaboration with
the National Center for Chronic Disease Prevention and Health Promotion (2000).
http://www.cdc.gov/growthcharts

SAFER · HEALTHIER · PEOPLE™

Figure 6.7
Example of a growth chart developed by the U.S. Centers for Disease Control and Prevention.
This one assesses both length-for-age and weight-for-age in U.S. females birth to 36 months of age.

2 to 20 years: Boys
Body mass index-for-age percentiles

NAME _____

RECORD # _____

Date	Age	Weight	Stature	BMI*	Comments

*To Calculate BMI: Weight (kg) ÷ Stature (cm) ÷ Stature (cm) x 10,000
or Weight (lb) ÷ Stature (in) ÷ Stature (in) x 703

SOURCE: Developed by the National Center for Health Statistics in collaboration with
the National Center for Chronic Disease Prevention and Health Promotion (2000).
http://www.cdc.gov/growthcharts

Figure 6.8

The body mass index-for-age growth charts developed by the CDC are an important advancement over the 1977 NCHS charts, which did not include BMI as an assessment variable. This chart is for males ages 2 to 20 years. The one for females is included in Appendix N.

The CDC growth charts are based primarily on anthropometric measurements performed on nationally representative samples of infants, children, and adolescents during a series of national health examination surveys conducted by the NCHS between 1963 and 1994. These include cycle II of the National Health Examination Survey (NHES) (1963–65), cycle III of the NHES (1966–70), the first National Health and Nutrition Examination Survey (NHANES I) (1971–74), NHANES II (1976–80), and NHANES III (1988–94).[8]

The CDC growth charts are an improvement over the 1977 NCHS charts, particularly the charts for birth to 36 months. The data used to develop the 1977 NCHS charts for birth to 36 months were collected between 1929 and 1975 as part of the Fels Longitudinal Study at the Fels Research Institute in Yellow Spring, Ohio. The infants in this study were primarily formula-fed, white, and middle-class, and they were from a limited geographical area of southwestern Ohio. Although the Fels Longitudinal Study provided the best available data on infants and young children at the time, there were problems with the data set. The population studied was not representative of the ethnically diverse U.S. population. The Fels data were collected at 3-month intervals and were inadequate for developing reference data at the 1-month intervals used in the charts. Median birth weights between 1929 and 1975 were approximately 125 g less than current median birth weights and do not represent recent national birth weight distributions. The anthropometric procedures used in the Fels Study systematically overestimated the recumbent length of infants and young children. Recumbent length data used in the current charts were collected using a more accurate measuring procedure. The infants in the Fels Study were primarily formula-fed. In recent decades, infant feeding practices in the United States have changed. Approximately 50% of U.S. infants are breast-fed, and about one-third are breast-fed for at least 3 months.

The current charts for birth to 36 months are based primarily on data sets from NHANES I (1971–74), NHANES II (1976–80), and NHANES III (1988–94). In order to provide sufficient data for revising the 1977 NCHS charts, NHANES III was specifically designed to "oversample" infants and preschool children ages 2 months through 5 years. In other words, a disproportionate number of infants and children in this age category were surveyed to provide the necessary data. However, because none of the NHES or NHANES surveys collected data on infants birth to 2 months of age, supplemental data from other sources were incorporated to create the infant growth chart data set. These included vital statistics data from Wisconsin and Missouri, data from the Pediatric Nutrition Surveillance System, and head circumference data from the Fels Longitudinal Study. In order to better assess children growing at the extremes of the distribution, the percentile curves of the current charts

for both age categories were extended to include the 3rd and 97th percentiles.

Several important changes were made in the charts for children and adolescents 2 to 20 years of age. The age range of the charts now extends to 20 years, whereas the 1977 NCHS charts did not extend beyond 17 completed years of age. Body mass index-for-age charts were added and an 85th percentile curve was added to the BMI-for-age charts and to the weight-for-stature charts. Additional data generated by NHANES II (1976–80) and NHANES III (1988–94) were used in the revised charts.[8] From among these changes, the most notable is the addition of the BMI-for-age charts. Data collected between 1963 and 1994 were used to develop these charts, except that NHANES III weight data for children ages ≥ 6 years were excluded. This was done to prevent the observed increases in body weight between NHANES II and NHANES III from inappropriately influencing the charts. Including these data would elevate the upper percentile curves used to identify children who are at risk of overweight (≥ 85th percentile and < 95th percentile) or who are overweight (≥ 95th percentile). If the NHANES III data were included, some children and adolescents who are overweight or at risk of overweight would not be classified as such.[8] The BMI-for-age charts replace the 1977 NCHS weight-for-stature charts that were limited to prepubescent males < 11.5 years of age and < 57 in. (145 cm) tall and to prepubescent females < 10.0 years of age and < 54 in. (137 cm) tall.[8] The 85th percentile curve was added to the BMI-for-age charts to assist clinicians in identifying children and adolescents in the upper 15% of the distribution. There is general agreement among experts that children and adolescents having a BMI-for-age ≥ 95th percentile are overweight, while those ≥ 85th percentile but < 95th percentile are considered at risk of overweight.[8]

The revised weight-for-stature charts benefited from additional data from NHANES II and NHANES III. These were developed for children 2 to 5 years of age who might be evaluated only during the preschool years—for example, children participating in the Special Supplemental Nutrition Program for Women, Infants, and Children (WIC). The revised charts are intended to apply to all racial and ethnic groups. Although racial and ethnic differences in growth exist (for example, BMI-for-age), the CDC decided that the available scientific evidence suggests that these differences are more likely a result of environmental factors and socioeconomic disparities, rather than genetics. In addition, there are insufficient data on specific racial and ethnic groups to create growth charts for these populations.

To use the charts properly, measurements for length, stature, head circumference, and weight must be carefully taken following the standardized methods originally used in collecting the data from which the charts were developed. The approaches outlined in this book conform to those standardized methods and therefore are appropriate. Because chronological age is the most influential variable in rapidly growing children, it is essential that the subject's exact age be known before plotting age-dependent variables (for example, weight for age).[2] Age should be calculated to the nearest month when using the birth-to-36-month charts and to the nearest quarter year when using the 2- to 18-year charts.[2]

To plot the data, first locate the subject's age on the chart's horizontal axis (see Figure 6.7). Then locate the subject's length, stature, weight, or head circumference on the vertical axis. Draw a small circle on the chart where the lines representing these two values intersect. Check to make sure that the circle you have drawn is at the correct point in reference to the two variables. A complete growth chart should include data that are both recorded numerically and plotted on the chart. If you plot the data while the subject is still present, you may repeat the measurements if unusual or changed values appear.[2]

Variables on the chart, shown in Figure 6.7, are presented as seven **percentile** curves: 5, 10, 25, 50, 75, 90, and 95. A child's length for age, for example, would be considered average when, once it was plotted, it was on or near the 50th percentile curve. In other words, the 50th percentile is considered the average, or **median,** value for the specific population of interest. If the plotted length for age were on the 75th percentile curve, 75% of girls her age would be shorter than she would. If a child's height for age were at the 10th percentile, only 10% of children of the same age and sex would be shorter. Ranking persons this way is appropriate if they are part of the reference population from which the data were obtained. Values less than the 5th percentile and greater than the 90th percentile warrant evaluation. If, over time, a person's plotted values change markedly (i.e., cross two percentile lines), the reasons for that change should be investigated.

The values displayed in the charts are called "reference data" rather than "standards." Reference data represent a cross-sectional description of a population and describe "what is." Standards, on the other hand, describe "what should be" and imply that the values are "ideals" or "goals" associated with maximum health and longevity.[12]

WEIGHT STANDARDS

Overweight is defined as a body weight above some reference point of acceptable weight that usually is defined in relation to height.[13] **Obesity** is defined as an excess of body fat in relation to lean body mass.[14,15] There is good evidence that overweight persons, as a group, tend to die sooner than average-weight persons, especially those who are overweight at younger ages.[16–19] As seen in Figure 6.9, risk of death increases as body mass index (a weight-height index discussed later in this chapter in the "Height-Weight Indices" section) increases above about

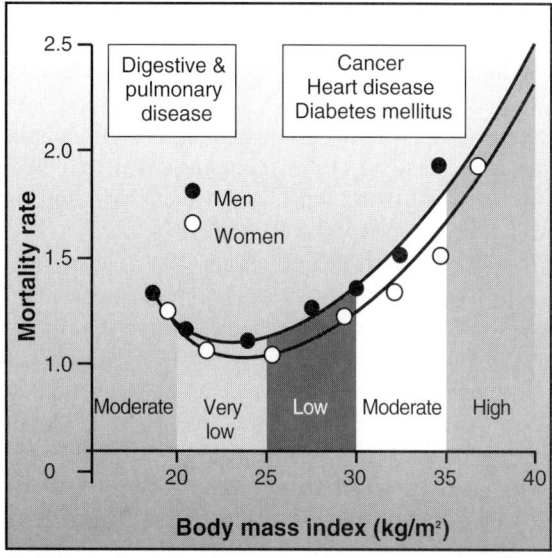

Body mass index and mortality risk

Figure 6.9

Risk of death from certain cancers, coronary heart disease, and diabetes mellitus increases as body mass index increases. Digestive disease and pulmonary diseases increase risk of death and often result in marked weight loss.

Source: Data from the American Cancer Society (adapted from Lew and Garfinkel).

25 kg/m².[15] Some researchers believe that the lowest mortality rates in the United States (and many other Western nations) is associated with body weights somewhat below the average weight of the population under consideration.[18,19] In other words, the "average" body weights of middle-aged Americans may not be the most healthy.

At the same time, however, dietitians and nutritionists should be cautioned against encouraging weight loss when it is not indicated. There is no question that a body weight that is too low is unhealthy and increases risk of death. This is seen in persons suffering starvation or anorexia nervosa. A person whose BMI is < 25 kg/m² probably does not have a weight problem and probably does not need to lose weight. Figure 6.9 shows the relationship between body mass index (BMI) and risk of death to be curvilinear instead of linear. It suggests that, as BMI falls below about 20 kg/m², risk of death increases. This relationship is referred to as a "J-shaped" curve. But what actually increases risk of mortality in persons with low BMI? Is it low body weight itself or certain diseases (e.g., chronic obstructive pulmonary disease, cancers of the gastrointestinal tract, and lung cancer) that, in addition to markedly increasing risk of death, often causes marked weight loss? A 26-year mortality study of nearly 9000 nonsmoking, nondrinking men did not show this curvilinear relationship, even among the 5% of men whose BMI was < 20 kg/m².[20] However, questions have been raised about this analysis. Some research suggests that the observed increased risk of death at a low BMI may result from loss of lean body mass rather than low body weight per se. Other research suggests that, when differences in fat loss are controlled for, weight loss is associated with an increased mortality rate. When differences in weight loss are controlled for, fat loss is associated with a decreased mortality rate.[19]

A variety of approaches exist for determining a person's recommended body weight. A very simple one frequently used by dietitians in the clinical setting, and known as the Hamwi equation, is to allow 100 lb (45.5 kg) for the first 60 in. (152 cm) of stature for females and then add 5 lb (2.3 kg) for each additional 1 in. (2.54 cm). For males, allow 106 lb (48 kg) for the first 60 in. (152 cm) of stature and then add 6 lb (2.7 kg) for each additional 1 in. (2.54 cm). By creating a range of ±10%, allowance for the effects of frame size can be made. Consider, for example, a female who is 68 in. tall. Based on this approach, her recommended body weight range would be 126 to 154 lb (140 lb ±10%).

Height-Weight Tables

Body weight can be assessed through the use of height-weight tables and the use of **relative weight** and **height-weight indices.** Height-weight tables are convenient, quick, easy to use, and understood by practically every adult. However, because of their limitations, they are being supplanted by better approaches, such as body mass index (kg/m^2).

The life insurance industry has been in the forefront of developing height-weight tables because of its access to the data necessary for generating them. The tables were developed by comparing the heights and weights of life insurance policyholders with statistical data (known as actuarial data) on mortality rates and/or longevity of policyholders. Actuarial data were compiled on literally millions of insured persons in the United States and Canada in an attempt to define weights associated with the greatest longevity and lowest mortality rates.[14,18,19,21] The insurance industry has used data from the tables to help screen applicants to avoid insuring persons who are poor risks. Good reviews of the topic have been published by Weigley,[21] Harrison,[13] and Manson and coworkers.[22]

The Metropolitan Life Insurance Company published the Ideal Weight Tables in 1942 and 1943,[23,24] the Desirable Weight Tables in 1959,[25] and the Height-Weight Tables in 1983.[26] Table 6.1 is the 1983 Metropolitan Life table. Table 6.2 compares the 1959 and 1983 Metropolitan tables with average weights from several studies.[22] The 1959 and 1983 Metropolitan tables were based on data from the Build and Blood Pressure Study 1959 and Build Study 1979, respectively. The American Cancer Society Study examined data on body weight and longevity on about 750,000 adult males and females from 1959 to 1973. In this study, the lowest mortality rates occurred among nonsmokers weighing 80% to 89% of

average weight.[22] Data from the first National Health and Nutrition Examination Survey show average weights for a representative sampling of the U.S. population between 1971 and 1974.

For a given stature, the weights defined by the Metropolitan tables as recommended were *less than the average* weights of the population under study. Although limitations with much of the existing data preclude a valid assessment of optimal weight, it appears that minimum mortality occurs at weights approximately 10% below the U.S. average.[22] Such terms as *ideal* and *desirable* were used to identify those weights, for a given stature, that were associated with greatest longevity or the least mortality from diabetes and diseases of the gallbladder, heart, kidneys, and blood.[18,21,22]

Age-Specific Weight Standards

Some researchers have suggested that weight in early adulthood should not be used as a standard of "desirable" or "healthy" weight throughout the remainder of life. They suggest that data on body weight and morbidity and mortality indicate that overweight during early adult life is more dangerous than a similar degree of overweight in later adult life.[27] Some of the same researchers think that weight standards should be more liberal for older adults than for younger adults. To support this view, they cite statistics showing that, as people age from their 20s to their 60s, the body weight associated with lowest mortality tends to increase about 4.5 kg, or 10 lb, per decade.[27-29]

Table 6.3 shows the height-weight table published in the 1990 revision of the *Dietary Guidelines for Americans.* Note that the suggested weights are considered applicable to both male and female adults and no reference is made to frame size. Also unique is the greater allowable weight range for persons 35 years of age or older, compared with those 19 to 34 years old. This represented a substantial increase over earlier weight recommendations. For example, compare the upper weight limit for a 68-in. female from Table 6.3 with the upper weight limit for a 68-in. female with medium frame from the 1983 Metropolitan table (Table 6.1). The maximum suggested weight from the 1990 *Dietary Guidelines for Americans* allowed this person to weigh 14 lb more (if ages 19 to 34 years) and 28 lb more (if 35 years or older) than the 1983 Metropolitan table. The appropriateness of higher allowable weights for older persons is discussed in the section "Limitations of Height-Weight Tables."

Limitations of Height-Weight Tables

Height-weight tables have several limitations, which are summarized in Box 6.1.[13,19,22,29] Because tables are formulated from data drawn from specific groups or populations, they may not be applicable to other groups or populations. This is especially true of tables based on insurance industry data, which are derived from people

TABLE 6.1	1983 Metropolitan Life Insurance Company Height-Weight Table for Persons Ages 25 to 59 Years (Height Without Shoes, Weight Without Clothing*)						
Height		**Small Frame**		**Medium Frame**		**Large Frame**	
in.	cm	lb	kg	lb	kg	lb	kg
Men							
61	155	123–129	56–59	126–136	57–62	133–145	60–66
62	157	125–131	57–60	128–138	58–63	135–148	61–67
63	160	127–133	58–60	130–140	59–64	137–151	62–69
64	163	129–135	59–61	132–143	60–65	139–155	63–70
65	165	131–137	60–62	134–146	61–66	141–159	64–72
66	168	133–140	60–64	137–149	62–68	144–163	65–74
67	170	135–143	61–65	140–152	64–69	147–167	67–76
68	173	137–146	62–66	143–155	65–70	150–171	68–78
69	175	139–149	63–68	146–158	66–72	153–175	70–80
70	178	141–152	64–69	149–161	68–73	156–179	71–81
71	180	144–155	65–70	152–165	69–75	159–183	72–83
72	183	147–159	67–72	155–169	70–77	163–187	74–85
73	185	150–163	68–74	159–173	72–79	167–192	76–87
74	188	153–167	70–76	162–177	74–80	171–197	78–90
75	191	157–171	71–78	166–182	75–83	176–202	80–92
Women							
57	145	99–108	45–49	106–118	48–54	115–128	52–58
58	147	100–110	45–50	108–120	49–55	117–131	53–60
59	150	101–112	46–51	110–123	50–56	119–134	54–61
60	152	103–115	47–52	112–126	51–57	122–137	55–62
61	155	105–118	48–54	115–129	52–59	125–140	57–64
62	157	108–121	49–55	118–132	54–60	128–144	58–65
63	160	111–124	50–56	121–135	55–61	131–148	60–67
64	163	114–127	52–58	124–138	56–63	134–152	61–69
65	165	117–130	53–59	127–141	58–64	137–156	62–71
66	168	120–133	55–60	130–144	59–65	140–160	64–73
67	170	123–136	56–62	133–147	60–67	143–164	65–75
68	173	126–139	57–63	136–150	62–68	146–167	66–76
69	175	129–142	59–65	139–153	63–70	149–170	68–77
70	178	132–145	60–66	142–156	65–71	152–173	69–79
71	180	135–148	61–67	145–159	66–72	155–176	70–80

Adapted from 1983 Metropolitan Height and Weight Tables. 1983. *Statistical Bulletin of the Metropolitan Life Insurance Company* 64 (Jan.–June):3. Courtesy of the Metropolitan Life Insurance Company.

*Height without shoes obtained by subtracting 1 in. from heights with shoes for males and females. Weight without clothes obtained by subtracting 5 lb and 3 lb from weight with clothes for males and females, respectively.

who apply for life insurance—predominantly white, middle-class adults. African Americans, Asians, Native Americans, Hispanics, and low-income persons are not proportionally represented.[10]

The quality of the data on height and weight is variable.[13] The same care in obtaining the NHANES data was not used in collecting data for the Metropolitan tables, where approximately 10% of the heights and weights were self-reported. Self-reporting of height and weight has been shown to be inaccurate, and the error is influ-

enced by such factors as sex, actual height, and actual weight.[30–32] Rowland,[31] for example, showed that errors in self-reported weight were directly related to a person's overweight status and increased directly with the magnitude of overweight. The frequency of overreporting height increases with increasing height and is more common in males than females.[33]

There is often inadequate documentation and control of certain variables known to confound the relationships between weight and mortality.[13,22] Most important among

Table 6.2	Comparison of Metropolitan Desirable Weights with Average Weights from U.S. Cohorts

			Average Weight for Ages 40–49 Years kg (lb)			
Height (Without Shoes), cm (ft. in.)	Metropolitan Tables* (Medium Frame), Weight in Kilograms (Pounds) (Without Clothing)		Insured Lives		American Cancer Society Study 1979§ (1959)‡	National Health and Nutrition Examination Survey (NHANES I, 1979‖ (1971–1974)‡
	1959	1983	Build and Blood Pressure Study 1959† (1935–1953)‡	Build Study 1979† (1950–1971)‡		
Men						
156 (5 1)	50–55 (111–122)	57–62 (126–136)	60 (133)	61 (135)	———	———
159 (5 2)	52–57 (114–126)	58–63 (128–138)	62 (137)	63 (139)	67 (148)	66 (145)#
162 (5 3)	53–59 (117–129)	59–64 (130–140)	64 (141)	65 (144)	68 (149)	68 (150)#
164 (5 4)	54–60 (120–132)	60–65 (132–143)	66 (145)	68 (149)	69 (153)	73 (162)
167 (5 5)	56–62 (123–136)	61–66 (134–146)	68 (149)	69 (153)	71 (156)	72 (159)
169 (5 6)	58–64 (127–140)	62–68 (137–149)	70 (154)	72 (158)	73 (160)	75 (166)
172 (5 7)	59–66 (131–145)	64–69 (140–152)	72 (158)	73 (162)	74 (163)	78 (173)
174 (5 8)	61–68 (135–149)	65–70 (143–155)	73 (162)	76 (167)	77 (169)	79 (174)
177 (5 9)	63–69 (139–153)	66–72 (146–158)	76 (167)	78 (171)	78 (173)	79 (175)
179 (5 10)	65–72 (143–158)	68–73 (149–161)	78 (171)	80 (176)	80 (177)	83 (184)
182 (5 11)	67–74 (147–163)	69–75 (152–165)	80 (176)	82 (181)	83 (182)	85 (188)
185 (6 0)	68–76 (151–168)	70–77 (155–169)	82 (180)	85 (187)	85 (187)	88 (194)
187 (6 1)	70–78 (155–173)	72–78 (159–173)	84 (185)	87 (192)	87 (192)	92 (203)
190 (6 2)	73–81 (160–178)	73–80 (162–177)	86 (190)	90 (198)	90 (198)	92 (203)#
192 (6 3)	75–83 (165–183)	75–83 (166–182)	89 (196)	92 (203)	92 (203)#	———
Women						
146 (4 9)	43–48 (94–106)	48–54 (106–118)	54 (120)	52 (115)	———	58 (127)#
149 (4 10)	44–49 (97–109)	48–54 (106–120)	56 (123)	54 (118)	52 (115)	59 (131)#
151 (4 11)	45–51 (100–112)	50–56 (110–123)	57 (126)	54 (120)	55 (121)	62 (136)
154 (5 0)	47–52 (103–115)	51–57 (112–126)	59 (129)	56 (124)	57 (126)	64 (141)
156 (5 1)	48–54 (106–118)	52–59 (115–129)	60 (132)	57 (126)	58 (128)	63 (138)
159 (5 2)	49–55 (109–122)	54–60 (118–132)	62 (136)	59 (130)	60 (132)	64 (141)
162 (5 3)	51–57 (112–126)	55–61 (121–135)	63 (139)	60 (133)	62 (136)	67 (148)
164 (5 4)	53–59 (116–131)	56–63 (124–138)	65 (143)	62 (136)	63 (139)	68 (151)
167 (5 5)	54–61 (120–135)	58–64 (127–141)	67 (147)	64 (140)	64 (142)	71 (156)
169 (5 6)	56–63 (124–139)	59–65 (130–144)	68 (151)	65 (144)	66 (146)	71 (156)
172 (5 7)	58–65 (128–143)	60–67 (133–147)	70 (155)	67 (147)	68 (150)	72 (158)
174 (5 8)	60–67 (132–147)	62–68 (136–150)	73 (160)	70 (152)	71 (156)	78 (172)
177 (5 9)	62–68 (136–151)	63–69 (139–153)	75 (165)	70 (155)	73 (161)	———
179 (5 10)	64–70 (140–155)	64–71 (142–156)	77 (170)	72 (159)	75 (165)	

Used with permission from Manson JE, Stampfer, MJ, Henniker CH, and Willett WC. 1987. Body weight and longevity: A reassessment. *Journal of the American Medical Association* 257:353–358. Copyright 1987, American Medical Association.

*Not age specific: 1959 tables recommended for ages 25 years and older, 1983 tables for ages 25 to 59 years.

†Without shoes or clothing.

‡Years when measurements were taken.

§Values are means for age groups 40 to 44 years and 45 to 49 years. Self-reported heights without shoes and weights with indoor clothing.

‖Values are means for age groups 35 to 44 years and 45 to 54 years. Measured without shoes; clothing ranged from 0.20 to 0.62 lb (not deducted from weights shown).

#Estimated values obtained from linear regression equations.

these confounding variables is cigarette smoking. Smokers tend to weigh less than nonsmokers but have higher mortality rates because of smoking-related diseases. Including data on smokers in height-weight tables tends to make lower weights appear less healthy and higher weights appear more healthy.[34]

Table 6.3	Suggested Weights for Adults	
	Weight (lb)[†]	
Height* (in.)	**19 to 34 Years**	**35 Years or Older**
60	97–128[‡]	108–138
61	101–132	111–143
62	104–137	115–148
63	107–141	119–152
64	111–146	122–157
65	114–150	126–162
66	118–155	130–167
67	121–160	134–172
68	125–164	138–178
69	129–169	142–183
70	132–174	146–188
71	136–179	151–194
72	140–184	155–199
73	144–189	159–205
74	148–195	164–210
75	152–200	168–216
76	156–205	173–222
77	160–211	177–228
78	164–216	182–234

1990. *Nutrition and your health: Dietary guidelines for Americans,* 3rd ed. U.S. Department of Agriculture and U.S. Department of Health and Human Services.

*Without shoes.

[†]Without clothes.

[‡]The higher weights in the ranges generally apply to men, who tend to have more muscle and bone; the lower weights more often apply to women, who have less muscle and bone.

There have been problems associated with frame measurements.[29] The 1959 Metropolitan tables never defined how frame size was determined. The frame size measurements used in the 1983 Metropolitan tables are based on NHANES I and NHANES II data and are so devised that 25% of the population is classified as having a small frame, 50% as having a medium frame, and 25% as having a large frame. Within the range of body weights considered acceptable for a given height and sex, the lower end of the weight range was assumed to be for small-framed persons, the middle of the range for medium-framed persons, and the upper end of the range for large-framed persons. This practice may not be appropriate because data on height/weight and frame size were obtained from two distinct population groups.

The weight measurements used in compiling the data were only those taken when the subjects initially applied for life insurance.[29] If weight changed between issuance of the policy and death, this was not taken into account. Age also was not taken into account.

Finally, weight tables fail to provide information on actual body composition—the proportions of fat and lean tissue—or on the distribution of body fat. This is a critical weakness because the quantity of weight (a person's actual weight) is considerably less important than the quality of weight (how much of that weight is fat and how much is lean tissue). An unusually muscular person with a low body fat content (for example, a football player or weight lifter) may be overweight according to a height-weight table but not obese. Body composition can be estimated from measurements of skinfolds, densitometry (hydrostatic or underwater weighing), and other methods.

The more liberal suggested weights for older persons have been called into question by several leading authorities on the health consequences of obesity and overweight.[19,34,35] Based on the limitations of height-weight tables, Willett and coworkers[34] regard the height-weight standards in the 1990 revision of the *Dietary Guidelines for Americans* as "fundamentally invalid" and state that there is "no biologic rationale for recommending that persons increase their weight as they grow older; indeed, there is much evidence to the contrary." The height-weight

 ***Box* 6.1**   **Strengths and Limitations of Height-Weight Tables**

Strengths

Weight is an important distinguishing feature of identification.

Weight and height can be accurately measured.

Height-weight tables are easily understood and used by many.

Height-weight tables are a part of our culture.

Limitations

The data on which height-weight tables are based are not representative of the entire population.

Quality of the data is variable.

Some of the data are cross-sectional and do not allow associations between weight and mortality to be drawn.

There is inadequate control of potentially confounding variables, especially smoking.

It is not always clear how frame size was determined.

Tables do not provide information on body composition.

standards suggest an average weight gain of approximately 16 lb between early and later adulthood. A weight gain of this magnitude has been shown to be associated with a 50% increase in risk of diabetes and a 30% increase in coronary heart disease risk.[36,37] Higher blood pressure and lower concentrations of high-density lipoprotein also would likely result. The researchers suggest that the only probable benefit would be increased bone density and reduced risk of hip fracture.[34] In a study of nearly 9000 nonsmoking, nondrinking men, there was no evidence for a "J-shaped" relationship between BMI and mortality in these males. Although the protective effect associated with a lower BMI decreased somewhat with increasing age, persons with a lower BMI still had a lower risk of death than persons with a higher BMI at all ages.[20]

Strengths of Height-Weight Tables

Height-weight tables have some strengths.[13] Body weight is an important concept, and next to age, sex, and race it is regarded as the most distinguishing feature of identification. Height and weight are easily measured, and most adults and many adolescents and children are able to understand and use height-weight tables. The tables have become ingrained in the medical and nonmedical culture of North America.[13]

Despite these strengths, height-weight tables are essentially obsolete. They have been replaced by body mass index (BMI), which is regarded as a better measure of adiposity.[19] A notable instance where BMI has replaced height-weight tables as the recommended approach for determining healthy weight is the *Dietary Guidelines for Americans,* as discussed in Chapter 2.

MEASURING FRAME SIZE

The classification of subjects on the basis of frame size has been a common feature of the Metropolitan height-weight tables. However, it was not until the 1983 tables that a technique for determining frame size (elbow breadth) was even specified. Additionally, the data on which the 1983 tables were based included no physical measurements of frame size.[18] In preparing the Metropolitan tables, classification of frame size apparently relied as much on subject self-appraisal as on any other method.[38]

Several approaches to determining frame size have been proposed,[39] including biacromial breadth (distance between the tips of the biacromial processes at the top of the shoulders) and bitrochanteric breadth (distance between the most lateral projections of the greater trochanter of the two femurs),[38,40–42] the ratio of stature to wrist circumference;[43] breadth of the chest based on chest X rays,[44] knee and wrist breadth,[45] and elbow breadth.[46] Measuring elbow breadth appears to be the most practical way of determining frame size and was taken into consideration when the 1983 Metropolitan tables were developed. The other methods are limited by such factors as lack of population norms, difficulty in obtaining measurements, and the influence of adiposity.[18,29,38]

When measuring elbow breadth, the subject stands erectly, with the right upper arm extended forward perpendicular to the body, as shown in Figure 6.10. The forearm is then flexed until the elbow forms a 90-degree angle, with fingers up, palm facing the subject. The measurer then should feel for the widest bony width of the elbow and place the heads of a flat-blade sliding caliper at those points. Pressure should be firm enough to compress soft tissues. The measurement should be read to the nearest 0.1 cm or ⅛ in.[40] Elbow breadth classifications for males and females of various stature are given in Table 6.4. Some data suggest that frame measurements do not materially improve the ability to predict body fat from body weight.[45,47] Other researchers suggest avoiding frame-adjusted tables because of the lack of data on the relationship of frame size to body weight.

The following formula can be used to determine frame size from the ratio of body height to wrist circumference,[43]

$$r = \frac{H}{C}$$

where r = the ratio of body height to wrist circumference; H = body height in centimeters; and C = circumference

Elbow flexed
90 degrees

Caliper blades measure
widest part of elbow.

Upper arm parallel to floor

Figure 6.10
Elbow breadth is sometimes used for determining frame size. With the arm and hand in this position, a sliding caliper can be used to measure the widest point at the elbow.

Table 6.4		**Elbow Breadth Classifications for Males and Females of Various Stature**						
Height*		**Small Frame**		**Medium Frame**		**Large Frame**		
in.	cm	in.	mm	in.	mm	in.	mm	
Males								
61–62	155–158	< 2½	< 64	2½–2⅞	64–73	> 2⅞	> 73	
63–66	159–168	< 2⅝	< 67	2⅝–2⅞	67–73	> 2⅞	> 73	
67–70	169–178	< 2¾	< 70	2¾–3	70–76	> 3	> 76	
71–74	179–188	< 2¾	< 70	2¾–3⅛	70–90	> 3⅛	> 79	
≥ 75	≥ 189	< 2⅞	< 73	2⅞–3¼	73–83	> 3¼	> 83	
Females								
57–58	145–148	< 2¼	< 57	2¼–2½	57–64	> 2½	> 64	
59–62	149–158	< 2¼	< 57	2¼–2½	57–64	> 2½	> 64	
63–66	159–168	< 2⅜	< 60	2⅜–2⅝	60–67	> 2⅝	> 67	
67–70	169–178	< 2⅜	< 60	2⅜–2⅝	60–67	> 2⅝	> 67	
≥ 71	≥ 79	< 2½	< 64	2½–2¾	64–70	> 2¾	> 70	

Courtesy of the Metropolitan Life Insurance Company.

*Table adapted to represent height without shoes.

Table 6.5	**Determining Frame Size from the Ratio of Body Height to the Circumference of the Right Wrist**	
	r Value	
Frame Size	**Women**	**Men**
Small	> 10.9	> 10.4
Medium	10.9–9.9	10.4–9.6
Large	< 9.9	< 9.6

Adapted from Grant JP, Custer PB, Thurlow J. 1981. Current techniques of nutritional assessment. *Surgical Clinics of North America* 61:437–463.

of the right wrist in centimeters. Compare the value for r with those in Table 6.5 to determine frame size.[43]

To measure the right wrist circumference, the arm should be flexed at the elbow with the palm facing upward and the hand muscles relaxed. Place the measuring tape around the wrist crease just distal to (beyond) the styloid processes of the radius and ulna (the two bony prominences at the wrist). The measuring tape must be no wider than 0.7 cm, so that it can fit into the depressions between the styloid processes and the bones of the hand. The tape should be perpendicular to the long axis of the forearm. The tape should be touching the skin but not compressing the soft tissues. Record the measurement to the nearest 0.1 cm.[48]

HEIGHT-WEIGHT INDICES

In view of the shortcomings of height-weight tables, particularly their inability to provide information on actual body composition, investigators have sought better approaches to assessing body weight and fatness, (or adi-

posity) that can be derived from easily obtainable anthropometric measures, such as weight and stature. This has led to the development of various height-weight indices or body mass indices which are shown in Table 6.6. An index is simply a ratio of one dimension (e.g., weight) to another dimension (e.g., height). The height-weight indices are of two types: relative weight and power-type indices.

Relative Weight

Relative weight is a person's *actual weight* divided by some *reference weight* for that person's height and multiplied by 100, so that it can be expressed as a percentage.

Table 6.6	**Height-Weight Indices***
Relative weight:	$\dfrac{\text{Actual weight}}{\text{Reference weight}} \times 100$
Weight/height ratio:	$\dfrac{\text{Weight}}{\text{Height}}$
Quetelet's index:	$\dfrac{\text{Weight}}{\text{Height}^2}$
Khosla-Lowe index:	$\dfrac{\text{Weight}}{\text{Height}^3}$
Ponderal index:	$\dfrac{\text{Height}}{\text{Weight}^{1/3}}$
Benn's index:†	$\dfrac{\text{Weight}}{\text{Height}^p}$

Data from Lee J, Kolonel LN, Hinds MW. 1981. Relative merits of the weight-corrected-for-height indices. *American Journal of Clinical Nutrition* 34:2521–2529.

*The numerical values of the indices depend on the values used (for example, kilograms and meters or pounds and inches).

†"p" is a population-specific exponent derived from height-weight data of the population sample. Consequently, its value changes from sample to sample.

The Framingham Heart Study, for example, used an index called Metropolitan relative weight, which uses as its reference weight the midpoint of the "desirable" weight range for a person of medium frame, as given in the 1959 Metropolitan tables.[18]

To calculate the Metropolitan relative weight (MRW), take as an example a 35-year-old male whose stature is 70 in., or 179 cm, and who weighs 181 lb, or 82 kg. The midpoint of the weight range for a 70-in. person with a medium frame from the 1959 Metropolitan height-weight table (Table 6.2) would be 151 lb, or 69 kg. The MRW for this person would be calculated as follows:

$$\frac{181 \text{ lb (actual weight)}}{151 \text{ lb (reference weight)}} \times 100 = 120\% \text{ MRW}$$

Thus, this man's MRW is 120%, or his weight is 20% greater than the reference weight. Depending as it does on height-weight tables, relative weight is subject to the same limitations of height-weight tables. A relative weight within the range of 90% to 120% is generally considered acceptable.

Power-Type Indices

As shown in Table 6.6, several power-type indices are available for assessing body weight relative to height.[49–52] The preferred index should be maximally correlated with body mass (weight) and should be minimally correlated with stature. In other words, it should be equally good at indicating body mass, no matter how tall or short a person is. Of those indices shown in Table 6.6, there is general agreement among researchers and expert panels that Quetelet's index is preferred for assessing the body weight of children, adolescents, and adults.[19,53–55]

The most widely used height-weight index is the **Quetelet's index** (W/H^2), which is more commonly known as **body mass index (BMI).**[19,53–56] Because all the power-type indices are body mass indices, the more technically correct name for W/H^2 is Quetelet's index. Quetelet's index is obtained by dividing weight in kilograms by height in meters squared. Consider a male weighing 70 kg (154 lb) and standing 178 cm, or 1.78 m, (70 in.) tall. His body mass index would be

$$\frac{70 \text{ kg (weight in kilograms)}}{3.17 \text{ m}^2 \text{ (height in meters squared)}} = 22 \text{ kg/m}^2$$

Body mass index has a relatively high correlation with estimates of body fatness and a low correlation with stature.[53] Garrow and Webster,[52] for example, showed that Quetelet's index correlated well with estimates of body composition from three methods—body density, total body water, and total body potassium—and concluded that Quetelet's index "is both a convenient and reliable indicator of obesity." The National Institutes of Health[19] has recommended that physicians use Quetelet's index in evaluating patients. Many scientists consider Quetelet's index to be an appropriate way to assess body weight in children and adolescents.[57–60] Roche and coworkers[61] have found Quetelet's index to be the best single indicator of total body fat in girls and adults and the best single indicator of percent body fat in men. Of the other height-weight indices shown in Table 6.6, Quetelet's index has shown the closest correlation with estimates of body fatness by skinfold measurements and densitometry.[62,63]

Frisancho and Flegel[64] have shown Quetelet's index to correlate well with estimates of body fatness based on skinfold measurements, and they recommend combining Quetelet's index with skinfold measurements whenever possible. Investigators have suggested combining Quetelet's index with the rather easily obtained waist circumference as an improved means of assessing increased risk in adults for heart disease, stroke, type 2 diabetes, and premature death.[19,53,65,66]

A **nomogram** for determining Quetelet's index is shown in Figure 6.11. To use the nomogram, place a straightedge on the point of the height scale that corresponds to height in centimeters or inches and on the point of the weight scale that corresponds to weight in kilograms or pounds. Then read the Quetelet's index on the center scale. Use nomograms with caution. In some publications, nomograms may be inadvertently modified and thus rendered inaccurate.[67] This occurred in two highly

Figure 6.11

The Quetelet index (kg/m^2) is calculated from this nomogram by placing a straightedge on the measurements for height and body weight and reading the point at which the straightedge intersects the central scale.

Source: Adapted with permission from Nieman DC. 1995. *Fitness and sports medicine: A health-related approach,* ed 3. Palo Alto: Bull Publishing Co.

respected reports: *The Surgeon General's Report on Nutrition and Health* and the National Research Council's *Diet and Health.*

Table 6.7 shows classifications of overweight and obesity and associated disease risk based on Quetelet's index (BMI) and waist circumference in adults. In Table 6.7, it should be noted that even in persons with a "normal" BMI, increased waist circumference can be a marker for increased risk of type 2 diabetes, hypertension, and cardiovascular disease.[65] There is no standard approach for using anthropometric measures to assess regional fat distribution in children. Consequently, use of waist circumference in conjunction with BMI is not recommended for children at this time.[54] The recommended approach for use of BMI for evaluating body weight in children and adolescents is use of the BMI-for-age growth charts developed by the CDC, discussed in the section "CDC Growth Charts."

As BMI increases above 20 kg/m^2, there is a gradual increase in risk of morbidity from such conditions as type 2 diabetes, hypertension, coronary heart disease, stroke, gallbladder disease, osteoarthritis, sleep apnea and other respiratory problems, and some types of cancer (prostate, colon, endometrial, and breast).[53,65] However, risk of morbidity and mortality from these conditions increases precipitously when BMI is greater than 25 kg/m^2. This observation resulted in *overweight* being defined as having a BMI of 25.0 to 29.9 kg/m^2 and in *obesity* being defined as a BMI of 30.0 or greater.

Based on data from NHANES III, for example, the prevalence of hypertension in adults with a BMI < 25 kg/m^2 is 18.2% and 16.5% for males and females, respectively. At a BMI ≥ 30 kg/m^2, the prevalence of hypertension is 38.4% and 32.2% in males and females, respectively.[65] Data from the Nurses' Health Study show that risk for colon cancer is twice as high in women with a BMI > 29 kg/m^2 than in women with a BMI < 21 kg/m^2.[68] This observed increase in morbidity and mortality with increased BMI is seen across all population groups. However, the specific degree of increased risk associated with any given level of overweight varies with race/ethnicity, age, gender, societal condition, and family history of disease or presence of other disease risk factors. Consequently, the classifications of overweight and obesity and associated disease risks shown in Table 6.7 are approximations based on the best available data and are influenced by a variety of factors, which must be carefully considered by the clinician.[65]

How do the BMIs of American adults compare with these standards? Figure 6.12 shows how the percent of American men and women classified as overweight (BMI of 25.0 to 29.9 kg/m^2) and classified as obese (BMI ≥ 30 kg/m^2) changed between 1960 and 1994, based on data from four nationally representative surveys, NHES I, NHANES I, NHANES II, and NHANES III. Between 1960 and 1994, the percent of overweight American men and women increased slightly from 37.8% to 39.4% in men and from 23.6% to 24.7% in women. During the same period, however, the prevalence of obesity increased from 10.4% to 19.9% in men and from 15.1% to 24.9% in women, and most of this increase occurred between NHANES II and NHANES III.[19,65]

As discussed in the section "CDC Growth Charts," age- and sex-specific BMI cutpoints are used to classify children as "at risk of overweight" or "overweight." Charts giving BMI-for-age percentiles have been developed by the CDC for children and adolescents ages 2 to 20 years (for example, Figure 6.8). Those with a BMI-for-age ≥ 85th percentile but < 95th percentile are classified as at risk for overweight. A BMI-for-age ≥ 95th

| TABLE 6.7 | Classification of Overweight and Obesity by Body Mass Index (BMI), Waist Circumference, and Associated Disease Risk* in Adults |

			Disease Risk* Relative to Normal Weight and Waist Circumference	
	BMI (kg/m^2)	Obesity Class	Men ≤ 40 in. (≤ 102 cm); Women ≤ 35 in. (≤ 88 cm)	Men > 40 in. (> 102 cm); Women > 35 in. (> 88 cm)
Underweight	< 18.5		——	——
Normal†	18.5–24.9		——	——
Overweight	25.0–29.9		Increased	High
Obesity	30.0–34.9	I	High	Very high
	35.0–39.9	II	Very high	Very high
Extreme obesity	≥ 40.0	III	Extremely high	Extremely high

Adapted from National Heart, Lung, and Blood Institute. 1998. *Clinical guidelines on the identification, evaluation, and treatment of overweight and obesity in adults.* Washington, DC: National Institutes of Health, U.S. Department of Health and Human Services.

*Disease risk for type 2 diabetes, hypertension, and cardiovascular disease.

†Increased waist circumference can also be a marker for increased risk even in persons of normal weight.

Figure 6.12 Change in the percent of American men and women classified as overweight (BMI 25.0 to 29.9 kg/m²) and obese (BMI ≥ 30 kg/m²) between 1960 and 1994.

Although the percent classified as overweight increased slightly during this time, the percent classified as obese increased substantially, particularly between NHANES II and NHANES III.

Source: National Heart, Lung, and Blood Institute. 1998. *Clinical guidelines on the identification, evaluation, and treatment of overweight and obesity in adults.* Washington, DC: National Institutes of Health, U.S. Department of Health and Human Services.

percentile is used to define overweight and identifies those children and adolescents with a significant likelihood of persistence of obesity into adulthood.[54] A BMI-for-age ≥ 95th percentile is associated with elevated blood pressure and lipid and lipoprotein profiles that increase the risk for obesity-related disease and mortality. Pediatric obesity experts recommend that these children and adolescents have an in-depth medical assessment and possibly undergo treatment for weight loss.[54] Figure 6.13 shows how the percent of overweight American males and females ages 6 to 11 years and 12 to 17 years changed between 1963 and 1994. These percentages are based on data from four nationally representative surveys, NHES cycles II and III, NHANES I, NHANES II,

Figure 6.13 Change in the percent of American children and adolescents classified as overweight between 1963 and 1994.

In this figure, the definition of overweight is a BMI-for-age ≥ 95th percentile for children and adolescents from cycles II and III of the National Health Examination Survey (NHES) conducted between 1963 and 1970. A particularly dramatic increase in the prevalence of overweight occurred between the administration of NHANES II and NHANES III.

Source: Data from the Centers for Disease Control and Prevention, National Center for Health Statistics.

and NHANES III. It's important to note that the "reference population" used to establish the 95th percentile for BMI-for-age was the data set from NHES cycles II and III.[54,69] This was the earliest available nationally representative data set for height and weight of children and adolescents and was chosen to be the standard against which data from the subsequent three surveys were compared. As can be seen in Figure 6.13, the percent of children and adolescents having a BMI-for-age ≥ 95th percentile (based on data from NHES II and III) increased in the decades since the early 1970s.

Although height-weight indices tend to be better predictors of obesity than height-weight tables or relative weight (they are more closely associated with percent of body fat than height-weight tables or relative weight), they still do not distinguish between overweight resulting from obesity and that resulting from muscular development. This requires the use of indirect and direct measurements of body composition, such as densitometry, total body water, and total body potassium. These measurements and the concept of body composition are discussed in the next sections.

Body Fat Distribution

Body fat distribution is an important concept in considering the health implications of obesity.[15,19,65] Where fat is placed, or distributed, within the body may actually be more important than quantity of body fat. Body fat distribution can be classified into two types: (1) upper body, android, or male type, and (2) lower body, gynoid, or female type.[19] Obese persons having a greater proportion of fat within the upper body, especially within the abdomen, compared with that within the hips and thighs, have **android obesity.** Obese persons with most of their fat within the hips and thighs have **gynoid obesity.** Android obesity is generally (but not always) seen in obese males, whereas females generally carry a greater proportion of their body fat on the hips and thighs.[19]

Numerous studies have shown that risk for insulin resistance, hyperinsulinemia (elevated blood insulin levels), noninsulin-dependent (type 2) diabetes mellitus, hypertension, hyperlipidemia (elevated blood cholesterol and triglyceride levels), and stroke, as well as risk for death are increased in persons with android obesity. Although the approaches used to assess fat distribution varied somewhat among these studies, they consistently showed that disease risk is associated with upper-body placement of body fat.[19,70] They also showed that fat distribution is a more important risk factor for morbidity and mortality than is obesity per se.[19,71] In obese adolescent females, android obesity tends to be associated with elevated levels of triglyceride, serum cholesterol, and low-density lipoprotein (LDL) cholesterol. Android obesity in

adolescent males tends to be associated with lower levels of high-density lipoprotein (HDL) cholesterol, a higher ratio of total cholesterol to HDL cholesterol, and higher levels of LDL cholesterol.[72]

Total abdominal fat has been described as the sum of the fat, or adipose tissue, present in three compartments of the body's abdominal region: subcutaneous (just under the skin), visceral (surrounding the organs within the peritoneal cavity), and retroperitoneal (outside of and posterior to the peritoneal cavity). Research suggests that excessive fat in the visceral compartment is most strongly correlated with increased risk for morbidity and mortality; however, this is a matter of debate and remains to be determined. What is certain is that the presence of increased total abdominal fat is an independent risk predictor, even when BMI is not markedly increased.[65,73] Total abdominal fat can be most accurately measured using magnetic resonance imaging or computed tomography. However, these approaches are expensive and not readily available in the clinical setting. Two other approaches for assessing total abdominal fat that are relatively easy to perform in the clinical setting are the waist-to-hip ratio and waist circumference. The waist-to-hip ratio (WHR) is calculated by dividing the waist circumference by the hip (or gluteal) circumference. Because of the increased risk for hypertension, type 2 diabetes, and hyperlipidemia associated with increased abdominal fat and the lower risks associated with fat placement in the hips and thighs, it is preferred that the waist circumference be less than the hip circumference, and consequently the WHR be somewhat less than 1. Some authorities recommend that the WHR be < 0.9 and < 0.8 for adult males and females, respectively, and that when WHR is greater than these cutpoints the risk for disease rises steeply.[15] In recent years, researchers have shown that waist circumference is actually a better predictor of total abdominal fat content than the WHR and a better predictor of disease risk.[74–76] For example, a team of Canadian researchers used computed tomography to measure abdominal fat content in nearly 800 adult males and females.[74] When they compared these measurements with estimates of abdominal fat content derived from WHR and waist circumference measurements, they found that waist circumference was the best overall predictor of abdominal visceral obesity and that, in women, WHR was a poor predictor and its use should be avoided. Because of this and other research, the National Institutes of Health (NIH) recommends using waist circumference to assess abdominal fat content.[65,73] The NIH has concluded that waist circumference is an easy and practical method for assessing regional body fat distribution. It is a valuable guide in assessing health risk in persons categorized as normal or overweight (in terms of BMI) and provides an independent prediction of risk over and above that of BMI.[65,73] Waist circumference has been shown to be positively correlated with the amount of fat within the abdomen and to serve as a good indicator of abdominal visceral obesity.[74]

Figure 6.14 illustrates how waist circumference is measured in adults.[65,73] Ask the subject to remove any outer clothing restricting easy access to the abdomen and waist or interfering with placement of the measuring tape against the bare skin or interfering with measurement accuracy (by compressing the abdomen or distorting the natural shape of the subject's abdomen and waist). The subject should be undressed to light underclothing and wearing a gown or smock to maintain his or her modesty. Locate the right iliac crest by using the fingertips to gently feel for the highest point of the hip bone on the subject's right side. Using a soft-tipped, washable pen, draw a short horizontal mark just above the uppermost lateral border of the right iliac crest. Then cross this with a vertical mark along the midaxillary line. Place an inelastic, flexible tape measure in a horizontal plane (parallel to the floor) around the abdomen at the level of this marked

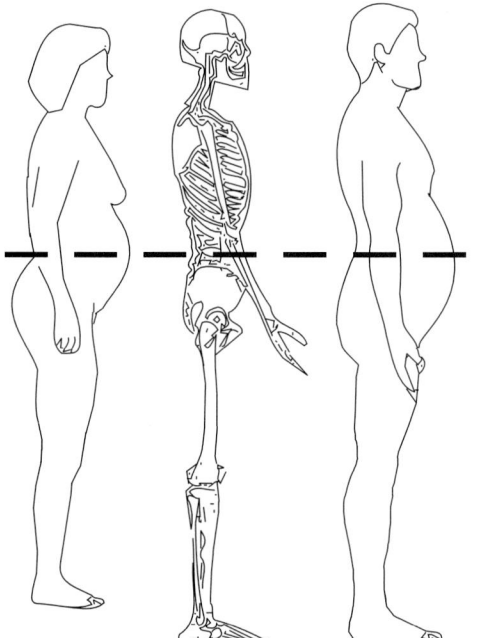

Figure 6.14

To measure waist circumference in adults, locate the top of the right iliac crest, the highest point of the hip bone on the right side. Place a measuring tape in a horizontal plane (parallel to the floor) around the abdomen at the level of the iliac crest. The tape should be snug but should not compress the skin. Take the reading at the end of a normal expiration. Repeat the measurement to ensure accuracy.

Source: National Heart, Lung, and Blood Institute. 1998. *The practical guide: Identification, evaluation, and treatment of overweight and obesity in adults.* Washington, DC: National Institutes of Health, U.S. Department of Health and Human Services.

point on the right side of the subject. The subject should stand erectly, abdominal muscles relaxed, arms at the side, and feet together. The tape should be snug against the skin but not so tight as to compress the skin. Take the reading at the end of a normal expiration. Repeat the measurement once or twice to ensure that an accurate measurement has been obtained and record the measurement to the nearest 0.1 cm.

As shown in Table 6.8, a "high-risk" waist circumference in adults is defined as > 40 in. (> 102 cm) in males and > 35 in. (> 88 cm) in females.[65,73] In addition to being used in the initial assessment of body weight and risk for disease, waist circumference is also useful for evaluating the success of weight loss treatment. Note that waist circumference has little predictive value in subjects having a BMI $\geq$ 35 kg/m^2 and that, in these persons, waist circumference does not need to be measured. Also, the cutpoints in Table 6.8 may not be applicable to persons whose height is < 60 in. (< 152 cm). The waist circumference cutpoints shown in Table 6.8 generally apply to all adult racial and ethnic groups in North America, although there are ethnic and age-related differences in regional body fat distribution that may influence the accuracy of waist circumference as a surrogate measure of abdominal fat content. For example, waist circumference is a better predictor of disease risk than is BMI for persons of Asian descent. In older persons, waist circumference is more valuable at estimating obesity-related disease risk.[65,73]

BODY COMPOSITION

Interest in human body composition has grown over the past several decades, largely because obesity has been associated with such diseases as diabetes mellitus, hypertension, and coronary heart disease.[16,17,77–79] Overweight is one of the most prevalent diet-related problems in the United States. As shown in Figures 6.12 and 6.13, the prevalence of overweight and obesity in the United States has markedly increased. In other countries with established market economies (e.g., Canada, Australia, western European countries), the prevalence of obesity, generally defined as a BMI $\geq$ 30 kg/m^2, averages in the range of 15% to 20%.[80] Obesity is relatively common in Latin America but much less so in sub-Saharan Africa and Asia. Globally, the prevalence of obesity is increasing, as is the prevalence of obesity-linked disease, such as type 2 diabetes.

TABLE 6.8	High-Risk Waist Circumferences for Adult Males and Females
Males	> 40 in. (> 102 cm)
Females	> 35 in. (> 88 cm)

Source: National Institutes of Health.

Measurements of body fat are important in studying the nature of obesity and the obese person's response to treatment. As previously mentioned, the percent of body fat, as well as its placement, can have profound effects on health.

Estimating fat and protein reserves is a common practice in assessing a patient's nutritional status. During nutritional deprivation, these stores are depleted, leading to increased morbidity and mortality, caused at least in part by nutrition-related impairment of the body's immune system.[81,82] Simple techniques to screen fat and protein reserves of patients are critical in the light of reports that malnutrition is seen in as many as half of all hospitalized patients in the United States, Canada, and other industrialized countries.[83–85]

Body composition can be an important factor in certain athletic events. For example, carrying excess fat can be detrimental to the performance of runners and gymnasts. Body composition measurements can help these athletes maintain body fat at levels that are neither too high nor too low.[4] Too low a percent body fat can adversely affect metabolism and health. Female athletes will experience oligomenorrhea (abnormally infrequent menstruation) and amenorrhea (absence or abnormal cessation of menstruation) when their percent body fat is too low. This, in turn, can result in bone demineralization and increased risk of osteoporosis and bone fractures. Inadequate body fat may indicate disease, starvation, or an eating disorder, such as anorexia nervosa.

The perspective that the body consists of two chemically distinct compartments forms the model on which most body composition methods are based.[86,87] In the two-compartment model, the body can be divided into fat mass and fat-free mass, or, according to an alternative approach, into adipose tissue and lean body mass. In the former view, developed by Keys and Brozek,[88] the fat mass includes all the solvent-extractable lipids contained in both adipose tissue and other tissues, and the residual is the fat-free mass. The fat-free mass is composed of muscle, water, bone, and other tissues devoid of fat and lipid. For example, the solvent ether could be used to extract all the fat and lipid from a minced animal carcass. That remaining after all the fat and lipid were extracted would be the fat-free mass. The lean body mass of the latter approach is similar to the fat-free mass except that lean body mass includes a small amount of lipid that our bodies must have—for example, lipid that serves as a structural component of cell membranes or lipid contained in the nervous system.[89] This essential lipid constitutes about 1.5% to 3% of the weight of the lean body.

Body composition often is defined as the *ratio of fat to fat-free mass* and frequently is expressed as a percentage of body fat. Adipose tissue contains about 14% water, is nearly 100% free of the electrolyte potassium, and is assumed to have a density of 0.90 g/cm^3.[4,86] The less

homogenous *fat-free compartment* is primarily composed of bone, muscle, other fat-free tissue, and body water. Its chemical composition is assumed to be relatively constant, with a water content of 72% to 74%, a potassium content of 60 to 70 mmol/kg in males and 50 to 60 mmol/kg in females, and a density of 1.10 g/cm^3 at normal body temperature.[86] However, several factors can affect the density of the fat-free compartment. Among these are age (the fat-free compartment in children is less dense than that of middle-aged persons, and bone density is decreased in elderly persons, especially those with osteoporosis), the degree of fitness (athletes have denser bone and muscle), and the body's state of hydration.[4] The use of anthropometry (measures of skinfold thicknesses, bone dimensions, and limb circumferences), determination of whole-body density (most commonly by underwater weighing), electrical conductance and impedance, and other methods to estimate body composition are based on the two-compartment model.[86]

An alternative approach to the two-compartment model is the four-compartment model, which views the human body as composed of four chemical groups: water, protein, mineral, and fat.[86] Methods for estimating body composition based on the four-compartment model include neutron activation analysis, isotope dilution techniques, bioelectrical impedance, total body electrical conductivity, and absorptiometry.[86]

A variety of methods exist for estimating body composition, and each has its strengths and limitations. Except for cadaveric studies, all of the following techniques are *indirect* measures.

CADAVERIC STUDIES

Only by analyzing cadavers can direct measurement of human body composition be made.[4] The most comprehensive direct study of body composition was the Brussels Cadaver Analysis Study (CAS), in which more than 30 cadavers were studied from 1979 to 1983.[90] The CAS helped validate various in vivo methods for estimating body composition and collected data for developing new anthropometric models for determining body composition.[90] Recumbent length, hydrostatic (underwater) weight, numerous girths and breadths, and skin surface area were measured. Skinfolds were measured at 14 standard sites. The skin and subcutaneous tissue then were cut open and carefully measured, so that skinfold measurements could be directly compared with measurements of skin and subcutaneous adipose tissue thickness. The skin, adipose tissue, skeletal muscle, bone, and viscera were dissected out and weighed in air and under water to determine density of the organs and tissues. The CAS allowed examination of several assumptions underlying the use of skinfold measurements and hydrostatic weighing to determine body composition. A major assumption of the CAS was that anthropometric measures and body composition in cadavers are similar to those of living subjects.[90,91]

SKINFOLD MEASUREMENTS

The most widely used method of indirectly estimating percent body fat in clinical settings is to measure skinfolds—the thickness of a double fold of skin and compressed subcutaneous adipose tissue (Figure 6.15).[5,91] Although more accurate methods for assessing percent body fat exist, skinfold measurement has these advantages: the equipment needed is inexpensive and requires little space; measurements are easily and quickly obtained; and, when correctly done, skinfold measurement provides estimates of body composition that correlate well with those derived from hydrostatic weighing,

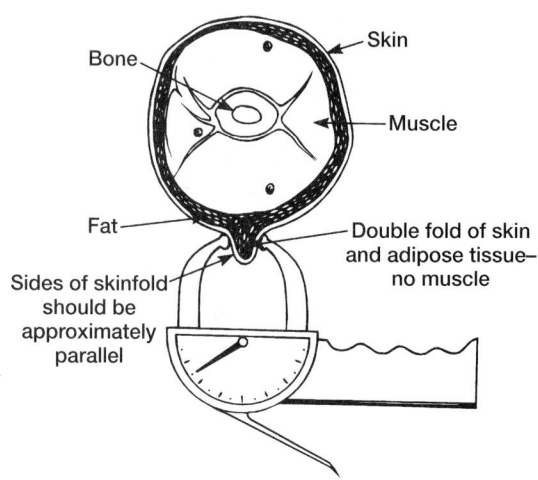

Figure 6.15

The double fold of skin and adipose tissue between the tips of the skinfold caliper should be large enough to form approximately parallel sides. Care should be taken to elevate only skin and adipose tissue, not muscle.

the most widely used laboratory method for determining body composition.

Assumptions in Using Skinfold Measurements

Estimating body fat from skinfold thickness measurements involves several assumptions, outlined in Box 6.2, that may not always hold true.[91] When a caliper is initially applied to a skinfold, the caliper reading decreases as its tips compress the fold of skin and subcutaneous adipose tissue. Thus, it is recommended to read the caliper dial about 4 seconds after the caliper tips have been applied to the skinfold.[92] Research has shown significant differences in skinfold compressibility at a particular site among individuals (interindividual variation) and at different sites on one individual (intraindividual variation).[91,93] Even after the timing of caliper readings has been standardized, similar thicknesses of adipose tissue may yield different caliper readings because of differences in compressibility.[91] Alternatively, compressibility differences may result in skinfolds of different thicknesses yielding similar caliper readings.[38] Of all the assumptions considered in this section, this probably has the greatest potential for being a significant source of error in estimating body composition from skinfold measurements.[91]

The CAS showed that skin thickness as a percent of total caliper reading varies at different sites and that "while the contribution of skin to total skinfold thickness is generally not large, it may lead to significant error especially in lean subjects."[91]

Thickness of subcutaneous adipose tissue varies widely among different skinfold sites within individuals and for the same skinfold site between individuals.[90,91,94] Consequently, overall subcutaneous adipose tissue is best assessed by measuring multiple skinfold sites. A minimum of three is recommended. Proper site selection is critical because subcutaneous fat layer thickness can vary significantly within a 2- to 3-cm proximity of certain sites.[86,95] Research has shown that certain skinfold sites are highly correlated to total subcutaneous adipose tissue

 Box 6.2 **Assumptions Involved in Using Skinfold Thickness Measurements to Predict Body Fat**

1. The double thickness of skin and subcutaneous adipose tissue has a constant compressibility.
2. Thickness of the skin is negligible or a constant fraction of the skinfold.
3. The thickness of subcutaneous adipose tissue is constant or predictable within and between individuals.

4. The fat content of adipose tissue is constant.
5. The proportion of internal to external fat is constant.
6. Body fat is normally distributed.

Adapted from Martin AD, Ross WD, Drinkwater DT, Clarys JP. 1985. Prediction of body fat by skinfold caliper: Assumptions and cadaver evidence. *International Journal of Obesity* 9(suppl 1):31–39.

and that sites from the lower limbs should be included in body composition prediction formulas.[91,96]

Adipose tissue can be divided into external, or subcutaneous (what lies directly under the skin), and internal portions (that within and around muscles and surrounding organs).[95] The only direct data on the relationship of external-to-internal adipose tissue comes from the CAS. These data show that each kilogram of subcutaneous adipose tissue is associated with approximately 200 g of internal adipose tissue and that skinfolds are significantly correlated with total adiposity.[90]

Although estimating body composition by skinfold measurements fails to meet all the assumptions of Box 6.2, it is preferred over use of other anthropometric variables and is certainly better than height-weight indices.[97] Thus, skinfold measurement is the most widely used method of indirectly estimating percent body fat in clinical settings.

Measurement Technique

Proper measurement of skinfolds requires careful attention to site selection and strict adherence to the following protocol, which is standard among researchers who have developed the prediction equations for determining body fatness from skinfold measurements.

1. Most North American investigators (including those conducting large national surveys from which reference data are derived) take skinfold measurements on the right side of the body. European investigators typically perform measurements on the left side.[98] From a practical standpoint, it matters little on which side measurements are taken. However, the authors of this textbook suggest that North American students be taught to take all measurements on the right side (except where indicated otherwise) to coincide with the efforts of most U.S. and Canadian researchers.

2. As a general rule, those with little experience in skinfold measurement should mark the site to be measured once it has been carefully identified. A flexible, nonstretchable tape measure can be used to locate midpoints on the body.[92]

3. The skinfold should be firmly grasped by the thumb and index finger of the left hand about 1 cm or ½ in. **proximal** to the skinfold site and pulled away from the body. This is usually easy with thin people, but it may be difficult with the obese and may be somewhat uncomfortable. The amount of tissue grasped must be enough to form a fold with approximately parallel sides. The thicker the fat layer under the skin, the wider the necessary fold.

4. The caliper is held in the right hand, perpendicular to the long axis of the skinfold and with the caliper's dial facing up and easily readable. The caliper tips should be placed on the site and should be about 1 cm or ½ in. **distal** to the fingers holding the skinfold, so that pressure from the fingers will not affect the measured value, as shown in Figure 6.16.

5. The caliper should not be placed too deeply into the skinfold or too close to the tip of the skinfold. The measurer should try to visualize where a true double fold of skin thickness is and place the caliper tips there. It is a good practice to position the caliper arms one at a time on the skinfold.

6. The dial is read approximately 4 seconds after the pressure from the measurer's hand has been released on the lever arm of the caliper. If caliper tips exert force for longer than 4 seconds, the reading will gradually become smaller as fluids are forced from the compressed tissues. The measurer's eyes and caliper dial should be positioned to avoid errors caused by parallax. Readings should be recorded to the nearest 1 mm.

7. A minimum of two measurements should be taken at each site. Measurements should be at least 15 seconds apart to allow the skinfold site to return to normal. If consecutive measurements vary by more than 1 mm, more should be taken until there is consistency.

8. The measurer should maintain pressure with the thumb and index finger throughout each measurement.

9. When measuring the obese, it may be impossible to elevate a skinfold with parallel sides, particularly over the abdomen. In this situation, the measurer should use both hands to pull the skinfold away while a partner attempts to measure the width. If the skinfold is too wide for the calipers, underwater weighing or another technique will have to be used.

10. Measurements should not be taken immediately after exercise or when the person being measured is overheated because the shift in body fluid to the skin will inflate normal skinfold size.

11. It takes practice to consistently grasp skinfolds at the same location every time. Accuracy can be tested by having several technicians take the same measurements and comparing results. It may take up to 50 practice sessions to become proficient in measuring skinfolds.

Several types of skinfold calipers are available (see Figure 6.17). The Lange skinfold caliper is most popular among U.S. researchers, whereas the Harpenden and Holtain are commonly used in Great Britain and Europe. Several less expensive plastic calipers are available, such as the Slim Guide and the Fat-Control Caliper. Some of the plastic calipers have been shown to give results comparable to the more expensive calipers.[99,100] The Slim Guide, which is being used increasingly, may be an acceptable caliper for those who cannot afford a more

Grasp a double fold of skin and subcutaneous adipose tissue with the thumb and index finger of the left hand.

Place the caliper tips on the site where the sides of the skinfold are approximately parallel and 1 cm distal to where the skinfold is grasped.

Position the caliper dial so that it can be read easily. Obtain the measurement about 4 sec after placing the caliper tips on the skinfold.

Figure 6.16
Accurate skinfold measurements require careful site selection and proper technique in placing and reading the caliper.

Figure 6.17 Examples of commercially available skinfold calipers. Back row, left to right: Lange, Slim Guide, Holtain. Front: Harpenden.
Source: Photo by M. Ware.

expensive instrument. Currently, the Lange and Harpenden calipers are highly recommended because these were used in developing prediction equations and reference values. Whatever the caliper used, the jaw tips should exert a pressure of 10 g/mm^2 throughout the caliper's full measurement range. The calipers should be calibrated periodically (for example, before measuring skinfolds on groups of subjects) by checking the dial reading against a graduated calibration block. Caliper readings should be within at least ±1 mm at each 5-mm interval from 5 to 50 mm.[101]

Site Selection

This section describes eight of the most commonly used skinfold sites following the Airlie Consensus Conference protocol as outlined in the *Anthropometric Standardization Reference Manual.*[96]

Chest

The chest, or pectoral skinfold site, is measured using a skinfold with its long axis running from the top of the anterior axillary fold to the nipple. The skinfold is grasped as high as possible on the anterior axillary fold, and the thickness of the fat fold is measured 1 cm or ½ in. below the fingers along the axis, as shown in Figures 6.18 and 6.19. The skinfold site is the same for males and females. Other than to help determine the long axis of the skinfold, the nipple is not used as a landmark for either males or females. This site can be measured on a female wearing a brassiere or two-piece bathing suit.

Triceps

Because of its accessibility, the triceps is the most commonly measured site. The triceps skinfold site is on the posterior aspect of the right arm, over the triceps muscle, midway between the lateral projection of the acromion process of the scapula and the inferior margin of the olecranon process of the ulna. These bony landmarks are shown in Figure 6.20. The midpoint between the acromion and olecranon processes should be marked

Figure 6.18
The location of the pectoral or chest skinfold site is the same for males and females.

Figure 6.19 **Measurement of the pectoral or chest skinfold.**
Note that the caliper is held perpendicular to the long axis of the skinfold. The blade tips are approximately 1 cm distal to the fingers grasping the skinfold.

Figure 6.20
The triceps skinfold site is located midway between the lateral projection of the acromion process of the scapula, **a,** and the olecranon process of the ulna, **b,** with the elbow flexed 90 degrees.

Figure 6.21 **Measurement of the triceps skinfold.**

along the *lateral* side of the arm with the elbow flexed 90 degrees, as shown in Figure 6.21. The subject's arm should now hang loosely at the side, with the palm of the hand facing *anteriorly* to properly determine the posterior midline. The skinfold site should be marked along the posterior midline of the upper arm at the same level as the previously marked midpoint. The measurer should stand behind the subject, grasp the skinfold with the thumb and index finger of the left hand about 1 cm or ½ in. proximal to the skinfold site, as shown in Figure 6.21. Again, notice in Figure 6.21 that the caliper tips are about 1 cm or ½ in. from the thumb and finger, the caliper is perpendicular to the long axis of the skinfold, and the dial can be easily read.

Subscapular

The subscapular site is 1 cm below the lowest, or inferior, angle of the scapula, as shown in Figure 6.22. The long axis of the skinfold is on a 45-degree angle directed down and to the right side. The site can be located by gently feeling for the inferior angle of the scapula or by having the subject place his or her right arm behind the back. It is measured with the subject standing with arms relaxed to the sides. The skin is grasped 1 cm above and medial to the site along the axis (see Figure 6.23).

Midaxillary

As shown in Figure 6.24, this site is at the right midaxillary line (a vertical line extending from the middle of the

Figure 6.22
The subscapular skinfold site is just below the inferior border of the scapula. The long axis of the site runs at 45 degrees of horizontal.

Figure 6.23 Measurement of the subscapular skinfold site.

Figure 6.24
The midaxillary site is a horizontal skinfold along the midaxillary line at the level of the xiphisternal junction.

Figure 6.25 Measurement of the midaxillary skinfold.

axilla) level with the xiphisternal junction (at the bottom of the sternum where the xiphoid process begins). It is measured with the subject standing erectly and with the right arm slightly abducted (moved away from center of the body) and flexed (bent posteriorly), as in Figure 6.25.

Suprailiac

This skinfold is measured just above the iliac crest at the midaxillary line (see Figure 6.26 and Figure 6.27). The

long axis follows the natural cleavage lines of the skin and runs diagonally. The subject should stand erectly with feet together and arms hanging at the sides, although the right arm can be abducted and flexed slightly to improve access to the site. The measurer should grasp the skinfold about 1 cm posterior to the midaxillary line and measure the skinfold at the midaxillary line.

Abdomen

The subject stands erectly with the body weight evenly distributed on both feet, abdominal muscles relaxed, and breathing quietly. A horizontal skinfold 3 cm to the right of and 1 cm below the midpoint of the umbilicus is measured (Figure 6.28).

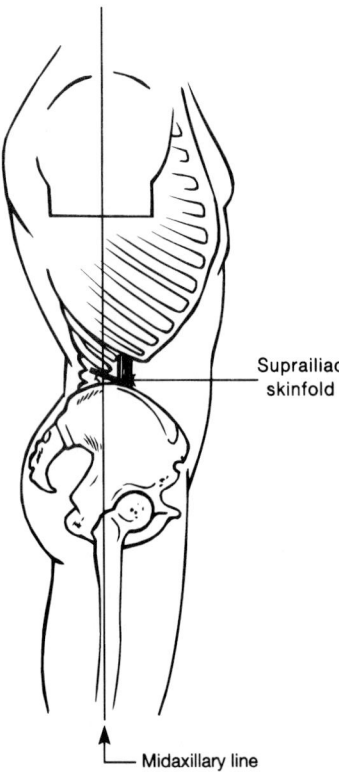

Figure 6.26
The suprailiac skinfold is measured just above the iliac crest at the midaxillary line. The long axis of the skinfold follows the natural cleavage lines of the skin.

Figure 6.27 Measurement of the suprailiac skinfold.

Figure 6.28 Measurement of the abdominal skinfold.

Thigh

This site is a vertical skinfold along the midline of the anterior aspect of the thigh midway between the junction of the midline and the inguinal crease and the proximal (upper) border of the patella, or knee cap (Figure 6.29). Flexing the subject's hip helps locate the inguinal crease. The subject shifts the weight to the left foot and relaxes the leg being measured by slightly flexing the knee with the foot flat on the floor. The skinfold is measured as shown in Figure 6.30.

Medial Calf

With the subject sitting, the right leg is flexed about 90 degrees at the knee with the sole of the foot flat on the

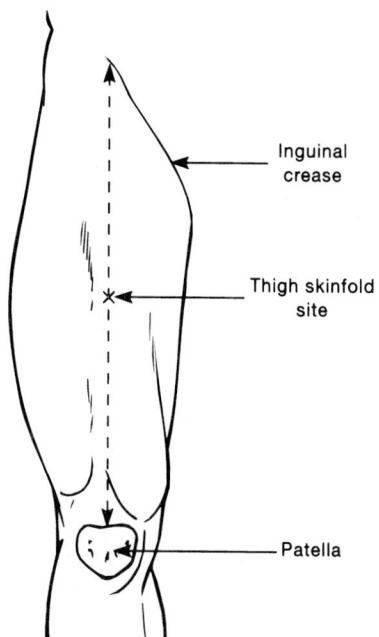

Figure 6.29
The thigh skinfold lies along the anterior midline of the thigh halfway between the inguinal crease and the proximal border of the patella.

Figure 6.30 Measurement of the thigh skinfold.

floor. The measurement also may be taken with the subject standing with the foot resting on a platform, so that the knee and hip are flexed about 90 degrees. The point of maximum calf circumference is marked at the medial (inner) aspect of the calf. A vertical skinfold is grasped about 1 cm proximal to the marked site and measured at the site (Figure 6.31).

Figure 6.31 Measurement of the medial calf skinfold.

Single-Site Skinfold Measurements

The triceps is the most commonly used single site for assessing body composition. The ease by which it is accessed and measured has made it popular in large population studies, such as NHANES. Although single-site skinfold measurements cannot be used to estimate percent body fat, they are useful for making comparisons among subjects for which reference data are available. For example, the triceps skinfold measurements of a child can be compared with reference data on triceps skinfolds taken from a large group of children of a similar sex and age. Reference data derived from NHANES II are shown in Appendixes O and P. Using the tables, the 50th percentile represents the median value for each age/sex group. If a subject had a skinfold thickness at the 85th percentile for his or her age/sex group, 85% of the subjects studied in that group would have smaller measurements, and only 15% would have larger measurements.

Using single skinfold measurements has certain limitations: investigators disagree about what is the best single site to use as an index of body composition; no equations exist for estimating body fat using just the triceps skinfold measurement; and multiple anthropometric measures are required to achieve reasonably accurate body composition estimates because of variations in subcutaneous adipose tissue distribution. Therefore, single-site skinfold measurements must be interpreted with caution and should be used only as a rough approximation of total body fat percentage or to compare individuals for which reference data exist.

Two-Site Skinfold Measurements

The most commonly used approach to assessing body composition for young people age 6 years through the mid-20s uses the sum of the triceps and subscapular sites.[101,102] These sites have the following advantages: they are highly correlated with other measures of body fatness; they are more reliably and objectively measured than most other sites; and national norms are available for them. Figure 6.32 outlines skinfold and body fat standards developed for persons ages 6 to 17 years using the sum of the triceps and subscapular skinfolds.[102]

Because measurement of the subscapular skinfold may be embarrassing to some children and youth or may raise ethical questions about male teachers touching female students, norms using the sum of the triceps and medial calf skinfold measurements have been developed.[102,103] This sum has proved to be a reasonably valid and reliable indicator of body composition. The medial calf site is easily accessible and can be measured without raising concerns about modesty. In some persons, the skin at the site may be quite taut, making it difficult to measure the site. Figure 6.33 provides standards based on the sum of triceps and medial calf skinfold measurements for persons 6 to 17 years old.[102] Using Figures 6.32 and 6.33, obesity for 6- to 17-year-old males

Figure 6.32 Body fat standards for persons 6 to 17 years old based on the sum of triceps and subscapular skinfold measurements.

Source: From the *Journal of Physical Education, Recreation & Dance,* November–December 1987, pp. 98–102.

Figure 6.33 Body fat standards for persons 6 to 17 years old based on the sum of triceps and medial calf skinfold measurements.

Source: From the *Journal of Physical Education, Recreation & Dance,* November–December 1987, pp. 98–102.

and females is greater than 25% body fat and greater than 32% body fat, respectively. An alternate approach for estimating percent body fat in children is to calculate the sum of biceps, triceps, subscapular, and suprailiac skinfold measurements (discussed in the section "Multiple-Site Skinfold Measurements").

Multiple-Site Skinfold Measurements

Predicting body density and then percent of body fat from skinfold measurements requires regression equations. These formulas have been developed by comparing a variety of skinfold and other anthropometric measures with measurements of body density (usually by hydrostatic weighing) to see which anthropometric measures are best at predicting body density. A statistical process called multiple-regression analysis is used.[4,97,104–106] The measure or combinations of measures most highly correlated with body density as determined by a separate method are then used in the regression equation.

The more than 100 different regression equations that have been developed can be classified as either population-specific equations or generalized equations.[95,97] Population-specific equations are derived from data on groups of people sharing certain characteristics, such as age and gender. The first valid regression equations, for example, were developed in 1951 for young and middle-aged men.[107] Numerous other population-specific equations have been developed since then, but their use is limited. Equations developed from data on middle-aged females, for example, may not be valid for females of other ages.

More recently, generalized equations have been developed that are applicable to persons varying greatly in age and body fatness. The primary advantage of this approach is that one generalized equation can replace several population-specific equations with no loss in prediction accuracy.[5,97] Table 6.9 shows several generalized prediction equations for calculating body density or percent body fat. Because fat placement differs between males and females, separate equations are given for each sex.

Table 6.10 shows equations for estimating body density developed by Durnin and Womersley.[108] These have

TABLE 6.10	Age- and Sex-Specific Body Composition Equations Developed by Durnin and Womersley
Age Range (Years)	**Equation**
Males	
17–19	Body density = $1.1620 - 0.0630 \times (\log \Sigma)^*$
20–29	Body density = $1.1631 - 0.0632 \times (\log \Sigma)$
30–39	Body density = $1.1422 - 0.0544 \times (\log \Sigma)$
40–49	Body density = $1.1620 - 0.0700 \times (\log \Sigma)$
50+	Body density = $1.1715 - 0.0779 \times (\log \Sigma)$
Females	
17–19	Body density = $1.1549 - 0.0678 \times (\log \Sigma)$
20–29	Body density = $1.1599 - 0.0717 \times (\log \Sigma)$
30–39	Body density = $1.1423 - 0.0632 \times (\log \Sigma)$
40–49	Body density = $1.1333 - 0.0612 \times (\log \Sigma)$
50+	Body density = $1.1339 - 0.0645 \times (\log \Sigma)$

Equations from Durnin JVGA, Womersley J. 1974. Body fat assessment from total body density and its estimation from skinfold thickness: Measurements on 481 men and women aged 16–72 years. *British Journal of Nutrition* 32:77–97.

*Σ = sum of the triceps, subscapular, suprailiac, and biceps skinfolds.

been used by many researchers and differ according to sex and age. The equations are based on the logarithm of the sum of four skinfolds—triceps, subscapular, suprailiac, and biceps. The biceps skinfold is a vertical fold on the anterior aspect of the arm, over the belly of the biceps muscle, directly opposite the triceps skinfold site.[92]

The equations in Table 6.9 and Table 6.10 predict either body fat percent or body density. Body density formulas require an additional calculation to estimate percent body fat. Two formulas are available for this step: the Brozek and the Siri equations:

TABLE 6.9	Generalized Body Composition Equations for Male and Female Adults*

Males

Body density = $1.11200000 - 0.00043499(X_1) + 0.00000055 (X_1)^2 - 0.00028826 (X_8)$

Percent body fat = $0.29288 (X_2) - 0.00050 (X_2)^2 + 0.15845 (X_8) - 5.76377$

Body density = $1.1093800 - 0.0008267 (X_3) + 0.0000016 (X_3)^2 - 0.0002574 (X_8)$

Body density = $1.1125025 - 0.0013125 (X_4) + 0.00000055 (X_4)^2 - 0.0002440 (X_8)$

Percent body fat = $0.39287 (X_5) - 0.00105 (X_5)^2 + 0.15772 (X_8) - 5.18845$

Females

Body density = $1.0970 - 0.00046971 (X_1) + 0.00000056 (X_1)^2 - 0.00012828 (X_8)$

Percent body fat = $0.29699 (X_2) - 0.00043 (X_2)^2 + 0.02963 (X_8) + 1.4072$

Percent body fat = $0.41563 (X_6) - 0.00112 (X_6)^2 + 0.03661 (X_8) + 4.03653$

Body density = $1.0994921 - 0.0009929 (X_7) + 0.0000023 (X_7)^2 - 0.0001392 (X_8)$

Data from Jackson AS, Pollock ML. 1985. Practical assessment of body composition. *Physician and Sportsmedicine* 13(5):76–90; Golding LA, Myers CR, Sinning WE. 1989. *The Y's way to physical fitness*, 3rd ed. Champaign, IL: Human Kinetics Books.

*X_1 = sum of chest, midaxillary, triceps, subscapular, abdomen, suprailiac, and thigh skinfolds; X_2 = sum of abdomen, suprailiac, triceps, and thigh skinfolds; X_3 = sum of chest, abdomen, and subscapular skinfolds; X_4 = sum of chest, triceps, and subscapular skinfolds; X_5 = sum of abdomen, suprailiac, and triceps skinfolds; X_6 = sum of triceps, abdomen, and suprailiac skinfolds; X_7 = sum of triceps, suprailiac, and thigh skinfolds; X_8 = age in years.

Brozek: Percent body fat =
(457 ÷ body density) − 414

Siri: Percent body fat =
(495 ÷ body density) − 450

A programmable calculator will help in the use of these equations. The nomogram shown in Figure 6.34 greatly simplifies calculating percent body fat from the sum of three skinfold thicknesses.[109] For males, the sum of the chest, abdomen, and thigh skinfold measurements should be used. For females, the sum of the triceps, suprailiac, and thigh skinfold measurements should be used. The nomogram was developed from data on males from 18 to 61 years old and females 18 to 55 years old, with the sum of skinfold measurements ranging from 14 to 118 mm and 16 to 126 mm for males and females, respectively.[109] The nomogram should be used with caution for subjects outside these ranges.

Investigators in The Netherlands have proposed regression equations for estimating body density and percent body fat in persons from infancy to age 18 years.[110] Based on their equations, they have formulated a table (Table 6.11) allowing the estimation of percent body fat of persons in this age range from the sum of biceps, triceps, subscapular, and suprailiac skinfold measurements.

What Is a Desirable Level of Fatness?

Determining with certainty just what constitutes a desirable level of body fatness is difficult. However, suggested percent body fat norms are given in Table 6.12. Note that the values are given in a range. This allows for error in measurement and for individual differences; what may be appropriate for one person may not be appropriate for another.[89,97]

Using the values in Table 6.12, the form shown in Figure 6.35, and the following formulas, a person can calculate a target weight necessary to achieve a certain percent body fat.[29]

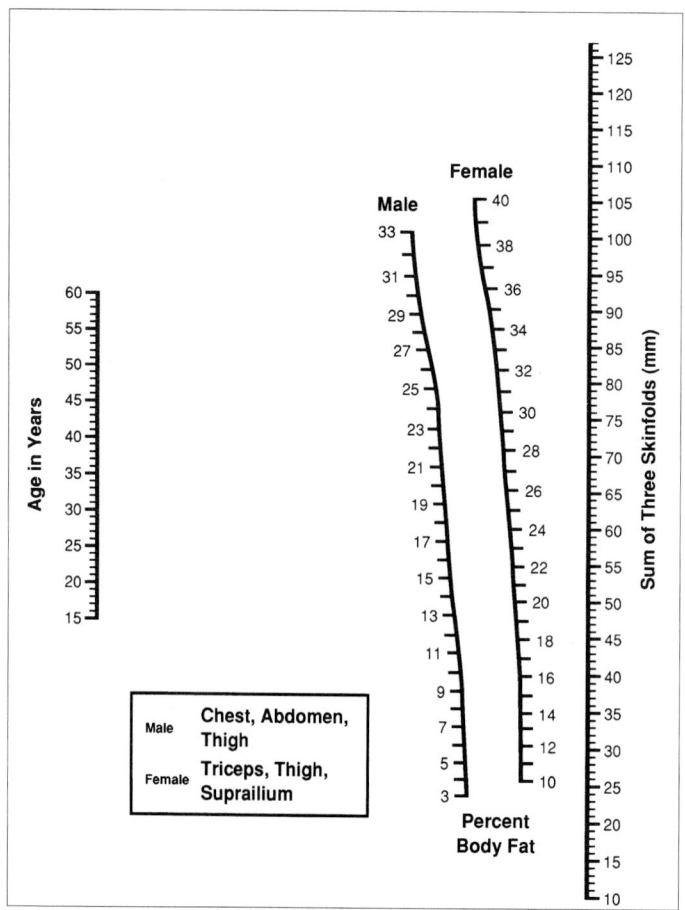

Figure 6.34 Nomogram for calculating percent of body fat from the sum of three skinfolds.
Use a straightedge to connect the subject's age (left axis) with the skinfold value (right axis). The percent body fat is read where the straightedge crosses the line representing the subject's sex.
Source: From the *Research Quarterly for Exercise and Sport* 52(3), 1981.

| Table 6.11 | Percent Body Fat Estimated from the Sum of Skinfold Thickness Measurements* in Persons from Infancy to Age 18 Years |

Percent Body Fat

Age (Years)	15%	20%	25%	30%	35%
Male					
0†	17	22	30	40	52
1‡	18	24	32	43	58
2	18	25	34	45	60
4	20	27	37	51	68
6	22	30	41	57	78
8	32	33	46	64	88
10	25	36	51	72	101
12	27	40	57	81	115
14	27	44	63	92	132
16	32	48	71	104	152
18	34	52	79	117	175
Female					
0†	17	22	30	40	52
1‡	18	24	32	43	58
2	18	25	34	45	60
4	18	25	34	46	62
6	19	25	35	47	63
8	19	26	35	48	65
10	19	27	37	51	69
12	21	30	42	58	80
14	23	33	47	66	92
16	25	37	53	75	106
18	27	40	58	85	122

From Westrate JA, Deurenberg P. 1989. Body composition in children: Proposal for a method for calculating body fat percentage from total body density or skinfold-thickness measurements. *American Journal of Clinical Nutrition* 50:1104–1115.

*Sum of biceps, triceps, subscapular, and suprailiac skinfold measurements, given in millimeters.

†Mean age used was 6 months.

‡Mean age used was 18 months.

| Table 6.12 | Body Fat Ranges for Persons 18 Years of Age and Older |

Classification	Males	Females
Unhealthy range (too low)	≤ 5%	≤ 8%
Acceptable range (lower end)	6–15%	9–23%
Acceptable range (upper end)	16–24%	24–31%
Unhealthy (too high)	≥ 25%	≥ 32%

Adapted from Nieman DC. 1999. *Exercise testing and prescription: A health-related approach,* 4th ed. Mountain View, CA: Mayfield.

Figure 6.35 Skinfold recording and calculation form.

Weight of fat = Total body weight × Percent body fat

Fat-free weight = Total body weight − Fat weight

Target weight = Present fat-free weight
÷ (100 − desired percent body fat)

For example, take a subject who weighs 200 lb, has 25% body fat, and desires to have a 15% body fat:

Weight of fat = 200 lb × 0.25 = 50 lb

Fat-free weight = 200 lb − 50 lb = 150 lb

Target weight = 150 lb ÷ 0.85 = 176 lb

DENSITOMETRY

Densitometry is assessing body composition by measuring the density of the entire body.[86,87] Density is expressed as mass per unit volume and usually is obtained through **hydrostatic,** or underwater, weighing, although other methods have been developed as described in the section "Air Displacement Plethysmography."[111]

Underwater Weighing

The most widely used technique of determining whole-body density is hydrostatic, or underwater, weighing.[86,87] The technique is based on **Archimedes' principle,** which states that the volume of an object submerged in water equals the volume of water the object displaces. Thus, if the mass and the volume of a body are known, the density of that body can be calculated. Using another formula, percent body fat can be calculated from body density.

This approach is based on the two-compartment model of body composition: the fat and fat-free mass. The fat-free mass is assumed to have a constant level of hydration and a constant proportion of bone mineral to muscle. The approach also assumes a constant fat mass density of 0.90 g/cm^3 and a density of the fat-free mass of 1.10 g/cm^3.[86,87] The densities of bone and muscle tissue are greater than the density of water (density of distilled water = 1.00 g/cm^3), whereas fat is less dense than water. Thus, muscular subjects having a low percentage of body fat tend to weigh more submerged in water than do subjects having a higher percentage of body fat.[29]

Body density can be calculated from the following formula,[4]

$$\text{Body density} = \frac{\text{WA}}{\dfrac{(\text{WA} - \text{WW})}{\text{DW}} - (\text{RV} + \text{VGI})}$$

where WA = body weight in air; WW = body weight submerged in water; DW = density of water; RV = residual lung volume; VGI = volume of gas in the gastrointestinal tract.

Equipment

The necessary equipment for underwater weighing includes a tank, tub, or pool of water of sufficient size for total body submersion; a scale or another method of determining the subject's underwater weight; and, attached to the scale, a chair or frame lowered into the water on which the subject sits (Figure 6.36).

The water should be comfortably warm, filtered, chlorinated, and undisturbed by wind or other activity in the water during testing.[29] A method of underwater weighing in a swimming pool using a wooden shell placed within the pool to reduce water movement, which can adversely affect weighing, has been described by Katch.[111]

The chair should be constructed so that the subject can sit under the water with legs slightly bent and the water at neck level, as shown in Figure 6.36. Weights should be attached to the chair, so that its empty or tare weight while under water is at least 3 kg for subjects of moderate body fatness and at least 4 to 6 kg for obese subjects.[10] Some researchers use a frame on which the subject lies submerged in the prone (face down) position while breathing through a snorkel.[4,111] They think that this position results in less up-and-down movement of the body in the water, thus resulting in fewer fluctuations of the scale.

Typically, an autopsy scale (such as the 9-kg capacity Chatillon autopsy scale shown in Figure 6.36) is used in underwater weighing. A strain gauge, or force cell, gives more precise measurements.[4,86,112] These instru-

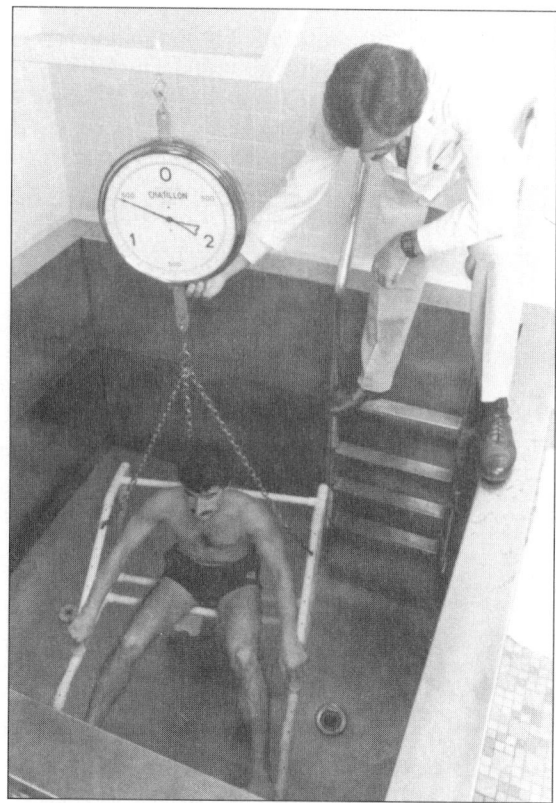

Figure 6.36
Equipment for underwater weighing includes a tank of sufficient size and shape for total human submersion, an accurate scale for measuring weight with 10-gram divisions, a method of measuring water temperature, and a chair that is weighted to prevent flotation.

ments can be interfaced with a computer, which, with the appropriate software, can easily determine the midpoint of fluctuations and can use that as the basis for further calculations.[4]

Procedure[4,29]

1. Obtaining basic data: name, date, age, sex, stature, and weight (in kilograms) in air should be collected and recorded on a form such as the one shown in Figure 6.37. The tester should record the tare weight—the underwater weight of the chair (and any attached weights)—before the subject sits in it. The subject should be several hours **postprandial,** clean, wearing only a swimsuit. The subject should have urinated and defecated immediately before weighing. Carbonated beverages and flatus-causing foods should be avoided before the procedure because gastrointestinal tract gas will decrease the subject's underwater weight, resulting in erroneously low measurements of body density.

2. Measuring skinfolds: skinfold measurements can help verify results from underwater weighing. These can be recorded on the form shown in Figure 6.37.

Body Composition Worksheet

Name _____ Date _____

Age _____ Sex _____ Height _____

Skinfolds (mm)

_____ Chest   _____ Suprailiac

_____ Triceps   _____ Abdominal

_____ Subscapular   _____ Thigh

_____ Midaxillary   _____ Medial calf

Hydrostatic Measurements

_____ Weight in air (Wa)

_____ Tare weight

_____ Average gross weight (average of best two trials)

Underwater weighing trials

1 _____   2 _____   3 _____   4 _____   5 _____

6 _____   7 _____   8 _____   9 _____   10 _____

_____ Weight in water (Ww) (average gross weight— tare weight)

_____ Density of water (Dw)

_____ Residual volume (RV)

Calculations

$$\text{Density} = \frac{Wa}{\dfrac{(Wa - Ww)}{Dw} - (RV + 100\ ml)}$$

_____ Percent body fat = (495 ÷ density) − 450

_____ Fat weight (weight in the air x fat%)

_____ Lean body weight (weight in the air − fat weight)

_____ Classification

Figure 6.37 Body composition worksheet.

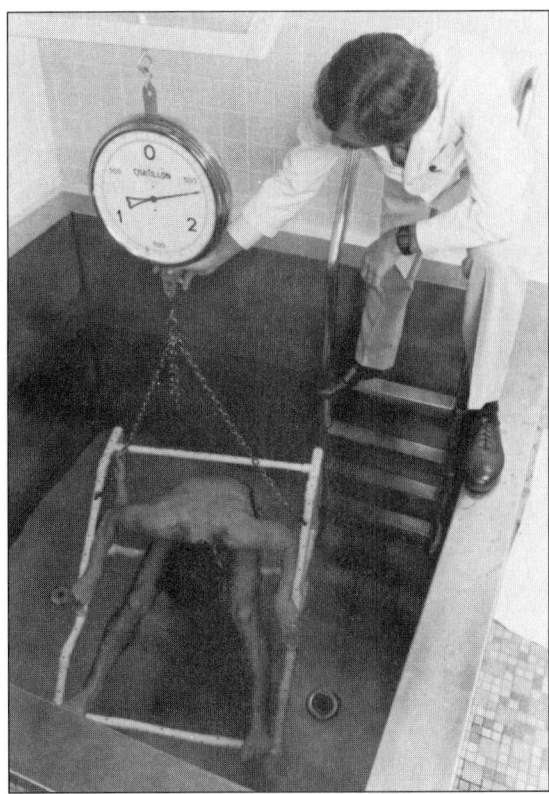

Figure 6.38 Subject's body position while submerged during underwater weighing. The water should be kept as calm as possible to get a good reading on the scale. Note how the tester is steadying the scale with his hand. Once the scale is relatively steady, the tester should remove the hand and take the reading.

3. Submerging: while comfortably seated in the chair, the subject exhales as fully as possible and slowly leans forward until the head is completely under the water, as shown in Figure 6.38. The subject continues to press as much air from the lungs as possible. After exhaling fully, the subject remains motionless and counts for 5 to 7 seconds before coming up for air. This allows the tester time to read the scale. While in the water, the subject should move slowly and deliberately to prevent water turbulence, which can make the subject bob up and down and make scale reading difficult. When the subject submerges, the tester can keep one hand on the scale to steady it, as shown in Figure 6.38.

4. Recording underwater weight: several trials usually are necessary before the subject becomes accustomed to the procedure and consistent readings are obtained. Katch and coworkers[111] weighed subjects 9 or 10 times and took the average of the last 3 underwater readings as the "true" underwater weight. Underwater weight should be recorded on the Body Composition Worksheet (Figure 6.37) as the gross weight in water. The net body weight in water is the gross weight in water minus the tare weight. The temperature of the water should be measured, and water density should be determined from standard tables.

5. Determining residual volume: residual volume (RV) is the amount of air remaining in the lungs after a maximal exhalation. All other things being equal, a subject with a large RV will be more buoyant (have a lower underwater weight) than one with a smaller RV. Although RV often is estimated, whenever possible it should be measured directly. When RV is estimated, hydrostatically determined percent body fat is no more accurate than when derived from skinfold measurements.[29] Techniques for measuring RV include nitrogen washout, helium dilution, and oxygen dilution. The choice of technique is generally a matter of which is available to the

investigator.[4] Whether RV should be measured at the same time as underwater weighing or immediately before or after is a point of contention among investigators.[4] Currently, there seems to be no clear advantage of one approach over the other.

If equipment for measuring RV is not available, it can be estimated from vital lung capacity.[113] RV is approximately 24% of vital lung capacity, provided the vital capacity is measured while the subject is in water.[4] Another approach is to use the following sex-specific formulas,[114]

$$\text{Male RV} = 0.017\,A + 0.06858\,S - 3.477$$
$$\text{Female RV} = 0.009\,A + 0.08128\,S - 3.900$$

where A = age in years and S = stature in inches. Because measuring gastrointestinal tract gas is impossible using conventional methods, it is nearly always estimated to be 100 mL in adults.[4,86] The value is likely smaller in children and larger in subjects who consumed flatus-producing foods or carbonated beverages before being measured.[4] The volume of gastrointestinal gas can range from 50 to 300 mL.[86]

6. Calculating density and percent body fat: using the formulas or the Body Composition Worksheet (Figure 6.37), you can calculate estimates of body density and percent body fat. The remainder of the calculations on the Body Composition Worksheet are the same as those discussed in the section "What Is a Desirable Level of Fatness?"

Weaknesses of Underwater Weighing

Underwater weighing has several weaknesses. It is not practical for testing large numbers of people. Subjects must be willing and able to remain submerged and motionless long enough for an accurate measurement of weight to be made. This requires considerable subject cooperation and training.[86,115,116] Consequently, about 10% to 20% of subjects find it difficult to be weighed under water. The technique requires some special equipment, experience, and financial investment. In many situations, skinfold measurements may be more practical.[29]

Densitometry is based on several assumptions. Perhaps the most tenuous of these is a constant density of the fat-free compartment.[4,86,90] A number of factors can affect the density of the fat-free mass, and these can influence the accuracy of body density measurement by 3% to 4%.[10] Athletes, for example, tend to have denser bone and muscle tissue, which may result in underestimation of body fat (possibly even *negative* body fat values), whereas the tendency of older persons to have less dense bones will likely result in overestimation of body fat.[4] Fat-free tissue density values for adults are probably not appropriate for use with children. Another concern is gas trapped in the gut, the amount of which can only be esti-

mated. Other factors affecting the accuracy of body density measurements include the consumption of food and carbonated beverages shortly before underwater weighing, fluid loss during intensive training, fluid retention before menstruation, and the degree of forcible exhalation while submerged.[4] Despite these weaknesses, underwater weighing remains the standard laboratory technique for determining body density and percent body fat.[29,115,116]

Air Displacement Plethysmography

As an alternative to underwater weighing, body volume (and, consequently, body density and percent body fat) can be measured using a technique known as air displacement plethysmography. The fundamental principle behind air displacement plethysmography is that, when a subject enters a chamber of known volume, the subject's body volume is equal to the reduction in chamber volume.[117,118] An example of a commercially available air displacement plethysmograph (what the manufacturer calls the "Bod Pod®") is shown in Figure 6.39. Figure 6.40 illustrates the major components of the plethysmo-

Figure 6.39 An air displacement plethysmograph.
Source: Photo by M. Ware.

Figure 6.40 **The major components of the air plethysmograph.**

Source: Adapted from Dempster P, Aitkens S. 1995. *Medicine and Science in Sports and Exercise.* 27:1692–1697. Ellis KJ. 2000. *Physiological Reviews* 80:649–680.

graph. The unit is constructed of fiberglass and consists of two chambers (front and rear), which are separated by a wall, which also serves as a molded seat on which the subject sits during testing. The subject enters and exits the front chamber of the unit through a hinged door containing a large acrylic window, giving the subject a comfortable sense of openness when the door is closed. The rear chamber houses electronic instruments, an air circulation system, valves, pressure transducers, and a breathing circuit. Attached to the wall separating the two chambers is a diaphragm, which, when moved during calibration and subject measurement, slightly alters the volume of the two chambers. These volume alterations during calibration and subject measurement are used, along with other values, to calculate the subject's volume. Connected to but outside the unit are a scale for weighing the subject and a computer for controlling the system and for collecting, analyzing, and outputting data.[115,117] In order to accurately measure body volume, it is necessary to minimize or account for the effects of clothing, hair, body surface area, and thoracic (lung and airway) gas volume. The effects of clothing and hair are minimized by having the subject dress in a tight-fitting swimsuit and wear a swimcap to compress the hair. Body surface area is calculated using a formula and accurate measurement of height and weight. Thoracic gas volume is measured during the final step of the measurement process.[117,119]

After voiding, the subject is weighed on the system's scale, and height is measured using a stadiometer. A two-step calibration process is performed, first with the front chamber empty and the door closed and then with a 50-liter calibration cylinder in the front chamber with the door closed. During each step of the calibration process, the electronically controlled diaphragm oscillates back and forth to alter the volume in the two chambers.[117] The subject then enters the front chamber, the door is closed, and the subject relaxes and breathes normally while the diaphragm oscillates back and forth. At the end of this 20-second measurement, the door is momentarily opened and then closed and the measurement process is repeated. If these two volume measurements are within 150 mL of each other, the measurements are accepted and the mean value is used for calculations. If they are not within 150 mL, a third measurement is taken. Any two of the three measurements that are within 150 mL of each other are averaged, and that value is used in calculations of body volume. Pressure differences within the front chamber when it is empty and when the subject is present are used in calculating the subject's body volume.[117–119]

The final step is measurement of the subject's thoracic gas volume, which includes all air in the lungs and airways. The door is opened and the subject is given a single-use, disposable breathing tube, which is connected to a breathing circuit housed in the unit's rear chamber. The subject's nostrils are sealed with a nose clip and the subject is instructed to breathe quietly through the mouth. The door is then closed. After several normal breaths, a valve in the breathing circuit momentarily closes at the midpoint of an exhalation. As previously instructed, the subject compresses and then relaxes the diaphragm muscle. This produces small pressure fluctuations within the subject's airway and in the chamber, which are used to calculate thoracic gas volume. The final body volume is calculated based on the initial volume measurement, corrected for thoracic gas volume and the subject's body surface area. This is then used to calculate percent body fat mass and percent body lean mass.[118,119]

Measurements of body composition derived from the Bod Pod® among different groups of subjects have been compared with those derived from other criterion methods, such as underwater weighing and dual-energy X-ray absorptiometry.[118–124] In general, these validation studies show good agreement between measurements of body composition based on air displacement plethysmography and these two other criterion methods when group means are compared. However, in some instances, air displacement plethysmography has been shown to provide significantly different estimates of body composition, and further research is needed.[119,121,122,124] Overall, air displacement plethysmography is a promising technique for body composition analysis in the clinical setting. Most noteworthy is the fact that plethysmography overcomes some of the methodological and technical constraints of underwater weighing. It is fairly quick and easy and is much more suitable for use with children, the elderly, and the disabled than is underwater weighing.[119,122,124] Like underwater weighing, calculations of body density from volume measurements derived from air displacement plethysmography are dependent on the assumption that fat-free tissue has a constant density.[115]

TOTAL BODY WATER

Water is normally the largest component of the human body. It composes approximately 60% and 50% of the weight of the adult male and female body, respectively. As much as 90% of the weight of neonates is water.[4,115,116] Because fat is free of water, all the water in the body is found in the fat-free mass. It has been assumed that fat-free tissue has an average water content of approximately 73.2%. Based on this assumption, a measure of total body water (TBW) should allow calculation of total body fat from the following formula.[47,86]

$$\text{Total body fat} = (\text{Body weight}) - \frac{\text{TBW}}{0.732}$$

Total body water is measured indirectly using **dilution techniques** where a known concentration and volume of a certain substance (a tracer) is given orally or parenterally to a subject, time is allowed for the tracer to equilibrate with water in the subject's body, and the concentration of the tracer in a sample of the subject's blood, urine, or saliva is analyzed. From this data, TBW is measured using the following relationship:

$$C_1 V_1 = C_2 V_2$$

where C_1 and V_1 = the concentration and volume, respectively, of tracer given to the subject; C_2 = the concentration of tracer in the body fluid sample taken from the subject; and V_2 = the volume of water in the body, or TBW.[86]

Of the numerous tracers used throughout the years, three are currently in common use: water labeled with either **tritium** (^3H_2O), **deuterium** (^2H_2O), or the stable isotope of oxygen ($H_2^{18}O$). Of these three, the tritium and deuterium isotopes of water are the most frequently used.[4,47,86,115] A tracer at a specified concentration and volume is either ingested orally or injected intravenously. This is followed by an equilibration period and then a sampling period.[86]

Deuterium is a stable isotope of hydrogen (does not emit radiation) that has a mass twice that of ordinary hydrogen. Lukaski[125] has described TBW measurement using deuterium-labeled water (deuterium oxide, or D_2O). After a subject had fasted 10 hours overnight, blood and saliva samples were obtained. A 10-g oral dose of D_2O in fruit juice or deionized water was given to each subject. During the next 4 hours, the subjects remained in a quiet state. Blood and saliva samples were taken at 30, 60, 90, 120, 180, and 240 minutes following the dose. Concentrations of D_2O in samples were determined by infrared absorption.

The concentration of D_2O in blood or saliva also can be determined by gas chromatography and mass spectrometry.[86,115] The use of D_2O has been found to be simple, accurate, noninvasive (if saliva collections are used), and suitable for field studies.[4] In healthy subjects, the tracer equilibrates in the body's water within 2 hours after ingestion and remains at a constant concentration for the next 3 hours. In subjects experiencing edema, ascites, or some other form of water accumulation, 4 to 6 hours may be required for the D_2O to equilibrate.[85] Because deuterium is a stable isotope, its use is safe and ethical, even with children and females of childbearing age. Major drawbacks of the method are the cost of the equipment necessary to measure the D_2O in samples and the tedious work involved in preparing samples for analysis.[4,115,116]

Tritium (^3H) is a radioactive isotope of hydrogen with a mass three times that of ordinary hydrogen. Its use in measuring TBW is similar to that of deuterium oxide. Its radioactivity, however, makes it unsuitable in research involving children and females of childbearing age, or in studies requiring repeated administration of the tracer over a short period (for example, every 2 weeks or less).[86] The concentration of the isotope in body fluids is determined by a liquid scintillation counter, which measures the radioactive emission from the sample.[47,115,116]

The use of water labeled with the heavy isotope of oxygen (^{18}O) as a tracer in dilution studies is gaining popularity among researchers. It has the advantage of being a stable (nonradioactive) isotope, and exhaled carbon dioxide in the form of $C^{18}O_2$ is in isotopic equilibrium with body water and can be used as the sample for easy analysis by mass spectrometry.[47,115,116] These advantages are offset somewhat by the higher cost of $H_2^{18}O$ compared with that of the hydrogen isotopes.[47]

The three main sources of error in measuring total body water are failure to administer an accurately measured dose; consumption of beverages by subjects during the equilibration period, which may prevent equilibration from being reached; and contamination of the samples by atmospheric water before analysis. Calculation of the fat mass from TBW is based on the assumption that fat-free tissue has a constant water content that averages approximately 73%. This average value is based on analyses of a limited number of cadavers with actual values ranging from 67.4% to 77.5%. These variations can result in considerable error in calculating total body fat from TBW.[47] It also appears that fatter subjects tend to have a higher water content in their fat-free tissues. Failure to account for this will lead to an underestimation of fat mass based on TBW.

Total Body Potassium

Two factors make measurements of total body potassium of interest to those studying body composition. More than 90% of all the body's potassium is located within fat-free tissues (as an intracellular cation), and 0.012% of all potassium is the naturally occurring potassium-40 (^{40}K) isotope, which emits a very small yet detectable amount of high-energy gamma radiation.[4,47,86,115]

Measurement of total body potassium (TBK) requires a specially constructed counter fitted with multiple gamma-ray detectors, which are interfaced with a computer for data collection and processing. Because of the low levels of gamma radiation emitted from a subject, very sensitive detectors are required. The counter must be large enough to admit a subject and to be screened from external radiation (cosmic and local sources of ionizing radiation) by massive shields of lead or steel, thus making it very expensive.[47,115] The counting process requires about 30 minutes. Recently developed counters yield an estimate of TBK with a precision of about ±3%.[47]

A major assumption of TBK measurement is that fat-free tissue has a known and constant potassium content. Researchers disagree on the concentration of potassium in fat-free tissue and whether there is a difference between the sexes.[4,47] The most widely published estimates are 66 and 60 mmol/kg of potassium in men and women, respectively.[47,115] It has been reported that the fat-free tissues of obese subjects tend to have a lower potassium content than the tissues of lean subjects. This may be due to actual differences in potassium content between obese and lean subjects. Another explanation may be that obese subjects have a thicker layer of potassium-poor fat surrounding a potassium-rich core of fat-free tissue,

absorbing some of the radiation and thus leading to an underestimation of actual TBK and an overestimation of fat content in the obese.[47,115] It also has been reported that the potassium content of fat-free tissues decreases with increasing age.[47] Another factor affecting the performance of the counters is the presence of radioactive contamination on the subject's body and clothing from atmospheric radon gas.[4,86] Therefore, it is recommended that subjects shower, wash their hair, and wear clean clothes before undergoing TBK measurements.[86]

Despite the reported precision of ±3%, the high cost and inherent limitations of the technique limit its use in estimating body composition. However, the technique does have value when used in conjunction with other measures. Combining the use of TBW measurements (which tend to underestimate body fat in obese subjects) with TBK measurements (which tend to overestimate body fat in the obese) may lead to more reliable estimates of body fat than either method alone.

Neutron Activation Analysis

Neutron activation analysis allows measurement of the body's content of calcium, iodine, hydrogen, sodium, chloride, phosphorus, carbon, and nitrogen.[4,86,115,126] Also known as in vivo neutron activation analysis, the method delivers a beam of neutrons to the subject, which interacts with the body's elements in several characteristic ways. In the most important of these (in terms of neutron activation analysis), atoms of target elements are activated, creating unstable isotopes, such as calcium-49 (^{49}Ca), nitrogen-15 (^{15}N), and sodium-24 (^{24}Na).[115,126,127] As these unstable isotopes revert back to their stable forms, gamma radiation of a characteristic energy is emitted from each. This is received by the system's detectors and analyzed by its computers. The unique energy level of the γ radiation identifies the element, and the radiation's level of activity represents its abundance. Gamma-ray emission can occur almost immediately (in which case, the technique is referred to as *prompt γ analysis*) or over a several-minute period (in which case, it is known as *delayed γ analysis*).[115,127]

Because a major component of muscle is nitrogen, the ability to measure nitrogen using neutron activation analysis allows the body's muscle and nonmuscle mass to be estimated.[86,115,126] The precision of repeated nitrogen determinations in healthy humans has been shown to be between 2% and 3%.[86]

Bone mineral content is of considerable interest to those studying osteoporosis, and neutron activation analysis is useful in measuring total body calcium, which is then used to quantitate total body bone mineral. The precision of repeated calcium measurements in healthy adults using neutron activation analysis has been 2.5%, making the method suitable for longitudinal studies of bone mass.[86] A more recent study of calcium content in phantoms (representations of the human body used for precision and accuracy testing) as measured by neutron activation analysis resulted in values within 3.6% of their known composition.[128]

Neutron activation analysis has been used successfully in clinical studies to assess the time required for body nitrogen to return to preoperative levels following aortic reconstruction surgery and to assess nutritional status in patients receiving continuous ambulatory peritoneal dialysis.[129,130] The accuracy and precision of the method are as good as, if not better than, those of other methods. It is preferable to isotope dilution techniques in patients requiring continuous intravenous fluid therapy and in those with large increases in body water. Newer, lighter-weight, portable units are making neutron activation analysis more available for body composition analysis in the clinical setting.[126] Neutron activation analysis is noninvasive and is not based on certain assumptions concerning ratios of major body compartments or their density, as are some of the methods used to assess body fat.[127]

The method has several drawbacks. It exposes subjects to ionizing radiation, is costly, and requires skilled operators.[82,115]

CREATININE EXCRETION

The amount of creatinine excreted in the urine over a 24-hour period can be used in estimating body muscle mass.[4,86] Creatinine is the only metabolite of creatine, a nitrogenous compound synthesized from amino acids in the liver and taken up by many tissues, but primarily by muscle. Ninety-eight percent of the body's creatine is found in muscle, primarily in the form of creatine phosphate (bound to adenosine triphosphate, where it serves as an immediate source of energy).[4,86] Creatine spontaneously dehydrates to form creatinine, which is then excreted unaltered in the urine. Therefore, measurement of creatinine in a 24-hour urine collection should reflect the level of total body creatinine and consequently total body muscle mass.[4]

Several problems are associated with this approach. The most notable of these are the influence of meat consumption on urinary creatinine levels and the large intraindividual variability in daily urinary creatinine excretion (about ±11%) in persons consuming a meat-free diet.[86] Dietary creatine can influence urinary creatinine independently of muscle mass. Therefore, the diets of subjects undergoing urinary creatinine measurements should be meat free or be of a constant composition.[4] Urine collections must be complete because an error of 15 minutes in the timing of 24-hour urine collections can affect results of creatinine measurements by 1%.[4,86] Some researchers advise making three consecutive 24-hour urine collections to assure a representative creatinine excretion for an individual.[86] The precision of automated procedures for determining creatinine concentration in urine is approximately 1% to 2%, introducing further error.[86]

Despite these potential sources of error, estimates of fat-free mass based on 24-hour urinary excretion of creatinine have been shown to correlate reasonably well with those derived from measurements of body density, total body nitrogen, and total body potassium.[131,132] More accurate estimates of fat-free mass can be obtained from measurement of body density, total body nitrogen, and total body potassium. However, when the necessary facilities or resources are unavailable or when subjects are too ill to undergo such testing, urinary creatinine may be the most acceptable approach. Another urinary metabolite that appears better correlated with densitometrically determined fat-free mass is 3-methylhistidine.

3-METHYLHISTIDINE

3-Methylhistidine is an amino acid found in actin and myosin, the contractile proteins of muscle. 3-Methylhistidine is a *derived amino acid;* it is formed by the addition of methyl groups to histidine present in actin and myosin after these contractile proteins have been synthesized. When these proteins are catabolized, the 3-methylhistidine is released, not reutilized for protein synthesis, but excreted quantitatively in the urine. Assuming that muscle protein synthesis and degradation are balanced during steady-state periods, urinary 3-methylhistidine should be proportional to muscle mass.[4]

Lukaski and coworkers[131] have shown 24-hour urinary excretion of 3-methylhistidine to be well correlated to fat-free mass, determined by densitometry in healthy males age 23 to 52 years consuming a meat-free diet. In a later study, Lukaski and coworkers[132] assessed skeletal muscle mass in 14 healthy adult males on a meat-free diet using measurements of 3-methylhistidine, total body nitrogen, and total body potassium. Urinary excretion of 3-methylhistidine was significantly related to skeletal muscle mass and appeared to be a valid index of muscle and fat-free mass.

Measurement of urinary 3-methylhistidine excretion is subject to the same potential errors as are possible in measurement of urinary creatinine excretion.[4,86] Intraindividual variability is reported to range from 10% to 20%. Subjects should refrain from eating meat during the measurement period. Twenty-four-hour urine collections should be accurately timed and complete.[86] Before 3-methylhistidine can be used as a routine indicator of muscle mass, however, the effects of sex, age, maturity, fitness status, recent intense exercise, disease, and injury on 3-methylhistidine levels must be better understood.

ELECTRICAL CONDUCTANCE

The use of electrical conductance to assess body composition is based on the marked difference in electrolyte content between fat and fat-free tissue.[115,133,134] Electrolytes such as sodium, chloride, potassium, and bicarbonate are found primarily in the fat-free tissues, whereas concentrations of these ions in adipose tissue are very low. Because electrolytes in body water are capable of conducting electricity, the body's fat-free mass has a greater electrical conductivity than its fat mass. This difference in conductivity is the basis of two body assessment methods: bioelectrical impedance and total body electrical conductivity.

Bioelectrical Impedance

When an electrical current is passed through the body, it is opposed by the nonconducting tissues (principally, fat and cell membranes) and is transmitted by electrolytes dissolved in water (largely found in the fat-free tissues, although adipose tissue contains about 14% water).[4,115,133,134] This opposition to an alternating current is called impedance, which is composed of two elements: resistance and reactance. In bioelectrical impedance analysis (BIA), an electronic instrument (Figure 6.41) generates an alternating current, which is passed through the body by means of four electrodes placed on the hand and foot. The current (50 kHz, 800 μA) is harmless and cannot be felt by the subject. The body's resistance to this current is measured by the instrument. Some BIA instruments simply provide the operator with a value for resistance, which is then used (along with the subject's stature, weight, and sex) to manually calculate total body water, fat-free mass, and percent of body fat. More sophisticated BIA instruments contain a computer and printer and are capable of automatically performing these calculations and providing a printed record.

Bioelectrical impedance analysis yields values for TBW that are very close to those obtained by dilution techniques.[115,116,133,134] One of the primary weaknesses of BIA, however, is estimating fat-free mass and percent of body fat from the value for TBW using regression equations. Because BIA relies on regression equations for calculating fat-free mass and percent of body fat, the method is only as good as the equation used.[115,135] Earlier equations tended to give inaccurate estimates of fat-free mass and percent of body fat; more recent equations are considerably better. Another weakness is that BIA assumes that subjects are normally hydrated. Dehydration caused by insufficient water intake, excessive perspiration, heavy exercise, or caffeine or alcohol use (which stimulates urine production, possibly leading to dehydration) will result in overestimation of fat mass. To prevent this, subjects are advised to drink plenty of water, refrain from consuming caffeine and alcohol the day before testing, and avoid heavy exercise 12 hours before testing.

When compared with estimates of percent body fat derived from underwater weighing, BIA has been shown to be as good as (if not slightly better than) skinfold measurements in predicting percent body fat.[133,134] The method has the advantage of being safe, convenient to use, portable, rapid, and noninvasive. Bioelectrical impedance was among the procedures used in NHANES III. The only drawback is the instrument's cost, which can range from $2,000 to $3,000.

Total Body Electrical Conductivity

The degree to which an object placed in an electromagnetic field will tend to disrupt that field depends on the quantity of conducting material in the object. Because electrolytes within the fat-free mass are capable of conducting electricity, the degree to which a body placed in an electromagnetic field (EMF) disrupts that field is closely related to the amount of fat-free mass.[115,135] The instrument for measuring total body electrical conductivity (TOBEC) consists of a large solenoid coil driven by an oscillating radio-frequency current, which generates an EMF. The subject is placed on a table, which is slowly rolled into the coil. Changes in the EMF are measured between the conditions when the subject is inside the coil and when the coil is empty.[115] These changes are proportional to the total electrical conductivity of the subject's body. Using the statistical process of multiple-regression analysis, regression equations have been developed allowing TBW, TBK, fat-free mass, and percent body fat to be predicted from these changes.[115] Although TOBEC has been shown to compare favorably with other body composition assessment methods, the bulkiness and high cost of the units (approaching $100,000) seriously limit their use in nutritional assessment.

Figure 6.41

Bioelectrical impedance offers a convenient, rapid, noninvasive, and safe approach for assessing body composition. In this unit, four electrodes are built into the top of a digital scale (shown on the left). The subject stands on the scale, which simultaneously measures body weight and bioelectrical impedance. The microprocessor/printer (on the right) performs the calculations and provides visual and written output of body composition.

Source: Photo courtesy of Tanita Corporation of America.

INFRARED INTERACTANCE

When a material is exposed to infrared light, the light is absorbed, reflected, or transmitted, depending on the scattering and absorption properties of the material.[86] For example, water, protein, and fat have specific infrared absorption characteristics because of the stretching and bending of hydrogen bonds associated with the carbon, oxygen, and nitrogen they contain.[136] Information about the chemical composition (for example, water, protein, and fat content) of a material is contained in the infrared light reflected from the material.[86] Infrared instruments have been used successfully since about 1965 to determine the amount of moisture, protein, fat, and starch in grains and oil seeds.[86,136]

In human body composition analysis, a battery-powered, computerized infrared spectrophotometer has been developed. A probe, or "light wand," which acts as both an infrared transmitter and a detector, is attached to the unit by an electrical cord. The probe is placed on the subject's skin, and infrared light of two wavelengths is transmitted through the skin from the probe. Infrared light reflected from the skin and underlying tissues is detected by the probe. Estimates of body composition are made by analyzing certain characteristics of the reflected light (the shape of the interactance spectrum).[86,136,137] The instrument does not provide a measurement of fat thickness.

As an approach to estimating body composition, infrared interactance is marketed as safe, noninvasive, rapid, and convenient to use. These advantages have made infrared interactance a popular body composition technique at some hospitals, health clubs, and weight loss clinics.[138] Recent validation studies have raised questions about the accuracy of infrared interactance to estimate body composition.[138–141] When compared with other body composition methods (underwater weighing, skinfold measurements, and bioelectrical impedance analysis), infrared interactance overestimated percent body fat in lean subjects ($< 8\%$ body fat) and underestimated body fat in obese subjects ($> 30\%$ body fat).[138,141]

As a method for estimating body composition, most researchers report that infrared interactance is inferior to skinfold measurements and bioelectrical impedance.[138–142] At this time, it is not a recommended approach for determining body composition.

ULTRASOUND

Ultrasound is a widely used medical imaging method and has been studied as a possible tool in nutritional assessment. The heart of the technique is the transducer.[143] The transducer converts electrical energy into high-frequency sound and then converts that sound back into electrical energy; in other words, it acts as both a transmitter and a receiver. When the transducer is applied to the body surface, the ultrasound is transmitted into the body in the form of short pulses. As the ultrasound perpendicularly strikes the interface between two tissues differing in density (for example, adipose tissue and muscle), some of the sound is reflected and received by the transducer. The first reflection occurs at the transducer-skin interface. Each succeeding tissue interface results in a reflection, the intensity of which is reduced by the depth of the patient's tissues. This reflected sound is visually displayed on a video screen.[4,86,143]

In most published studies, ultrasonography has been compared with use of skinfold calipers. The results have been mixed and may be due to differences in instrumentation, technique, and interpretation.[144–146] Considerable skill is required in using the method and interpreting its results. The transducer must be applied to the skin surface with uniform and constant pressure to prevent differences in adipose and other soft tissue compression.[86,147] Differences in study populations could partly explain the conflicting results. For example, ultrasound may be preferable to skinfold calipers in measuring very obese individuals because of difficulty in accurately measuring skinfolds on them.[135,147]

Ultrasound has several advantages. It is noninvasive, nonradioactive, safe, and relatively portable, although less so than skinfold calipers. It may be a more appropriate technique for assessing persons whose skinfolds are thick and/or difficult to measure. Compared with the use of skinfold calipers, ultrasound is much more expensive and requires more training for its operation and interpretation.[86,135]

COMPUTED TOMOGRAPHY

Computed tomography (CT) is an imaging technique producing highly detailed cross-sectional images of the body resulting from differences in the transmission of an X-ray beam through body tissues of differing density.[135] Although its role in medicine is primarily for diagnostic purposes, it has proved to be a valuable research tool in assessing body composition and nutritional status. The CT system consists of an X-ray source aligned opposite an array of radiation detectors. In some CT scanners, the beam and detectors rotate in a plane perpendicular to the subject. Some instruments have a full circle of detectors, and only the X-ray source moves.[115,143]

As the X-ray beam passes through the subject, it is weakened, or attenuated, by the body's tissues and eventually picked up by the detectors. The response of the detectors is then transmitted to a computer, which also considers the spatial arrangement of the subject and X-ray beam. From these data, the computer reconstructs the subject's cross-sectional anatomy, using mathematic equations adapted for computer processing.[115,143]

CT has been particularly useful in studying the relative deposition of subcutaneous and intraabdominal fat.[148–150] CT images can be used to differentiate among various types of lean tissue, such as skeletal muscle, visceral mass, or organ mass; to provide data on the amount and distribution of adipose tissue in skeletal muscle; and to discriminate between cortical and trabecular bone.[115,154] Estimates of subcutaneous and intraabdominal fat from CT have been shown to compare very closely with direct measurements in cadavers and laboratory animals.[151,152] CT scans at three sites—lower chest, abdomen, and midthigh—have been shown to be effective in estimating body fat mass in premenopausal obese women.[153]

The potential for using CT in assessing body composition and nutritional status has been limited by problems of radiation exposure and the high cost and limited availability of the instrument.[86,115] Multiple scans of the same individual, whole-body scans, and use of CT with children and women of childbearing age are not encouraged because of the exposure to ionizing radiation. The use of the technology in nutritional assessment is restricted, for the most part, to special research applications. Recently, however, techniques have been used to reduce radiation exposure without compromising the accuracy of measurements of abdominal fat volume and distribution.[115,150,155]

MAGNETIC RESONANCE IMAGING

Magnetic resonance imaging (MRI) is a technology that allows both imaging of the body and in vivo chemical analysis without hazard to the subject.[115,156] Originally referred to as nuclear magnetic resonance, this approach is based on the fact that the nucleus of an atom acts as a magnet; it has north and south poles and is said to be a *magnetic dipole.* Ordinarily, nuclei or magnetic dipoles are oriented randomly. However, if a subject is placed in a large bore magnet generating a very strong magnetic field, the magnetic dipoles become aligned in relation to the magnetic field. If a radio-frequency wave is then directed into the subject's body, some of the nuclei will absorb energy from the radio wave and change their orientation with respect to the magnetic field. When the radio wave is discontinued, the nuclei gradually return to their equilibrium state (relaxation) and emit a signal that can be received by the system. These data are then processed by computer to generate an image much the same way as in CT.[86,115,135]

The hydrogen nucleus is particularly well suited for analysis because of its high concentration and abundance in the body and its easy detection by MRI. Tissue levels of phosphorus also can be detected in tissues using MRI. This allows investigators to quantify the relative amounts of ATP, phosphocreatine, and inorganic phosphorus in the body's tissues.[115] MRI allows researchers to monitor the metabolic functions of certain tissues and organs in response to certain treatments, including various nutritional regimens.[115,156]

MRI is a valuable tool for assessing muscle mass and regional fat distribution, giving accurate and precise measurements of muscle and adipose tissue content, when compared with direct measures in cadavers. For example, MRI was used to measure the intraabdominal, retroperitoneal, and subcutaneous adipose tissue content in three unembalmed cadavers, which were subsequently dissected so that the adipose tissue in these three compartments could be accurately weighed.[157] MRI was shown to be an accurate technique to evaluate the content of the adipose tissue in these compartments. In a similar study, MRI was used to measure adipose tissue–free skeletal muscle cross-sectional area, adipose tissue embedded in muscle (interstitial adipose tissue), and adipose tissue surrounding muscle (subcutaneous adipose tissue) in nearly 120 arms and legs of cadavers.[158] The limbs were then carefully dissected and the corresponding tissues weighed. Values obtained from MRI compared favorably with those obtained from direct analysis of the tissues involved. The accuracy and precision with which MRI can make these measurements has made MRI the "method of choice for calibration of field methods designed to measure body fat and skeletal muscle *in vivo.*"[156]

The advantages of MRI are several. It is totally noninvasive, uses no ionizing radiation (thus, it is safe for children, females of childbearing age, and multiple studies on the same subject), produces high-quality images of the body, allows the amount and distribution of body fat to be studied, and can be used to study the metabolic activity of tissues or organs. MRI can image hydrogen, phosphorus, carbon, fluoride, sodium, and potassium.[115] The low-contrast resolution of MRI is much better than that of CT. Drawbacks of the method are its restricted availability and high cost.[86]

DUAL-ENERGY X-RAY ABSORPTIOMETRY

Dual-energy X-ray absorptiometry (DXA) is discussed in Chapter 8 as a means of assessing bone mineral density, an area in which it is particularly well suited because of its high precision in measuring bone mineral density. In recent years, considerable attention has been given to using DXA to measure fat and nonbone lean tissue.[159] DXA has the advantage of being safe (because of the low-radiation dose subjects receive) and relatively quick (a whole-body scan takes 20 to 35 minutes). The fact that the procedure requires little cooperation from patients makes it an attractive body composition assessment method for the very young, the very old, and the sick. The use of effective and user-friendly software allows personnel with minimal training to operate the instrument and produce high-quality output.[159] Estimates of percent body fat from DXA have been found to be highly correlated with those from underwater weighing.[160,161]

As with any relatively new technology, DXA has some limitations. Marked differences in the hydration of lean tissue from that seen in healthy adults may adversely affect the accuracy of body composition measures. Consequently, concerns have been raised about the appropriateness of using DXA for assessing body composition in infants (who tend to have a higher degree of lean tissue hydration than adults) and persons with acute or chronic alterations in body water. Body composition measurements may be affected by the thickness of the body part being scanned, possibly resulting in systemat-ic differences between thin and obese persons or affecting the accuracy of serial measurements in persons losing or gaining weight. The accuracy of regional soft tissue measurements can be adversely affected by the presence of bone (especially by ribs in the thorax) and the calcification of soft tissues (as is seen in the aortas of older people).[159]

Dual-energy X-ray absorptiometry has considerable promise as a body composition assessment technique, but further research and development is necessary before it can be considered a "gold standard."[159]

SUMMARY

1. Anthropometry is the measurement of body size, weight, and proportions. Adherence to proper technique is critical to obtaining accurate and precise measurements. Among children, length, stature, weight, and head circumference are the most sensitive and commonly used anthropometric indicators of health.

2. Body weight, one of the most important measurements in nutritional assessment, should be obtained using an electronic or balance-beam scale with nondetachable weights that is appropriate for the subject. Attention must be given to regular calibration of balance-beam scales, especially after they have been moved.

3. Standards for assessing physical growth of persons from birth to age 20 years have been developed by the Centers for Disease Control and Prevention. These growth charts allow a child's development to be easily categorized relative to the development of other children of similar age and sex.

4. Overweight is a body weight above some reference weight, which usually is defined in relation to stature. Obesity is an excess of body fat in relation to lean body mass. Overweight persons tend to die sooner than average-weight persons, especially those who are overweight at younger ages. The lowest mortality in the United States is associated with body weights that are somewhat below average for a given group based on sex and stature.

5. Approaches to assessing body weight include height-weight tables, relative weight, and height-weight indices. The life insurance industry, a leader in the development of height-weight tables, has attempted to define body weights for a given sex and stature that are associated with the lowest mortality.

6. Height-weight tables fail to provide information on body composition. Their data are not drawn from representative population samples and are sometimes self-reported. They inadequately control for confounding variables, such as cigarette smoking, which tend to make lower body weights appear less healthy.

7. Relative weight is a person's actual weight divided by some reference weight for that person's height, multiplied by 100, and expressed as a percentage of reference weight. Relative weights between 90% and 120% are considered within normal limits.

8. Of the various body mass indices available, the most common is Quetelet's index—weight in kilograms divided by height in meters squared. Although body mass indices tend to be better predictors of obesity than height-weight tables or relative weight, they still do not distinguish between overweight resulting from obesity and that resulting from unusual muscular development.

9. The distribution of body fat may be as important a consideration as total quantity of fat. Body fat distribution can be classified into two types: upper body (android, or male, type) and lower body (gynoid, or female, type). Android obesity is associated with increased risk of insulin resistance, hyperinsulinemia, noninsulin-dependent (type 2) diabetes mellitus, hypertension, hyperlipidemia, stroke, and death. The waist-to-hip ratio and waist circumference are valuable indices of regional body fat distribution.

10. Body composition analysis can provide estimates of the body's reserves of fat, protein, water, and several minerals. The two-compartment model divides the body into fat and fat-free masses. The four-compartment model views the human body as composed of four chemical groups: water, protein, mineral, and fat. Most approaches to determining body composition are indirect measures.

11. Measurement of skinfolds is the most widely used method of indirectly estimating percent body fat. What is actually measured is the thickness of a

double fold of skin and compressed subcutaneous adipose tissue.

12. Skinfold measures have several advantages. The equipment is inexpensive and portable. Measurements can be easily and quickly obtained, and they correlate well with body density measurements. Proper measurement of skinfolds requires careful site selection and strict adherence to the standardized techniques outlined in this chapter.

13. The triceps is the most commonly used single skinfold site. Single-site skinfold measurements must be interpreted with caution and should be used only as a rough approximation of total body fat percentage. Results should be compared with reference data derived from large population surveys, such as NHANES III.

14. For assessing body composition of young people, the sum of two sites (triceps and subscapular or triceps and medial calf) often is used. These sites correlate with other measures of body fatness and are more reliably and objectively measured than most other sites, and reference data are available.

15. Regression equations allow body density and percent body fat to be estimated from multiple skinfold measures. These equations were developed by seeing which combination of anthropometric measures best predict body density. Generalized equations can be applied to groups varying greatly in age and body fatness and can replace several population-specific equations with little loss in prediction accuracy.

16. Densitometry involves measuring the density of the entire body, usually by hydrostatic (underwater) weighing. If mass and volume of the body are known, its density can be calculated. However, hydrostatic weighing is not practical for testing large groups. It requires considerable subject cooperation, special equipment, experience, and financial investment.

17. Despite its weaknesses, underwater weighing remains the standard laboratory technique for determining body density and percent body fat. Compared with other body density methods and more sophisticated body composition techniques, the costs are low.

18. Air displacement plethysmography involves using a specially designed two-chambered unit for measuring the body's volume, which is then used to calculate body density and composition. Subjects better tolerate this method than underwater weighing. It requires less subject cooperation, and residual lung volume measurements are not needed. It appears as accurate and precise as underwater

weighing, but the equipment is considerably more complex and costly.

19. Total body water is measured indirectly using dilution techniques where a tracer of known concentration and volume is given to a subject, time is allowed for the tracer to equilibrate with the subject's body water, and the concentration of the tracer in a sample of the subject's blood, urine, or saliva is analyzed. Commonly used tracers include deuterium oxide and water labeled with the heavy isotope of oxygen.

20. Measurement of total body potassium can also be used to evaluate body composition. More than 90% of body potassium is located within fat-free tissues, and 0.012% of potassium is potassium-40 isotope, which emits gamma radiation.

21. Neutron activation analysis is based on the response of elements (e.g., nitrogen, calcium, and carbon) to neutron beam irradiation and is particularly useful in estimating total body muscle. The method's drawbacks include ionizing radiation exposure, high cost, and limited availability.

22. Measurement of creatinine in a 24-hour urine collection reflects total body muscle mass. Despite limitations by such factors as dietary creatine, intraindividual variation, and timing of urine collections, estimates of fat-free mass based on urinary creatinine correlate reasonably well with estimates derived from measurements of body density, total body nitrogen, and total body potassium.

23. 3-Methylhistidine is an amino acid found in the contractile proteins actin and myosin. When these proteins are catabolized, 3-methylhistidine is released and excreted in the urine. Urinary excretion has been shown to be a valid index of muscle and fat-free mass. However, its measurement is subject to the same potential errors as those in measurements of urinary creatinine excretion.

24. The marked difference in electrolyte content between fat and fat-free tissues is a basic principle behind body composition estimates from bioelectrical impedance analysis (BIA) and total body electrical conductivity (TOBEC). In BIA, the body's resistance to a minute electrical current is used to calculate total body water, from which the percentages of body fat and fat-free mass are calculated using various formulas.

25. In TOBEC, the degree to which a body placed in an electromagnetic field (EMF) disrupts that field is closely related to the amount of fat-free mass. TOBEC uses an instrument consisting of a large solenoid coil driven by an oscillating radio-frequency current, which generates an EMF. Like

BIA, the accuracy of total body water estimates can be affected by dehydration. It appears to be an acceptable technique for body composition assessment, but its use is limited by high cost.

26. When infrared light is projected through the skin, some of the energy is reflected from the skin and underlying tissues. Estimates of body composition are made by analyzing certain characteristics of this reflected energy. The approach tends to overestimate percent body fat in lean subjects and underestimate percent body fat in obese subjects. This method is inferior to skinfold measurements and is not recommended for determining body composition.

27. In ultrasound, high-frequency sound waves are transmitted into the body from a transducer applied to the skin surface. As ultrasound strikes the interface between two tissues differing in density (for example, adipose tissue and muscle), some of it is reflected and received by the transducer. The time lag between reflections allows tissue layer depth to be calculated. Ultrasound compares favorably with skinfold measurements but may be preferable to skinfold measurements when evaluating very obese people.

28. Computed tomography is an imaging technique producing highly detailed cross-sectional images of the body caused by differences in the transmission of an X-ray beam through body tissues of differing density.

29. Magnetic resonance imaging is a technology allowing both imaging of the body and in vivo chemical analysis without radiation hazard to the subject.

30. Body composition estimates derived from dual-energy X-ray absorptiometry (DXA) compare favorably with those from underwater weighing. DXA has the advantage of requiring little subject cooperation, being relatively quick, and having a low radiation dose. Differences in hydration and the presence of bone or calcified soft tissues may affect the accuracy of body composition measurements.

REFERENCES

1. Chumlea WC, Roche AF, Mukherjee D. 1987. *Nutritional assessment of the elderly through anthropometry.* Columbus, OH: Ross Laboratories.

2. Moore WM, Roche AF. 1983. *Pediatric anthropometry,* 2nd ed. Columbus, OH: Ross Laboratories.

3. Heymsfield SB, Casper K. 1987. Anthropometric assessment of the adult hospitalized patient. *Journal of Parenteral and Enteral Nutrition* 11(suppl):36S–41S.

4. Brodie DA. 1988. Techniques of measurement of body composition. Part I. *Sports Medicine* 5:11–40.

5. Pollock ML, Jackson AS. 1984. Research progress in validation of clinical methods of assessing body composition. *Medicine and Science in Sports and Exercise* 16:606–613.

6. Chumlea WC, Roche AF, Steinbaugh ML. 1985. Estimating stature from knee height for persons 60 to 90 years of age. *Journal of the American Geriatrics Society* 33:116–120.

7. Gordon CC, Chumlea WC, Roche AF. 1988. Stature, recumbent length, and weight. In Lohman TG, Roche AF, Martorell R, eds. *Anthropometric standardization reference manual.* Champaign, IL: Human Kinetics Books.

8. Kuczmarski RJ, Ogden CL, Grummer-Strawn LM, Flegal KM, Guo SS, et al. 2000. *CDC growth charts: United States. Advance data from vital and health statistics; no. 314.* Hyattsville, MD: National Center for Health Statistics.

9. Winick M, Rosso P. 1969. Head circumference and cellular growth of the brain in normal and marasmic children. *Journal of Pediatrics* 74:774–778.

10. Roche AF, Himes JH. 1980. Incremental growth charts. *American Journal of Clinical Nutrition* 33:2041–2052.

11. Chumlea WC, Guo S, Roche AF, Steinbaugh ML. 1988. Prediction of body weight for the nonambulatory elderly from anthropometry. *Journal of the American Dietetic Association* 88:564–568.

12. National Center for Health Statistics. 1993. *Executive summary of the growth chart workshop, 1992.* Hyattsville, MD: U.S. Department of Health and Human Services, Public Health Service, Centers for Disease Control.

13. Harrison GG. 1985. Height-weight tables. *Annals of Internal Medicine* 103:989–994.

14. Food and Nutrition Board, National Research Council. 1989. *Diet and health: Implications for reducing chronic disease risk.* Washington, DC: National Academy Press.

15. Bray GA, Gray DS. 1988. Obesity. Part I: Pathogenesis. *Western Medical Journal* 149:429–441.

16. Must A, Spadano J, Coakley EH, Field AE, Colditz G, Dietz WH. 1999. The disease burden associated with overweight and obesity. *Journal of the American Medical Association* 282:1523–1529.

17. Koplan JP, Dietz WH. 1999. Caloric imbalance and public health policy. *Journal of the American Medical Association* 282:1579–1581.

18. Simopoulos AP, VanItallie TB. 1984. Body weight, health, and

longevity. *Annals of Internal Medicine* 100:285–295.

19. National Task Force on the Prevention and Treatment of Obesity. 2000. Overweight, obesity, and health risk. *Archives of Internal Medicine* 160:898–904.

20. Lindsted K, Tonstad S, Kuzma JW. 1991. Body mass index and patterns of mortality among Seventh-day Adventist men. *International Journal of Obesity* 15:397–406.

21. Weigley ES. 1984. Average? Ideal? Desirable? A brief overview of height-weight tables in the United States. *Journal of the American Dietetic Association* 84:417–423.

22. Manson JE, Stampfer MJ, Hennekens CH, Willett WC. 1987. Body weight and longevity: A reassessment. *Journal of the American Medical Association* 257:353–358.

23. Ideal weights for women. 1942. *Statistical bulletin of the Metropolitan Life Insurance Company* 23(October):6–8.

24. Ideal weights for men. 1943. *Statistical bulletin of the Metropolitan Life Insurance Company* 24(June):6–8.

25. New weight standards for men and women. 1959. *Statistical bulletin of the Metropolitan Life Insurance Company* 40(November–December):1–3.

26. Metropolitan height and weight tables. 1983. *Statistical bulletin of the Metropolitan Life Insurance Company* 64(January–June):2.

27. Andres R. 1985. Mortality and obesity: The rationale for age-specific height-weight tables. In Andres R, Bierman EL, Hazzard WR, eds. *Principles of geriatric medicine.* New York: McGraw Hill.

28. Andres R, Elahe D, Tobin JD, Muller DC, Brant L. 1985. Impact of age on weight goals. *Annals of Internal Medicine* 103:1030–1033.

29. Nieman DC. 1999. *Exercise testing and prescription: A health-related approach,* 4th ed. Mountain View, CA: Mayfield.

30. Pirie P, Jacobs D, Jeffery R, Hannan P. 1981. Distortion in self-reported height and weight data. *Journal of the American Dietetic Association* 78:601–606.

31. Rowland ML. 1991. Self-reported weight and height. *American Journal of Clinical Nutrition* 52:1125–1133.

32. Schlichting PF, Hoilund-Carlsen PF, Quaade F, Lauritzen SL. 1981. Comparison of self-reported height and weight with controlled height and weight in women and men. *International Journal of Obesity* 5:67–76.

33. DelPrete LR, Caldwell M, English C, Banspach SW, Lefebvre C. 1992. Self-reported and measured weights and heights of participants in community-based weight loss programs. *Journal of the American Dietetic Association* 92:1483–1486.

34. Willett WC, Stampfer M, Manson J, VanItallie T. 1991. New weight guidelines for Americans: Justified or injudicious? *American Journal of Clinical Nutrition* 53:1102–1103.

35. Marwick C. 1993. Obesity experts say less weight still best. *Journal of the American Medical Association* 269:2617–2618.

36. Colditz GA, Willett WC, Stampfer MJ, Manson JE, Hennekens CH, Arky RA, Speizer FE. 1990. Weight as a risk factor for clinical diabetes in women. *American Journal of Epidemiology* 132:501–513.

37. Manson JE, Colditz GA, Stampfer MJ, Willett WC, Rosner B, Monson RR, Speizer FE, Hennekens CH. 1990. A prospective study of obesity and risk of coronary heart disease in women. *New England Journal of Medicine* 322:882–889.

38. Frisancho AR. 1990. *Anthropometric standards for the assessment of growth and nutritional status.* Ann Arbor: University of Michigan Press.

39. Novascone MA, Smith EP. 1989. Frame size estimation: A comparative analysis of methods based on height, wrist circumference, and elbow breadth. *Journal of the American Dietetic Association* 89:964–966.

40. Wilmore JH, Frisancho RA, Gordon CC, Himes JH, Martin AD, Martorell R, Seefeldt VD. 1988. Body breadth equipment and measurement techniques. In Lohman TG, Roche AF, Martorell R, eds. *Anthropometric standardization reference manual.* Champaign, IL: Human Kinetics Books.

41. Katch VL, Freedson PS. 1982. Body size and shape: Derivation of the HAT frame size model. *American Journal of Clinical Nutrition* 36:669–675.

42. Katch VL, Freedson PS, Katch FI, Smith L. 1982. Body frame size: Validity of self-appraisal. *American Journal of Clinical Nutrition* 36:676–679.

43. Grant JP, Custer PB, Thurlow J. 1981. Current techniques of nutritional assessment. *Surgical Clinics of North America* 61:437–463.

44. Garn SM, Pesick SD, Hawthorne VM. 1983. The bony chest breadth as a frame size standard in nutritional assessment. *American Journal of Clinical Nutrition* 37:315–318.

45. Baecke JAH, Burema J, Deurenberg P. 1982. Body fatness, relative weight and frame size in young adults. *British Journal of Nutrition* 48:1–6.

46. Frisancho AR, Flegel PN. 1983. Elbow breadth as a measure of frame size for U.S. males and females. *American Journal of Clinical Nutrition* 37:311–314.

47. Garrow JS. 1983. Indices of adiposity. *Nutrition Abstracts and Reviews* 53:697–708.

48. Callaway CW, Chumlea WC, Bouchard C, Himes JH, Lohman GT, Martin AD, Mitchell CD, Mueller WH, Roche AF, Seefeldt VD. 1988. Circumferences. In Lohman TG, Roche AF, Martorell R, eds. *Anthropometric standardization reference manual.* Champaign, IL: Human Kinetics Books.

49. Lee J, Kolonel LN, Hinds MW. 1981. Relative merits of the weight-corrected-for-height indices. *American Journal of Clinical Nutrition* 34:2521–2529.

50. Lee J, Kolonel LN, Hinds MW. 1982. Relative merits of old and new indices of body mass: A commentary. *American Journal of Clinical Nutrition* 36:727–728.

51. Lee J, Kolonel LN. 1983. Body mass indices: A further commentary. *American Journal of Clinical Nutrition* 38:660–661.

52. Garrow JS, Webster J. 1985. Quetelet's index (w/h^2) as a measure of fatness. *International Journal of Obesity* 9:147–153.

53. Willett WC, Dietz WH, Colditz GA. 1999. Guidelines for healthy weight. *New England Journal of Medicine* 341:427–434.

54. Barlow SE, Dietz WH. 1998. Obesity evaluation and treatment: Expert committee recommendations. *Pediatrics* 102:e29.

55. Flegal KM. 1999. The obesity epidemic in children and adults: Current evidence and research issues. *Medicine and Science in Sports and Exercise* 31(suppl):S509–S514.

56. Smalley KJ, Knerr AN, Kendrick ZV, Colliver JA, Owen OE. 1990. Reassessment of body mass indices. *American Journal of Clinical Nutrition* 52:405–408.

57. Dietz WH, Robinson TN. 1998. Uses of the body mass index as a measure of overweight in children and adolescents. *Journal of Pediatrics* 132:191–193.

58. Killeen J, Vanderburg D, Harlan W. 1978. Application of weight-height ratios and body mass indices to juvenile populations—the National Health Examination Survey data. *Journal of Chronic Diseases* 31:529–537.

59. Dietz WH, Bellizzi MC. 1999. Introduction: The use of body mass index to assess obesity in children. *American Journal of Clinical Nutrition* 70(suppl):S123–S125.

60. Bellizzi MC, Dietz WC. 1999. Workshop on childhood obesity: Summary of the discussion. *American Journal of Clinical Nutrition* 70(suppl):S173–S175.

61. Roche AF, Siervogel RM, Chumlea WC, Webb P. 1981. Grading body fatness from limited anthropometric data. *American Journal of Clinical Nutrition* 34:2831–2838.

62. Keys A, Fidanza F, Karvonen MJ, Kimura N, Taylor HL. 1972. Indices of relative weight and obesity. *Journal of Chronic Diseases* 25:329–343.

63. Norgan NG, Ferro-Luzzi A. 1982. Weight-height indices as estimators of fatness in men. *Human Nutrition: Clinical Nutrition* 36C:363–372.

64. Frisancho AR, Flegel PN. 1982. Relative merits of old and new indices of body mass with reference to skinfold thickness. *American Journal of Clinical Nutrition* 36:697–699.

65. National Institutes of Health. 1998. *Clinical guidelines on the identification, evaluation, and treatment of overweight and obesity in adults.* National Heart, Lung, and Blood Institute. NIH publication number 98-4083.

66. U.S. Department of Agriculture/U.S. Department of Health and Human Services. 2000. *Nutrition and your health: Dietary guidelines for Americans,* 5th ed. Hyattsville, MD: U.S. Department of Agriculture, Center for Nutrition Policy and Promotion. Home and Garden Bulletin no. 232.

67. Kahn HS. 1991. A major error in nomograms for estimating body mass index. *American Journal of Clinical Nutrition* 54:435–437.

68. Giovannucci E, Colditz GA, Stampfer MJ, Willett WC. 1996. Physical activity, obesity, and risk of colorectal adenoma in women (United States). *Cancer Causes and Control* 7:253–263.

69. Troiano RP, Flegal KM. 1999. Overweight prevalence among youth in the United States: Why so many different numbers? *International Journal of Obesity* 23(suppl 2):S22–S27.

70. Kaye SA, Folsom AR, Prineas RJ, Potter JD, Gapstur SM. 1990. The association of body fat distribution with lifestyle and reproductive factors in a population study of postmenopausal women. *International Journal of Obesity* 14:583–591.

71. Troisi RJ, Weiss ST, Segal MR, Cassano PA, Vokonas PS, Landsberg L. 1990. The relationship of body fat distribution to blood pressure in normotensive men: The normative aging study. *International Journal of Obesity* 14:515–525.

72. Zwiauer K, Widhalm K, Kerbl B. 1990. Relationship between body fat distribution and blood lipids in obese adolescents. *International Journal of Obesity* 14:271–277.

73. National Institutes of Health. 2000. *The practical guide; identification, evaluation, and treatment of overweight and obesity in adults.* National Heart, Lung, and Blood Institute. NIH publication number 00-4084.

74. Rankinen T, Kim SY, Perusse L, Despres JP, Bouchard C. 1999. The prediction of abdominal visceral fat level from body composition and anthropometry: ROC analysis. *International Journal of Obesity and Related Metabolic Research* 23:801–809.

75. Turcato E, Bosello O, Francesco VD, Harris TB, Zoico E, et al. 2000. Waist circumference and abdominal sagittal diameter as surrogates of body fat distribution in the elderly: Their relation with cardiovascular risk factors. *International Journal of Obesity and Related Metabolic Research* 24:1005–1010.

76. Clasey JL, Bouchard C, Teates CD, Riblett JE, Thorner MO, et al. The use of anthropometric and dual-energy x-ray absorptiometry (DXA) measures to estimate total abdominal and abdominal visceral fat in men and women. *Obesity Research* 7:256–264.

77. Must A, Strauss RS. 1999. Risk and consequences of childhood and adolescent obesity. *International Journal of Obesity and Related Metabolic Disorders* 23(suppl 2): S2–S11.

78. Flegal KM. 1999. The obesity epidemic in children and adults: Current evidence and research issues. *Medicine and Science in Sports and Exercise* 31(suppl): S509–S514.

79. Colditz GA. 1999. Economic costs of obesity and overweight.

Medicine and Science in Sports and Exercise 31(suppl):S663–S667.

80. Seidell JC. 2000. Obesity, insulin resistance and diabetes—a worldwide epidemic. *British Journal of Nutrition* 83(suppl 1): S5–S8.

81. Chandra RK. 1981. Immunodeficiency in undernutrition and overnutrition. *Nutrition Reviews* 39:225–231.

82. Chandra RK. 1991. 1990 McCollum Award lecture. Nutrition and immunity: Lessons from the past and new insights into the future. *American Journal of Clinical Nutrition* 53:1087–1101.

83. Bistrian BR, Blackburn GL, Hallowel E, Heddle R. 1974. Protein status of general surgical patients. *Journal of the American Medical Association* 230:858–860.

84. Bistrian BR, Blackburn GL, Vitale J, Cochran D, Naylor J. 1976. Prevalence of malnutrition in general medical patients. *Journal of the American Medical Association* 235:1567–1570.

85. Coats KG, Morgan SL, Bartolucci AA, Weinsier RL. 1993. Hospital-associated malnutrition: A reevaluation 12 years later. *Journal of the American Dietetic Association* 93:27–33.

86. Lukaski HC. 1987. Methods for the assessment of human body composition: Traditional and new. *American Journal of Clinical Nutrition* 46:537–556.

87. Wang J, Thornton JC, Kolesnik S, Pierson RN. 2000. Anthropometry in body composition. An overview. *Annals of the New York Academy of Sciences* 904:317–326.

88. Keys A, Brozek J. 1953. Body fat in adult man. *Physiological Reviews* 33:245–325.

89. Wilmore JH, Buskirk ER, DiGirolamo M, Lohman TG. 1986. Body composition: A round table. *Physician and Sportsmedicine* 14:144–162.

90. Clarys JP, Martin AD, Drinkwater DT, Marfell-Jones MJ. 1987. The skinfold: Myth and reality. *Journal of Sports Sciences* 5:3–33.

91. Martin AD, Ross WD, Drinkwater DT, Clarys JP. 1985. Prediction of body fat by skinfold caliper: Assumptions and cadaver evidence. *International Journal of Obesity* 9:31–39.

92. Harrison GG, Buskirk EB, Carter JEL, Johnston JE, Lohman TG, Pollock ML, Roche AF, Wilmore J. 1988. Skinfold thicknesses and measurement technique. In Lohman TG, Roche AF, Martorell R, eds. *Anthropometric standardization reference manual.* Champaign, IL: Human Kinetics Books.

93. Himes JH, Roche AF, Siervogel RM. 1979. Compressibility of skinfolds and the measurement of subcutaneous fatness. *American Journal of Clinical Nutrition* 32:1734–1740.

94. Siervogel RM, Roche AF, Himes JH, Chumlea WC, McCammon R. 1982. Subcutaneous fat distribution in males and females from 1 to 39 years of age. *American Journal of Clinical Nutrition* 36:162–171.

95. Lohman TG. 1981. Skinfolds and body density and their relation of body fatness: A review. *Human Biology* 53:181–225.

96. Lohman TG. 1988. Anthropometry and body composition. In Lohman TG, Roche AF, Martorell R, eds. *Anthropometric standardization reference manual.* Champaign, IL: Human Kinetics Books.

97. Jackson AS, Pollock ML. 1985. Practical assessment of body composition. *Physician and Sportsmedicine* 13(5):76–90.

98. Martorell R, Mendoza F, Mueller WH, Pawson IG. 1988. Which side to measure: Right or left? In Lohman TG, Roche AF, Martorell R, eds. *Anthropometric standardization reference manual.* Champaign, IL: Human Kinetics Books.

99. Leger LA, Lambert J, Martin P. 1982. Validity of plastic skinfold caliper measurements. *Human Biology* 54:667–675.

100. Burgert SL, Anderson CF. 1979. A comparison of triceps skinfold values as measured by the plastic McGaw caliper and Lange caliper. *American Journal of Clinical Nutrition* 32:1531–1533.

101. Ross JG, Pate RR, Delpy LA, Gold RS, Svilar M. 1987. New health-related fitness norms. *Journal of Physical Education, Recreation, and Dance* 58:(9)66–70.

102. Lohman TG. 1987. The use of skinfolds to estimate body fatness on children and youth. *Journal of Physical Education, Recreation, and Dance* 58(9):98–102.

103. American Alliance for Health, Physical Education, Recreation, and Dance. 1985. *Norms for college students: Health-related physical fitness test.* Reston, VA: American Alliance for Health, Physical Education, Recreation, and Dance.

104. Jackson AS, Pollack ML, Ward A. 1980. Generalized equations for predicting body density of women. *Medicine and Science in Sports and Exercise* 12:175–182.

105. Pollock ML, Laughridge EE, Coleman B, Linnerud AC, Jackson A. 1975. Prediction of body density in young and middle-aged women. *Journal of Applied Physiology* 38:745–749.

106. Jackson AS, Pollock ML. 1978. Generalized equations for predicting body density in men. *British Journal of Nutrition* 40:497–504.

107. Brozek J, Keys A. 1951. The evaluation of leanness-fatness in man: Norms and intercorrelations. *British Journal of Nutrition* 5:194–205.

108. Durnin JVGA, Womersley J. 1974. Body fat assessment from total body density and its estimation from skinfold thickness: Measurements on 481 men and women aged 16–72 years. *British Journal of Nutrition* 32:77–97.

109. Baun WB, Baun MR, Raven PB. 1981. A nomogram for the estimate of percent body fat from generalized equations. *Research Quarterly for Exercise and Sport* 52:380–384.

110. Westrate JA, Deurenberg P. 1989. Body composition in children: Proposal for a method for calculating body fat percentage from total body

density or skinfold-thickness measurements. *American Journal of Clinical Nutrition* 50:1104–1115.

111. Katch F, Michael ED, Horvath SM. 1967. Estimation of body volume by underwater weighing: Description of a simple method. *Journal of Applied Physiology* 23:811–813.

112. Akers R, Buskirk ER. 1969. An underwater weighing system utilizing "force cube" transducers. *Journal of Applied Physiology* 26:649–652.

113. Wilmore JH. 1969. A simplified method for determination of residual volumes. *Journal of Applied Physiology* 27:96–100.

114. Goldman HI, Becklake MR. 1959. Respiratory function tests: Normal values at median altitudes and the prediction of normal results. *American Review of Tuberculosis and Pulmonary Diseases* 79:457–467.

115. Ellis KJ. 2000. Human body composition: In vivo methods. *Physiological Reviews* 80:649–680.

116. Wagner DR, Heyward VH. 1999. Techniques of body composition assessment: A review of laboratory and field methods. *Research Quarterly for Exercise and Sport* 70:135–149.

117. Dempster P, Aitkens S. 1995. A new air displacement method for the determination of human body composition. *Medicine and Science in Sports and Exercise* 27:1692–1697.

118. McCrory MA, Gomez TD, Bernauer EM, Molé PA. 1995. Evaluation of a new air displacement plethysmograph for measuring human body composition. *Medicine and Science in Sports and Exercise* 27:1686–1691.

119. Sardinha LB, Lohman TG, Teixeira PJ, Guedes DP, Going SB. 1998. Comparison of air displacement plethysmography with dual-energy x-ray absorptiometry and 3 field methods for estimating body composition in middle-aged men. *American Journal of Clinical Nutrition* 68:786–793.

120. Fields DA, Hunter GR, Goran MI. 2000. Validation of the Bod Pod with hydrostatic weighing: Influence of body clothing. *International Journal of Obesity* 24:200–205.

121. Collins MA, Millard-Stafford ML, Sparling PB, Snow TK, Rosskopf LB, Webb SA, Omar J. 1999. Evaluation of the Bod Pod for assessing body fat in collegiate football players. *Medicine and Science in Sports and Exercise* 31:1350–1356.

122. Dewit O, Fuller NJ, Fewtrell MS, Wells JCK. 2000. Whole body air displacement plethysmography compared with hydrodensitometry for body composition analysis. *Archives of Disease in Childhood* 82:159–164.

123. Biaggi RR, Vollman MW, Nies MA, Brener CE, Flakoll PJ, et al. 1999. Comparison of air-displacement plethysmography with hydrostatic weighing and bioelectrical impedance analysis for the assessment of body composition in healthy adults. *American Journal of Clinical Nutrition* 69:898–903.

124. Nunez C, Kovera AJ, Pietrobelli A, Heshka S, Horlick M, Kehayias JJ, et al. 1999. Body composition in children and adults by air displacement plethysmography. *European Journal of Clinical Nutrition* 53:382–387.

125. Lukaski HC, Johnson PE. 1985. A simple, inexpensive method of determining total body water using a tracer dose of D_2O and infrared absorption of biological fluids. *American Journal of Clinical Nutrition* 41:363–370.

126. Kehayias JJ, Valtuena S. 1999. Neutron activation analysis determination of body composition. *Current Opinion in Clinical Nutrition and Metabolic Care* 2:453–463.

127. Beddoe AH, Hill GL. 1985. Clinical measurement of body composition using *in vivo* neutron activation analysis. *Journal of Parenteral and Enteral Nutrition* 9:504–520.

128. Ryde SJ, Morgan WD, Compston J, Evans CJ. 1990. Measurements of total body calcium by prompt-gamma neutron activation analysis using a 252Cf source. *Biological Trace Element Research* 26-27:429–437.

129. Fletcher JP, Allen BJ, Blagojevic N. 1990. Changes in body protein composition following aortic reconstruction. *Australian and New Zealand Journal of Surgery* 60:209–211.

130. Pollock CA, Allen BJ, Warden RA, Caterson RJ, Blagojevic N, Cocksedge B, Mahoney JF, Waugh DA, Ibels LS. 1990. Total body nitrogen by neutron activation in maintenance dialysis. *American Journal of Kidney Diseases* 16:38–45.

131. Lukaski HC, Mendez J. 1980. Relationship between fat free weight and urinary 3-methylhistidine excretion in man. *Metabolism* 29:758–761.

132. Lukaski HC, Mendez J, Buskirk ER, Cohn SH. 1981. Relationship between endogenous 3-methylhistidine excretion and body composition. *American Journal of Physiology* 240:E302–307.

133. Segal KR, Gutin B, Presta E, Wang J, VanItallie TB. 1985. Estimation of human body composition by electrical impedance methods: A comparative study. *Journal of Applied Physiology* 58:1565–1571.

134. Lukaski HC, Bolonchuk WW, Hall CB, Siders WA. 1986. Validation of tetrapolar bioelectrical impedance method to assess human body composition. *Journal of Applied Physiology* 60:1327–1332.

135. Brodie DA. 1988. Techniques of measurement of body composition. Part II. *Sports Medicine* 5:74–98.

136. Conway JM, Norris KH. 1987. Noninvasive body composition in humans by near infrared interactance. In Ellis KJ, Yasumura S, Morgan WD, eds. *In vivo body composition studies*. London, England: Institute of Physical Sciences in Medicine.

137. Conway JM, Norris KH, Bodwell CE. 1984. A new approach for the estimation of body composition: Infrared interactance. *American Journal of Clinical Nutrition* 40:1123–1130.

138. Mclean KP, Skinner JS. 1992. Validity of Futrex-5000 for body composition determination. *Medicine and Science in Sports and Exercise* 24:253–258.

139. Williams DP, Going SB, Milliken LA, Hall MC, Lohman TG. 1995. Practical techniques for assessing body composition in middle-aged and older adults. *Medicine and Science in Sports and Exercise* 27:776–783.

140. Thomas DW, Ryde SJ, Ali PA, Birks JL, Evans CJ, Saunders NH, et al. 1997. The performance of an infra-red interactance instrument for assessing total body fat. *Physiological Measurement* 18:305–315.

141. Brooke-Wavell K, Jones PR, Norgan NG, Hardman AE. 1995. Evaluation of near infra-red interactance for assessment of subcutaneous and total body fat. *European Journal of Clinical Nutrition* 49:57–65.

142. Wilmore KM, McBride PJ, Wilmore JH. 1994. Comparison of bioelectrical impedance and near-infrared interactance for body composition assessment in a population of self-perceived overweight adults. *International Journal of Obesity* 18:375–381.

143. Bushong SC. 1993. *Radiologic science for technologists: Physics, biology, and protection,* 5th ed. St. Louis, MO: Mosby.

144. Borkan GA, Hults DE, Cardarelli JC, Burrows BA. 1982. Comparison of ultrasound and skinfold measurements in assessment of subcutaneous and total fatness. *American Journal of Physical Anthropology* 58:307–313.

145. Fanelli MT, Kuczmarski RJ. 1984. Ultrasound as an approach to assessing body composition. *American Journal of Clinical Nutrition* 39:703–709.

146. Chiba T, Lloyd DA, Bowen A, Condon-Meyers A. 1989. Ultrasonography as a method of nutritional assessment. *Journal of Parenteral and Enteral Nutrition* 13:529–534.

147. Booth RAD, Goddard A, Paton A. 1966. Measurement of fat thickness in man: A comparison of ultrasound, Harpenden calipers and electrical conductivity. *British Journal of Nutrition* 20:719–725.

148. Weits T, van der Beek EJ, Wedel M, Hubben MW, Koppeschaar HP. 1989. Fat patterning during weight reduction: A multimodal investigation. *Netherlands Journal of Medicine* 35:174–184.

149. Seidell JC, Bakker CJG, van der Kooy K. 1990. Imaging techniques for measuring adipose-tissue distribution—A comparison between computed tomography and 1.5-T magnetic resonance. *American Journal of Clinical Nutrition* 51:953–957.

150. Rogalla P, Meiri N, Hoksch B, Boeing H, Hamm B. 1998. Low-dose spiral computed tomography for measuring abdominal fat volume and distribution in a clinical setting. *European Journal of Clinical Nutrition* 52:597–602.

151. Rössner S, Bo WJ, Hiltbrandt E, Hinson W, Karstaedt N, Santago P, Sobol WT, Crouse JR. 1990. Adipose tissue determinations in cadavers—A comparison between cross-sectional planimetry and computed tomography. *International Journal of Obesity* 14:893–902.

152. Weingand KW, Hartke GT, Noordsy TW, Ledeboer DA. 1988. A minipig model of body adipose tissue distribution. *International Journal of Obesity* 13:347–355.

153. Ferland M, Despres JP, Tremblay A, Pinault S, Nadeau A, Moorjani S, Lupien PJ, Theriault G, Bouchard C. 1989. Assessment of adipose tissue distribution by computed axial tomography in obese women: Association with body density and anthropometric measurements. *British Journal of Nutrition* 61:139–148.

154. Goodpaster BH, Thaete FL, Kelley DE. 2000. Composition of skeletal muscle evaluated with computed tomography. *Annals of the New York Academy of Sciences* 904:18–24.

155. Starck G, Lonn L, Cederblad A, Alpsten M, Sjostrom L, Ekholm S. 1998. Dose reduction for body composition measurements with CT. *Applied Radiation and Isotopes* 49:561–563.

156. Ross R, Goodpaster B, Kelley D, Boada F. 2000. Magnetic resonance imaging in human body composition research. *Annals of the New York Academy of Sciences* 904:12–17.

157. Abate N, Burns D, Peshock RM, Garg A, Grundy SM. 1994. Estimation of adipose tissue mass by magnetic resonance imaging: Validation against dissection in human cadavers. *Journal of Lipid Research* 35:1490–1496.

158. Mitsiopoulos N, Baumgartner RN, Heymsfield SB, Lyons W, Gallagher D, Ross R. 1998. Cadaver validation of skeletal muscle measurement by magnetic resonance imaging and computerized tomography. *Journal of Applied Physiology* 85:115–122.

159. Roubenoff R, Kehayias JJ, Dawson-Hughes B, Heymsfield SB. 1993. Use of dual-energy x-ray absorptiometry in body composition studies: Not yet a "gold standard." *American Journal of Clinical Nutrition* 58:589–591.

160. Going SB, Massett MP, Hall MC, Bare LA, Root PA, Williams DP, Lohman TG. 1993. Detection of small changes in body composition by dual-energy x-ray absorptiometry. *American Journal of Clinical Nutrition* 57:845–850.

161. Wellens R, Cameron W, Guo S, Roche AF, Reo NV, Siervogel RM. 1994. Body composition in white adults by dual-energy x-ray absorptiometry, densitometry, and total body water. *American Journal of Clinical Nutrition* 59:547–555.

ASSESSMENT ACTIVITY 6.1

Assessment and Classification of Body Weight

Successful treatment of overweight begins with the assessment and classification of body weight. This assessment activity explains how to assess and classify body weight, waist circumference, and risk status using the approaches recommended by the U.S. National Institutes of Health in its publication *The Practical Guide; Identification, Evaluation, and Treatment of Overweight and Obesity in Adults.*[73] Although several accurate methods exist for measuring body fat, most of these methods are not readily available in the clinical setting. Body mass index (BMI) is recommended as the most practical approach for assessing body weight in the clinical setting and can be used as a surrogate method for assessing body fat content. Table 6.7 gave classifications of overweight and obesity, based on BMI. It should be noted that BMI overestimates body fat in very muscular persons and in

patients with edema. It can underestimate body fat in persons who have lost muscle mass (such as the elderly). Waist circumference is recommended as the most practical tool for assessing a person's abdominal fat content. The cutpoints for high-risk waist circumference were given in Table 6.8. BMI and waist circumference also can be used to monitor response to weight management treatment in persons whose BMI is < 35 kg/m^2.

Begin this assessment activity by accurately measuring your stature, body weight, and waist circumference and then calculating your body mass index (BMI), following the instructions in this chapter. Classify your BMI and waist circumference (high-risk or low-risk) using Tables 6.7 and 6.8 and Figure 6.42; if applicable, classify your disease risk ("increased," "high," "very high," or "extremely high") using Table 6.7. Record your results in the following spaces:

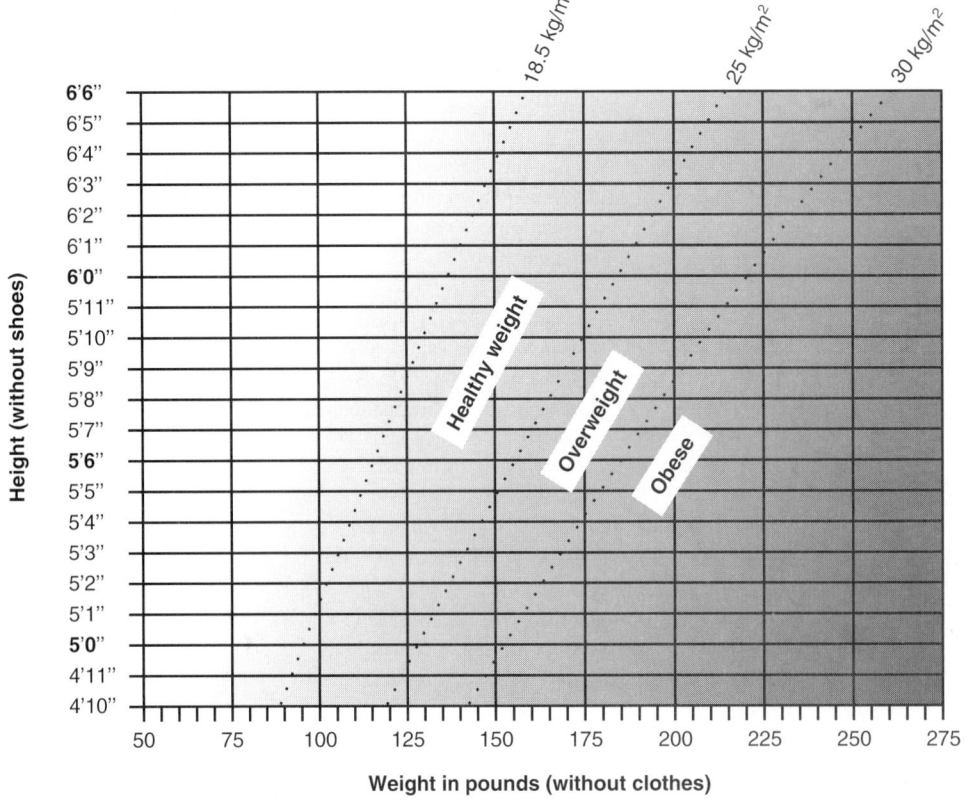

Figure 6.42

Using body mass index (BMI), body weight can be grouped into three categories. Healthy weight is defined as a BMI of 18.5 kg/m^2 up to 25 kg/m^2, overweight is a BMI of 25 kg/m^2 up to 30 kg/m^2, and obese is a BMI of 30 kg/m^2 or greater.

Source: Adapted from U.S. Department of Agriculture/U.S. Department of Health and Human Services. 2000. *Nutrition and Your Health: Dietary Guidelines for Americans,* 5th ed. Hyattsville, MD: U.S. Department of Agriculture, Center for Nutrition Policy and Promotion.

Body weight:

_____ lb _____ kg (pounds ÷ 2.2 = kg)

Body stature:

_____ in. _____ m (inches × 0.0254 = m)

Waist circumference:

_____ in. _____ cm (inches × 2.54 = cm)

Body mass index:

_____ kg/m²

BMI classification:

_____

Waist circumference classification:

_____

Disease risk classification:

_____

Elevated BMI, high-risk waist circumference, or both suggest the need for weight loss but do not indicate the required intensity of intervention. Patients who have certain obesity-related diseases (*comorbidities*) or who have cardiovascular disease risk factors (Table 6.13) are at a higher risk for mortality than those who do not have these diseases or risk factors. Consequently, patients need to be screened for these diseases and risk factors and, when present, placed on a program of intense risk-factor modification and weight management intervention.

TABLE 6.13	Diseases and Risk Factors That Place Patients at Increased Risk for Mortality

Diseases Placing Patients at Very High Risk for Mortality

- Established coronary heart disease
- Atherosclerotic diseases other than coronary heart disease (e.g., peripheral arterial disease, abdominal aortic aneurysm, symptomatic carotid artery disease)
- Type 2 diabetes (fasting plasma glucose ≥ 126 mg/dL or 2-hour postprandial plasma glucose ≥ 200 mg/dL)
- Sleep apnea

Cardiovascular Disease Risk Factors

- Cigarette smoking
- Hypertension (systolic blood pressure ≥ 140 mm Hg or diastolic blood pressure ≥ 90 mm Hg) or current use of antihypertensive medication
- High-risk low-density lipoprotein cholesterol (≥ 160 mg/dL) or borderline high-risk (130 to 159 mg/dL), along with two or more other risk factors
- Low high-density lipoprotein cholesterol (< 35 mg/dL)
- Impaired fasting glucose (between 110 and 125 mg/dL)
- Family history of premature coronary heart disease
- Age (if male, ≥ 45 years; if female, ≥ 55 years or postmenopausal)
- Physical inactivity

ASSESSMENT ACTIVITY 6.2

Body Composition Evaluation Using Skinfold Measurements

This assessment activity gives you an opportunity to use skinfold measurements to estimate percent body fat and to evaluate body composition.

Step 1

Photocopy the "Skinfold Measurements" form in Figure 6.35. Using the information described in this chapter, have your instructor or a classmate measure the thickness of three of your skinfolds (chest, abdomen, and thigh for men; triceps, suprailiac, and thigh for women), and record the values on the "Skinfold Measurements" form.

Step 2

Total the values of the three skinfold measurements and enter this number on the appropriate line in the "Skinfold Measurements" form.

Step 3

Estimate percent body fat using the nomogram in Figure 6.34. Enter this percentage on the appropriate line in the "Skinfold Measurements" form. Using Table 6.12, classify your percent body fat and write that classification on the appropriate line in the "Skinfold Measurements" form.

Step 4

Calculate your fat weight, lean body weight, and desired body weight, as indicated in the "Skinfold Measurements" form and the text.

ASSESSMENT OF THE HOSPITALIZED PATIENT

INTRODUCTION

In today's cost-conscious health care environment, the desire to control health care costs supports the assessment of the nutritional status of hospitalized patients. Recent estimates of the prevalence of protein-energy malnutrition (PEM) among hospitalized patients typically range from 20% to 50%.[1] These estimates vary, depending on the measures used to define PEM and the population studied (elderly and more acutely ill patients are more likely to have PEM than younger and less acutely ill patients). Compared with their well-nourished counterparts, patients with PEM have a greater risk of postoperative infection, with an increased length of hospital stay, a higher risk for mortality, and a greater likelihood of readmission to the hospital following discharge.[1] Appropriate nutritional support of these patients can result in faster recovery and shorter hospital stays, which translate into reduced health care expenditures. Another reason that nutritional assessment of hospitalized patients is important is our increasing capability to provide nutritional support to these patients through enteral and parenteral routes.

This chapter discusses approaches to assessing the nutritional status of hospitalized patients. It brings together many of the various assessment techniques discussed in previous chapters (e.g., anthropometric and dietary) and shows how they are used to evaluate nutritional status in hospitalized patients. It also builds on Chapter 6 by introducing several new anthropometric techniques that are unique to the acute-care setting.

ASSESSING NUTRITIONAL STATUS

Assessing the nutritional status of the hospitalized patient involves four goals.[2,3] First, patients who are nutritionally at risk need to be identified through a process known as *nutritional screening.* Once a patient is shown to be at nutritional risk, a more in-depth nutritional assessment should be done to determine the severity and causes of the patient's nutritional impairment. Although both undernutrition and overnutrition can negatively affect health, most frequently it is undernutrition (particularly, protein-energy malnutrition) that is of greatest concern in hospitalized patients. The risk of the patient's undernutrition worsening his or her condition, causing a related disease, or possibly resulting in death should then be ascertained. Finally, the patient should be monitored to ensure an appropriate response to nutritional support.

Nutritional Screening

Nutritional screening "is the process of identifying characteristics known to be associated with nutrition problems. Its purpose is to pinpoint individuals who are malnourished or at nutritional risk."[4] The standards for nutrition care established by the Joint Commission on the Accreditation of Health Care Organizations (JCAHO) do not require that nutritional screening be done within a specific time following admission but, rather, indicate

that it be carried out "in a timely, effective, and efficient manner." Considering the emphasis given to short hospitalizations in order to contain health care costs, it is reasonable to expect that a nutritional screen be done on all patients within the first 24 to 48 hours following admission, although, the earlier the screen is performed and acted on, the sooner the patient will, if necessary, receive and benefit from nutritional support. Nutritional screening can be done by any member of the health care team. Because it does not require the high degree of nutrition knowledge and expertise of a registered dietitian, it is best done by a dietetic technician. Box 7.1 outlines the characteristics of the nutritional screening process.[4] The Nutrition Screening Initiative and its outstanding screening forms are discussed in the Nutrition Screening Initiative section.

Screening can be greatly facilitated by using a checklist or form on which pertinent patient information can be entered. Once completed, this form can be placed in the patient's medical record (often referred to as the patient's "chart") for other members of the health care team to refer to. An example of a nutritional screening form is shown in Figure 7.1.[5] Information required to complete the form includes anthropometric, biochemical, clinical, and dietary data. Much of this information can be obtained from the patient's medical record. To use the screening form in Figure 7.1, place a check in every box that applies to the patient and, when appropriate, enter pertinent patient data on the line next to certain items.

Suppose your patient's serum albumin were 2.5 mg/dL. Check the box following number 1 to indicate that the serum albumin level is $\leq$ 2.9 mg/dL. Then enter the patient's serum albumin level on the line following that item. Enter the patient's anthropometric data next (Ht = height; Admit Wt = body weight on admission; DBW = desirable body weight). A patient's usual weight is his or her stable weight in the past 6 to 12 months. It can be determined by asking the patient or a significant other or looking in the nurses' notes or in the medical

---

 Box 7.1   **Characteristics of the Nutritional Screening Process**

- It can be completed in any setting, either through personal contact with the patient or by collecting data from the patient's chart.
- It facilitates completion of early intervention.
- It includes the collection of relevant data on risk factors and the interpretation of data for intervention and treatment.

- It determines the need for a more in-depth nutritional assessment.
- It is cost-effective.

Adapted from Posthauer ME, Dorse B, Foiles RA, et al. 1994. ADA's definitions for nutrition screening and nutrition assessment. *Journal of the American Dietetic Association* 94:838–839.

Nutritional Screening Form

Laboratory Values

1. ☐ Albumin ≤ 2.9 mg/dl _____   6. ☐ Albumin < 3.5 mg/dl _____

Anthropometrics

Ht _____   Admit Wt _____   Usual Wt _____   DBW _____

BMI _____   % DBW _____   % Wt Lost _____

2. ☐ <80% DBW   7. ☐ 80%-90% of Usual Wt

3. ☐ >10% Wt Lost   8. ☐ 5%-10% Wt Lost

Feeding

4. ☐ TPN/PPN or Tube Feeding   9. ☐ Loss of appetite (<1/2 trays)

                                            10. ☐ Chewing or swallowing difficulty

                                            11. ☐ >3 days of NPO, dextrose, and/or clear liquids only

Nutrition-Related Problems/Diagnoses

5. ☐ Malnutrition   ☐ Sepsis   12. ☐ Nutrition-related diagnosis/problems _____

☐ Decubitus ulcers   ☐ AIDS   13. ☐ Serum cholesterol ≥ 200 mg/dL

☐ Dysphagia/renal/hepatic diet restrictions 14. ☐ Random glucose ≥ 200 mg/dL

                                            15. ☐ BMI ≥ 27 kg/m^2 women; ≥ 28 kg/m^2 men

☐ No further nutrition evaluation recommended at this time

☐ Patient may benefit from further nutritional evaluation and will be seen by a Registered Dietitian or Dietetic Technician

☐ Care Level I   ☐ Care Level II   ☐ Care Level III

☐ Diet counseling/education/classes recommended (1 risk in criteria 13-15), which requires a physician order

Patient Information

Current diet order: _____

Screened by: _____

Date: _____

Figure 7.1 **An example of a form that can be used to screen patients for nutritional risk.**

Source: Adapted from Hedberg AM, Garcia N, Trejus IJ, Weinmann-Winkler S, Gabriel ML, Lutz AL. 1988. Nutritional risk screening: Development of a standardized protocol using dietetic technicians. *Journal of the American Dietetic Association* 88:1553–1556.

records of previous hospitalizations, if these are available. Desirable (or reference) body weight can be obtained from a height-weight chart. The particular height-weight chart used varies among health care facilities. Calculate the percent of desirable weight (or relative weight) and percent of weight lost (these are discussed in the section on Physical Examination. Enter the values in the appropriate lines and place checks in the appropriate boxes. Check on the form whether the patient is on total parenteral nutrition (TPN) or peripheral parenteral nutrition (PPN), is receiving tube feedings, has experienced loss of appetite (eating less than one-half of the food on meal trays), has been NPO ("non per os," meaning "nothing by mouth"), or has received only intravenous fluids (e.g., 5% dextrose in water) or clear liquids for more than 3 days. Certain diagnoses, such as decubitus ulcer, sepsis,

AIDS, diet restrictions because of dysphagia, renal or hepatic disease, and, of course, a diagnosis of malnutrition, place a patient at nutritional risk. Nutritional risk is increased when serum cholesterol, random (or nonfasting) serum glucose, and body mass index are above certain cutpoints. Nutritional risk can also be elevated in certain nutrition-related diagnoses and problems, as listed in Box 7.2

A patient receiving one check for items 6 through 12 (found along the right side of the form) falls in Care Level I. Follow-up for these patients can be done by a registered dietitian or a dietetic technician. A patient having one or more checks for items 1 through 5 (found on the left side of the form) or two or more checks for items 6 through 12 falls within Care Level II and should receive further evaluation by a registered dietitian. Patients receiving enteral or parenteral nutritional support are placed in Care Level III and are further evaluated by a registered dietitian. A patient not meeting these criteria requires no further nutritional evaluation unless a change in his or her condition warrants it. If a patient receives a check for items 13 through 15, he or she would likely benefit from diet counseling or education. A check is placed in the appropriate box (diet counseling/education/classes and so on) to signal the patient's physician, who can then order any necessary intervention.

Nutritional Assessment

Once nutritional screening has identified a patient to be at nutritional risk, a nutritional assessment should be done to determine the severity and causes of the patient's nutritional impairment, to evaluate whether the nutritional impairment is a factor contributing to the worsening of the patient's medical condition, and to monitor the patient's response to nutritional support. If the nutritional impairment is identified and documented as a factor appreciably worsening the patient's health (what is called a comorbidity and complicating condition), it could increase the reimbursement the health care facility receives for that patient's care.[4,6,7] This is an important consideration for dietitians who want to document the revenue-generating ability and cost-effectiveness of nutrition services rather than being a nonreimbursable service and easy target of draconian budget cuts.

Because no single measurement or test by itself is capable of providing information sufficient to evaluate a patient's nutritional status, a variety of available measurements and tests must be used. Much of the basic information needed to assess a patient's nutritional status is fairly easy to obtain by simply asking the patient (or a close friend or relative of the patient) or by using relatively inexpensive tests or measurements. It is important to note that some of this information is routinely collected by the medical and nursing staff and is recorded in the patient's medical record. This basic information includes the patient's stature, usual and present weight, and past and current dietary practices; any significant changes in eating habits; and the presence of any nutrition-related problems. The medical record can provide much relevant information from the physician's history and physical exam, relevant information about previous hospitalizations, reports from consulting physicians, and results of various X-ray, imaging, and diagnostic tests, including routine laboratory tests, such as a complete blood count and chemistry profile (see Chapter 9 for additional information about laboratory tests). Important information can be obtained from the notes recorded by nurses and allied health professionals. In many instances, this information is sufficient to assess the nutritional status of less critically ill patients or those with more obvious nutritional deficits.

Box 7.2 Diagnoses and Problems That Can Increase Risk of Malnutrition

Trauma: fracture, burn, closed head injury, gunshot wound, spinal cord injury, motor vehicle accident

Dysphagia

Bowel resection

Short bowel syndrome

Small bowel obstruction

Hypoglycemia

Failure to thrive

Congenital heart disease

Chronic obstructive pulmonary disease

Anorexia

Cancer

Diarrhea

Vomiting

Anemia

Stroke or hemiparesis

Gastrointestinal bleeding

Crohn's disease

Dumping syndrome

Decubitus ulcers

Organ transplant

Diabetes mellitus

Coronary artery disease

Pancreatitis

For more critically ill patients or those with less obvious nutritional deficits, more detailed anthropometric, laboratory, and dietary information may need to be collected. Included among anthropometric measures are skinfold measurements (usually only triceps and subscapular), and measurements of midarm and midcalf circumferences. Additional biochemical measurements include 24-hour urinary creatinine (for calculating the creatinine-height index), 24-hour urine urea nitrogen (for estimating nitrogen balance), serum proteins (which are more sensitive indicators of protein nurture and repletion than serum albumin), and tests of delayed cutaneous hypersensitivity. Indirect calorimetry may be used to measure energy expenditure and energy needs. Dietary assessment may include calorie counts, more extensive patient interviewing, and questioning of surrogates having knowledge of the patient's dietary intake.

In addition, more sophisticated and specialized nutritional assessment techniques are available. These include neutron activation analysis, isotope dilution, whole-body potassium measurement, computed tomography, and magnetic resonance imaging to determine body composition and response to nutritional therapy. Because of high cost, restricted availability, and other drawbacks, these methods are infrequently used in assessing the critically ill. Instead, their use is limited to research applications.

History

Obtaining a patient's history is the first step in clinical assessment of nutritional status.[8] Data on the patient's history can be obtained from the medical record and from interviews with the patient or others knowledgeable about the patient's habits. Parts of the medical record that are particularly helpful include the medical history; entries made by physicians, nurses, social workers, and other members of the health care team; and medical records from previous admissions.[9] Other essential components of a patient's history include pertinent facts about past and current health, use of medications, and personal and household information. Components of the medical history and psychosocial factors to consider in nutritional assessment are discussed in Chapter 10.

Dietary Information

Dietary information includes the patient's food preferences, allergies and intolerances, and usual eating pattern (timing and location of meals and snacks). Data should also be collected about the amount of money available for purchasing food, ability to obtain and prepare food, eligibility for and access to food assistance programs, and use of vitamin, mineral, and other supplements (if not obtained in the history).

A 24-hour recall or simple food frequency questionnaire can provide important data on usual eating patterns and can help generate additional questions on dietary intake. Patients sent home to return for later follow-up visits can be asked to complete a food frequency questionnaire or a multiple-day (usually a 3-day) diet record. Hospitalized patients' food intake can be evaluated by a calorie count, in which the caloric and nutrient value of foods eaten from the patient's tray for 1 or more days are calculated and recorded.

Physical Examination

Two of the most important measurements to obtain are body weight and stature (or length, in the case of infants and young children unable to stand without assistance). Weight is a gross measure of the body's fluid and tissue mass, and serial weighings indicate changes in those body constituents. Marked weight loss is generally viewed as a manifestation of serious disease.[1] Weight is an important variable in equations predicting energy expenditure and in Quetelet's index.[10] Stature is necessary for determining weight for stature and for calculating Quetelet's index, the creatinine height index, body surface area, and energy expenditure.[11]

Body weight gain can indicate repletion of lean and fat tissues, development of obesity, or abnormal accumulation of body fluids, as in edema, ascites, pleural effusion, or fluid overload in a patient receiving excessive intravenous fluid. Loss of body weight can represent the presence, severity, or progress of a disease or nutritional impairment. It can also be seen in patients receiving diuretics. Depletion of lean body mass can be masked by the simultaneous retention of fluid. For these reasons, body weight measurements need to be carefully scrutinized.

One way to evaluate body weight is to compare it to some reference, or "desirable," weight. This can be expressed as a percent of desirable body weight. This is the same as relative weight, which was discussed in Chapter 6. The following equation is used for calculating percent of desirable weight (relative weight):

$$\text{Percent desirable body weight} = \frac{\text{Current weight}}{\text{"Desirable," or reference, weight}} \times 100$$

The value for reference weight depends on what a particular health care facility has chosen for its standard. Usually, this is a height-weight table similar to the ones shown in Chapter 6. If the patient's percent of desirable body weight (%DBW) is 80%, he or she is 20% below desirable body weight. Many authors regard a %DBW of < 80% as substandard.[8]

Recent changes in body weight are a better indicator of nutritional status than are static weight measurements.[1] One way to assess change in body weight is to calculate percent of usual weight. This can be done using the following equation:

$$\% \text{ usual weight} = \frac{\text{Current or admit weight}}{\text{Usual weight}} \times 100$$

Information about usual weight can be obtained from the patient, a person close to the patient, nurses' notes, or medical records of previous admissions. An alternate approach to assessing recent changes in body weight is to calculate percent of weight change using the following equation:

$$\frac{\% \text{ weight}}{\text{change}} = \frac{\text{Usual weight} - \text{Current weight}}{\text{Usual weight}} \times 100$$

A weight loss $< 5\%$ is considered small. A 5% to 10% weight loss is considered potentially significant. A weight loss $> 10\%$ is considered definitely significant.[1,12] Rapid changes in body weight should be interpreted with caution. A change in body weight > 1 lb/d (0.5 kg/d) indicates fluid shifts and not a true change in body weight.

The rate of weight loss is as important to consider as the amount lost. A 12% weight loss during the past 6 months is more significant than a similar weight loss during the past 12 months. The pattern of weight loss is also important to consider. Imagine two patients, Patient A and Patient B. Patient A lost 12% of her usual weight over a period 6 months to 1 month prior to admission but regained half that weight in the month just before admission and is continuing to regain. Consequently, she has a net loss of 6% of her body weight. Patient B lost 6% of his usual weight during the 6 months prior to admission and is continuing to lose weight. Some health care professionals would consider the nutritional status of Patient A to be better than that of Patient B.[12]

Because important clinical decisions are based on the patient's weight and stature, it is important to obtain measurements that are as accurate and precise as possible. This can be done by following the techniques outlined in Chapter 6. Although the patient should be asked about his or her weight history, actual weight and stature should be measured or estimated using the appropriate equation, rather than relying on the patient's stated weight and stature. If stated weight and stature are recorded in the patient's chart, they should be labeled as such.

Weighing can be complicated by the patient's condition and the presence of casts, traction devices, and life-support equipment. Nonambulatory patients, for example, can be weighed using bed or wheelchair scales (see Chapter 6), or weight can be estimated from various anthropometric measures, including subscapular skinfold, calf circumference, knee height, and midarm circumference. (explained later in this chapter).[13] When patients cannot stand for stature measurements or when stature is likely to be inaccurate because of skeletal deformity, it can be estimated from knee height, as explained in the section "Knee Height."[11,13] As discussed in Chapter 6, body weight for stature can be compared with height-weight charts, and relative weight and Quetelet's index can be calculated and compared with various standards.

Another valuable indicator of nutritional status is arm muscle area. Arm muscle area is calculated from measures of the triceps skinfold and the midarm circumference.[14] Arm muscle area has been shown to be a useful index of total body muscle in young children[8] and in adults.[14]

Besides weight, stature, and other anthropometric measures, the physical examination involves numerous measurements and observations, including measurement of heart and respiratory rate and body temperature; observation of heart, respiratory, and bowel sounds; examination of the head, neck, thorax, abdomen, extremities, and integument (skin, hair, and nails); and examination of the nervous and circulatory systems. This information is gathered during the physical examination and initial work-up on admission and is available in the patient's chart.

Knee Height

Knee height is measured with the subject in the supine position (lying facing up), using one of several commercially available large, broadblade sliding calipers (see Appendix M for sources).[11,13,15,16]

Measurements are made on the *left leg* because this side was used by researchers in developing the equations given in Table 7.1.[11] The knee and ankle of the left leg are

TABLE 7.1	Equations for Estimating Stature from Knee Height for Various Groups	
Age[*]	**Equation**[†]	**Error**[‡]
Black Females		
> 60	$S = 58.72 + (1.96 \text{ KH})$	8.26 cm
19–60	$S = 68.10 + (1.86 \text{ KH}) - (0.06 \text{ A})$	7.60 cm
6–18	$S = 46.59 + (2.02 \text{ KH})$	8.78 cm
White Females		
> 60	$S = 75.00 + (1.91 \text{ KH}) - (0.17 \text{ A})$	8.82 cm
19–60	$S = 70.25 + (1.87 \text{ KH}) - (0.06 \text{ A})$	7.20 cm
6–18	$S = 43.21 + (2.14 \text{ KH})$	7.80 cm
Black Males		
> 60	$S = 95.79 + (1.37 \text{ KH})$	8.44 cm
19–60	$S = 73.42 + (1.79 \text{ KH})$	7.20 cm
6–18	$S = 39.60 + (2.18 \text{ KH})$	9.16 cm
White Males		
> 60	$S = 59.01 + (2.08 \text{ KH})$	7.84 cm
19–60	$S = 71.85 + (1.88 \text{ KH})$	7.94 cm
6–18	$S = 40.54 + (2.22 \text{ KH})$	8.42 cm

Adapted from Chumlea WC, Guo SS, Steinbaugh ML. 1994. Prediction of stature from knee height for black and white adults and children with application to mobility-impaired or handicapped persons. *Journal of the American Dietetic Association* 94:1385–1388.

[*]Age in years rounded to the nearest year

[†]S = stature; KH = knee height; A = age in years.

[‡]Estimated stature will be within this value for 95% of persons within each age, sex, race group.

Figure 7.2
When knee height is being measured, the knee and ankle
of the left leg should be bent at 90-degree angles.

Figure 7.4
The fixed blade of the caliper is placed under the heel, and
the moveable shaft is positioned parallel to the fibula, over
the lateral malleolus, and just behind the head of the fibula.

positioned at a 90-degree angle, as shown in Figure 7.2.
These angles should be verified by a right triangle,
square, or other appropriate device. The fixed blade of
the caliper is placed under the heel of the left foot, and
the moveable blade is placed on the anterior surface
of the left thigh. The caliper shaft is positioned parallel to
the fibula (the outside bone of the lower leg), over the lateral malleolus (the most prominent bony projection on
the outer side of the left ankle), and just posterior to the
head of the fibula (Figure 7.3 and Figure 7.4). Pressure is
applied to the two blades to compress the soft tissues.[13,15,16] The measurement is recorded to the nearest
0.1 cm. Two measurements made in quick succession
should agree to within 0.5 cm.

Estimating Stature

For most patients, stature can be easily obtained. However, for persons who are nonambulatory or who have contractures, severe arthritis, paralysis, amputations, or other
conditions limiting their ability to stand erectly, stature
may have to be estimated. The most common approach is
to estimate stature from knee height because knee height
has been shown to correlate highly with stature.[11,17,18] An
alternate approach is estimating stature from either
upper-arm or lower-arm length as described by Jarzem.[19]

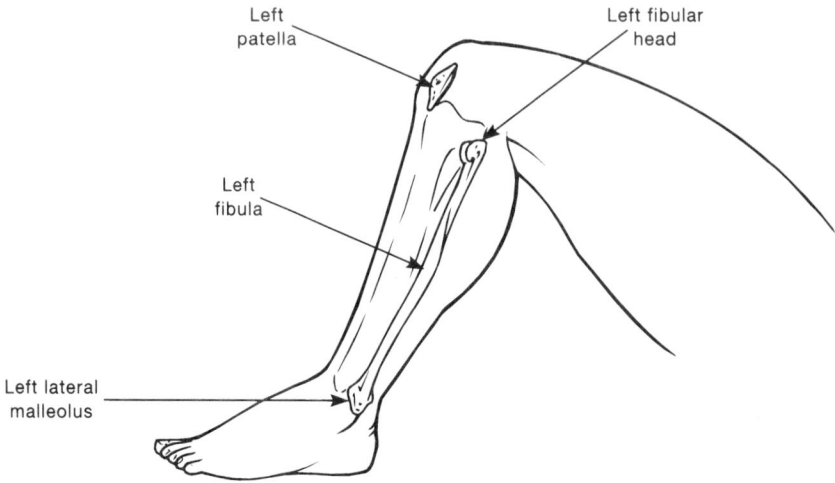

Left
patella

Left fibular
head

Left
fibula

Left lateral
malleolus

Figure 7.3 Anatomical landmarks for proper placement of the knee height caliper.

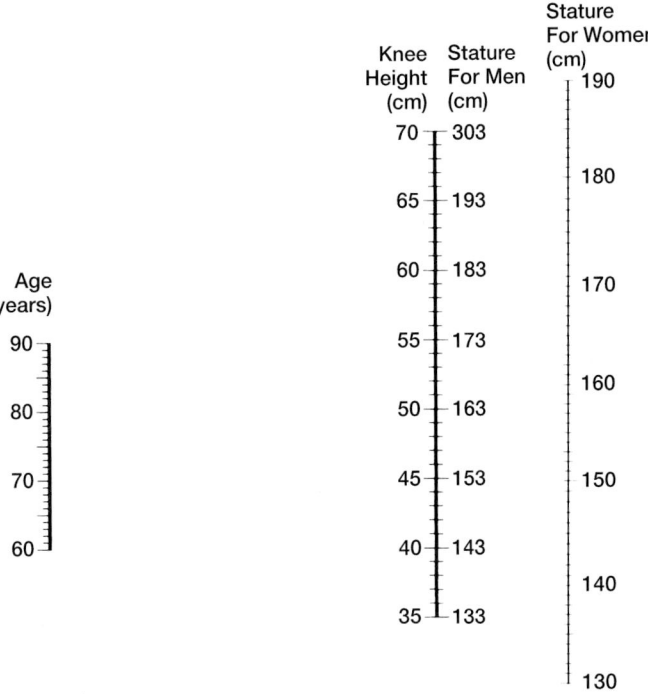

Figure 7.5 **Nomogram for estimating stature from knee height in persons ages 60 to 90 years.**

To use, locate the patient's age and knee height on the appropriate columns and connect these points with a straightedge. The estimated stature can be read where the straightedge crosses the appropriate sex-specific column.

Source: Adapted with permission of Ross Laboratories, Columbus, OH 43216, from Chumlea WC, Roche AF, Mukherjee D. 1987. *Nutritional assessment of the elderly through anthropometry.* Columbus, OH: Ross Laboratories.

The sex-, age-, and race-specific equations in Table 7.1 can be used for estimating stature in children, adults, and older persons. Data from national surveys of healthy, able-bodied persons were used to develop these equations, and they reflect normal patterns of growth and development. The nomogram in Figure 7.5 can be used for estimating stature from age and knee height in persons 60 to 90 years old.

An alternative approach to measuring the stature of a bedridden patient who has no skeletal abnormalities or contractures is to align his or her body so that the lower extremities, trunk, shoulders, and head are in a straight line and mark on the bedsheet the position of the base of the heels and top of the crown, as shown in Figure 7.6.

The distance between these two lines can then be measured using a suitable tape measure.

When done carefully, this approach is somewhat more accurate than estimates derived from knee height in patients without skeletal abnormalities or contractures. However, it is always preferable to obtain standing measurements of stature when patients are able to stand and when these measurements are not contraindicated by the patient's condition.

Midarm Circumference

Midarm circumference (MAC), also known as upper midarm circumference, can be used in equations for calculating arm muscle area and estimated body

Figure 7.6

An alternative approach to measuring recumbent length in the bedridden patient is simply to place a mark on the bed sheet at the top of the patient's head and at the bottom of the heel. With the patient out of bed or rolled to one side, measure the distance.

weight.[2,13,16] As an indicator of muscle and subcutaneous adipose tissue, it is an accepted measure of nutritional status. It and related upper-arm anthropometric measurements can be obtained quickly and noninvasively.[20] MAC is the circumference of the upper arm at the triceps skinfold site. In the ambulatory patient, the triceps skinfold site is measured and marked as described in Chapter 6. The arm is relaxed to the side with the palm of the hand facing the thigh. A nonstretchable measuring tape is placed around the arm, perpendicular to the long axis of the arm, and at the level of the triceps skinfold site (see Figure 7.7). The tape should be placed in contact with the arm but without compressing the soft tissues. The measurement should be recorded to the nearest 0.1 cm.[15]

In the nonambulatory patient, MAC is measured while the patient is in the supine position.[11,21] Either the right or left side can be used for this and subsequent recumbent measurements.[15] With the upper arm approximately parallel to the body, the forearm is placed palm down across the middle of the body with the elbow bent 90 degrees. Using a nonstretchable tape measure, the midpoint of the upper arm is located between the tip of the acromion process and the olecranon process and marked, as shown in Figure 7.8[13,21] (These are the same anatomical landmarks used for determining the triceps skinfold site described in Chapter 6.)

Once the midpoint of the upper arm is properly marked, the arm is returned to the patient's side with the palm facing upward. The arm is then raised slightly off the surface of the examination table by placing a folded pillow or towel under the patient's elbow. A nonstretchable tape measure is placed around the upper arm at the level of the marked midpoint and perpendicular to the long axis of the arm (Figure 7.9). The tape should come in contact with the skin of the arm but should not be pulled so tight that it indents or compresses the soft tissues. The measurement should be recorded to the nearest 0.1 cm.[13,21]

Figure 7.7
Midarm circumference is measured with the subject standing. The tape is placed around the arm, perpendicular to the long axis, and at the level of the triceps skinfold site.

Figure 7.8
When the subject cannot stand, midarm circumference is measured by first locating and marking the midpoint of the upper arm between the tip of the acromion process and the olecranon process.

Figure 7.9 Measurement of the midarm circumference of the recumbent subject.
A folded towel under the elbow raises the arm off the surface of the table. The tape is perpendicular to the long axis of the arm and touches the arm without compressing soft tissues.

Calf Circumference

Calf circumference is used in some equations for estimating body weight and is a measure of muscle and subcutaneous adipose tissue. In elderly men, it is significantly correlated with lean body mass.[22] Calf circumference can be measured with the subject standing, sitting, or lying in the supine position. If ambulatory, the subject can either sit on an examination table with the right or left leg hanging freely or stand with the feet about 20 cm (8 in.) apart, with the body weight equally distributed on both feet.[21] A nonstretchable measuring tape should be looped horizontally around the calf and moved up and down until the greatest calf circumference is found. The tape should be tightened around the calf so that it contacts the skin without indenting or compressing the soft tissues. The circumference should be recorded to the nearest 0.1 cm.[21]

If nonambulatory, the subject should be in the supine position with the knee bent at a 90-degree angle. The tape

Figure 7.10 Measurement of calf circumference of the recumbent subject.
The tape measure is kept in a plane perpendicular to the long axis of the lower leg.

measure should be looped around the calf in a plane perpendicular to the long axis of the lower leg (Figure 7.10) and moved up and down. When the greatest cirumference of the lower leg is found, the tape should be tightened around the calf so that it contacts the skin without indenting or compressing the soft tissues. The circumference should be recorded to the nearest 0.1 cm.[13,15]

Recumbent Skinfold Measurements

In the recumbent patient, the triceps and subscapular skinfolds can be measured with the patient lying on the right or left side.[15] Apart from differences in body positioning, the techniques for measuring skinfolds in the recumbent patient are essentially the same as those described in Chapter 6.

The subject is positioned as shown in Figure 7.11. The right arm is in front of the body at a 45-degree angle, the trunk is in a straight line, the shoulders are perpendicular to the spine and examination table, and the arm to be measured is lying on the trunk with the palm down. The legs are slightly flexed at the hips and knees.[13,15]

As in the standing ambulatory patient, the triceps skinfold is measured at the back of the upper arm at the level of the marked midpoint. With the thumb and index finger of the left hand, the measurer grasps a double fold of skin and adipose tissue about 1 cm (½ in.) above the marked midpoint of the upper arm. The long axes of the skinfold and arm must be parallel. Holding the skinfold, the measurer places the caliper tips on the skinfold and reads the dial after about 4 seconds (Figure 7.12). The measurer's eyes should be in line with the needle and dial of the caliper to avoid errors caused by parallax.[13,15]

For measuring the subscapular skinfold, the body is positioned as shown in Figure 7.11. The same site is used as when the subject is standing, and the skinfold is grasped and measured along the same axis (see Chapter 6). Because the subject is lying on the right side, however, the measurement technique is somewhat different. The subscapular skinfold site is just distal to the inferior angle of the left scapula. As shown in Figure 7.13, the measurer grasps the double layer of skin and adipose tissue

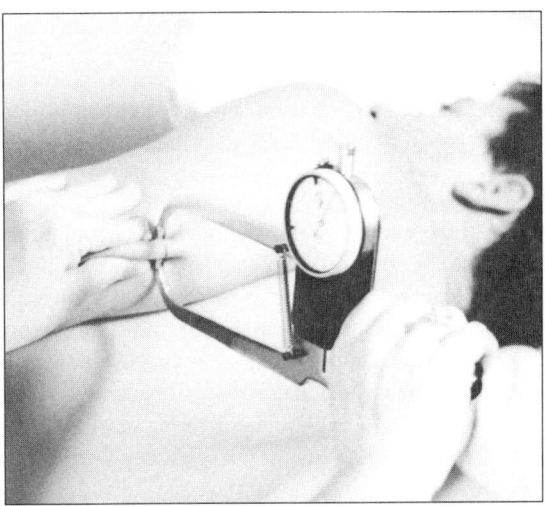

Figure 7.12 Measurement of triceps skinfold of the recumbent subject.

Figure 7.11 Body position for measurement of triceps and subscapular skinfolds of the recumbent subject.

Figure 7.13 Measurement of subscapular skinfold of the recumbent subject.

along the axis of the skinfold, so that the thumb and index finger of the left hand are about 1 cm (½ in.) from the actual measurement site. Note that the left hand is distal and lateral to the skinfold site. Holding the skinfold, the measurer places the caliper tips at the site and reads the dial after about 4 seconds. The measurer should look directly at the dial of the caliper to avoid errors caused by parallax.[13,15] A minimum of two measurements should be taken at each site. Successive measurements should be at least 15 seconds apart from each other to allow the skinfold site to return to normal. If consecutive measurements vary by more than 1 mm, additional measurements should be taken until the readings are consistent.

The sum of the triceps and subscapular skinfold thicknesses can be used as an indicator of the body's energy reserves. Appendix Q provides percentiles for the sum of triceps and subscapular skinfold thicknesses for males and females ages 1 to 74 years. Although researchers disagree about which standards are the most appropriate, the guidelines in Table 7.2 can be used for interpreting these age-, sex-, and race-specific percentile values.[1] The cutoff point for excess fat was chosen as greater than the 85th percentile because it has been observed that persons above this point are at significantly greater risk of hypertension and hypercholesterolemia than persons at or below the 85th percentile.[23]

Estimating Body Weight

Most patients can be weighed on scales, but sometimes it is difficult or impossible to obtain a patient's weight. This may be because of the patient's medical condition, equipment attached to the patient (for example, life support devices, traction equipment, casts, or braces), or lack of a suitable bed or wheelchair scale. Despite the critical importance of body weight in delivering nutritional therapy, it is estimated that about 22% of hospitalized adults receiving nutritional support have no record of body weight.[24]

TABLE 7.2	Guidelines for Interpreting the Age-, Sex-, and Race-Specific Percentile Values for the Sum of Triceps and Subscapular Skinfold Thicknesses for Males and Females Given in Appendix Q

Percentile	Category
≤ 5th	Lean
> 5th but ≤ 15th	Below average
> 15th but ≤ 75th	Average
> 75th but ≤ 85th	Above average
> 85th	Excess fat

From Frisancho AR. 1990. *Anthropometric standards for the assessment of growth and nutritional status.* Ann Arbor: University of Michigan Press.

When it is difficult or impossible to obtain a patient's body weight directly, it can be estimated from various anthropometric measures (that is, knee height, midarm circumference, calf circumference, and subscapular skinfold thickness) using the equations given in Tables 7.3 and 7.4. The decision of which equation to use will depend on the patient's age and the anthropometric measures that can be obtained or are available.

From Tables 7.3 and 7.4, it can be noted that a certain amount of error is inherent in the process of estimating body weight from anthropometric measures. This error can be minimized by using an equation requiring a larger number of variables (four as opposed to two) and by paying strict attention to measurement technique. Although estimates of body weight may be as much as 14 kg greater than or less than actual body weight, an estimate of body weight recorded on a patient's chart is better than no weight recorded. The use of estimated

TABLE 7.3	Equations for Estimating Body Weight in Persons 65 Years of Age and Older from Anthropometric Measures

	SEE[†]
Females[*]	
Weight = (MAC × 1.63) + (CC × 1.43) − 37.46	±4.96 kg
Weight = (MAC × 0.92) + (CC × 1.50) + (SSF × 0.42) − 26.19	±4.21 kg
Weight = (MAC × 0.98) + (CC × 1.27) + (SSF × 0.40) + (KH × 0.87) − 62.35	±3.80 kg
Males[*]	
Weight = (MAC × 2.31) + (CC × 1.50) − 50.10	±5.37 kg
Weight = (MAC × 1.92) + (CC × 1.44) + (SSF × 0.26) − 39.97	±5.34 kg
Weight = (MAC × 1.73) + (CC × 0.98) + (SSF × 0.37) + (KH × 1.16) − 81.69	±4.48 kg

From Chumlea WC, Guo S, Roche AF, Steinbaugh ML. 1988. Prediction of body weight for the nonambulatory elderly from anthropometry. *Journal of the American Dietetic Association* 88:564–568.

[*]Weight is in kg; MAC = midarm circumference, in cm; CC = calf circumference, in cm; SSF = subscapular skinfold thickness, in mm; KH = knee height, in cm.
[†]SEE = standard error of the estimate.

TABLE 7.4	Equations for Estimating Body Weight from Knee Height (KH) and Midarm Circumference (MAC) for Various Groups		

Age[*]	Race	Equation[†]	Accuracy[‡]
Females			
6–18	Black	Weight = (KH × 0.71) + (MAC × 2.59) − 50.43	±7.65 kg
6–18	White	Weight = (KH × 0.77) + (MAC × 2.47) − 50.16	±7.20 kg
19–59	Black	Weight = (KH × 1.24) + (MAC × 2.97) − 82.48	±11.98 kg
19–59	White	Weight = (KH × 1.01) + (MAC × 2.81) − 66.04	±10.60 kg
60–80	Black	Weight = (KH × 1.50) + (MAC × 2.58) − 84.22	±14.52 kg
60–80	White	Weight = (KH × 1.09) + (MAC × 2.68) − 65.51	±11.42 kg
Males			
6–18	Black	Weight = (KH × 0.59) + (MAC × 2.73) − 48.32	±7.50 kg
6–18	White	Weight = (KH × 0.68) + (MAC × 2.64) − 50.08	±7.82 kg
19–59	Black	Weight = (KH × 1.09) + (MAC × 3.14) − 83.72	±11.30 kg
19–59	White	Weight = (KH × 1.19) + (MAC × 3.21) − 86.82	±11.42 kg
60–80	Black	Weight = (KH × 0.44) + (MAC × 2.86) − 39.21	±7.04 kg
60–80	White	Weight = (KH × 1.10) + (MAC × 3.07) − 75.81	±11.46 kg

From Ross Laboratories, Columbus, OH 43210.

*Age (in years) is rounded to the nearest year.

†Weight is in kg: lb ÷ 2.2 = kg; kg × 2.2 = lb. Knee height is in cm; in. × 2.54 = cm; cm ÷ 2.54 = in.

‡For persons within each group, estimated body weight should be within the stated value for 95% of the subjects.

weights should be reserved for patients who cannot be weighed or for whom weights would be inaccurate, and every reasonable effort should be made to obtain direct measurements of body weights on patients.

If a patient has had an amputation, the patient's current body weight can be adjusted to account for the weight of the amputated body part. Table 7.5 shows the percent of total body weight contributed by individual body parts that are frequently amputated. These values are then used in the following equation to calculate adjusted body weight.[8,25]

TABLE 7.5	Percent of Total Body Weight Contributed by Individual Body Parts

Body Part	Contribution to Body Weight (%)
Entire arm	6.5
Upper arm	3.5
Forearm	2.3
Hand	0.8
Entire leg	18.5
Upper leg	11.6
Lower leg	5.3
Foot	1.8

From Brunnstrom S. 1983. *Clinical kinesiology*, 4th ed. Philadelphia: Davis.

$$\text{Adjusted wt} = \frac{\text{Current weight}}{100 - \% \text{ of amputation}} \times 100$$

Suppose you have a patient whose current weight is 157 lb and whose leg has been amputated at the right knee (right lower leg and foot removed). From Table 7.5, it can be seen that the lower leg and foot contribute approximately 7.1% of total body weight. Given this information and the equation, adjusted body weight can be calculated:

$$\text{Adjusted wt} = \frac{157 \text{ lb}}{100 - 7.1} \times 100$$

$$\text{Adjusted wt} = 169 \text{ lb}$$

Thus, this patient's adjusted body weight (approximately what it would be without the amputation) is 169 lb.

Arm Muscle Area

Arm muscle area (AMA) is used as an index of lean tissue or muscle in the body.[13,26] This is based on the observation that an organism facing nutritional deprivation draws on its nutritional reserves in the form of adipose tissue, visceral protein, and skeletal protein. In the case of upper-arm anthropometry, thickness of the triceps skinfold is used as an index of fat stores, and arm muscle size is used to represent muscle protein reserves.[26]

As the size of arm muscle changes in response to growth, development, and nutritional status, the resulting change in arm muscle area is greater than the change in midarm circumference. Consequently, changes in upper-arm musculature are not as easily detected by measurement of midarm circumference as by measurement of AMA. Therefore, AMA is the preferred nutritional index.[26]

AMA is correlated with creatinine excretion in children[9] and is related to total body muscle mass in adults.[14] It is particularly valuable in assessing persons with edema, whose body weights would be augmented by increased intracellular water, and in assessing persons who have undergone amputation.

AMA is estimated from the triceps skinfold measurement and midarm circumference.[13,14,26] The standard equation for calculating arm muscle area is[26]

$$AMA = \frac{[MAC - (\pi \times TSF)]^2}{4\pi}$$

where AMA = arm muscle area in mm^2; MAC = midarm circumference in mm; and TSF = triceps skinfold thickness in mm. Use of this formula is based on the following assumptions. In cross section, both the midarm and midarm muscle compartment are circular; the triceps skinfold thickness is twice the average thickness of the subcutaneous fat layer; bone atrophies in proportion to muscle wasting in protein-energy malnutrition; and the cross-sectional area of bone and the sheath containing the nervous and vascular tissues of the upper arm are small and insignificant.[14] In reality, however, several of these factors are significant sources of error in estimating AMA. When estimates of AMA derived from this equation were compared with AMA measured by computed tomography (see Chapter 6), the equation overestimated AMA by 20% to 25%.[14]

Heymsfield and coworkers[14] have developed the following revised equations, which partially correct for the overestimation of AMA by subtracting a constant that accounts for the presence of bone, nervous tissue, and vascular tissue in the upper arm:

$$cAMA \text{ for females} = \frac{[MAC - (\pi \times TSF)]^2}{4\pi} - 6.5$$

$$cAMA \text{ for males} = \frac{[MAC - (\pi \times TSF)]^2}{4\pi} - 10$$

where cAMA = corrected arm muscle area in cm^2; MAC = midarm circumference in cm; and TSF = triceps skinfold thickness in cm. Note that these equations call for all measurements to be made in *centimeters*. The nomogram in Figure 7.14 facilitates calculation of cAMA. Estimates of cAMA have been shown to be within ±8% of actual AMA, based on computed tomography. It should be noted that measurements must be carefully taken by trained observers and that the equations and nomogram for cAMA have not been validated for use with elderly persons.[14] In the obese, all of the equations tend to overestimate AMA when compared with values derived from computed tomography, and the magnitude of overestimation is proportional to the degree of adiposity. Heymsfield[14] recommends that AMA prediction equations not be used for persons having a relative weight of ≥ 125 per-

TABLE 7.6	Guidelines for Interpreting the Age/Sex Percentile Values for Arm Muscle Area Given in Appendix R
Percentile	Category
≤ 5th	Wasted
> 5th but ≤ 15th	Below average
> 15th but ≤ 85th	Average
> 85th but ≤ 95th	Above average
> 95th	High muscle

From Frisancho AR. 1990. *Anthropometric standards for the assessment of growth and nutritional status.* Ann Arbor: University of Michigan Press.

cent, but Frisancho[23] suggests they not be used for persons whose triceps skinfold thickness exceeds the 85th age and sex percentile. Despite these limitations, estimates of muscle mass derived from anthropometry can be collected inexpensively and easily and are helpful in assessing nutritional status and response to nutritional support.

Appendix R provides means and percentiles of AMA for males and females ages 1 to 74 years. For persons ages 18 years and older, the values are for corrected AMA. The guidelines in Table 7.6 can be used for interpreting these age/sex percentile values. No single index (for example, AMA) can be used as a reliable indicator of nutritional status. Basic assumptions inferred from anthropometry should be corroborated by data derived from dietary, biochemical, and clinical observations.[23]

DETERMINING ENERGY REQUIREMENTS

Twenty-four-hour energy expenditure is primarily determined by resting energy expenditure, the thermic effect of food, the thermic effect of exercise, and whether disease or injury is present.[27] As Sims and Danforth[27] pointed out, these "components of energy expenditure are not entirely discrete but are useful divisions when attempting to investigate factors that might regulate or control them."

Twenty-four-hour energy expenditure can be represented by the following equation:

$$24\text{-}EE = REE + TEF + TEE + TED$$

where 24-EE = 24-hour energy expenditure; REE = resting energy expenditure; TEF = thermic effect of food; TEE = thermic effect of exercise; and TED = thermic effect of disease and injury.

Basal metabolic rate (BMR) is defined as the lowest rate of energy expenditure of an individual. It is calculated from oxygen consumption measured over a 6- to 12-minute period when the subject is in a postabsorptive state (no food consumed during the previous 12 hours) and has rested quietly during the previous 30 minutes in a thermally neutral environment (room temperature is perceived as neither hot nor cold). To be precise, however,

Figure 7.14 **Nomogram for estimating corrected arm muscle area.**
To use, locate the patient's midarm circumference and triceps skinfold in the
appropriate columns. Connect these points with a straightedge. The corrected
arm muscle area is read where the straightedge crosses the arm muscle area
column. Note that there are values for females and males.

Source: Adapted with permission of Ross Laboratories, Columbus, OH 43216, from Chumlea WC,
Roche AF, Mukherjee D. 1989. *Nutritional assessment of the elderly through anthropometry.*

the point of lowest energy expenditure—the true BMR—
occurs in the early morning hours of deep sleep. Obtaining a truly basal metabolic measurement is impractical in
most instances. Therefore, a more appropriate term for
metabolic rate or energy expenditure in the awake, resting, postabsorptive subject is *resting energy expenditure
(REE),* also known as resting metabolic rate.

In the clinical setting, achieving optimal conditions
for determining REE can be difficult sometimes because
of the continuous care patients undergo. In these situations, the term *REE* is used in the scientific literature to
represent energy expenditure measured by indirect
calorimetry under conditions that are as controlled as the
clinical situation allows.[28,29] As shown in Figure 7.15,
REE is the largest component of 24-hour energy expenditure, accounting for roughly 65% to 75% of 24-hour
energy expenditure in healthy persons.

The second largest contributor to 24-hour energy
expenditure is the energy expended for muscular work,
or the thermic effect of exercise (TEE).[27] Of all the
components of a healthy person's 24-hour energy
expenditure, it is the most variable. For most North

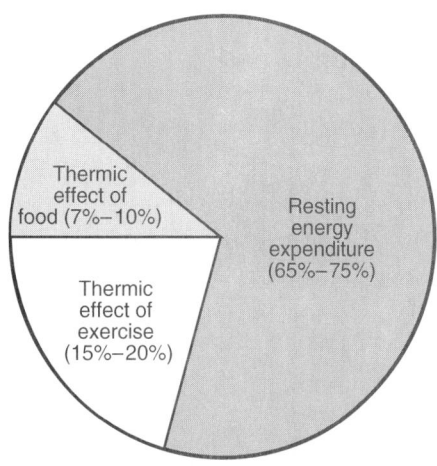

Figure 7.15 The components of 24-hour energy expenditure in healthy persons.

Americans, it accounts for about 15% to 20% of 24-hour energy expenditure but can increase by a factor of two or more with regular, high-intensity, long-duration physical activity.[27] Energy expended in exercise generally exceeds the REE in athletes who train several hours daily.

The thermic effect of food (TEF), also known as diet-induced thermogenesis or the specific dynamic action of food, is the increased energy expenditure following food consumption or administration of parenteral or enteral nutrition. The TEF is the energy cost of nutrient absorption, transport, storage, and metabolism. It accounts for about 7% to 10% of 24-hour energy expenditure.[27]

The energy needs of patients can be determined in two ways: measuring energy expenditure or estimating these needs using a variety of guidelines.[2,28,30]

Measuring Energy Expenditure

Calorimetry is the measurement of energy expenditure. Direct calorimetry measures the body's heat output, whereas indirect calorimetry determines energy expenditure by measuring the body's oxygen consumption and carbon dioxide production. Because energy expenditure measurements using direct and indirect calorimetry are performed in a laboratory, they may not accurately represent energy expenditure of free-living subjects (i.e., persons living at home and engaged in typical work and leisure-time activities). To more accurately measure the energy expenditure of free-living subjects, researchers can use two other methods: doubly labeled water and the bicarbonate-urea method.

Direct Calorimetry

Although simple in theory, direct calorimetry is cumbersome and expensive in practice.[31,32] It requires a highly sophisticated chamber or specially designed suit, which allows measurement of both the sensible heat given off by the body and the latent heat of vaporized water from the lungs and skin.[28,33,34] Measurements may require a subject to be confined within the chamber or suit for 24 hours or longer. Consequently, this approach is not suitable for critically ill patients. The USDA Human Nutrition Research Center in Beltsville, Maryland, has a direct calorimeter, which it uses for nutrition research requiring highly accurate measurements of energy expenditure. This is shown in Figures 7.16a and 7.16b.

Indirect Calorimetry

Indirect calorimetry is based on the fact that energy metabolism ultimately depends on oxygen utilization (VO_2) and carbon dioxide production (VCO_2).[31,32,35] Thus, expired air contains less oxygen and more carbon dioxide than inspired air. When the volume of expired air is known and the differences in oxygen and carbon dioxide concentrations in inspired and expired air are known, the body's energy expenditure can be calculated. Estimations of energy expenditure by indirect calorimetry have been shown to be practically identical to those derived from direct calorimetry.

Several techniques can be used in indirect calorimetry. In *closed circuit calorimetry*, the subject is connected via a mouthpiece, mask, or endotracheal tube to a spirometer filled with a known amount of 100% oxygen.[29,33,35] The subject rebreathes only the gas within the spirometer—a closed system. Carbon dioxide is removed from the system by a canister of soda lime (potassium hydroxide) placed in the breathing circuit. The subject's VO_2 is determined either from the amount of oxygen consumed from the spirometer or from the amount of added oxygen needed to maintain a constant volume within the spirometer.[29] The closed circuit technique is neither portable nor suitable to use on exercising subjects. During exercise, the apparatus offers excessive resistance to gas flow, and the removal of carbon dioxide is inadequate.

In *open circuit calorimetry*, the subject breathes through a two-way valve in which room air is inspired from one side of the valve, and expired air passes through the opposite side to where it is either analyzed immediately or collected for later analysis. In the *Douglas bag method* of open circuit calorimetry, the expired air is collected in large vinyl bags or latex rubber meteorologic balloons for later analysis. A lightweight, portable apparatus strapped to the subject's back also can be used to measure ventilation and can periodically collect samples of expired air for later analysis.[28,33]

A more common approach to open circuit indirect calorimetry in clinical settings is use of a *computerized metabolic monitor*, which can be taken to the bedside for measuring energy expenditure of patients who are either spontaneously breathing or breathing with the assistance of a mechanical ventilator.[28,31] The portable computerized

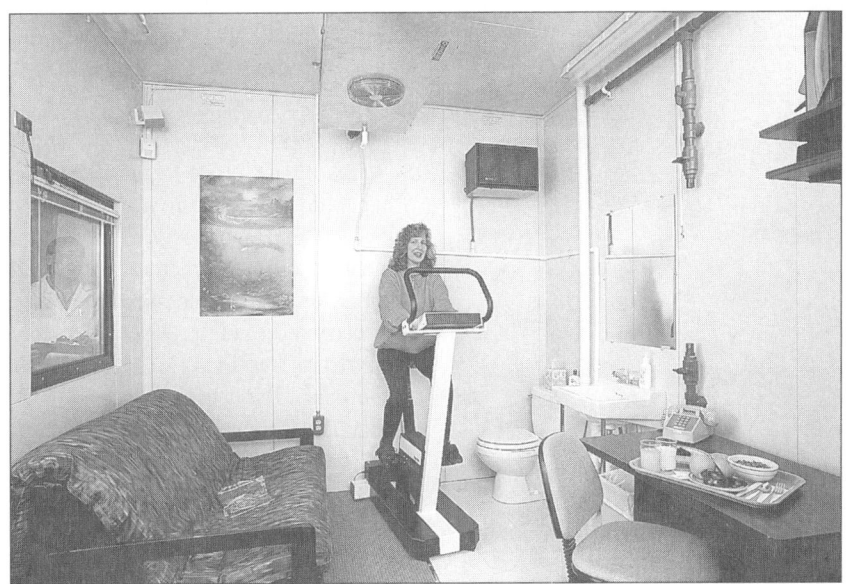

Figure 7.16a The USDA Human Nutrition Research Center's direct calorimeter.
Two researchers are shown operating the calorimeter while a subject can be seen inside the unit.

Source: Photo courtesy of Dr. James L. Seale, U.S. Department of Agriculture, Agriculture Research Service, Beltsville Human Nutrition Research Center, Energy and Protein Research Laboratory, Beltsville, MD.

Figure 7.16b
The interior of the USDA Human Nutrition Research Center's direct calorimeter provides a small but comfortable living space to subjects undergoing energy expenditure measurements lasting as long as 24 hours.

Source: Photo courtesy of Dr. James L. Seale, U.S. Department of Agriculture, Agriculture Research Service, Beltsville Human Nutrition Research Center, Energy and Protein Research Laboratory, Beltsville, MD.

metabolic monitor shown in Figure 7.17 has a ventilated hood, which can be placed over the face of a patient while in bed and can be made air-tight with a snugly fitting collar. The volume of inspired and expired air (known as minute ventilation) is typically measured using a pneumotachograph. Gas analyzers in the unit determine the oxygen and carbon dioxide content of both inspired and expired air, and they determine the caloric requirements and substrate utilization. Data can be displayed on the unit's video screen, recorded on an optional printer, or downloaded to a computer for storage and/or further analysis. Use of a mouthpiece or face mask often results in discomfort and stress to the patient, which can affect test results. The hood on the monitor in Figure 7.17 avoids this problem and can result in an accurate and representative measurement of metabolic rate in the critically ill patient.[28,31]

In terms of the accuracy and reproducibility of energy expenditure measurements, computerized metabolic monitors have been shown to compare favorably with more time-consuming approaches. They are relatively easy to operate, and they analyze data quickly. Because of their complexity, however, they are much more expensive to purchase and maintain.

Doubly Labeled Water

Another approach to measuring energy expenditure is the doubly labeled water (DLW) method. Using this ap-

Figure 7.17 An example of a computerized metabolic monitor in operation.
This unit uses indirect calorimetry to determine a patient's resting energy expenditure. The plastic hood allows expired air to be collected without the annoyance of a mask or mouthpiece.
Source: Photo courtesy of SensorMedics Corporation.

proach, a subject drinks a known amount of two stable isotopes of water, ^2H_2O and $H_2^{18}O$. The two isotopes mix with the body's water and are gradually eliminated from the body. The ^2H_2O is lost from the body only as water, whereas the $H_2^{18}O$ is lost from the body in water and as $C^{18}O_2$.[31,32,36,37] The subject then provides periodic samples of urine over the next 3 weeks, which allow monitoring of the body's elimination of the ^2H and ^{18}O. The difference between the rates at which deuterium and ^{18}O are lost from the body is an index of the body's carbon dioxide production. Using standard indirect calorimetric techniques, researchers can calculate energy expenditure with considerable accuracy and precision.

The method has been validated in humans by use of carefully performed energy balance studies and by direct and indirect calorimetry.[37,38] In laboratory testing, DLW has demonstrated an accuracy of 1% and a coefficient of variation of 3% to 6%.[36] The DLW technique is considered the best available method for providing average estimates of the 24-hour energy expenditure of free-living subjects (those outside a controlled setting) over an extended period of time of 1 to 3 weeks. Although it does not provide a direct measurement of energy expended in physical activity (thermic effect of exercise), this can be calculated by subtracting estimates of resting metabolic rate and the thermic effect of food from measured 24-hour energy expenditure. Use of DLW is limited by the expense of the isotopes and its dependence on isotope ratio mass spectrometry for analysis of urine samples and consequently is unsuitable for use in large, epidemiologic studies.[31,37–39] As mentioned in Chapter 3, comparisons of energy expenditure determined by DLW with reported energy intake from 24-hour recalls and food records have raised serious questions about the accuracy of reported energy intakes in dietary studies.[32,36,40–42]

Bicarbonate-Urea Method

A recently developed approach to measuring total energy expenditure in free-living subjects over relatively short periods of time (several hours to several days) is the bicarbonate-urea method.[31,37,43] Like doubly labeled water, the bicarbonate-urea method relies on an estimate of carbon dioxide production to calculate energy expenditure in free-living subjects. However, in this newer approach, the isotope used is ^{14}C administered intravenously or subcutaneously in the form of bicarbonate ($H^{14}CO_3^-$). The labeled bicarbonate mixes freely with and becomes diluted by the endogenous CO_2 produced by the body. Most of the labeled carbon is eliminated from the body through expired CO_2, while some is eliminated as urea in urine. The amount of labeled carbon in the urea is used to estimate CO_2 production from which energy expenditure is estimated.[37,44]

British researchers have shown that energy expenditure estimates based on the bicarbonate-urea method compare favorably with those derived from whole-body calorimetry in apparently healthy subjects and those with HIV infection and lung cancer.[44–46] The researchers used an insulin pump to continuously administer the labeled bicarbonate via subcutaneous injection to each free-living subject over a several-day study period. Compared with doubly labeled water, the bicarbonate-urea method has the advantages of being less costly and providing estimates of total energy expenditure over shorter periods of time (several hours to several days), allowing the day-to-day variations in energy expenditure to be studied.[37]

Estimating Energy Needs

In most clinical settings, energy expenditure usually is not measured. Instead, it is estimated using one of numerous available formulas, of which two of the most common are shown in Table 7.7.

Harris-Benedict Equations

There are approximately 190 published guidelines for estimating the nonprotein energy requirements of hospitalized patients.[30] The most widely used equations for predicting REE are those published in 1919 by Harris and Benedict.[47] Indirect calorimetry was used to determine the REE of 239 healthy young adults (136 males and 103 females with a

mean age of 27 and 31 years, respectively). From these data, Harris and Benedict derived regression equations (Table 7.7) that best predicted REE using the variables weight, stature, age, and sex.[47,48] Recent research has shown the Harris-Benedict equations' accuracy of prediction among healthy, adequately nourished persons to be within ±14% of REE measured by indirect calorimetry.[48,49] In malnourished, ill patients, however, the Harris-Benedict equations tend to underestimate REE by as much as 22%.[48] Despite these shortcomings, the Harris-Benedict equations are the most widely used in estimating the energy needs of most patients in clinical settings.

World Health Organization Equations

Numerous other equations for predicting REE in healthy populations are available.[49–51] Some are derived from original research,[33,34] and others are based on a reanalysis of data published by Harris and Benedict between 1919 and 1935.[48,52] The WHO equations were developed by a group of experts and are probably the best equations currently available.[53] Because stature was not found to significantly improve the predictive ability of the equations, it was omitted from those developed by the WHO.

The Harris-Benedict and WHO equations predict *resting energy expenditure* in kilocalories. To arrive at estimates of 24-hour energy expenditure, the REE must be increased to account for TEE. This is done by multiplying REE by one of the activity factors shown in Box 7.3 to arrive at TEE. Theoretically, REE includes TEF as well as TEE. In most clinical settings, however, no additional allowance is made for TEF. However, use of an additional factor to account for increased metabolism caused by disease, injury, and surgery is often necessary to estimate the 24-hour energy expenditure of patients.

A major decision in developing prediction equations is which variables to include. The major determinant of REE is fat-free mass—what some researchers call the *active protoplasmic tissue* or the *body cell mass*.[34,48,49,51] These are the body's metabolically active, energy-consuming cells. Statistical analysis of the data

TABLE 7.7	Examples of Equations for Estimating Resting Energy Expenditure in Healthy Persons*		

Harris-Benedict

Females	REE = 655.096 + 9.563 W + 1.850 S − 4.676 A	
Males	REE = 66.473 + 13.752 W + 5.003 S − 6.755 A	

Harris-Benedict (Values Rounded for Simplicity)

Females	REE = 655.1 + 9.6 W + 1.9 S − 4.7 A	
Males	REE = 66.5 + 13.8 W + 5.0 S − 6.8 A	

World Health Organization (WHO)			SD†
Females	3–10 years old	22.5 W + 499	±63
	10–18 years old	12.2 W + 746	±117
	18–30 years old	14.7 W + 496	±121
	30–60 years old	8.7 W + 829	±108
	> 60 years old	10.5 W + 596	±108
Males	3–10 years old	22.7 W + 495	±62
	10–18 years old	17.5 W + 651	±100
	18–30 years old	15.3 W + 679	±151
	30–60 years old	11.6 W + 879	±164
	> 60 years old	13.5 W + 487	±148

From Harris JA, Benedict FG. 1919. *A biometric study of basal metabolism in man.* 279. Washington, DC: Carnegie Institution of Washington; World Health Organization; *Energy and protein requirements. Report of a Joint FAO/WHO/UNU expert consultation.* Technical Report Series 724. Geneva, Switzerland: World Health Organization. 1985.

*REE = resting energy expenditure in kilocalories (kcal); W = body weight in kg; S = stature in cm; A = age.

†SD = standard deviation of the differences between actual and computed values—68% of the time, actual REE will be within ±1 standard deviation of the predicted REE.

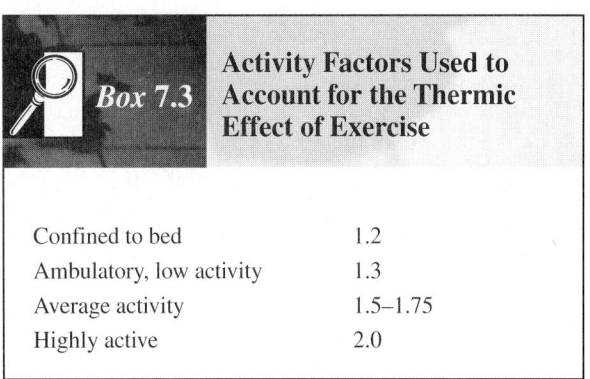

	Box 7.3	**Activity Factors Used to Account for the Thermic Effect of Exercise**
Confined to bed		1.2
Ambulatory, low activity		1.3
Average activity		1.5–1.75
Highly active		2.0

From Zeman FJ. 1991. *Clinical nutrition and dietetics.* New York: Macmillan; Long CL. 1984. The energy and protein requirements of the critically ill patient. In Wright RA, Heymsfield SB, eds. *Nutritional assessment.* Boston: Blackwell Scientific Publications.

(stepwise multiple-regression analysis) has shown that stature and body weight are reasonably well correlated with REE, and, because these measures can be easily and accurately performed, one or both are included in most equations. Stature was not found to improve the predictability of the WHO equations. Some of the earlier REE equations used body surface area as a variable.

When using these equations, keep in mind that there is a large interindividual variability in REE. Even though a particular equation may be able to predict the *mean* REE for a given *group* of people with a rather high degree of accuracy, the accuracy of that same equation in predicting *one individual's* REE may be quite low. Thus, it should be remembered that even the best prediction equation provides only an approximation of REE.

Should actual body weight or desirable body weight be used to predict energy expenditure? This is primarily a concern when working with obese patients. Use of actual body weight has been shown to be better at predicting energy expenditure than use of a patient's desirable body weight.[54] However, if it is the practice of a particular facility to adjust body weight for obese patients, the following equation can be used.[55]

$$\text{Adjusted body weight}$$
$$= (\text{actual body weight} - \text{DBW})$$
$$\times\ 0.25 + \text{DBW}$$

Energy Expenditure in Disease and Injury

Surgery, trauma, infection, burns, and various diseases can cause 24-hour energy expenditure and urinary nitrogen excretion to increase markedly.[28,29] The effect of various stresses on REE in hospitalized patients is shown in Figure 7.18.[28] The normal range of resting energy expenditure is represented by the light horizontal bar across the middle of the figure. Starvation in the unstressed person results in a hypometabolic state (below average metabolic rate) as the body attempts to conserve its energy reserves. The time when peak energy expenditure occurs in response to stress varies, depending on the severity of the illness or injury, and energy needs gradually return to normal during recovery. Figure 7.18 represents average values for both males and females of varying ages and body sizes and assumes no secondary complications, which can prolong periods of increased energy needs. The clinical course of individual patients can be expected to vary somewhat from these average values.

A common approach to estimating a patient's energy needs is to calculate the 24-hour energy expenditure, as outlined in Box 7.4, and then to increase this value by the appropriate injury factors shown in Table 7.8. This second step is necessary because the prediction equations given in Table 7.7 are based on data collected from healthy subjects.

Of all the conditions in Table 7.8, burns have the greatest potential for increasing energy expenditure.[56–59] When caloric intake fails to adequately meet energy

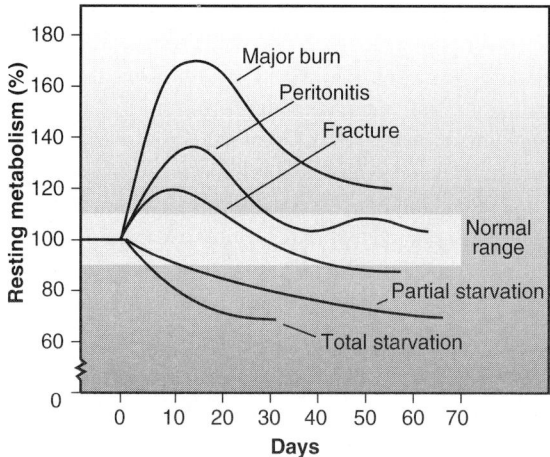

Figure 7.18 **Effect of various stresses on resting energy expenditure in hospitalized patients.**

Source: From Long CL, Schaffel N, et al. 1979. Metabolic response to injury and illness: Estimation of energy and protein needs from indirect calorimetry and nitrogen balance. *Journal of Parenteral and Enteral Nutrition* 3:452–456.

expenditure in burn patients, weight loss, delayed wound healing, and poor clinical outcome will result. A number of equations or approaches have been proposed for estimating the energy and protein needs of burn patients.[56–58,60–63] Several of these are shown in Table 7.9. An approach to estimating the energy requirements of a burn patient is to simply calculate his or her REE using the Harris-Benedict equation and then increase this value by an injury factor (1.6 to 2.2) and possibly an activity factor to account for energy the patient expends while in therapy.[63] A very simple approach, shown in Table 7.9, is merely to double the REE derived from the Harris-Benedict equation.[60]

The equations developed by Curreri and coworkers, shown in Table 7.9, have been frequently used for calculating the energy needs of burned patients.[56,64] In these equations, energy requirements for patients of different ages are estimated by adding resting energy expenditure (REE) as predicted by the Harris-Benedict equation to the product of the percent of body surface area burned (%BSAB) and an age-dependent constant. In the originally published equation for adults, resting or basal energy requirement was estimated by multiplying the patient's body weight in kilograms by 25.[64] This is based on the observation that REE is approximately 25 kcal/kg of body weight. The Curreri equations have the advantage of linking energy estimates with percent of body surface area burned. However, studies comparing the energy needs of severely burned patients as measured by indirect calorimetry and as estimated by the Curreri equations show that the equations tend to overestimate energy needs, resulting in overfeeding.[58,65,66] One explanation for this may be that recent advances in the management of severe burns result in less of a hypermetabolic response to the thermal injury as when the Curreri formula[58] was originally developed in the early 1970s.[58]

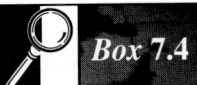

Box 7.4 Estimating Resting Energy Expenditure (REE) and 24-Hour Energy Expenditure Using the World Health Organization (WHO) Equations

Using the WHO equations (or the Harris-Benedict equations from Table 7.7) is quite easy. As an example, take a 23-year-old female with a body weight of 64 kg (141 lb). Begin by selecting the proper equation for the subject's sex and age. Then calculate the predicted REE using the subject's weight of 64 kg.

$$REE = 14.7\ W + 496$$
$$REE = (14.7 \times 64) + 496$$
$$REE = 941 + 496$$
$$REE = 1437\ kcal$$

To arrive at an estimate of 24-hour energy expenditure, the value for REE (1437 kcal) is then multiplied by an activity factor (Box 7.3) that accounts for the thermic effect of exercise—the calories expended during physical activity. Assuming this person has an activity level at the low end of the average activity category, the activity factor of 1.5 will be used.

$$1437\ kcal \times 1.5 = 2156\ kcal$$

This gives an estimated 24-hour energy expenditure of 2156 kcal. How do these values compare with those derived from the Harris-Benedict equation in Table 7.7, assuming the subject is 168 cm (66 in.) tall?

Condition	Injury Factor*
Minor surgery	1.0–1.1
Major surgery	1.1–1.3
Mild infection	1.0–1.2
Moderate infection	1.2–1.4
Severe infection	1.4–1.8
Skeletal or blunt trauma	1.2–1.4
Skeletal or head trauma (steroid treated)	1.6–1.8
Burns involving ≤ 20% BSA†	1.2–1.5
Burns involving 20% to 40% BSA	1.5–1.8
Burns involving > 40% BSA	1.8–2.0

TABLE 7.8 Injury Factors Used to Account for the Thermic Effect of Disease and Injury

From Long CL. 1984. The energy and protein requirements of the critically ill patient. In Wright RA, Heymsfield SB, eds. *Nutritional assessment.* Boston: Blackwell Scientific Publications.

*Multiply the predicted resting energy expenditure adjusted for the thermic effect of food and the thermic effect of exercise by the appropriate injury factor to arrive at an estimate of the patient's 24-hour energy expenditure. The range in values allows adjustment depending on the severity of the disease or injury.

†BSA = body surface area.

The equation in Table 7.9 developed by Allard and coworkers[61] has been shown to fairly accurately predict the energy requirements of burned patients, compared with energy expenditure measured by indirect calorimetry. Referred to as the "Toronto formula," it was derived by multiple-regression analysis of data collected from 23 patients with a mean burned body surface area of 39%.[67] Energy requirement is estimated by beginning with a negative value of 4343 kcal and adding or subtracting to this value various products. The equation requires information on the percent body surface area burned (estimated on

admission and corrected where amputation was performed); the number of kilocalories the patient received in the previous 24 hours, including all dextrose infusions, parenteral and enteral feedings; REE calculated from the Harris-Benedict equation; the average of the hourly rectal temperatures from the previous 24 hours expressed in degrees Celsius; and the number of postburn days as of the previous day. The Toronto formula has been shown to more closely predict the energy requirements of severely burned patients than the modified Curreri or the practice of doubling REE derived from the Harris-Benedict equation, both of which tend to overestimate energy requirements.[61] Energy expenditure predictions derived from the Toronto formula have also been shown to compare favorably with measured resting energy expenditure of clinically stable, mechanically ventilated burn patients.[68] The Toronto formula is unique in that it considers the thermic effect of food (which tends to be elevated in critically ill patients), the increased metabolic rate caused by elevations in body temperature, and the gradual fall in metabolic rate with time.

Energy Needs: Estimated or Measured?

Estimates of energy expenditure obtained from equations are just that—estimates. They are approximate and should be used only as rough guidelines.[58,69] However, for most hospital patients, estimates of energy expenditure are acceptable in providing the care their conditions demand. For these patients, the time and financial costs of measuring energy needs are not warranted. However, in some instances, it may be cost-effective to determine energy expenditure rather than to rely solely on estimates. The use of total parenteral nutrition (TPN) is quite expensive; not only are the solutions themselves costly but their administration requires a considerable time investment by nurses, pharmacists, physicians, and registered dietitians. Basing the administration of TPN solutions on

TABLE 7.9	Equations for Estimating the Energy Requirements of Patients with Burns*

Age	Equation
Allard[67]	
Adults	$kcal = -4343 + (10.5 \times \%BSAB) + (0.23\ CI) + (0.84\ REE) + (114\ T) - (4.5\ PBD)$
Cunningham[60]	
0–3 yr	$kcal = 2 \times REE$
Curreri[64]	
0–1 yr	$kcal = REE + (15 \times \%BSAB)$
1–3 yr	$kcal = REE + (25 \times \%BSAB)$
4–15 yr	$kcal = REE + (40 \times \%BSAB)$
16–59 yr	$kcal = REE + (40 \times \%BSAB)$
≥ 60 yr	$kcal = REE + (65 \times \%BSAB)$
Hildreth[62]	
Child	$kcal = (1800 \times m^2\ BSA) + (2200 \times m^2\ BSAB)$
Adolescent	$kcal = (1500 \times m^2\ BSA) + (1500 \times m^2\ BSAB)$
Long	
Any age	$kcal = REE \times injury\ factor \times activity\ factor$

*kcal = estimated daily energy requirement in kilocalories; REE = resting energy expenditure as predicted by the Harris-Benedict equation; BSA = body surface area in m^2; BSAB = body surface area burned in m^2; %BSAB = percent of body surface area burned; CI = the number of kilocalories the patient received in the previous 24 hours; T = average rectal temperature of the previous 24 hours in degrees Celsius; PBD = the number of postburn days prior to the day the energy requirements are calculated; see Box 7.3 for activity factors and Table 7.8 for injury factors.

measured energy expenditure may help prevent excessive use of TPN.[30] Not only is undernutrition associated with increased morbidity and mortality, but overnutrition can have negative clinical outcomes as well.[30] Measuring energy expenditure allows administration of TPN solutions to be based on physiologic need and promotes patient recovery. Thus, the cost of indirect calorimetry may be justified by both improved patient care and savings resulting from more judicious use of costly resources, such as TPN solutions and staff time and savings to the hospital because of shorter hospital stays.[30] In the case of burn patients, routine use of indirect calorimetry allows tailoring of nutritional support and is valuable in the early detection of significant undernutrition or overnutrition.[65] Considering the seriousness of thermal injury and the importance of nutritional support in its management, measuring the energy expenditure of severely burned patients should be standard practice.[69]

DETERMINING PROTEIN REQUIREMENTS

Protein serves as a functional component of body tissues and enzymes and as a fuel source. The protein needs of healthy, nonpregnant, nonlactating adults generally can be met with an intake of 0.8 g/kg body weight per day. In trauma or burn patients, protein catabolism increases markedly, as does protein loss, as indicated by urinary nitrogen excretion. Nitrogen makes up about 16% of protein and serves as a convenient way of measuring protein intake and losses.

Protein Losses in Disease and Injury

Figure 7.19 shows how urinary nitrogen losses vary over time among different conditions.[28] The normal range of urinary nitrogen loss is represented by the figure's light horizontal bar. Partial or total starvation in the unstressed person often results in *reduced* nitrogen losses as the body attempts to spare protein. The opposite is true in trauma or burn patients, even though their energy and protein intake often are reduced substantially. Trauma and burns are usually associated with increased protein catabolism and urinary nitrogen losses, although the patient's nutritional status before injury can affect the extent of loss. All other factors being equal, nitrogen losses after trauma and thermal injury are less in depleted persons and the elderly. Under these conditions, the protein reserves may be so depleted that the response is blunted or may not even be observed.

As with changes in REE seen in response to injury and illness (Figure 7.18), urinary nitrogen losses vary in degree and duration with the severity of the injury, may take several days after onset of the disease or trauma to reach their peak, and gradually return to the normal range.

Estimating Protein Needs

In practice, there is no single best method for conclusively determining the amount of protein that should be in the diet of patients suffering from trauma, burns, and other injuries. The protein requirements of these patients can only be estimated. Three approaches are commonly

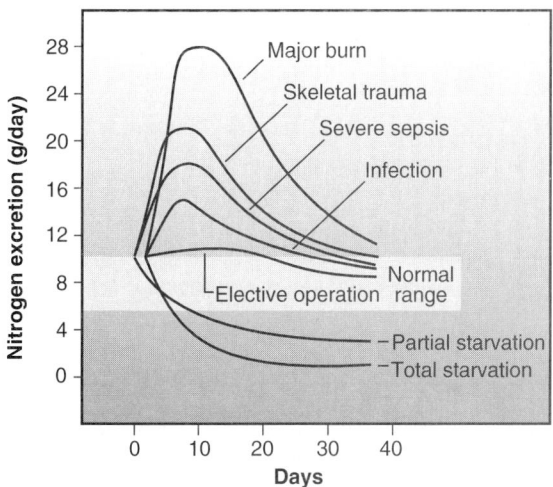

Figure 7.19 Effect of various stresses on urinary nitrogen excretion in hospitalized patients.

Source: Used with permission from Long CL, Schaffel N, et al. 1979. Metabolic response to injury and illness: Estimation of energy and protein needs from indirect calorimetry and nitrogen balance. *Journal of Parenteral and Enteral Nutrition* 3:452–456.

TABLE 7.10	Suggested Ranges of Protein Intake per Kilogram of Body Weight During Peak Catabolic Response for Various Injuries and Conditions in Adults

Stress Level	Condition	Protein (g/d)
Normal	Healthy	0.8
Mild	Minor surgery, mild infection	0.8–1.2
Moderate	Major surgery, moderate infection, moderate skeletal trauma	1.2–1.8
Severe	Severe infection, multiple injuries, severe trauma, major burns	1.6–2.2

From Ireton-Jones CS, Hasse JM. 1992. Comprehensive nutritional assessment: The dietitian's contribution to the team effort. *Nutrition* 8:75–81; Long CL. 1984. The energy and protein requirements of the critically ill patient. In Wright RA, Heymsfield SB, eds. *Nutritional assessment.* Boston: Blackwell Scientific Publications; Waymack JP, Herndon DN. 1992. Nutritional support of the burned patient. *World Journal of Surgery* 16:80–86; Mentegut WJ, Lowry SF. 1993. Nutrition in burn patients. *Seminars in Nephrology* 13:400–408.

used—basing protein intake on body weight, caloric intake, or nitrogen balance.[28] Table 7.10 provides some suggested ranges of protein intake per kilogram of body weight for various injuries and situations. If the energy needs of a patient are reasonably well defined, these can be used to estimate protein requirements. Some authorities consider 1 g of nitrogen (or 6.25 g of protein) for every 150 nonprotein kilocalories to be an adequate daily protein intake for critically ill adults and adults with burns when the percent body surface area burned is ≤ 10.[28] When injuries are very severe or the burn involves more than 10% body surface area, 1 g of nitrogen is recommended for every 100 nonprotein kilocalories.

Nitrogen balance (discussed in Chapter 9) involves 24-hour measurement of protein intake and an estimate of nitrogen losses where N Bal = nitrogen balance; protein intake = protein intake in g/24 hours; and UUN = urine urea nitrogen in g/24 hours.

$$\text{N Bal} = \frac{\text{Protein intake}}{6.25} - \text{UUN} - 4$$

Protein intake is divided by 6.25 to arrive at an estimate of nitrogen intake. Because protein is 16% nitrogen, dividing grams of protein by 6.25 gives you grams of nitrogen. Nitrogen loss is *estimated* by measuring urine urea nitrogen (which accounts for 85% to 90% of total urinary nitrogen) and subtracting a constant (4 g in the equation, although this value can vary from 2 to 4 g) to account for dermal, fecal, and nonurea nitrogen losses, which cannot be easily measured.[70,71]

Measuring total urinary nitrogen (TUN) is more difficult, expensive, and time consuming than measuring urinary urea nitrogen (UUN). Consequently, estimating TUN from measurements of UUN is standard practice. However, some researchers question the appropriateness of this practice, suggesting that in trauma and burn patients UUN represents only about 65% of TUN, as opposed to 80% to 90% in healthy persons.[72,73] They suggest that TUN should be measured directly rather than estimated from UUN. Other researchers report that estimates of TUN based on UUN are significantly different from direct measures of TUN but that the differences are small and clinically insignificant to justify the added expense and trouble of directly measuring TUN.[74]

Despite the problems associated with measuring protein intake and nitrogen excretion, nitrogen balance is generally accepted as an appropriate and cost-effective way of monitoring the protein status of burn and other critically ill patients.[28,58,72,74] Although not an exact indicator of nutritional adequacy, nitrogen balance studies serve as an excellent guide to nutritional support when used in conjunction with changes in body weight and energy expenditure measured by indirect calorimetry.[74] However, even if more protein is provided a patient than is calculated from losses in the urine, nitrogen balance is difficult to achieve in the early stage of severe trauma and thermal injury. The catabolism associated with the stress of trauma and thermal injury, as well as the atrophy of muscle caused by immobilization and disuse, result in considerable urinary nitrogen losses. Given time and the provision of adequate energy and protein, the patient gradually will begin to retain more protein than is excreted and will replace lost body protein.[28,58]

NUTRITION SCREENING INITIATIVE

The Nutrition Screening Initiative (NSI) is an endeavor begun in 1989 to encourage routine nutritional screening and better nutrition care in America's health and medical care settings.[75,76] It is a joint project of the American Dietetic Association, the American Academy of Family

Physicians, and the National Council on the Aging. Also playing a pivotal role in guiding the NSI is a Blue Ribbon Advisory Committee composed of more than 25 organizations and professionals from the fields of nutrition, medicine, and aging.[76]

The focus of the NSI is older Americans—the most rapidly growing segment of the U.S. population and a group at disproportionate risk for poor nutritional status.[77] Among the major goals of the NSI is determining the best way to identify potential risk factors and major indicators of poor nutritional status among older adults and raising public and professional awareness of poor nutritional status.[77] The NSI defines a risk factor as "a characteristic or occurrence that increases the likelihood that an individual has or will have problems with nutritional status."[76] Risk factors associated with poor nutritional status (Box 7.5) include inappropriate food intake, poverty, social isolation, dependency and disability, acute or chronic diseases or conditions, chronic medication use, and advanced age.[78]

The NSI defines an indicator as "an observable, recordable phenomenon such as a physical sign, specific symptom, syndrome, or measurable parameter that indicates that poor nutritional status is already present in the individual and is causing some effect."[76] Major and minor indicators of poor nutritional status are shown in Box 7.6. These can be identified through interviews, observation, physical examination, anthropometric measurements, and laboratory tests.

Public Awareness Checklist

Before people will seek screening for nutritional status, they must be aware that a potential problem exists. This

---

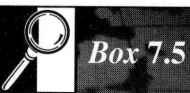

| **Box 7.5** | **Risk Factors for Poor Nutritional Status** |

- Inappropriate food intake
- Poverty
- Social isolation
- Dependency/disability
- Acute/chronic diseases or conditions
- Chronic medication use
- Advanced age ($\geq$ 80 years)

From the Nutrition Screening Initiative, a project of the American Academy of Family Physicians, the American Dietetic Association, and the National Council on Aging, and funded in part by a grant from Ross Laboratories, a division of Abbott Laboratories.

---

requires increased public awareness that poor nutritional status is a common problem. The NSI developed a public awareness checklist (Figure 7.20) to help identify individuals at greater than average risk for poor nutritional status. The checklist is intended to serve two purposes. The first is to provide people with basic nutrition information regarding the characteristics that may increase the likelihood of poor nutritional status. The second is to encourage the public to talk with health and social service providers about their nutritional concerns.[75]

The checklist uses the mnemonic "DETERMINE" to convey basic nutrition information and to help users recall the major risk factors and indicators of poor nutritional status. The checklist is not intended to be used as a diagnostic device.

 Box 7.6   **Major and Minor Indicators of Poor Nutritional Status in Older Americans**

MAJOR INDICATORS

- Weight loss $\leq$ 10 lb
- Underweight or overweight
- Serum albumin $<$ 3.5 g/dL
- Change in functional status
- Inappropriate food intake
- Midarm muscle circumference $<$ 10th percentile
- Triceps skinfold $<$ 10th percentile or $>$ 95th percentile
- Obesity
- Nutrition-related disorders
- Osteoporosis
- Osteomalacia
- Folate deficiency
- Vitamin B$_{12}$ deficiency

MINOR INDICATORS

- Alcoholism
- Cognitive impairment
- Chronic renal insufficiency
- Multiple concurrent medications
- Malabsorption syndromes
- Anorexia, nausea, dysphagia
- Change in bowel habits
- Fatigue, apathy, memory loss
- Poor oral/dental status
- Dehydration
- Poorly healing wounds
- Loss of subcutaneous fat or muscle mass
- Fluid retention
- Reduced iron, ascorbic acid, zinc

From the Nutrition Screening Initiative, a project of the American Academy of Family Physicians, the American Dietetic Association, and the National Council on Aging, and funded in part by a grant from Ross Laboratories, a division of Abbott Laboratories.

The Warning Signs of poor nutritional health are often overlooked. Use this checklist to find out if you or someone you know is at nutritional risk.

Read the statements below. Circle the number in the "yes" column for those that apply to you or someone you know. For each "yes" answer, score the number in the box. Total your nutritional score.

DETERMINE YOUR NUTRITIONAL HEALTH

	YES
I have an illness or condition that made me change the kind and/or amount of food I eat.	2
I eat fewer than 2 meals per day.	3
I eat few fruits or vegetables or milk products.	2
I have 3 or more drinks of beer, liquor or wine almost every day.	2
I have tooth or mouth problems that make it hard for me to eat.	2
I don't always have enough money to buy the food I need.	4
I eat alone most of the time.	1
I take 3 or more different prescribed or over-the-counter drugs a day.	1
Without wanting to, I have lost or gained 10 pounds in the last 6 months.	2
I am not always physically able to shop, cook and/or feed myself.	2
	TOTAL

Total Your Nutritional Score. If it's –

0-2   **Good!** Recheck your nutritional score in 6 months.

3-5   **You are at moderate nutritional risk.** See what can be done to improve your eating habits and lifestyle. Your office on aging, senior nutrition program, senior citizens center or health department can help. Recheck your nutritional score in 3 months.

6 or more   **You are at high nutritional risk.** Bring this checklist the next time you see your doctor, dietitian or other qualified health or social service professional. Talk with them about any problems you may have. Ask for help to improve your nutritional health.

Remember that warning signs suggest risk, but do not represent a diagnosis of any condition. Turn the page to learn more about the Warnings Signs of poor nutritional health.

These materials are developed and distributed by the Nutrition Screening Initiative, a project of:

 AMERICAN ACADEMY OF FAMILY PHYSICIANS

 THE AMERICAN DIETETIC ASSOCIATION

NC OA   NATIONAL COUNCIL ON THE AGING, INC.

 The Nutrition Screening Initiative • 1010 Wisconsin Avenue, NW • Suite 800 • Washington, DC 20007
The Nutrition Screening Initiative is funded in part by a grant from Ross Products Division of Abbott Laboratories.

Figure 7.20 The "Determine Your Nutritional Health" checklist developed by the Nutrition Screening Initiative to identify persons at increased risk of poor nutritional status.

Source: From the Nutrition Screening Initiative, a project of the American Academy of Physicians, the American Dietetic Association, and the National Council on Aging, and funded in part by a grant from Ross Laboratories, a division of Abbott Laboratories.

continued

The Nutrition Checklist is based on the Warning Signs described below. Use the word <u>DETERMINE</u> to remind you of the Warning Signs.

Disease

Any disease, illness or chronic condition which causes you to change the way you eat, or makes it hard for you to eat, puts your nutritional health at risk. Four out of five adults have chronic diseases that are affected by diet. Confusion or memory loss that keeps getting worse is estimated to affect one out of five or more of older adults. This can make it hard to remember what, when or if you've eaten. Feeling sad or depressed, which happens to about one in eight older adults, can cause big changes in appetite, digestion, energy level, weight and well-being.

Eating Poorly

Eating too little and eating too much both lead to poor health. Eating the same foods day after day or not eating fruit, vegetables, and milk products daily will also cause poor nutritional health. One in five adults skip meals daily. Only 13% of adults eat the minimum amount of fruit and vegetables needed. One in four older adults drink too much alcohol. Many health problems become worse if you drink more than one or two alcoholic beverages per day.

Tooth Loss/Mouth Pain

A healthy mouth, teeth and gums are needed to eat. Missing, loose or rotten teeth or dentures which don't fit well, or cause mouth sores, make it hard to eat.

Economic Hardship

As many as 40% of older Americans have incomes of less than $6,000 per year. Having less -- or choosing to spend less -- than $25-30 per week for food makes it very hard to get the foods you need to stay healthy.

Reduced Social Contact

One-third of all older people live alone. Being with people daily has a positive effect on morale, well-being and eating.

Multiple Medicines

Many older Americans must take medicines for health problems. Almost half of older Americans take multiple medicines daily. Growing old may change the way we respond to drugs. The more medicines you take, the greater the chance for side effects such as increased or decreased appetite, change in taste, constipation, weakness, drowsiness, diarrhea, nausea, and others. Vitamins or minerals, when taken in large doses, act like drugs and can cause harm. Alert your doctor to everything you take.

Involuntary Weight Loss/Gain

Losing or gaining a lot of weight when you are not trying to do so is an important warning sign that must not be ignored. Being overweight or underweight also increases your chance of poor health.

Needs Assistance In Self Care

Although most older people are able to eat, one of every five have trouble walking, shopping, buying and cooking food, especially as they get older.

Elder Years Above Age 80

Most older people lead full and productive lives. But as age increases, risk of frailty and health problems increase. Checking your nutritional health regularly makes good sense.

 The Nutrition Screening Initiative • 1010 Wisconsin Avenue, NW • Suite 800 • Washington, DC 20007
The Nutrition Screening Initiative is funded in part by a grant from Ross Products Division of Abbott Laboratories.

Figure 7.20 *Continued.*

A nutrition score of 0 to 2 is considered good, and a recheck in 6 months is recommended. A recheck in 3 months and a self-help approach to improving nutritional status is encouraged for persons scoring between 3 and 5 points, which is considered moderate nutritional risk. Persons with a nutrition score of 6 or more are regarded at high nutritional risk and are encouraged to take the checklist with them the next time they visit their physician, dietitian, or other health or social service provider.

Screening Tools

A practical approach to nutritional screening recommended by the NSI is outlined in Figure 7.21. The first step is completing the checklist. Persons at increased risk for poor nutritional status then can be screened at one of two screening levels. The Level I Screen (Figure 7.22) is a basic nutrition evaluation instrument that can be administered in a community setting by a social service or health care professional or another trained person. It is designed to distinguish between persons at high risk and those at moderate risk for poor nutritional status. High-risk individuals are those with a documented, significant change in body weight. They should be referred to a physician for more in-depth assessment. Persons at moderate risk may benefit from dietary counseling, dental evaluation, food stamps, home-delivered or congregate meals, economic assistance programs, shopping or transportation assistance, increased socialization, and increased physical activity.[75] The Level I Screen should be repeated annually or if a major change in status occurs.

The Level II Screen (Figure 7.23) is administered by a health professional and requires the input of a physician and dietitian. In addition to the items covered by the Level I Screen, the Level II Screen requires data from laboratory tests, anthropometric measures, physical examination, and tests of mental and cognitive status.[75] Potential problems that may be identified by this screen include unintentional weight loss, protein-energy malnutrition, osteoporosis, vitamin or mineral deficiency, obesity, and elevated serum cholesterol. If potential problems are identified, the person should be referred to the appropriate health care professional.

SCHEMATIC—A PRACTICAL APPPROACH TO NUTRITIONAL SCREENING

Figure 7.21 Outline of a practical approach to nutritional screening recommended by the Nutrition Screening Initiative.

Source: Reprinted with permission by the Nutrition Screening Initiative, a project of the American Academy of Family Physicians, the American Dietetic Association, and the National Council on Aging, and funded in part by a grant from Ross Laboratories, a division of Abbott Laboratories.

Level 1 Screen

Body Weight

Measure height to the nearest inch and weight to the nearest pound. Record the values below and mark them on the Body Mass Index (BMI) scale to the right. Then use a straight edge (ruler) to connect the two points and circle the spot where this straight line crosses the center line (body mass index). Record the number below.

Healthy older adults should have a BMI between 24 and 27.

Height (in): _____
Weight (lbs): _____
Body Mass Index: _____
(number from center column)

Check any boxes that are true for the individual:

❑ Has lost or gained 10 pounds (or more) in the past 6 months.

❑ Body mass index < 24

❑ Body mass index > 27

For the remaining sections, please ask the individual which of the statements (if any) is true for him or her and place a check by each that applies.

NOMOGRAM FOR BODY MASS INDEX

WEIGHT
KG LB

BODY
MASS
INDEX
$[WT/(HT)^2]$

WOMEN   MEN

OBESE   OBESE

OVERWEIGHT   OVERWEIGHT

ACCEPTABLE   ACCEPTABLE

HEIGHT
CM IN

© George A Bray 1978

Eating Habits

❑ Does not have enough food to eat each day

❑ Usually eats alone

❑ Does not eat anything on one or more days each month

❑ Has poor appetite

❑ Is on a special diet

❑ Eats vegetables two or fewer times daily

❑ Eats milk or milk products once or not at all daily

❑ Eats fruit or drinks fruit juice once or not at all daily

❑ Eats breads, cereals, pasta, rice, or other grains five or fewer times daily

❑ Has difficulty chewing or swallowing

❑ Has more than one alcoholic drink per day (if woman); more than two drinks per day (if man)

❑ Has pain in mouth, teeth, or gums

continued

Figure 7.22 The Level I Screen developed by the Nutrition Screening Initiative; it is designed to distinguish between persons at high and moderate risk of poor nutritional status and to be administered by a social service or health care professional.

Source: From the Nutrition Screening Initiative, a project of the American Academy of Family Physicians, the American Dietetic Association, and the National Council on Aging, and funded in part by a grant from Ross Laboratories, a division of Abbott Laboratories.

A physician should be contacted if the individual has gained or lost 10 pounds unexpectedly or without intending to during the past 6 months. A physician should also be notified if the individual's body mass index is above 27 or below 24.

Living Environment

☐ Lives on an income of less than $6000 per year (per individual in the household)

☐ Lives alone

☐ Is housebound

☐ Is concerned about home security

☐ Lives in a home with inadequate heating or cooling

☐ Does not have a stove and/or refrigerator

☐ Is unable or prefers not to spend money on food (<$25-$30 per person spent on food each week)

Functional Status

Usually or always needs assistance with (check each that apply):

☐ Bathing

☐ Dressing

☐ Grooming

☐ Toileting

☐ Eating

☐ Walking or moving about

☐ Traveling (outside the home)

☐ Preparing food

☐ Shopping for food or other necessities

If you have checked one or more statements on this screen, the individual you have interviewed may be at risk for poor nutritional status. Please refer this individual to the appropriate health care or social service professional in your area. For example, a dietitian should be contacted for problems with selecting, preparing, or eating a healthy diet, or a dentist if the individual experiences pain or difficulty when chewing or swallowing. Those individuals whose income, lifestyle, or functional status may endanger their nutritional and overall health should be referred to available community services: home-delivered meals, congregate meal programs, transportation services, counseling services (alcohol abuse, depression, bereavement, etc.), home health care agencies, day care programs, etc.

Please repeat this screen at least once each year--sooner if the individual has a major change in his or her health, income, immediate family (e.g., spouse dies), or functional status.

These materials developed by the Nutrition Screening Initiative.

Figure 7.22 *Continued.*

Level II Screen

Complete the following screen by interviewing the patient directly and/or by referring to the patient chart. If you do not routinely perform all of the described tests or ask all of the listed questions, please consider including them but do not be concerned if the entire screen is not completed. Please try to conduct a minimal screen on as many older patients as possible, and please try to collect serial measurements, which are extremely valuable in monitoring nutritional status. Please refer to the manual for additional information.

Anthropometrics

Measure height to the nearest inch and weight to the nearest pound. Record the values below and mark them on the Body Mass Index (BMI) scale to the right. Then use a straight edge (paper, ruler) to connect the two points and circle the spot where this straight line crosses the center line (body mass index). Record the number below; healthy older adults should have a BMI between 24 and 27; check the appropriate box to flag an abnormally high or low value.

NOMOGRAM FOR BODY MASS INDEX

© George A Bray 1978

Height (in):_____
Weight (lbs):_____
Body Mass Index
(weight/height²):____ _____

Please place a check by any statement regarding BMI and recent weight loss that is true for the patient.

❑ Body mass index < 24

❑ Body mass index > 27

❑ Has lost or gained 10 pounds (or more) of body weight in the past 6 months

Record the measurement of mid-arm circumference to the nearest 0.1 centimeter and of triceps skinfold to the nearest 2 millimeters.

Mid-arm circumference (cm):_____
Triceps skinfold (mm):_____
Mid-arm muscle circumference (cm):_____

Refer to the table and check any abnormal values:

❑ Mid-arm muscle circumference <10th percentile

❑ Triceps skinfold < 10th percentile

❑ Triceps skinfold > 95th percentile

Note: mid-arm circumference (cm) - {0.314 x triceps skinfold (mm)}= mid-arm *muscle* circumference (cm)

For the remaining sections, please place a check by any statements that are true for the patient.

Laboratory Data

❑ Serum albumin below 3.5 g/dl

❑ Serum cholesterol below 160 mg/dl

❑ Serum cholesterol above 240 mg/dl

Drug Use

❑ Three or more prescription drugs, OTC medications, and/or vitamin/mineral supplements daily

continued

Figure 7.23 The Level II Screen developed by the Nutrition Screening Initiative; it is designed to identify common problems, such as protein-energy malnutrition, obesity, elevated serum cholesterol levels, and osteoporosis.

Source: From the Nutrition Screening Initiative, a project of the American Academy of Family Physicians, the American Dietetic Association, and the National Council on Aging, and funded in part by a grant from Ross Laboratories, a division of Abbott Laboratories.

Clinical Features

Presence of (check each that apply):

☐ Problems with mouth, teeth, or gums

☐ Difficulty chewing

☐ Difficulty swallowing

☐ Angular stomatitis

☐ Glossitis

☐ History of bone pain

☐ History of bone fractures

☐ Skin changes (dry, loose, nonspecific lesions, edema)

	Men		Women	
Percentile	55-65 y	65-75 y	55-65 y	65-75 y
Arm circumference (cm)				
10th	27.3	26.3	25.7	25.2
50th	31.7	30.7	30.3	29.9
95th	36.9	35.5	38.5	37.3
Arm muscle circumference (cm)				
10th	24.5	23.5	19.6	19.5
50th	27.8	26.8	22.5	22.5
95th	32.0	30.6	28.0	27.9
Triceps skinfold (mm)				
10th	6	6	16	14
50th	11	11	25	24
95th	22	22	38	36

From Frisancho AR. 1981 New norms of upper limb fat and muscle areas for assessment of nutritional status. Am J Clin Nutr: 34:2540-2545. American Society for Clinical Nutrition.

Eating Habits

☐ Does not have enough food to eat each day

☐ Usually eats alone

☐ Does not eat anything on one or more days each month

☐ Has poor appetite

☐ Is on a special diet

☐ Eats vegetables two or fewer times daily

☐ Eats milk or milk products once or not at all daily

☐ Eats fruit or drinks fruit juice once or not at all daily

☐ Eats breads, cereals, pasta, rice, or other grains five or fewer times daily

☐ Has more than one alcoholic drink per day (if woman); more than two drinks per day (if man)

Living Environment

☐ Lives on an income of less than $6000 per year (per individual in the household)

☐ Lives alone

☐ Is housebound

☐ Is concerned about home security

☐ Lives in a home with inadequate heating or cooling

☐ Does not have a stove and/or refrigerator

☐ Is unable or prefers not to spend money on food (<$25-$30 per person spent on food each week)

Functional Status

Usually or always needs assistance with (check each that apply):

☐ Bathing

☐ Dressing

☐ Grooming

☐ Toileting

☐ Eating

☐ Walking or moving about

☐ Traveling (outside the home)

☐ Preparing food

☐ Shopping for food or other necessities

Mental/Cognitive Status

☐ Clinical evidence of impairment, e.g., Folstein < 26

☐ Clinical evidence of depressive illness, e.g., Beck Depression Inventory > 15, Geriatric Depression Scale > 5

Patients in whom you have identified one or more major indicator of poor nutritional status require immediate medical attention; if minor indicators are found, ensure that they are known to a health professional or to the patient's own physician. Patients who display risk factors of poor nutritional status should be referred to the appropriate health care or social service professional (dietitian, nurse, dentist, case manager, etc.).

These materials developed by the Nutrition Screening Initiative.

Figure 7.23 *Continued.*

SUMMARY

1. Assessing the nutritional status of hospitalized patients involves at least four goals: identifying those at nutritional risk, determining the severity and causes of nutritional impairment, determining the patient's risk of dying from the undernutrition or developing a related disease condition, and monitoring to evaluate response to nutrition therapy.

2. The purpose of nutritional screening is to identify potentially malnourished individuals at nutritional

risk. Screening should be done on all patients within the first 24 to 48 hours following admission. It is best done by a dietetic technician.

3. Because no single measurement or test is capable of evaluating a patient's nutritional status, a variety of data must be used. The most fundamental include the patient's stature, usual and present weight, and past and current dietary practices; significant changes in eating habits; and the presence of any

nutrition-related problems. Some of this information is routinely collected by the nursing and medical staff and can be found in the patient's medical record. For critically ill patients or those with less obvious nutritional deficits, detailed anthropometric, laboratory, and dietary information may need to be collected.

4. The history includes facts about past and current health, use of medications, and personal and household information as it pertains to nutritional status. Dietary information relates to food intake, food preferences, intolerances and allergies, usual eating pattern, use of supplements, and resources for purchasing and preparing food. Physical examination includes anthropometric data as well as findings from the physical examination available from the patient's chart.

5. Stature and body weight are important measures to be obtained from hospitalized patients. Under certain conditions they may have to be calculated from such variables as the patient's knee height, calf circumference, age, and sex, or they may be obtained by measuring body length while the patient is lying in bed. When calculations are performed, care should be exercised in selecting the proper equation.

6. Midarm circumference is the circumference of the upper arm at the triceps skinfold site. It is an indicator of muscle and subcutaneous adipose tissue and can be obtained quickly and noninvasively in both ambulatory and nonambulatory patients. Arm muscle area, calculated from the triceps skinfold measurement and midarm circumference, is used as an index of lean tissue or muscle in the body.

7. Calf circumference is used in estimating body weight and as an indicator of muscle and subcutaneous adipose tissue. Obtaining calf circumference and measures of skinfold thickness in bedridden patients is somewhat different than in ambulatory persons, and the standardized protocol outlined in this chapter should be strictly followed.

8. Energy needs are based on an individual's 24-hour energy expenditure, which is determined by resting energy expenditure, the thermic effect of food, energy expended in physical activity, and whether disease or injury is present. Resting energy expenditure is the largest component of 24-hour energy expenditure.

9. Twenty-four-hour energy expenditure can be determined through indirect calorimetry or roughly approximated from a variety of equations. Indirect calorimetry involves measurement of the body's oxygen consumption and carbon dioxide production and often uses a computerized metabolic monitor. The energy expenditure of patients usually is estimated. In critically ill persons or those receiving parenteral or enteral feedings, indirect calorimetry may be preferable to estimating energy expenditure.

10. Surgery, trauma, infection, burns, and various diseases can cause 24-hour energy expenditure and urinary excretion of nitrogen to increase markedly. Energy expenditure in patients can be obtained through indirect calorimetry or estimates using a variety of equations.

11. The degree and duration of increased protein catabolism following injury vary with the trauma's severity. Protein catabolism may take several days to peak before gradually returning to normal. Recommended protein intake can be based on nitrogen balance, body weight, or energy intake.

12. The Nutrition Screening Initative (NSI) was begun in 1989 to encourage routine nutritional screening and better nutrition care in America's health and medical care settings. The goals of the NSI include raising public and professional awareness of poor nutritional status and developing assessment tools to identify potential risk factors and major indicators of poor nutritional status, especially among older adults. Assessment tools developed include a public awareness checklist and screening instruments for assessing nutritional status at two levels.

REFERENCES

1. Corish CA, Kennedy NP. 2000. Protein-energy undernutrition in hospital in-patients. *British Journal of Nutrition* 83:575–591.

2. Klein S, Kinney J, Jeejeebhoy K, Alpers D, Hellerstein M, Murray M, Twomey P. 1997. Nutrition support in clinical practice: Review of published data and recommendations for future research directions. *American Journal of Clinical Nutrition* 66:683–706.

3. McMahon K, Brown JK. 2000. Nutritional screening and assessment. *Seminars in Oncology Nursing* 16:106–112.

4. Posthauer ME, Dorse B, Foiles RA, et al. 1994. ADA's definitions for nutrition screening and nutrition assessment. *Journal of the American Dietetic Association* 94:838–839.

5. Hedberg AM, Garcia N, Trejus IJ, Weinmann-Winkler S, Gabriel ML, Lutz AL. 1988. Nutritional risk screening: Development of a standardized protocol using dietetic technicians. *Journal of the American Dietetic Association* 88:1553–1556.

6. Trimble JM. 1992. Reimbursement enhancement in a New Jersey hospital: Coding for malnutrition in prospective payment systems. *Journal of the American Dietetic Association* 92:737–738.

7. Sayarath VG. 1993. Nutrition screening for malnutrition: Potential economic impact at a community hospital. *Journal of the American Dietetic Association* 93:1440–1442.

8. Ireton-Jones CS, Hasse JM. 1992. Comprehensive nutritional assessment: The dietitian's contribution to the team effort. *Nutrition* 8:75–81.

9. Hopkins B. 1993. Assessment of nutritional status. In Gottschlich MM, Matarese LE, Shronts EP, eds. *Nutrition support dietetics core curriculum,* 2nd ed. Silver Spring, MD: American Society for Parenteral and Enteral Nutrition.

10. Chumlea WC, Guo S, Roche AF, Steinbaugh ML. 1988. Prediction of body weight for the nonambulatory elderly from anthropometry. *Journal of the American Dietetic Association* 88:564–568.

11. Chumlea WC, Guo SS, Steinbaugh ML. 1994. Prediction of stature from knee height for black and white adults and children with application to mobility-impaired or handicapped persons. *Journal of the American Dietetic Association* 94:1385–1388.

12. Detsky AS, Smalley PS, Change J. 1994. Is this patient malnourished? *Journal of the American Medical Association* 271:54–58.

13. Chumlea WC, Roche AF, Mukherjee D. 1987. *Nutritional assessment of the elderly through anthropometry.* Columbus, OH: Ross Laboratories.

14. Heymsfield SB, McManus C, Smith J, Stevens V, Nixon DW. 1982. Anthropometric measurement of muscle mass: Revised equations for calculating bone-free arm muscle area. *American Journal of Clinical Nutrition* 36:680–690.

15. Chumlea WC. 1988. Methods of nutritional anthropometric assessment for special groups. In Lohman TG, Roche AF, Martorell R, eds. *Anthropometric standardization reference manual.* Champaign, IL: Human Kinetics Books.

16. Chumlea WC, Roche AF. 1988. Assessment of the nutritional status of healthy and handicapped adults. In Lohman TG, Roche AF, Martorell R, eds. *Anthropometric standardization reference manual.* Champaign, IL: Human Kinetics Books.

17. Cockram DB, Baumgartner RN. 1990. Evaluation of accuracy and reliability of calipers for measuring recumbent knee height in elderly people. *American Journal of Clinical Nutrition* 52:397–400.

18. Muncie HL, Sobal J, Hoopes JM, Tenney JH, Warren JW. 1987. A practical method of estimating stature of bedridden female nursing home patients. *Journal of the American Geriatrics Society* 35:285–289.

19. Jarzem PF, Gledhill RB. 1993. Predicting height from arm measurements. *Journal of Pediatric Orthopaedics* 13:761–765.

20. Falciglia G, O'Conner J, Gedling E. 1988. Upper arm anthropometric norms in elderly white subjects. *Journal of the American Dietetic Association* 88:569–574.

21. Callaway CW, Chumlea WC, Bouchard C, Himes JH, Lohman TG, Martin AD, Mitchell CD, Mueller WH, Roche AF, Seefeldt VD. 1988. Circumferences. In Lohman TG, Roche AF, Martorell R, eds. *Anthropometric standardization reference manual.* Champaign, IL: Human Kinetics Books.

22. Chumlea WC, Roche AF, Webb P. 1984. Body size, subcutaneous fatness and total body fat in older adults. *International Journal of Obesity* 8:311–317.

23. Frisancho AR. 1990. *Anthropometric standards for the assessment of growth and nutritional status.* Ann Arbor: University of Michigan Press.

24. Guenter PA, Moore K, Crosby LO, Buzby GP, Mullen JL. 1982. Body weight measurement of patients receiving nutritional support. *Journal of Parenteral and Enteral Nutrition* 6:441–443.

25. Brunnstrom S. 1983. *Clinical kinesiology,* 4th ed. Philadelphia: Davis.

26. Frisancho AR. 1981. New norms of upper limb fat and muscle areas for assessment of nutritional status. *American Journal of Clinical Nutrition* 34:2540–2545.

27. Sims AH, Danforth E. 1987. Expenditure and storage of energy in man. *Journal of Clinical Investigation* 79:1019–1025.

28. Long CL. 1984. The energy and protein requirements of the critically ill patient. In Wright RA, Heymsfield SB, eds. *Nutritional assessment.* Boston: Blackwell Scientific Publications.

29. Damask MC, Schwarz Y, Weissman C. 1987. Energy measurements and requirements of critically ill patients. *Critical Care Clinics* 3:71–96.

30. Foster GD, Knox LS, Dempsey DT, Mullen JL. 1987. Caloric requirements in total parenteral nutrition. *Journal of the American College of Nutrition* 6:231–253.

31. Poelman ET, Horton ES. 1998. Energy needs: Assessment and requirements in humans. In Shils ME, Olson JA, Shike M, Ross AC, eds. *Modern nutrition in health and disease,* 9th ed. Baltimore, MD: Williams & Wilkins.

32. Murgatroyd PR, Shetty PS, Prentice AM. 1993. Techniques for the measurement of human energy expenditure: A practical guide. *International Journal of Obesity* 17:549–568.

33. Ravussin E, Burnand B, Schutz Y, Jéquier E. 1982. Twenty-four-hour energy expenditure and resting metabolic rate in obese, moderately obese, and control subjects. *American Journal of Clinical Nutrition* 35:566–573.

34. Ravussin E, Lillioja S, Anderson TE, Christin L, Bogardus C. 1986. Determinants of 24-hour energy expenditure in man. *Journal of Clinical Investigation* 78:1568–1578.

35. McClave SA, Snider HL. 1992. Use of indirect calorimetry in

clinical nutrition. *Nutrition in Clinical Practice* 7:207–221.

36. Schoeller DA. 1990. How accurate is self-reported dietary energy intake? *Nutrition Reviews* 48:373–379.

37. Gibney ER. 2000. Energy expenditure in disease: Time to revisit? *Proceedings of the Nutrition Society* 59:199–207.

38. Seale JL, Rumpler WV, Conway JM, Miles CW. 1990. Comparison of doubly labeled water, intake-balance, and direct- and indirect-calorimetry methods for measuring energy expenditure in adult men. *American Journal of Clinical Nutrition* 52:66–71.

39. Livingstone MBE, Prentice AM, Coward AW, Ceesay SM, Strain JJ, McKenna PG, Nevin GB, Barker ME, Hickey RJ. 1990. Simultaneous measurement of free-living energy expenditure by the doubly labeled water method and heart-rate monitoring. *American Journal of Clinical Nutrition* 52:59–65.

40. Bandini LG, Schoeller DA, Dietz WH. 1990. Energy expenditure in obese and nonobese adolescents. *Pediatric Research* 27:198–202.

41. Prentice AM, Black AE, Coward WA, Davies HL, Goldberg GR, Murgatroyd PR, Ashford J, Sawyer M, Whitehead RG. 1986. High levels of energy expenditure in obese women. *British Medical Journal* 292:983–987.

42. Johnson RK, Goran MI, Poehlman ET. 1994. Correlates of over- and underreporting of energy intake in healthy older men and women. *American Journal of Clinical Nutrition* 59:1286–1290.

43. Elia M, Fuller N, Murgatroyd P. 1988. The potential use of the labelled bicarbonate method for estimating energy expenditure in man. *Proceedings from the Nutrition Society* 47:247–258.

44. Elia M, Jones MG, Jennings G, Poppitt SD, Fuller NJ, Murgatroyd PR, Jebb SA. 1995. Estimating energy expenditure from specific activity of urine urea during lengthy subcutaneous NaH^{14}CO$_3$ infusion. *American Journal of Physiology* 269:E172–E182.

45. Gibney E, Elia M, Jebb SA, Murgatroyd P, Jennings G. 1997. Total energy expenditure in patients with small-cell lung cancer: Results of a validated study using the bicarbonate-urea method. *Metabolism* 46:1412–1417.

46. Paton NI, Elia M, Jebb SA, Jennings G, Macallan DC, Griffin GE. 1996. Total energy expenditure and physical activity measured with the bicarbonate-urea method in patients with human immunodeficiency virus infection. *Clinical Science* 91:241–245.

47. Harris JA, Benedict FG. 1919. *A biometric study of basal metabolism in man.* Publication 279. Washington, DC: Carnegie Institution of Washington.

48. Roza AM, Shizgal HM. 1984. The Harris Benedict equation reevaluated: Resting energy requirements and the body cell mass. *American Journal of Clinical Nutrition* 40:168–182.

49. Owen OE, Holup JL, D'Alessio DA, Craig ES, Polansky M, Smalley KJ, Karle EC, Bushman MC, Owen LR, Mozzoli MA, Kedrick ZV, Boden GH. 1987. A reappraisal of the caloric requirement of men. *American Journal of Clinical Nutrition* 46:875–885.

50. de Boer JO, van Es AJH, van Raaij JMA, Hautvast JGAJ. 1987. Energy requirements and energy expenditure of lean and overweight women, measured by indirect calorimetry. *American Journal of Clinical Nutrition* 46:13–21.

51. Mifflin MD, St Jeor ST, Hill LA, Scott BJ, Daugherty SA, Koh YO. 1990. A new predictive equation for resting energy expenditure in healthy individuals. *American Journal of Clinical Nutrition* 51:241–247.

52. Cunningham JJ. 1980. A reanalysis of the factors influencing basal metabolic rate in normal adults. *American Journal of Clinical Nutrition* 33:2372–2374.

53. World Health Organization. 1985. *Energy and protein requirements. Report of a joint FAO/WHO/UNU expert consultation.* Technical Report Series 724. Geneva, Switzerland: World Health Organization.

54. Ireton-Jones CS, Turner WW. 1991. Actual or ideal body weight: Which should be used to predict energy expenditure? *Journal of the American Dietetic Association* 91:193–195.

55. Parenteral and Enteral Nutrition Team. 1994. *Parenteral and enteral nutrition manual,* 7th ed. Ann Arbor, MI: University of Michigan Medical Center, p. 14.

56. Curreri PW. 1990. Assessing nutritional needs for the burned patient. *Journal of Trauma* 30(12 suppl):S20–S23.

57. Bell SJ, Wyatt J. 1986. Nutrition guidelines for burned patients. *Journal of the American Dietetic Association* 86:648–653.

58. Waymack JP, Herndon DN. 1992. Nutritional support of the burned patient. *World Journal of Surgery* 16:80–86.

59. Montegut WJ, Lowry SF. 1993. Nutrition in burn patients. *Seminars in Nephrology* 13:400–408.

60. Cunningham JJ, Lydon MK, Russell WE. 1990. Calorie and protein provision for recovery from severe burns in infants and young children. *American Journal of Clinical Nutrition* 51:533–537.

61. Allard JP, Pichard C, Hoshino E, Stechison S, Fareholm L, Peters WJ, Jeejeebhoy KN. 1990. Validation of a new formula for calculating the energy requirements of burn patients. *Journal of Parenteral and Enteral Nutrition* 14:115–118.

62. Hildreth MA, Herndon DN, Parks KH. 1987. Evaluation of a caloric requirement formula in burned children treated with early excision. *Journal of Trauma* 27:188–189.

63. Hansbrough JF. 1998. Enteral nutritional support in burn patients. *Gastrointestinal Endoscopy Clinics of North America* 8:645–667.

64. Curreri PW, Richmond D, Marvin J, Baxter CR. 1974. Dietary requirements of patients with major burns. *Journal of the American Dietetic Association* 65:415–417.

65. Saffle JR, Medina E, Raymond J, Westenskow D. 1985. Use of indirect calorimetry in the nutritional management of burned patients. *Journal of Trauma* 25:32–39.

66. Turner WW, Ireton CS, Hunt JL, Baster CR. 1985. Predicting energy expenditure in burned patients. *Journal of Trauma* 25:11–16.

67. Allard JP, Jeejeebhoy KN, Whitwell J, Pashutinski L, Peters WJ. 1988. Factors influencing energy expenditure in patients with burns. *Journal of Trauma* 28:199–202.

68. Royall D, Fairholm L, Peters WJ, Jeejeebhoy KJ, Allard JP. 1994. Continuous measurement of energy expenditure in ventilated burn patients: An analysis. *Critical Care Medicine* 22:399–406.

69. Mancusi-Ungaro HR, Van Way CW, McCool C. 1992. Caloric and nitrogen balance as predictors of nutritional outcome in patients with burns. *Journal of Burn Care and Rehabilitation* 13:695–702.

70. Benjamin DR. 1989. Laboratory tests and nutritional assessment:

Protein-energy status. *Pediatric Clinics of North America* 36:139–161.

71. Alcock NW. Laboratory tests for assessing nutritional status. In Shils ME, Olson JA, Shike M, Ross AC, eds. *Modern nutrition in health and disease,* 9th ed. Baltimore, MD: Williams & Wilkins.

72. Konstantinides FN, Radmer WJ, Becker WK, Herman VK, Warren WE, Solem LD, Williams JB, Cerra FB. 1992. Inaccuracy of nitrogen balance determinations in thermal injury with calculated total urinary nitrogen. *Journal of Burn Care and Rehabilitation* 13:254–260.

73. Loder PB, Kee AJ, Horsburgh R, Jones M, Smith RC. 1989. Validity of urinary urea nitrogen as a measure of total urinary nitrogen in adult patients requiring parenteral nutrition. *Critical Care Medicine* 17:309–312.

74. Milner EA, Cioffi WG, Mason AD, McManus WF, Pruitt BA. 1993. Accuracy of urinary urea nitrogen for predicting total urinary nitrogen

in thermally injured patients. *Journal of Parenteral and Enteral Nutrition* 17:414–416.

75. White JV, Ham RJ, Lipschitz DA, Dwyer JT, Wellman NS. 1991. Consensus of the Nutrition Screening Initative: Risk factors and indicators of poor nutritional status in older Americans. *Journal of the American Dietetic Association* 91:783–787.

76. White JV, Ham RJ, Lipschitz DA. 1991. *Report of nutrition screening 1: Toward a common goal.* Washington, DC: Nutrition Screening Initiative.

77. Dwyer JT. 1991. *Screening older Americans' nutritional health: Current practices and future possibilities.* Washington, DC: Nutrition Screening Initiative.

78. White JV, Dwyer JT, Possner BM, Ham RJ, Lipschitz DA, Wellman NS. 1992. Nutrition Screening Initiative: Development and implementation of the public awareness checklist and screening tools. *Journal of the American Dietetic Association* 92:163–167.

ASSESSMENT ACTIVITY 7.1

Estimating Stature and Body Weight

Although stature and body weight usually can be easily obtained by direct measurement, there are times when they have to be estimated. Stature can be estimated from knee height, age, sex, and race using the equations in Table 7.1. Body weight can be estimated from knee height, age, sex, race, and midarm circumference using the equations in Tables 7.3 and 7.4. In this assessment activity, you will have an opportunity to practice measuring knee height, midarm circumference, stature, and body weight. You will use the appropriate formulas in Tables 7.1, 7.3, and 7.4 for calculating estimates of stature and body weight and then will compare these estimates with values obtained by direct measurement.

Your class can divide into groups of two or three students and measure each other's knee height and midarm circumference as outlined in this chapter. Two consecutive measurements of knee height should agree with each other to within 0.5 cm and be recorded. Measurements of midarm circumference should be recorded to within

0.1 cm. Be sure to mark the triceps skinfold site (where the midarm circumference is measured) if you plan to measure the triceps skinfold site in Assessment Activity 7.2. These values then can be substituted into the appropriate equations to obtain estimates of stature and body weight. Stature and body weight then can be measured directly following the guidelines in Chapter 6.

Once all students have completed their measurements and calculations, these can be listed on the board or on a sheet of paper distributed to all students. The means and standard deviations of all estimates and measures can be quickly calculated using a pocket calculator with statistical functions. In addition, the differences between estimated and measured values for stature and body weight can be calculated, and the mean and standard deviations of these can be calculated as well.

What was the difference between the estimated and measured values? Although it is clearly better to directly measure stature and body weight, estimates are generally better than no values at all.

Arm Muscle Area

Arm muscle area is used as an index of lean tissue or muscle in the body and represents muscle protein reserves. This assessment activity will help familiarize you with the anthropometric measurements and calculations required in arriving at estimates of arm muscle area.

In addition to midarm circumference (already obtained in Assessment Activity 7.1), the formula for arm muscle area requires measurement of the triceps skinfold. If you marked the triceps skinfold site in Assessment Activity 7.1, it will be easy to make this measurement. Review the section on triceps skinfold measurement in Chapter 6 if necessary. A pocket calculator and the following equations can be used for calculating corrected arm muscle area:

$$\text{cAMA for females} = \frac{[\text{MAC} - (\pi \times \text{TSF})]^2}{4\pi} - 6.5$$

$$\text{cAMA for males} = \frac{[\text{MAC} - (\pi \times \text{TSF})]^2}{4\pi} - 10$$

where cAMA = corrected arm muscle area in cm^2; MAC = midarm circumference in cm; and TSF = triceps skinfold thickness in cm. Note that these equations call for all measurements to be made in *centimeters*. **The nomogram in** Figure 7.14 also can be used to calculate corrected arm muscle area.

Appendix R provides means, standard deviations, and percentiles of arm muscle area for males and females ages 1 to 74 years. For persons ages 18 years and older, the values are for corrected arm muscle area. Table 7.6 can be used for interpreting these age/sex percentile values. No single index (for example, arm muscle area) is a reliable indicator of nutritional status. Basic assumptions inferred from anthropometry should be corroborated by data derived from dietary, biochemical, and clinical observations.

NUTRITIONAL ASSESSMENT IN DISEASE PREVENTION

INTRODUCTION

The prominent role of diet and nutritional status in several leading causes of death for Americans gives nutritional assessment an important role to play in disease prevention. This chapter addresses nutritional assessment as it relates to three major causes of death and disability: coronary heart disease, osteoporosis, and diabetes.

Several risk factors of coronary heart disease, the leading cause of death for Americans, are related to diet. Among these are elevated serum total and low-density-lipoprotein cholesterol (LDL-C), low levels of high-density-lipoprotein cholesterol (HDL-C), obesity, hypertension, and diabetes. This chapter also discusses issues in measuring lipid and lipoprotein levels, which apply to practically all measurements in nutritional assessment.

Osteoporosis, a loss of mineral from bones that leaves them weakened and more likely to fracture, is a major cause of disability and death among older persons. Available methods for assessing bone mineral content are discussed. We conclude the chapter with a discussion of criteria for diagnosing diabetes.

Reducing the individual and societal burden imposed by these and other diseases lies in our ability to prevent their premature onset through early diagnosis and research into more effective preventive measures. Nutritional assessment plays a prominent role in each of these.

CORONARY HEART DISEASE

Coronary heart disease, also referred to as coronary artery disease, is one of more than 50 different diseases affecting the heart and blood vessels, which collectively are known as cardiovascular diseases. Coronary heart disease results when the coronary arteries supplying the heart with vital oxygen and nutrients become narrowed and inelastic because of atherosclerosis. Evidence supports the view that atherosclerosis begins in childhood with the formation of a fatty streak as lipids (primarily cholesterol and its esters) become deposited in macrophages (large phagocytic cells located within connective tissue) and smooth muscle cells within the inner lining of large elastic and muscular arteries. These early lesions do not disturb blood flow in the affected artery. As more lipid collects within the artery wall during adolescence and early adulthood, a fibrous plaque develops that projects into the channel, or lumen, of the artery, resulting in ischemia, or impaired blood flow. Ischemia within the heart muscle or myocardium can result in angina pectoris, which is chest pain caused by insufficient blood flow to the heart. If the impaired blood flow is severe enough, the tissues fed by the obstructed artery may die. This is known as an infarct. When this process affects the coronary arteries, a heart attack, or myocardial infarction, occurs. When the cerebral arteries are affected (known as cerebrovascular disease), a stroke results. Atherosclerotic changes within the aorta and iliac and femoral arteries can result in peripheral vascular disease.

Coronary heart disease (CHD) is the leading cause of death of American males and females.[1] More than 6 million Americans alive today have CHD. According to American Heart Association estimates, about 1.1 million Americans have heart attacks each year. Each year, nearly 500,000 people die of heart attack. Nearly half of these deaths occur before the victims reach the hospital. This is due in part to the unfortunate fact that about half of all heart attack victims wait more than 2 hours before seeking help. Everyone should be familiar with the warning signs of heart attack (outlined in Box 8.1) and promptly seek medical care if they occur. Despite a more than 26% decline in the death rate from CHD since 1988, it remains the leading cause of death in the United States and many other Western nations.[1]

Coronary Heart Disease Risk Factors

As discussed in Chapter 1, several factors or traits influence a person's risk of developing CHD and how rapidly atherosclerosis progresses.[1,2] The risk factors other than

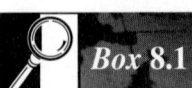
Box 8.1   **Warning Signals of a Heart Attack**

- Uncomfortable pressure, fullness, squeezing, or pain in the center of the chest that lasts more than a few minutes or goes away and comes back
- Pain spreading to the shoulders, neck, or arms

- Chest discomfort with lightheadedness, fainting, sweating, nausea, or shortness of breath

Not all of these warning signs occur in every heart attack. If some start to occur, however, don't wait. Get help immediately. Adapted from *Heart stroke and facts.* 2000. Dallas, TX: American Heart Association.

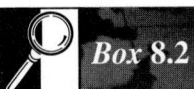

Box 8.2   Major Coronary Heart Disease Risk Factors Other Than LDL Cholesterol*

POSITIVE RISK FACTORS

- Current cigarette smoking
- Hypertension (blood pressure ≥ 140/90 mm Hg or on antihypertensive medication)
- Low HDL cholesterol (< 40 mg/dL)
- Family history of premature CHD (CHD in a male first-degree relative < 55 years old or CHD in a female first-degree relative < 65 years old)**
- Presence of CHD risk equivalents†
- Age (men ≥ 45 years old; women ≥ 55 years old)

NEGATIVE RISK FACTORS‡

- HDL cholesterol ≥ 60 mg/dL

**A first-degree relative is one's parent, sibling, or offspring.
†CHD risk equivalents include diabetes mellitus; clinical forms of atherosclerotic disease (other than CHD), such as peripheral arterial disease, abdominal aortic aneurysm, and symptomatic carotid artery disease; and the presence of multiple risk factors, which together confer a 10-year risk for CHD that is greater than 20%.

*The presence of one or more risk factors influences low-density lipoprotein treatment goals. Age (defined differently for men and women) is treated as a risk factor because rates of CHD are higher in the elderly than in the young, and higher in men than in women of the same age. Obesity is not listed as a risk factor because it operates through other risk factors that are included (hypertension, hyperlipidemia, decreased HDL-C), but it should be considered a target for intervention. Physical inactivity is similarly not listed as a risk factor, but it, too, should be considered a target for intervention, and physical activity is recommended as desirable for everyone.
‡If HDL-C is ≥ 60 mg/dL, subtract one risk factor because high HDL-C decreases CHD risk.

Adapted from National Cholesterol Education Program. 2001. *Third report of the expert panel on detection, evaluation, and treatment of high blood cholesterol in adults.* Bethesda, MD: U.S. Department of Health and Human Services, Public Health Service; National Institutes of Health; National Heart, Lung, and Blood Institute.

LDL-C levels are shown in Box 8.2. The "positive" risk factors are those that increase CHD risk. An HDL-C level ≥ 60 mg/dL is considered a "negative" risk factor because it decreases risk of CHD. Some of these risk factors are modifiable (e.g., cigarette smoking and, to a somewhat lesser degree, hypertension) while others are obviously not modifiable (e.g., age, male sex, and family history of premature CHD).

Serum Lipids and Lipoproteins

Cholesterol is a lipid, or fatlike, substance present only in foods of animal origin and synthesized by the body. It serves as a structural component of cell membranes and a precursor for steroid hormones and vitamin D, and it is used by the liver to form bile acids, which facilitate fat digestion and absorption. About 93% of the body's cholesterol is present in cell membranes, whereas only about 7% circulates in the blood. Triglyceride, a compound consisting of three fatty acids esterified to a molecule of glycerol, is the usual storage form of lipid in humans and animals.

There is a strong causal relationship between elevated low-density-lipoprotein cholesterol (LDL-C) and incidence of and mortality from CHD.[1–5] As serum LDL-C concentration increases, risk of CHD rises proportionally. CHD is rare in groups having a low serum LDL-C concentration, even when other CHD risk factors, such as cigarette smoking, hypertension, and diabetes mellitus, are relatively common.[3,4] The National Cholesterol Education Program has concluded that elevated LDL cholesterol is a major cause of CHD and, in its *Third Report of the National Cholesterol Education Program Expert*

Panel on Detection, Evaluation, and Treatment of High Blood Cholesterol in Adults (referred to as the *Adult Treatment Panel III* or *ATP III*), the primary goals for the prevention and treatment of CHD are stated in terms of serum concentration of LDL-C.[2]

Because lipids such as cholesterol and triglycerides are fat soluble, they must be transported within the bloodstream from sites of absorption or synthesis to sites of storage or metabolism by lipoproteins. The major lipid-transporting lipoproteins are chylomicrons, very low-density lipoprotein (VLDL), low-density lipoproteins (LDL), and high-density lipoprotein (HDL).[3,6] Lipoproteins are spherical macromolecular complexes of lipids (triglycerides, cholesterol, cholesterol esters, and phospholipids) and proteins known as apoproteins. Apoproteins control the interaction and metabolic fate of lipoproteins. They activate enzymes that modify the composition and structure of lipoproteins, they are involved in the binding and ingestion of lipoproteins by cells, and they participate in the exchange of lipids among lipoproteins of different classes.[6] Figure 8.1 shows the relative size and the lipid composition of the three major lipoprotein particles.

Chylomicrons are the largest lipoproteins, containing about 90% triglycerides by weight. They are synthesized in the intestine and transport dietary triglycerides from the small intestine to adipose tissue, muscle, and the liver. The dietary cholesterol they carry is taken up by the liver for production of bile acids or later incorporation into VLDL. Chylomicrons are not found in fasting serum, except in certain disease states.[6]

VLDL is 60% triglyceride by weight and contains 10% to 15% of the serum's total cholesterol. It is

High-density lipoprotein

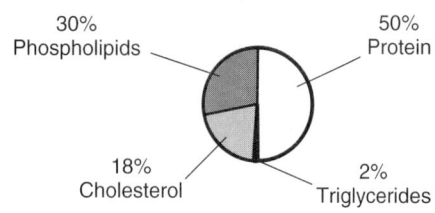

30%
Phospholipids

50%
Protein

18%
Cholesterol

2%
Triglycerides

Low-density lipoprotein

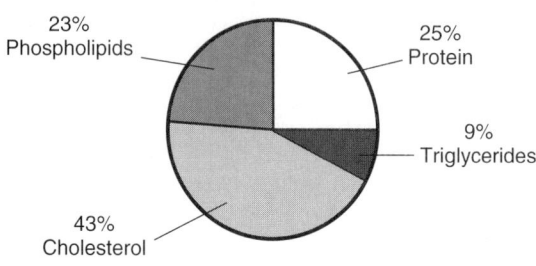

23%
Phospholipids

25%
Protein

9%
Triglycerides

43%
Cholesterol

Very low-density lipoprotein

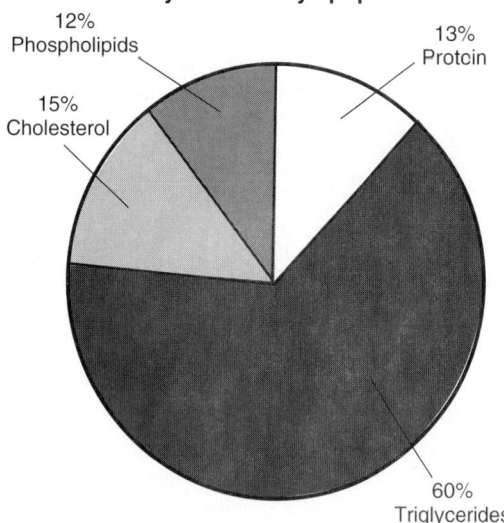

12%
Phospholipids

13%
Protein

15%
Cholesterol

60%
Triglycerides

Figure 8.1 **The relative size and the lipid composition of the three major lipoprotein particles found in fasting serum.**

Source: From Haskell WL. 1994. The influence of exercise on the concentrations of triglyceride and cholesterol in human plasma. *Exercise and Sports Science Review* 12:205–244.

synthesized in the liver and primarily carries triglyceride to the cells for storage and metabolism. Removal of triglyceride from VLDL results in smaller, denser particles known as intermediate-density lipoprotein (IDL). The density of IDL falls between that of VLDL and LDL. About half the IDL is catabolized by the liver, and the remaining IDL undergoes additional changes (for example, uptake of cholesterol) that transforms it into LDL.

Thus, LDL levels are linked to hepatic VLDL production and IDL catabolism.

The primary role of LDL is to transport cholesterol to the various cells of the body. LDL contains approximately 70% of the serum's total cholesterol, is considered the most atherogenic (atherosclerosis-producing) lipoprotein, and *is the prime target of attempts to lower serum cholesterol.* Clinical trials have shown, for example, that, for every 1% decrease in serum total cholesterol (most of which is found in the LDL particle), CHD risk falls roughly 2%. About 70% to 80% of LDL is removed from the serum by LDL receptors located on the plasma membranes of hepatic and peripheral cells. The remaining 20% to 30% is degraded by macrophages.

Most clinical laboratories do not measure LDL-C directly. Instead, they calculate it based on measurements of total cholesterol, HDL-C, and triglyceride. In this procedure, VLDL cholesterol (VLDL-C) is estimated by dividing triglyceride by 5. The following equation is recommended by the National Cholesterol Education Program:[2]

$$\text{LDL-C} = \text{TC} - \text{HDL-C} - (\text{TG} \div 5)$$

where TC = total cholesterol and TG = triglyceride. This formula cannot be used when the triglyceride level is > 300 mg/dL.

HDL is the smallest and densest of the lipoproteins. Secreted by the liver and small intestine in a disc-shaped form, HDL eventually assumes a spherical shape as it takes up phospholipids and cholesterol from other lipoproteins and body cells. As serum HDL levels *rise,* risk of CHD *decreases.* In other words, higher serum levels of HDL are protective against risk for CHD.[2,5]

Data from several studies have shown that a 1% increase in serum HDL cholesterol (the cholesterol carried by the HDL particle) translates into a 1.5% to 2% reduction in CHD risk.

HDL is thought to be involved in the reverse transport of cholesterol.[3–5] It is currently hypothesized that HDL picks up cholesterol from the bloodstream and various cells of the body and transports it to the liver and other lipoproteins, where it is excreted in the bile, converted to bile acids, or reprocessed into VLDL. It is theorized that this reverse transport process is responsible, at least in part, for the strong inverse relationship between serum HDL-C and CHD risk, although it is likely that other mechanisms are involved as well.[3–5]

A more recently discovered lipoprotein, and one in which there is currently considerable interest, is lipoprotein(a) [Lp(a)] or "lipoprotein small a." Lp(a) is a low-density lipoprotein-like particle that shares many characteristics with plasminogen.[7–9] Some research suggests that Lp(a) may promote blood coagulation by interfering with the action of plasminogen and plasmin, which are involved in the lysis, or dissolution, of blood clots and inhibition of blood clotting. This could lead to thrombus formation in atherosclerotic arteries and increased risk of heart attack or stroke. However, the role of Lp(a) in blood coagulation is not clear. Studies investigating the relationship of Lp(a) to CHD risk have yielded conflicting results. In those studies suggesting that Lp(a) is an independent risk factor for CHD, the mechanism underlying its association with CHD has not been defined. Simple and accurate methods for measuring Lp(a) have yet to be developed, and its potential use as a marker of increased risk for CHD is still in the research stage. In addition, there is no effective therapy for lowering elevated Lp(a) levels.

Lipoproteins, Cholesterol, and Coronary Heart Disease

The relationship between serum total cholesterol and CHD mortality is shown in Figure 8.2.[2] It can be noted that CHD risk steadily increases as serum cholesterol rises. The increase in CHD risk is particularly steep after serum cholesterol rises above 200 mg/dL (5.17 mmol/L). For example, men whose cholesterol levels are at or above the 90th percentile have four times the risk of CHD compared with men whose cholesterol levels are at or below the 10th percentile.[2,10]

Guidelines developed by the National Cholesterol Education Program (NCEP) for classifying total cholesterol and HDL-C levels in adults are shown in Table 8.1. The cutoff point that defines "high blood cholesterol" (total cholesterol of 240 mg/dL) is the value above which risk of CHD rises steeply and corresponds to approximately the 80th percentile for the adult U.S.

TABLE 8.1	Classification of LDL, Total, and HDL Cholesterol*

LDL Cholesterol

	mg/dL	mmol/L
Optimal	< 100	< 2.59
Near optimal/above optimal	100–129	2.59–3.35
Borderline high	130–159	3.36–4.13
High	160–189	4.14–4.90
Very high	≥ 190	≥ 4.91

Total Cholesterol

Desirable	< 200	< 5.17
Borderline high	200–239	5.17–6.19
High	≥ 240	≥ 6.20

HDL Cholesterol

Low	< 40	< 1.03
High	≥ 60	≥ 1.55

From National Cholesterol Education Program. 2001. *Third report of the expert panel on detection, evaluation, and treatment of high blood cholesterol in adults.* Bethesda, MD: U.S. Department of Health and Human Services, Public Health Service; National Institutes of Health; National Heart, Lung, and Blood Institute

*LDL = low-density lipoprotein; HDL = high-density lipoprotein.

population based on data from the third National Health and Nutrition Examination Survey (NHANES III). Reference values for serum levels of total cholesterol, LDL cholesterol, and HDL cholesterol and the ratio of total cholesterol to HDL cholesterol (TC/HDL-C) are given in Appendix S.

The atherosclerotic process begins in childhood and progresses slowly into adulthood.[2,11,12] There is also evidence that children and adolescents with elevated serum cholesterol frequently come from families whose adult members have a high incidence of CHD or elevated serum cholesterol levels.[11] For these reasons, the NCEP has established guidelines for classifying total cholesterol and LDL-C levels in children and adolescents from families with elevated serum cholesterol levels or premature CHD. These are shown in Table 8.2. The average total cholesterol and LDL-C levels in persons ages 1 to 19 years are approximately 160 mg/dL (4.14 mmol/L) and 100 mg/dL (2.59 mmol/L), respectively. The cutoff points for the "borderline" (170 mg/dL) and "high" (200 mg/dL) values in this age group correspond to the 75th and 95th percentiles, respectively.

How do mean (average) cholesterol levels for adult Americans compare with these standards? According to data from NHANES III, shown in Figure 8.3, the mean total cholesterol levels for all U.S. males and females ages 20 years and over are 205 mg/dL and 207 mg/dL, respectively. Mean total cholesterol levels for males ages 20 to 34 years and for females ages 20 to 44 years are within the range considered as "desirable" by the NCEP. For the rest of adult Americans, mean levels are greater

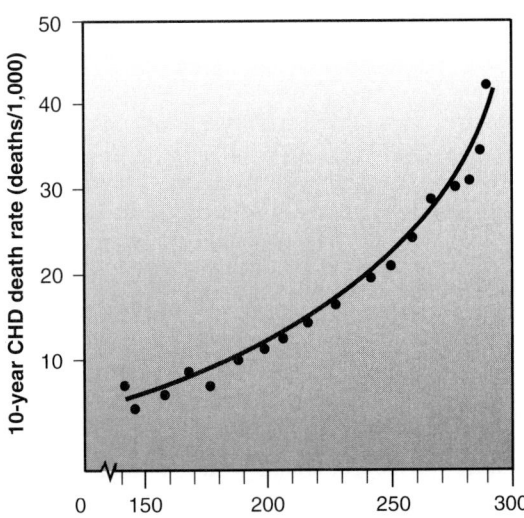

Figure 8.2 **The relationship between serum total cholesterol and coronary heart disease (CHD) mortality in men.**

Source: From National Cholesterol Education Program. 1993. *Second report of the expert panel on detection, evaluation, and treatment of high blood cholesterol in adults.* Bethesda, MD: U.S. Department of Health and Human Services, Public Health Service; National Institutes of Health; National Heart, Lung, and Blood Institute.

| TABLE 8.2 | The National Cholesterol Education Program's Classification of Total Cholesterol and LDL-C Levels in Children and Adolescents from Families with Hypercholesterolemia or Premature Coronary Heart Disease |

	Total Cholesterol		Low-Density-Lipoprotein Cholesterol	
	mg/dL	mmol/L	mg/dL	mmol/L
Acceptable	< 170	< 4.40	< 110	< 2.84
Borderline-high	170–199	4.40–5.16	110–129	2.84–3.35
High	≥ 200	≥ 5.17	≥ 130	≥ 3.36

From National Cholesterol Education Program. 1991. *Report of the expert panel on blood cholesterol levels in children and adolescents.* Bethesda, MD: U.S. Department of Health and Human Services, Public Health Service; National Institutes of Health; National Heart, Lung, and Blood Institute.

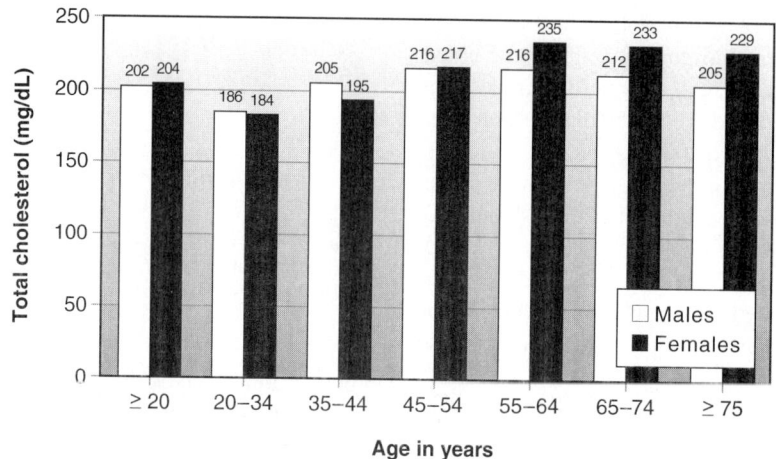

Figure 8.3 Mean total cholesterol levels of adult Americans, 1988–1994.
As Americans age, their mean serum total cholesterol levels rise. After about age 35, serum total cholesterol levels for most Americans are greater than that recommended by the National Cholesterol Education Program.
Source: Data from the National Center for Health Statistics.

than desirable. Thus, the majority of Americans could benefit from lower serum cholesterol.

In contrast to total cholesterol and LDL-C levels, CHD risk *falls* as HDL-C levels *rise*.[2–5] According to data from the Framingham Heart Study, in the presence of high serum HDL-C levels, the risk of CHD is relatively low, even in subjects with increased serum total cholesterol or LDL-C. In contrast, persons with low HDL-C levels are at increased CHD risk, even if their total cholesterol and LDL-C levels are within the "desirable" range.

According to the NCEP, an HDL-C level below 40 mg/dL (1.03 mmol/L) is defined as a "low" serum level and is considered a major risk factor. An HDL-C level ≥ 60 mg/dL (≥1.55 mmol/L) is considered a "negative risk factor," which decreases CHD risk.[2]

Lipoprotein Ratios

Another approach to evaluating HDL-C levels that is suggested by some investigators is to calculate the ratio of two lipid values—for example, the LDL-C/HDL-C ratio (LDL-C level divided by HDL-C level) and the TC/HDL-C ratio (total cholesterol level divided by HDL-C level).[12–16] Data from the Framingham Heart Study show that, the higher a person's TC/HDL-C ratio, the greater is his or her risk of having symptomatic CHD. In other words, as total cholesterol increases in proportion to HDL-C, CHD risk increases as well. According to Framingham data, 50- to 70-year-old men having a TC/HDL-C ratio of 4.4 have an average risk for CHD, compared with men their age. This cutoff point roughly corresponds to a total cholesterol of 200 mg/dL (5.17 mmol/L) and an HDL-C of 45 mg/dL (1.16 mmol/L). Those having a TC/HDL-C ratio of 3.0 have half the risk, and those with a ratio of 6.2, 7.7, or 9.5 have two, three, or four times the average risk, respectively.[15] Although not a substitute for measurements of individual lipid and lipoprotein levels, the TC/HDL-C ratio appears, in many instances, to be a valuable adjunct to evaluating CHD risk.[10]

Figure 8.4 illustrates the relationship between the total cholesterol/HDL-C ratio and risk of myocardial infarction. The figure is based on data collected by Harvard University researchers as part of the Health Professionals Follow-Up Study.[17] The researchers considered a ratio of less than 3.0 to be optimal. As a subject's ratio increased above 3.0, relative risk of myocardial infarction increased. The average American male has a ratio of 4.6, while the average American female's ratio is 4.0.

Triglyceride and Coronary Heart Disease

The connection between serum triglyceride levels and CHD risk is controversial.[2,18-20] Most population studies show serum plasma triglyceride levels to be positively associated with increased CHD risk. However, in most of these studies, triglyceride was not shown to act independently to increase CHD risk after statistical adjustments were made for closely associated factors, such as total cholesterol, HDL-C, high blood pressure, cigarette smoking, and obesity. Some researchers argue that elevated triglyceride levels reflect certain lipoprotein alterations (elevated VLDL-C and LDL-C and decreased HDL-C) or accompany other disease states known to increase CHD risk, such as diabetes mellitus, nephrotic syndrome, and chronic renal disease.[2,15] More recent meta-analyses of prospective studies, however, suggest that elevated serum triglyceride is an independent risk factor for CHD, particularly in persons with low HDL-C.[21,22] Consequently, the NCEP, in its *Adult Treatment Panel III,* now recognizes elevated triglyceride as an independent risk factor for CHD

and has identified VLDL cholesterol as a target for cholesterol-lowering therapy. Table 8.3 provides NCEP guidelines for classifying serum triglyceride.

Estimating CHD Risk

The National Cholesterol Education Program has developed charts for estimating the actual likelihood (or "absolute risk") that one will develop CHD within the next 10 years.[2,23] Table 8.4 shows the chart for adult males, and Table 8.5 shows the chart for adult females. The charts are based on data collected from the Framingham Study and use the following variables: age, total serum cholesterol, serum HDL cholesterol, systolic blood pressure, whether one is being treated for hypertension, and cigarette smoking. Total and HDL cholesterol measurements should be the average of at least two measurements obtained from lipoprotein analysis. Although the charts use total and HDL cholesterol as variables, LDL cholesterol remains the primary target of cholesterol-lowering therapy. Systolic blood pressure should be based on the average of several blood pressure measurements. Note that the number of points assigned for systolic blood pressure depends on whether one is taking medication to treat hypertension ("treated") or not receiving any antihypertensive treatment ("untreated"). The term *smoker* applies to any cigarette smoking in the past month.

To estimate the likelihood that one will develop CHD in the next 10 years, select the appropriate chart (male or female), determine the points for each variable, enter these in the appropriate spaces, and then determine the point total. By comparing the point total with the values in the table at the bottom left corner of each chart, it is possible to determine one's "absolute" 10-year risk for CHD—in other words, the person's actual likelihood of developing coronary heart disease. For example, if one's absolute 10-year risk is > 20%, then there is a greater than 1 in 5 chance of developing CHD in the next 10 years. The *ATP III* guidelines recommend that this assessment of absolute 10-year risk be used in determining the intensity of therapy for reducing CHD risk for persons with two or more CHD risk factors.[2,23] In persons

Figure 8.4 **Total cholesterol/HDL-C ratio and risk for myocardial infarction.** As the total cholesterol/HDL cholesterol ratio increases, the risk of myocardial infarction (MI) increases.

Source: Data from Stampfer MJ, Sacks FM, Salvini S, Willett WC, Hennekens CH. 1991. A prospective study of cholesterol, apolipoproteins, and the risk of myocardial infarction. *New England Journal of Medicine* 325:373–381.

TABLE 8.3	**Classification of Serum Triglyceride**	
	mg/dL	mmol/L
Normal	< 150	< 1.69
Borderline-high	150–199	1.69–2.25
High	200–499	2.26–5.64
Very high	≥ 500	≥ 5.65

From National Cholesterol Education Program. 2001. *Third report of the expert panel on detection, evaluation, and treatment of high blood cholesterol in adults.* Bethesda, MD: U.S. Department of Health and Human Services, Public Health Service; National Institutes of Health; National Heart, Lung, and Blood Institute.

TABLE 8.4 | **Estimating Risk of CHD in the Next 10 Years, Men**

Ages	Points
20–34	–9
35–39	–4
40–44	0
45–49	3
50–54	6
55–59	8
60–64	10
65–69	11
70–74	12
75–79	13

Total Cholesterol*	Points at Ages 20–39	Points at Ages 40–49	Points at Ages 50–59	Points at Ages 60–69	Points at Ages 70–79
< 160	0	0	0	0	0
160–199	4	3	2	1	0
200–239	7	5	3	1	0
240–279	9	6	4	2	1
≥ 280	11	8	5	3	1

	Points at Ages 20–39	Points at Ages 40–49	Points at Ages 50–59	Points at Ages 60–69	Points at Ages 70–79
Nonsmoker	0	0	0	0	0
Smoker	8	5	3	1	1

HDL*	Points
≥ 60	–1
50–59	0
40–49	1
< 40	2

Systolic BP†	Untreated	Treated
< 120	0	0
120–129	0	1
130–139	1	2
140–159	1	2
≥ 160	2	3

Point Total	10-Year Risk (%)
< 0	< 1
0–4	1
5–6	2
7	3
8	4
9	5
10	6
11	8
12	10
13	12
14	16
15	20
16	25
≥ 17	≥ 30

How to Use This Risk-Prediction Chart

1. Determine the points for each variable and then total the points in the spaces below:

Age	+	Total Cholesterol	+	HDL	+	Smoking	+	Systolic BP	=	Point Total

2. Compare point total with the chart to the left to determine one's risk of developing CHD in the next 10 years.

Adapted from National Cholesterol Education Program. 2001. *Third report of the expert panel on detection, evaluation, and treatment of high blood cholesterol in adults.* Bethesda, MD: U.S. Department of Health and Human Services, Public Health Service; National Institutes of Health; National Heart, Lung, and Blood Institute.
*Measured in mg/dL
†Measured in mmHg

TABLE 8.5 | Estimating Risk of CHD in the Next 10 Years, Women

Ages	Points
20–34	−7
35–39	−3
40–44	0
45–49	3
50–54	6
55–59	8
60–64	10
65–69	12
70–74	14
75–79	16

Total Cholesterol*	Points at Ages 20–39	Points at Ages 40–49	Points at Ages 50–59	Points at Ages 60–69	Points at Ages 70–79
<160	0	0	0	0	0
160–199	4	3	2	1	1
200–239	8	6	4	2	1
240–279	11	8	5	3	2
≥280	13	10	7	4	2

	Points at Ages 20–39	Points at Ages 40–49	Points at Ages 50–59	Points at Ages 60–69	Points at Ages 70–79
Nonsmoker	0	0	0	0	0
Smoker	9	7	4	2	1

HDL*	Points
≥60	−1
50–59	0
40–49	1
<40	2

Systolic BP†	Untreated	Treated
<120	0	0
120–129	1	3
130–139	2	4
140–159	3	5
≥160	4	6

Point Total	10-Year Risk (%)	Point Total	10-Year Risk (%)
<9	<1	19	8
9–12	1	20	11
13–14	2	21	14
15	3	22	17
16	4	23	22
17	5	24	27
18	6	≥25	≥30

How to Use This Risk-Prediction Chart

1. Determine the points for each variable and then total the points in the spaces below:

Age	+	Total Cholesterol	+	HDL	+	Smoking	+	Systolic BP	=	Point Total

2. Compare point total with the chart to the left to determine one's risk of developing CHD in the next 10 years.

Adapted from National Cholesterol Education Program. 2001. *Third report of the expert panel on detection, evaluation, and treatment of high blood cholesterol in adults.* Bethesda, MD: U.S. Department of Health and Human Services, Public Health Service; National Institutes of Health; National Heart, Lung, and Blood Institute.
*Measured in mg/dL
†Measured in mmHg

with 0 to 1 risk factor, short-term and long-term CHD is so low that use of the charts is not considered necessary.

National Cholesterol Education Program's Guidelines

The NCEP was created by the National Heart, Lung, and Blood Institute in November 1985 with the overall goal of reducing the prevalence of high blood cholesterol in the United States. It has issued reports, written by different panels of experts, that address elevated cholesterol levels in several populations. These reports recommend the *patient-based approach* and/or the *population-based, or public health, approach*.[2,24] The former establishes guidelines for the identification and treatment by physicians of individuals with elevated cholesterol levels. The latter approach emphasizes dietary and lifestyle changes that can be made by all people to lower average cholesterol levels in the entire population. The two approaches are complementary, and together they represent a coordinated strategy for reducing coronary risk.

Two somewhat related concepts are primary prevention and secondary prevention. Primary prevention involves risk factor reduction (smoking cessation, lowering of elevated total and LDL cholesterol levels, control of high blood pressure, and so on) in patients with no evidence or diagnosis of CHD. Secondary prevention involves risk factor reduction in patients who have evidence of CHD and in whom CHD or some other atherosclerotic disease has been diagnosed. The National Cholesterol Education Program considers primary prevention to be the most effective approach for reducing the prevalence of CHD in the United States.[2]

In 1988, the NCEP published the *Report of the Expert Panel on Detection, Evaluation, and Treatment of High Blood Cholesterol in Adults.*[25] This report outlined a patient-based strategy for the primary prevention of coronary heart disease in persons with "high" LDL-C ($\geq$ 160 mg/dL) and in persons having a "borderline-high" LDL-C (130–159 mg/dL) and two or more CHD risk factors. This report was revised in 1993, when the NCEP published its *Second Report of the Expert Panel on Detection, Evaluation, and Treatment of High Blood Cholesterol in Adults.*[24] This report affirmed the conclusions of the previous one and added the recommendation that persons with established CHD maintain a somewhat more rigorous LDL-C goal of $\leq$ 100 mg/dL. Another revision, the *Third Report of the Expert Panel on Detection, Evaluation, and Treatment of High Blood Cholesterol in Adults* (the *ATP III*), was published in 2001.[2] This report continues to build on the foundation of the two previous reports while making several new recommendations, as outlined in Box 8.3. In 1990, the *Report of the Expert Panel on Population Strategies for Blood Cholesterol Reduction* was published.[26] As the title indicates, this report took a population-based, or public health,

approach to the problem of elevated blood cholesterol levels among Americans. The *Report of the Expert Panel on Blood Cholesterol Levels in Children and Adolescents,* published by the NCEP in 1991, made recommendations that were both patient-based and population-based.[11] All of these reports make similar dietary and other lifestyle recommendations.

Assessing Risk for Coronary Heart Disease

The *Third Report of the Expert Panel on Detection, Evaluation, and Treatment of High Blood Cholesterol in Adults* (also known as the *Adult Treatment Panel III* or *ATP III*), identifies risk assessment as the first step to be taken in reducing one's risk for CHD. Risk assessment is the basis for establishing the goal for serum LDL cholesterol and other targets for CHD risk reduction, such as dietary change, blood pressure control, smoking cessation, weight reduction, and increased physical activity. Risk assessment involves three components: (1) a complete lipoprotein profile (measurement of serum total cholesterol, LDL cholesterol, HDL cholesterol, and triglycerides); (2) identification of the presence of clinical CHD as well as what the *ATP III* calls "CHD risk equivalents"; and (3) identification of the major, independent CHD risk factors other than elevated LDL-C (review Box 8.2).

The *ATP III* recommends that all adults ages 20 years or more have a fasting lipoprotein profile performed at least once every 5 years. Because of potential analytical errors, the profile should be done twice within a period of 1 to 8 weeks and the values averaged. If the values for LDL-C from the two profiles differ by more than 30 mg/dL, a third profile should be performed and the three values averaged. Fasting is necessary for the accurate measurement of triglyceride, which is required for the calculation of LDL-C. However, total cholesterol and HDL-C can be accurately measured in the nonfasting state. If the nonfasting total cholesterol is $\geq$ 200 mg/dL or HDL-C is < 40 mg/dL, then measurement of LDL-C is warranted, and a fasting lipoprotein profile is recommended for proper management of serum lipids and lipoprotein values based on LDL-C. The *ATP III* classifications of total cholesterol, LDL-C, and HDL-C were shown in Table 8.1. Results of the lipoprotein profile must be interpreted with caution in persons recovering from a recent heart attack or unstable angina. When LDL-C is > 100 mg/dL, a clinical evaluation should be done to rule out a genetic disorder or secondary causes.

A prior diagnosis of CHD (the presence of preexisting CHD) markedly increases one's risk of recurrent CHD. The presence of CHD risk equivalents also markedly increases one's risk for coronary heart disease. CHD risk equivalents are conditions or combinations of CHD risk factors that increase the risk of CHD to a level

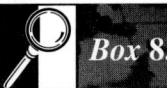

Box 8.3 New Features of the *ATP III*

INCREASED FOCUS ON MULTIPLE RISK FACTORS

- Diabetes is regarded as a "CHD risk equivalent." Persons diagnosed with diabetes but who are not diagnosed with CHD have a markedly elevated risk for CHD, which is roughly equivalent to those already diagnosed with CHD. Other CHD risk equivalents include peripheral arterial disease, abdominal aortic aneurysm, symptomatic carotid artery disease, and any combination of other CHD risk factors that confer an absolute 10-year risk of CHD that is greater than 20%.
- Data from the Framingham Heart Study are used to predict one's likelihood of having CHD in the next 10 years ("absolute 10-year risk"), using the charts shown in Tables 8.4 and 8.5. Persons with a higher absolute 10-year risk should make more intensive therapeutic lifestyle changes.
- Persons with multiple metabolic risk factors, such as abdominal obesity, hypertension, insulin resistance, low HDL-C, and elevated triglycerides (characteristics of the "metabolic syndrome"), are identified as candidates for more intensive therapeutic lifestyle changes.

MODIFICATIONS OF LIPID AND LIPOPROTEIN CLASSIFICATIONS

- *ATP III* creates an "optimal" level of LDL-C (< 100 mg/dL)

- *ATP III* changes definition of "low" HDL-C from < 35 mg/dL to < 40 mg/dL. The latter value is considered a better indicator of depressed HDL-C.
- *ATP III* lowers the cutpoints for classifying triglyceride to give more attention to moderate triglyceride elevations

SUPPORT FOR IMPLEMENTATION

- The preferred initial blood test is now a complete lipoprotein profile, which includes serum measurements of total cholesterol, LDL cholesterol, HDL cholesterol, and triglycerides.
- *ATP III* encourages the use of plant stanols and sterols and viscous (soluble) dietary fiber as therapeutic dietary options to enhance the lowering of LDL cholesterol.
- *ATP III* presents strategies for promoting a person's adherence to the therapeutic lifestyle changes and drug therapies.
- *ATP III* recommends treatment beyond LDL cholesterol lowering for persons with triglycerides ≥ 200 mg/dL.

Adapted from National Cholesterol Education Program. 2001. *Third report of the expert panel on detection, evaluation, and treatment of high blood cholesterol in adults.* Bethesda, MD: U.S. Department of Health and Human Services, Public Health Service; National Institutes of Health; National Heart, Lung, and Blood Institute.

equivalent to that of diagnosed CHD. CHD risk equivalents include clinical forms of atherosclerotic disease other than CHD (e.g., peripheral arterial disease, abdominal aortic aneurysm, and symptomatic carotid artery disease), diabetes, and CHD risk factors that together result in an absolute 10-year CHD risk of greater than 20%.[2] It is important to note that diabetes is considered a CHD risk equivalent due to the markedly elevated risk of CHD in persons with diabetes.

The presence of other CHD risk factors that were shown in Box 8.2 should then be assessed. Persons with two or more of these risk factors should have their absolute 10-year (short-term) CHD risk evaluated, using the charts in Tables 8.4 and 8.5. A 10-year CHD risk greater than 20% is considered a CHD risk equivalent. Those with zero to one CHD risk factor do not need to have their absolute CHD risk assessed because their CHD risk is likely to be so low as to make this additional step unnecessary.

Results of the assessment are then used to determine the goal for serum LDL-C, as shown in Table 8.6. Persons having zero to one of the major, independent risk factors listed in Box 8.2 have an LDL-C goal of < 160 mg/dL.

Those with two or more of these risk factors have an LDL-C goal of < 130 mg/dL. Persons at the greatest risk for CHD, those already diagnosed with CHD or having a CHD risk equivalent, have an LDL-C goal of < 100 mg/dL.

Besides the major, independent risk factors listed in Box 8.2, the *ATP III* recognizes two additional categories of factors that potentially increase one's risk for CHD:

TABLE 8.6	Three Categories of Risk that Modify LDL Cholesterol Goals
Risk Category	**LDL Goal (mg/dL)**
Zero to one risk factor	< 160
Multiple (two or more) risk factors[*]	< 130
Presence of CHD or CHD risk equivalents	< 100

Adapted from National Cholesterol Education Program. 2001. *Third report of the expert panel on detection, evaluation, and treatment of high blood cholesterol in adults.* Bethesda, MD: U.S. Department of Health and Human Services, Public Health Service; National Institutes of Health; National Heart, Lung, and Blood Institute.

[*]Risk factors that modify the LDL goal were shown in Table 8.2.

life-habit risk factors and emerging risk factors.[2] The life-habit risk factors include obesity, physical inactivity, and an atherogenic diet. Although the LDL-C goals shown in Table 8.6 are not necessarily lowered when a person is found to have one or more of these life-habit risk factors, they are regarded as "direct targets for clinical intervention." The emerging risk factors include the elevated serum levels of lipoprotein(a) and homocysteine and the presence of factors that increase the formation of blood clots (prothrombotic factors) or that may inflame the arterial wall (proinflammatory factors). The emerging risk factors do not categorically alter the LDL-C treatment goals but may be considered when determining the intensity of risk reduction therapy.[2]

Many persons at higher risk for CHD likely have various combinations of major risk factors, life-habit risk factors, and emerging risk factors, which together constitute what is known as the "metabolic syndrome." The metabolic syndrome is characterized by abdominal obesity (discussed in Chapter 6), atherogenic dyslipidemia (elevated triglyceride, small LDL particles, low HDL-C), elevated blood pressure, insulin resistance (with or without glucose intolerance), and prothrombotic and proinflammatory factors. The *ATP III* considers the metabolic syndrome to be a "secondary target" of risk reduction therapy after serum LDL-C, the primary risk reduction target. Table 8.7 lists the clinical determinants of the metabolic syndrome as identified by the *ATP III*. A diagnosis of metabolic syndrome can be made when three or more of these risk factors are present.[2]

TABLE 8.7	Clinical Determinants of the Metabolic Syndrome
Risk Factor	**Defining Level**
Abdominal obesity*	Waist circumference:[†] males > 40 in (> 102 cm) females > 35 in (> 88 cm)
Triglycerides	≥ 150 mg/dL
HDL cholesterol	Males < 40 mg/dL Females < 50 mg/dL
Blood pressure	Systolic ≥ 130 mm Hg Diastolic ≥ 85 mm Hg
Fasting plasma glucose	≥ 110 mg/dL

Adapted from National Cholesterol Education Program. 2001. *Third report of the expert panel on detection, evaluation, and treatment of high blood cholesterol in adults.* Bethesda, MD: U.S. Department of Health and Human Services, Public Health Service; National Institutes of Health; National Heart, Lung, and Blood Institute.

*Overweight and obesity are associated with insulin resistance and the metabolic syndrome. However, the presence of abdominal obesity is more highly correlated with risk for the metabolic syndrome than is an elevated body mass index (BMI). Therefore, the simple measure of waist circumference is recommended to identify the presence of abdominal obesity.

†Some male patients can develop multiple metabolic risk factors when the waist circumference is only marginally increased (e.g., 37–39 in. or 94–102 cm). Such patients may have a strong genetic contribution to insulin resistance. They should benefit from changes in life habits, similarly to men with categorical increases in waist circumference.

Therapeutic Lifestyle Changes

The term *therapeutic lifestyle changes* is used by the *ATP III* to identify multifaceted lifestyle approaches to reduce risk for CHD. Included among the therapeutic lifestyle changes (TLC) are various dietary recommendations, as shown in Table 8.8, increased consumption of plant stanols/sterols (2 g/d) and viscous (soluble) dietary fiber (10–25 g/d), weight reduction when indicated, and increased physical activity. The TLC dietary recommendations shown in Table 8.8 are similar to the *Dietary Guidelines for Americans* (discussed in Chapter 2) but differ in some respects. Among these are the recommendations for saturated fat, dietary cholesterol, and percent of total calories from fat. The *Dietary Guidelines for Americans* recommend that all persons ages 2 years and older limit their intake of saturated fat to no more than about 10% of calories. Because the TLC diet is targeted to persons with increased risk of CHD, especially elevated LDL-C, it makes the more conservative recommendation of no more than 7% of calories from saturated fat. This reflects the fact that, of any dietary component, saturated fat has the greatest impact on serum total and LDL cholesterol levels. The second most important factor influencing serum total and LDL cholesterol levels is dietary cholesterol. The *Dietary Guidelines for Americans* recommend < 300 mg/d, compared with the TLC's recommendation of < 200 mg/d. The *Dietary Guidelines for Americans* recommend limiting total fat intake to < 30% of calories, while the TLC diet has a more liberal recommendation of up to 35% of calories from fat but with the majority of total fat coming from monounsatu-

TABLE 8.8	Nutrient Composition of the Therapeutic Lifestyle Change Diet
Nutrient	**Recommended Intake**
Saturated fat*	Less than 7% of total calories
Polyunsaturated fat	Up to 10% of total calories
Monounsaturated fat	Up to 20% of total calories
Total fat	25% to 35% of total calories
Carbohydrate†	50% to 60% of total calories
Fiber	20 to 30 g/d
Protein	Approximately 15% of total calories
Cholesterol	Less than 200 mg/day
Total calories (energy)‡	Balance energy intake and expenditure to maintain healthy body weight or to prevent weight gain.

From National Cholesterol Education Program. 2001. *Third report of the expert panel on detection, evaluation, and treatment of high blood cholesterol in adults.* Bethesda, MD: U.S. Department of Health and Human Services, Public Health Service; National Institutes of Health; National Heart, Lung, and Blood Institute.

Trans fatty acids are another LDL-raising fat that should be kept at a low intake.

†Carbohydrate should be derived predominantly from foods rich in complex carbohydrates, including grains, especially whole grains, fruits, and vegetables.

‡Daily energy expenditure should include at least moderate physical activity (contributing approximately 200 kcal per day).

rated fats. This modest increase in the proportion of energy from fat (primarily from monounsaturated fats) with a commensurate decrease in energy from carbohydrate may help reduce elevated triglycerides in some persons. Despite this more liberal fat recommendation, total energy intake should be balanced with energy expenditure to maintain a healthy weight or to prevent unhealthful weight gain.

Once CHD risk has been assessed and found to be elevated, application of lifestyle therapy should begin. A model of steps to follow in applying the various therapeutic lifestyle changes is shown in Figure 8.5. At the first visit with the health care provider following risk assessment, the therapeutic lifestyle changes are initiated, with an emphasis on reducing intake of saturated fat and dietary cholesterol to levels indicated in Table 8.8. Referral to a registered dietitian competent in medical nutrition therapy of CHD and related risk factors should be considered. Physical activity level should be assessed, and, if necessary, moderate physical activity should be encouraged. After 6 weeks, the lipoprotein profile should be repeated to evaluate any changes in serum LDL-C in response to therapeutic lifestyle changes. If the LDL-C goal is not achieved at this point, application of the therapeutic lifestyle changes should be intensified, reduction of saturated fat and dietary cholesterol intake should be reinforced (preferably with the help of a dietitian), and consideration should be given to other options for further lowering LDL-C, such as increasing intake of viscous

(soluble) dietary fibers and including plant stanols/sterols in the diet.

Another 6 weeks are given for determining the maximum effect of dietary therapy on reducing LDL-C. If dietary therapies alone are not effective at achieving the LDL-C goal, increased attention should be given to managing body weight, maintaining adequate physical activity, and, if necessary, addressing any of the clinical determinants of the metabolic syndrome (shown in Table 8.7). Administration of cholesterol-lowering drugs should also be considered at this point. However, in the presence of markedly increased levels of LDL-C and multiple CHD risk factors or CHD equivalents, it may be necessary to begin drug treatment simultaneously with therapeutic lifestyle changes. Table 8.9 outlines the LDL-C goals and cutpoints at which therapeutic lifestyle changes and drug therapy are initiated. For example, consider a person previously diagnosed with CHD or who had CHD risk equivalents and an LDL-C level of greater than 130 mg/dL. Therapeutic lifestyle changes and cholesterol-lowering drug therapy would begin simultaneously. If this person had an LDL-C level between 100 and 129 mg/dL, cholesterol lowering drug therapy would be considered optional.

Therapeutic lifestyle change is considered the cornerstone of therapy to reduce blood cholesterol levels. The general aim of dietary therapy is to reduce serum total and LDL cholesterol while providing a nutritionally adequate diet. The rationale for the TLC dietary recommendations

Figure 8.5 A model for applying therapeutic lifestyle changes.

Source: From National Cholesterol Education Program. 2001. *Third report of the expert panel on detection, evaluation, and treatment of high blood cholesterol in adults.* Bethesda, MD: U.S. Department of Health and Human Services, Public Health Service; National Institutes of Health; National Heart, Lung, and Blood Institute.

TABLE **8.9**	**LDL-C Goals and Cutpoints for Therapeutic Lifestyle Changes and Drug Therapy in Different Risk Categories**		
Risk Category	**LDL Goal**	**LDL Level at Which to Initiate Therapeutic Lifestyle Changes (TLC)**	**LDL Level at Which to Consider Drug Therapy**
CHD or CHD risk equivalents 10-year risk > 20%	< 100 mg/dL	≥ 100 mg/dL	≥ 130 mg/dL (100–129 mg/dL: drug optional)*
Two or more risk factors 10-year risk 10–20%	< 130 mg/dL	≥ 130 mg/dL	≥ 130 mg/dL
Two or more risk factors 10-year risk < 10%	< 130 mg/dL	≥ 130 mg/dL	≥ 160 mg/dL
Zero to one risk factor†	< 160 mg/dL	≥ 160 mg/dL	≥ 190 mg/dL (160–189 mg/dL: drug optional)

From National Cholesterol Education Program. 2001. *Third report of the expert panel on detection, evaluation, and treatment of high blood cholesterol in adults.* Bethesda, MD: U.S. Department of Health and Human Services, Public Health Service; National Institutes of Health; National Heart, Lung, and Blood Institute.

*Some authorities recommend use of LDL-lowering drugs in this category if an LDL cholesterol < 100 mg/dL cannot be achieved by therapeutic lifestyle changes. Others prefer use of drugs that primarily modify triglycerides and HDL, such as nicotinic acid or fibrate. Clinical judgment also may call for deferring drug therapy in this subcategory.

†Almost all people with zero to one risk factor have a 10-year risk < 10%; thus, 10-year risk assessment in people with zero to one risk factor is not necessary.

given in Table 8.8 is thoroughly discussed in the *ATP III* report and in the American Heart Association's dietary guidelines, and they are briefly reviewed later in this chapter in Dietary Treatment in Coronary Heart Disease.[27] It is important to assess the patient's current eating habits before initiating medical nutrition therapy for CHD risk reduction. This can be done using the MEDFICTS dietary assessment questionnaire, discussed in Chapter 3 and shown in Appendix G. A simple approach for assessing a patient's eating habits is to simply ask about his or her intake of foods known to be major contributors of saturated fat and cholesterol. The *ATP III* has developed what it calls the *Dietary CAGE*, as shown in Box 8.4. The acronym CAGE represents four groups of foods that are common sources of saturated fat and cholesterol. These include cheese and other high-fat dairy foods, foods rich in animal fats, high-fat foods purchased away from home, and miscellaneous high-fat commercial foods.[2] If greater

detail and accuracy are needed, other methods, such as multiple 24-hour recalls, a 3-day food record, or a food frequency questionnaire, can be used. With adequate training, physicians or members of their staffs can assist patients in nutritional education and behavioral change. However, some patients may need counseling from a registered dietitian from the outset. It should be emphasized to patients that the goal is not a temporary "diet" but, rather, a permanent change in eating behavior.[2]

Inadequate lowering of cholesterol levels can result from several factors.[2] Inherited metabolic disorders of lipid metabolism (for example, absent or dysfunctional LDL receptors or hepatic lipoprotein overproduction) can result in severe elevations of serum cholesterol that are resistant to lowering, no matter how strict the diet. Some patients are biologically resistant to LDL lowering by dietary modification and will not achieve the cholesterol-lowering goal despite good adherence to diet.

 Box 8.4   **Dietary CAGE for Assessing Intakes of Saturated Fat and Cholesterol**

- C—Cheese (and other sources of dairy fats—whole milk, 2% milk, ice cream, cream, whole fat yogurt)
- A—Animal fats (hamburger, ground meat, frankfurters, bologna, salami, sausage, fried foods, fatty cuts of meat)
- G—Got it away from home (high-fat meals either purchased and brought home or eaten in restaurants)
- E—Eat (extra) high-fat commercial products: candy, pastries, pies, doughnuts, cookies

Adapted from National Cholesterol Education Program. 2001. *Third report of the expert panel on detection, evaluation, and treatment of high blood cholesterol in adults.* Bethesda, MD: U.S. Department of Health and Human Services, Public Health Service; National Institutes of Health; National Heart, Lung, and Blood Institute.

Some patients refuse to change their eating habits despite the intensive efforts of the physician and counselors. However, a concerted effort by health professionals to promote behavioral change should minimize the size of this patient group. It may take up to a year, or even longer, for some patients to adopt the recommended dietary changes. Thus, adequate time should be allowed for patients to attempt to modify their diets to achieve the desired therapeutic goals.[2]

Lowering Cholesterol in the Population

In the *Report of the Expert Panel on Population Strategies for Blood Cholesterol Reduction,* similar CHD risk factors are identified as in the *ATP III* report and similar total cholesterol and LDL-C cutoff points are used in classifying persons.[26] The Expert Panel has recommended that all healthy Americans about age 2 years and older adopt a diet similar to the one outlined in Table 8.8. The rationale for this diet is outlined in the section "Dietary Treatment in Coronary Heart Disease."

Will population strategies be successful in lowering the average serum cholesterol levels of Americans? Even before government agencies made a concerted effort to promote a heart-healthy diet, the average cholesterol level of Americans was declining, as shown in Figure 8.6. A comparison of data from the first National Health Examination Survey (1960–62) with data collected from NHANES III (1988–94) shows that mean serum total cholesterol levels of U.S. males and females ages 20 to 74 years have declined 12 mg/dL in males and 17 mg/dL in females, respectively. This fact, along with a decrease in cigarette smoking and a possible increase in leisure-time physical activity, have no doubt contributed to the nearly 60% decline in heart disease mortality between 1950 and 2000, as shown in

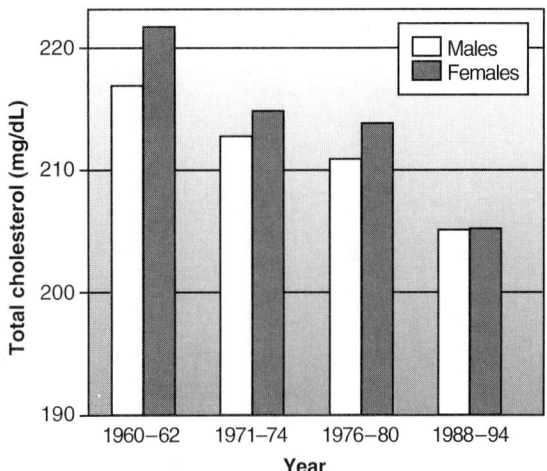

Figure 8.6 **Mean total serum cholesterol in U.S. adults, 1960–1994.**
Since between 1960 and 1962, mean serum cholesterol levels of U.S. males and females ages 20 through 74 years have declined 12 mg/dL and 17 mg/dL, respectively. Values shown are age-adjusted.
Source: Data from the National Center for Health Statistics.

Figure 8.7. During the same period, there was 70% reduction in age-adjusted stroke mortality, as shown in Figure 8.8. Despite these reductions, heart disease mortality is 50% greater for blacks than it is for whites. Stroke mortality is nearly twice as high for blacks as for whites.

Not only is there good evidence that lowering serum cholesterol levels reduces CHD risk, but several studies have shown that cholesterol lowering can slow the progression of and even reverse atherosclerotic narrowing.[28–34] According to the NCEP, "the conclusion now seems inescapable that definite regression can be expected in 16% to 47% of patients, provided that large

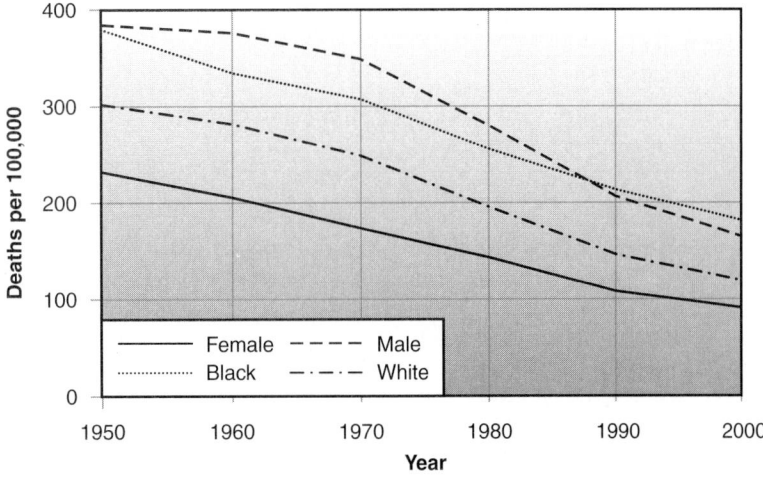

Figure 8.7 **Age-adjusted death rate (per 100,000 resident population) for heart disease by race and sex, United States, 1950–2000.**
Source: Data from the National Center for Health Statistics.

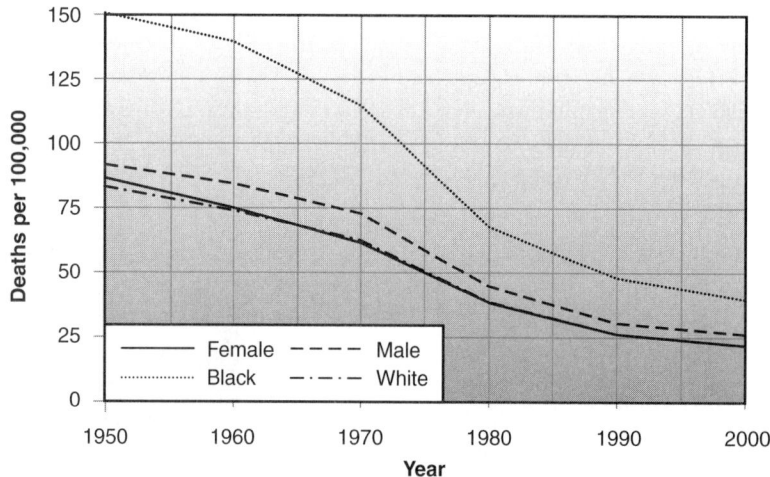

Figure 8.8 Age-adjusted death rate (per 100,000 resident population) for stroke by race and sex, United States, 1950–2000.

Source: Data from the National Center for Health Statistics.

decreases in LDL-cholesterol (of the order of 34% to 48%) are induced for a period of 2 to 5 years."[11]

Coronary Heart Disease in Children and Adolescents

There is considerable scientific evidence that CHD begins in childhood. For example, there are good data indicating that atherosclerosis was present in the coronary arteries of U.S. soldiers killed in the Korean and Vietnam wars.[35,36] These studies showed lesions and narrowing consistent with CHD in 77% of the soldiers whose average age was 22 years. Data from a number of researchers studying the development and progression of coronary artery lesions in infants and children support the view that atherosclerosis begins in childhood and progresses slowly into adulthood.[37–40] Evidence from the Pathobiological Determinants of Atherosclerosis in Youth study, for example, indicates that early atherosclerotic lesions in the coronary arteries of adolescents and young adults are associated with smoking, high serum total cholesterol, LDL-C and VLDL-C levels, and low HDL-C levels. Data from the study have provided strong justification for reducing CHD risk factors in young persons.[41–45]

Other research has shown that children and adolescents in the United States have higher cholesterol levels than their counterparts in many other countries.[46–49] This probably is because children in the United States and children in other countries who have higher total cholesterol levels have a higher intake of saturated fatty acids and dietary cholesterol. In Table 8.10 it can be seen that, as the percent of kilocalories from saturated fatty acids increases, serum total cholesterol increases as well. One exception is the country of Ghana, where intake of dietary cholesterol is low.

Reducing Cholesterol Levels in Children and Adolescents

Clearly, prevention of CHD needs to begin in childhood. A convenient and apparently effective starting place is

TABLE 8.10 | **Dietary Saturated Fatty Acids and Cholesterol Intake and Serum Total Cholesterol in Boys Ages 7 to 9 Years in Six Countries**

	Dietary Intake		
Country	Saturated Fatty Acids (% of Energy)	Cholesterol (mg/1000 kcal)	Serum Total Cholesterol (mg/dL)
Philippines	9.3	97	147
Italy	10.4	159	159
Ghana	10.5	48	128
United States	13.5	151	167
Netherlands	15.1	142	174
Finland	17.7	157	190

From National Cholesterol Education Program. 1991. *Report of the expert panel on blood cholesterol levels in children and adolescents.* Bethesda, MD: U.S. Department of Health and Human Services, Public Health Service; National Institutes of Health; National Heart, Lung, Blood Institute.

the cholesterol levels of children and adolescents. The *Report of the Expert Panel on Blood Cholesterol Levels in Children and Adolescents* makes both patient-based and population-based recommendations for reducing cholesterol levels in these age groups.[11]

The goal of the population-based recommendations is "to lower average population levels of blood cholesterol in children and adolescents in order to reduce the incidence of adult CHD and generally to improve health."[11] These recommendations are similar to those suggested for most adults—adoption of the American Heart Association's dietary guidelines beginning at about age 2 years.[27] The panel suggested that "nutritional adequacy be achieved by eating a wide variety of foods," that energy "be adequate to support growth and development and to reach or maintain desirable body weight," that dietary cholesterol intake be less than 300 mg/day, and that no more than 10% and 30% of calories be derived from saturated fatty acids and total fat, respectively.[11] The rationale for these recommendations is given in the section "Dietary Treatment in Coronary Heart Disease." You may want to refer to the Expert Panel's report for its outstanding suggestions for implementing the population approach.[11]

The goal of the patient-based approach is to identify those children and adolescents with elevated serum cholesterol levels or with other CHD risk factors that are likely to increase their risk for CHD as adults.[11] The Expert Panel did not recommend that all U.S. children and adolescents have their cholesterol levels measured (that is, universal screening). They did recommend, however, that serum cholesterol be measured in a specific subgroup of youth (that is, selective screening)—those at greatest risk of having high blood cholesterol as adults and an increased risk for CHD. Elevated serum cholesterol levels and other CHD risk factors tend to aggregate, or cluster, in families as a result of both shared environments and genetic factors. Children with high cholesterol levels often have high levels as adults, but not always. There are many instances when an adult's cholesterol level is not as high as would be expected based on childhood levels. The Expert Panel suggested that the following children and adolescents, ages 2 years or older, be screened for elevated cholesterol and other risk factors:[11]

- Those whose parents or grandparents, by age 55 years or less, underwent diagnostic coronary arteriography and were found to have coronary atherosclerosis or had balloon angioplasty or coronary artery bypass surgery
- Those whose parents or grandparents, by age 55 years or less, suffered documented myocardial infarction, angina pectoris, peripheral vascular disease, cerebrovascular disease, or sudden cardiac death
- Those with a parent having high serum cholesterol ($\geq$ 240 mg/dL)
- Those whose parental or grandparental history is unknown, especially if the youth has other CHD risk factors, as outlined in Box 8.5.
- Health care providers may decide to screen youth judged at high risk for CHD—for example, youth who are overweight; are cigarette smokers; have high blood pressure or diabetes; are on certain medications, such as isotretinoin (Accutane) or steroids; or who consume excessive amounts of saturated fatty acids, total fat, and cholesterol.

Figure 8.9 outlines the steps for risk assessment. The panel recommended that a child's total cholesterol be measured when his or her parent has high blood cholesterol. Once a borderline-high or high blood cholesterol is established (review Table 8.2), then lipoprotein analysis is recommended. In youth having a positive family history for CHD (Box 8.5), lipoprotein analysis is recommended at the outset. Classification, education, and follow-up are based on LDL-C levels, as shown in Figure 8.10. As is the case with elevated LDL-C levels in adults, the suggested dietary approach to treating elevated cholesterol levels in children and adolescents is to begin by applying the American Heart Association's dietary guidelines, as indicated in Figure 8.11 and as discussed in the section "Dietary Treatment in Coronary Heart Disease."[27]

Dietary Treatment in Coronary Heart Disease

In the past 3 decades, government agencies and private organizations have developed a variety of dietary and lifestyle recommendations for promoting healthy levels

Box 8.5 Risk Factors That May Contribute to Early Onset of CHD

- Family history of premature CHD, cerebrovascular or occlusive peripheral vascular disease (definite onset before age 55 in a sibling, parent, or sibling of a parent)
- Cigarette smoking

- Elevated blood pressure
- Low HDL-C (< 40 mg/dL)
- Overweight (BMI > 95th percentile BMI for age)
- Diabetes mellitus
- Physical inactivity

From National Cholesterol Education Program. 1991. *Report of the expert panel on blood cholesterol levels in children and adolescents.* Bethesda, MD: U.S. Department of Health and Human Services, Public Health Service; National Institutes of Health; National Heart, Lung, and Blood Institute.

*Defined as a history of premature (before age 55 years) cardiovascular disease in a parent or grandparent.

Figure 8.9 **Steps in assessing cholesterol and lipoprotein levels in children and adolescents.**

Source: From National Cholesterol Education Program. 1991. *Report of the expert panel on blood cholesterol levels in children and adolescents.* Bethesda, MD: U.S. Department of Health and Human Services, Public Health Service; National Institutes of Health; National Heart, Lung, and Blood Institute.

of serum lipids and lipoproteins and for reducing overall coronary heart disease risk. Several of these are discussed at length in Chapter 2. Consistent features among these various recommendations have been limiting consumption of foods rich in total fats, saturated fatty acids, and dietary cholesterol; maintaining a healthy body weight by balancing energy intake with energy expenditure; and keeping sodium intake moderate.

Of these recommendations, the most widely advocated in North America have been the "Step-One" and "Step-Two" diets, which, until recently, have been a standard feature of recommendations from the National Cholesterol Education Program and the American Heart Association. Better understanding of the complex relationships among numerous dietary and lifestyle factors and various coronary heart disease and stroke risk factors has led to the creation of broader recommendations, which allow a more individualized approach to risk reduction and "place greater emphasis on foods and an overall eating pattern and the need for all Americans to achieve and maintain a healthy body weight."[27] This broader set of recommendations is embodied in the

recently revised American Heart Association's dietary guidelines, as well as the *ATP III*'s "therapeutic lifestyle change" diet, which was outlined in Table 8.8.

The American Heart Association's dietary guidelines are intended for individuals in the general population greater than 2 years of age. These collectively replace the Step-One diet and are outlined in Box 8.6. These guidelines may have to be modified to accommodate medical nutrition therapy for individuals presenting with such conditions as preexisting cardiovascular disease, specific lipid disorders (e.g., elevated serum triglyceride, low serum HDL-C, or the presence of chylomicrons in fasting serum), diabetes mellitus, insulin resistance, congestive heart failure, and kidney disease.[27]

Saturated Fatty Acids

Saturated fatty acids (SFA) are the most important dietary determinant of serum total cholesterol and LDL-C levels.[2,27] One exception to this rule is stearic acid (18:0), an SFA that appears to have a neutral effect on serum cholesterol and lipoprotein levels.[50] Moderation should still be practiced in the consumption of fats high in stearic acid, such as beef fat

*AHA = American Heart Association.

Figure 8.10 Classification, education, and follow-up of children and adolescents based on their low-density lipoprotein (LDL) cholesterol levels.

Source: From National Cholesterol Education Program. 1991. *Report of the expert panel on blood cholesterol levels in children and adolescents.* Bethesda, MD: U.S. Department of Health and Human Services, Public Health Service; National Institutes of Health; National Heart, Lung, and Blood Institute.

and cocoa butter, because these fats contain a substantial amount of the other SFAs that raise serum cholesterol.[51]

The American Heart Association recommends that members of the general population (ages > 2 years) limit their intake of SFA to < 10% of energy. Persons with elevated LDL-C or preexisting cardiovascular disease are advised to limit SFA intake to < 7% of energy. According to data from NHANES III, SFAs provide, on average, 12% of energy. According to data from the 1994–96 Continuing Survey of Food Intakes by Individuals, estimated average SFA intake for all Americans was 11.5% of energy. Data from the 1994–96 and the 1998 Continuing

Survey of Food Intakes by Individuals showed that average intake for persons ages 19 years and younger was 12%.

During the past several decades, average SFA intake among Americans has declined from a high of nearly 20% of energy to the current level of 12%.[27] This is recognized as a major factor in the decline of mean total serum cholesterol levels. However, more progress is needed in further reducing SFA intake to meet the American Heart Association's goals. This can be done by identifying foods rich in saturated fat and substituting foods containing less saturated fat. Major food sources of

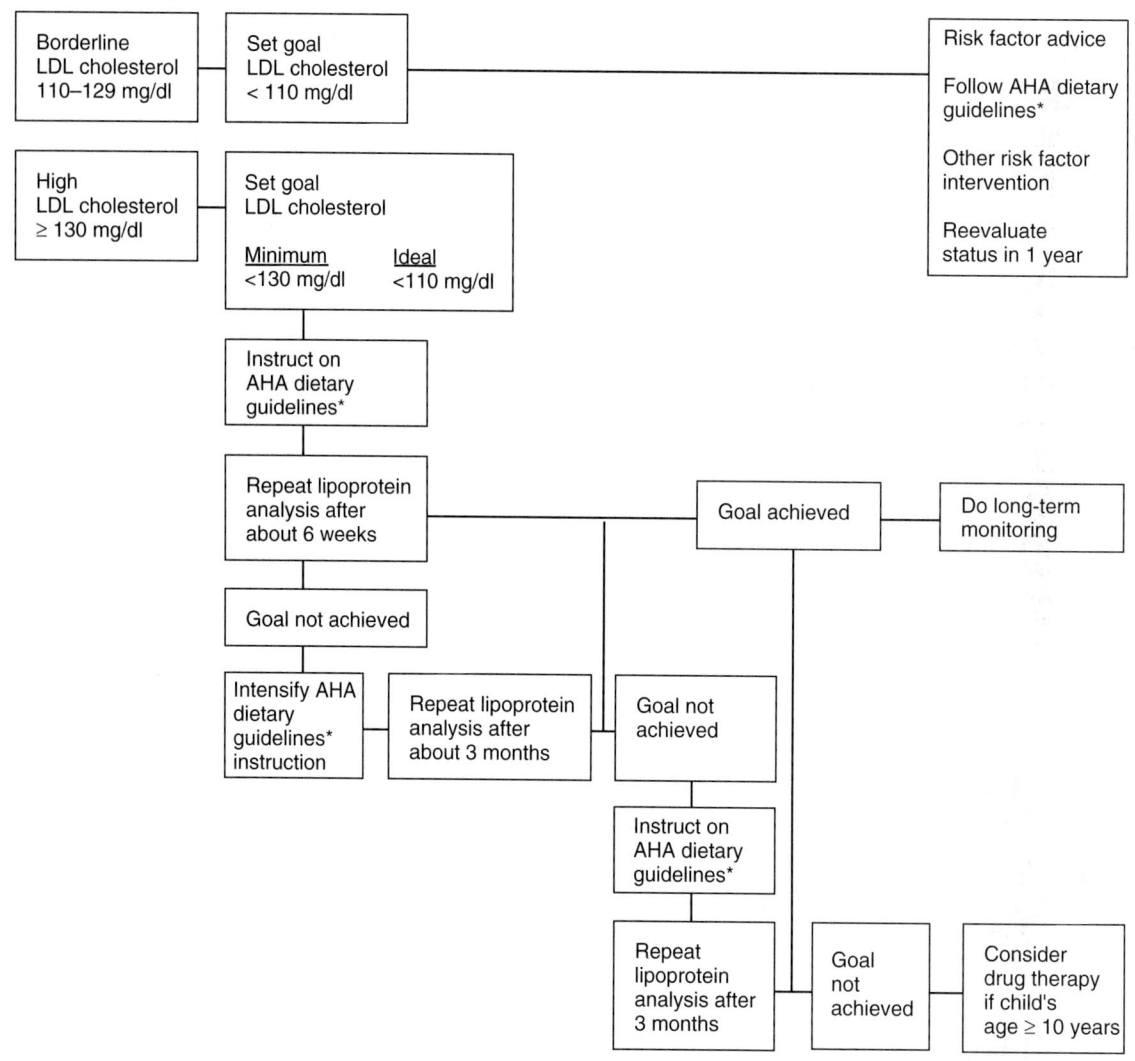

*AHA = American Heart Association.

Figure 8.11   Recommended approach to dietary treatment of elevated low-density lipoprotein (LDL) cholesterol levels in children and adolescents.

Source: Adapted from National Cholesterol Education Program. 1991. *Report of the expert panel on blood cholesterol levels in children and adolescents.* Bethesda, MD: U.S. Department of Health and Human Services, Public Health Service; National Institutes of Health; National Heart, Lung, and Blood Institute.

saturated fat in the diets of U.S. adults include full-fat dairy products, beef, poultry, stick margarine, pastries, cookies, and quick breads made with meat fats and hydrogenated vegetable fats.[52] Particular attention should be given to monitoring the intake of these foods when evaluating the diets of persons with elevated serum levels of total cholesterol and LDL-C.

Trans *Fatty Acids*

A growing body of evidence shows that consumption of dietary *trans* unsaturated fatty acids increases LDL-C and reduces HDL-C.[53–55] Although saturated fatty acids appear to increase LDL-C to a somewhat greater extent than an equal amount of dietary *trans* unsaturated fatty acids, the detrimental effects of dietary *trans* unsaturated fatty acids on serum lipid and lipoprotein levels has led to recommen-

dations to limit intake of foods rich in *trans* unsaturated fatty acids.[2,27,56] The American Heart Association, for example, recommends that total intake of "cholesterol-raising fatty acids" not exceed 10% of energy.[27] The *ATP III*'s therapeutic lifestyle change diet recommends that intake of *trans* unsaturated fatty acids be kept low.[2]

Trans fatty acids are unsaturated fatty acids containing at least one double bond in the *trans* configuration. In most naturally occurring unsaturated fatty acids (particularly those found in vegetable oils), double bonds are typically in the *cis* configuration. However, unsaturated *trans* fatty acids naturally occur at relatively low levels in meat and dairy foods as by-products of fermentation in ruminant animals.[57] The richest sources of *trans* fatty acids are hydrogenated and partially hydrogenated vegetable fats, such as vegetable shortening and some mar-

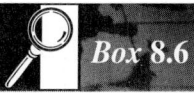

Box 8.6   Major Components of the American Heart Association Dietary Guidelines

A HEALTHY EATING PATTERN, INCLUDING FOODS FROM ALL MAJOR FOOD GROUPS

- Consume a variety of fruits, vegetables, and grain products, including whole grains.
- Include fat-free and low-fat dairy products, fish, legumes, poultry, and lean meats.

A HEALTHY BODY WEIGHT

- Match energy intake to overall energy needs; limit consumption of foods with a high caloric density and/or low nutritional quality, including those with a high sugar content.
- Maintain a level of physical activity that achieves fitness and balances energy expenditure with energy intake; for weight reduction, expenditure should exceed intake.

A DESIRABLE BLOOD CHOLESTEROL AND LIPOPROTEIN PROFILE

- Limit the intake of foods high in saturated fatty acids and cholesterol.
- Substitute grains and unsaturated fatty acids from vegetables, fish, legumes, and nuts.

A DESIRABLE BLOOD PRESSURE

- Limit intake of salt (sodium chloride) to < 6 g per day (< 2400 mg sodium per day).
- Limit alcohol consumption (no more than one drink per day for women and two drinks per day for men).
- Maintain a healthy body weight and a dietary pattern emphasizing vegetables, fruits, and low-fat or fat-free dairy products.

Adapted from Krauss RM, Eckel RH, Howard B, Appel LJ, Daniels SR, Deckelbaum RJ, et al. 2000. AHA dietary guidelines: revision 2000. *Circulation* 102:2296–2311.

garines. Foods prepared with hydrogenated vegetable fats (i.e., vegetable shortening) are generally high in *trans* fatty acids. These foods include cookies, crackers, doughnuts, and other baked goods, as well as commercially prepared fried foods. The vegetable shortening used for deep fat frying by the food service industry makes French fries a particularly common source of dietary *trans* fatty acids.[58]

Dietary Cholesterol

Dietary cholesterol (cholesterol in food) also raises serum total cholesterol and LDL-C levels (especially the latter), although the elevations are not as great as those seen in diets high in SFA.[2,27,59–61] As is the case with intake of saturated fatty acids, the response of serum total cholesterol and LDL-C to dietary intake of cholesterol varies widely among individuals.[2,27,62] Epidemiologic studies suggest that dietary cholesterol intake is also associated with increased risk for coronary heart disease.[63–66] In several studies, researchers have found dietary cholesterol to be an independent predictor of CHD, *apart from its effects on serum cholesterol.*[63,67]

According to data from NHANES III, mean dietary cholesterol intake for American males and females is 322 mg and 221 mg per day, respectively. However, mean dietary cholesterol intake for males and females ages 20 to 49 years is approximately 369 mg and 243 mg per day, respectively. According to data from the 1994–96 Continuing Survey of Food Intakes by Individuals, mean daily dietary cholesterol intakes for males and females ages 20 years and older is 331 mg and 213 mg, respectively. The American Heart Association recommends that members of the general population (age > 2 years) limit their intake of dietary cholesterol to < 300 mg per day and that persons with elevated LDL-C or preexisting cardiovascular disease limit their intake to < 200 mg per day.[27] Persons following the *ATP III*'s therapeutic lifestyle change diet are advised to limit their dietary cholesterol intake to < 200 mg per day.[2] Identification of foods containing dietary cholesterol is relatively easy, given the fact that dietary cholesterol is found only in foods of animal origin. Particularly rich sources include egg yolk, full-fat dairy products, and organ meats (e.g., liver, kidney, and brain). Most foods high in saturated fat are also sources of dietary cholesterol. Consequently, reducing consumption of these foods results in a double benefit of reduced intake of saturated fat and dietary cholesterol.

Confusion about dietary cholesterol's influence on serum cholesterol is primarily due to the high variability of response of serum total cholesterol and LDL-C to consumption of dietary cholesterol.[2] A report of an 88-year-old man having a plasma total cholesterol level of 200 mg/dL (5.17 mmol/L) despite eating about 25 eggs per day for more than 15 years is a case in point.[68] Amazingly, he was almost completely free of any clinically important atherosclerosis. He absorbed only 18% of the cholesterol he ate (people normally absorb 45% to 55%), he had twice the normal rate of bile acid synthesis, and his body synthesized less than average amounts of cholesterol. Despite this *one* individual's highly unusual cholesterol metabolism, it remains prudent for the rest of us with more normal cholesterol metabolism to follow a low-cholesterol diet.

Total Calories

Another significant dietary factor is total caloric intake, with its implications for obesity. Because obesity is associated with elevated serum LDL-C, increased risk for hypertension and type 2 diabetes mellitus, and is an independent risk factor for CHD, the *ATP III* and American Heart Association recommend balancing energy intake with energy expenditure to prevent weight gain once an adult has attained his or her healthy weight or to maintain a healthy body weight.[2,27] For many adults, this can be accomplished by modestly reducing energy intake (consuming 500 to 1000 fewer kilocalories per day) and increasing energy expenditure through moderate physical activity on most days of the week. Emphasizing foods with a low energy density (e.g., fruits, vegetables, legumes, whole-grain products, fat-free dairy products, and lean meats) is recommended.[27] Dietary approaches to weight management for children and adolescents must be consistent with appropriate growth and development. The American Heart Association does not recommend the use of very low-fat diets or high-protein diets for weight management in the general population.[27] In overweight persons, weight reduction has been shown to lower serum LDL-C and triglycerides, to raise HDL-C, to assist in the control of hypertension, and to improve glycemic control in persons with type 2 diabetes.[2,27]

Total and Unsaturated Fat

Most people in the general population older than 2 years will benefit from a diet providing a moderate intake of total fat while saturated and *trans* fatty acids and dietary cholesterol are kept low and polyunsaturated fatty acids do not exceed 10% of energy.[2,27] The American Heart Association recommends that saturated and *trans* unsaturated fats not exceed 10% of energy.[27] A diet providing no more than 30% of energy from fat and moderately restricted in total energy (a daily deficit of 500 to 1000 kilocalories) can be particularly beneficial for overweight and obese individuals when combined with regular physical activity of moderate intensity and duration. However, in persons with the metabolic syndrome and type 2 diabetes, the amount of carbohydrate (50% to 60% of energy) in a moderately fat-restricted diet ($\leq$ 30% of energy) may elevate serum triglyceride and depress serum HDL-C.[2,27] Consequently, a dietary treatment strategy for patients presenting with elevated triglycerides and low HDL-C is to moderately restrict percent of energy from carbohydrate and increase the proportion of energy from monounsaturated fats, while keeping intake of dietary cholesterol and polyunsaturated, saturated, and *trans* fatty acids low.[2,27] Weight reduction is also recommended by keeping total energy intake moderate while increasing physical activity. Individuals with severe hypertriglyceridemia ($\geq$ 1000 mg/dL) may benefit from a very low-fat diet ($<$ 10% of energy from all forms of fat) and pharmacologic treatment.[27]

Protein and Carbohydrate

The *ATP III* recommends that protein compose about 15% of total calories and that emphasis be given to plant-and soy-based sources of protein.[2] The American Heart Association dietary guidelines also recommend consumption of soy protein, particularly for persons at high risk for CHD and with elevated total and LDL-cholesterol.[27] Plant foods contain no cholesterol (unless prepared with some type of animal product) and tend to be low in both total and saturated fat. Mortality from CHD is higher in nonvegetarians than in vegetarians, who generally rely heavily on plant foods for protein, energy, and other nutrient needs.[69,70] Most of the decreased CHD mortality rate in vegetarians is likely due to the differences in the types and amounts of fat found in plants compared with foods of animal origin; however, several nondietary factors no doubt play a role as well. There is convincing evidence that dietary substitution of soy protein for animal proteins lowers blood levels of total cholesterol, LDL-C, and triglycerides without lowering HDL-C.[71-75] This cholesterol-lowering effect appears to require the presence of the naturally occurring soy isoflavones, which may be removed in some commercial soy protein concentrates prepared by ethanol washing, which removes most of the isoflavones and other potentially active soy components. Plants also contain phytochemicals, some of which have antioxidant and other beneficial properties that confer protection against heart disease, stroke, and cancer.

An intake of carbohydrates at 55% or more of total calories is generally recommended. This includes simple sugars (monosaccharides and disaccharides), complex digestible carbohydrates (starches), and complex indigestible carbohydrates (fiber). To ensure that adequate vitamins, minerals, and fiber are consumed, intake of complex digestible carbohydrates should be kept high and that of simple sugars relatively low. In most people, when digestible carbohydrates are substituted for saturated fatty acids, serum LDL-C generally falls to about the same extent as when oleic and linoleic acids are substituted in this manner.[2]

Fiber can be defined as plant materials in the diet that are resistant to digestion by enzymes produced by the human intestinal tract.[76] Fiber can be divided into the soluble and insoluble fractions. The soluble fibers (gums, pectins, mucilages, and some hemicelluloses) are effective in lowering serum total cholesterol and LDL-C levels, although these effects are not as pronounced in persons with lower serum total cholesterol as it is in those having higher levels.[76-78]

Probable mechanisms for this effect include soluble fiber's ability to bind bile acids and promote their excretion in the feces and the reduction of cholesterol absorption by fiber's interference with micelle formation.[79,80] The release of short-chain fatty acids (especially propionate) from the bacterial fermentation of dietary fiber may decrease hepatic cholesterol synthesis, thus lowering serum cholesterol levels and providing several other beneficial effects.[81,82]

General Principles

The goal of the *ATP III*'s therapeutic lifestyle change diet for the treatment of elevated cholesterol levels is not a temporary "diet" but, rather, a permanent change in eating behavior that is consistent with good overall nutrition. Consumption of a variety of foods is important because no single food item provides all the essential nutrients in the amounts needed. One of the best ways to ensure an adequate diet is to include in one's meals a variety of foods from all food groups.

Although preventing obesity by controlling energy consumption is a major concern of many people, supplying the nutrient and energy needs of growing and developing children and adolescents must not be overlooked. For example, the energy needs of 2- to 3-year-old children per unit of body weight are particularly high. In addition, the capacity of a child's gastrointestinal tract for food at any one time is limited. Consequently, children's diets should include foods that are good sources of energy and nutrients and yet low in SFA and cholesterol. Some young children may need snacks to help them meet their energy and nutrient needs, and suitable selections are available that will keep children's diets within the recommended guidelines.

Issues in Measuring Lipid and Lipoprotein Levels

The public health impact of cardiovascular disease and the causal relationships between cardiovascular disease and serum lipid and lipoprotein levels make measurement of total cholesterol, low-density-lipoprotein cholesterol, and high-density-lipoprotein cholesterol among the most important in the clinical laboratory.[83] The presence of specific and detailed guidelines for detecting, evaluating, and treating elevated blood cholesterol levels in adults (e.g., the *Adult Treatment Panel III*) require that serum lipid and lipoprotein measurement meet certain standards for *precision, accuracy,* and *total analytical error.* Although these three particularly important aspects apply to any measurement, whether a clinical laboratory test (such as serum total cholesterol) or measurement of weight or stature, they are discussed in this section as they relate to measurement of lipid and lipoprotein levels.

Precision (or reproducibility) relates to the difference in results when the same measurement is repeatedly performed. The difference, or variability, in results from repeated, or replicate, measurements should be within acceptable limits. *Accuracy* relates to the difference between the measured value as reported by a clinical laboratory and the "true," or "real," measurement value obtained by using the definitive analytical process known as the "reference method" of measurement. Accuracy is often expressed in terms of *bias,* which is defined as the average deviation of the measured value from the true, or real, value. *Total analytical error* is the National Cholesterol Education's primary criterion for evaluating the performance of an analytical test (e.g., measuring serum cholesterol), and it accounts for both accuracy and precision.[83,84]

Precision

Precision and its relationship to bias are illustrated in Figure 8.12. Precision is high when multiple analyses of the same sample result in values that are reasonably close. In Figure 8.12, high precision can be thought of as multiple shots at the target being in close proximity of each other, as seen in Figure 8.12a and 8.12b. Precision is low when multiple analyses performed on one sample result in values differing considerably, as illustrated in Figure 8.12c and 8.12d. Ideally, replicate analyses of a single sample would yield the same measurement result, but the reality is that these replicate measurements vary somewhat because of potential variation in sample preparation (some analyses require precipitation and ultracentrifugation of the serum or plasma) and analytical variation inherent in the automatic analyzers used in clinical laboratories. Automatic analyzers are subject to slight variation in function over time. In addition, the reagents used in the analyzers can vary slightly from lot to lot. Obviously, the challenge to the clinical laboratory and the reagent manufacturer is to minimize such fluctuations.[84]

The importance of precision in diagnosing and monitoring persons with high cholesterol levels is illustrated in Figure 8.13. The figure shows the effect of differing degrees of imprecision (sometimes referred to as "random error" or "analytical noise") in cholesterol measurement. If a person's serum sample has a true cholesterol value of 240 mg/dL (6.21 mmol/L), values from replicate analyses of that sample could be scattered over a wide range, depending on the precision of the analytical

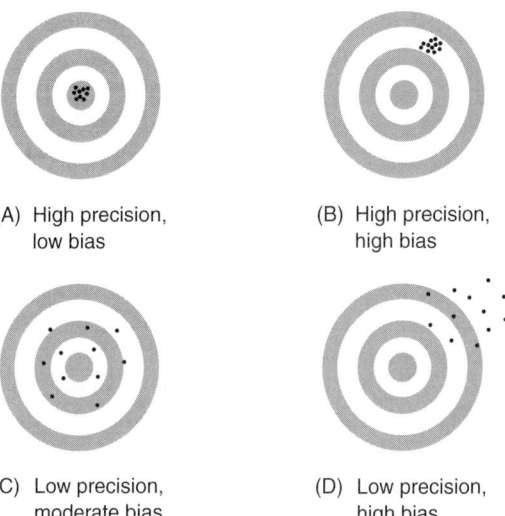

(A) High precision, low bias

(B) High precision, high bias

(C) Low precision, moderate bias

(D) Low precision, high bias

Figure 8.12
Multiple shots at a target can be used to illustrate precision and bias. Note that high precision is necessary for low bias to exist.

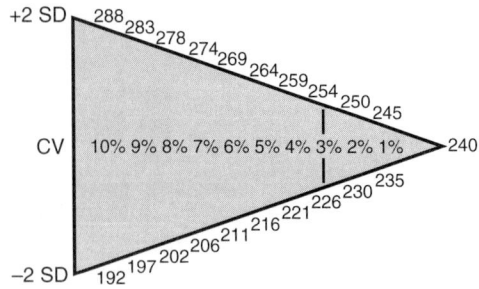

Figure 8.13 Effect of differing degrees of imprecision in analysis of a blood specimen with a true cholesterol value of 240 mg/dL.
An analytic method having a precision consistent with a coefficient of variation (CV) of 3% would yield, on repeat measurements of the same sample, values ranging from 226 to 254 mg/dL SD = standard deviation.

Source: From National Cholesterol Education Program. 1988. *Current status of blood cholesterol measurement in clinical laboratories in the United States: A report from the Laboratory Standardization Panel of the National Cholesterol Education Program.* Bethesda, MD: U.S. Department of Health and Human Services, Public Health Service; National Institutes of Health; National Heart, Lung, and Blood Institute.

TABLE 8.11	Analytical Performance Goals for Lipid and Lipoprotein Measurements Established by the National Cholesterol Education Program

	Imprecision[*]	Bias[†]	Total Analytical Error[‡]
Total cholesterol	CV ≤ 3%	≤ ±3%	≤ 8.9%
Triglyceride	CV ≤ 5%	≤ ±5%	≤ 15.0%
HDL cholesterol	CV ≤ 6%	≤ ±10%	≤ 22.0%
LDL cholesterol	CV ≤ 4%	≤ ±4%	≤ 12.0%

Adapted from National Cholesterol Education Program. 1995. *Recommendations on lipoprotein measurement from the working group on lipoprotein measurement.* Bethesda, MD: U.S. Department of Health and Human Services, Public Health Service; National Institutes of Health; National Heart, Lung, and Blood Institute.

[*]CV = coefficient of variation.

[†]Percent difference between the measured value and the true value when analyzed using the reference method.

[‡]Total analytical error = percent bias + (1.96 × CV). Total analytical error is the National Cholesterol Education Program's primary criterion for analytical performance.

method. Replicate analyses of a single specimen allow calculation of the measurement as represented by the coefficient of variation (CV). CV is a measure of imprecision and is calculated by dividing the standard deviation (SD) of replicate analyses by the mean of those replicate analyses and then multiplying them by 100 (CV = SD ÷ mean × 100).[83]

Figure 8.13 shows, for example, that, if the precision of an analytical method for serum total cholesterol were such that the CV were 10%, replicate cholesterol analyses of a single specimen having a true value of 240 mg/dL would yield values ranging from 192 to 288 mg/dL. Obviously, with this degree of imprecision, it would be very difficult to properly identify persons with elevated serum cholesterol. Recent surveys indicate that the analytical CV of clinical laboratories is in the range of 3% to 7%, with an average of 4%.[84] The National Cholesterol Education Program believes that a modern, well-controlled clinical laboratory should be able to maintain analytical CVs of less than 4%.[84] Analytical performance goals established by the National Cholesterol Education Program are shown in Table 8.11.

Accuracy

Accuracy and bias (also referred to as systematic error or overall inaccuracy) and their relationship to precision were illustrated in Figure 8.12. Bias is low when multiple shots at the target repeatedly hit the "bull's eye," as shown in Figure 8.12a. When bias is low, precision is simultaneously high. However, it is impossible for bias to be low when precision is low; thus, precision is a prerequisite for accuracy. Note, also, that high precision does not ensure accuracy, as illustrated in Figure 8.12b. Accu-

racy is necessary to correctly identify patients with elevated lipid and lipoprotein levels and to monitor their response to treatment. Clinical misdiagnosis can occur from inaccurate measurements, resulting in the reporting of false positive values (measurement results falsely classifying a person as having a condition) or false negative values (measurement results falsely classifying a person as not having a condition).

The true value of a measurement is determined using the reference method, which can be thought of as the "gold standard" measurement process. The U.S. Centers for Disease Control and Prevention (CDC) has established reference methods for measuring each of the lipids and lipoproteins. The CDC-sponsored Cholesterol Reference Method Laboratory Network has established a formal certification program for clinical laboratories, manufacturers of automated analyzers, and organizations providing laboratory standardization and proficiency testing. Laboratory standardization and proficiency testing programs provide clinical laboratories with an opportunity to determine the precision and accuracy of their instruments. The bias of a particular analytical method or automated analyzer can be determined by comparing the mean value of replicate analyses performed on the particular analyzer with the mean value of replicate analyses of the same sample performed using the reference method. The percentage difference between the mean results of the clinical laboratory undergoing evaluation and that of the reference method is known as the relative bias.[83]

If a laboratory's particular analytical method of measuring serum total cholesterol has a *positive bias* of 10% and a subject's true cholesterol value is

200 mg/dL (5.17 mmol/L), the laboratory's reported value is 220 mg/dL (5.69 mmol/L), or 10% greater than the true value. If a person's true value is 240 mg/dL (6.21 mmol/L), a 10% negative bias results in a reported value of 216 mg/dL (5.59 mmol/L), or 10% less than the true value. If the true value is 240 mg/dL (6.21 mmol/L), a 10% positive bias yields a reported value of 264 mg/dL (6.83 mmol/L). Thus, at a given bias, the higher the true cholesterol value, the greater the magnitude of the error. The National Cholesterol Education Program's goals for bias were shown in Table 8.11.

Total Analytical Error

The National Cholesterol Education Program's primary criterion for analytical performance is expressed in terms of *total analytical error*, which takes into account both accuracy (represented as bias) and precision (represented as the coefficient of variation).[84] Total analytical error is calculated using the following equation: total analytical error = percent bias + (1.96 × coefficient of variation).[84] Because calculation of total analytical error includes both bias and the coefficient of variation, a greater inaccuracy (larger bias) can be tolerated if the measurements are very precise.[84] On the other hand, if the measurements are more accurate (bias is low), then a greater degree of imprecision (larger coefficient of variation) can be tolerated. The National Cholesterol Education Program's goals for total analytical error were shown in Table 8.11.

Sources of Error in Cholesterol Measurement

Approximately one-third of within-individual variability in cholesterol analyses is due to laboratory errors. These factors are beyond the scope of this text and will not be addressed.

The remaining two-thirds of within-individual variability is due to a variety of factors occurring before the sample is actually analyzed. These can be referred to as *preanalytical factors*.[83–85] Preanalytical factors operate before or during blood sampling or during sample storage or shipment to the laboratory. They can be divided into biological factors contributing to the patient's usual cholesterol level and those factors altering the patient's usual cholesterol level (Table 8.12).

As can be seen in Table 8.12, numerous factors have the potential for altering usual cholesterol level. Some of these can be controlled by those persons involved in the drawing, preparation, storage, and shipment of blood specimens. In addition, certain conditions call for postponing measurement of serum lipid and lipoprotein levels. Among those identified by the National Cholesterol Education Program are recent myocardial infarction, stroke, trauma, acute infections, and pregnancy.

Fasting Total cholesterol and HDL-C levels can be measured in nonfasting persons. Recent food intake affects plasma total cholesterol levels by only about 1.5% or less.[86] The NCEP recommended that plasma triglyceride concentrations be measured only after a fast of at least 12 hours because absorption of fat after a meal elevates blood triglyceride levels. When a patient's LDL-C value is desired, a fast of at least 12 hours also is necessary because LDL-C typically is calculated from measurements of triglyceride, cholesterol, and HDL-C. If the triglyceride concentration is > 400 mg/dL (> 4.52 mmol/L), the LDL-C should be measured directly instead of being calculated.[86]

TABLE 8.12	**Preanalytical Factors Affecting Within-Individual Variability in Cholesterol Levels**			
Biological	**Behavioral**	**Clinical (Disease-Induced)**	**Clinical (Drug-Induced)**	**Sample Collecting and Handling**
Age	Usual diet	Acute and transient: burns, infections, recent myocardial infarction, recent stroke, trauma	Antihypertensives: beta-blockers, chlorothalidone, thiazides	Anticoagulants/preservatives
Individual biology	Alcohol			Fasting status
Race	Caffeine		Immunosupressives: cyclosporine, prednisolone, tacrolimus	Diurnal variation/time of day
Sex	Exercise	Endocrine: diabetes mellitus, hypothyroidism, hypopituitarism, pregnancy		Hemoconcentration
	Smoking		Steroids: estrogen, progestin	Posture
	Stress	Hepatic: congenital biliary atresia		Specimen storage
		Renal: chronic renal failure, nephrotic syndrome		Venous vs. capillary blood
		Storage diseases: Gaucher disease, glycogen storage disease, Tay-Sachs disease		Venous occlusion
		Other: anorexia nervosa, systemic lupus erythematosus		

Adapted from Rifai N, Dufour R, Cooper GR. 1997. Preanalytical variation in lipid, lipoprotein, and apolipoprotein testing. In Rifai N, Warnick GR, Dominiczak MH, eds. *Handbook of lipoprotein testing.* Washington, DC: American Association of Clinical Chemistry, pp. 75–97; Warnick GR. 2000. Measurement of cholesterol and other lipoprotein constituents in the clinical laboratory. *Clinical Chemistry and Laboratory Medicine* 38:287–300.

Posture   When a person sits or lies down after standing for several minutes, his or her plasma volume increases, and the concentration of cholesterol (and other non-diffusible plasma components) decreases. Compared with values in blood drawn while a person is standing, cholesterol levels can be significantly lower in blood drawn from the same person after he or she has been lying down for 5 minutes and may be as much as 10% to 15% lower in blood drawn after the person has been lying down for 20 minutes. Cholesterol levels in blood drawn after a person has been sitting for 10 to 15 minutes have been shown to be 6% lower than those in blood drawn from the same person while standing. It is recommended that blood sampling conditions be standardized to the sitting position. The patient should sit quietly for about 5 minutes before the sample is drawn.[86]

Venous Occlusion   If a tourniquet is applied to a vein for a prolonged period, the concentration of cholesterol (and other nondiffusible plasma components) will increase. The cholesterol concentration of blood drawn from a vein following a 2-minute tourniquet application can be 2% to 5% higher than that of venous blood drawn after a 30- to 60-second tourniquet application. A 10% to 15% average increase can result from a 5-minute tourniquet application. Venipuncture should be completed as rapidly as possible, preferably within 1 minute.[86]

Anticoagulants   Plasma is derived from whole blood, which is treated with an anticoagulant. The anticoagulants heparin and ethylenediamine tetraacetic acid are preferred. Fluoride, citrate, and oxalate anticoagulants should not be used because they cause plasma components to be diluted (cholesterol concentration is lower when these are used).[86,87]

Recent Heart Attack and Stroke   When a person has suffered a heart attack or stroke, his or her total cholesterol and LDL-C should not be measured for 8 weeks following the attack. These levels fall considerably in a heart attack or stroke victim and remain low for several weeks.

Trauma and Acute Infections   Cholesterol levels can fall by as much as 40% in a person who has suffered severe trauma and can fall temporarily in response to severe pain, surgery, and short-term physical strain. Cholesterol measurements should be performed no sooner than 8 weeks after such conditions have occurred.

Pregnancy   Increases in LDL and VLDL during pregnancy can lead to increases in cholesterol levels by as much as 35%. It is recommended that lipid measurements not be made until 3 to 4 months after delivery.

Hypertension

Hypertension (high blood pressure) is one of the most common risk factors for cardiovascular and renal diseases. It is associated with increased risk of developing CHD, stroke, congestive heart failure, renal insufficiency, and peripheral vascular disease.[88,89] Figure 8.14 shows that, as systolic blood pressure (SBP) or diastolic blood pressure (DBP) increase, there is an increased risk of death from cardiovascular disease.

Arterial blood pressure is measured using a device called a sphygmomanometer ("blood pressure cuff") and is expressed in millimeters of mercury (mm Hg). Systolic blood pressure is the blood pressure following systole, the phase of cardiac contraction. Diastolic blood pressure is that following diastole, the phase of cardiac relaxation. Blood pressure is expressed as two numbers, as in 120/80. The first number (120 mm Hg) is systolic blood pressure, and the second is diastolic blood pressure (80 mm Hg). From the standpoint of cardiovascular disease, an "optimal" blood pressure is one that is less than 120/80, although unusually low blood pressure readings should be evaluated for clinical significance.

Table 8.13 shows the guidelines developed by the National High Blood Pressure Education Program for classifying blood pressure. For blood pressure to be considered within the "normal" range, systolic pressure must be < 130 mm Hg and diastolic pressure must be < 85 mm Hg. An "optimal" blood pressure is defined as a systolic pressure < 120 mm Hg and diastolic pressure < 80 mm Hg.[88] According to NHANES III data, approximately 50 million Americans, or 25% of the U.S. adult population, have hypertension or are taking antihypertensive medications.[1,88] Roughly 50% of the U.S. adult population and 80% of those 50 years of age and older have a higher than optimal blood pressure. These individuals are at markedly increased risk for cardiovascular disease and stroke.

The prevalence of hypertension, based on NHANES III data collected between 1988 and 1994, for different age and sex groups is shown in Figure 8.15. The figure clearly shows that hypertension is much more common among older Americans. Because of the cross-sectional nature of NHANES III, these estimates are based on reported use of antihypertensive medication or on blood pressure measurements obtained at a single visit to a mobile examination center (see Chapter 4).

More conservative estimates based on two or more evaluations of blood pressure or use of antihypertensive medication place the prevalence of hypertension at 30 to 40 million Americans. Regardless of which estimate is used, hypertension is a very common problem. Hypertension is more common in black males and females than in white males and females, as shown in Figure 8.16. The figure also shows that the percentage of black and white males and females with hypertension decreased from the 1970s to 1994.

Figure 8.14

The bars in this figure represent the distribution of systolic blood pressure (chart on the left) and diastolic blood pressure (chart on the right) for males ages 35 to 57 years participating in the Multiple Risk Factor Intervention Trial ($N = 347{,}978$). The curved lines represent the 12-year rate of cardiovascular mortality for each level of systolic blood pressure (SBP) and diastolic blood pressure (DBP). As either SBP or DBP increases, risk of death from cardiovascular disease increases.

Source: Adapted from National High Blood Pressure Education Program Working Group. 1993. National High Blood Pressure Education Program Working Group report on primary prevention of hypertension. *Archives of Internal Medicine* 153:186–208.

TABLE 8.13	Classification of Blood Pressure for Persons Ages 18 Years and Older[*]		
	Systolic BP (mm Hg)		**Diastolic BP (mm Hg)**
Optimal[†]	< 120	and	< 80
Normal	< 130	and	< 85
High-normal	130–139	or	85–89
Hypertension[‡]			
Stage 1	140–159	or	90–99
Stage 2	160–179	or	100–109
Stage 3	≥ 180	or	≥ 110

Adapted from National High Blood Pressure Education Program. 1997. *The sixth report of the Joint National Committee on Prevention, Detection, Evaluation, and Treatment of High Blood Pressure.* Washington, DC: National Institutes of Health; National Heart, Lung, and Blood Institute.

[*]Not taking antihypertensive drugs and not acutely ill. When systolic and diastolic blood pressures fall into different categories, the higher category should be selected to classify the individual's blood pressure status. For example, 160/92 mm Hg should be classified as Stage 2 hypertension, and 174/120 mm Hg should be classified as Stage 3 hypertension. Isolated systolic hypertension is defined as SBP of 140 mm Hg or greater and DBP below 90 mm Hg and is staged appropriately (e.g., 170/82 mm Hg is defined as Stage 2 isolated systolic hypertension). In addition to classifying stages of hypertension on the basis of average blood pressure levels, clinicians should specify presence or absence of target organ disease and additional risk factors. This specificity is important for risk classification and treatment.

[†]Optimal blood pressure with respect to cardiovascular risk is below 120/80 mm Hg. However, unusually low readings should be evaluated for clinical significance.

[‡]Based on the average of two or more readings taken at each of two or more visits after an initial screening.

Efforts to reduce morbidity and mortality related to hypertension can be grouped into two broad categories: the patient-based, or clinical, approach and the population-based, or public health, approach. Early efforts to reduce hypertension-related morbidity and mortality centered on the patient-based approach, which involves clinicians detecting and treating individual cases of hypertension. More recently, greater attention has been given to the population-based approach, which stresses increased public awareness of hypertension and encourages every adult to know his or her blood pressure and to avoid those behaviors identified as risk factors for hypertension. These efforts have been quite successful, as demonstrated by the dramatic decline in deaths from coronary heart disease and stroke, as was shown in Figures 8.7 and 8.8.

Another indicator of success is shown in Figure 8.17. Using data from NHANES II (1976–80), NHANES III Phase 1 (1988–91), and NHANES III Phase 2 (1991–94), Figure 8.17 shows general improvement during those years in the percentage of persons with hypertension who are aware of their condition, who are being treated, and whose hypertension is under control. However, since 1991, this progress has reversed somewhat, as shown by data from NHANES III Phase 2 (1991–94). According to the latest data shown in Figure 8.17, less than 70% of persons with hypertension are aware of their condition, roughly half are treated, and fewer than 30% have adequate control of their blood pressure. This lack of awareness and inadequate control can result in significant

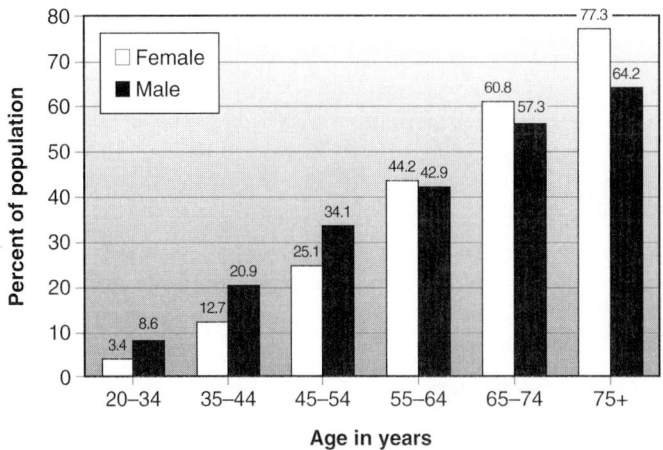

Figure 8.15

Data from NHANES III (1988–94) show that the prevalence of hypertension in the United States varies by age and sex. Between 20 and 54 years of age, hypertension is more common in males than in females. After age 54, prevalence is greater in females than in males. Hypertension is defined by either elevated blood pressure (systolic pressure $\geq$ 140 mm Hg or diastolic pressure $\geq$ 90 mm Hg) or the need to take medication to control blood pressure.

Source: Data from the National Center for Health Statistics.

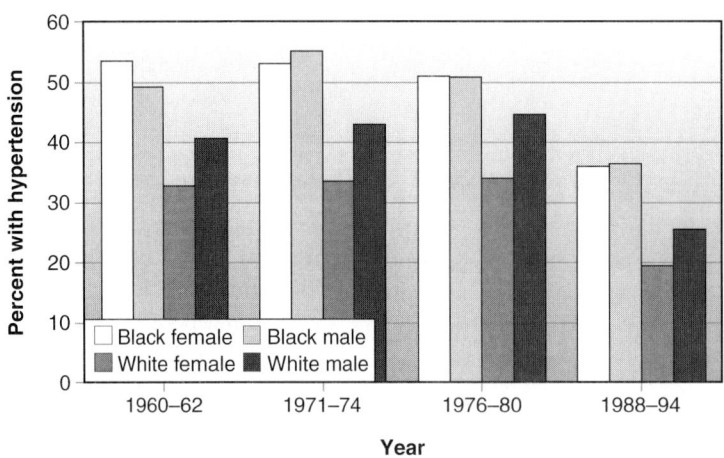

Figure 8.16 **The prevalence of hypertension among persons 20 years of age and older, according to sex and race, United States, 1960–62, 1971–74, 1976–80, 1988–1994.**

Non-Hispanic black females and males are more likely to have hypertension than white females and males. However, prevalence rates for all groups have generally declined since the 1970s. Hypertension is defined by either elevated blood pressure (systolic pressure $\geq$ 140 mm Hg or diastolic pressure $\geq$ 90 mm Hg) or the need to take medication to control blood pressure.

Source: Data from the National Center for Health Statistics.

vascular damage to the eyes, heart, kidneys, and brain. Although pharmacologic therapy for hypertension markedly reduces mortality and morbidity from cardiovascular disease and stroke, long-term pharmacologic therapy involves the expense of ongoing medical supervision and carries with it undesirable side effects. Even with optimal blood pressure control, persons with hyper-

tension still have a higher morbidity and mortality than persons with normal or optimal blood pressure.[88] Thus, there remains a need to increase efforts to promote hypertension awareness and to identify and modify risk factors leading to high blood pressure.

Increasing attention is being given to primary prevention of hypertension using the population-based approach by

Figure 8.17

Data collected from national surveys show that high blood pressure awareness, treatment, and control in the U.S. have generally improved, except in recent years, and that more work needs to be done to improve blood pressure awareness, treatment, and control.

Source: Data from the National Center for Health Statistics.

modifying risk factors associated with hypertension. The most important of these risk factors are a high sodium intake, excessive consumption of energy, physical inactivity, excessive alcohol consumption, and inadequate potassium intake. Box 8.7 lists lifestyle factors having proven efficacy in preventing and managing hypertension. Clinical trials have shown that lifestyle modifications involving these lifestyle factors can lower elevated blood pressure at little cost, with minimal risk, and to an extent equal to or greater than single-drug therapy.[88,90–92] Even when these modifications fail to control hypertension, they can reduce the number and dosage of antihypertensive medications needed to manage the condition—what is referred to as a "step-down" in therapy. Primary prevention is particularly helpful in lowering the elevated blood pressures of persons in groups at higher risk of hypertension,

such as African Americans, older persons, and persons with hypertension or diabetes.[88]

Body Weight

The evidence linking body weight to blood pressure and overweight to hypertension is strong and consistent. A body mass index ≥ 27 kg/m^2 is closely correlated with increased blood pressure. Excess adipose tissue within the abdomen (abdominal fat) has been associated with increased risk of hypertension, dyslipidemia, type 2 diabetes, and coronary heart disease.[88] As discussed in Chapter 6, the best clinical approach to assessing abdominal adiposity is measuring waist circumference. The *Dietary Guidelines for Americans* define high-risk waist circumference in adult males and females as > 40 in. and > 35 in., respectively. Several studies have shown that loss of excess body weight reduces both SBP and DBP and that the degree of blood pressure reduction is related to the extent of weight loss. A weight reduction of as little as 10 pounds is effective at reducing elevated blood pressure in overweight persons with hypertension, while enhancing the effectiveness of antihypertensive drugs and reducing cardiovascular disease risk by enhancing the management of type 2 diabetes and dyslipidemia.[88]

The largest randomized controlled trial to evaluate the impact of weight loss in persons with high-normal blood pressure, the Trials of Hypertension Prevention, showed that an average weight loss of 8.4 lb (3.8 kg) resulted in a 2.9 mm Hg and 2.3 mm Hg reduction in SBP and DBP, respectively.[90,93] Although this may seem like an insignificant decline in blood pressure, it has been estimated that a 2-mm Hg decline in the population mean SBP might reduce the annual mortality from stroke, CHD, and all causes by 6%, 4%, and 3%, respectively.[88,94] Not only is weight loss an effective means of lowering blood pressure, but it also tends to improve the lipid and lipoprotein profile and reduce the risk of developing noninsulin-dependent diabetes mellitus and possibly breast cancer.

  Box 8.7   **Lifestyle Modifications for Hypertension Prevention and Management**

- Lose weight if overweight.
- Limit alcohol intake to no more than two drinks per day or to no more than one drink per day for women and lighter-weight people.
- Increase aerobic physical activity (30 to 45 minutes most days of the week).
- Reduce sodium intake to no more than 2400 mg per day (100 mmoL sodium or 6 g sodium chloride).

- Maintain adequate intake of dietary potassium (approximately 3500 mg or 90 mmoL per day).
- Maintain adequate intake of dietary calcium and magnesium for general health.
- Stop smoking and reduce intake of dietary saturated fat and cholesterol for overall cardiovascular health.

Adapted from National High Blood Pressure Education Program. 1997. *The sixth report of the Joint National Committee on Prevention, Detection, Evaluation, and Treatment of High Blood Pressure.* Washington, DC: National Institutes of Health; National Heart, Lung, and Blood Institute.

Sodium

Research on the association between sodium intake and blood pressure has been hampered by several methodologic challenges. These include difficulty in measuring sodium intake, variable adherence to the prescribed reduction in sodium, the large day-to-day intraindividual (within-person) variation in sodium intake, the wide range of blood pressure values at any level of sodium intake, the small interindividual (between-person) variation in sodium intakes within a given population group, inadequate trial design, small numbers of subjects, and limitations in analysis and presentation of research findings. Despite these challenges, there is unequivocal evidence of a direct association between sodium intake and risk for hypertension.[83,84]

Based on data from NHANES III, the estimated average sodium intake of American adults is in excess of 3.4 g per day.[88] This estimate is similar for all racial and ethnic groups but does not include discretionary sodium use, such as table salt (sodium chloride) added in cooking or at the table. Consequently, average sodium intake by adults is probably closer to 4.0 g per day. This is far in excess of human physiologic need and is much greater than the typical intakes of people in less industrialized societies, who do not experience North America's age-related increase in blood pressure. Research clearly shows that, for most people, a modest reduction in sodium intake to the current recommendation of 2.4 g per day is a safe and effective way to reduce risk for hypertension.[88,91,95] The blood pressures of African Americans, older persons, and those with hypertension are more responsive to changes in dietary sodium. A modest reduction in sodium intake to the current recommendation of 2.4 g per day and the other modest risk factor modifications that were shown in Box 8.6 are sufficient to control mild hypertension in many patients. For those still needing antihypertensive medication, these steps will reduce their requirement for medication.[88,91,95]

Recent data from the Dietary Approaches to Stop Hypertension (DASH) trial show that a further reduction in sodium intake to 1.5 g per day provides a safe and effective way to further reduce risk for hypertension. The DASH trial was a multicenter, randomized feeding trial testing the effects of certain dietary patterns on blood pressure. These and other data provide a scientific basis for a lower goal for dietary sodium than the level currently recommended.[91,95] Achieving even the current sodium recommendation is challenging, given the fact that 75% of all sodium in the North American diet comes from processed foods. Success in achieving this modest goal will depend on consumers being better informed about the risks of high-sodium foods and avoiding high-sodium foods and food preparation methods, improved sodium labeling of foods (e.g., labeling foods as "high," "moderate," or "low" in sodium), and consumers demanding that the food industry increase the availability of low-sodium products.

Alcohol

Despite the difficulty of measuring the alcohol intake of study participants, there is consistent evidence of a strong positive relationship between alcohol consumption and blood pressure. It is estimated that as much as 5% to 7% of the overall prevalence of hypertension in the United States can be attributed to an alcohol intake of three drinks or more per day.[88] One drink of alcohol (0.5 fluid ounce of ethanol) is equivalent to 12 fluid ounces of beer, 4 fluid ounces of wine, or 1 ounce of 100-proof spirits. Furthermore, when alcohol intake is reduced, there is a subsequent reduction in blood pressure. A reduction in alcohol intake has been shown to be effective in lowering blood pressure in both hypertensive and normotensive individuals, and it may help prevent hypertension. Persons with hypertension should be advised to limit their alcohol intake to no more than two drinks per day.[94]

Physical Activity

Numerous studies have shown an inverse relationship between leisure-time and work-related physical activity and blood pressure. Other studies have shown that blood pressure tends to be lower in physically fit individuals. Although these studies have certain design limitations, they provide consistent evidence that increased physical activity results in an average reduction of approximately 6 to 7 mm Hg for both SBP and DBP. This reduction is not dependent on weight loss. A low to moderate exercise intensity (40% to 60% of maximum oxygen consumption) is as effective at lowering blood pressure in patients with mild to moderate hypertension as higher-intensity exercise. This can be achieved by brisk walking for 30 to 45 minutes most days of the week.[88]

Dietary Pattern

A number of studies have identified an inverse relationship between blood pressure and consumption of foods providing potassium, calcium, and magnesium. Persons consuming vegetarian diets, for example, tend to have a lower blood pressure than nonvegetarians. Aspects of the vegetarian diet believed to reduce blood pressure include minerals (potassium, calcium, and magnesium), reduced fat content, and possibly dietary fiber.[96,97] In studies investigating individual nutrients, often when provided in supplemental form, the reduction in blood pressure is typically small and inconsistent, probably because the blood pressure–lowering effect of a single nutrient is too small to detect in clinical trials. However, when these nutrients are consumed together, the cumulative effect is sufficient to bring about a statistically and clinically significant lowering of blood pressure. Food is incredibly complex and contains countless nutrients and components other than those few being examined in trials or measured in observational studies. When evaluating the blood pressure–lowering effects of foods, these nutrients and food components and the complex interactions among them must be considered.[96,97]

Consequently, increased attention is being given to the overall dietary pattern, rather than to a few individual nutrients. This is in large part due to results from the Dietary Approaches to Stop Hypertension (DASH) trial.[91,97] The DASH trial showed that a diet rich in fruits, vegetables, and fat-free or low-fat dairy products lowers elevated blood pressure, particularly when sodium intake is kept moderate.[91,97] The DASH diet, combined with a moderate sodium restriction and sustained efforts to modify the other factors associated with hypertension, which were listed in Box 8.7, is a safe, effective, and low-cost nonpharmacologic approach for promoting optimal to normal blood pressure.

OSTEOPOROSIS

Osteoporosis is a bone disorder characterized by inadequate bone strength, leading to increased risk for bone fracture. Bone strength is a function of two factors: bone mineral density and bone quality. Bone mineral density accounts for approximately 70% of bone strength and is expressed as grams of mineral per area or volume of bone. Bone density is determined by peak bone mass and the amount of bone loss. Bone quality relates to bone architecture, bone turnover, mineralization, and the accumulation of damage to the bone (e.g., microfractures). Figure 8.18 illustrates how bone architecture and density can differ between normal bone and that from an individual with osteoporosis. When sufficient force is applied to osteoporotic bone, a fracture occurs, making osteoporosis a significant risk factor for fracture. A fracture can occur not only from a traumatic event, such as a fall, but also from the stress placed on bone during normal lifting and bending.[98]

Osteoporosis is a major public health problem affecting nearly 30 million Americans and each year resulting in more than 1.5 million fractures, including 700,000 vertebral fractures, 300,000 fractures of the proximal femur (hip), 250,000 distal forearm (wrist) fractures, and more than 300,000 fractures at other sites. Hip fractures have the greatest morbidity, mortality, and socioeconomic impact. Of those persons having a hip fracture, 20% die within 1 year, 28% require long-term care, and 50% never recover the ability to walk without assistance.[98–100] Hip and vertebral fractures often result in serious depression as patients grapple with pain, physical limitations, and lifestyle changes. Vertebral fractures result in back pain, height loss, and kyphosis, an abnormal backward curvature of the spine. Postural and height changes associated with kyphosis can limit activity (e.g., bending and reaching), cause restrictive lung disease, and alter abdominal anatomy, leading to constipation, abdominal pain, reduced appetite, and premature satiety.[101] The annual economic burden of health care costs is estimated to be as high as $15 billion. The National Institutes of Health estimates that 10 million Americans already have osteoporosis and that nearly 20 million more have low bone density, placing them at increased risk for the disease.[98] American women are four times more likely than men to develop osteoporosis. Along with heart disease and breast cancer, it is one of the three most serious diseases affecting women.[100] Among Americans ages 50 years and older, 50% of females and 12% of males will have a osteoporosis-related fracture in their lifetime. For any given age, osteoporotic fractures are twice as common in females than in males, and, because they live longer than males, females experience an even higher absolute incidence during their lifetime.[98]

A

B

Figure 8.18 Scanning electron micrographs of bone biopsy specimens from the iliac crest: A is normal, and B is from a person with osteoporosis.

At about age 20 or 25 years, the bones of the human skeleton reach 90% to 95% of their *peak bone mass* (the point of maximum bone mineralization). Over the next 10 years, the final 5% to 10% of bone mineral is added, in a process known as *consolidation.* There is considerable interindividual variation in peak bone mass because of such factors as heredity, sex, race, and environmental factors. On average, males have 10% to 15% greater peak bone mass than females, and the bones of black persons are about 10% denser than those of white persons. Black males have the most dense bones, followed by white males, black females, and white females.[98,100]

Once peak mass is reached, bone mineral content begins to decline in both sexes at an annual rate of 0.3% to 0.5%.[102] In males, this gradual decline remains fairly constant, resulting in a lifetime bone mineral loss of 20% to 30%. In females, around the time of menopause (generally occurring at age 45 to 55 years) or following surgical removal of both ovaries, the rate of bone mineral loss temporarily accelerates to as high as 4% to 8% annually. Lifetime losses in females may be 40% to 50% or more of peak bone mass. The major factor in the higher rate of bone demineralization in the years immediately following menopause is apparently due to estrogen deficiency.[99]

Bones: Structure and Remodeling

Bones can be classified as being composed of two types of structural tissue: *cortical,* or *compact,* tissue and *trabecular,* or *cancellous,* tissue. The very dense cortical tissue forms the outer shells of bones, encasing the trabecular tissue, which is composed of a fine, spongelike mesh with numerous small voids. The marrow elements occupy these voids.[99] The total skeleton is composed of 80% cortical bone and 20% trabecular bone. Cortical bone is found primarily in the appendicular skeleton (bones of the limbs), whereas most of the trabecular bone is found in the axial skeleton (the skull and vertebral bones).[103]

Bone is a dynamic tissue and is constantly undergoing change in a process known as *remodeling.* The bone resorption cells, or osteoclasts, are active at numerous points within bone. They secrete enzymes that dissolve bone before it is reformed and provide a source of blood calcium when dietary intake is inadequate. The bone-forming cells, or osteoblasts, secrete an organic matrix composed largely of collagen. This matrix then becomes hardened by deposits of calcium and phosphate crystals known as *hydroxyapatite.* The rate of remodeling, or turnover rate, is approximately eight times faster in trabecular bone than in cortical bone, leading to a faster decline in bone mineral content in trabecular bone.[103] Consequently, symptoms of osteoporosis appear earlier in trabecular bone—in for example the spine (vertebral bodies) and wrist (distal radius).[99,103]

Osteoporosis: Classification and Risk Factors

Osteoporosis can be classified as either primary (not related to other disease) or secondary (when an identifiable cause other than age or menopause is present). Osteoporosis can be secondary to such conditions as Cushing's syndrome, malignancies of the bone (myeloma), hyperthyroidism, hyperparathyroidism, male hypogonadism, and amenorrhea. Certain inherited diseases, such as osteogenesis imperfecta, can also result in osteoporosis, as can long-term use of such medications as thiazide diuretics and heparin.[99,102] The most common form is primary osteoporosis, in which no other disease is apparent. This is most frequently seen in middle-aged and older females and older males. In these age groups, Type I and Type II primary osteoporosis are most commonly seen.[99,102]

Type I is seen in postmenopausal females between 51 and 75 years of age and primarily involves loss of trabecular bone. Low estrogen levels accompanying menopause lead to increased bone remodeling and accelerated bone loss. Production of vitamin D_3 and intestinal absorption of calcium often are decreased in postmenopausal women, exacerbating bone loss. This leads to fractures at sites where trabecular bone predominates (for example, vertebral bodies and the distal radius).[99,102]

Type II osteoporosis is seen in both sexes after age 70 years. It is related to several age-related changes, such as decreased osteoblast function, decreased calcium absorption, decreased vitamin D_3 synthesis, and decreased levels of calcitonin (calcitonin inhibits bone resorption).[99] In Type II osteoporosis, bone mineral is lost from both trabecular and cortical bone. The most common sites of fractures are the hip and vertebrae. Multiple fractures of the vertebrae can lead to a marked curvature of the thoracic spine known as *thoracic kyphosis* or "dowager's hump." Other sites include the proximal humerus (bone of the upper arm), pelvis, and proximal tibia (large bone of the lower leg).

Various risk factors are associated with the development of osteoporosis. These are shown in Table 8.14. Compared with leaner persons, obese persons tend to be at lower risk for osteoporosis because of the greater density of their bones, which must support a greater body weight. Early menopause, either natural or surgically induced by removal of both ovaries (bilateral oophorectomy), shortens the time that a woman experiences estrogen's protective effects and thus increases risk. Risk is also increased by menstrual irregularities (oligomenorrhea or amenorrhea) resulting from an unhealthfully low percent body fat. This may be due to excessive physical activity coupled with caloric restriction (as seen in some long-distance runners, gymnasts, and ballet dancers) or from eating disorders, such as anorexia nervosa or bulimia.

Peak bone mass is a major factor determining risk of developing osteoporosis. At any given age, risk for fracture is less in people who have achieved a greater peak

TABLE 8.14	Risk Factors for Osteoporosis and Their Scientific Validity

Well-Established Evidence	Moderate Evidence
Obesity (−)	Alcohol (+)
African ancestry (−)	Cigarette smoking (−)
Estrogen use (−)	Thiazide diuretic use (+)
High peak bone mass (−)	Moderate exercise (−)
Heavy exercise (−)	Caffeine use (+)
Female (+)	Fluoridated water use (−)
Caucasian/Asian (+)	
Age (+)	
Early menopause (+)	
Menstrual irregularities (+)	
Family history (+)	
Bilateral oophorectomy (+)	
Low dietary calcium (+)	
Corticosteroid use (+)	
Bed rest (+)	

From McBean LD, Forgac T, Finn SC. 1994. Osteoporosis: Visions for care and prevention—A conference report. *Journal of the American Dietetic Association* 94:668–671; National Osteoporosis Foundation. 2000. *Physician's guide to prevention and treatment of osteoporosis.* Washington, DC: National Osteoporosis Foundation; U.S. Department of Health and Human Services. 2000. *Consensus Development Conference statement: Osteoporosis prevention, diagnosis, and therapy.* Bethesda, MD: National Institute of Arthritis and Musculoskeletal and Skin Diseases, National Institutes of Health.

(−) = decreased risk; (+) = increased risk.

bone mass during the period of bone development than in those with a lower peak bone mass. Because they have the greatest average peak bone mass, black males tend to develop osteoporosis least often of any sex/race group. Compared with white females, black females have a higher peak bone mass and, consequently, less incidence of osteoporosis.[99]

Bone Densitometry

Bone densitometry, the measurement of bone mineral content, is important in the early detection and treatment of osteoporosis and in monitoring its progression and response to treatment.[103,107] Currently, there is no accurate measure of overall bone strength. However, because bone mineral density accounts for approximately 60% to 80% of the variation in bone strength, it is generally used as a proxy measure of bone strength.[98,103–107] Consequently, the most common approach to diagnosing osteoporosis and predicting fracture risk is bone densitometry, the measurement of bone mineral density, which is primarily determined by bone mineral content.[98,104] Bone mineral density measurements correlate strongly with the load-bearing capacity of the hip and spine and with fracture risk.[98] In addition to radiogrammetry, five basic approaches are used to quantify bone density. These include single-photon absorptiometry, dual-photon absorptiometry, dual-energy X-ray absorptiometry, quan-

titative computed tomography, and quantitative ultrasound. Other techniques, such as neutron activation analysis, Compton scattering, ultrasonic transmission velocity or attenuation, and magnetic resonance, are either not widely available or are in the early stages of development.[103–107]

Single-photon absorptiometry primarily measures content of cortical bone in the peripheral appendicular skeleton (for example, the bones of the forearm, wrist, and hands).[103] Dual-photon absorptiometry and dual-energy X-ray absorptiometry are capable of measuring both cortical and trabecular bone in the spine, hip, and total skeleton. Quantitative computed tomography provides a measure of trabecular bone in the vertebrae and other sites.[103] Quantitative ultrasound, a more recently introduced approach, shows considerable promise for assessing skeletal status in osteoporosis.[104–106] The various features of each are summarized in Table 8.15.

Radiogrammetry

Radiogrammetry uses standard X rays of bones, from which measurements of cortical bone thickness are obtained using a caliper or other measuring device. It usually is performed on the bones of the hands (metacarpals) and is widely available, easy to perform, reproducible, and backed by a large body of normative data.[103,107] Measurements of bone mineral content within the appendicular skeleton, however, fail to reflect mineral status of the axial skeleton. Therefore, this method is of limited value in assessing early osteoporosis and fracture and in assessing bones in which improvements in mineral content caused by treatment are likely to be seen.[103,107]

TABLE 8.15	Comparison of Bone Densitometry Techniques*			
	SPA	DPA	QCT	DXA
Precision (%)	2–3	2–4	2–5	1–2
Accuracy (%)	5	4–10	5–20	3–5
Duration of examination (min)	15	20–45	10–20	5
Absorbed dose (mrem)	10	5	100–1,000	1–3
Radiation source	Iodine-125	Gadolinium-153	X-ray	X-ray
Source renewal (months)	6	12–18	N/A	N/A
Cost	Low	Moderate	High	Low

From Sartoris DJ, Resnick D. 1990. Current and innovative methods for noninvasive bone densitometry. *Orthopedics* 28:257–278; U.S. Dept. of Health and Human Services. 1991. *Osteoporosis research, education, and health promotion.* Bethesda, MD: National Institute of Arthritis and Musculoskeletal and Skin Diseases, National Institutes of Health.

*SPA = single-photon absorptiometry; DPA = dual-photon absorptiometry; QCT = quantitative computerized tomography; DXA = dual-energy X-ray absorptiometry; N/A = not applicable.

Single-Photon Absorptiometry

In single-photon absorptiometry (SPA), a single-energy beam of photons from a radioisotope (iodine-125) is directed through the bone and overlying soft tissue and is received by a detector and counter. The measured transmission rate of the photon beam is inversely proportional to the bone mineral content, which is expressed as bone mineral per square centimeter scanned.[107] The method involves a low radiation dose, and individual examinations are inexpensive. The instruments are portable and thus suited to epidemiologic studies in remote populations.

Usual sites for SPA measurements are those within the appendicular skeleton—the distal third of the radius, the calcaneus (the heel bone), and the distal femur.[103,105–107] Results from SPA are influenced by the variable thicknesses of soft tissue. Renewal of the radiation source every 6 months requires additional attention and expense. Thus, the general consensus is that SPA primarily measures cortical bone and consequently is not well suited for predicting bone strength and fracture risk at typical osteoporotic fracture sites or for monitoring change caused by osteoporosis treatment.[103,105–108] Experts in metabolic bone disease have little or no use today for appendicular bone densitometry, even by sophisticated methods.[109]

Dual-Photon Absorptiometry

Dual-photon absorptiometry (DPA) is similar in concept to SPA except it uses photon beams at two different energy levels derived from a radioisotopic source (gadolinium-153). This allows measurement of bone mineral content that is independent of the thickness or density of soft tissues in the photon path, which is a drawback of SPA.[103,105–108] However, DPA measurements can be adversely affected by calcification of blood vessels, other soft tissue calcification, and abnormal outgrowths of bones. Bone mineral content is expressed in grams per centimeter, which is an expression based on area rather than density.[103]

Usual sites for measurement with DPA are the spine, hip, upper femur, and total body. Measurements express both cortical and trabecular bone. The main advantages of DPA are low radiation dose, sufficient accuracy for making clinical judgments, a large number of accessible anatomic sites, and independence from the effects of soft tissues. Limiting factors include DPA's long scanning time (20 to 45 minutes), the expense involved in replacing the radiation source every 12 to 18 months, and low short-term precision that is insufficient for detecting bone mineral changes over the follow-up periods typically used in clinical studies of treatments for osteoporosis.[103,107] DPA is a significant improvement over SPA, but overall it appears that measurements by quantitative CT and dual-energy X-ray absorptiometry are better at assessing the mineral content of trabecular bone and are more predictive of vertebral fracture than is DPA.[103,107]

Quantitative Computed Tomography

Quantitative computed tomography (QCT) uses a device consisting of an array of X-ray sources and radiation detectors aligned opposite each other. As the X-ray beams pass through the subject, they are weakened, or attenuated, by the body's tissues and eventually picked up by the detectors. Data from the detectors then are transmitted to a computer, which reconstructs the subject's cross-sectional anatomy using mathematic equations adapted for computer processing.[110]

QCT can provide a quantitative measure of mineral content in cortical and/or trabecular bone within either the appendicular or axial skeleton.[103,107] In measurements of the axial skeleton, it has several advantages over dual-photon absorptiometry. It distinguishes between cortical and trabecular bone and is unaffected by mineral deposits outside the skeleton. Dual-energy QCT has been shown to measure changes in trabecular mineral content in the spine, radius, and tibia with considerable precision. However, it requires sophisticated calibration and positioning and careful technical monitoring.[103] The accuracy of single-energy QCT is more variable, depending on the amount of fat in the bone marrow.[108] The potential for using QCT in assessing bone mineral content is limited by problems of high radiation exposure, high cost, and limited availability of the method.[108,111] However, technical advances are resulting in lower radiation doses, lower costs, and greater availability, thus making QCT increasingly important in evaluating bone diseases.[105–107]

Dual-Energy X-Ray Absorptiometry

Dual-energy X-ray absorptiometry (DXA) is currently the leading technique for measuring bone density because of its capacity to measure bone mineral content at axial and appendicular sites, its superior capabilities for monitoring changes in the skeleton over time and in response to osteoporosis treatment, and its superior quality-control procedures.[103–107] An example of a commercially available DXA unit is shown in Figure 8.19. It is similar in concept to dual-photon absorptiometry but has several advantages. In DXA, the energy source is an X-ray tube, which provides an energy beam of greater intensity than the radioisotope used with DPA.[103–107] DXA has a much shorter scanning time (5 minutes versus 20 minutes), which reduces errors from patient movement, allows better use of instruments, reduces patient costs, and shortens the duration of discomfort in patients with osteoporosis who are experiencing back pain.[103,108] Radiation exposure from DXA is substantially less than in QCT. A major advantage over DPA is the improved precision, which allows

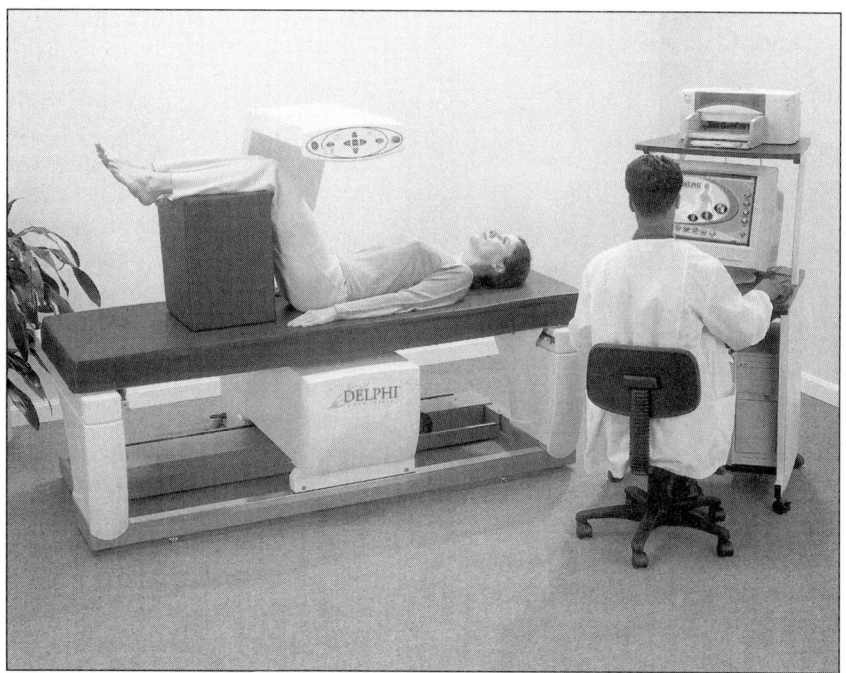

Figure 8.19 An example of a commercially available dual-energy X-ray absorptiometry (DXA) unit in operation.
Source: Photo courtesy of Hologic Incorporated.

changes in bone mineral content to be detected over short periods.[103–109] Development of new software has permitted measurement of total and regional body calcium and body composition.[112]

Of all the methods compared, DXA has the lowest precision error and is the most sensitive method for detecting changes in bone mineral density in the axial skeleton, where the earliest losses of bone mineral and their consequences occur. This, coupled with its speed, ease of use, and low radiation dose, has made DXA the clinical method of choice for studying bone changes associated with metabolic diseases.[103–107]

Quantitative Ultrasound

For years, ultrasound has been successfully used for non-destructive material testing. Characteristic changes in the transmission of ultrasound have been used to evaluate mechanical competence and to detect the presence of damage in both materials and structures.[104] Only recently has ultrasound been used to assess osteoporotic fracture risk. Quantitative ultrasound (QUS) assesses skeletal status using high-frequency sound waves transmitted through bone by measuring two characteristics of the transmitted sound waves: changes in the intensity of the sound waves (attenuation) and the velocity of the transmitted sound.[104,105] These characteristics reflect the mechanical properties of cortical and trabecular bone, which in turn determine bone stiffness, failure load, and fracture risk.[104,113]

Sonometers have been designed for assessing bone at different anatomic sites, such as the tibia and the phalanges (bones of the fingers), but the most common measurement site is the calcaneus (heel bone). The calcaneus is easily accessible, has a high percentage of trabecular bone, is weight bearing, and has a pattern of osteoporotic loss similar to that of the spine.[106] When using a sonometer, the heel of the foot is positioned between two transducers, which transmit and receive the ultrasound signals (typically in the frequency range of 0.1 to 1.0 MHz) as illustrated in Figure 8.20. The ultrasonic wave is transmitted from one transducer, through the heel, and is received by the other transducer. Maintaining good acoustic contact between the transducers and the skin of the heel is essential to allow high transmission of the ultrasound between the transducers and the tissues of the foot. Two methods are used to accomplish this. A "wet system" utilizes a temperature-stabilized water bath in which the patient's foot is immersed. A more recently developed "dry system" uses silicone pads and ultrasound gel to directly couple the transducers to the heel.[105,106] The commercially available dry systems have the advantage of processing patients at a faster rate, and they are more convenient to use (no water bath is necessary). When the ultrasonic wave is transmitted through the tissues of the heel, the intensity of the sound wave is dampened, or weakened, depending on various physical characteristics of the bone. This is referred to as broadband ultrasound attenuation (BUA). The other characteristic of ultrasound transmission is the velocity at which

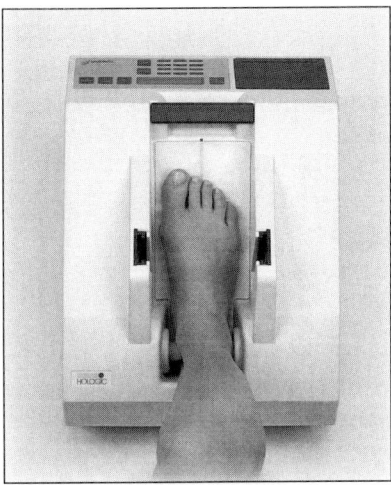

Figure 8.20 **Quantitative ultrasound measurement on the calcaneus (heel bone).**
The heel lies between two transducers: one transmits the ultrasonic wave through the calcaneus while the other receives the wave. A foot-positioning aide (not shown in this illustration) ensures precise placement of the foot and heel within the unit.
Source: Photo courtesy of Hologic Incorporated.

the sound waves pass through bone and surrounding soft tissue. This is referred to as the speed of sound (SOS) and is considered an index of bone strength. A high SOS suggests that the bone is strong and less susceptible to fracture. In some commercial QUS units, BUA and SOS are used to calculate a third parameter shown to be related to fracture risk. Depending on the manufacturer of the unit, this third parameter is referred to as "stiffness" or a "quantitative ultrasound index."[104-106,113]

Exactly what QUS measures is still under investigation.[105] QUS does not actually measure bone mineral content. Rather, it assesses bone mass and several aspects of bone microarchitecture, such as the connectivity, spacing, thickness, and number of trabeculae in bone, all of which appear to be important determinants of fracture risk. It has been suggested that QUS assesses factors important to osteoporotic fracture risk other than bone mineral density, which cannot be assessed using DXA.[105,113,117] Measures of BUA and SOS derived from QUS closely correlate with measures of bone mineral content derived from DXA.[114] In addition, several studies have shown that QUS assessment of the calcaneus is capable of identifying persons at increased risk for osteoporotic fracture nearly as well as assessments using SXA and DXA.[104,113-116] Two large prospective studies have shown QUS capable of predicting future risk for osteoporotic fracture risk in older females as well as DXA.[113,117] However, in these two studies, ultrasound measurements were done using devices employing the wet system, and the

more recently available commercial units employing a dry system need additional evaluation before they can be expected to have the same predictive value as the wet systems. DXA remains the definitive method for evaluating bone density, risk of fracture, and response to treatment for osteoporosis. However, QUS does have several advantages over DXA. It is less expensive and more portable than DXA and does not expose patients to ionizing radiation. Consequently, QUS instruments can be conveniently located in rooms that do not have radiation shielding. The regulations for training and licensing operators of QUS instruments are considerably less stringent than those required for DXA. QUS is a promising new technique for bone assessment, but because of limited experience in applying this new technology it cannot yet be recommended as the sole means of assessing fracture risk and monitoring skeletal changes in response to treatment. At this time, it appears that QUS is better suited as a screening method and that abnormal QUS values should be followed up by a regular DXA measurement to confirm the presence of osteoporosis.[104,105,115]

Prevention and Treatment

Preventing and treating osteoporosis involves attaining the greatest genetically possible bone mineral density and then minimizing its loss. The three major interacting factors influencing bone health are diet, exercise, and estrogen.[98-100] Calcium, phosphorus, and vitamins D and C are particularly important in achieving optimal bone mineral density. High intake of protein, sodium, and caffeine appear to increase risk of osteoporosis. More research is needed on the roles of vitamin K, manganese, copper, and zinc.[118] Primary prevention of osteoporosis begins in childhood and continues throughout adolescence and into the mid-30s, when the skeleton is acquiring its genetically programmed peak mineral mass. Secondary prevention is also critical to reducing morbidity and mortality. Although lost bone mineral cannot be replaced, the rate at which losses occur can be reduced by diet, exercise, and estrogen replacement therapy. It is estimated that adequate nutrition can reduce the impact of osteoporosis by one-half or more. Exercise by older adults can also help maintain muscular strength, stability, and balance, which will help reduce falls and risk for osteoporosis-related injury.[100]

Studies show that adequate calcium intake during childhood and adolescence is associated with improved bone mineral density, thus contributing to peak bone mineral density.[119,120] In adult women at least 5 years following menopause, adequate calcium intake has been shown to slow the rate of bone demineralization.[118,121] In an 18-month study of 1765 women ages 69 years and over, women increased their calcium intake from 500 mg to 1700 mg per day and consumed 20 μmg of vitamin D (cholecalciferol). Nonvertebral fractures were reduced by

32% and hip fractures were reduced by 43%.[122] Finnish researchers studied the influence of supplemental vitamin D given to males and females ages 75 years and older who had a vitamin D deficiency but had adequate calcium intake. Participants received annual injections of 3750 μmg or 7500 μmg of vitamin D (ergocalciferol) over a period of 2 to 5 years. For females receiving supplemental vitamin D, fractures of the upper limb and ribs were approximately half of that seen for females in the control group. There was no significant difference in the rate of fractures of the lower limbs in females. Among males, the fracture rate in those receiving vitamin D did not differ significantly from that of the control group.[123] Thus, the benefits of increased calcium and vitamin D intake can be seen in younger persons as well as in older persons. Although there is not uniform agreement among studies, the weight of evidence clearly shows the efficacy of increased calcium intake in slowing the rate of bone mineral loss and markedly reducing the risk for fracture in older adults.[121–124] The lack of agreement stems from the difficulty of measuring dietary calcium intake and the fact that diet and exercise appear to have little, if any, effect on slowing the rate of bone demineralization during the first 5 years following menopause.[121]

Because osteoporosis is a multifactorial disease, measures such as estrogen replacement therapy for post-menopausal women, weight-bearing exercise, and smoking cessation should be included along with dietary attempts to delay the rate of bone demineralization.

DIABETES MELLITUS

Diabetes mellitus is a group of diseases characterized by a defect in insulin secretion and/or increased cellular resistance to insulin, resulting in elevated plasma (or serum) glucose levels, abnormalities of carbohydrate and lipid metabolism, characteristic pathologic changes in the nerves and small blood vessels, and aggravation of atherosclerosis.[125,126] Since 1932, diabetes mellitus has been among the top 10 leading causes of death in America. It is a major cause of blindness, renal failure, congenital malformation, and lower extremity amputation. The prevalence of coronary artery disease and peripheral vascular disease is twice as common among persons with diabetes, compared with those without diabetes. It afflicts more than 20 million Americans, or approximately 8% of the population.[126]

Types of Diabetes

There are five categories of patients with diabetes, or impaired glucose metabolism: type 1 diabetes, type 2 diabetes, gestational diabetes mellitus, impaired fasting glucose, and impaired glucose tolerance. The vast majority of diabetes cases fall into two broad categories, type 1 diabetes and type 2 diabetes.[126] Type 1 diabetes is

that form resulting from the destruction of the insulin-secreting beta cells of the pancreas. The beta cells are typically destroyed by an autoimmune process in which antibodies produced by the patient's own immune system destroy these insulin-secreting cells.[126,127] Although the rate and extent of beta cell destruction can vary considerably among persons with type 1 diabetes, most patients eventually become dependent on insulin injections for survival and to prevent life-threatening ketoacidosis.[126] Type 1 diabetes is generally diagnosed in children and young adults and accounts for 5% to 10% of diabetes cases.

Type 2 diabetes is that form resulting from insulin resistance and a "relative" insulin deficiency. *Insulin resistance* refers to abnormalities in the binding of insulin to the insulin receptor located within the cell's plasma membrane, to defects in glucose transport into the cell, and to abnormalities in other intracellular processes involved in glucose metabolism, including insulin-stimulated glycogen synthesis.[128] Although blood insulin levels in patients with type 2 diabetes may appear normal or even elevated, they are inadequate to compensate for insulin resistance, and a relative insulin deficiency is said to exist. Type 2 is the most common form of diabetes, seen in 90% to 95% of persons with diabetes. Historically, type 2 was generally diagnosed in persons older than 30 years of age but is now seen in all age groups, and its incidence is rising fastest in children and young adults, in large part due to the high prevalence of obesity and physical inactivity among youth. Most patients with type 2 diabetes are obese or have increased amounts of adipose tissue in the abdominal region. The major risk factors for type 2 diabetes are shown in Box 8.8. Type 2 frequently goes undiagnosed for years because hyperglycemia develops gradually. Ketoacidosis seldom occurs spontaneously and generally arises only in response to the stress of another illness, such as an acute infection.[126]

Gestational diabetes mellitus (GDM) is a class of diabetes defined by any degree of glucose intolerance with onset or first recognition during pregnancy, notwithstanding the possibility that unrecognized impaired glucose tolerance may have existed prior to conception.[126,129,130] The classification of GDM is used regardless of whether insulin or diet modification is used for treatment or whether the condition persists after delivery. Patients with GDM should be reevaluated 6 weeks postpartum, by which time most patients exhibit normal glucose regulation.[126] About 7% of all pregnancies are complicated by GDM, although the prevalence ranges from 1% to 14%, depending on the population studied. Of all pregnancies complicated by diabetes, 90% involve GDM, making it the most common medical disorder affecting pregnancy. Early diagnosis and effective management of GDM is important to reduce the risk of perinatal morbidity and mortality and to reduce the risk for cesarean

Box 8.8   **Major Risk Factors for Type 2 Diabetes**

- History of diabetes in a parent or sibling
- Obesity (BMI $\geq$ 27 kg/m^2)
- Habitual physical inactivity
- Race/ethnicity (African, Hispanic, Asian, Pacific Islander, Native American)
- Previously identified IFG* or IGT*
- Hypertension ($\geq$ 140/90 mm Hg in adults or on antihypertensive therapy)

- HDL cholesterol $\leq$ 35 mg/dL and/or triglyceride level $\geq$ 250 mg/dL
- History of gestational diabetes or delivery of a child with birth weight > 9 lb
- Polycystic ovary syndrome

*IFG = impaired fasting glucose; IGT = impaired glucose tolerance.

Adapted from American Diabetes Association. 2001. Screening for diabetes. *Diabetes Care* 24(suppl):S21–S24.

delivery.[126,130] *Impaired fasting glucose (IFG)* and *impaired glucose tolerance (IGT)* refer to a metabolic stage between normal glucose homeostasis and diabetes. Impaired fasting glucose occurs when fasting plasma glucose levels are greater than the upper limit of "normal" ($\geq$ 110 mg/dL) but are not sufficiently elevated to be diagnostic for diabetes (i.e., < 126 mg/dL). Approximately 13.4 million people in the United States, or about 7% of the population, have IFG. Individuals with impaired glucose tolerance often have normal blood glucose levels (are euglycemic) in their daily lives and may exhibit hyperglycemia only when tested for diabetes using an oral glucose tolerance test.[126] IGT is diagnosed when the plasma glucose level is < 200 mg/dL 2 hours after a person is given a drink containing 75 grams of glucose.

Diagnosis of Diabetes

Despite the public health significance of diabetes, data from NHANES III show that about 50% of people with diabetes are not diagnosed. Three testing criteria are recognized for diagnosing diabetes, as shown in Box 8.9.[126] Repeat testing on a subsequent day using any one of the three criteria must be positive to confirm a diagnosis of diabetes. For example, if a patient presents with the classic symptoms of diabetes and has a casual plasma glucose $\geq$ 200 mg/dL, a diagnosis of diabetes can be con-

firmed only by testing on a subsequent day, revealing (1) the classic symptoms with a casual plasma glucose $\geq$ 200 mg/dL, (2) fasting plasma glucose (FPG) $\geq$ 126 mg/dL, or (3) an oral glucose tolerance test (OGTT) with a 2-hour plasma glucose $\geq$ 200 mg/dL.

Blood Glucose

Diagnosis of diabetes mellitus is not difficult when a person has the classic signs and symptoms of diabetes and a markedly elevated blood glucose level. It is also relatively easy when a patient with no symptoms has persistently elevated fasting plasma glucose levels. In other instances, the diagnosis of diabetes may rest on use of the oral glucose tolerance test (OGTT).

A normal fasting plasma glucose level is considered < 110 mg/dL. For the purpose of some glucose measurements, fasting can be defined as no consumption of food or beverage other than water for at least 8 hours before testing.[126]

Oral Glucose Tolerance Test

The oral glucose tolerance test (OGTT) involves having the patient drink a beverage containing a known amount of glucose, usually 75 grams for adults or 1.75 g/kg for children. Venous blood is drawn immediately before the glucose beverage is consumed and then at set intervals following consumption to monitor changes in blood sugar

Box 8.9   **Diagnostic Criteria for Diabetes Mellitus***

1. Presence of the classic symptoms of diabetes plus a casual plasma glucose $\geq$ 200 mg/dL; *casual* is defined as testing at any time of the day regardless of time since last meal
2. Fasting plasma glucose (FPG) $\geq$ 126 mg/dL; fasting is defined as no caloric intake for at least 8 hours

3. An oral glucose tolerance test (OGTT) with a 2-hour plasma glucose $\geq$ 200 mg/dL

*Classic symptoms of diabetes include polyuria (excessive urination), polydipsia (excessive thirst), polyphagia (excessive consumption of food), unexplained weight loss, blurred vision, and recurrent infections.

Adapted from American Diabetes Association. 2001. Report of the Expert Committee on the Diagnosis and Classification of Diabetes Mellitus. *Diabetes Care* 24(suppl):S5–S20.

level. In preparing for the OGTT, it is best for the patient to consume more than 150 g of carbohydrate per day, abstain from alcohol, and have unrestricted activity for 3 days before the test.[126] On the morning of the test, the fasting subject consumes the glucose beverage within a 5- to 10-minute period. Plasma glucose is measured while fasting and usually at 1-hour intervals for 2 or 3 hours.

A plasma glucose level ≥ 200 mg/dL (≥ 11.1 mmol/L) at 2 hours is diagnostic of diabetes. Figure 8.21 shows examples of how plasma glucose might respond to an OGTT in a person with diabetes, a person with impaired glucose tolerance, and a person without diabetes. In the curve representing the person with diabetes, the plasma glucose exceeds 200 mg/dL at 2 hours after consuming the glucose load.

The 2-hour, 75-g OGTT can be used as a one-step screening test for GDM. At the first prenatal visit, pregnant women should be screened for risk factors. Those women having a high risk for GDM (i.e., marked obesity, personal history of GDM, family history of diabetes, or glycosuria) should undergo glucose testing at their earli-

est convenience. If glucose testing does not indicate GDM, these patients should be retested at 24 to 28 weeks of gestation. Woman of average risk should be tested at 24 to 28 weeks of gestation. The only group not requiring glucose testing are women at low risk who meet all the criteria listed in Box 8.10. In order for a positive diagnosis of GDM to be made, two or more of the following plasma glucose values for the 75-g OGTT must be met or exceeded: fasting 95 mg/dL; 1-hour 180 mg/dL; 2-hour 155 mg/dL.

Self-monitoring of Blood Glucose

In self-monitoring of blood glucose (SMBG), persons with diabetes periodically measure the amount of glucose in a small sample of their blood. This process is critical to glycemic control—maintaining blood glucose levels within an acceptable range. Self-monitoring of blood glucose allows a person with diabetes to evaluate how various combinations of diet, exercise, and medication affect blood glucose levels and determine the best combinations for optimal blood glucose control.

Figure 8.21 **Diagnosis of diabetes using the oral glucose tolerance test (OGTT).**
Normally, plasma glucose should be < 140 mg/dL 2 hours after ingesting 75 g of glucose (the so-called glucose challenge). A diagnostic criterion for impaired glucose tolerance (IGT) is a 2-hour plasma glucose ≥ 140 mg/dL and < 200 mg/dL. A 2-hour plasma glucose ≥ 200 mg/dL is a diagnostic criterion for diabetes.

 Box 8.10   **Factors Associated with Low Risk of Gestational Diabetes Mellitus**

- Age < 25 years
- Normal weight before pregnancy
- Not a member of a group at high risk for GDM[*]
- No known history of diabetes in a first-degree relative[†]

- No history of abnormal glucose tolerance
- No history of poor obstetric outcome

[*]Includes Hispanic American, Native American, Asian American, African American, Pacific Islander.
[†]A first-degree relative is a parent, a sibling, or an offspring.

Adapted from American Diabetes Association. 2001. Gestational diabetes mellitus. *Diabetes Care* 24(suppl):S77–S79.

Self-monitoring of blood glucose can be accurately and precisely done using specially designed reagent strips, small pieces of plastic with a test pad affixed to one end. The test pad is impregnated with an enzyme and chemicals that react to the glucose in a drop of blood applied to the test pad. The finger is first pricked using a lancet. A drop of blood from the finger is applied to the test pad of the reagent strip and then wiped away after a certain number of seconds. The enzymatic and chemical reaction results in the test pad's changing color. The change in color is proportional to the amount of glucose in the blood. To determine blood glucose level, the color change can be compared with a color chart included with the reagent strips, or the reagent strip can be inserted into a small, battery-operated meter, which optically "reads" the color on the test pad and indicates the blood glucose level on the meter's electronic display (see Figure 8.22).

The frequency of SMBG depends primarily on the type of diabetes and a person's overall therapy. In some instances, monitoring as often as seven times a day is appropriate. For persons with type 1 diabetes, it is recommended that SMBG be done before each meal and at bedtime. In some instances, it is appropriate to do additional testing 1 to 2 hours after meals and occasionally in the middle of the night to monitor glycemic control. Recom-

mendations for type 2 diabetes depend on the type of therapy. For type 2 diabetes controlled by diet and exercise alone, SMBG can be done one or two times per week. For persons using diet and exercise along with oral hypoglycemic agents (medications taken orally to help control blood glucose levels), SMBG should be done daily at different times during the day. If glycemic control is good, these individuals can reduce the frequency of SMBG to one or two times per week. For those with type 2 diabetes who also take insulin, it is recommended that SMBG be done at least twice a day at different times. Testing should be more frequent when there are changes in a person's schedule, exercise habits, medications, diet, and body weight and when illness occurs.[126,131]

Glycosylated Hemoglobin

One drawback of blood glucose measurements is that they are an index of glycemic control only at the time the testing is done. For example, a person with diabetes who ordinarily runs a high blood glucose might be extra careful about maintaining glycemic control just before his or her visit with a physician. To assess mean glucose levels for the past 8 to 12 weeks, a physician can use a test measuring the amount of hemoglobin that is glycosylated. During the life span of a red blood cell, glucose in the blood binds to the major form of hemoglobin (Hb) in the red blood cell, hemoblogin A (HbA). When this occurs, the hemoglobin is said to be glycosylated. There are several forms of HbA in the red blood cell. The form of glycosylated HbA that most closely correlates with mean blood glucose levels is referred to as hemoglobin A_{1C} (HbA_{1C}). This binding of glucose to HbA is almost irreversible during the life span of the red blood cell. Consequently, HbA_{1C} reflects average blood glucose levels during the past 8 to 12 weeks. The proportion of HbA_{1C} does not decline with a temporary fall in blood glucose. It decreases only when glycemic control has been consistent over a period of several weeks, and older red blood cells with a high proportion of HbA_{1C} gradually die and are replaced by new red blood cells with a low proportion of HbA_{1C}. Consequently, the test is a good way to assess a patient's adherence to his or her program of blood glucose control.

In persons without diabetes, HbA_{1C} accounts for about 4% to 8% of the total hemoglobin. In persons with diabetes, blood glucose levels are usually elevated, more of the Hb becomes glycosylated, and the proportion of HbA_{1C} is greater. The American Diabetes Association recommends that the goal of therapy be an HbA_{1C} value < 7%. Patients with an HbA_{1C} value consistently > 8% should have their treatment plan reevaluated.[131] The American Association of Clinical Endocrinologists recommends the somewhat lower target HbA_{1C} value of < 6.5%. These target HbA_{1C} values apply only when assays are traceable to the reference method used by researchers conducting the Diabetes Control and

Figure 8.22 **Example of a portable, battery-operated glucose meter for performing self-monitoring of blood glucose.**

Source: Photo courtesy of LifeScan, a Johnson & Johnson Company.

Complications Trial (DCCT), a prospective clinical study investigating the effects of glycemic control on the incidence of microvascular complications, such as neuropathy (nerve damage), retinopathy (damage to the retina that can lead to blindness), and nephropathy (damage to the nephron of the kidney). In the DCCT, 1441 persons ages 13 to 39 years who had type 1 diabetes were randomly assigned to either a standard treatment group or an experimental treatment group.[132,133] The standard treatment group received conventional treatment for their type 1 diabetes—one or two insulin injections per day, periodic self-monitoring of urine or blood glucose, clinic appointments every 3 months, and nutrition education as requested by the participant. Those in the experimental treatment group received intensive therapy that involved continuous subcutaneous insulin infusion with an insulin pump or multiple insulin injections and monthly clinic appointments. Insulin adjustments were guided by self-monitoring of blood glucose done at least four times per day and at 3 A.M. once per week.

Persons in the standard treatment group had a mean glucose level of 231 mg/dL and a mean HbA_{1C} of 9%. Those in the experimental treatment group had a mean glucose level of 155 mg/dL and a mean HbA_{1C} of 7%. Compared with those in the standard treatment group, persons in the experimental group receiving intensive therapy had a dramatic reduction in the incidence of microvascular complications related to diabetes. There was a 76% reduction in retinopathy, a 60% reduction in neuropathy, and a 39% reduction in microalbuminuria (a sign of kidney disease).[132,133] Thus, frequent SMBG and periodic monitoring of HbA_{1C} are useful for persons with diabetes who wish to maintain glycemic control.

Medical Nutrition Therapy

In 1994, the American Diabetes Association published a major revision of its nutrition recommendations and principles for people with diabetes.[134] These recommendations presented two major philosophical changes in the nutritional management of diabetes. One was that the focus of therapy for persons with type 1 diabetes should include reasonable goals for the control of blood glucose and lipid levels, in addition to weight loss, if necessary. The other philosophical change was that a client's diet should be individually tailored according to his or her lifestyle and nutritional and metabolic needs. Rather than clients merely receiving and following a generic set of instructions from health professionals through the process of "diabetes patient education," they are encouraged to become more fully informed of and involved in the management of their condition through the process of "self-management training." Instead of "diet therapy" for persons with diabetes, the new recommendations use "medical nutrition therapy."[134] These principles were reaffirmed by the American Diabetes Association in its most recent nutrition recommendations for people with diabetes.[135,136]

Medical nutrition therapy is a four-part approach that involves assessing an individual's nutritional, metabolic, and lifestyle needs; identifying nutritional and lifestyle goals; designing an intervention to achieve these goals; and evaluating therapeutic outcomes.[135,136] This four-step model is outlined in Figure 8.23. The American Diabetes Association has identified four goals of medical nutrition therapy that apply to all persons with diabetes and six additional goals of medical nutrition therapy that apply to specific situations.[137] These are shown in Box 8.11.

Medical nutrition therapy is assessment-based; goal setting, intervention, and evaluation depend in large part on data collected through nutritional assessment. Assessment begins with establishing rapport with the client and then proceeds with collecting pertinent clinical data, obtaining a diet history, and assessing current nutrient intake. The types of information included in these three components are shown in Box 8.12. Nutritional assessment shows what the client is currently doing, suggests what he or she is able and willing to do, and determines how likely he or she will be to adhere to

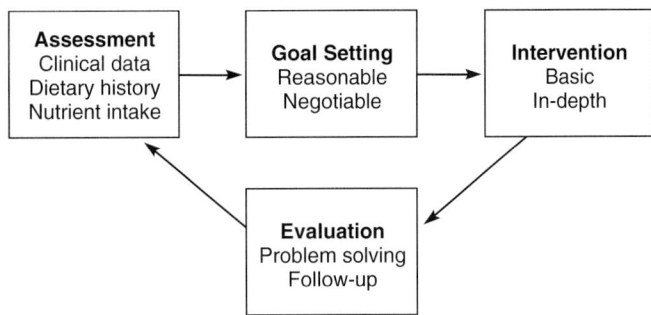

Figure 8.23 **The four-step model for medical nutrition therapy for diabetes.**

Source: From Tinker LF, Heins JM, Holler HJ. 1994. Commentary and translation: 1994 nutrition recommendations for diabetes. *Journal of the American Dietetic Association* 94:507–511.

Box 8.11   Goals of Medical Nutrition Therapy for Diabetes

GOALS OF MEDICAL NUTRITION THERAPY THAT APPLY TO
ALL PERSONS WITH DIABETES

1. Attain and maintain optimal metabolic outcomes
   including:
   • Blood glucose levels in the normal range or as close
     to normal as is safely possible to prevent or reduce
     the risk for complications of diabetes.
   • Lipid and lipoprotein profiles that reduce the risk for
     macrovascular disease.
   • Blood pressure levels that reduce the risk for
     vascular disease.
2. Prevent and treat the chronic complications of diabetes.
   Modify nutrient intake and lifestyle as appropriate for
   the prevention and treatment of obesity, dyslipidemia,
   cardiovascular disease, hypertension, and nephropathy.
3. Improve health through healthy food choices and
   physical activity.
4. Address individual nutritional needs, taking into
   consideration personal and cultural preferences and
   lifestyle while respecting the individual's wishes and
   willingness to change.

GOALS OF MEDICAL NUTRITION THERAPY THAT APPLY TO
SPECIFIC SITUATIONS

1. For youth with type 1 diabetes, provide adequate
   energy to ensure normal growth and development,
   integrate insulin regimens into usual eating and
   physical activity habits.
2. For youth with type 2 diabetes, facilitate changes in
   eating and physical activity habits that reduce insulin
   resistance and improve metabolic status.
3. For pregnant and lactating women, provide adequate
   energy and nutrients needed for optimal outcomes.
4. For older adults, provide for the nutritional and
   psychological needs of an aging individual.
5. For individuals treated with insulin or insulin
   secretagogues, provide self-management education for
   treatment and prevention of hypoglycemia, acute
   illnesses, and exercise-related blood glucose problems.
6. For individuals at risk for diabetes, decrease risk by
   encouraging physical activity and promoting food
   choices that facilitate moderate weight loss or at least
   prevent weight gain.

Adapted from American Diabetes Association. 2002. Position statement: Evidence-based nutrition principles and recommendations for the treatment and prevention of
diabetes and related complications. *Diabetes Care* 25(suppl):S50–S60.

Box 8.12   Components of Nutritional Assessment for People with Diabetes

Clinical Data

Obtain height and weight

Determine body frame size

Determine desirable or healthy weight

Measure blood pressure

Assess laboratory values:

   blood glucose levels

   blood lipid levels

   glycosylated hemoglobin

   protein in urine

Identify diabetes medication:

   insulin

   oral hypoglycemic agents

Dietary History

Determine usual food intake

Assess nutrition and health attitudes

Assess previous dietary education and outcomes

Nutritional Intake

Assess overall nutritional adequacy

Assess energy intake

Assess nutrient distribution

Assess type of carbohydrate, protein, and fat

Determine appropriate nutrition intervention

Adapted from American Diabetes Association. 1994. Nutrition recommendations and principles for people with diabetes mellitus. *Diabetes Care* 17:519–522; Tinker LF,
Heins JM, Holler HJ. 1994. Commentary and translation: 1994 nutrition recommendations for diabetes. *Journal of the American Dietetic Association* 94:507–511.

nutritional recommendations. Once data from the
assessment are discussed with the client, the process of
goal setting can begin. Goal setting allows the client to
set his or her own goals that are reasonable, specific,
and measurable. Although goal setting is the responsi-

bility of the client, the dietitian can negotiate with the
client, so that goals promote positive changes in eating
and other lifestyle habits, resulting in improvements in
blood glucose and lipid levels and nutrient intake.
Remember that, as a client's metabolic control changes

over time (e.g., glucose and lipid levels improve), goals will also change.

Rather than prescribing a set energy level and percentage of energy from carbohydrates, protein, and fat, the nutrition intervention should be individually tailored to address any metabolic abnormality. Through self-management training, the intervention should help the client acquire the knowledge and meal planning skills necessary to adapt diet and lifestyle to achieve his or her goals, despite the various situations demanded by modern life.

Over the course of the twentieth century, nutrition recommendations for diabetes changed markedly, as shown in Table 8.16. Overall, the recommended proportion of energy from carbohydrate has increased while the recommended proportion of energy from fat, particularly saturated fat, has decreased. Because carbohydrate has a much greater impact on blood glucose level than protein or fat, considerable attention has been given to the amounts and types of carbohydrate in the diets of persons with diabetes. Scientific evidence supports the concept that the total amount of carbohydrate in meals and snacks is more important than the source or type of carbohydrate.[137] Sucrose (e.g., table sugar) does not increase blood glucose level to a greater extent than does an isocaloric amount of starch. Consequently, sucrose and sucrose-containing foods do not necessarily need to be restricted by people with diabetes, as long as they are substituted, gram for gram, for other carbohydrate sources. If sucrose and sucrose-containing foods are added to the meal plan, the administration of insulin or other glucose-lowering medication may need adjustment to cover the increased carbohydrate intake. When selecting carbohydrate sources, emphasis should be given to whole grains, fruits, vegetables, and nonfat dairy products because these foods have a high nutrient density, are relatively low in kilocalories, and provide vitamins, minerals, dietary fiber, and numerous other dietary components necessary for good health.[137] Dietary fiber is a beneficial food component and useful in preventing and treating constipation, and soluble fiber has the potential to lower elevated serum lipid levels. However, the American Diabetes Association's dietary fiber recommendation for people with diabetes is the same as for the general population: 20 to 35 g of dietary fiber per day from a wide variety of food sources.[137] Although fructose produces a lower postprandial glycemic response when used in place of sucrose or starch, its use may increase blood lipid levels. Consequently, the American Diabetes Association does not recommend the use of added fructose as a sweetening agent. Sugar alcohols (polyols) also produce a lower postprandial glycemic response than do sucrose, fructose, or glucose, but there is no evidence that the amounts of sugar alcohols typically consumed by persons with diabetes result in a significant improvement in glycemic control. Four different non-nutritive sweeteners have received approval by the U.S. Food and Drug Administration for use in the United States: saccharin, aspartame, acesulfame potassium, and sucralose. All four provide a sweet taste to foods and beverages, contain little, if any, energy, and appear safe for use by all persons, including persons with diabetes and women who are pregnant or lactating.[137]

Because of the importance of maintaining optimal serum lipid and lipoprotein levels, persons with diabetes are advised to limit their intake of saturated fat to less than 10% of kilocalories. Persons with elevated low-density lipoprotein levels ($\geq$ 100 mg/dL) are advised to limit saturated fat intake to less than 7% of kilocalories. Intake of polyunsaturated fatty acids should not exceed 10% of kilocalories, and intake of *trans*-unsaturated fatty acids should be minimized.[137]

Apart from these restrictions, the amount of energy derived from fat should be based on the nutritional

TABLE 8.16	Changes in Dietary Recommendations for Persons with Diabetes During the Twentieth Century		
	Distribution of Energy		
Year	**Carbohydrate (% kcal)**	**Fat (% kcal)**	**Protein (% kcal)**
Pre-1921		Starvation diets	
1921	20	70	10
1950	40	40	20
1971	45	35	20
1986	50–60	30	12–20
1994	Based on assessment	< 10% SFA* Up to 10% PUFA* Based on assessment	15–20

Adapted from American Diabetes Association. 2001. Nutrition recommendations for people with diabetes mellitus. *Diabetes Care* 24(suppl):S44–S47; Franz MJ, Bantle JP. 1999. *American Diabetes Association guide to medical nutrition therapy for diabetes.* Alexandria, VA: American Diabetes Association.

*SFA = saturated fatty acids; PUFA = polyunsaturated fatty acids.

assessment and treatment goals. Persons with hyper-triglyceridemia may be sensitive to carbohydrate and may want to lower their carbohydrate and saturated fat intake and modestly increase their intake of monounsaturated fat. Evidence is mounting that a high-fat diet contributes to obesity and that a low-fat diet, independent of energy reduction, is beneficial in weight loss.[135–137] Therefore, it may be prudent for obese persons with diabetes to reduce fat and increase carbohydrate intake. Dietary cholesterol should be limited to 300 mg/d per day or less; however, persons with elevated levels of LDL-C ($\geq$ 100 mg/dL) may want to adopt the more stringent recommendations for both dietary cholesterol and saturated fat of the National Cholesterol Education Program's therapeutic lifestyle changes diet.

When diabetes is well controlled, blood glucose levels are not generally affected by an alcohol intake of no more than two drinks per day ingested with and in addition to the usual meal plan. Because alcohol consumption may increase the risk of hypoglycemia in persons treated with insulin and oral hypoglycemic agents, if consumed, it should be consumed with meals. Abstention is advised during pregnancy and for persons with a history of alcohol abuse. Abstention or reduced intake may be advisable for individuals with pancreatitis, dyslipidemia, or nephropathy.

Energy supplied by protein can range between 15% and 20%, although with the onset of nephropathy, a protein intake approaching the RDA (0.8 g/kg of body weight per day, or about 10% of energy) should be considered. Reducing sodium intake lowers blood pressure in both normotensive and hypertensive persons. However, the blood pressure response to sodium reduction is generally greater in those with diabetes and hypertension. The goal is to reduce sodium intake to less than 2400 mg per day or sodium chloride (table salt) intake to less than 6000 mg per day.[137] Potassium supplementation may be required in some persons taking diuretics. Vitamin and mineral supplementation is not necessary for most people with diabetes when dietary intake is adequate. There appears to be no benefit in taking chromium and magnesium supplements unless a documented deficiency of these nutrients exists.[135–137]

SUMMARY

1. Coronary heart disease (CHD) remains the leading cause of death in the United States despite a more than 26% decline in CHD death rates since 1988. CHD is causally associated with several risk factors, especially elevated blood cholesterol levels, high blood pressure, and cigarette smoking.

2. Because cholesterol, triglycerides, and other lipids are fat soluble, they are transported in the blood by lipoproteins. CHD risk is directly related to serum levels of total cholesterol and low-density-lipoprotein cholesterol (LDL-C) and inversely related to levels of high-density-lipoprotein cholesterol (HDL-C). The National Cholesterol Education Program (NCEP) has set desirable levels of total cholesterol in adults at < 200 mg/dL.

3. Atherosclerosis begins in childhood and progresses slowly into adulthood. Children and adolescents with elevated serum cholesterol frequently come from families whose adult members have a high incidence of CHD or elevated serum cholesterol levels. According to the NCEP, acceptable levels of total cholesterol and LDL-C in children and adolescents are < 170 mg/dL and < 110 mg/dL, respectively.

4. Two ways of addressing the problem of high serum cholesterol levels are the population-based and the patient-based approaches. The former emphasizes dietary and lifestyle changes for all people to lower average cholesterol levels in the entire population. The latter promotes identification and treatment of individuals with elevated cholesterol levels by physicians.

5. The *Third Report of the National Cholesterol Education Program Expert Panel on Detection, Evaluation, and Treatment of High Blood Cholesterol in Adults* uses a multifaceted lifestyle approach called *therapeutic lifestyle changes* as a component of CHD risk reduction. The therapeutic lifestyle changes diet recommends that saturated fat intake be limited to < 7% of total calories, that dietary cholesterol intake be less than 200 mg/day, and that polyunsaturated and monounsaturated fat provide no more than 10% and 20% of calories, respectively. The recommendation for total fat is liberalized somewhat to 25% to 35% of calories, recognizing that a slight decrease in calories from carbohydrate and a slight increase in calories from monounsaturated fat will lower serum triglycerides in some patients.

6. After about age 2 years, children can safely follow the therapeutic lifestyle changes diet. Although the NCEP discourages cholesterol screening for all children, it advises cholesterol testing for children whose parents or grandparents have elevated cholesterol and lipoprotein levels or who have definite CHD or other cardiovascular disease by age 55 years, as well as cholesterol testing for children at high risk for CHD because of overweight, cigarette smoking, high blood pressure, diabetes, and so on.

7. A number of dietary factors can influence serum cholesterol and lipoprotein levels. Saturated fatty acids tend to raise total cholesterol and LDL-C levels, whereas substitution of saturated fats with polyunsaturated and monounsaturated fats tends to lower total cholesterol and LDL-C. Dietary cholesterol tends to raise serum cholesterol, but it is not as potent an elevator as saturated fats. Obesity elevates total cholesterol and LDL-C levels and depresses HDL-C levels. Consumption of soluble dietary fiber tends to lower elevated total cholesterol and LDL-C levels.

8. Precision, or reproducibility, relates to the difference in results when the same blood sample is measured repeatedly. The coefficient of variation (CV) is a measure of precision and is calculated by dividing the standard deviation (SD) by the mean and multiplying by 100 ($CV = SD \div mean \times 100$). The NCEP recommends that laboratories achieve a $CV \leq 3\%$.

9. Accuracy relates to the difference between the measured value reported by the clinical laboratory and the true, or real, value that has been previously established by comparison with a known standard (reference material) and/or a definitive measurement method. Bias is a measure of inaccuracy, or departure from accuracy. Inaccurate measurement leads to clinical misdiagnosis caused by reporting of false positive or false negative values.

10. Hypertension is one of the most common risk factors for cardiovascular and renal diseases. One of every four Americans has hypertension or is taking antihypertensive medication. As systolic blood pressure increases above 120 mm Hg and diastolic blood pressure increases above 80 mm Hg, risk for death from cardiovascular disease increases.

11. The most important risk factors for hypertension are high sodium intake, excessive energy consumption and physical inactivity (both promoting obesity), excessive alcohol consumption, and inadequate potassium intake.

12. Osteoporosis is a condition in which bone mineral content is decreased, resulting in greater susceptibility to fracture. Common fracture sites include the pelvis, vertebrae, hip, distal forearm, and humerus. Osteoporotic fractures are twice as common in females than in males, and, because they live longer than males, females experience an even higher absolute incidence during their lifetime.

13. Peak bone mass, a major factor determining risk of osteoporosis development, varies considerably among individuals because of heredity, sex, race, and environmental factors. On average, males have 20% to 30% greater peak bone mass than females, and the bones of black males and females are about 10% denser than those of white males and females.

14. Bone densitometry, the measurement of bone mineral content, is important in early detection and treatment of osteoporosis and in monitoring its progression and response to treatment. Approaches to bone densitometry include radiogrammetry, single-photon absorptiometry, dual-photon absorptiometry, quantitative computed tomography, dual-energy X-ray absorptiometry, and quantitative ultrasound.

15. In children and adolescents, optimal calcium intake increases bone mineral density. In postmenopausal women, calcium and vitamin D supplementation and estrogen replacement therapy decrease the rate of bone demineralization and reduce fracture risk.

16. Diabetes is a group of diseases characterized by lack of insulin secretion and/or increased insulin resistance, elevated plasma glucose levels, abnormal carbohydrate and lipid metabolism, pathologic changes in the nerves and small blood vessels, and aggravation of atherosclerosis. Among the diseases classified as diabetes are type 1 diabetes, type 2 diabetes, gestational diabetes mellitus, impaired fasting glucose, and impaired glucose tolerance.

17. Despite its public health significance, diabetes is undiagnosed in about 50% of people who have the disease. Diagnostic criteria for diabetes include the presence of symptoms of diabetes and fasting glucose measurements of > 140 mg/dL (> 7.8 mmol/L) on two occasions. The oral glucose tolerance test also can be used to diagnose diabetes.

18. Glycosylated hemoglobin (HbA_{1C}) is a useful test for assessing a person's mean glucose levels during the past 8 to 12 weeks. Self-monitoring blood glucose is an accurate and precise way to monitor how changes in diet, exercise, and medications affect glycemic control. Glycemic control has been shown to be effective in reducing the risk of microvascular complications in persons with type 1 diabetes.

19. The American Diabetes Association's nutrition recommendations for people with diabetes encourages people with diabetes to become better informed about diabetes and its nutritional management, rather than simply follow a standard "diabetic diet."

20. Medical nutrition therapy is an approach involving nutritional assessment, goal setting, intervention, and evaluation. Its goals are to control blood glucose, blood lipids, and blood pressure; to provide adequate calories for normal growth and development, pregnancy, and lactation; to prevent delay, or treat nutrition-related complications of diabetes; and to improve health through optimal nutrition.

REFERENCES

1. American Heart Association. 2001. *Heart and Stroke Statistical Update.* Dallas, TX: American Heart Association.

2. National Cholesterol Education Program. 2001. *Third report of the expert panel on detection, evaluation, and treatment of high blood cholesterol in adults.* Bethesda, MD: U.S. Department of Health and Human Services, Public Health Service; National Institutes of Health; National Heart, Lung, and Blood Institute.

3. Grundy SM. 1999. Nutrition and diet in the management of hyperlipidemia and atherosclerosis. In Shils ME, Olson JA, Shike M, Ross CE, eds. *Modern nutrition in health and disease,* 9th ed. Baltimore: Williams & Wilkins.

4. Stamler J, Daviglus ML, Garside DB, Dyer AR, Greenland P, Neaton JD. 2000. Relationship of baseline serum cholesterol levels in 3 large cohorts of younger men to long-term coronary, cardiovascular, and all-cause mortality and to longevity. *Journal of the American Medical Association* 284:365–367.

5. Jeppesen J, Hein HO, Suadicani P, Gyntelberg F. 2001. Low triglycerides-high high-density lipoprotein cholesterol and risk of ischemic heart disease. *Archives of Internal Medicine* 161:361–366.

6. Smmenkovich CF. 1999. Nutrient and genetic regulation of lipoprotein metabolism. In Shils ME, Olson JA, Shike M, Ross CE, eds. *Modern nutrition in health and disease,* 9th ed. Baltimore: Williams & Wilkins.

7. Hahmann HW, Schatzer-Klotz D, Bunte T, Becker D, Schieffer HJ. 1999. The significance of high levels of lipoprotein(a) compared with established risk factors in premature coronary artery disease: Differences between men and women. *Atherosclerosis* 144:221–228.

8. Scanu AM. 1991. Lipoprotein(a) and atherosclerosis. *Annals of Internal Medicine* 115:209–218.

9. Schaefer EJ, Lamon-Fava S, Jenner JL, McNamara JR, Ordovas JM, Davis E, Abolafia JM, Lippel K, Levy RI. 1994. Lipoprotein(a) levels and risk of coronary heart disease in men. *Journal of the American Medical Association* 271:999–1003.

10. Martin MJ, Hulley SB, Browner WS, Kuller LH, Wentworth D. 1986. Serum cholesterol, blood pressure, and mortality: Implications from a cohort of 361,622 men. *Lancet* 2:933–936.

11. National Cholesterol Education Program. 1991. *Report of the expert panel on blood cholesterol levels in children and adolescents.* Bethesda, MD: U.S. Department of Health and Human Services, Public Health Service; National Institutes of Health; National Heart, Lung, and Blood Institute.

12. Linn S, Fulwood R, Carroll M, Brook JG, Johnson C, Kalsbeek WD, Rifkind BM. 1991. Serum total cholesterol: HDL cholesterol ratios in U.S. white and black adults by selected demographic and socioeconomic variables (HANES II). *American Journal of Public Health* 81:1038–1043.

13. Kinosian B, Glick H, Garland G. 1994. Cholesterol and coronary heart disease: Predicting risk by levels and ratios. *Annals of Internal Medicine* 121:641–647.

14. Castelli WP, Anderson K, Wilson PW, Levy D. 1992. Lipids and risk of coronary heart disease: The Framingham Study. *Annals of Epidemiology* 2:23–28.

15. Grundy SM, Greenland P, Herd A, Huebsch JA, Jones RJ, Mitchell JH, Schlant RC. 1987. Cardiovascular and risk factor evaluation of healthy American adults. *Circulation* 75:1339A–1362A.

16. Assmann G, Cullen P, Fruchart C, Lewis B, Mancini M, Carmena R. 1999. Coronary heart disease prevention task force. *European Heart Journal* 20:841–844.

17. Stampfer MJ, Sacks FM, Salvini S, Willett WC, Hennekens CH. 1991. A prospective study of cholesterol, apolipoproteins, and the risk of myocardial infarction. *New England Journal of Medicine* 325:373–381.

18. National Institutes of Health Consensus Development Panel on Triglyceride, High-Density Lipoprotein, and Coronary Heart Disease. 1993. Triglyceride, high-density lipoprotein, and coronary heart disease. *Journal of the American Medical Association* 269:505–510.

19. Criqui MH, Heiss G, Cohn R, Cowan LD, Suchindran CM, Bangdiwala S, Kritchevsky S, Jacobs DR Jr, O'Grady HK, Davis CE. 1993. Plasma triglyceride level and mortality from coronary heart disease. *New England Journal of Medicine* 328:1220–1225.

20. Avins AL, Neuhaus JM. 2000. Do triglycerides provide meaningful information about heart disease risk? *Archives of Internal Medicine* 160:1903–1904.

21. Tenkanen L, Pietila K, Manninen V, Manttari M. 1994. The triglyceride issue revisited. Findings from the Helsinki Heart Study. *Archives of Internal Medicine* 154:2714–2720.

22. Assmann G, Schulte H, Funke H, von Eckardstein A. 1998. The emergence of triglycerides as a significant independent risk factor in coronary heart disease. *European Heart Journal* 19 (suppl M):M8–M14.

23. Lauer MS, Fontanarosa PB. 2001. Updated guidelines for cholesterol management. *Journal of the American Medical Association* 285:2508–2509.

24. National Cholesterol Education Program. 1993. *Second report of the expert panel on detection, evaluation, and treatment of high blood cholesterol in adults.* Bethesda, MD: U.S. Department of Health and Human Services, Public Health Service; National Institutes of Health; National Heart, Lung, and Blood Institute.

25. National Cholesterol Education Program. 1988. *Report of the expert panel on detection,*

evaluation, and treatment of high blood cholesterol in adults. Bethesda, MD: U.S. Department of Health and Human Services, Public Health Service; National Institutes of Health; National Heart, Lung, and Blood Institute.

26. National Cholesterol Education Program. 1990. *Report of the expert panel on population strategies for blood cholesterol reduction.* Bethesda, MD: U.S. Department of Health and Human Services, Public Health Service; National Institutes of Health; National Heart, Lung, and Blood Institute.

27. Krauss RM, Eckel RH, Howard B, Appel LJ, Daniels SR, Deckelbaum RJ, et al. 2000. AHA dietary guidelines: Revision 2000. *Circulation* 102:2296–2311.

28. Blankenhorn DH, Johnson RL, Mack WJ, El Zein HA, Vailas LI. 1990. The influence of diet on the appearance of new lesions in human coronary arteries. *Journal of the American Medical Association* 263:1646–1652.

29. Buchwald H, Varco RL, Matts JP, Long JM, Fitch LL, Campbell GS, POSCH Group. 1990. Effect of partial ileal bypass surgery on mortality and morbidity from coronary heart disease on patients with hypercholesterolemia: Report of the Program on the Surgical Control of Hyperlipidemias (POSCH). *New England Journal of Medicine* 323:946–955.

30. Kane JP, Mallory MJ, Ports TA, Phillips R, Diehl JC, Havel RJ. 1990. Regression of coronary atherosclerosis during treatment of familial hypercholesterolemia with combined drug regimens. *Journal of the American Medical Association* 264:3007–3012.

31. Ornish D, Brown SE, Scherwitz LW, Billings JH, Armstrong WT, Ports TA, McLanahan SM, Kirkeeide RL, Brand RJ, Gould KL. 1990. Can lifestyle changes reverse coronary heart disease? *Lancet* 336:129–133.

32. Ornish D, Scherwitz LW, Billings JH, Gould KL, Merritt TA, Sparler S, et al. 1998. Intensive lifestyle change for reversal of coronary

heart disease. *Journal of the American Medical Association* 280:2001–2007.

33. Stampfer MJ, Hu FB, Manson JE, Rimm EB, Willett WC. 2000. Primary prevention of coronary heart disease in women through diet and lifestyle. *New England Journal of Medicine* 343:16–22.

34. Haskell WL, Alderman EL, Fair JM, Maron DJ, Mackey SF, Superko HR, et al. 1994. Effects of intensive multiple risk factor reduction on coronary atherosclerosis and clinical events in men and women with coronary artery disease. The Stanford Coronary Risk Intervention Project (SCRIP). *Circulation* 89:975–990.

35. Enos WF, Beyer JC, Holmes RH. 1955. Pathogenesis of coronary disease in American soldiers killed in Korea. *Journal of the American Medical Association* 158:912–914.

36. McNamara JJ, Molot MA, Stremple JF, Cutting RT. 1971. Coronary artery disease in combat casualties in Vietnam. *Journal of the American Medical Association* 216:1185–1187.

37. Stary HC. 1989. Evolution and progression of atherosclerotic lesions in coronary arteries of children and young adults. *Arteriosclerosis* 9(suppl):I19–I32.

38. Stary HC. 1990. The sequence of cell and matrix changes in atherosclerotic lesions of coronary arteries in the first forty years of life. *European Heart Journal* 11(suppl):E3–E19.

39. McGill HC, McMahan CA. 1998. Determinants of atherosclerosis in the young. Pathobiological Determinants of Atherosclerosis in Youth (PDAY) Research Group. *American Journal of Cardiology* 82(suppl):30T–36T.

40. Wissler RW, Strong JP, and the PDAY Research Group. Risk factors and progression of atherosclerosis in youth. *American Journal of Pathology* 153:1023–1033.

41. McGill HC, McMahan CA, Zieske AW, Sloop GD, Walcott JV, Troxclair DA, et al. 2000. Associations of coronary heart disease risk factors with the

intermediate lesion of atherosclerosis in youth. The Pathobiological Determinants of Atherosclerosis in Youth (PDAY) Research Group. *Arteriosclerosis, Thrombosis, and Vascular Biology* 20:1998–2004.

42. Wissler RW. 1995. An overview of the quantitative influence of several risk factors on progression of atherosclerosis in young people in the United States. Pathobiological Determinants of Atherosclerosis in Youth (PDAY) Research Group. *The American Journal of the Medical Sciences* 310(suppl):S29–S36.

43. McGill HC, McMahan CA, Zieske AW, Malcom GT, Tracy RE, Strong JP. 2001. Effects of nonlipid factors on atherosclerosis in youth with a favorable lipoprotein profile. *Circulation* 103:1546–1550.

44. Strong JP. 1995. Natural history and risk factors for early human atherogenesis. Pathobiological Determinants of Atherosclerosis in Youth (PDAY). *Clinical Chemistry* 41:134–138.

45. Wissler RW. 1994. New insights into the pathogenesis of atherosclerosis as revealed by PDAY. Pathobiological Determinants of Atherosclerosis in Youth. *Atherosclerosis* 108(suppl):S3–S20.

46. National Center for Health Statistics. 1983. Dietary intake source data: United States 1976–80. *Vital and Health Statistics,* Series 11, No. 231. Hyattsville, MD: U.S. Department of Health and Human Services, Public Health Service; National Center for Health Statistics.

47. National Center for Health Statistics. 1978. *Total serum cholesterol levels in children 4–17 years: United States, 1971–74.* Hyattsville, MD: U.S. Department of Health and Human Services, Public Health Service; National Center for Health Statistics.

48. Knuiman JT, Hermus RJ, Hautvast JG. 1980. Serum total and high density lipoprotein (HDL) cholesterol concentrations in rural and urban boys from 16 countries. *Atherosclerosis* 36:529–537.

49. Knuiman JT, Westenbrink S, van der Heyden L, West CE, Burema J, DeBoer J, et al. 1983. Determinants of total and high density lipoprotein cholesterol in boys from Finland, the Netherlands, Italy, the Philippines and Ghana with special reference to diet. *Human Nutrition: Clinical Nutrition* 37C:237–254.

50. Bonanome A, Grundy SM. 1988. Effect of dietary stearic acid on plasma cholesterol and lipoprotein levels. *New England Journal of Medicine* 318:1244–1248.

51. Rosenberg IH, Schaefer EJ. 1988. Dietary saturated fatty acids and blood cholesterol. *New England Journal of Medicine* 318:1270–1271.

52. Subar AF, Krebs-Smith SM, Cook A, Kahle LL. 1998. Dietary sources of nutrients among US adults, 1989–1991. *Journal of the American Dietetic Association* 98:537–547.

53. Mensink RP, Katan MB. 1990. Effect of dietary *trans* fatty acids on high-density and low-density lipoprotein cholesterol in healthy subjects. *New England Journal of Medicine* 323:439–445.

54. Judd JT, Clevidence BA, Muesing RA, Wittes J, Sunkin ME, Podczasy JJ. 1994. Dietary trans fatty acids: Effects on plasma lipids and lipoproteins of healthy men and women. *American Journal of Clinical Nutrition* 59:861–868.

55. Lichtenstein AH, Ausman LM, Jalbert SM, Schaefer EJ. 1999. Effects of different forms of dietary hydrogenated fats on serum lipoprotein cholesterol levels. *New England Journal of Medicine* 340:1933–1940.

56. U.S. Department of Agriculture/ U.S. Department of Health and Human Services. 2000. Nutrition and Your Health: Dietary Guidelines for Americans, 5th ed. Hyattsville, MD: U.S. Department of Agriculture, Center for Nutrition Policy and Promotion.

57. Lichtenstein AH. 2000. Dietary trans fatty acid. *Journal of Cardiopulmonary Rehabilitation* 20:143–146.

58. Katan MB. 2000. Trans fatty acids and plasma lipoproteins. *Nutrition Reviews* 58:188–191.

59. Hegsted DM, Ausman LM, Johnson JA, Dallal GE. 1993. Dietary fat and serum lipids: An evaluation of the experimental data. *American Journal of Clinical Nutrition* 57:875–883.

60. Beynen AC, Katan MB. 1985. Effect of egg yolk feeding on the concentration and composition of serum lipoprotein in man. *Atherosclerosis* 54:157–166.

61. Schonfeld G, Patsch W, Rudel LL, Nelson C, Epstein M, Olson RE. 1982. Effects of dietary cholesterol and fatty acids on plasma lipoproteins. *Journal of Clinical Investigation* 69:1072–1080.

62. Beynen AC, Katan MB. 1985. Reproducibility of the variations between humans in the response of serum cholesterol to cessation of egg consumption. *Atherosclerosis* 57:19–31.

63. Shekelle RB, Stamler J. 1989. Dietary cholesterol and ischaemic heart disease. *Lancet* 1:1177–1179.

64. McGee DL, Reed DM, Yano K, Kagan A, Tillotson J. 1984. Ten-year incidence of coronary heart disease in the Honolulu Heart Program. Relationship to nutrient intake. *American Journal of Epidemiology* 119:667–676.

65. Kromhout D, de Lezenne Coulander C. 1984. Diet, prevalence and 10-year mortality from coronary heart disease in 871 middle-aged men. The Zutphen Study. *American Journal of Epidemiology* 119:733–741.

66. Kushi LH, Lew RA, Stare FJ, Ellison CR, Lozy M, Bourke G, Daly L, Graham I, Hickey N, Mulcahy R, Kevaney J. 1985. Diet and 20-year mortality from coronary heart disease. The Ireland-Boston Diet-Heart Study. *New England Journal of Medicine* 312:811–818.

67. Gotto AM. 1991. Cholesterol intake and serum cholesterol level. *New England Journal of Medicine* 324:912–913.

68. Kern F. 1991. Normal plasma cholesterol in an 88-year-old man who eats 25 eggs a day. *New England Journal of Medicine* 312:896–899.

69. Burr ML, Sweetnam PM. 1982. Vegetarianism, dietary fiber, and mortality. *American Journal of Clinical Nutrition* 36:873–877.

70. Phillips RL, Kuzma JW, Beeson WL, Lotz T. 1980. Influence of selection versus lifestyle on risk of fatal cancer and cardiovascular disease among Seventh-day Adventists. *American Journal of Epidemiology* 112:296–314.

71. Carroll KK. 1991. Review of clinical studies on cholesterol-lowering response to soy protein. *Journal of the American Dietetic Association* 91:820–827.

72. Anderson JW, Johnstone BM, Cook-Newell ME. 1995. Meta-analysis of the effects of soy protein intake on serum lipids. *New England Journal of Medicine* 333:276–282.

73. Teixeira SR, Potter SM, Weigel R, Hannum S, Erdman JW, Hasler CM. 2000. Effects of feeding 4 levels of soy protein for 3 and 6 wk on blood lipids and apolipoproteins in moderately hypercholesterolemic men. *American Journal of Clinical Nutrition* 71:1077–1084.

74. Crouse JR, Morgan T, Terry JG, Ellis J, Vitolins M, Burke GL. 1999. A randomized trial comparing the effect of casein with that of soy protein containing varying amounts of isoflavones on plasma concentrations of lipids and lipoproteins. *Archives of Internal Medicine* 159:2070–2076.

75. Potter SM, Baum JA, Teng H, Stillman RJ, Shay NF, Erdman JW. 1998. Soy protein and isoflavones: Their effects on blood lipids and bone density in postmenopausal women. *American Journal of Clinical Nutrition* 68(suppl): 1375S–1379S.

76. Life Sciences Research Office. 1987. *Physiological effects and health consequences of dietary fiber.* Bethesda, MD: Life Sciences Research Office, Federation of American Societies for Experimental Biology.

77. Ludwig DS, Pereira MA, Kroenke CH, Hilner JE, Van Horn L,

Slattery ML, Jacobs DR. 1999. Dietary fiber, weight gain, and cardiovascular disease risk factors in young adults. *Journal of the American Medical Association* 282:1539–1546.

78. Van Horn L. 1997. Fiber, lipids, and coronary heart disease. A statement for healthcare professionals from the Nutrition Committee, American Heart Association. *Circulation* 95:2701–2704.

79. Story JA, Kritchevsky D. 1976. Comparison of the binding of various bile acids and bile salts in vitro by several types of fiber. *Journal of Nutrition* 106:1292–1294.

80. Story JA. 1985. Dietary fiber and lipid metabolism. *Proceedings of the Society for Experimental Biology and Medicine* 180:447–452.

81. Chen WJL, Anderson JW, Jennings D. 1984. Propionate may mediate the hypocholesterolemic effects of certain soluble plant fibers in cholesterol-fed rats. *Proceedings of the Society for Experimental Biology and Medicine* 175:215–218.

82. Cummings JH, Englyst HN. 1987. Fermentation in the human large intestine and the available substrates. *American Journal of Clinical Nutrition* 45:1243–1255.

83. Warnick GR. 2000. Measurement of cholesterol and other lipoprotein constituents in the clinical laboratory. *Clinical Chemistry and Laboratory Medicine* 38:287–300.

84. National Cholesterol Education Program. 1995. *Recommendations on Lipoprotein Measurement from the Working Group on Lipoprotein Measurement.* Bethesda, MD: U.S. Department of Health and Human Services, Public Health Service; National Institutes of Health; National Heart, Lung, and Blood Institute.

85. Rifai N, Dufour R, Cooper GR. 1997. Preanalytical variation in lipid, lipoprotein, and apolipoprotein testing. In Rifai N, Warnick GR, Dominiczak MH, eds. *Handbook of lipoprotein testing.* Washington, DC: American Association of Clinical Chemistry, pp. 75–97.

86. National Cholesterol Education Program. 1990. *Recommendations for improving cholesterol measurement: A report from the Laboratory Standardization Panel of the National Cholesterol Education Program.* Bethesda, MD: U.S. Department of Health and Human Services, Public Health Service; National Institutes of Health; National Heart, Lung, and Blood Institute.

87. Cooper GR, Myers GL, Smith SJ, Schlant RC. 1992. Blood lipid measurements: Variations and practical utility. *Journal of the American Medical Association* 267:1652–1660.

88. National High Blood Pressure Education Program. 1997. *Sixth report of the Joint National Committee on Detection, Evaluation, and Treatment of High Blood Pressure.* Bethesda, MD: U.S. Department of Health and Human Services, Public Health Service; National Institutes of Health; National Heart, Lung, and Blood Institute.

89. Gorelick PB, Sacco RL, Smith DB, Alberts M, et al. 1999. *Prevention of a first stroke: A review of guidelines and a multidisciplinary consensus statement from the National Stroke Association.* Englewood, CO: National Stroke Association. See also *Journal of the American Medical Association* 281(1999):1112–1120.

90. Stevens VJ, Obarzanek E, Cook NR, Lee IM, Appel LJ, et al. 2001. Long-term weight loss and changes in blood pressure: Results of the Trials of Hypertension Prevention, phase II. *Annals of Internal Medicine* 134:1–11.

91. Sacks FM, Svetkey LP, Vollmer WM, Appel LJ, et al. 2001. Effects on blood pressure of reduced sodium and the Dietary Approaches to Stop Hypertension (DASH) diet. *New England Journal of Medicine* 344:3–10.

92. Appel LJ, Espeland MA, Easter L, Wilson AC, Folmar S, Lacy CR. 2001. Effect of reduced sodium intake on hypertension control in older individuals. *Archive of Internal Medicine* 161:685–693.

93. The Trials of Hypertension Prevention Collaborative Research Group. 1992. The effects of nonpharmacologic interventions on blood pressure of persons with high normal levels: Results of the Trials of Hypertension Prevention. Phase I. *Journal of the American Medical Association* 267:1213–1220.

94. National High Blood Pressure Education Program Working Group. 1993. National High Blood Pressure Education Program Working Group report on primary prevention of hypertension. *Archives of Internal Medicine* 153:186–208.

95. Greenland P. 2001. Beating high blood pressure with low-sodium DASH. *New England Journal of Medicine* 344:53–55.

96. Kotchen TA, McCarron DA. 1998. Dietary electrolytes and blood pressure. A statement for healthcare professionals from the American Heart Association Nutrition Committee. *Circulation* 98:613–617.

97. Appel LJ, Moore TJ, Obarzanek E, Vollmer WM, Svetkey LP, Sacks FM, et.al. 1997. A clinical trial of the effects of dietary patterns on blood pressure. *New England Journal of Medicine* 336:1117–1124.

98. U.S. Department of Health and Human Services. 2000. *Consensus Development Conference Statement: Osteoporosis Prevention, Diagnosis, and Therapy.* Bethesda, MD: National Institute of Arthritis and Musculoskeletal and Skin Diseases, National Institutes of Health.

99. Gillespy T, Gillespy MP. 1991. Osteoporosis. *Radiologic Clinics of North America* 29:77–84.

100. McBean LD, Forgac T, Finn SC. 1994. Osteoporosis: Visions for care and prevention—A conference report. *Journal of the American Dietetic Association* 94:668–671.

101. National Osteoporosis Foundation. 2000. *Physician's*

Guide to Prevention and Treatment of Osteoporosis. Washington, DC: National Osteoporosis Foundation.

102. Krane SM, Holick MF. 1994. Metabolic bone disease. In Isselbacher KJ, Braunwald E, Wilson JD, Martin JB, Fauci JB, Kasper DL, eds. *Harrison's principles of internal medicine,* 13th ed. New York: McGraw-Hill.

103. Lang P, Steiger P, Faulkner K, Glüer C, Genant HK. 1991. Osteoporosis: Current techniques and recent developments in quantitative bone densitometry. *Radiologic Clinics of North America* 29:49–76.

104. Gluer CC. 1997. Quantitative ultrasound techniques for the assessment of osteoporosis: Expert agreement on current status. The International Quantitative Ultrasound Consensus Group. *Journal of Bone and Mineral Research* 12:1280–1288.

105. Maricic M, Chen Z. 2000. Bone densitometry. *Clinics in Laboratory Medicine* 20:469–488.

106. Blake GM, Gluer CC, Fogelman I. Bone densitometry: Current status and future prospects. *British Journal of Radiology* 70(Special Number):S177–S186.

107. Sartoris DJ, Resnick D. 1990. Current and innovative methods for noninvasive bone densitometry. *Orthopedics* 28:257–278.

108. Sartoris DJ, Moscona A, Reskick D. 1990. Progress in radiology: Dual-energy radiographic absorptiometry for bone density. *Annals New York Academy of Sciences* 592:307–325.

109. Mazess RB, Barden HS, Bisek JP, Hanson J. 1990. Dual-energy x-ray absorptiometry for total-body and regional bone-mineral and soft-tissue composition. *American Journal of Clinical Nutrition* 51:1106–1112.

110. Bushong SC. 1993. *Radiologic science for technologists: Physics, biology, and protection,* 5th ed. St. Louis, MO: Mosby.

111. Lukaski HC. 1987. Methods for the assessment of human body composition: Traditional and new. *American Journal of Clinical Nutrition* 46:537–556.

112. Roubenoff R, Kehayias JJ, Dawson-Hughes B, Heymsfield SB. 1993. Use of dual-energy x-ray absorptiometry in body composition studies: Not yet a "gold standard." *American Journal of Clinical Nutrition* 58:589–591.

113. Bauer DC, Gluer CC, Cauley JA, Vogt TM, Ensrud KE, Genant HK, Black DM. 1997. Broadband ultrasound attenuation predicts fractures strongly and independently of densitometry in older women. *Archives of Internal Medicine* 157:629–634.

114. Prins SH, Jorgensen HL, Jorgensen LV, Hassager C. 1998. The role of quantitative ultrasound in the assessment of bone: A review. *Clinical Physiology* 18:3–17.

115. Sorensen HA, Jorgensen NR, Jensen JE, Rasmussen AM, Hansen B, Nielsen SP, Sorensen OH. 2001. Comparison of quantitative ultrasound and dual X-ray absorptiometry in estrogen-treated early postmenopausal women. *Journal of Clinical Densitometry* 4:97–104.

116. Frost ML, Blake GM, Fogelman I. 2001. Quantitative ultrasound and bone mineral density are equally strongly associated with risk factors for osteoporosis. *Journal of Bone and Mineral Research* 16:406–416.

117. Hans D, Dargent-Molina P, Schott AM, Sebert JL, Cormier C, Kotzki PO, Delmas PD, Pouilles JM, Breart G, Meunier PJ. 1996. Ultrasonographic heel measurements to predict hip fracture in elderly women: The EPIDOS prospective study. *Lancet* 348:511–514.

118. Heaney RP. 1993. Nutritional factors in osteoporosis. *Annual Review of Nutrition* 13:287–316.

119. Johnston CC, Miller JZ, Slemenda CW, Reister TK, Hui

S, Christian JC, Peacock M. 1992. Calcium supplementation and increases in bone mineral density in children. *New England Journal of Medicine* 327:82–87.

120. Lloyd T, Andon MB, Rollings N, Martel JK, Landis JR, Demers LM, Eggli DF, Kieselhorst K, Kulin HE. 1993. Calcium supplementation and bone mineral density in adolescent girls. *Journal of the American Medical Association* 270:841–844.

121. Dawson-Hughes B, Sallal GE, Krall EA, Sadowski L, Sahyoun N, Tannenbaum S. 1990. A controlled trial of the effect of calcium supplementation on bone density in postmenopausal women. *New England Journal of Medicine* 323:878–883.

122. Chapuy MC, Arlot ME, Duboeuf F, Brun J, Crouzet B, Arnaud S, Delmas PD, Meunier PJ. 1992. Vitamin D3 and calcium to prevent hip fractures in elderly women. *New England Journal of Medicine* 327:1637–1642.

123. Heikinheimo RJ, Inkovaara JA, Harju EJ, Haavisto MV, Kaarela RH, Kataja JM, Kokko AM, Kolho LA, Rajala SA. 1992. Annual injection of vitamin D and fractures of aged bones. *Calcified Tissue International* 51:105–110.

124. Matkovic V, Heaney RP. 1992. Calcium balance during human growth: Evidence for threshold behavior. *American Journal of Clinical Nutrition* 55:992–996.

125. American Diabetes Association. 2001. Screening for diabetes. *Diabetes Care* 24(suppl):S21–S24.

126. American Diabetes Association. 2001. Report of the Expert Committee on the Diagnosis and Classification of Diabetes Mellitus. *Diabetes Care* 24(suppl):S5–S20.

127. American Diabetes Association. 1998. Medical Management of Type 1 Diabetes, 3rd ed. Alexandria, VA: American Diabetes Association.

128. American Diabetes Association. 1998. Medical Management of Type 2 Diabetes, 4th ed.

Alexandria, VA: American Diabetes Association.

129. American Diabetes Association. 2000. Medical management of pregnancy complicated by diabetes, 3rd ed. Alexandria, VA: American Diabetes Association.

130. American Diabetes Association. 2001. Gestational diabetes mellitus. *Diabetes Care* 24(suppl):S77–S79.

131. American Diabetes Association. 2001. Tests of glycemia in diabetes. *Diabetes Care.* 24(suppl):S80–S82.

132. DCCT Research Group. 1993. Expanded role of the dietitian in the Diabetes Control and Complications Trial: Implications for clinical practice. *Journal of the American Dietetic Association* 93:758–767.

133. American Diabetes Association. 2001. Implications of the Diabetes Control and Complications Trial. *Diabetes Care* 24(suppl):S25–S27.

134. American Diabetes Association. 1994. Nutrition recommendations and principles for people with diabetes mellitus. *Diabetes Care* 17:519–522.

135. American Diabetes Association. 2001. Nutrition recommendations for people with diabetes mellitus. *Diabetes Care.* 24(suppl):S44–S47.

136. Franz MJ, Bantle JP. 1999. American Diabetes Association Guide to Medical Nutrition Therapy for Diabetes. Alexandria, VA: American Diabetes Association.

137. American Diabetes Association. 2002. Position statement: Evidence-based nutrition principles and recommendations for the treatment and prevention of diabetes and related complications. *Diabetes Care.* 25(suppl):S50–S60.

ASSESSMENT ACTIVITY 8.1

Lipid and Lipoprotein Levels and Coronary Heart Disease Risk

The National Cholesterol Education Program recommends that all adults 20 years of age or older know their serum total cholesterol. Values < 200 mg/dL (5.17 mmol/L) can be repeated at least every 5 years. Values of 200 mg/dL (5.17 mmol/L) or greater should be verified by a repeat measurement within 1 to 8 weeks. If the second value is within 30 mg/dL (0.8 mmol/L) of the first, the average of the two can be used as a guide for subsequent decisions. Otherwise, a third test should be obtained in another 1 to 8 weeks and the average of the three values used.

You are encouraged to have your blood lipid and lipoprotein levels measured and to know these values. There are several ways you can do this. Your professor may be able to arrange with student health services or a local hospital or clinical laboratory to have cholesterol and lipoprotein measurements performed on all interested students in your class. If measurements are done on several members of your class, they may be done at a reduced price; for example, triglycerides, total cholesterol, low-density-lipoprotein cholesterol, and high-density-lipoprotein cholesterol may be measured for $20 or less, or you may want to have your cholesterol or lipid and lipoprotein levels measured on your own. Some hospitals offer low-priced testing as a community service.

When you receive your results, answer the following questions:

1. What are the highest, lowest, mean, and median values for each of the lipids and lipoproteins measured?

2. How do these compare with the population norms given in Appendix S?

3. What are the highest, lowest, mean, and median values for the ratio of total cholesterol to high-density-lipoprotein cholesterol?

4. How do these compare with the values shown in Appendix S?

5. Is there anyone in your class needing follow-up testing, according to the National Cholesterol Education Program's guidelines given in this chapter?

ASSESSMENT ACTIVITY 8.2

Calculating 10-Year Coronary Heart Disease Risk

Using data obtained from the Framingham Heart Study, the National Cholesterol Education Program has developed tables for calculating the likelihood of a person's having a myocardial infarction or dying from coronary heart disease (CHD) within the next 10 years (review Tables 8.4 and 8.5). The values for total cholesterol and high-density-lipoprotein cholesterol (HDL-C) used to score risk should be the average of at least two measurements obtained from lipoprotein analysis. The average of several blood pressure measurements is needed for an accurate assessment of baseline systolic blood pressure. A person taking medication for hypertension is considered treated and at increased risk for CHD, as reflected in a higher risk score. The designation "smoker" means any cigarette smoking in the past month.

Consider, for example, a nonsmoking, 45-year-old male who has a total cholesterol of 223 mg/dL, a high-density-lipoprotein cholesterol (HDL-C) level of 43 mg/dL, and a systolic blood pressure of 127 mm Hg. Also assume that this individual is not being treated for hypertension. In Table 8.4, this male would receive 0 points for being a nonsmoker, 3 points for age, 5 points

for total cholesterol at age 45 years, 1 point for HDL-C, and 0 points for systolic blood pressure. The total of all points would be 9, giving this individual a 10-year risk for myocardial infarction or death from CHD of 5%. You are encouraged to estimate your own 10-year risk and that of several hypothetical patients.

In Tables 8.4 and 8.5, the points assigned for total cholesterol and cigarette smoking decline with advancing age, suggesting that the risk for CHD from these two variables decreases with advancing age. However, this decline is more apparent than real because of the exponential rise in risk with mounting Framingham points. For example, for males, a change in total points from 9 to 10 increases the 10-year risk a mere 1%, but a change from 15 to 16 points increases risk by 5%. Thus, in older persons who have several points due to age alone, the addition of fewer points for high total cholesterol or smoking increases absolute risk as much as or more than do more points at a younger age. Thus, Tables 8.4 and 8.5 should not be misconstrued to mean that risk contributed by total cholesterol and smoking declines in importance with advancing age.

BIOCHEMICAL ASSESSMENT OF NUTRITIONAL STATUS

INTRODUCTION

Compared with the other methods of nutritional assessment (anthropometric, clinical methods, and dietary), biochemical tests provide the most objective and quantitative data on nutritional status. Biochemical tests often can detect nutrient deficits long before anthropometric measures are altered and clinical signs and symptoms appear. Some of these tests are useful indicators of recent nutrient intake and can be used in conjunction with dietary methods to assess food and nutrient consumption.

This chapter discusses the topic of biochemical methods in nutritional assessment, reviews the more commonly encountered tests for those nutrients of public health importance, and provides examples of various biochemical techniques in nutritional assessment.

Nutritional science is a relatively young discipline, and use of biochemical methods as indicators of nutritional status is still in its early development. This, along with all that yet remains unknown about the human body, makes the use of these measures in nutritional assessment a rapidly developing field and one with many research opportunities.

USE OF BIOCHEMICAL MEASURES

Biochemical tests available for assessing nutritional status can be grouped into two general and somewhat arbitrary categories: *static tests* and *functional tests.* These are sometimes referred to as *direct* and *indirect tests,* respectively.[1] Other, more detailed classification schemes also may be encountered.[2]

Static tests are based on measurement of a nutrient or its metabolite in the blood, urine, or body tissue—for example, serum measurements of albumin, calcium, or vitamin A. These are among the most readily available tests, but they have certain limitations. Although they indicate nutrient levels in the particular tissue or fluid sampled, they often fail to reflect the overall nutrient status of an individual or whether the body as a whole is in a state of nutrient excess or depletion.[3] For example, the amount of calcium in serum can be easily determined, but that single static measurement is a poor indicator of the body's overall calcium status or of bone mineral content.

Functional tests of nutritional status are based on the idea that "the final outcome of a nutrient deficiency and its biologic importance are not merely a measured level in a tissue or blood, but the failure of one or more physiologic processes that rely on that nutrient for optimal performance."[2] Included among these functional tests are measurement of dark adaptation (assesses vitamin A status), urinary excretion of xanthurenic acid in response to consumption of tryptophan (assesses vitamin B$_6$ status), and impairment of immune status resulting from protein-energy malnutrition and other nutrient deficits. Although many functional tests remain in the experimental stage, this is an area of active research and one that is likely to be fruitful.[2] One drawback of some functional tests, however, is a tendency to be nonspecific; they may indicate general nutritional status but not allow identification of specific nutrient deficiencies.[2]

Biochemical tests can also be used to examine the validity of various methods of measuring dietary intake or to determine if respondents are underreporting or overreporting what they eat. The ability of a food frequency questionnaire to accurately measure protein intake, for example, can be assessed by 24-hour urine nitrogen excretion. When properly used, this method is sufficiently accurate to use as a validation method in dietary surveys. As with any test requiring a 24-hour urine sample, however, each collection must be complete (i.e., respondents must collect all urine during an exact 24-hour period).

Urinary nitrogen is best estimated using multiple 24-hour urine samples, and any extrarenal nitrogen losses must be accounted for.[4] The doubly labeled water technique, as mentioned in Chapters 3 and 7, is another biochemical test useful for determining validity and accuracy of reporting. It can be an accurate way of measuring energy expenditure without interfering with a respondent's everyday life.[5] If reported energy and protein consumption fail to match estimates of energy and protein intake derived from these properly performed biochemical tests, then the dietary assessment method may be faulty or the respondent did not accurately report food intake.

Biochemical tests are a valuable adjunct in assessing and managing nutritional status; however, their use is not without problems. Most notable among these is the influence that nonnutritional factors can have on test results. A variety of pathologic conditions, use of certain medications, and technical problems in a sample collection or assay can affect test results in ways that make them unusable. Another problem with some biochemical tests is their nonspecificity. A certain test may indicate that a patient's general nutritional status is impaired yet lack the specificity to indicate which nutrient is deficient. Additionally, no single test, index, or group of tests by itself is sufficient for monitoring nutritional status. Biochemical tests must be used in conjunction with measures of dietary intake, anthropometric measures, and clinical methods.

PROTEIN STATUS

The importance of assessing protein status has been well summarized by Phinney:

> Protein is the principal compound upon which body structure and function is based. Unlike the major fuels, fat and carbohydrate, it is not stored to any degree in a non-functional form awaiting use. In this context, a gain or loss of protein represents an equivalent gain or loss of function, and thus evaluation of a patient's protein nutriture can be very important.[6]

Assessing protein status can be approached by use of anthropometric (Chapters 6 and 7), biochemical, clinical (Chapter 10), and dietary data (Chapters 3 and 4). Although each of these approaches has its strengths and limitations, biochemical methods have the potential of being the most objective and quantitative.[7]

Biochemical assessment of protein status has typically been approached from the perspective of the two-compartment model: evaluation of somatic protein and visceral protein status. The body's somatic protein is found within skeletal muscle. Visceral protein can be regarded as consisting of protein within the organs or viscera of the body (liver, kidneys, pancreas, heart, and so on), the erythrocytes (red blood cells), and the granulocytes and lymphocytes (white blood cells), as well as the serum proteins.[8] The somatic and visceral pools contain

the metabolically available protein (known as body cell mass), which can be drawn on, when necessary, to meet various bodily needs. The somatic and visceral protein pools comprise about 75% and 25% of the body cell mass, respectively.[6] Together, they comprise about 30% to 50% of total body protein.[8] The remaining body protein is found primarily in the skin and connective tissue (bone matrix, cartilage, tendons, and ligaments) and is not readily exchangeable with the somatic and visceral protein pools.[6] Division of the body's protein into these two compartments is somewhat arbitrary and artificial. Although the somatic compartment is homogeneous, the visceral protein pool is composed of hundreds of different proteins serving many structural and functional roles.

Although protein is not considered a public health issue among the general population of developed nations, protein-energy malnutrition (PEM), also known as protein-calorie malnutrition, can be a result of certain diseases and is clearly a pressing concern in many developing nations. Protein-energy malnutrition can be seen in persons with cancer and acquired immune deficiency syndrome (AIDS), children who fail to thrive, and homeless persons.

Because of its high prevalence and relationship to infant mortality and impaired physical growth, PEM is considered the most important nutritional disease in developing countries.[9] It is also of concern in developed nations. According to some reports, PEM has been observed in nearly half of the patients hospitalized in medical and surgical wards in the United States. In more recent studies, the prevalence of PEM ranged from 30% to 40% among patients with hip fractures, patients undergoing thoracic surgery for lung cancer, patients receiving ambulatory peritoneal dialysis, and children and adolescents with juvenile rheumatoid arthritis.[10–13]

Assessment of protein status is central to the prevention, diagnosis, and treatment of PEM. The causes of PEM can be either primary (inadequate food intake) or secondary (other diseases leading to insufficient food intake, inadequate nutrient absorption or utilization, increased nutritional requirement, and increased nutrient losses).[7,9] The protein and energy needs of hospitalized patients can be two or more times those of healthy persons as a result of hypermetabolism accompanying trauma, infection, burns, and surgical recovery.[14] PEM can result in kwashiorkor (principally a protein deficiency), marasmus (predominantly an energy deficiency), or marasmic kwashiorkor (a combination of chronic energy deficit and chronic or acute protein deficiency).[9] Clinical findings pertinent to kwashiorkor and marasmus are discussed in Chapter 10.

As Young and coworkers[7] have written, "no single test or group of tests can be recommended at this time as a routine and reliable indicator of protein status." Each of the approaches discussed has certain limitations.

Densitometry, total body potassium, and total body nitrogen (discussed in Chapter 6) stand out as relatively precise and accurate methods of assessing protein status but have limited clinical application because of their expense, limited availability, and problems with patient tolerance. Total body nitrogen as measured by neutron activation analysis and total body potassium as measured by either potassium-40 counting or neutron activation analysis are limited by the expense of the procedures and the availability of equipment. Body weight is a readily obtained indicator of energy and protein reserves. However, it must be carefully interpreted because it fails to distinguish between fat mass and fat-free mass, and losses of skeletal muscle and adipose tissue can be masked by water retention resulting from edema and ascites. The creatinine-height index is also well suited to the clinical setting but has limited precision and accuracy. Use of midarm muscle circumference and midarm muscle area are two other approaches to assessing somatic protein status. These are discussed in Chapter 7.

Rather than relying on any single indicator, a combination of measures can produce a more complete picture of protein status. The choice of approaches depends on methods available to the particular facility. Biochemical data on nutritional status constitute only part of the necessary information to properly quantitate nutritional depletion and PEM. Data relating to dietary intake, pertinent anthropometric measures, and clinical findings are necessary as well.

Creatinine Excretion and Creatinine-Height Index

A biochemical test sometimes used for estimating body muscle mass is 24-hour urinary creatinine excretion. Creatinine, a product of skeletal muscle, is excreted in a relatively constant proportion to the mass of muscle in the body. It is readily measured by any clinical laboratory. Lean body mass can be estimated by comparing 24-hour urine creatinine excretion with a standard based on stature (Table 9.1) or from reference values of 23 and 18 mg/kg of recommended body weight for males and females, respectively. Another approach is using the creatinine-height index (CHI), a ratio of a patient's measured 24-hour urinary creatinine excretion and the expected excretion of a reference adult of the same sex and stature. The CHI is expressed by the following formula:

$$\text{CHI} = \frac{\text{24-hr urine creatinine (mg)} \times 100}{\text{Expected 24-hr urine creatinine (mg)}}$$

Expected 24-hour urine creatinine values are shown in Table 9.1. These should be matched to the subject's sex and height.

The CHI is expressed as a percent of expected value. A CHI of 60% to 80% is considered indicative of mild protein depletion; 40% to 60% reflects moderate protein depletion; and a value under 40% represents severe depletion.[2]

As mentioned in the section "Use of Biochemical Measures," a major concern when using any test requiring a 24-hour urine sample is obtaining a complete urine

TABLE 9.1	**Expected 24-Hour Urinary Creatinine Values for Height for Adult Males and Females**

Adult Males[*]		Adult Females[†]	
Height (cm)	Creatinine (mg)	Height (cm)	Creatinine (mg)
157.5	1288	147.3	830
160.0	1325	149.9	851
162.6	1359	152.4	875
165.1	1386	154.9	900
167.6	1426	157.5	925
170.2	1467	160.0	949
172.7	1513	162.6	977
175.3	1555	165.1	1006
177.8	1596	167.6	1044
180.3	1642	170.2	1076
182.9	1691	172.7	1109
185.4	1739	175.3	1141
188.0	1785	177.8	1174
190.5	1831	180.3	1206
193.0	1891	182.9	1240

Adapted from Blackburn GL, Bistrian BR, Maini BS, Schlamm HT, Smith MR. 1977. Nutritional and metabolic assessment of the hospitalized patient. *Journal of Parenteral and Enteral Nutrition* 1:11–12.

[*]Creatinine coefficient for males = 23 mg/kg of "ideal" body weight.
[†]Creatinine coefficient for females = 18 mg/kg of "ideal" body weight.

sample collected during an exact 24-hour period. The value of protein status measurements based on urinary creatinine measurements can also be compromised by the effect of diet on urine creatinine levels, variability in creatinine excretion, and the use of height-weight tables for determining expected creatinine excretion based on sex and stature.[6] These limitations are discussed in Chapter 6.

3-methylhistidine

Measurement of urinary excretion of 3-methylhistidine is another potential approach for assessing muscle mass. It is subject to many of the same problems as assessment of urinary creatinine excretion (see Chapter 6), and values can be affected by a variety of factors, such as age, sex, maturity, hormonal status, degree of physical fitness, recent intense exercise, injury, and disease.[2,7] There also appears to be a significant pool of 3-methylhistidine outside of skeletal muscle, further complicating its use as an index of skeletal muscle protein breakdown.[15] Additional research into this approach is needed. However, it is doubtful that this method will become a routine biochemical assessment technique.

Nitrogen Balance

A person is said to be in nitrogen balance when the amount of nitrogen (consumed as protein) equals the amount excreted by the body. Nitrogen balance is the expected state of the healthy adult. It occurs when the rate of protein synthesis, or anabolism, equals the rate of protein degradation or catabolism. Positive nitrogen balance occurs when nitrogen intake exceeds nitrogen loss and is seen in periods of anabolism, such as childhood or recovery from trauma, surgery, or illness. Negative nitrogen balance occurs when nitrogen losses exceed nitrogen intake and can result from insufficient protein intake, catabolic states (for example, sepsis, trauma, surgery, and cancer), or during periods of excessive protein loss (as a result of burns or certain gastrointestinal and renal diseases characterized by unusual protein loss). Nutritional support can help return a patient to positive nitrogen balance or at least prevent severe losses of energy stores and body protein.[2,14]

Nitrogen balance studies involve 24-hour measurement of protein intake and an estimate of nitrogen losses from the body. The following formula is used:

$$N_2 \text{ Balance} = \frac{PRO}{6.25} - UUN - 4$$

where N_2 Balance = nitrogen balance; PRO = protein intake (g/24 h); and UUN = urine urea nitrogen (g/24 h).

Protein intake, measured by dietary assessment methods, is divided by 6.25 to arrive at an estimate of nitrogen intake. Nitrogen loss is generally estimated by measuring urine urea nitrogen (which accounts for 85% to 90% of nitrogen in the urine) and adding a constant (for example, 4 g) to account for nitrogen losses from the skin, stool, wound drainage, nonurea nitrogen, and so on, which cannot be easily measured.[2,14]

Problems associated with measuring protein intake and nitrogen excretion limit the usefulness of this approach. For example, it is difficult to account for the unusually high nonurine nitrogen losses seen in some patients with burns, diarrhea, vomiting, or fistula drainage. In such cases, this approach to calculating nitrogen balance may not yield accurate results.

Serum Proteins

Serum protein concentrations can be useful in assessing protein status, in determining whether a patient is at risk of experiencing medical complications, and for evaluating a patient's response to nutritional support. The serum proteins of primary interest in nutritional assessment are shown in Table 9.2.[14] In most instances, their measurement is simple and accurate. Use of serum protein measurements is based on the assumption that decreases in serum concentrations are due to decreased liver production (the primary site of synthesis). This is considered a consequence of a limited supply of amino acids from which the serum proteins are synthesized or a decrease in the liver's capacity to synthesize serum proteins. The extent to which nutritional status or liver function affects

serum protein concentrations cannot always be determined. A number of factors other than inadequate protein intake affect serum protein concentrations. These are noted in Table 9.2

Albumin

The most familiar and abundant of the serum proteins, as well as the most readily available clinically, is albumin. Serum albumin level has been shown to be an indicator of depleted protein status and decreased dietary protein intake. Measured over the course of several weeks, it has been shown to correlate with other measures of protein status (for example, measures of immunocompetence) and to respond to protein repletion. Low concentrations of serum albumin are associated with increased morbidity and mortality in hospitalized patients.[7,16,17] Despite these correlations, the value of albumin as a protein status indicator is limited by several factors. Its relatively long half-life (14 to 20 days) and large body pool (4 to 5 g/kg of body weight) cause serum levels to respond slowly to nutritional change, making it a poor indicator of early protein depletion and repletion.[2,7,14]

Serum albumin level is determined by several factors: the rate of synthesis, its distribution in the body, the rate at which it is catabolized, abnormal losses from the body, and altered fluid status.[14] These are summarized in Table 9.3. About 60% of the body's albumin is found outside the bloodstream. When serum concentrations begin falling during early PEM, this extravascular albumin moves into the bloodstream, helping maintain normal serum concentrations despite protein and energy deficit.[2,7,14] During the acute catabolic phase of an injury, an infection, or surgery, there is increased synthesis of substances known as acute-phase reactants. Included among these are C-reactive protein, fibrinogen, haptoglobin, and Á1-glycoprotein. Acute-phase reactants decrease synthesis of albumin, prealbumin, and transferrin. Consequently, levels of these serum proteins may remain low during this catabolic phase despite the provision of adequate nutritional support.[14] The practice of administering albumin to severely ill patients also can interfere with its use as an indicator of protein status.[4]

Transferrin

Serum transferrin is a β-globulin synthesized in the liver that binds and transports iron in the plasma. Because of its smaller body pool and shorter half-life, it has been considered a better index of changes in protein status compared with albumin.[2] Although serum transferrin has been shown to be associated with clinical outcome in children with kwashiorkor and marasmus, its use to predict morbidity and mortality outcomes in hospitalized patients has produced conflicting results.[8]

Serum transferrin can be measured directly (by radial immunodiffusion and nephelometry), but it is frequently estimated indirectly from total iron-binding

TABLE 9.2 | Serum Proteins Used in Nutritional Assessment

Serum Protein	Normal Value, Mean ±SD or (Range)[*]	Half-Life	Function	Comments[†]
Albumin	45 (35–50)	18–20 days	Maintains plasma oncotic pressure; carrier for small molecules	In addition to protein status, other factors affect serum concentrations.
Transferrin	2.3 (2.6–4.3)	8–9 days	Binds iron in plasma and transports to bone marrow	Iron deficiency increases hepatic synthesis and plasma levels; increases during pregnancy, during estrogen therapy, and in acute hepatitis; reduced in protein-losing enteropathy and nephropathy, chronic infections, uremia, and acute catabolic states; often measured indirectly by total iron-binding capacity; equations for indirect prediction should be developed locally.
Prealbumin	0.30 (0.2–0.4)	2–3 days	Binds T_3 and, to a lesser extent, T_4; carrier for retinol-binding protein	Level is increased in patients with chronic renal failure on dialysis due to decreased renal catabolism; reduced in acute catabolic states, after surgery, in hyperthyroidism, in protein-losing enteropathy; increased in some cases of nephrotic syndrome; serum level determined by overall energy balance as well as nitrogen balance.
Retinol-binding protein (RBP)	0.372 ±0.0073[‡]	12 hours	Transports vitamin A in plasma; binds noncovalently to prealbumin	It is catabolized in renal proximal tubular cell; with renal disease, RBP increases and half-life is prolonged; low in vitamin A deficiency, acute catabolic states, after surgery, and in hyperthyroidism.
Insulin-like growth factor-1 (IGF-1)	0.83 IU/mL (0.55–1.4)	2–6 hours	One of a family of insulin-like peptides that have anabolic actions on fat, muscle, cartilage, and cultured cells	It was referred to earlier as somatomedin-C; levels fall rapidly with fasting and quickly recover during refeeding; low values in hypothyroid patients, with estrogen administration, and possibly in obesity; may be a valid nutritional marker during acute-phase response.
Fibronectin	Plasma: 2.92 ±0.2 Serum: 1.82 ±0.16	4–24 hours	A glycoprotein found in many tissues; a soluble form appears in blood and behaves as an opsonic glycoprotein; may exert chemotactic activity and be involved in wound healing	Plasma fibronectin deficiency may contribute to host defense suppression with malnutrition; may be a sensitive marker during nutritional depletion and repletion; levels may be influenced by acute-phase response; more clinical studies needed; reference ranges not well studied.

Adapted from Heymsfield SB, Tighe A, Wang ZM. 1994. Nutritional assessment by anthropometric and biochemical methods. In Shils ME, Olson JA, Shike M, eds. *Modern nutrition in health and disease,* 8th ed. Philadelphia: Lea & Febiger.

[*]All units are g/L. Normal range varies among centers; check local values.

[†]All the listed proteins are influenced by hydration and the presence of hepatocellular dysfunction.

[‡]Normal values are age- and sex-dependent. Table value is for pooled subjects.

TABLE 9.3	Factors Determining Serum Albumin Levels
Rate of synthesis	Biosynthesis is decreased by lack of dietary protein, physiologic stress, liver disease, hypothyroidism, and the presence of excessive levels of serum cortisol.
Distribution in body	Normally, 30% to 40% of the body's albumin is found in the blood and lymphatic vessels (the intravascular space) with the remainder in lean tissues outside the blood and lymphatic vessels (the extravascular space), especially the skin. Following surgery or thermal injury, albumin shifts from the intravascular space to the extravascular space, with a concomitant fall in serum albumin levels. In semistarvation, albumin shifts from the extravascular space to the intravascular space.
Rate of catabolism	The catabolic rate is decreased in semistarvation and hypometabolism and increased by physiologic stress, hypermetabolism, Cushing's syndrome, and some malignant tumors.
Abnormal losses from the body	Causes of abnormal losses include thermal burns, nephrotic syndrome, and protein-losing enteropathies.
Altered fluid status	Levels decline when blood volume increases from such causes as congestive heart failure, fluid overload, and renal failure. Dehydration decreases blood volume and results in increased albumin levels.

capacity (TIBC) using a prediction formula suited to the particular facility's method for measuring TIBC.[8]

The use of transferrin as an index of nutritional status and repletion is limited by several factors other than protein status that affect its serum concentration. As was outlined in Table 9.2, transferrin levels decrease in chronic infections, protein-losing enteropathy, chronically draining wounds, nephropathy, acute catabolic states (e.g., surgery and trauma), and uremia. Serum levels can be increased during pregnancy, estrogen therapy, and acute hepatitis.[14,18]

Prealbumin

Prealbumin, also known as transthyretin and thyroxine-binding prealbumin, is synthesized in the liver and serves as a transport protein for thyroxine (T_4) and as a carrier protein for retinol-binding protein. Because of its short half-life (2 to 3 days) and small body pool (0.01 g/kg body weight), it is considered a more sensitive indicator of protein nutriture and one that responds more rapidly to changes in protein status than albumin or transferrin.

Prealbumin decreases rapidly in response to deficits of either protein or energy and is sensitive to the early stages of malnutrition. Because serum concentration quickly returns to expected levels once adequate nutritional therapy begins, it is not recommended as an endpoint for terminating nutritional support. It may prove to be better suited as an indicator of recent dietary intake than as a means of assessing nutritional status.[2] Serum concentration also will return to expected levels in response to adequate energy in the absence of sufficient protein intake. Its use as an indicator of protein status appears to be preferable to the use of albumin or transferrin. However, like the other serum proteins outlined in Table 9.2, several factors other than protein status affect its concentration in serum. Levels are reduced in liver disease, sepsis, protein-losing enteropathies, hyperthyroidism, and acute catabolic states (e.g., following surgery or trauma). Serum prealbumin can be increased in

patients with chronic renal failure who are on dialysis due to decreased renal catabolism.[14,18]

Retinol-Binding Protein

Retinol-binding protein, a liver protein, acts as a carrier for retinol (vitamin A alcohol) when complexed with prealbumin. It circulates in the blood as a 1:1:1 trimolecular complex with retinol and prealbumin.[19] Retinol-binding protein shares several features with prealbumin. It responds quickly to protein-energy deprivation and adequate nutritional therapy, as well as to ample energy in the absence of sufficient protein. Like prealbumin, it may be a better indicator of recent dietary intake than of overall nutritional status. It has a much shorter half-life (about 12 hours) than prealbumin. Its smaller body pool (0.002 g/kg body weight), however, complicates its precise measurement. There is no convincing evidence that its use in nutritional assessment is preferred over prealbumin. Because it is catabolized in the renal proximal tubule cell, serum levels are increased in renal disease and its half-life is prolonged. Serum levels can be decreased in vitamin A deficiency, acute catabolic states, and hyperthyroidism.[14]

Insulin-like Growth Factor-1

Also referred to as somatomedin C, insulin-like growth factor-1 (IGF-1) is a growth-promoting peptide produced by the liver in response to growth hormone stimulation.[20] Although technically not a serum protein, it is included in this section for the sake of convenience. Decreased serum concentration of IGF-1 is seen in PEM.[7] Unlike prealbumin, its concentration in serum is restored by adequate administration of protein, but not when ample energy is present in the absence of protein deficit. Low serum concentrations of IGF-1 in patients with PEM were shown to return to expected levels after 3 to 16 days of nutritional therapy. During the same period, no significant changes were seen in serum albumin, transferrin, prealbumin, and retinol-binding protein, suggesting that IGF-1 is a more sensitive indicator of protein status.[22] IGF-1 may be a valid indicator of nutritional status during the acute-phase response.[14]

The combination of low serum concentration of IGF-1 and normal or elevated concentration of growth hormone indicates the presence of PEM. Although this pattern of IGF-1 and growth hormone can result from several other conditions as well (for example, hypothyroidism, renal failure, cirrhosis of the liver, and peripheral growth hormone resistance), most of these conditions can be ruled out by other biochemical tests or physical examination.[2,14]

IGF-1 shows promise as an indicator of protein status, but additional research is required before it becomes a routine test in the clinical setting.[7]

Fibronectin

Fibronectin is a glycoprotein synthesized by many cell types, including liver cells, endothelial cells, and fibroblasts. In contrast to the previously discussed serum proteins, the nonliver sources appear to be most important. Fibronectin functions in cell adhesion, wound healing, hemostasis, and macrophage function.[2] Nutritional deprivation results in decreased serum concentrations, which return to expected levels with nutritional therapy.[21–25] In malnourished children, low serum concentrations of fibronectin respond to nutritional therapy more readily than other signs.[21] Children with PEM who receive intravenous administration of fibronectin as an adjunct to nutritional therapy have decreased mortality and faster normalization of albumin, transferrin, and prealbumin serum concentrations, compared with children in a control group.[24]

Other factors affecting serum concentrations of fibronectin include trauma, burns, shock, and sepsis. Fibronectin holds promise as a useful indicator of nutritional status, but additional research is required before it becomes a routine part of clinical care.[2]

Immunocompetence

A close and complex relationship exists between nutrition and immunity. Nutritional deficits can lead to impaired immunocompetence, infection, and inflammation, which in turn can have profound effects on nutrition and nutrient metabolism.[2,25] Tests of immunocompetence can be useful functional indicators of nutritional status. Because changes in immune response can occur early in nutritional deficiency, immunocompetence can be used as an early functional indicator of nutritional status and as an index of response to nutritional support.[25,26]

Anergy and other immunological changes can be used as prognostic indicators for complications, duration of hospitalization, and mortality in medical and surgical patients.[26] Immune responses may be useful in determining safe upper and lower limits of nutrient intake.

Although sensitive to impaired nutritional status, they often lack specificity: they are good indicators of general nutritional deficit but can rarely identify the specific nutritional deficiency.[2,7,25] A variety of factors other than nutritional status also can affect immunocompetence.

Nonspecific and Antigen-Specific Immunity

The immune system's defense mechanisms can be divided into two broad categories: nonspecific and antigen-specific.[26] The nonspecific defenses include the skin, mucous membranes, phagocytic cells, mucus, cilia, complement, lysozyme, and interferon. These are naturally present defenses that act as the first line of protection against infection and are not influenced by prior contact with infectious agents. The antigen-specific defenses act in response to exposure to specific infectious agents and antigens (molecules that stimulate antibody production) and involve the B-lymphocytes and T-lymphocytes. B-lymphocytes, responsible for humoral immunity, secrete antibodies. T-lymphocytes, responsible for cell-mediated immunity, attack host cells that have become infected with viruses or fungi, transplanted human cells, and cancerous cells.[27] Compared with other parts of the immune system, the effects of malnutrition on cell-mediated immunity are more frequent, develop earlier, and are more clinically significant.[2] A variety of responses to nutrient deficiency, especially PEM, have been identified and used as indicators of nutritional status.

Total Lymphocyte Count

The total number of lymphocytes can be derived from a routine complete blood count that includes a *differential count*. The differential gives the percentage of different white blood cells in the sample examined. The percentage of lymphocytes in the sample is multiplied by the number of white blood cells (WBCs) and divided by 100:

$$\text{TLC} = \frac{\% \text{ lymphocytes} \times \text{WBC count}}{100}$$

where TLC = total lymphocyte count; % lymphocytes = percentage of lymphocytes from the differential count; and WBC count = white blood cell count (cells/mm^3).

Mild nutritional depletion would be represented by a total lymphocyte count within the range of 1200 to 1800 lymphocytes/mm^3, moderate depletion would be in the range of 800 to 1199 lymphocytes/mm^3, and less than 800 lymphocytes/mm^3 would represent severe depletion.

Factors affecting total lymphocyte count besides nutritional status include cancer, inflammation, infection, stress, sepsis, and certain drugs, such as steroids, chemotherapeutic agents, and immunosuppressive agents.

Delayed Cutaneous Hypersensitivity

Delayed cutaneous hypersensitivity (DCH) involves the injection of a small amount of antigen within the skin (intradermally) to determine the subject's reaction. Because the degree of reactivity to the antigen is a function of the subject's cell-mediated immunity (the T-lymphocytes),[28] the test is sometimes referred to as cell-mediated hypersensitivity.[29] Under normal conditions, the injection site should become inflamed, with a characteristic hardening (induration) and redness (erythema) noted between 24 and 72 hours after injection. In persons with compromised cell-mediated immunity, the response would be less than expected or absent (known as *anergy*). Antigens used include streptokinase-streptodornase, candidin, trichophyton, tuberculin (purified protein derivative), and mumps.[29]

DCH is reported to be decreased in PEM and deficiencies of vitamins B_6 and A, zinc, and iron. As summarized by Twomey and coworkers,[30] a subject's reactivity also is affected by a variety of technical factors (including antigen source and batch, method of administration, and reader variability), patient factors (such as age, prior exposure to antigen, and psychologic state), several drugs, and a number of diseases (including infection, inflammation, immune alterations, and cancers).

IRON STATUS

Iron deficiency is the most common single nutrient deficiency in the United States and the most common cause of anemia. Although the prevalence of iron deficiency appears to have declined in recent years, it remains relatively high in vulnerable groups, such as women of childbearing age.[31]

Iron deficiency results when ingestion or absorption of dietary iron is inadequate to meet iron losses or iron requirements imposed by growth or pregnancy. Considerable iron can be lost from heavy menstruation, frequent blood donations, early feeding of cow's milk to infants, frequent aspirin use, or disorders characterized by gastrointestinal bleeding. Risk of iron deficiency increases during periods of rapid growth—notably, in infancy (especially in premature infants), adolescence, and pregnancy. The consequences of iron deficiency include reduced work capacity, impaired body temperature regulation, impairments in behavior and intellectual performance, increased susceptibility to lead poisoning, and decreased resistance to infections.[31]

Anemia is a hemoglobin level below the normal reference range for individuals of the same sex and age. Descriptive terms such as *microcytic, macrocytic,* and *hypochromic* are sometimes used to describe anemias. *Microcytic* refers to abnormally small red blood cells defined by a mean corpuscular volume (MCV) < 80 femtoliters (fL), whereas *macrocytic* describes unusually large red blood cells defined as an MCV > 100 fL. Hypochromic cells are those with abnormally low levels of hemoglobin as defined by a mean corpuscular hemoglobin concentration < 320 g of hemoglobin/L or by a mean corpuscular hemoglobin < 27 picograms (pg, 10^{-12} grams).

Although the most common cause of anemia is iron deficiency, it also may result from infection, chronic disease, and deficiencies of folate and vitamin B_{12}. Of particular concern to physicians working with individual patients and nutritional epidemiologists attempting to estimate the prevalence of iron deficiency in populations is differentiating iron-deficiency anemia from anemia caused by inflammatory disease, infection, chronic diseases, and thalassemia traits.[32]

Stages of Iron Depletion

The risk of iron deficiency increases as the body's iron stores are depleted. Iron depletion can be divided into three stages. These stages and the biochemical tests used in identifying them are shown in Table 9.4. Figure 9.1 illustrates how values for these tests change throughout the stages of iron deficiency.

The first stage of iron depletion, depleted iron stores, is not associated with any adverse physiologic effects, but it does represent a state of vulnerability.[31,33] Low stores occur in healthy persons and appear to be the usual physiologic condition for growing children and menstruating women.[31,34] As shown in Figure 9.1, during this first stage, low iron stores are reflected by decreased serum ferritin levels, but values for the other biochemical tests remain within normal limits.

The second stage of iron depletion, iron deficiency without anemia, can be considered representative of early or mild iron deficiency because, at this point, adverse

TABLE 9.4	Stages of Iron Depletion and the Laboratory Tests Used to Identify Them	
Stage	**Descriptive Term**	**Biochemical Test**
First	Depleted iron stores	Serum ferritin level
Second	Iron deficiency (without anemia)	Transferrin saturation Erythrocyte protoporphyrin
Third	Iron-deficiency anemia	Hemoglobin Mean corpuscular

From Life Sciences Research Office, Federation of American Societies of Experimental Biology. 1989. *Nutrition monitoring in the United States: An update report on nutrition monitoring.* Washington, DC: U.S. Department of Health and Human Services, Public Health Service.

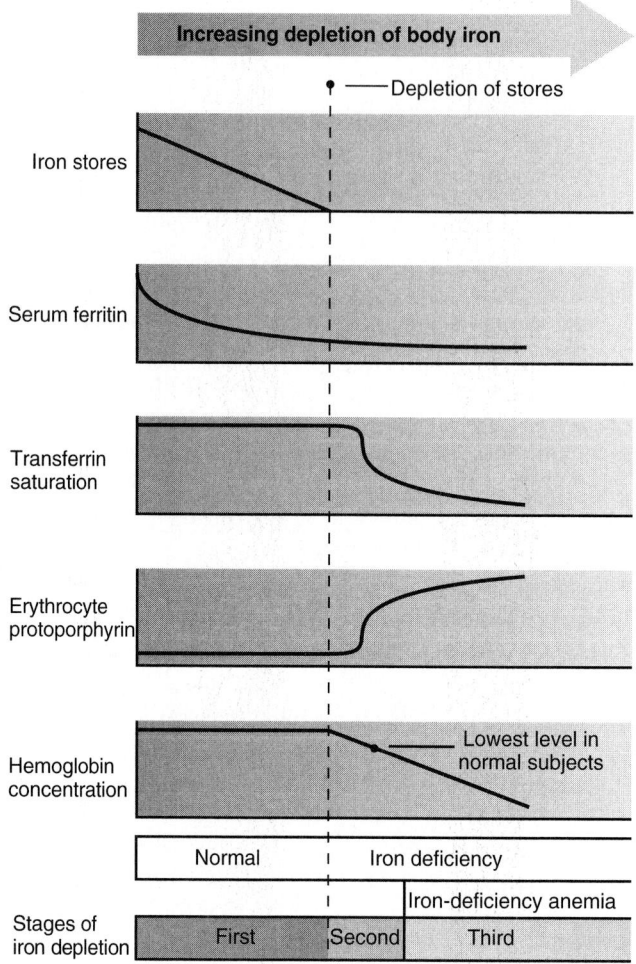

Figure 9.1 **Changes in body iron compartments and laboratory assessments of iron status during the stages of iron depletion.**

Source: From Life Sciences Research Office, Federation of American Societies for Experimental Biology. 1989. *Nutrition monitoring in the United States: An update report on nutrition monitoring.* Washington, DC: U.S. Department of Health and Human Services, Public Health Service.

physiologic consequences can begin to occur. This stage is characterized by changes indicating insufficient iron for normal production of hemoglobin and other essential iron compounds (for example, myoglobin and iron-containing enzymes).[31,33] As shown in Figure 9.1, this stage is assessed by decreased transferrin saturation and increased erythrocyte protoporphyrin levels. A precursor of hemoglobin, erythrocyte protoporphyrin increases when too little iron is available for optimal hemoglobin synthesis. Although hemoglobin may be decreased at this stage, it may not fall below the lowest levels seen in normal subjects. Consequently, hemoglobin is not a useful indicator of either stage 1 or stage 2 iron depletion.[31]

The third stage of iron depletion, iron-deficiency anemia, is characterized by decreased serum ferritin, transferrin saturation, hemoglobin, and MCV and increased erythrocyte protoporphyrin.[31,33]

No single biochemical test is diagnostic of impaired iron status. Several different static tests used together provide a much better measure of iron status.[31]

Serum Ferritin

When the protein apoferritin combines with iron, ferritin is formed. Ferritin, the primary storage form for iron in the body, is found primarily in the liver, spleen, and bone marrow. In healthy persons, approximately 30% of all iron in the body is in the storage form, most of this as ferritin but some as hemosiderin. As iron stores become depleted, tissue ferritin levels decrease. This is accompanied by a fall in serum ferritin concentration.[35] Measurement of serum ferritin concentration is the most sensitive test available for detecting iron deficiency, and decreases occur before morphologic changes are seen in red blood

Figure 9.2 **Sequence of events in developing iron deficiency and overload.**
The shaded areas indicate the relative quantities of iron in each compartment (e.g., in stores, in circulation, and in the erythrocytes). The sequence of increasingly unshaded areas shows its proportional disappearance during successive stages of iron deficiency. RE = reticuloendothelial; IBC = iron-binding capacity; RBC = red blood cell. To convert μg to SI units (nmol), multiply by 17.9.

Source: From Herbert V. 1987. The 1986 Herman Award Lecture. Nutrition science as a continually unfolding story: The folate and vitamin B$_{12}$ paradigm. *American Journal of Clinical Nutrition* 46:387–402.

cells, in the other indicators (shown in Figure 9.1), or before anemia occurs.[35] From Figures 9.1 and 9.2 it can also be noted that, once serum stores are depleted, serum ferritin levels no longer reflect the severity of iron deficiency. Cutoff values for serum ferritin and other tests used to indicate the presence of iron deficiency in the second National Health and Nutrition Examination Survey (NHANES II) are shown in Table 9.5.[31]

Serum ferritin levels can be increased by the presence of inflammation, infection, trauma, certain chronic

TABLE 9.5	Cutoff Values Indicative of Iron Deficiency Developed for Use with Data from the Second National Health and Nutrition Examination Survey*			
Age (yr)	Serum Ferritin (μg/L)	Transferrin Saturation (%)	Erythrocyte Protoporphyrin (μmol/L RBC)	MCV (fL)
1–2	———	< 12	> 1.42	< 73
3–4	< 10	< 14	> 1.33	< 75
5–10	< 10	< 15	> 1.24	< 76
11–14	< 10	< 16	> 1.24	< 78
15–74	< 12	< 16	> 1.24	< 80

From Life Sciences Research Office, Federation of American Societies for Experimental Biology. 1989. *Nutrition monitoring in the United States: An update report on nutrition monitoring.* Washington, DC: U.S. Department of Health and Human Services, Public Health Service.

*RBC = red blood cell; MCV = mean corpuscular volume; fL = femtoliter, 10^{-15} liter.

diseases, iron overload (excessive iron stores), viral hepatitis, and certain cancers (for example, Hodgkin's disease).[35]

Transferrin, Serum Iron, and Total Iron-Binding Capacity

Iron is transported in the blood bound to transferrin, a β-globulin protein molecule synthesized in the liver. Transferrin accepts iron from sites of hemoglobin destruction (the primary source for iron bound to transferrin) and from storage sites and iron absorbed through the intestinal tract. It then delivers the iron to sites where it is used—primarily the bone marrow for hemoglobin synthesis, as well as to storage sites, to the placenta for fetal needs, and to all cells for incorporation into iron-containing enzymes. Each molecule of transferrin has the capacity to transport two atoms of iron, but under most circumstances only about 30% of the available iron-binding sites are occupied or saturated.[34]

Because iron is carried in the blood by transferrin, serum iron level is a measure of the amount of iron bound to transferrin. Levels fall sometime between depletion of tissue iron stores and development of anemia, although they may actually be normal in persons with iron deficiency.[34,35]

Total iron-binding capacity measures the amount of iron capable of being bound to serum proteins and provides an estimate of serum transferrin. It is usually measured by adding an excess of iron to serum (thus saturating iron-binding proteins in serum), removing all iron not bound to protein in the serum, and then measuring serum iron. Because it is assumed that most serum iron is bound to transferrin, TIBC is an indirect measure of serum transferrin. Because other serum proteins can bind iron, TIBC is not an exact measure of transferrin, especially in cases of iron overload and certain other conditions. In about 30% to 40% of persons with iron-deficiency anemia, TIBC is not elevated.[35]

Transferrin saturation is the ratio of serum iron to TIBC and is calculated using the following formula:

$$TS = \frac{\text{Serum iron } (\mu \text{ mol/L})}{\text{TIBC } (\mu \text{ mol/L})} \times 100$$

where TS = percent transferrin saturation and TIBC = total iron-binding capacity.

Transferrin saturation is the percent of transferrin that is saturated with iron. In uncomplicated iron-deficiency anemia, serum iron levels decrease and TIBC increases, resulting in a decreased transferrin saturation. Cutoff values for transferrin saturation that are indicative of the presence of iron deficiency are shown in Table 9.5.

Measures of serum iron, TIBC, transferrin saturation, and serum ferritin concentration are useful in distinguishing iron deficiency from other disorders capable of causing microcytic anemias (anemias in which the erythrocytes are smaller than normal).[34] Transferrin saturation, however, is considered to be a more sensitive indicator of iron deficiency than either serum iron or TIBC.[35]

A variety of factors can affect these measures.[34,35] There is a considerable diurnal (cyclic changes within a 24-hour period) and day-to-day variation in serum iron concentrations. Serum iron can be as much as 50% greater in the morning than in the evening, and values taken at the same time of day can vary as much as 30% from one day to the next. The primary factor affecting TIBC is the status of body iron stores. TIBC is increased with depletion of iron stores and decreased in iron overload and in response to inflammation. There is no diurnal variation in TIBC.

Erythrocyte Protoporphyrin

Protoporphyrin is a precursor of heme and accumulates in red blood cells (erythrocytes) when the amount of heme that can be produced is limited by iron deficiency. Protoporphyrin concentration is generally reported in the range of 0.622 ± 0.27 μmol/L of red blood cells, although the value can vary depending on the analytic method. As can be seen from Table 9.5, iron deficiency can lead to a more than twofold increase over normal values. Erythrocyte protoporphyrin increases as iron depletion worsens, as can be seen in Figures 9.1 and 9.2. Lead poisoning also can result in increased erythrocyte protoporphyrin levels.

Hemoglobin

Hemoglobin is an iron-containing molecule capable of carrying oxygen and is found in red blood cells. Grams of hemoglobin per liter (or deciliter) of blood is an index of the blood's oxygen-carrying capacity. Measurement of hemoglobin in whole blood is the most widely used screening test for iron-deficiency anemia.

The amount of hemoglobin in blood primarily depends on the number of red blood cells and to a lesser extent on the amount of hemoglobin in each red blood cell.[35] Reference values are 14 to 180 g/L (14 to 18 g/dL) for men and 120 to 160 g/L (12 to 16 g/dL) for women. Hemoglobin levels for black men and women average 5 to 10 g/L less than levels for white men and women at most ages.[35] Hemoglobin and hematocrit values useful for defining anemia and iron-deficiency anemia are shown in Table 9.6. These were developed by the U.S. Centers for Disease Control and Prevention and are based on the 5th percentile values for a reference population from NHANES II. During pregnancy, the plasma volume increases, leading to a condition known as hemodilution, resulting in lower hemoglobin levels.[35] Depending on the trimester of pregnancy, hemoglobin levels as low as 105 g/L (10.5 g/dL) are considered within normal limits. As can be seen in Table 9.6, boys and girls have similar

TABLE 9.6	Hemoglobin and Hematocrit Values for Determining Anemia and Iron-Deficiency Anemia	
	Hemoglobin (g/L)	Hematocrit (%)
Age (years)		
1.0–1.9	110	33
2.0–4.9	112	34
5.0–7.9	114	35
8.0–11.9	116	36
12.0–14.9 (females)	118	36
12.0–14.9 (males)	123	37
15.0–17.9 (females)	120	36
15.0–17.9 (males)	126	38
18+ (females)	120	36
18+ (males)	135	40
Pregnancy		
1st trimester	110	33
2nd trimester	105	32
3rd trimester	110	33

From Life Sciences Research Office, Federation of American Societies for Experimental Biology. 1989. *Nutrition monitoring in the United States: An update report on nutrition monitoring.* Washington, DC: U.S. Department of Health and Human Services, Public Health Service.

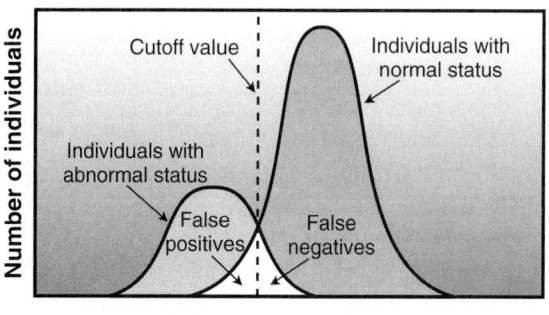

Figure 9.3 **Effect of applying a cutoff value for an indicator of nutritional status to the distributions of values for individuals with adequate status and individuals with inadequate status.**

Source: From Life Sciences Research Office, Federation of American Societies for Experimental Biology. 1989. *Nutrition monitoring in the United States: An update report on nutrition monitoring.* Washington, DC: U.S. Department of Health and Human Services, Public Health Service.

hemoglobin levels up until about age 11 years, after which values for males tend to be 5 to 15 g/L higher than for females, depending on age.[35]

Although hemoglobin and hematocrit values are useful in diagnosing anemia, they tend not to become abnormal until the late stages of iron deficiency and are not good indicators of early iron deficiency.

The use of cutoff points (as in Table 9.6) to classify laboratory values inevitably results in some degree of misclassification. For example, no matter where the cutoff value is placed in Figure 9.3, there will be some individuals with adequate iron status whose hemoglobin levels fall below the cutoff value. These are the false positives. There will be some, on the other hand, with an inadequate iron status whose hemoglobin levels fall above the cutoff value. These are the false negatives.

Hematocrit

Hematocrit (also known as *packed cell volume*) is defined as the percentage of red blood cells making up the entire volume of whole blood. It can be measured manually by comparing the height of whole blood in a capillary tube

with the height of the RBC column after the tube is centrifuged. In automated counters, it is calculated from the RBC count (number of RBCs per liter of blood) and the mean corpuscular volume. Hematocrit depends largely on the number of red blood cells and to a lesser extent on their average size. Normal ranges for hematocrit are 40% to 54% and 37% to 47% for males and females, respectively.[35]

Mean Corpuscular Hemoglobin

The mean corpuscular hemoglobin (MCH) is the amount of hemoglobin in red blood cells. It is calculated by dividing hemoglobin level by the red blood cell count. Reference values are approximately 26 to 34 pg. MCH is influenced by the size of the red blood cell and the amount of hemoglobin in relation to the size of the cell.[35]

A similar measure, mean corpuscular hemoglobin concentration (MCHC) is the average concentration of hemoglobin in the average red blood cell. It is calculated by dividing the hemoglobin value by the value for hematocrit. Normal values lie in the range of 320 to 360 g/L (32 to 36 g/dL).[35]

Mean Corpuscular Volume

Mean corpuscular volume (MCV) is the volume of the average red blood cell. It is calculated by dividing the hematocrit value by the RBC count. Values for MCV are normally in the range of 80 to 100 fL for both males and females.

Factors increasing MCV (resulting in macrocytosis) include deficiencies of folate or vitamin B_{12}, chronic liver disease, alcoholism, and cytotoxic chemotherapy. Among factors decreasing MCV (resulting in microcytosis) are chronic iron deficiency, thalassemia, anemia of chronic diseases, and lead poisoning.[35] Reference blood cell values for adults are shown in Table 9.7.

TABLE 9.7	Reference Blood Cell Values for Adults		
		Males	**Females**
Hemoglobin (g/L of blood)		140–180	120–160
Hematocrit (%)		40–54	37–47
Red cell count ($\times 10^{12}$/L blood)		4.5–6.0	4.0–5.5
Mean corpuscular hemoglobin (pg)		26–34	26–34
Mean corpuscular hemoglobin concentration (g/L of blood)		320–360	320–360
Mean corpuscular volume (fL)		80–100	80–100

From Ravel R. 1994. *Clinical laboratory medicine: Clinical application of laboratory data,* 6th ed. St. Louis: Mosby.

Models Assessing Impaired Iron Status

Because no single biochemical test exists for reliably assessing impaired iron status, several different indicators should be used together.[19,31,33] Different models using multiple biochemical values have been developed for evaluating iron status (Table 9.8).[31-33] The *ferritin model* uses three indicators: serum ferritin, transferrin saturation, and erythrocyte protoporphyrin. The *MCV model* uses MCV, transferrin saturation, and erythrocyte protoporphyrin as indicators. Both models require that at least two of the three indicators be abnormal. The ferritin model tends to overestimate the presence of iron defi-

TABLE 9.8	Laboratory Measurements Used in Four Models for Assessing Iron Deficiency
Model	**Measurements Used**
Ferritin model[*]	Serum ferritin Transferrin saturation Erythrocyte protoporphyrin
Mean corpuscular volume (MCV) model[*]	MCV Transferrin saturation Erythrocyte protoporphyrin
Four-variable model[†]	MCV or serum ferritin Transferrin saturation Erythrocyte protoporphyrin
Hemoglobin percentile shift model[‡]	Hemoglobin Transferrin saturation Erythrocyte protoporphyrin

From Life Sciences Research Office, Federation of American Societies for Experimental Biology. 1989. *Nutrition monitoring in the United States: An update report on nutrition monitoring.* Washington, DC: U.S. Department of Health and Human Services, Public Health Service; Johnson MA. 1990. Iron: Nutrition monitoring and nutrition status assessment. *Journal of Nutrition* 120:1486–1491.

[*]Two of three values must be abnormal.

[†]Values for either MCV or serum ferritin (or both) must be abnormal, in addition to at least one other abnormal value.

[‡]The hemoglobin percentile shift model estimates the median change in hemoglobin of a population after excluding individuals with low transferrin saturation and/or high erythrocyte protoporphyrin.

ciency because it includes ferritin, which reflects stores in the first stage of iron depletion. The MCV model, on the other hand, includes three biochemical tests, all of which reflect altered red blood cell formation.[31] Both models are capable of identifying persons in the second and third stages of iron depletion.

A concern about these models is that iron status indicators sometime fail to distinguish iron-deficiency anemia from the other common causes of anemia. When data from all four indicators (serum ferritin, erythrocyte protoporphyrin, transferrin saturation, and MCV) are combined in what is called the *four-variable model,* anemias caused by inflammatory conditions are better distinguished from iron-deficiency anemia. The model is considered diagnostic for iron-deficiency anemia when either the value for serum ferritin or for MCV plus one additional value are abnormal according to the values in Table 9.5.[31]

When estimating the prevalence of iron-deficiency anemia in populations from data derived from such studies as NHANES, two other approaches are helpful in discriminating between anemias related to inflammatory conditions and those caused by iron deficiency. One is the hemoglobin percentile shift, which estimates the median change in hemoglobin of a population after excluding individuals with low transferrin saturation ($<$ 16%) and/or high concentrations of erythrocyte protoporphyrin ($>$ 1.2 µmol/L of red blood cells).[32,33]

Another approach is to consider values from one of several nonspecific indicators of infection, inflammatory disease, and malignancy when evaluating indicators of iron status. These include erythrocyte sedimentation rate (ESR), zeta-sedimentation rate (ZSR), and C-reactive protein (CRP).

ESR and ZSR measure the rate at which red blood cells sediment in anticoagulated blood under a given set of conditions.[32,35] CRP is a glycoprotein found only in trace amounts in healthy people but elevated during acute inflammation or tissue destruction. It is not influenced by anemia or plasma protein changes and begins to rise about 4 to 6 hours after the onset of inflammation. CRP is considered by many to be the best indicator of acute inflammation, whereas ESR is the preferred indicator of chronic inflammation. These indicators are of value both in clinical practice and in population studies to help distinguish iron-deficiency anemia from anemia resulting from chronic disease.[32]

CALCIUM STATUS

Calcium is essential for bone and tooth formation, muscle contraction, blood clotting, and cell membrane integrity.[31] Of the 1200 g of calcium in the adult body, approximately 99% is contained in the bones. The remaining 1% is found in extracellular fluids, intracellular structures, and cell membranes.[19]

Osteoporosis, a calcium-related health condition of concern, is discussed in Chapter 8. Interest in osteoporosis prevention and treatment, coupled with data showing low calcium intakes in certain groups, especially women, has made calcium a current public health issue. This has sparked interest in assessing the body's calcium status.

At the current time, there are no appropriate biochemical indicators for assessing calcium status. This is due in large part to the biological mechanisms that tightly control serum calcium levels despite wide variations in dietary intake.[31,36] Potential approaches to assessing calcium status can be categorized in three areas: bone mineral content measurement, biochemical markers, and measures of calcium metabolism.[36] Of these three approaches, measurement of bone mineral content by such methods as quantitative computed tomography, single- and dual-photon absorptiometry, and dual-energy X-ray absorptiometry is currently the most feasible approach to assessing calcium status. These techniques are discussed in Chapter 8. However, fewer biochemical markers and measures of calcium metabolism are available. Attempts to identify a calcium status indicator in blood have been unsuccessful.[36]

Serum Calcium Fractions

Serum calcium exists in three fractions: protein-bound, ionized, and complexed.[37] These and other values for calcium in body fluids are shown in Table 9.9. The protein-bound calcium is considered physiologically inactive, whereas the ionized fraction is considered physiologically active and functions as an intracellular regulator.[36–38] Complexed calcium is complexed with small negative ions, such as citrate, phosphate, and lactate. Its biological role is uncertain. Because the ionized and complexed calcium are diffusible across semipermeable membranes, these two fractions can be collectively referred to as *ultrafilterable calcium.* Serum levels of calcium are so tightly controlled by the body that there is little, if any, association between dietary calcium intake and serum levels.[38] Altered serum calcium levels are rare and indicate serious metabolic problems rather than low or high dietary intakes. Low serum calcium, or hypocalcemia (serum calcium concentration < 2.3 mmol/L), can result from a variety of conditions, including hypoparathyroidism (deficient or absent levels of parathyroid hormone), renal disease, and acute pancreatitis. High serum calcium concentrations, or hypercalcemia (serum calcium > 2.75 mmol/L), can be due to increased intestinal absorption, bone resorption, or renal tubular reabsorption resulting from such conditions as hyperparathyroidism, hyperthyroidism, and hypervitaminosis D (excessive intake of vitamin D).[36]

TABLE 9.9	Normal Values for Calcium in Body Fluids	
	Mean	Normal Range
Plasma		
Total calcium (mmol/L)	2.5	2.3–2.75
Ionized (mmol/L)	1.18	1.1–1.28
Complexed (mmol/L)		0.15–0.30
Protein-bound (mmol/L)		0.93–1.08
Urine		
24-hour calcium (mmol/L)		
Women	4.55	1.25–10
Men	6.22	1.25–12.5
Fasting calcium: creatinine ratio (molar)		
Postmenopausal women	$0.341 \pm 0.183^*$	
Men	$0.169 \pm 0.099^*$	

From Weaver CM. 1990. Assessing calcium status and metabolism. *Journal of Nutrition* 120:1470–1473.

*Mean ± SD.

The association between total serum calcium and blood pressure has been investigated, although results have been somewhat conflicting. Several studies[39,40] have found ultrafilterable calcium to be negatively correlated with hypertension but have found no significant correlation between total serum calcium and the presence of hypertension. Other investigators,[41,42] however, have reported positive associations between total serum calcium and blood pressure. Clearly, more research is needed to sort out these apparent discrepancies.

Increased levels of complexed calcium and ionized calcium in postmenopausal women have been reported, suggesting that these have potential as markers of low bone mass.[38,43]

Urinary Calcium

Urinary calcium levels are more responsive to changes in dietary calcium intake than are serum levels.[36] However, urinary calcium is affected by a number of other factors, including those factors leading to hypercalcemia. When serum levels are high, more calcium is available to be excreted through the urine. There is a diurnal variation in urinary calcium, with concentrations higher during the day and lower in the evening.[37] Calcium output tends to be increased when the diet is rich in dietary protein and is low in phosphate and tends to be decreased by high-protein diets rich in phosphate.[37] Urinary calcium losses are increased when the volume of urine output is higher and when the kidneys' ability to reabsorb calcium is impaired.[36,37] Hypocalciuria can result from those factors leading to hypocalcemia as well as from renal failure.[36,37]

Use of the ratio of calcium to creatinine calculated from 2-hour fasting urine samples has been suggested as a possible indicator of calcium status but requires further research. The calcium level in an overnight urine sample shows potential as an indicator of compliance with calcium supplementation.[36]

ZINC STATUS

Zinc's most important physiologic function is as a component of numerous enzymes.[55] Consequently, zinc is involved in many metabolic processes, including protein synthesis, wound healing, immune function, and tissue growth and maintenance. Severe zinc deficiency characterized by hypogonadism and dwarfism has been observed in the Middle East. Evidence of milder forms of zinc deficiency (detected by biochemical and clinical measurements) has been found in several population groups in the United States. In humans and laboratory animals, a reduction or cessation of growth is an early response to zinc deficiency, and supplementation in growth-retarded infants and children who are mildly zinc deficient can result in a growth response.[45–47]

Because there is concern about the adequacy of zinc intake among certain groups, especially females, zinc is considered a potential public health issue for which further study is needed. Nutrient intake data and other specific findings suggest that several U.S. population groups may have marginal zinc intakes. According to NHANES III data, the average intake of zinc among females ages 20 to 49 years (approximately 9.6 mg/d) is roughly 80% of the RDA. Biochemical and clinical data derived from U.S. government nutritional monitoring activities, however, show no impairment of zinc status.

Serum Zinc Concentrations

There is currently no specific sensitive biochemical or functional indicator of zinc status.[45] Static measurements of serum zinc are available, but their use is complicated by the body's homeostatic control of zinc levels and by factors influencing serum zinc levels that are unrelated to nutritional status.[44,45]

There is little, if any, functional reserve of zinc in the body, as there is of some other nutrients (for example, iron, calcium, and vitamin A). The body's zinc levels are maintained by both conservation and redistribution of tissue zinc. In mild zinc deficiency, conservation is manifested by reduction or cessation of growth in growing organisms and by decreased excretion in nongrowing organisms. In most instances of mild deficiency, this

appears to be the extent of clinical and biochemical changes. If the deficiency is severe, however, additional clinical signs soon appear.[45]

Mature animals and humans have a remarkable capacity to conserve zinc when intakes are low. As a result, inducing zinc deficiency in full-grown animals can be difficult.[45] Several mechanisms are responsible for this. Fecal zinc excretion, for example, can be cut by as much as 60% when dietary intake is low. Not only is the efficiency of intestinal absorption of zinc increased, but losses via the gastrointestinal tract, urine, and sweat are diminished.[45,48,49]

In laboratory animals, deficiency can lead to selective redistribution of zinc from certain tissues to support other, higher-priority tissues. In mild zinc deficiency, plasma zinc levels apparently can be maintained at the expense of zinc from other tissues.[48,50] Some evidence suggests that redistribution of total body zinc also occurs in humans.

The result of the body's conservation of and ability to redistribute zinc is that measurements of serum zinc are not a reliable indicator of dietary zinc intake or changes in whole-body zinc status.[31,45] This is especially the case in mild zinc deficiency. For example, serum zinc concentrations in growth-retarded children whose growth responded to zinc supplementation were not significantly different from concentrations in normally developed children either before or after supplementation.[61] Despite these limitations, measurement of serum zinc concentration may be a useful, albeit late, indicator of the size of the body's exchangeable zinc pool. Less than expected values may signal a loss of zinc from bone and liver and increased risk for clinical and metabolic signs of zinc deficiency.[45]

Several factors unrelated to nutritional status can influence serum zinc levels. Decreased levels can result from stress, infection or inflammation, and use of estrogens, oral contraceptives, and corticosteroids.[44,45] Serum zinc can fall by 15% to 20% following a meal.[45] Increased serum zinc concentrations can result from fasting and red blood cell hemolysis.

Metallothionen and Zinc Status

Metallothionen is a protein found in most tissues but primarily in the liver, pancreas, kidney, and intestinal mucosa. Metallothionen holds promise as a potential indicator of zinc status, particularly when used in conjunction with serum zinc levels.[45] Measurable amounts are found in serum and in red blood cells. Metallothionen has the capacity of binding zinc and copper, and tissue metallothionen concentrations often are proportional to zinc status. In animals, levels are almost undetectable in zinc deficiency and are responsive to zinc supplementation. Whereas serum zinc levels fall in response to acute stimuli (for example, stress, infection, and inflammation), hepatic and serum metallothionen levels are increased in response to these stimuli. Thus, when serum levels of zinc fall and of metallothionen rise, it is likely that tissue zinc has been redistributed in response to acute stimuli and that a zinc deficiency is not present because metallothionen is not responsive to acute stimuli in zinc-deficient animals. If serum zinc and metallothionen are both below expected levels, it is likely that zinc deficiency is present. Erythrocyte metallothionen (which is not affected by stress) also can be used as an indicator of zinc status.[45]

Hair Zinc

Several researchers have investigated the use of zinc in hair as an indicator of body zinc status.[67,68] Decreased concentration of zinc in hair has been reported in zinc-deficient dwarfs, in marginally deficient children and adolescents, and in conditions related to zinc deficiency, such as celiac disease, acrodermatitis enteropathica, and sickle-cell disease.[53] Because hair grows slowly (about 1 cm per month), levels of zinc and other trace elements in hair reflect nutritional status over many months and thus are not affected by diurnal variations or short-term fluctuations in nutritional status. Because of this, hair zinc levels may not be correlated with measurements of zinc in serum or erythrocytes, which reflect shorter-term zinc status.[53] Obtaining a sample is noninvasive, and analyzing hair for zinc and other trace elements is relatively easy.

It is important to note that trace elements in hair can come from endogenous sources (those that are ingested or inhaled by the subject and then enter the hair through the hair follicle) and exogenous sources (contamination from trace elements in dust, water, cosmetics, and so on).[51–53] A major drawback in using hair as an indicator of trace element status is its susceptibility to contamination from these exogenous sources. Some exogenous contaminants can be removed by carefully washing the hair sample before analysis, and several standardized washing procedures have been suggested.[53] However, some contaminants may be difficult or impossible to remove. Selenium, an ingredient in some antidandruff shampoos, is known to increase the selenium content of hair and cannot be removed by the recommended washing procedures.[54]

A variety of other nonnutritional factors may affect the trace element content of hair. Included among these are certain diseases, rate of hair growth, hair color, sex, pregnancy, and age.[49,51,53] It has been reported, for example, that higher concentrations of zinc, iron, nickel, and copper can be found in red hair, compared with brown hair, and that iron and manganese are found in higher concentrations in brown hair than in blonde hair.[55] These factors limit the usefulness of hair as an index of zinc and other trace element status.

Urinary Zinc

Lower than expected concentrations of zinc have been reported in the urine of zinc-depleted persons.[53] However, factors other than nutritional status can influence urinary zinc levels, such as liver cirrhosis, viral hepatitis, sickle-cell anemia, surgery, and total parenteral nutrition. Problems associated with obtaining 24-hour urine collections can also complicate use of this indicator. Consequently, urine measurements of zinc are not the preferred approach to assessing zinc status.

Functional Indicators

Several functional indicators have been proposed for assessing zinc status. These are listed in Table 9.10. Although some of these indicators are sensitive to nutritional status in general and zinc status in particular, a positive response when applied could be indicative of a lack of one of several nutrients, protein, and/or energy. Some of the tests are cumbersome to use and are limited by inter- and intraobserver error and a lack of standardized protocols for their administration and interpretation.

VITAMIN A STATUS

Vitamin A status can be grouped into five categories: deficient, marginal, adequate, excessive, and toxic. In the deficient and toxic states, clinical signs are evident, while biochemical or static tests of vitamin A status must be relied on in the marginal, adequate, and excessive states.[56] Biochemical assessment of vitamin A status generally involves static measurements of vitamin levels in serum, breast milk, and liver tissue and functional tests, such as dose-response tests, examination of epithelial cells of the conjunctiva, and assessment of dark adaptation.[56–58]

TABLE 9.10	**Functional Tests That May Be Indicative of Zinc Status**
Experimental wound healing	Growth response to zinc supplementation
Nitrogen retention	Collagen accumulation in implant sponge
Lymphocyte (T-cell) blastogenesis	Delayed cutaneous hypersensitivity
Zinc uptake by erythrocyte	Platelet aggregation
Sperm count	Dark adaptometry
Olfactory acuity	Taste acuity

From King JC, Keen CL. 1994. Zinc. In Shils ME, Olson JA, Shike M, eds. *Modern nutrition in health and disease,* 8th ed. Philadelphia: Lea & Febiger; King JC. 1990. Assessment of zinc status. *Journal of Nutrition* 120:1474–1479.

Serum Levels

Measurement of serum vitamin A is the most common biochemical measure of vitamin A status.[57] Under normal conditions, about 95% of serum vitamin A is in the form of retinol and bound to retinol-binding protein, and about 5% is unbound and in the form of retinyl esters.[58] Serum measurements are predictive of vitamin A status only when the body's reserves are either critically depleted or overfilled. Because serum vitamin A may be within the expected range despite low vitamin A concentrations within the liver, some investigators do not recommend serum measurements as a screening test for vitamin A status.[59] However, data from serum measurements can be of some value in drawing conclusions about the relationship of serum measurements to clinical signs of deficiency, dietary intake data, and various socioeconomic factors. Serum concentrations < 10 μg/dL $(0.35$ μmol/L) have generally been considered deficient, and values < 20 μg/dL $(0.70$ μmol/L) have been considered low.[56,57] Serum values > 30 μg/dL $(> 1.05$ μmol/L) are indicative of adequate status, while serum levels > 100 μg/dL are diagnostic of hypervitaminosis A, particularly when 50% or more of the vitamin is found in the form of retinyl ester.[56] Guidelines based on data from NHANES suggest that some persons within the population surveyed, particularly postadolescents, are likely vitamin A deficient even when their serum concentrations are in the range of 20 to 29 μg/dL $(0.70$ to 1.05 μmol/L), as shown in Table 9.11.[60]

Vitamin A levels in breast milk can also be used as an index of vitamin A status. Levels < 10 μg/dL $(0.35$ μmol/L) suggest the nursing child is at risk for vitamin A deficiency. Adequate vitamin A for growth and development will be provided when levels in breast milk are > 20 μg/dL $(0.70$ μmol/L). The nursing child's body reserves will increase when breast milk levels are > 40 μg/dL $(1.40$ μmol/L).[56]

Relative Dose Response

The relative dose-response test (RDR) and modified relative dose-response test (MRDR) are based on the principle that, "when stores of retinol are high, plasma retinol concentration is little affected by oral administration of vitamin A. But when reserves are low, the plasma retinol concentration increases markedly, reaching a peak 5 h after an oral dose."[59] As hepatic vitamin A stores become depleted, retinol-binding protein (RBP) accumulates in the liver in an unbound state known as *apo-RBP*. When vitamin A is given to a subject whose stores are depleted, the vitamin A is absorbed from the intestinal tract; is taken up by the liver, where it binds to the apo-RBP; and then is released from the liver in the form of *holo-RBP* (the complex of RBP and vitamin A). In the RDR, a fasting blood sample is taken, followed by oral administration of vitamin A as retinyl palmitate. Another blood sample is drawn 5 hours later. Comparison of the fasting and postdosing holo-RBP measurements represents the extent of apo-RBP accumulation, which is directly related to the shortage of vitamin A.[3,61]

The RDR is calculated using the following formula:[57]

$$RDR = \frac{\text{Vit A}_5 - \text{vit A}_0}{\text{Vit A}_5} \times 100$$

where vit A_5 = serum vitamin A level 5 hours after receiving the dose of vitamin A and vit A_0 = fasting serum vitamin A level.

TABLE 9.11	Guidelines for Interpretation of Serum Total Vitamin A Levels in Selected Low Ranges in Populations		
Serum Vitamin A Levels (μg/dL)	3–11 Years	12–17 Years	18–74 Years
< 10	Vitamin A status[*] is very likely to improve with increased consumption of vitamin A; impairment of function[†] is likely.		
< 20	Vitamin A status is likely to improve with increased consumption of vitamin A.	Vitamin A status is likely to improve with increased consumption of vitamin A; some individuals may exhibit impairment of function.	Vitamin A status is very likely to improve with increased consumption of vitamin A; impairment of function is likely.
20–29	Vitamin A status of some individuals may improve with increased consumption of vitamin A; improvement is most likely in those with values 20–24 μg/dL.	Vitamin A status may improve with increased consumption of vitamin A; improvement is more likely in those with values 20–24 μg/dL.	Vitamin A status may improve with increased consumption of vitamin A; some individuals may exhibit impairment of function.

From Pilch SM. 1987. Analysis of vitamin A data from the Health and Nutrition Examination Surveys. *Journal of Nutrition* 117:636–640.

[*]*Vitamin A status* refers to serum vitamin A levels and tissue levels of the nutrient.

[†]Impairment of function may include impaired dark adaptation, night blindness, ocular lesions, and possibly impaired immune function.

An RDR > 50% is considered indicative of acute deficiency, values between 20% and 50% indicate marginal status, and values < 20% suggest adequate intake.[56]

Limitations of the RDR include the 5-hour waiting period and the need to draw two blood samples.[3]

The MRDR is based on the same principle but uses only one blood sample 5 hours after administration of the test dose of dehydroretinol, a naturally occurring form of vitamin A but one rarely present in most diets.[3] The measured response is the molar ratio of dehydroretinol to retinol in the serum sample. A ratio > 0.06 indicates marginal or poorer vitamin A status. A ratio < 0.03 indicates adequate vitamin A status.[56]

The assay is limited by the fact that there currently is no commercial source of dehydroretinol, and the assay requires the use of high-pressure liquid chromatography to distinguish between the two forms of vitamin A. The assay is still under development but does have the advantage of requiring only one blood sample.[3]

Conjunctival Impression Cytology

Vitamin A deficiency can result in morphologic changes in epithelial cells covering the body and lining its cavities. It can result in a decline in the number of mucus-producing goblet cells in the epithelium of the conjunctiva of the eye. The epithelial cells also may take on a more squamous appearance—flatter cells, smaller nuclei, and with the cytoplasm making up a greater proportion of the total cell.[57] The conjunctival impression cytology test involves the microscopic examination of the conjunctival epithelial cells to determine morphologic changes indicative of vitamin A deficiency.[57,62]

A minute sample of epithelial cells can be obtained by touching a strip of cellulose ester filter paper to the outer portion of the conjunctiva for 3 to 5 seconds and then gently removing it. The filter paper with the adherent epithelial cells is placed in a fixative solution, where it can be stored until being stained and examined by ordinary light microscopy.[57,63]

The test is limited by several factors. It is difficult to get tissue samples from children under 3 years of age, and the cytologists must follow standardized criteria in evaluating samples. The sensitivity of the test is limited by conjunctival and systemic infections and possibly by severe malnutrition.[57] Theoretically, test results allow the vitamin A status of persons to be categorized in one of four groups: normal, marginal (+), marginal (−), and deficient. Because of difficulty in interpreting the two intermediate categories, conjunctival impression cytology is primarily used to detect populations at risk for deficiency. A population would be considered at risk for vitamin A deficiency if more than 50% of persons in a sample selected from the population had results that were not in the normal category.[56]

Dark Adaptation

The best-defined function of vitamin A is its role in the visual process. The visual pigment rhodopsin is generated when the protein opsin in the rods of the retina combines with a *cis*-isomer of retinol. When light strikes the eye, rhodopsin is split into opsin and a *trans*-isomer of retinol, generating the visual-response signal. The *trans*-isomer is then converted back to the *cis*-isomer, which then combines with opsin to reform rhodopsin. During this process, some of the retinol isomer is lost and must be replaced by vitamin A present in the retina. Under normal conditions, sufficient retinol is present, and rhodopsin is readily formed. When vitamin A is in short supply, less rhodopsin is formed, and the eye fails to adapt as readily to low light levels after exposure to bright light levels.[56,57]

Tests are available to directly measure the level of rhodopsin and its rate of regeneration. Field tests measuring visual acuity in dim light after exposure to bright light also can be used.[57] However, the relative dose response, when available, is a more specific and objective test of vitamin A status and is preferred over functional tests of dark adaptation.

Direct Measurement of Liver Stores

Direct measurement of hepatic vitamin A stores in liver tissue can be used as an indicator of vitamin A status.[56] In many countries, the median vitamin A concentration in liver tissue of well-nourished persons is approximately 100 μg of retinol/g of liver tissue. A concentration > 20 μg of retinol/g of liver tissue is considered adequate for both children and adults of all ages.[56] Concentrations < 5 μg of retinol/g of liver tissue are associated with vitamin A deficiency.

The assay can be done on a very small amount of liver tissue obtained by inserting a biopsy needle through the abdominal wall. Because of the invasiveness of the biopsy procedure, assaying liver tissue for vitamin A is limited to situations when a liver biopsy is necessary for diagnostic purposes or when liver tissue can be obtained from postmortem examinations.[57]

VITAMIN C STATUS

Vitamin C is a generic term for compounds exhibiting the biological activity of *ascorbic acid,* the reduced form of vitamin C. The oxidized form of vitamin C is known as *dehydroascorbic acid.* The sum of ascorbic acid and dehydroascorbic acid constitutes all the naturally occurring biologically active vitamin C.[64] When used in this chapter, the term *vitamin C* refers to total vitamin C—the sum of ascorbic acid and dehydroascorbic acid.

Vitamin C is necessary for the formation of collagen; the maintenance of capillaries, bone, and teeth; the promotion of iron absorption; and the protection of vitamins and minerals from oxidation. Some evidence suggests a protective effect against certain cancers. Deficiency of vitamin C results in scurvy, a condition characterized by weakness, hemorrhages in the skin and gums, and defects in bone development in children.

Data from NHANES III show that mean vitamin C intakes in the United States are well above the RDI.[65] However, intakes among women and children of lower socioeconomic status may be inadequate, causing vitamin C to be a potential public health issue for which more study is needed.[31]

Assessing vitamin C status is limited primarily to measuring levels in serum (or plasma) and in leukocytes (white blood cells).[64,66] Several functional tests of vitamin C status have been suggested, but these do not appear to be reliable or suitable for field use.[64,67,68]

Serum and Leukocyte Vitamin C

Measurement of serum (or plasma) vitamin C is the most commonly used biochemical procedure for assessing vitamin C status.[66,68] However, in recent years, there has been increasing interest in using the level of vitamin C in polymorphonuclear leukocytes (the granular leukocytes: neutrophils, eosinophils, and basophils) and the mononuclear leukocytes (the agranular leukocytes: lymphocytes and monocytes) as indicators of vitamin C status.[69–71] Serum levels of ascorbic acid have been shown to correlate with dietary vitamin C intake and with vitamin C levels in leukocytes (white blood cells).[72,73] However, research suggests that vitamin C concentration in serum is a better indicator of recent dietary intake of vitamin C than leukocyte levels and that leukocyte vitamin C levels better represent cellular stores and the total body pool of the vitamin.[72–74]

An obvious deficient state with biochemical and/or clinical symptoms exists when serum ascorbic acid values are < 11 μmol/L. Marginal vitamin C status with moderate risk of developing clinical signs of deficiency exists when serum ascorbic acid values are between 11 and 23 μmol/L. The lower limit of normal serum ascorbic acid is considered 28 μmol/L.[64]

Factors affecting vitamin C levels in tissues and fluids include cigarette smoking and sex.[64] Compared with nonsmokers, cigarette smokers tend to have lower vitamin C levels in serum and leukocytes even after correcting for vitamin C intake.[64,71,75] The metabolic turnover of vitamin C in smokers has been estimated to be 40% higher than that of nonsmokers. This finding led the Subcommittee on the 10th Edition of the RDAs to recommend that cigarette smokers ingest at least 100 mg of vitamin C daily, as opposed to the RDA for adults of 60 mg of vitamin C daily.[19] However, evidence suggests that smokers may need to ingest > 200 mg of vitamin C

daily to achieve serum ascorbic acid levels typically seen in nonsmokers meeting the RDI.[76]

After correcting for vitamin C intakes, females consistently show higher vitamin C levels in tissues and fluids than males.[64,71,75] Age does not appear to influence vitamin C levels in adults.[64,69]

Other Approaches

The requirement of vitamin C for a number of biochemical reactions within the body has resulted in a search for functional tests of the vitamin's status. The capillary fragility test was proposed as a functional test of vitamin C status during the early 1930s, but its results lack specificity for vitamin C because a number of factors other than vitamin C status affect capillary fragility.[67] The ascorbic acid saturation test can be a reliable index of vitamin C depletion.[64,66] The required 24-hour urine sample limits its usefulness to highly cooperative subjects in a clinical or research setting. At this time, no reliable functional indicator of vitamin C status exists, but, as our understanding of the role of vitamin C in human physiology unfolds, one or more may be developed.[64] Functional measures currently under investigation include markers of collagen metabolism, the urinary carnitine-to-creatinine ratio, and in vitro measurement of ascorbate-free radicals.[64]

Measurement of urinary vitamin C does not discriminate well between adequate and deficient vitamin C intakes.[73] This approach also is limited by difficulty in collecting urine samples and by the increase in urinary excretion of vitamin C in response to several drugs (aminopyrine, aspirin, barbiturates, and paraldehyde).[66] The ease with which saliva samples can be obtained has made measurement of salivary vitamin C a desirable assessment approach. Unfortunately, salivary vitamin C levels do not consistently reflect vitamin C intake; therefore, this does not appear to be a useful indicator of vitamin C status.[73]

In general, serum and leukocyte measurements are preferred over those in erythrocytes, urine, and saliva.[64,66,73] Serum levels appear more indicative of dietary intake, but leukocyte levels of vitamin C are a better index of cellular stores and the body's total vitamin C pool.[64,72,73]

VITAMIN B$_6$ STATUS

The vitamin B$_6$ group is composed of three naturally occurring compounds related chemically, metabolically, and functionally: pyridoxine (PN), pyridoxal (PL), and pyridoxamine (PM). Within the liver, erythrocytes, and other tissues of the body, these forms are phosphorylated into pyridoxal 5'-phosphate (PLP) and pyridoxamine phosphate (PMP). PLP and PMP primarily serve as coenzymes in a large variety of reactions.[19,77] Especially important among these are the transamination reactions in protein metabolism. PLP also is involved in other metabolic transformations of amino acids and in the metabolism of carbohydrates, lipids, and nucleic acids.[19,78,79] Because of its role in protein metabolism, the requirement for vitamin B_6 is directly proportional to protein intake.[19]

Data from NHANES III show that mean vitamin B_6 intakes for infants and children of both sexes and for adolescent and adult males (except those 80 years or older) are greater than the RDA. Mean intakes for adolescent and middle-aged females fall below the RDA.[65] The 1985–86 CSFII showed that vitamin B_6 intakes for about 75% of all American women were below the 1989 RDA. However, after adjusting for lower than expected protein intakes, many more women met the protein-based vitamin B_6 allowance than the RDA.[31] Another factor complicating the interpretation of vitamin B_6 intakes is the incomplete nutrient composition data; analytical values for vitamin B_6 were available for only 70% of the foods in CSFII 1985–86.[31]

Although frank vitamin B_6 deficiency resulting in clinical manifestations is not considered widespread in the general U.S. population, there is evidence of impaired status among certain groups—most notably, the elderly and alcoholic individuals. There is also concern about excessive vitamin B_6 intake and the possibility of resulting peripheral nervous system damage.[80] Because of these concerns, vitamin B_6 is being considered a potential public health issue for which further study is needed.[31]

Vitamin B_6 status can be assessed by several methods. Static measurements can be made of vitamin B_6 concentrations in blood or urine, and functional tests can measure the activity of several enzymes dependent on vitamin B_6.[1,19]

Plasma and Erythrocyte Pyridoxal 5′-Phosphate

The most frequently used biochemical indicator of vitamin B_6 status is plasma PLP.[1,78,79] PLP accounts for approximately 70% to 90% of the total vitamin B_6 present in plasma.[1] PL is the next most abundant form in plasma, followed by lower levels of PN and PM.[79]

Fasting measurements of plasma PLP are considered the single most informative indicator of vitamin B_6 status for healthy persons.[79] In rats, plasma PLP has been shown to be significantly correlated with muscle PLP.[1] In humans, muscle PLP accounts for more than 80% of the body's vitamin B_6 stores.[81] In response to changes in dietary intake of vitamin B_6, plasma PLP levels have been shown to plateau within 7 to 10 days when intake is in the range of 0.5 to 1.0 mg/day.[79]

Use of this single measure is limited by the fact that abnormally low concentrations of plasma PLP may result from asthma, coronary heart disease, and pregnancy and may not reflect a true vitamin B_6 deficiency.[79] Dietary intake of vitamin B_6 and protein can affect plasma PLP concentrations as well. As shown in Table 9.12, increases in dietary vitamin B_6 intake raise plasma PLP, and plasma levels fall in response to increased protein consumption.[1] Thus, although plasma PLP is a valuable measure, the assessment of vitamin B_6 status is best accomplished by using several indicators in conjunction with each other—for example, measures of other vitamin B_6 forms and/or functional tests.[1,82] Table 9.13 lists expected biochemical values for adults with adequate vitamin B_6 status for various measures of the vitamin.

Measurement of PLP in erythrocytes has been suggested as another approach to assessing vitamin B_6 status.[1,82] Certain characteristics of the erythrocyte may make it unrepresentative of other body tissues. The ability of hemoglobin to bind tightly to PLP and PL, along with the relatively long life of red blood cells (about 120 days), may make red blood cells a significant reservoir for vitamin B_6 and may complicate the use of erythrocyte PLP levels as a useful indicator of vitamin B_6 status.[1,79,82]

Plasma Pyridoxal

Measurement of plasma PL has been suggested as an additional indicator of B_6 status to use with plasma PLP.[1,82] PL is the major dietary form of the vitamin, crosses all membranes on absorption from the gastrointestinal tract, and comprises about 8% to 30% of the total plasma vitamin B_6. There are questions about how well plasma PL represents vitamin B_6 status, and further research is needed on this indicator. Despite these questions, plasma PL is recommended in the assessment of B_6 status.[1]

TABLE 9.12	Factors Affecting Plasma PLP* Concentrations
Factors	**Effect**
Increased vitamin B_6 intake	Increases
Increased protein intake	Decreases
Increased glucose	Decreases (a)†
Increased plasma volume	Decreases
Increased physical activity	Increases (a)
Decreased uptake into nonhepatic tissues	Increases
Increased age	Decreases

From Leklem JE. 1990. Vitamin B_6: A status report. *Journal of Nutrition* 120:1503–1507.

*PLP = pyridoxal 5′-phosphate.

†(a) indicates that the effect is an acute effect.

TABLE 9.13	Indices for Evaluating Vitamin B$_6$ Status and Suggested Values for Adequate Status in Adults

Indices	Suggested Values for Adequate Status*
Direct	
Blood	
Plasma pyridoxal 5′-phosphate (PLP)	> 30 nmol/L
Plasma pyridoxal	NV†
Plasma total vitamin B$_6$	> 40 nmol/L
Erythrocyte PLP	NV
Urine	
4-pyridoxic acid	> 3.0 μmol/day
Total vitamin B$_6$	> 0.5 μmol/day
Indirect	
Blood	
Erythrocyte alanine transaminase index	< 1.25‡
Erythrocyte aspartic transaminase index	< 1.80
Urine	
2-g tryptophan load; xanthurenic acid	< 65 μmol/day
3-g methionine load; cystathionine	< 350 μmol/day
Oxalate excretion	NV
Diet Intake	
Vitamin B$_6$ intake, weekly average	> 1.2–1.5 mg/day
Vitamin B$_6$: protein ratio	> 0.020
Other	
Electroencephalogram pattern	NV

From Leklem JE. 1990. Vitamin B$_6$: A status report. *Journal of Nutrition* 120:1503–1507.

*These values are dependent on sex, age, and, for most, protein intake.

†NV = no value established; limited data are available.

‡The index value for each transaminase represents the ratio of the enzyme activity with added PLP to the activity without PLP added.

Total Vitamin B$_6$

Total vitamin B$_6$ in plasma and urine can be measured by microbiological assay using *Saccharomyces uvarum* as the test organism.[1,82] Plasma levels of PL can be estimated from plasma measures of total vitamin B$_6$ and PLP because PL and PLP constitute about 90% of total vitamin B$_6$ in plasma.[1] Because plasma concentrations of total vitamin B$_6$ have not been frequently measured, the values given in Table 9.13 were derived by multiplying plasma PLP values by 1.25.[1]

Total vitamin B$_6$ in urine also can be measured by the same microbiological assay used for plasma.[1] However, urinary levels of vitamin B$_6$ are not considered a useful indicator for assessing B$_6$ status.[1] Urinary vitamin B$_6$ has been shown to correlate closely with intake levels in adults, making it a potentially useful indicator of recent dietary intake. Excretions below 0.5 μmol/day are considered indicative of deficiency.[1] Use of urinary levels, however, is complicated by limitations associated with urine collections. Leklem[78] recommends that vitamin B$_6$ assays be performed on several 24-hour urine samples collected over 1 to 3 weeks. Use of urinary vitamin B$_6$ measures is not valid in persons receiving vitamin B$_6$ antagonists, such as the drugs isoniazid, penicillamine, and cycloserine. The ingestion of oral contraceptives does not appear to affect urinary excretion of vitamin B$_6$.

Urinary 4-pyridoxic Acid

4-pyridoxic acid (4-PA) is the major urinary metabolite of vitamin B$_6$. Urinary excretion of 4-PA has been shown to change rapidly in response to alterations in vitamin B$_6$ intake[1] and to be indicative of immediate dietary intake. Thus, it is considered useful as a short-term index of vitamin B$_6$ status. In studies of subjects whose usual dietary intake of vitamin B$_6$ was known, males had a 4-PA excretion of 3.5 μmol/day, and females had a 4-PA excretion of > 3.2 μmol/day. Urinary excretions of 4-PA of ≥ 3.0 μmol/day appear to be indicative of acceptable vitamin B$_6$ status.[1] 4-PA is likely to be absent from urine of persons with a marked vitamin B$_6$ deficiency.

Tryptophan Load Test

Historically, the most widely used indicator of vitamin B$_6$ status has been the tryptophan load test.[1] This test is based on the requirement for PLP in the metabolism of the amino acid tryptophan (for example, conversion of the tryptophan to nicotinic acid). In the absence of PLP, tryptophan metabolism is altered, resulting in the production and eventual urinary excretion of several metabolites. Of these, xanthurenic acid is the easiest and most commonly measured. Usually, a test load of 2 g of L-tryptophan is administered to a subject, whose urine is then collected over a 24-hour period. Urinary levels of xanthurenic acid in subjects with adequate vitamin B$_6$ status usually range from 30 to 40 μmol/day in response to the 2 g of tryptophan. Urinary xanthurenic acid < 65 μmol/day is considered indicative of adequate vitamin B$_6$ status.[1]

Factors other than vitamin B$_6$ status can affect urinary excretion of xanthurenic acid. These include protein intake, exercise, lean body mass, individual variations, amount of tryptophan used in the test dose, use of estrogen and oral contraceptives, and pregnancy. For this reason, use of the tryptophan load test has been questioned as an appropriate index of vitamin B$_6$ status. With the more recent development of direct measures for assessing B$_6$ status, the tryptophan load test is used less often. However, when conditions that can adversely affect test outcome are absent, the procedure is regarded as a valid, although somewhat outdated, indicator of hepatic vitamin B$_6$ status.[1]

Methionine Load Test

The principle of the methionine load test is similar to that of the tryptophan load test. PLP is required in the metabolism of the amino acid methionine. Compared with persons with adequate vitamin B_6 status, those with impaired vitamin B_6 status have higher urine levels of the metabolites cystathionine and cysteine sulfonic acid following consumption of 3 g of methionine.[1]

Use of this test is limited by the required 24-hour urine sample and factors other than vitamin B_6 status that can affect test results (for example, protein intake). Because this test has been used in a limited number of studies, no definitive values for urinary cystathionine are available. The value of < 350 μmol/day given in Table 9.13 is based on three studies.[1]

Erythrocyte Transaminases

Another commonly used functional indicator of vitamin B_6 status is measurement of the activity of two enzymes known to be sensitive to B_6 status: erythrocyte alanine transaminase (EALT or EGPT) and erythrocyte aspartic acid transaminase (EAST or EGOT).[1] In persons whose vitamin B_6 reserves have been depleted, activity of these two enzymes is decreased and activity is increased after the in vitro addition of excess PLP. Consequently, measurements of the activity of EALT and EAST appear to be of value in assessing vitamin B_6 status.

The test uses two measurements: the activity of the enzymes at the unstimulated, or basal, level (as removed from the subject), and the stimulated level of enzyme activity (after the in vitro addition of excess PLP). From these data, two additional values are calculated. One is the stimulation index, which is the ratio of stimulated activity to unstimulated activity. The other is the percent stimulation, which is calculated from the following formula:[78]

$$\text{Percent stimulation} = \frac{(SA - UA) \times 100}{UA}$$

where SA = stimulated activity and UA = unstimulated activity.

Of the two measures, EALT appears to be the more responsive to changes in vitamin B_6 status and is considered a better indicator.[78]

The approach is limited by the considerable interindividual variation seen in the erythrocyte transaminase activities of persons with apparently adequate vitamin B_6 status, with or without stimulation by added PLP. This has been shown to vary by as much as 25% and 50% for EALT and EAST, respectively. Test results also may be adversely affected by a concomitant riboflavin deficiency. There are also limited data on the degree of stimulation and percent stimulation in response to varying levels of vitamin B_6 depletion and repletion over time. Because a uniform method of reporting data has not been followed, it is difficult to interpret data and compare results of studies using this method. A standardized approach to reporting results from this assay is needed.[1]

FOLATE STATUS

Folate, or folacin, is a group of compounds with properties and chemical structures similar to folic acid, or pteroylglutamic acid.[31,83] Folate functions as a coenzyme transporting single carbon groups from one compound to another in amino acid metabolism and nucleic acid synthesis. One of the most significant of folate's functions appears to be purine and pyrimidine synthesis. Folate deficiency can lead to inhibition of DNA synthesis, impaired cell division, and alterations in protein synthesis. These effects are especially seen in rapidly dividing cells (such as erythrocytes and leukocytes).[19,84]

Data from NHANES III show that the mean intake of folate is above the RDA for all groups, except for pregnant and lactating females.[65] Data from the 1985–86 CSFII showed that mean folate consumption was below the 1989 RDA for about 50% of women whose income was less than 130% of the Federal Poverty Income guidelines. About 25% of all women had folate intakes less than the RDI. Serum and RBC folate levels measured in subgroups of NHANES II indicated that women 20 to 44 years old were at greatest risk for folate deficiency. Other groups known to be at risk include premature infants and women during the last half of pregnancy. Because oral contraceptives may depress folate absorption, women taking them are also considered at risk for folate deficiency. However, NHANES II showed no significant difference between blood folate levels of oral contraceptive users and those of nonusers. Folate is considered to be a potential public health issue requiring further study.[31] A primary concern is extensive evidence showing that females with a marginal folate status have an increased risk of giving birth to infants with neural tube defects.[85–87] Neural tube defects include spina bifida, encephalocele, and anencephaly.

As shown in Figure 9.4, folate status can be characterized as being in positive balance, normal, or in negative balance.[83] Positive folate balance can be divided into two stages: stage I, early positive folate balance, and stage II, excess. Figure 9.4 lists several indices of folate status and gives values for these indices during these two stages of positive folate balance, as well as during other times.

Negative folate balance can be divided into four stages, as outlined in Figure 9.4.[83,84,88] Stage I of negative folate balance is called early negative folate balance. The earliest abnormality seen in this stage is a reduction in serum folate to levels < 3 ng/mL, with all other indices in Figure 9.4 being within normal limits. The earliest

Figure 9.4 **Sequential changes in the development of folate deficiency.**
The shaded areas indicate the relative quantities of folate in each compartment (e.g., in the liver, plasma, and erythrocytes). The sequence of increasingly unshaded areas shows its proportional disappearance during successive stages of folate deficiency. The earliest abnormalities in each stage are boxed. RBC = red blood cell; dU = dioxyuridine; MCV = mean corpuscular volume.

Source: From Herbert V, Das KC. 1994. Folic acid and vitamin B_{12}. In Shils ME, Olson JA, Shike M, eds. *Modern nutrition in health and disease,* 8th ed. Philadelphia: Lea & Febiger.

abnormalities seen in stage II of negative folate balance, folate depletion, are a less than expected red blood cell folate level and abnormally low serum folate levels. As folate status deteriorates, stage III, or folate deficiency erythropoiesis follows, as indicated by abnormal values for the deoxyuridine (dU) suppression test, evidence of hypersegmentation of the nuclei of the polymorphonuclear leukocytes (average number of lobes > 3.5), and liver folate < 1.2 μg/g. Stage IV, folate deficiency anemia, is characterized by morphologic changes in erythrocytes (red blood cells become macroovalocytic—MCV increases and the cells become oval in shape) and decreased hemoglobin concentration (anemia).[83,84]

The morphologic changes seen in erythrocytes, leukocytes, and bone marrow cells that accompany folate deficiency are identical to those caused by vitamin B_{12} deficiency. A comparison of values for erythrocyte folate and serum vitamin B_{12} is necessary to differentiate between the two deficiencies because folate deficiency can occur as a result of vitamin B_{12} deficiency.[83]

Serum Folate

After about 3 weeks of negative folate balance, serum folate falls below 7 nmol/L (3 ng/mL). This concentration is considered indicative of negative folate balance, but it fails to give useful information on body stores of folate when used alone.[84,89] Serum folate cannot discriminate between a transient fluctuation in serum concentration in response to recent dietary folate intake and chronic deficiency accompanied by depleted body stores and functional changes.[84] Nonnutritional factors that can increase serum folate concentrations include acute renal failure, active liver disease, and hemolysis of red blood cells. Alcohol consumption, cigarette smoking, and oral contraceptive use may lower serum folate levels.[8]

Approaches for measuring serum folate include radioisotope dilution assay and microbiological assay using *Lactobacillus casei*.[89,90]

Erythrocyte Folate

A reduction in erythrocyte folate stores is considered the best clinical index of depleted tissue stores. Erythrocyte folate levels reflect folate status at the time the erythrocyte was synthesized because only young cells in the bone marrow take up folate.[84,89] Values less than 360 nmol/L (160 ng/mL) are considered indicative of tissue folate depletion.[88] Unlike serum folate, erythrocyte folate is less subject to transient fluctuations in dietary intake. It decreases after tissue stores are depleted because erythrocytes have a 120-day average life span and reflect folate status at the time of their synthesis. It has been shown to correlate with liver folate stores and to reflect total body stores.[8]

As with serum folate, erythrocyte folate concentrations can be determined either by the microbiological assay or by radioisotope dilution.[90]

Deoxyuridine Suppression Test

The deoxyuridine (dU) suppression test is a functional indicator of folate status.[84] It is an in vitro biochemical test that not only defines the presence of megaloblastosis but helps identify which nutrient deficiency is responsible (folate or vitamin B_{12}). The dU suppression test is conducted in bone marrow or other DNA-synthesizing cells by measuring the incorporation of radioactive thymidine into DNA in the absence versus the presence of large amounts of deoxyuridine, which should suppress the incorporation of this tracer material to 10% to 20% of the control value.[89] Although the dU suppression test correlates fairly well with plasma and erythrocyte folate concentrations, erythrocyte folate is a superior indicator of folate status.[91]

VITAMIN B_{12} STATUS

Vitamin B_{12}, or cobalamin, include a group of cobalt-containing molecules that can be converted to methylcobalamin or 5′-deoxyadenosylcobalamin, the two coenzyme forms of vitamin B_{12} that are active in human metabolism.[19] Vitamin B_{12} is synthesized by bacteria, fungi, and algae, but not by yeast, plants, and animals. Vitamin B_{12} synthesized by bacteria accumulates in the tissues of animals that are then consumed by humans. Thus, animal products serve as the primary dietary source of vitamin B_{12}. Although plants are essentially devoid of vitamin B_{12} (unless they are contaminated by microorganisms or soil containing vitamin B_{12}), foods such as breakfast cereals, soy beverages, and plant-based meat substitutes are sometimes fortified with vitamin B_{12}.[19,83]

The diets of most Americans supply more than adequate amounts of vitamin B_{12}. Data from NHANES III show that mean vitamin B_{12} intake is well above the RDI for all sex-age groups, including pregnant and lactating females.[65] Vegans, or strict vegetarians (persons eating no animal products), could become vitamin B_{12} deficient, although this is unlikely because of the practice of fortification. Despite these facts, vitamin B_{12} deficiency does occur, although rarely because of a dietary deficiency. More than 95% of the cases of vitamin B_{12} deficiency seen in the United States are due to inadequate absorption of the vitamin, generally because of pernicious anemia caused by inadequate production of intrinsic factor. Because most vitamin B_{12} absorption occurs in the distal ileum, B_{12} malabsorption could also result from surgical resection of the distal ileum, bacterial overgrowth in the small intestine ("blind loop" syndrome), or damage to the ileum from such causes as tropical sprue or regional enteritis.[92]

Intrinsic factor (Castle's intrinsic factor) is a glycoprotein produced by the parietal cells of the gastric glands, located in the body of the stomach. Intrinsic factor (IF) combines with vitamin B_{12} in the upper small intestine. The B_{12}-IF complex is carried to the ileum (the distal part of the small intestine), where it attaches to B_{12}-IF receptors on the brush border of ileal mucosal cells. The B_{12}-IF complex is then taken up by the ileal mucosal cells and makes its way into the blood for distribution to the rest of the body.[83] Under normal circumstances, most vitamin B_{12} is absorbed by this mechanism; however, approximately 1% of ingested vitamin B_{12} can be absorbed through passive diffusion along the entire length of the small intestine.[83] The usual cause of inadequate IF production is atrophy of the gastric mucosa, a condition most often seen in older persons. Thus, pernicious anemia is a disease of the elderly, with an average age at diagnosis of 60 years. Other causes of inadequate IF production include total gastrectomy and extensive damage to the gastric mucosa caused by ingestion of corrosive agents.[92]

Clinical features of vitamin B_{12} deficiency involve the blood, the gastrointestinal tract, and the nervous system. An early feature of vitamin B_{12} deficiency is megaloblastic anemia, which is characterized by the presence of abnormally large cells (megaloblasts) in the peripheral blood and a low hemoglobin level. A mean corpuscular volume (MCV) > 100 fL is suggestive of megaloblastic anemia. The tongue may become sore, smooth, and beefy red. Anorexia with moderate weight loss and diarrhea may also be present. The most troublesome consequences of B_{12} deficiency occur in the nervous system. Neurologic manifestations include demyelination and axonal degeneration of the peripheral nerves, spinal cord, and cerebrum. Eventually, irreversible neuronal death can occur in these areas. The earliest symptoms of these changes are numbness and paresthesias (abnormal sensations, such as burning, prickling, or the feeling that ants are crawling on the skin) in the extremities. This can progress to weakness, muscular incoordination (ataxia), irritability, forgetfulness, severe dementia, and even psychosis.[92]

As shown in Figure 9.5, vitamin B_{12} status can be characterized as being in positive balance, normal, or in negative balance.[83] Positive B_{12} balance can be divided into two stages: stage I, early positive B_{12} balance, and stage II, excess. Figure 9.5 lists several indices of vitamin B_{12} status and gives values for these indices during these two stages of positive B_{12} balance, as well as during other times.

As outlined in Figure 9.5, negative B_{12} balance can be divided into two states of depletion and two stages of deficiency. Stage I of negative B_{12} balance is called early negative B_{12} balance. The earliest abnormalities in this stage are decreased serum levels of holo-transcobalamin II (vitamin B_{12} complexed with its primary transport protein, transcobalamin II) and decreased saturation of transcobalamin II (a decreased percentage of transcobalamin II that is carrying or is saturated with cobalamin). These occur when decreased vitamin B_{12} absorption depletes the amount of vitamin B_{12} complexed with and

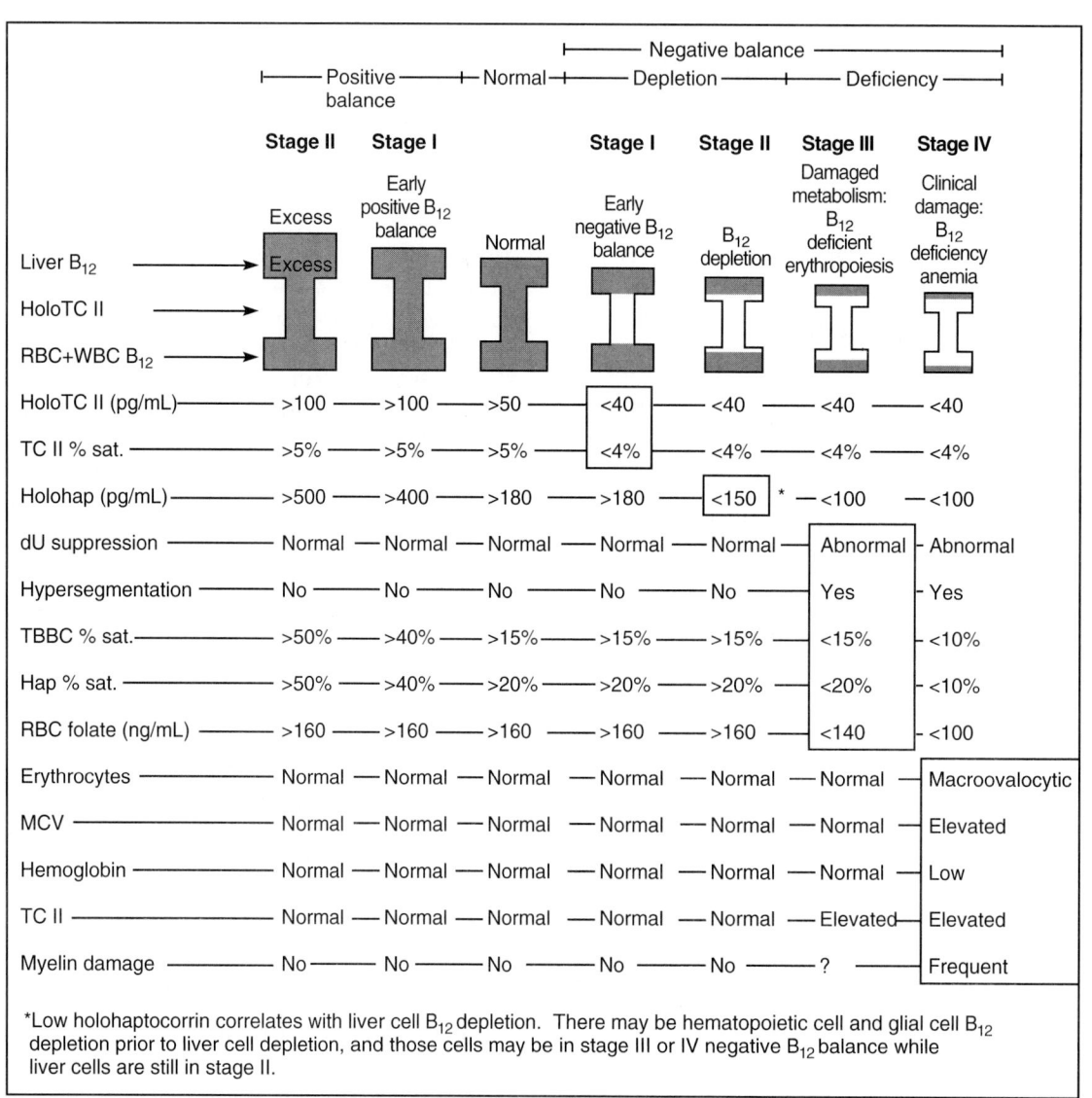

Figure 9.5 **Sequential changes in the development of vitamin B_{12} deficiency.**
The shaded areas indicate the relative quantities of vitamin B_{12} in each compartment (e.g., in the liver, that transported by transcobalamin II, and in the erythrocytes and leukocytes). The sequence of increasingly unshaded areas shows its proportional disappearance during successive stages of vitamin B_{12} deficiency. The earliest abnormalities in each stage are boxed. HoloTC II = the complex of vitamin B_{12} and transcobalamin II; TC II sat. = percent transcobalamin II saturation; holohap = holohaptocorrin; dU = deoxyuridine; TBBC % sat. = total B_{12}-binding capacity percent saturation; hap % sat. = percent saturation of haptocorrin; RBC = red blood cell; MCV = mean corpuscular volume.
Source: From Herbert V, Das KC. 1994. Folic acid and vitamin B_{12}. In Shils ME, Olson JA, Shike M, eds. *Modern nutrition in health and disease,* 8th ed. Philadelphia: Lea & Febiger.

carried by its transport protein, transcobalamin II. During this stage, however, total vitamin B_{12} level remains within normal limits. Stage II of negative B_{12} balance is B_{12} depletion. The earliest abnormality seen in this stage is a decreased level of holohaptocorrin (holohap).

Vitamin B_{12} deficiency is represented by stage III and stage IV of negative B_{12} balance. Stage III is known as B_{12} deficient erythropoiesis. This is characterized by abnormal values for the deoxyuridine (dU) suppression test, evidence of hypersegmentation of the nuclei of the polymorphonuclear leukocytes, decreased total B_{12}-binding capacity (TBBC), a lower than expected percent saturation of haptocorrin (hap), and decreased levels of folate in erythrocytes or red blood cells (RBC). This is characterized by enlarged erythrocytes (they appear macroovalocytic and have an increased MCV), low hemoglobin, elevated levels of transcobalamin II, and the frequent presence of myelin damage.[83]

Once vitamin B_{12} deficiency is discovered, the Schilling test can be used to determine its cause.[92,93] In the first stage of the Schilling test, a patient is given an oral dose of vitamin B_{12} labeled with a radioactive isotope of cobalt. A short time later, this is followed by an intramuscular or a subcutaneous injection of 1 mg of nonlabeled vitamin B_{12}. The patient then collects a 24-hour urine specimen. The amount of labeled vitamin B_{12} in the urine specimen is proportional to the amount of vitamin B_{12} absorbed. In pernicious anemia, < 5% of the administered dose of labeled B_{12} should be present in the urine specimen. In the second stage, the patient is given radioactively labeled B_{12} bound to intrinsic factor. Absorption of the vitamin will now approach normal if the patient has pernicious anemia or some other type of intrinsic factor deficiency. Urinary excretion of the labeled vitamin B_{12} should be > 10% of the administered dose. If urinary excretion is still low (< 5% of the administered dose), the patient likely has a defect in vitamin B_{12} absorption due to ileal dysfunction.

In another form of the Schilling test, a fasting patient is given an oral dose of vitamin B_{12} labeled with an isotope of cobalt (^{57}Co), which is bound to intrinsic factor, and, at the same time, a separate oral dose of vitamin B_{12} containing a different isotope of cobalt (^{58}Co), which is not bound to intrinsic factor. In 1 to 2 hours, the patient is given 1 mg of nonlabeled vitamin B_{12} by intramuscular or subcutaneous injection. A 24-hour urine specimen is collected. In pernicious anemia, the excretion of ^{58}Co is low (usually < 5% of the administered dose), while excretion of the ^{57}Co that was bound to the intrinsic factor is normal (> 10% of the administered dose). In intestinal malabsorption, excretion of both ^{58}Co and ^{57}Co is low. For the test to be valid, the patient must have a complete 24-hour urine specimen and normal renal function.[93]

BLOOD CHEMISTRY TESTS

Blood chemistry tests include a variety of assays performed on plasma or serum that are useful in the diagnosis and management of disease. They include electrolytes, enzymes, metabolites, and other miscellaneous substances, which are discussed in this section. When run at one time, blood chemistry tests often are known by such names as the *chemistry profile, chemistry panel, chem profile,* and *chem panel.* To perform these tests, clinical laboratories use an automated analyzer capable of performing several thousand blood tests per hour. The patient's plasma or serum sample is placed into the analyzer, which performs the desired tests and provides a printout of the patient's results, including reference ranges and flagged abnormal results. A related series of tests, often known as the *coronary risk profile,* measures levels of triglyceride, total cholesterol, and HDL-C (cholesterol carried by high-density lipoproteins) and calculates LDL-C (cholesterol carried by low-density lipoproteins) and, in some instances, the total cholesterol/HDL-C ratio. These are discussed in Chapter 8.

Following is a brief overview of the major blood chemistry tests. Normal adult serum levels (known as reference ranges) are given. These reference ranges vary, depending on the individual biochemical and analytic method used. It is generally best, however, to use reference ranges suggested by the laboratory performing the analyses.

Alanine Aminotransferase

Alanine aminotransferase (ALT), also known as serum glutamic pyruvic transaminase (SGPT), is an enzyme found in large concentrations in the liver and to a lesser extent in the kidneys, skeletal muscles, and myocardium (heart muscle).[94] Injury to the liver caused by such conditions as hepatitis (viral, alcoholic, and so on), cirrhosis, and bile duct obstruction or from drugs toxic to the liver is the usual cause of elevated serum ALT levels. Levels may be elevated to a lesser extent in myocardial infarction, musculoskeletal diseases, and acute pancreatitis. Decreased levels may result from chronic renal dialysis.[93] The adult reference range is 0.02 to 0.35 μkat/L (1 to 21 units/L).[94]

Albumin and Total Protein

Albumin is a serum protein produced in the liver. Total protein is the sum of all serum proteins, but the vast majority of total protein is composed of albumin and globulin. Once total protein and albumin are known, an estimate of globulin can be calculated. Levels of albumin and total protein reflect nutritional status, and alterations suggest the need for further diagnostic testing. The adult reference range for albumin is 35 to 50 g/L (3.5 to 5.0 g/dL); for globulin, 23 to 35 g/L (2.3 to 3.5 g/dL); and for total protein, 60 to 84 g/L (6.0 to 8.4 g/dL).[94]

Alkaline Phosphatase

Alkaline phosphatase (ALP) is an enzyme found in the liver, bone, placenta, and intestine and is useful in detecting diseases in these organs. Expected values are higher in children, during skeletal growth in adolescents, and during pregnancy.[94] Elevated levels can be seen in conditions involving increased deposition of calcium in bone (hyperparathyroidism, healing fractures, certain bone tumors) and certain liver diseases.[93] Low levels of ALP usually are not clinically significant. The adult reference range is 0.22 to 0.65 μkat/L (13 to 39 units/L).[94]

Aspartate Aminotransferase

Aspartate aminotransferase (AST), also known as serum glutamic oxaloacetic transaminase (SGOT), is an enzyme found in large concentrations in the myocardium, liver, skeletal muscles, kidneys, and pancreas. Within 8 to 12 hours following injury to these organs, AST is released into the blood. Serum levels peak in 24 to 36 hours and then return to normal in about 4 to 6 days following injury.[94] Elevated levels are seen in such conditions as myocardial infarction (blood levels reflect the size of the infarct), liver diseases (for example, acute viral hepatitis), pancreatitis, musculoskeletal injuries, and exposure to drugs toxic to the liver.[93] The adult reference range is 0.12 to 0.45 μkat/L (7 to 27 units/L).[94]

Bilirubin

Bilirubin, the major pigment of bile, is produced by the spleen, liver, and bone marrow from the breakdown of the heme portion of hemoglobin and is released into the blood. Most of the bilirubin combines with albumin to form what is called free, or unconjugated, bilirubin. Free bilirubin then is absorbed by the liver, where it is conjugated (joined) to other molecules to form what is called conjugated bilirubin and is then excreted into the bile. Serum bilirubin levels can be reported as direct bilirubin, indirect bilirubin, or total bilirubin. Direct bilirubin is a measure of conjugated bilirubin in serum. Indirect bilirubin is a measure of free, or unconjugated, bilirubin in serum. Total bilirubin is a measure of both direct and indirect bilirubin.[94]

Serum bilirubin rises when the liver is unable to either conjugate or excrete bilirubin. Elevated conjugated (direct) bilirubin suggests obstruction of bile passages within or near the liver. Elevated free, or unconjugated (indirect), bilirubin is indicative of excessive hemolysis (destruction) of red blood cells. Elevated indirect bilirubin also is seen in neonates whose immature livers are unable to adequately conjugate bilirubin. A serum bilirubin concentration greater than about 2 mg/dL results in jaundice. The adult reference ranges for adults are 1.7 to 20.5 μmol/L (0.1 to 1.2 mg/dL) for total, up to 5.1 μmol/L (up to 0.3 mg/dL) for direct (conjugated), and 1.7 to 17.1 μmol/L (0.1 to 1.0 mg/dL) for indirect (unconjugated) bilirubin.[94]

Blood Urea Nitrogen

Urea, the end product of protein metabolism and the primary method of nitrogen excretion, is formed in the liver and excreted by the kidneys in urine. An increased blood urea level usually indicates renal failure, although it may also result from dehydration, gastrointestinal bleeding, congestive heart failure, high protein intake, insufficient renal blood supply, or blockage of the urinary tract.[94] Blood urea nitrogen (BUN) is more easily measured than urea and is used as an index of blood urea levels. Elevated BUN is referred to as azotemia. Decreased BUN can result from liver disease, overhydration, malnutrition, or anabolic steroid use. In the absence of other signs elevated BUN is probably insignificant. The adult reference range is 8 to 25 mg/dL (2.9 to 9.8 mmol/L).[94]

Calcium

Serum levels of calcium, an important cation (positively charged ion), are helpful in detecting disorders of the bones and parathyroid glands, kidney failure, and certain cancers. Calcium is discussed at length in the earlier section "Calcium Status." The adult reference range for total calcium is 8.5 to 10.5 mg/dL (2.1 to 2.6 mmol/L), and for ionized calcium it is 2.0 to 2.4 mEq/L (1.0 to 1.2 mmol/L).[94]

Carbon Dioxide

Measurement of carbon dioxide (CO_2) in serum helps assess the body's acid-base balance. Elevated CO_2 is seen in metabolic alkalosis, and decreased levels reflect metabolic acidosis. The adult reference range in serum or plasma is 24 to 30 mEq/L (24 to 30 mmol/L).[94]

Chloride

Chloride, an electrolyte, is the primary anion (negatively charged ion) within the extracellular fluid. It works in conjunction with sodium to help regulate acid-base balance, osmotic pressure, and fluid distribution within the body. It often is measured along with sodium, potassium, and carbon dioxide. Low serum chloride levels (hypochloremia) are associated with alkalosis and low serum potassium levels (hypokalemia). Hypokalemia may not accompany hypochloremia if the patient receives a potassium supplement that does not contain chloride or takes a potassium-sparing diuretic. Hyperchloremia (elevated serum chloride) may be seen in kidney disease, overactive thyroid, anemia, or heart disease. The adult reference range is 100 to 106 mEq/L (100 to 106 mmol/L).[94]

Cholesterol

According to the National Cholesterol Education Program, a desirable serum total cholesterol level is < 200 mg/dL (5.17 mmol/L). Chapter 8 discusses recommended levels of serum cholesterol and its relationship to coronary heart disease. Population reference values for serum total cholesterol are shown in Appendix S.

Creatinine

Measurement of serum creatinine, like measurement of blood urea nitrogen, is used for evaluating renal function. Elevated serum levels are seen when 50% or more of the kidney's nephrons are destroyed. The reference range for adult males is 0.8 to 1.2 mg/dL (70 to 110 μmol/L), and for adult females it is 0.6 to 0.9 mg/dL (50 to 80 μmol/L).[93] Creatinine is discussed in greater detail in Chapter 6.

Glucose

Measurement of serum glucose is of interest in the diagnosis and management of diabetes mellitus. This is discussed in detail in Chapter 8. The adult reference range for fasting serum glucose is 60 to 115 mg/dL (3.3 to 6.4 mmol/L). Use of serum glucose to diagnose diabetes is discussed at length in Chapter 8. Serum glucose can also be used to diagnose hypoglycemia, or low blood sugar. Glycosylated hemoglobin (HbA$_{1C}$), an index of long-term blood sugar control, and the oral glucose tolerance test (OGTT) are also discussed in Chapter 8.

Lactic Dehydrogenase

Lactic dehydrogenase (LDH), an enzyme found in the cells of many organs (skeletal muscles, myocardium, liver, pancreas, spleen, and brain), is released into the blood when cellular damage to these organs occurs. Serum levels of LDH rise 12 to 24 hours following a myocardial infarction and are often measured to determine whether an infarction has occurred. Increased LDH may result from a number of other conditions, including hepatitis, cancer, kidney disease, burns, and trauma. Measurement of five forms of LDH, known as isoenzymes, allows a more definitive diagnosis to be made. Low serum LDH is of no clinical significance. The adult reference range for serum LDH is 45 to 90 units/L (0.75 to 1.50 μkat/L).[93,94]

Phosphorus

The serum level of phosphorus (also known as inorganic phosphorus) is closely correlated with serum calcium level. Elevated serum phosphorus (hyperphosphatemia) is seen in renal failure, hypoparathyroidism, hyperthyroidism, and increased phosphate intake (use of phosphate-containing laxatives and enemas). Low serum phosphorus (hypophosphatemia) can be seen in hyperparathyroidism, rickets, osteomalacia, and chronic use of antacids containing aluminum hydroxide or calcium carbonate, which binds phosphorus in the gastrointestinal tract and prevents its absorption. The adult reference range is 3.0 to 4.5 mg/dL (1.0 to 1.5 mmol/L).[94]

Potassium

Potassium, the major intracellular cation, is involved in the maintenance of acid-base balance, the body's fluid balance, and nerve impulse transmission. Elevated serum potassium (hyperkalemia) is most often due to renal failure but also may result from inadequate adrenal gland function (Addison's disease), severe burns, or crushing injuries. Low serum potassium (hypokalemia) can result from a number of causes, including use of diuretics or intravenous fluid administration without adequate potassium supplementation, vomiting, diarrhea, and eating disorders.[93,94] The reference range for adults is 3.5 to 5.0 mEq/L (3.5 to 5.0 mmol/L).

Sodium

Sodium, the major extracellular cation, is primarily involved in the maintenance of fluid balance and acid-base balance. Elevated serum levels (hypernatremia) are most frequently seen in dehydration resulting from insufficient water intake, excessive water output (for example, severe diarrhea or vomiting, profuse sweating, burns), or loss of antidiuretic hormone control. Hypernatremia suggests the need for water. Hyponatremia may be due to conditions resulting in excessive sodium loss from the body (vomiting, diarrhea, gastric suctioning, diuretic use), conditions resulting in fluid retention (congestive heart failure or renal disease), or water intoxication. The adult reference range is 135 to 145 mEq/L (135 to 145 mmol/L).[94]

Triglyceride

Triglyceride (TG) is a useful indicator of lipid tolerance in patients receiving total parenteral nutrition. Fasting serum TG provides a good estimate of very low-density lipoprotein levels. Factors contributing to increased fasting serum TG include genetic factors, obesity, physical inactivity, cigarette smoking, excess alcohol intake, very-high carbohydrate diets, type 2 diabetes, chronic renal failure, nephrotic syndrome, and use of such drugs as corticosteroids, protease inhibitors, beta-adrenergic blocking agents, and estrogen. Elevated serum TG is now considered a risk factor for coronary heart disease and an indicator of persons needing coronary heart disease risk-reduction intervention. According to the National Cholesterol Education Program, a normal serum TG is <150 mg/dL (< 1.69 mmol/L). Borderline-high and high TG are 150 to 199 mg/dL (1.69 to 2.25 mmol/L) and 200 to 499 mg/dL (2.26 to 5.63 mmol/L), respectively. Very-high serum TG is considered ≥ 500 mg/dL (5.64 mmol/L). Population reference values for serum TG are shown in Appendix S.

SUMMARY

1. Biochemical tests to assess nutritional status can be grouped into two general categories: static and functional tests. Static tests are based on measurement of a nutrient or specific metabolite in the blood, urine, or body tissue. Functional tests involve the physiologic processes that rely on the presence of adequate quantities of a nutrient.

2. The value of biochemical tests is limited by nonnutritional factors affecting test results and the occasional inability of tests to identify the nutrient deficiency. Monitoring nutritional status requires the use of several biochemical tests used in conjunction with each other and with data derived from dietary, anthropometric, and clinical methods. Compared with other assessment methods, biochemical tests have the advantage of being somewhat more objective and quantitative.

3. Protein-energy malnutrition can be either primary (insufficient intake of protein and calories) or secondary (resulting from other diseases). When severe, it results in kwashiorkor (principally a protein deficiency), marasmus (predominantly an energy deficiency), or marasmic kwashiorkor (a combination of chronic energy deficit and chronic or acute protein deficiency).

4. Creatinine and 3-methylhistidine are two muscle metabolites excreted in urine used to quantitate muscle mass. Creatinine is excreted in a relatively constant proportion to the body's muscle mass. Muscle mass can be estimated by comparing 24-hour urine creatinine excretion with certain standards. The creatinine-height index is a ratio of a patient's measured 24-hour urinary creatinine excretion and the expected excretion by a reference adult of the same sex and stature expressed as a percent of expected value. The use of creatinine and 3-methylhistidine is limited by problems associated with 24-hour urine collections, the effect of diet on urine concentrations, diurnal variations in excretion of creatinine and 3-methylhistidine, and a variety of other factors affecting their excretion.

5. Included among the serum proteins used to assess protein nutriture are albumin, transferrin, prealbumin, retinol-binding protein, and fibronectin. Considerations in their use include their body pool amount, half-life, and responsiveness to protein and energy depletion and repletion. Other considerations include how serum proteins are affected by nutritional and nonnutritional factors and how they correlate with morbidity and mortality.

6. Because nutrient deficiency often compromises immunity, tests of immunocompetence (e.g., total lymphocyte count and delayed cutaneous hypersensitivity) can be used to assess nutritional status. Although these tests can detect immune problems associated with general nutritional deficits, they often are unable to identify the specific nutrient that is deficient and are affected by a variety of nonnutritional factors.

7. Iron deficiency is the most common single nutrient deficiency in the United States and the most common cause of anemia. Serum ferritin is the most useful index of the body's iron stores. Hemoglobin is the most widely used screening test for iron-deficiency anemia but is not an early indicator of iron depletion. Hematocrit is defined as the percentage of red blood cells making up the entire volume of whole blood.

8. Models that combine several indicators of iron status are better at predicting the presence of iron deficiency. Among these are the ferritin model, the MCV model, the four-variable model, and the hemoglobin percentile shift model. These models allow better discrimination between iron-deficiency anemias and those caused by infection, inflammation, and chronic disease than do single measurements. This discrimination is enhanced when nonspecific measures of acute inflammation, such as erythrocyte sedimentation rate, zeta-sedimentation rate, or C-reactive protein, are included with the models.

9. Biochemical tests for assessing calcium status are hampered by the body's tight control of serum calcium levels. Measurement of urinary calcium, which is more responsive to dietary calcium change than serum calcium, is limited by the need for 24-hour urine samples and several nonnutritional factors that affect results.

10. Despite changes in dietary intake, the body maintains tight metabolic control of zinc status through conservation and redistribution of tissue zinc. Consequently, there are no sensitive biochemical or functional indicators of zinc status. Serum zinc level is not reflective of dietary changes and is only a late indicator of the body's exchangeable zinc pool size.

11. Assessing vitamin A status involves static measurements of vitamin levels in serum and liver, and functional tests, such as dose-response tests, conjunctival impression cytology, and dark adaptation. Serum measurements are predictive of vitamin A status only when the body's reserves are either critically depleted or overfilled.

12. The relative dose-response test (RDR) is based on the principle that, when a person's vitamin A reserves are low, plasma retinol concentration

increases markedly within 5 hours after administration of a dose of vitamin A. The RDR has the ability to identify persons with marginal vitamin A status. It is limited by a 5-hour wait and the need to draw two blood samples.

13. Measurements of vitamin C in serum and leukocytes can be used for assessing vitamin C status. Serum vitamin C is a good indicator of recent vitamin C intake, whereas leukocyte vitamin C better represents cellular stores and the total body pool. There is currently no reliable functional indicator of vitamin C status. Problems with measuring vitamin C in red blood cells, saliva, and urine make these poor indicators.

14. Assays for assessing vitamin B_6 status include measurement of plasma pyridoxal 5′-phosphate (PLP), plasma pyridoxal, plasma total vitamin B_6, erythrocyte PLP, urine 4-pyridoxic acid, and urine total vitamin B_6. Functional measures include determination of erythrocyte transaminase activity, the tryptophan load test, and the methionine load test.

15. Plasma PLP appears to be the single most informative indicator of vitamin B_6 status for healthy persons, but results must sometimes be interpreted with caution because values can be affected by several diseases. Measurement of plasma pyridoxal is recommended in the assessment of B_6 status despite concerns about how well it represents vitamin B_6 status. 4-pyridoxic acid is the major urinary metabolite of vitamin B_6. It is considered a useful indicator of immediate dietary intake and of short-term vitamin B_6 status.

16. When vitamin B_6 deficiency exists, unusually high concentrations of xanthurenic acid and cystathionine occur in 24-hour urine collections after administration of tryptophan and methionine, respectively. Direct measures of vitamin B_6 are replacing the tryptophan load test, which historically has been the most widely used indicator of vitamin B_6 status. The methionine load test is used less frequently, and no definitive reference values for urinary cystathionine are available. Both load tests are limited by the need for 24-hour urine collections and by nonnutritional confounders.

17. Erythrocyte alanine transaminase and erythrocyte aspartic acid transaminase are two enzymes whose activity is decreased in vitamin B_6 deficiency. Measurement of their activity before and after in vitro addition of vitamin B_6 can be a useful index of vitamin B_6 status, but the approach has certain limitations.

18. Measures for assessing folate status include measurement of serum folate and erythrocyte folate and the deoxyuridine suppression test. Serum folate is indicative of negative folate balance but cannot discriminate between transient fluctuations in serum folate and chronic deficiency and depleted body stores. Erythrocyte folate is considered to be the best clinical index of depleted tissue stores. The deoxyuridine suppression test is a useful index of plasma and erythrocyte folate concentrations but is not as good an indicator as erythrocyte folate measurement.

19. The primary cause of vitamin B_{12} deficiency is inadequate absorption, usually because of inadequate gastric production of intrinsic factor, although ileal resection or ileal dysfunction can also cause B_{12} malabsorption. Pernicious anemia is characterized by hematologic, gastrointestinal, and nervous system abnormalities. Once vitamin B_{12} deficiency has been diagnosed, the Schilling test is used to determine whether it is due to lack of intrinsic factor production or to ileal dysfunction.

20. Blood chemistry tests are assays performed on the substances in plasma or serum that are useful in diagnosing and managing disease. They include electrolytes, enzymes, metabolites, and other substances present in serum or plasma. These tests usually are performed using an automated chemistry analyzer capable of performing several thousand blood tests per hour.

REFERENCES

1. Leklem JE. 1990. Vitamin B_6: A status report. *Journal of Nutrition* 120:1503–1507.

2. Benjamin DR. 1989. Laboratory tests and nutritional assessment: Protein-energy status. *Pediatric Clinics of North America* 36:139–161.

3. Underwood BA. 1990. Dose-response tests in field surveys.

Journal of Nutrition 120:1455–1458.

4. Bingham SA. 1994. The use of 24-h urine samples and energy expenditure to validate dietary assessments. *American Journal of Clinical Nutrition* 59(suppl):S227–S231.

5. Black AE, Prentice SM, Goldberg GR, Jebb SA, Bingham SA,

Livingstone MBE, Coward WA. 1993. Measurements of total energy expenditure provide insights into the validity of dietary measurements of energy intake. *Journal of the American Dietetic Association* 93:572–579.

6. Phinney SD. 1981. The assessment of protein nutrition in the

hospitalized patient. *Clinics in Laboratory Medicine* 1:767–774.

7. Young VR, Marchini JS, Cortiella J. 1990. Assessment of protein nutritional status. *Journal of Nutrition* 120:1469–1502.

8. Gibson RS. 1990. *Nutritional assessment.* New York: Oxford University Press.

9. Torun B, Chew F. 1994. Protein-energy malnutrition. In Shils ME, Olson JA, Shike M, eds. *Modern nutrition in health and disease,* 8th ed. Philadelphia: Lea & Febiger.

10. Foster MR, Heppenstall RB, Friedenberg ZB, Hozack WJ. 1990. A prospective assessment of nutritional status and implications in patients with fractures of the hip. *Journal of Orthopedic Trauma* 4:49–57.

11. Bashir Y, Graham TR, Torrence A, Gibson GJ, Corris PA. 1990. Nutritional state of patients with lung cancer undergoing thoracotomy. *Thorax* 45:183–186.

12. Young GA, Kopple JD, Lindholm B, Vonesh EF, et al. 1991. Nutrition assessment of continuous ambulatory peritoneal dialysis patients: An international study. *American Journal of Kidney Diseases* 17:462–471.

13. Henderson CJ, Lovell DJ. 1989. Assessment of protein-energy malnutrition in children and adolescents with juvenile rheumatoid arthritis. *Arthritis Care and Research* 2:108–113.

14. Heymsfield SB, Tighe A, Wang ZM. 1994. Nutritional assessment by anthropometric and biochemical methods. In Shils ME, Olson JA, Shike M, eds. *Modern nutrition in health and disease,* 8th ed. Philadelphia: Lea & Febiger.

15. Rennie MJ, Millward DJ. 1983. 3-methylhistidine excretion and the urinary 3-methylhistidine/creatinine ratio are poor indicators of skeletal muscle protein breakdown. *Clinical Science* 65:217–225.

16. Herrmann FR, Safran C, Levkoff SE, Minaker KL. 1992. Serum albumin level on admission as a predictor of death, length of stay, and readmission. *Archives of Internal Medicine* 152:125–130.

17. Tuchschmid Y, Tschantz P. 1992. Complications in gerontologic surgery: Role of nutritional status and serum albumin. *Helvetica Chirurgica Acta* 58:771–774.

18. Kovacevich DS, Braunschweig CL, August DA, eds. 1994. *Parenteral and enteral nutrition manual,* 7th ed. Ann Arbor: University of Michigan Medical Center.

19. Food and Nutrition Board, National Research Council. 1989. *Recommended Dietary Allowances,* 10th ed. Washington, DC: National Academy Press.

20. Unterman TG, Vazquez RM, Slas AJ, Matryn PA, Phillips LS. 1985. Nutrition and somatomedin. XIII. Usefulness of somatomedin-C in nutritional assessment. *American Journal of Medicine* 78:228–234.

21. Sandberg L, VanReken D, Waiwaiku K, Martin-Yeboah P, Weiss C, Updegraff V, Hanson A, Schleman M, Lodhian B. 1985. Plasma fibronectin levels in acute and recovering malnourished children. *Clinical Physiology and Biochemistry* 3:257–264.

22. Yoder MC, Anderson DC, Gopalakrishna GS, Douglas SD, Polin RA. 1987. Comparison of serum fibronectin, prealbumin, and albumin concentrations during nutritional repletion in protein-calorie malnourished infants. *Journal of Pediatric Gastroenterology and Nutrition* 6:84–88.

23. McKone TK, Davis AT, Dean RE. 1985. Fibronectin: A new nutritional parameter. *American Surgeon* 51:336–339.

24. Sandberg LB, Owens AJ, VanReken DE, Horowitz B, Fredell JE, Takyi Y, Troko DM, Horowitz MS, Hanson AP. 1990. Improvement in plasma protein concentrations with fibronectin treatment in severe malnutrition. *American Journal of Clinical Nutrition* 52: 651–656.

25. Chandra RK. 1981. Immunodeficiency in undernutrition and overnutrition. *Nutrition Reviews* 39:225–231.

26. Chandra RK. 1991. 1990 McCollum Award Lecture. Nutrition and immunity: Lessons from the past and new insights into the future. *American Journal of Clinical Nutrition* 53:1087–1101.

27. VanDeGraf KM, Fox SI. 1992. *Concepts of human anatomy and physiology.* Dubuque, IA: Wm. C. Brown.

28. Chandra RK. 1981. Immunocompetence as a functional index of nutritional status. *British Medical Bulletin* 37:89–94.

29. Myrvik QN. 1994. Immunology and nutrition. In Shils ME, Olson JA, Shike M, eds. *Modern nutrition in health and disease,* 8th ed. Philadelphia: Lea & Febiger.

30. Twomey P, Ziegler D, Rombeau J. 1982. Utility of skin testing in nutritional assessment: A critical review. *Journal of Parenteral and Enteral Nutrition* 6:50–58.

31. Life Sciences Research Office, Federation of American Societies for Experimental Biology. 1989. *Nutrition monitoring in the United States: An update report on nutrition monitoring.* Washington, DC: U.S. Department of Health and Human Services, Public Health Service.

32. Johnson MA. 1990. Iron: Nutrition monitoring and nutrition status assessment. *Journal of Nutrition* 120:1486–1491.

33. Expert Scientific Working Group. 1985. Summary of a report on assessment of the iron nutritional status of the United States population. *American Journal of Clinical Nutrition* 42:1318–1330.

34. Fairbanks VF. 1994. Iron in medicine and nutrition. In Shils ME, Olson JA, Shike M, eds. *Modern nutrition in health and disease,* 8th ed. Philadelphia: Lea & Febiger.

35. Ravel R. 1989. *Clinical laboratory medicine: Clinical application of laboratory data,* 5th ed. St. Louis: Mosby.

36. Weaver CM. 1990. Assessing calcium status and metabolism. *Journal of Nutrition* 120:1470–1473.

37. Allen LH, Wood RJ. 1994. Calcium and phosphorus. In Shils ME, Olson JA, Shike M, eds. *Modern nutrition in health and disease,* 8th ed. Philadelphia: Lea & Febiger.

38. Nordin BEC, Need AG, Hartley TF, Philcox JC, Wilcox M, Thomas DW. 1989. Improved method for calculating calcium fractions in plasma: Reference values and effects of menopause. *Clinical Chemistry* 35:14–17.

39. McCarron DA. 1982. Low serum concentrations of ionized calcium in patients with hypertension. *New England Journal of Medicine* 307:226–228.

40. Resnick LM, Laragh JH, Sealey LE, Alderman MH, 1983. Divalent cations in essential hypertension: Relations between serum ionized calcium, magnesium, and plasma renin activity. *New England Journal of Medicine* 309:888–891.

41. Kesteloot H, Geboers J. 1982. Calcium and blood pressure. *Lancet* 1:813–815.

42. Robinson D, Bailey AR, Williams PT. 1982. Calcium and blood pressure. *Lancet* 2:1215–1216.

43. Marshall RW, Francis RM, Hodgkinson A. 1982. Plasma total and ionized calcium, albumin, and globulin concentrations in pre- and post-menopausal women and the effects of estrogen administration. *Clinica Chemica Acta* 122:283–287.

44. King JC, Keen CL. 1994. Zinc. In Shils ME, Olson JA, Shike M, eds. *Modern nutrition in health and disease,* 8th ed. Philadelphia: Lea & Febiger.

45. King JC. 1990. Assessment of zinc status. *Journal of Nutrition* 120:1474–1479.

46. Walravens PA, Krebs NF, Hambidge KM. 1983. Linear growth of low income preschool children receiving a zinc supplement. *American Journal of Clinical Nutrition* 38:195–201.

47. Walravens PA, Hambidge KM, Koepfer DM. 1989. Zinc supplementation in infants with a nutritional pattern of failure to thrive: A double-blind, controlled study. *Pediatrics* 83:532–538.

48. Giugliano R, Millward DJ. 1984. Growth and zinc homeostasis in the severely Zn-deficient rat. *British Journal of Nutrition* 52:545–560.

49. Taylor CM, Bacon JR, Aggett PJ, Bremner I. 1991. Homeostatic regulation of zinc absorption and endogenous losses in zinc-deprived men. *American Journal of Clinical Nutrition* 53:755–763.

50. Jackson MJ, Jones DA, Edwards RHT. 1982. Tissue zinc levels as an index of body zinc status. *Clinical Physiology* 2:333–343.

51. Hambidge KM. 1982. Hair analysis: Worthless for vitamins, limited for minerals. *American Journal of Clinical Nutrition* 36:943–949.

52. Taylor A. 1986. Usefulness of measurements of trace elements in hair. *Annals of Clinical Biochemistry* 23:364–378.

53. Jacob RA. 1981. Zinc and copper. *Clinics in Laboratory Medicine* 1:743–766.

54. Davies TS. 1982. Hair analysis and selenium shampoos. *Lancet* 2:935.

55. DeAntonio SM, Katz SA, Scheiner DM, Wood JD. 1982. Anatomically-related variations in trace-metal concentrations in hair. *Clinical Chemistry* 28:2411–2413.

56. Olson JA. 1994. Vitamin A, retinoids, and carotenoids. In Shils ME, Olson JA, Shike M, eds. *Modern nutrition in health and disease,* 8th ed. Philadelphia: Lea & Febiger.

57. Underwood BA. 1990. Methods for assessment of vitamin A status. *Journal of Nutrition* 120:1459–1463.

58. Garry PJ. 1981. Vitamin A. *Clinics in Laboratory Medicine* 1:699–711.

59. Amedee-Manesme O, Mourey MA, Hanck A, Therasse J. 1987. Vitamin A relative dose response test: Validation by intravenous injection in children with liver disease. *American Journal of Clinical Nutrition* 46:286–289.

60. Pilch SM. 1987. Analysis of vitamin A data from the health and nutrition examination surveys. *Journal of Nutrition* 117:636–640.

61. Amedee-Manesme O, Anderson D, Olson JA. 1984. Relation of the relative dose response to liver concentrations of vitamin A in generally well-nourished surgical patients. *American Journal of Clinical Nutrition* 39:898–902.

62. Amedee-Manesme O, Luzeau R, Wittepen JR, Hanck A, Sommer A. 1988. Impression cytology detects subclinical vitamin A deficiency. *American Journal of Clinical Nutrition* 47:875–878.

63. Luzeau R, Carlier C, Ellrodt A, Amedee-Manesme O. 1987. Impression cytology with transfer: An easy method of detection of vitamin A deficiency. *International Journal of Vitamin and Nutrition Research* 58:166–179.

64. Jacob RA. 1990. Assessment of human vitamin C status. *Journal of Nutrition* 120:1480–1485.

65. Alaimo K, McDowell MA, Briefel RR, Bischof AM, Caughman CR, Loria CM, Johnson CL. 1994. Dietary intake of vitamins, minerals, and fiber of persons ages 2 months and over in the United States: Third National Health and Nutrition Examination Survey, Phase 1, 1988–91. *Advance Data from Vital and Health Statistics* No. 258. Hyattsville, MD: U.S. Center for Health Statistics.

66. Sauberlich HW. 1981. Ascorbic acid (vitamin C). *Clinics in Laboratory Medicine* 1:673–684.

67. Solomons NW, Allen LH. 1983. The functional assessment of nutritional status: Principles, practice and potential. *Nutrition Reviews* 41:33–50.

68. Jacob RA. 1994. Vitamin C. In Shils ME, Olson JA, Shike M, eds. *Modern nutrition in health and disease,* 8th ed. Philadelphia: Lea & Febiger.

69. Blanchard J, Conrad KA, Watson RR, Garry PJ, Crawley JD. 1989. Comparison of plasma, mononuclear, and polymorphonuclear leukocyte

vitamin C levels in young and elderly women during depletion and supplementation. *European Journal of Clinical Nutrition* 43:97–106.

70. Schaus ES, Kutnink MA, O'Conner DK, Omaye ST. 1986. A comparison of leukocyte ascorbate levels measured by the 2,4-dinitrophenylhydrazine method with high-performance liquid chromatography using electrochemical detection. *Biochemical Medicine and Metabolic Biology* 36:369–376.

71. VanderJagt DJ, Garry PJ, Bhagavan HN. 1989. Ascorbate and dehydroascorbate: Distribution in mononuclear cells of healthy elderly people. *American Journal of Clinical Nutrition* 49:511–516.

72. Omaye ST, Schaus EE, Kutnink MA, Hawkes WC. 1987. Measurement of vitamin C in blood components by high-performance liquid chromatography. Implication in assessing vitamin C status. *Annals of the New York Academy of Science* 498:389–401.

73. Jacob RA, Skala JH, Omaye ST. 1987. Biochemical indices of human vitamin C status. *American Journal of Clinical Nutrition* 46:818–826.

74. Evans RM, Currie L, Campbell A. 1982. The distribution of ascorbic acid between various cellular components of blood in normal individuals, and its relation to the plasma concentration. *British Journal of Nutrition* 47:473–482.

75. Garry PJ, Goodwin JS, Hunt WC, Gilbert BA. 1982. Nutritional status in a healthy elderly population: Vitamin C. *American Journal of Clinical Nutrition* 36:332–339.

76. Schectman G, Byrd JC, Hoffman R. 1991. Ascorbic acid requirements for smokers: Analysis of a population survey. *American Journal of Clinical Nutrition* 53:1466–1470.

77. Sauberlich HE. 1985. Interaction of vitamin B_6 with other nutrients. In Reynolds RD, Leklem JE, eds. *Vitamin B_6: Its role in health and disease.* New York: Alan R. Liss.

78. Leklem JE. 1994. Vitamin B_6. In Shils ME, Olson JA, Shike M, eds. *Modern nutrition in health and disease,* 8th ed. Philadelphia: Lea & Febiger.

79. Leklem JE. 1988. Vitamin B_6 metabolism and function in humans. In Leklem JE, Reynolds RD, eds. *Clinical and physiological applications of vitamin B_6.* New York: Alan R. Liss.

80. Schaumberg H, Kaplan J, Windebank A, Vick N, Rasmus S, Pleasure D, Brown MJ. 1983. Sensory neuropathy from pyridoxine abuse: A new megavitamin syndrome. *New England Journal of Medicine* 309:445–448.

81. Coburn SP, Lewis DLN, Fink WJ, Mahuren JD, Schaltenbrand WD, Costill DL. 1988. Human vitamin B_6 pools estimated through muscle biopsies. *American Journal of Clinical Nutrition* 48:291–294.

82. Leklem JE. 1988. Challenges and directions in the search for clinical applications of vitamin B_6. In Leklem JE, Reynolds RD, eds. *Clinical and physiological applications of vitamin B_6.* New York: Alan R. Liss.

83. Herbert V, Das KC. 1994. Folic acid and vitamin B_{12}. In Shils ME, Olson JA, Shike M, eds. *Modern nutrition in health and disease,* 8th ed. Philadelphia: Lea & Febiger.

84. Bailey LB. 1990. Folate status assessment. *Journal of Nutrition* 120:1508–1511.

85. Reider MJ. 1994. Prevention of neural tube defects with periconceptual folic acid. *Clinical Perinatology* 21:483–503.

86. Rose NC, Mennuti MT. 1994. Periconceptual folate supplementation and neural tube defects. *Clinical Obstetrics and Gynecology* 37:605–620.

87. Rush D. 1994. Periconceptual folate and neural tube defect. *American Journal of Clinical Nutrition* 59(2 suppl):S511–S515.

88. Herbert V. 1987. The 1986 Herman Award Lecture. Nutrition science as a continually unfolding story: The folate and vitamin B_{12} paradigm. *American Journal of Clinical Nutrition* 46:387–402.

89. Colman N. 1981. Laboratory assessment of folate status. *Clinics in Laboratory Medicine* 1:775–796.

90. Bailey LB, Moyers S, Gregory JF. 2001. Folate. In Bowman BA, Russell RM, eds. *Present knowledge in nutrition,* 8th ed. Washington, DC: International Life Sciences Institute.

91. Tamura T, Soong SJ, Sauberlich HE, Hatch KD, Cole P, Butterworth CE. 1990. Evaluation of the deoxyuridine suppression test by using whole blood samples from folic acid–supplemented subjects. *American Journal of Clinical Nutrition* 51:80–86.

92. Babior BM, Bunn HF. 1994. Megaloblastic anemias. In Isselbacher KJ, Braunwald E, Wilson JD, Martin JB, Fauci AS, Kasper DL, eds. *Harrison's principles of internal medicine,* 13th ed. New York: McGraw-Hill.

93. Wallach J. 1992. *Interpretation of diagnostic tests,* 5th ed. Boston: Little, Brown.

94. Tilkian SM, Conover MB, Tilkian AG. 1987. *Clinical implications of laboratory tests,* 4th ed. St. Louis: Mosby.

95. National Cholesterol Education Program. 2001. *Third report of the expert panel on detection, evaluation, and treatment of high blood cholesterol in adults.* Bethesda, MD: U.S. Department of Health and Human Services, Public Health Service; National Institutes of Health; National Heart, Lung, and Blood Institute.

ASSESSMENT ACTIVITY 9.1

Visiting a Clinical Laboratory

Every hospital or clinic has a clinical laboratory where at least some of the facility's biochemical tests are performed. Specimens are sometimes sent to an outside clinical laboratory because it has specialized instruments and expertise or because its automated analyzers allow certain tests to be performed more economically. However, all hospitals have facilities for performing certain basic tests, especially those required in emergency situations. Among

these are tests for electrolytes, blood gases, enzymes diagnostic of cardiac or liver disease, and glucose.

Your class can arrange to visit a clinical laboratory to see how some of these tests are performed. You may be surprised by the capability of various automated instruments used to perform the chemistry profile and complete blood count on a single specimen of serum or whole blood.

ASSESSMENT ACTIVITY 9.2

Chemistry Profile, Complete Blood Count, and Coronary Risk Profile

The chemistry profile, complete blood count (CBC), and coronary risk profile are among the most basic series of tests performed by clinical laboratories. Generally included in the chemistry profile are those tests listed in the section entitled "Blood Chemistry Tests." Included in the CBC are the red blood cell count, white blood cell count, and measurements of hemoglobin, hematocrit, mean corpuscular volume, mean corpuscular hemoglobin, and mean corpuscular hemoglobin concentration. The coronary risk profile measures levels of triglyceride, total cholesterol, and HDL-C (cholesterol carried by high-density lipoproteins) and calculates LDL-C (cholesterol carried by low-density lipoproteins) and the total cholesterol/HDL-C ratio. These tests are discussed in Chapter 8. These measurements are routinely performed using automated instruments capable of performing several thousand tests per hour.

Members of your class may want to have their blood drawn by a qualified venipuncturist and have the samples sent to a clinical laboratory for analysis. Tests that might be performed include the CBC, chemistry profile, and coronary risk profile. One alternative is to perform some of these tests right in the classroom. A variety of desktop blood analyzers are available, which can perform several tests. Included among these are the Abbott Vision, the Kodak Ectakem DT 60, and the Boehringer Mannheim

Reflotron. You probably have seen one of these used for measuring total cholesterol at a health fair or shopping center. Your school's student health center may have one of these instruments and might be willing to bring it to your classroom for a demonstration.

Another example of a simple test that can be done in the classroom is the hematocrit. The necessary equipment includes a centrifuge, capillary tubes, lancets, alcohol wipes, gloves, and some way of comparing the volume of whole blood in the capillary tube with the volume of packed cells after the tube is spun down. Whatever approach your class takes, compare your test results with the reference values given in this chapter and Chapter 8. Obtain an average value for the class and compare this with the reference values.

Remember, in handling blood specimens or any bodily fluid, precautions must be taken to protect patients and laboratory staff from infectious agents, especially those causing hepatitis as well as the human immunodeficiency virus (HIV). All bodily fluids must be regarded as being infectious and handled with the utmost care. All syringes, lancets, needles, tubes, and other materials that have come in contact with blood or other bodily fluids must be handled safely and disposed of properly. Gloves should be worn whenever drawing blood or handling other bodily fluids.

10

CLINICAL ASSESSMENT OF NUTRITIONAL STATUS

time and cost of hospitalization. Signs are defined as observations, made by a qualified examiner, of which the patient is usually unaware. Symptoms are clinical manifestations reported by the patient. This chapter discusses clinical assessment of nutritional status and gives examples of clinical indicators of impaired nutritional status. As a dietitian or nutritionist, you will likely see some of the conditions discussed and illustrated in this chapter. For example, protein-energy malnutrition and severe wasting are common features of certain cancers, acquired immune deficiency syndrome (AIDS), and advanced disease of the gastrointestinal tract. However, some of the other conditions discussed in this chapter, such as clinical signs of advanced nutrient deficiency, are rarely seen in developed countries but occur more frequently in less industrialized nations. Despite their rare occurrence, these conditions and their clinical signs are still of interest to students and practitioners of nutrition. Because many of the clinical findings are not specific for a particular nutrient deficiency, they often must be integrated with anthropometric, biochemical, and dietary data before arriving at a definitive diagnosis.

INTRODUCTION

Clinical assessment of nutritional status involves a detailed history, a thorough physical examination, and the interpretation of the signs and symptoms associated with malnutrition. It can be an efficient and effective way for an experienced and astute clinician to evaluate a patient's nutritional status without having to depend entirely on laboratory and diagnostic tests that may delay initiation of nutritional support and increase the

MEDICAL HISTORY

Obtaining a patient's history is the first step in the clinical assessment of nutritional status.[1] A good way to begin is by reviewing the patient's medical record, giving careful attention to the patient's medical history.[2,3] Components from the medical history to consider in nutritional assessment are shown in Box 10.1.

| **Box 10.1** | **Components of the Medical History to Consider in Nutritional Assessment** |

- Past and current diagnoses of nutritional consequence
- Diagnostic procedures
- Surgeries
- Chemotherapy and radiation therapy
- History of nutrition-related problems
- Existing nutrient deficiencies

- Medications and their nutrient interactions
- Psychosocial history—alcohol, smoking, finances, social support
- Signs or symptoms suggestive of vitamin deficiency
- Signs or symptoms suggestive of mineral deficiency

Adapted from Phinney SD. 1981. The assessment of protein nutrition in the hospitalized patient. *Clinics in Laboratory Medicine* 1:767–774; McLaren DS. 1992. *A colour atlas and text of diet-related disorders,* 2nd ed. London: Mosby Europe; Jeejeebhoy KN. 1994. Clinical and functional assessments. In Shills ME, Olson, JA, Shike M, eds. *Modern nutrition in health and disease,* 8th ed. Philadelphia: Lea & Febiger.

Essential components of a patient's history include pertinent facts about past and current health and use of medications, as well as personal and household information.[1,2] A variety of diseases can affect nutritional status. Among these are diabetes, kidney disease, various cancers, coronary heart disease, stroke, liver disease (e.g., hepatitis and cirrhosis), gallbladder disease, AIDS, ulcers, and colitis, as well as recent or past surgical procedures. Other conditions affecting nutritional status also should be explored: the ability to chew and swallow; appetite; and the presence of vomiting, diarrhea, constipation, flatulence, belching, or indigestion. An inquiry should be made about the patient's usual weight and any recent changes (gains or losses) in weight. A systematic approach to the detection of deficiency syndromes based on findings from the history is shown in Table 10.1.

Information on the use of medications will provide clues about the patient's actual or perceived medical condition. This will include prescription and over-the-counter medications, vitamin and mineral supplements, and nontraditional medications, such as herbal and folk remedies.

Psychosocial factors include the patient's age; occupation; educational level; marital status; income; living arrangements; number of dependents; use of alcohol, tobacco, and illicit drugs; degree of social and emotional support; and access to and ability to pay for health care. These factors are summarized in Box 10.2.

The necessary detail of the history will vary depending on circumstances and will be influenced by the patient's ability to respond to questioning. In some instances, the necessary information might need to be obtained from a surrogate (a parent, a companion, a sibling, or another person knowledgeable about the patient's life habits). Much of this information can be obtained from the history and physical examination performed by the admitting physician, from the notes of nurses or social workers, and from previous medical records. Remember that this and all information about the patient

should be dealt with in a confidential and strictly professional manner.

DIETARY HISTORY

Included with the dietary history is information about the patient's eating practices. This includes a wide range of information about usual eating patterns (timing and location of meals and snacks), food likes and dislikes, intolerances and allergies, amount of money available for purchasing food, ability to obtain and prepare food, eligibility for and access to food assistance programs, and use of vitamin, mineral, and other supplements. These and other factors are included in Box 10.2.

For example, when inquiring about appetite, satiety, or discomfort, it is important to ask if the patient has experienced any changes in desire for food, if he or she experiences satiety earlier or later than usual, and if there is any pain or discomfort associated with eating. Questions about the ability to chew and swallow food are important. Are there dental or oral problems making it difficult to chew certain foods or to consume adequate energy to support normal body weight? If the patient wears dentures, are they well fitting? If swallowing is painful or difficult, for what foods?

Questioning the patient about bowel habits can often provide information pertinent to the diagnosis of gastrointestinal disease. The patient should be asked about changes in bowel habits, such as constipation, diarrhea, or unusual amounts of flatus (gas), and about stool consistency and color. Obviously, the presence of bright red blood in the stool is an important finding. Stools containing digested blood (e.g., from a bleeding peptic ulcer) may appear black or tarry. The finding of frothy, watery, and foul-smelling stools suggests the possibility of fat malabsorption. Table 10.2 gives a listing of clinical findings and links their presence with either an excess or a deficiency of various nutrients.

TABLE 10.1 | Nutritional History Screens—a Systematic Approach to the Detection of Deficiency Syndromes

Mechanism of Deficiency	If History Of	Suspect Deficiency Of
Inadequate intake	Alcoholism	Energy, protein, thiamin, niacin, folate, pyridoxine, riboflavin
	Avoidance of fruit, vegetables, grains	Vitamin C, thiamin, niacin, folate
	Avoidance of meat, dairy products, eggs	Protein, vitamin B_{12}
	Constipation, hemorrhoids, diverticulosis	Dietary fiber
	Isolation, poverty, dental disease, food idiosyncrasies	Various nutrients
	Weight loss	Energy, other nutrients
Inadequate absorption	Drugs (especially antacids, anticonvulsants, cholestyramine, laxatives, neomycin, alcohol)	Various nutrients, depending on drug/nutrient interaction
	Malabsorption (diarrhea, weight loss, steatorrhea)	Vitamins A, D, K; energy; protein; calcium; magnesium; zinc
	Parasites	Iron, vitamin B_{12} (fish tapeworm)
	Pernicious anemia	Vitamin B_{12}
	Surgery	
	Gastrectomy	Vitamin B_{12}, iron
	Small bowel resection	Vitamin B_{12}, (if distal ileum), others as in malabsorption
Decreased utilization	Drugs (especially anticonvulsants, antimetabolites, oral contraceptives, isoniazid, alcohol)	Various nutrients, depending on drug/nutrient interaction
	Inborn errors of metabolism (by family history)	Various nutrients
Increased losses	Alcohol abuse	Magnesium, zinc
	Blood loss	Iron
	Centesis (ascitic, pleural taps)	Protein
	Diabetes, uncontrolled	Energy
	Diarrhea	Protein, zinc, electrolytes
	Draining abscesses, wounds	Protein, zinc
	Nephrotic syndrome	Protein, zinc
	Peritoneal dialysis or hemodialysis	Protein, water-soluble vitamins, zinc
Increased requirements	Fever	Energy
	Hyperthyroidism	Energy
	Physiologic demands (infancy, adolescence, pregnancy, lactation)	Various nutrients
	Surgery, trauma, burns, infection	Energy, protein, vitamin C, zinc
	Tissue hypoxia	Energy (inefficient utilization)
	Cigarette smoking	Vitamin C, folic acid

From Weinsier RL, Morgan SL, Perrin VG. 1993. *Fundamentals of clinical nutrition.* St. Louis: Mosby.

 Box 10.2 | **Factors to Consider in Taking a Patient's Dietary History**

- Weight changes
- Usual meal pattern
- Appetite
- Satiety
- Discomfort after eating
- Chewing/swallowing ability
- Likes/dislikes
- Taste changes/aversions
- Allergies
- Nausea/vomiting

- Bowel habits—diarrhea, constipation, steatorrhea
- Living conditions
- Snack consumption
- Vitamin/mineral supplement use
- Alcohol/drug use
- Previous diet restrictions
- Surgery/chronic diseases
- Ability to purchase and prepare food
- Access to and ability to pay for health care

Adapted from Phinney SD. 1981. The assessment of protein nutrition in the hospitalized patient. *Clinics in Laboratory Medicine* 1:767–774; McLaren DS. 1992. *A colour atlas and text of diet-related disorders,* 2nd ed. London: Mosby Europe; Jeejeebhoy KN. 1994. Clinical and functional assessments. In Shills ME, Olson, JA, Shike M, eds. *Modern nutrition in health and disease,* 8th ed. Philadelphia: Lea & Febiger.

TABLE 10.2 | Clinical Nutrition Examination

Clinical Findings	Consider Deficiency Of	Consider Excess Of	Frequency
Hair, Nails			
Flag sign (traverse depigmentation of hair)	Protein		Rare
Easily pluckable hair	Protein		Common
Sparse hair	Protein, biotin, zinc	Vitamin A	Occasional
Corkscrew hairs and unemerged coiled hairs	Vitamin C		Common
Traverse ridging of nails	Protein		Occasional
Skin			
Scaling	Vitamin A, zinc, essential fatty acids	Vitamin A	Occasional
Cellophane appearance	Protein		Occasional
Cracking (flaky paint or crazy pavement dermatosis)	Protein		Rare
Follicular hyperkeratosis	Vitamins A, C		Occasional
Petechiae (especially perifollicular)	Vitamin C		Occasional
Purpura	Vitamins C, K		Common
Pigmentation, desquamation of sun-exposed areas	Niacin		Rare
Yellow pigmentation-sparing sclerae (benign)		Carotene	Common
Eyes			
Papilledema		Vitamin A	Rare
Night blindness	Vitamin A		Rare
Perioral			
Angular stomatitis	Riboflavin, pyridoxine, niacin		Occasional
Cheilosis (dry, cracking, ulcerated lips)	Riboflavin, pyridoxine, niacin		Rare
Oral			
Atrophic lingual papillae (slick tongue)	Riboflavin, niacin, folate, vitamin B_{12}, protein, iron		Common
Glossitis (scarlet, raw tongue)	Riboflavin, niacin, pyridoxine, folate, vitamin B_{12}		Occasional
Hypogeusesthesia, hyposmia	Zinc		Occasional
Swollen, retracted, bleeding gums (if teeth are present)	Vitamin C		Occasional
Bones, Joints			
Beading of ribs, epiphyseal swelling, bowlegs	Vitamin D		Rare
Tenderness (subperiosteal hemorrhage in child)	Vitamin C		Rare
Neurologic			
Headache		Vitamin A	Rare
Drowsiness, lethargy, vomiting		Vitamins A, D	Rare
Dementia	Niacin, vitamin B_{12}		Rare
Confabulation, disorientation	Thiamin (Korsakoff's psychosis)		Occasional
Ophthalmoplegia	Thiamin, phosphorus		Occasional
Peripheral neuropathy (e.g., weakness; paresthesia; ataxia; decreased tendon reflexes; fine tactile sense, vibratory sense, and position sense)	Thiamin, pyridoxine, vitamin B_{12}	Pyridoxine	Occasional
Tetany	Calcium, magnesium		Occasional
Other			
Parotid enlargement	Protein (also consider bulimia)		Occasional
Heart failure	Thiamin (wet beriberi), phosphorus		Occasional
Sudden heart failure, death	Vitamin C		Rare
Hepatomegaly	Protein	Vitamin A	Rare
Edema	Protein, thiamin		Common
Poor wound healing, pressure ulcers	Protein, vitamin C, zinc		Common

From Weinsier RL, Morgan SL, Perrin VG. 1993. *Fundamentals of clinical nutrition.* St. Louis: Mosby.

SUBJECTIVE GLOBAL ASSESSMENT

Subjective Global Assessment (SGA) is a clinical technique for assessing the nutritional status of a patient based on features of the patient's history and physical examination.[4] Unlike traditional methods that rely heavily on objective anthropometric and biochemical data, SGA is based on four elements of the patient's history (recent loss of body weight, changes in usual diet, presence of significant gastrointestinal symptoms, and the patient's functional capacity) and three elements of the physical examination (loss of subcutaneous fat, muscle wasting, and presence of edema or ascites).[5] Information obtained from the history and physical examination can be entered into a form, such as the one shown in Figure 10.1, to arrive at an SGA rating of nutritional status. Two excellent articles giving detailed descriptions of the approach have been published.[4,5]

HISTORY

1. Weight Change

Maximum body weight _____
Weight 6 months ago _____
Current weight _____
Overall weight loss in past 6 months _____
Percent weight loss in past 6 months _____
Change in 2 past weeks: _____ increase _____ no change _____ decrease

$$\% \text{ Wt change} = \frac{\text{wt 6 months ago} - \text{current wt}}{\text{wt 6 mos ago}} \times 100$$

2. Dietary Intake (relative to normal)

_____ No change
_____ Change Duration: _____ Weeks
         Type: _____ Increased intake
               _____ Suboptimal solid diet
               _____ Full liquid diet
               _____ IV or hypocaloric liquids
               _____ Starvation

3. Gastrointestinal Symptoms (lasting > 2 weeks)

_____ None
_____ Nausea   _____ Vomiting   _____ Diarrhea   _____ Anorexia

4. Functional Capacity

_____ No dysfunction
_____ Dysfunction Duration: _____ weeks
          Type: _____ Works suboptimally
                _____ Ambulatory
                _____ Bedridden

PHYSICAL EXAMINATION

(For each trait specify: 0 = normal; 1+ = mild; 2+ = moderate; 3+ = severe)

_____ Loss of subcutaneous fat (shoulders, triceps, chest, hands)
_____ Muscle wasting (quadriceps, deltoids)
_____ Ankle edema
_____ Ascites

Subjective Global Assessment Rating (select one)

_____ A = well nourished
_____ B = moderately (or suspected of being) malnourished
_____ C = severely malnourished

Figure 10.1 Form for rating nutritional status based on Subjective Global Assessment.

Source: From Detsky AS, McLaughlin JR, Baker JP, Johnston N, Whittaker S, Mendelson RA, Jeejeebhoy KN. 1987. What is Subjective Global Assessment of nutritional status? *Journal of Parenteral and Enteral Nutrition* 11:8–13; Detsky AS, Smalley PS, Change J. 1994. Is this patient malnourished? *Journal of the American Medical Association* 271:54–58.

Elements of the History

The first of the four elements of the SGA history is the percent and pattern of weight loss within 6 months prior to examination. A weight loss < 5% is considered small. A 5% to 10% weight loss is considered potentially significant. A weight loss > 10% is considered definitely significant. The pattern of weight loss is also important. A patient who has lost 12% of his or her weight in the past 6 months but has recently gained 6% of it back is considered better nourished than a patient who has lost 6% of his or her weight in the past 6 months and continues to lose weight. Information about the patient's maximum weight and what it was 6 months ago can be compared with the patient's current weight. Questions about changes in the way clothing fits may confirm reports of weight change. Information about changes in body weight in the past 2 weeks (increase, no change, decrease) should be elicited as well. These data can be entered or noted in the appropriate places in Figure 10.1.

Dietary intake, the second element of the history, is classified as either normal (i.e., what the patient usually eats) or abnormal (i.e., a change from the patient's usual diet). If intake is abnormal, the duration in weeks is entered, and the appropriate box is checked to indicate the type of dietary intake abnormality (i.e., increased intake, suboptimal solid, full-liquid, IV or hypocaloric liquids, or starvation). The patient can be asked if the amount of food consumed has changed and, if so, by how much and why. If the patient is eating less, it would be valuable to know what happens when he or she tries to eat more. Ask for a description of a typical breakfast, lunch, and dinner and how that compares with what the patient typically ate 6 or 12 months ago.

Information about any gastrointestinal symptoms persisting more than 2 weeks (the third history element) should be elicited and noted on the form. Diarrhea or occasional vomiting lasting only a few days is not considered significant. The presence or absence of any dysfunction in the patient's ability to attend to activities of daily living (the last history element) should also be noted on the form. If a dysfunction is present, its duration and type should be noted.

Elements of the Physical Examination

The first of the three elements of the physical examination is loss of subcutaneous fat. The four anatomic areas listed in Figure 10.1 (shoulders, triceps, chest, and hands) should be checked for loss of fullness or loose-fitting skin, although the latter may appear in older persons who are not malnourished. Illustrations of subcutaneous fat loss in the arm, chest wall, and hands are shown in Figure 10.2 and Figure 10.3. Loss of subcutaneous fat should be noted as normal (0), mild loss (1+), moderate loss (2+), or severe loss (3+).

According to Detsky, the presence of muscle wasting (the second element of the physical examination) is best assessed by examining the deltoid muscles (located

Figure 10.2 **Subcutaneous tissue loss from the arm and chest wall.**

Figure 10.3
Loss of subcutaneous tissue can be clearly seen in the hand on the left, compared with the hand of a healthy person on the right.

at the sides of the shoulders) and the quadriceps femoris muscles (the muscles of the anterior thigh).[4,5] Loss of subcutaneous fat in the shoulders and deltoid muscle wasting gives the shoulders a squared-off appearance, similar to that shown in Figure 10.4. These areas can be assessed as being normal or mildly, moderately, or severely wasted.

The presence of edema at the ankle or sacrum can also be assessed as absent, mild, moderate, or severe. The presence of "pitting" edema can be checked by momentarily pressing the area with a finger and then looking for a persistent depression (more than 5 seconds) where the finger was. Ankle edema and ascites can be assessed as absent, mild, moderate, or severe. When considerable edema or ascites are present, weight loss is a less important variable.

Figure 10.4

The squared-off appearance of the shoulders indicates the loss of subcutaneous tissue and wasting of the deltoid muscle.

The final step in SGA is arriving at a rating of nutritional assessment. Instead of an explicit numerical weighting scheme SGA depends on the clinician's subjectively combining the various elements to arrive at an overall, or global, assessment. Patients with weight loss > 10% that is continuing, poor dietary intake, and severe loss of subcutaneous fat and muscle wasting fall within

the severely malnourished category (class C rank). Patients with at least a 5% weight loss, reduced dietary intake, and mild to moderate loss of subcutaneous fat and muscle wasting fall within the moderately malnourished category (class B rank). Patients are generally ranked as well nourished when they have had a recent improvement in appetite or the other historical features of SGA. A class A rank would be given to patients having a recent increase in weight (that is not fluid retention), even if their net loss for the past 6 months was between 5% and 10%. Using this approach, very few well-nourished patients are classified as malnourished, but some patients with mild malnutrition may be missed.[4,5]

Despite this subjective nature, clinicians (nurses and residents) trained to use SGA tend to arrive at very similar rankings when comparing their evaluations of a series of 109 patients.[4] The method has also been shown to be a powerful predictor of postoperative complications.[5]

PROTEIN-ENERGY MALNUTRITION

Clinical Signs

In its most severe states, protein-energy malnutrition (PEM) takes the form of kwashiorkor or marasmus (also discussed in Chapter 9). Kwashiorkor is predominantly a protein deficiency, whereas marasmus is mainly an energy deficiency.[6] Kwashiorkor (Figure 10.5) is characterized by a relatively normal weight, generally intact skeletal musculature, and decreased concentrations of serum proteins.[6–8] A common feature

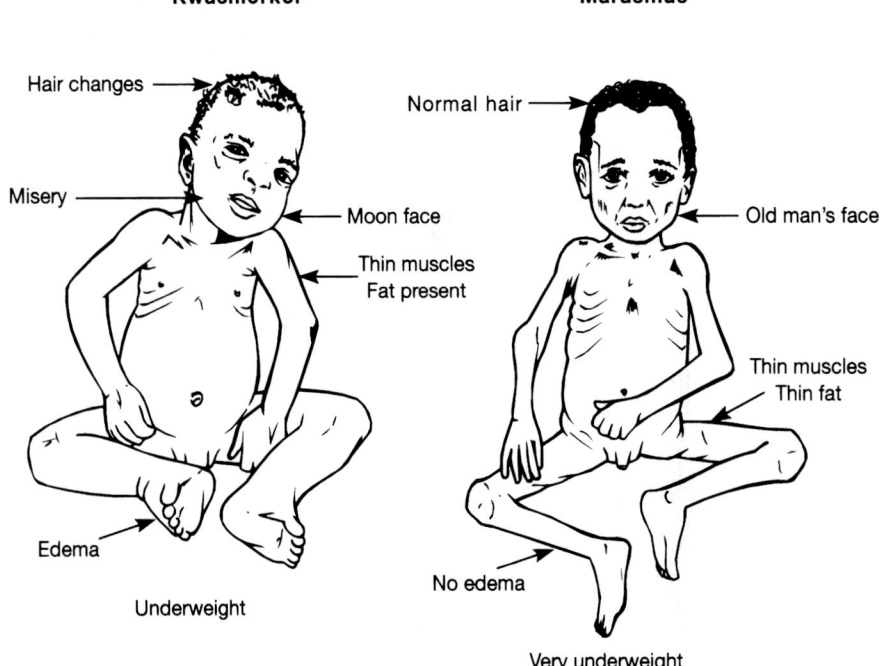

Figure 10.5 Differences in clinical signs between kwashiorkor and marasmus.

Source: Adapted from Jellife DB. 1968. *Clinical nutrition in developing countries.* Washington, DC: U.S. Department of Health, Education, and Welfare.

is soft, pitting, painless edema in the feet and legs, extending into the perineum, upper extremities, and face in severe cases. The hair can become dry, brittle, dull, and easily pulled out without pain. The marasmic patient typically presents with significant loss of body weight, skeletal muscle, and adipose tissue mass but with serum protein concentrations relatively intact. Patients are often seen at 60% or less of their expected weight for height, and marasmic children have a marked reduction in their longitudinal growth. Patients are described as having a "skin and bones" appearance. General characteristics of kwashiorkor and marasmus are outlined in Table 10.3.

Although such obvious cases of kwashiorkor and marasmus as illustrated in Figure 10.5 will not often be seen in developed countries, severe cases of protein-energy malnutrition and wasting still occur, especially as a result of AIDS, certain cancers, some gastrointestinal diseases, and alcoholism and other instances of substance abuse. The emaciated condition of the body and general ill health resulting from these and other diseases is also called *cachexia.* Many patients presenting with protein-energy malnutrition and wasting will have diagnostic features in common with either marasmus or kwashiorkor. For example, Figure 10.6 illustrates a case of severe protein-energy malnutrition having several diagnostic features common to marasmus. When this 29-year-old male presented for treatment (A and B), he had lost considerable skeletal muscle, adipose tissue, and body weight. There was no edema present. The wasting is particularly apparent in the neck, shoulders, and upper arm in A and B. After 3 months of nutritional support (C and D), there was an obvious increase in skeletal muscle, adipose tissue, and body weight. The face became fuller and there was considerably less wasting apparent in the neck, shoulders, and upper arm.

A   B

C   D

Figure 10.6 Marasmic-like severe protein-energy malnutrition in a 29-year-old male before treatment (A and B) and after 3 months of nutritional support (C and D).

TABLE 10.3	Characteristics of Kwashiorkor and Marasmus	
Variable	**Kwashiorkor**	**Marasmus**
Skeletal muscle	No major losses	Significant losses
Serum proteins	Significantly decreased	Relatively normal
Adipose tissue	Preserved	Significant loss
Body weight	Relatively normal	Significant loss
Edema	Pitting edema common	Absent
Predisposing factors	Ample energy with little or no protein	Starvation, lack of both protein and total energy

Data from McLaren DS. 1992. *A colour atlas and text of diet-related disorders,* 2nd ed. London: Mosby Europe; Torun B, Chew F. 1999. Protein-energy malnutrition. In Shils ME, Olson JA, Shike M, Ross AC, eds. *Modern nutrition in health and disease,* 9th ed. Baltimore, MD: Williams & Wilkins; Phinney SD. 1981. The assessment of protein nutrition in the hospitalized patient. *Clinics in Laboratory Medicine* 1:767–774.

An example of severe protein-energy malnutrition is illustrated in Figure 10.7. As is the case with kwashiorkor, edema can be clearly seen, especially in the legs and feet of this 46-year-old male (A and B). Some wasting can also be seen in the neck, shoulders, and upper arms. After 3 months of treatment (C and D), there was a fuller appearance to the face, neck, shoulders, and upper arms and no apparent edema.

Other clinical signs of PEM include the "flag sign" and growth failure. In the flag sign, there are alternating bands of depigmented and normal-colored hair produced by alternating periods of poor and relatively good protein intake. Hair grown during periods of poor protein intake can become depigmented and turn a dull brown, red, or even yellowish white. Hair grown during periods of more adequate protein intake returns to its normal color. The flag sign is especially noticeable in persons with long, dark-colored hair. An example of the flag sign is shown Figure 10.8.

Growth failure (or failure to thrive) is the most common sign of malnutrition in children. It is a failure to gain weight and height at the expected rate. Growth failure

A   B

C   D

Figure 10.7 **Kwashiorkor-like protein-energy
malnutrition in a 46-year-old male before treatment (A and
B) and after 3 months of nutritional support (C and D).**

Figure 10.8
The flag sign is characterized by bands of depigmented
hair that grew during periods of inadequate protein
intake. The normally colored hair grew during periods
of relatively adequate protein intake.

can result from one or any combination of factors, such
as inadequate nutrient intake, nutrient malabsorption,
failure to utilize nutrients, increased nutrient losses, and
increased nutrient requirements. Major contributing factors to growth failure include poverty, inadequate emotional and social nurturing, and infections, especially par-
asitic gut infestations. Figure 10.9 illustrates growth
failure. The ages of the children in this picture are, from
left to right, 2, 4.5, and 5.5 years. The child on the left
and the child in the center are of normal size for their age.
However, the child on the right has a markedly reduced
height for age and weight for age, although his weight-to-
height ratio is normal and there appear to be no other
signs of clinical malnutrition. Although he is 3.5 years
older than the child on the left, he is less than 5 cm taller.

Classifying Protein-Energy Malnutrition

The severity of PEM in children and adolescents can be
classified using records of age and measurements of
weight and height or length.[6] From these, weight for
height (or length) and height for age can be calculated.
Weight for height is a convenient index of current
nutritional status, while height for age better represents
past nutritional status. In this context of classifying the
severity of PEM, *wasting* has been suggested as a term
for a deficit in weight for height, and the term *stunting*
has been suggested for a deficit in height for age.
Patients with PEM can be placed in one of four categories: normal; wasted but not stunted (indicating acute
PEM); wasted and stunted (indicating acute and
chronic PEM); or stunted but not wasted (indicating
past PEM with adequate nutrition at present).[6] The
severity of wasting can be determined by calculating
weight as a percentage of the reference median weight
for height using the following equation:

$$\% \text{ weight for height} = \frac{\text{Actual body weight}}{\text{Reference weight for height}} \times 100$$

where reference weight for height = the median (or 50th
percentile) weight for height for the subject's age and
sex. To determine the severity of stunting, calculate the
height as a percentage of the reference height for age
using the following equation:

$$\% \text{ height for age} = \frac{\text{Actual height or length}}{\text{Reference height for age}} \times 100$$

Figure 10.9
An example of growth failure can be seen in the
child to the right, who is 5.5 years old and yet no
more than 5 cm taller than the child on the left,
who is 2 years old. The child in the middle is
4.5 years old. Less than expected height for age
(stunting) is the most common evidence of chronic,
mild PEM.

TABLE 10.4	Reference Values for Classifying Deficits in Weight for Height and Height for Age[*]

Classification	Weight for Height[†] (Deficit = Wasting)	Height for Age[†] (Deficit = Stunting)
Normal	90% to 110%	95% to 105%
Mild deficit	80% to 89%	90% to 94%
Moderate deficit	70% to 79%	85% to 89%
Severe deficit	< 70% or with edema	< 85%

Adapted from Torun B, Chew F. 1999. Protein-energy malnutrition. In Shils ME,
Olson JA, Shike M, Ross AC, eds. *Modern nutrition in health and disease*, 9th
ed. Baltimore, MD: Williams & Wilkins

[*]Reference values for classifying the severity of deficits in weight for height
(wasting) are derived using the percentage of reference median weight for height,
and deficits in height for age (stunting) are derived using the percentage of
reference median height for age. Median weight for height and median height for
age are derived from the NCHS growth charts (see Chapter 6).

[†]Percentage calculated from equations discussed in the text.

where reference height for age = the median (or 50th
percentile) height for the subject's age and sex. The values derived from these equations can then be compared
with the reference values shown in Table 10.4 to classify
the severity of wasting or stunting.

A simple approach to assessing the severity of
PEM in an adult is to compare his or her body mass
index (kg/m^2) (see Chapter 6) with the reference values
shown in Table 10.5. The table also gives values for
determining the presence of PEM in adolescents but
does not allow the severity of PEM in this age group to
be assessed.[9] These values can be used for either males
or females.

HIV INFECTION

Nutritional alterations are common in persons infected with
the human immunodeficiency virus (HIV), the recognized
cause of acquired immune deficiency syndrome, or AIDS.
Before the development of the protease inhibitor drugs for
treating HIV infection, a common feature of patients with
AIDS was PEM characterized by marked weight loss and
depletion of body cell mass, a condition known as HIV
wasting syndrome.[10,11] During this "pre-protease inhibitor
era," more than 60% of HIV-positive patients presented
with PEM, and, in roughly 80% of deaths attributed to

AIDS, protein-energy malnutrition was considered a concurrent cause of death.[12] Since AIDS was first recognized in
1981, remarkable progress has been made in developing
antiretroviral agents for treating HIV infection and AIDS.
These drugs have improved the quality and duration of life
of HIV-infected persons in the industrialized world and
have led to decreased incidence of the severe malnutrition
characteristic of HIV wasting syndrome, although altered
body fat distribution and metabolic alterations are still common in these HIV patients.[10,11]

HIV wasting syndrome is typically characterized
by the disproportionate loss of lean body mass and
muscle wasting with relative preservation of fat mass.
The U.S. Centers for Disease Control and Prevention's
definition of HIV wasting syndrome is shown in
Box 10.3. Wasting is of considerable concern because
it is associated with increased morbidity in people with

TABLE 10.5	Reference Values for Classifying the Severity of Protein-Energy Malnutrition (PEM) in Adult Males and Females and the Presence of PEM in Adolescent Males and Females

Subject Age	Body Mass Index	PEM
18 years and older	< 16.0	Severe
	16.0–16.9	Moderate
	17.0–18.4	Mild
	≥ 18.5	Normal
14–17 years	< 16.5	Present
11–13 years	< 15.0	Present

Adapted from Torun B, Chew F. 1999. Protein-energy malnutrition. In Shils ME,
Olson JA, Shike M, Ross AC, eds. *Modern nutrition in health and disease*, 9th
ed. Baltimore, MD: Williams & Wilkins.

Box 10.3 **HIV Wasting Syndrome as Defined by the U.S. Centers for Disease Control and Prevention**

1. Involuntary weight loss of more than 10% of weight
2. Chronic diarrhea (at least two loose stools a day for 30 days or more) or chronic weakness
3. Constant or intermittent fever for 30 days or more
4. Absence of a condition or an illness other than HIV infection that might cause symptoms

From Kurtzweil P. 1995. Warding off HIV wasting syndrome. *FDA Consumer* 29(3):16–20.

AIDS.[10–13] It results in physical impairment, psychologic stress, decreased tolerance of therapeutic agents, increased susceptibility to infection, and overall diminished quality of life. The known adverse effects of malnutrition on immune function also suggest that wasting may independently affect the progression of AIDS. Prevention of HIV wasting and preservation of body weight (both adipose tissue and lean tissue mass) may enhance survival, enhance physical and social functioning, and enrich the quality of life of people with AIDS.[10,11] Although HIV wasting is a multifactorial condition, the causes can be categorized under three general headings: decreased food intake, increased nutrient requirements, and nutrient malabsorption. These are outlined in Table 10.6.

With the introduction of protease inhibitors in 1996 and even newer antiretroviral therapies in more recent years, the number of patients dying from AIDS in developed countries has decreased by 67%, the prognosis of HIV-infected patients in these countries has dramatically improved, and HIV wasting syndrome is no longer the AIDS terminal phase.[12] Despite these dramatic improvements, some people with AIDS experience marked changes in body fat distribution and certain metabolic alterations, such as hyperlipidemia, insulin resistance, and diabetes mellitus.[12,14] These changes in body fat distribution include fat accumulation in the abdominal region (truncal and visceral obesity), in the axillary pads (bilateral symmetric lipomatosis), and in the dorsocervical pads at the posterior base of the neck (referred to by

TABLE 10.6 | **Causes of and Contributing Factors for HIV Wasting Syndrome**

Causes	Contributing Factors
Decreased Food Intake	
Loss of appetite	Nausea, vomiting, medications, altered taste; anorexia caused by the effects of cytokines, such as tissue necrosis factor, interleukin-1, and interferon; the presence of undigested micronutrients in ileum and colon may also depress appetite
Difficulty chewing and swallowing	Mouth and throat sores from Kaposi's sarcoma and opportunistic infections, such as candidiasis and herpes simplex; esophageal ulcers of viral, mycobacterial, and neoplastic origin; neurologic disease
Decreased interest in eating	Depression, ostracism, isolation, loneliness
Inability to prepare meals	Lack of access to food, poverty, profound weakness, AIDS-induced dementia
Increased Nutrient Requirements	
Hypermetabolism	Resting metabolic rate is generally increased in persons with AIDS unless severe wasting is present; loss of adipose tissue and negative nitrogen balance are exacerbated by near-normal serum levels of the thyroid hormone triiodothyronine (T_3) that ordinarily fall below normal in the presence of malnutrition and wasting
Fever	Opportunistic infections of viral, mycobacterial, and neoplastic origin
Nutrient Malabsorption	
Diarrhea	Occurs in > 50% of persons with AIDS; many cases apparently caused by protozoal infections
Inflammation of bowel mucosa	Protozoal infections (cryptosporidiosis and microsporidiosis) appear to result in malabsorption apart from diarrhea; deficiency of lactase and disaccharidase activity seen; HIV alone may affect the structure and function of the small bowel

Data from Oster MH, Enders SR, Samuels SJ, Cone LA, Hooton TM, Browder HP, Flynn NM. 1994. Megestrol acetate in patients with AIDS and cachexia. *Annals of Internal Medicine* 121:400–408; Von Roenn JH, Armstrong D, Kotler DP, Cohn DL, Klimas NG, Tchekmedyian NS, Cone L, Brennan PJ, Weitzman SA. 1994. Megestrol acetate in patients with AIDS-related cachexia. *Annals of Internal Medicine* 121:393–399; Hecker LM, Kotler DP. 1990. Malnutrition in patients with AIDS. *Nutrition Reviews* 48:393–401; Singer P, Katz DP, Dillon L, Kirvelä O, Lazarus T, Askanazi J. 1992. Nutritional aspects of the acquired immunodeficiency syndrome. *American Journal of Gastroenterology* 87:265–273.

Figure 10.10 **Increased adiposity in the dorsocervical fat pads of a patient receiving protease inhibitor therapy for AIDS.** This is referred to by some as "buffalo hump" or "bull neck" and is one of the alterations in body fat distribution seen in AIDS patients presenting with lipodystrophy syndrome.

Source: Reproduced with permission of *Canadian Journal of Plastic Surgery.* 1999; 7:129–131.

some as "buffalo hump" or "bull neck") and loss of fat in the arms, legs, and nasolabial and cheek pads (peripheral lipodystrophy).[12] An example of increased adiposity in the dorsocervical pads of a patient receiving protease inhibitor therapy for AIDS is shown in Figure 10.10. It appears that these alterations in body fat distribution are due, at least in part, to certain metabolic changes brought about by the multiple drugs used to treat HIV infection.[12,14,15] The so-called buffalo hump is also a clinical feature of Cushing's syndrome, a combination of symptoms and signs resulting from a persistent elevation of serum glucocorticosteroids. Unlike the loss of facial fat seen in patients presenting with peripheral lipodystrophy, a characteristic feature of Cushing's syndrome is a fullness or roundness of the face, which is referred to as "moon face."

EATING DISORDERS

Anorexia nervosa and bulimia nervosa are conditions in which a disturbance in eating behavior is seen. Both have clinical signs aiding in their diagnosis. Anorexia nervosa is characterized by a refusal to maintain a min-

imally normal body weight, an intense fear of gaining weight that is not alleviated by losing weight, and a distorted perception of body shape or size in which a person feels overweight (either globally or in certain body areas) despite being markedly underweight.[16] The American Psychiatric Association's diagnostic criteria for anorexia nervosa are shown in Box 10.4. A prominent clinical feature of persons with anorexia nervosa is marked weight loss, which in some instances can become extreme and life threatening. Figure 10.11 gives an example of the severe wasting commonly seen in persons with anorexia nervosa.

Bulimia nervosa is characterized by episodes of binging (eating unusually large amounts of food in a discrete period of time), followed by some behavior to prevent weight gain, such as purging (usually self-induced vomiting but also including misuse of laxatives, diuretics, enemas, or other medications), fasting, or excessive exercise.[16,17] The American Psychiatric Association's diagnostic criteria for bulimia nervosa are shown in Box 10.5. Persons with bulimia nervosa are usually within the normal weight range, although some may be slightly underweight or overweight. Recurrent vomiting may erode the teeth, especially the lingual surfaces of the

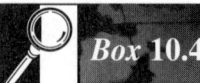

Box 10.4 **The American Psychiatric Association's Diagnostic Criteria for Anorexia Nervosa**

A. Refusal to maintain body weight at or above a minimally normal weight for age and height (e.g., weight loss leading to maintenance of body weight less than 85% of that expected or failure to make expected weight gain during period of growth, leading to body weight less than 85% of that expected)

B. Intense fear of gaining weight or becoming fat, even though underweight

C. Disturbance in the way in which one's body weight or shape is experienced, undue influence of body weight or shape on self-evaluation, or denial of the seriousness of the current low body weight

D. In postmenarcheal females, amenorrhea—i.e., the absence of at least three consecutive menstrual cycles

(a woman is considered to have amenorrhea if her periods occur only following hormone administration—e.g., estrogen)

TYPES OF ANOREXIA NERVOSA

Restricting type: During the current episode of anorexia nervosa, the person has not regularly engaged in binge-eating or purging behavior (i.e., self-induced vomiting or the misuse of laxatives, diuretics, or enemas).

Binge-eating/purging type: During the current episode of anorexia nervosa, the person has regularly engaged in binge-eating or purging behavior (i.e., self-induced vomiting or the misuse of laxatives, diuretics, or enemas).

From American Psychiatric Association. 2000. *Diagnostic and Statistical Manual of Mental Disorders,* 4th ed., text revision. Washington, DC: American Psychiatric Association.

front teeth, and increase the incidence of dental caries. An example of dental erosion in an 18-year-old female who had, from age 15 years, used vomiting as a purging method is shown in Figure 10.12. There may also be noticeable enlargement of the salivary glands, particularly the parotid glands. An example of asymmetrical hypertrophy of the parotid gland in a 20-year-old female who developed bulimia nervosa at age 17 years is shown in Figure 10.13.

A third category of disordered eating recognized by the American Psychiatric Association is called eating disorder not otherwise specified. This category is for eating disorders that fail to meet the criteria for either anorexia nervosa or bulimia nervosa.[16,17] Examples of disordered eating that fall under this category are outlined in Box 10.6.

MINI NUTRITIONAL ASSESSMENT

The Mini Nutritional Assessment (MNA) is a nutritional screening instrument using data that are relatively easy to obtain.[18,19] The MNA, shown in Figure 10.14, is designed to provide primary care health professionals with a single tool to efficiently identify elderly patients at nutritional risk who may subsequently need a more extensive nutritional assessment.[18] It is primarily intended for evaluating the so-called frail elderly—older persons exhibiting some kind of functional impairment, such as mobility, hearing, or cognitive disorders; those older persons living in nursing homes; and persons older than 85 living in the community. The instrument is also effective for screening the hospitalized elderly and those requiring surgery. It has been shown to be most useful at identifying persons at nutritional risk when included as part of a comprehensive assessment of an elderly person's cognition, independence, and mobility.[18] Approximately 10 to 15 minutes are needed to complete the instrument.[18,19] Most of the required information can be obtained from the physical examination and from a brief interview with the patient or someone knowledgeable about the

Figure 10.11 Severe wasting seen in a person with anorexia nervosa.

Box 10.5 | The American Psychiatric Association's Diagnostic Criteria for Bulimia Nervosa

A. Recurrent episodes of binge eating. An episode of binge eating is characterized by both of the following:
    (1) Eating, in a discrete period (e.g., within any 2-hour period), an amount of food that is definitely larger than most people would eat during a similar period of time and under similar circumstances
    (2) A sense of lack of control over eating during the episode (e.g., a feeling that one cannot stop eating or control what or how much one is eating)
B. Recurrent inappropriate compensatory behavior in order to prevent weight gain, such as self-induced vomiting; misuse of laxatives, diuretics, enemas, or other medications; fasting; or excessive exercise
C. The binge eating and inappropriate compensatory behaviors both occur, on average, at least twice a week for 3 months.

D. Self-evaluation is unduly influenced by body shape and weight.
E. The disturbance does not occur exclusively during episodes of anorexia nervosa.

TYPES OF BULIMIA NERVOSA

Purging type: During the current episode of bulimia nervosa, the person has regularly engaged in self-induced vomiting or the misuse of laxatives, diuretics, or enemas.

Nonpurging type: During the current episode of bulimia nervosa, the person has used other inappropriate compensatory behaviors, such as fasting or excessive exercise, but has not regularly engaged in self-induced vomiting or the misuse of laxatives, diuretics, or enemas.

From American Psychiatric Association. 2000. *Diagnostic and Statistical Manual of Mental Disorders,* 4th ed., text revision. Washington, DC: American Psychiatric Association.

patient's condition and dietary habits. In addition, some anthropometric data are necessary, including height and weight (for calculating body mass index), mid-arm circumference, and calf circumference.[18] The MNA was developed and thoroughly evaluated by researchers at Toulouse University Hospital, Toulouse, France; the University of New Mexico, Albuquerque; and the Nestlé Research Center in Lausanne, Switzerland.[18]

The MNA is completed by assigning points for each of the 18 items in the instrument, which are then summed to provide a "malnutrition indicator score." When the malnutrition indicator score is ≥ 24, the patient's nutritional status can be considered good, and

these patients should be given general dietary and lifestyle information about how to remain in good health. A patient whose malnutrition indicator score is < 17 is likely to be at high risk for protein-energy malnutrition and should be followed up with a comprehensive nutritional assessment. Those whose malnutrition indicator score is between 17 and 23.5 are at increased risk for malnutrition and should also receive further evaluation of their nutritional status. Research shows the MNA to be a practical, noninvasive, and cost-effective instrument for identifying elderly persons at risk for malnutrition.[20,21]

Figure 10.12 **Dental erosion in an 18-year-old female who had been vomiting to control her weight from the age of 15 years; note that her top incisors are markedly eroded.**

Figure 10.13 **Asymmetrical parotid gland enlargement in a 20-year-old female who developed bulimia nervosa at the age of 17 years; she was vomiting four times each day.**

Mini Nutritional Assessment
MNA®

Last name: _____ First name: _____ Sex: _____ Date: _____

Age: _____ Weight, kg: _____ Height, cm: _____ I.D. Number: _____

Complete the screen by filling in the boxes with the appropriate numbers.
Add the numbers for the screen. If score is 11 or less, continue with the assessment to gain a Malnutrition Indicator Score.

Screening

A Has food intake declined over the past 3 months due to loss of appetite, digestive problems, chewing or swallowing difficulties?
0 = severe loss of appetite
1 = moderate loss of appetite
2 = no loss of appetite ☐

B Weight loss during last months
0 = weight loss greater than 3 kg (6.6 lbs)
1 = does not know
2 = weight loss between 1 and 3 kg (2.2 and 6.6 lbs)
3 = no weight loss ☐

C Mobility
0 = bed or chair bound
1 = able to get out of bed/chair but does not go out
2 = goes out ☐

D Has suffered psychological stress or acute disease in the past 3 months
0 = yes   2 = no ☐

E Neuropsychological problems
0 = severe dementia or depression
1 = mild dementia
2 = no psychological problems ☐

F Body Mass Index (BMI) (weight in kg) / (height in m)^2
0 = BMI less than 19
1 = BMI 19 to less than 21
2 = BMI 21 to less than 23
3 = BMI 23 or greater ☐

Screening score (subtotal max. 14 points) ☐☐

12 points or greater	Normal – not at risk – no need to complete assessment
11 points or below	Possible malnutrition – continue assessment

Assessment

G Lives independently (not in a nursing home or hospital)
0 = no   1 = yes ☐

H Takes more than 3 prescription drugs per day
0 = yes   1 = no ☐

I Pressure sores or skin ulcers
0 = yes   1 = no ☐

J How many full meals does the patient eat daily?
0 = 1 meal
1 = 2 meals
2 = 3 meals ☐

K Selected consumption markers for protein intake
• At least one serving of dairy products (milk, cheese, yogurt) per day? yes ☐ no ☐
• Two or more serving of legumes or eggs per week? yes ☐ no ☐
• Meat, fish or poultry every day yes ☐ no ☐
0.0 = if 0 or 1 yes
0.5 = if 2 yes
1.0 = if 3 yes ☐.☐

L Consumes two or more servings of fruits or vegetables per day?
0 = no   1 = yes ☐

M How much fluid (water, juice, coffee, tea, milk...) is consumed per day?
0.0 = less than 3 cups
0.5 = 3 to 5 cups
1.0 = more than 5 cups ☐.☐

N Mode of feeding
0 = unable to eat without assistance
1 = self-fed with some difficulty
2 = self-fed without any problem ☐

O Self view of nutritional status
0 = view self as being malnourished
1 = is uncertain of nutritional state
2 = views self as having no nutritional problem ☐

P In comparison with other people of the same age, how do they consider their health status?
0.0 = not as good
0.5 = does not know
1.0 = as good
2.0 = better ☐.☐

Q Mid-arm circumference (MAC) in cm
0.0 = MAC less than 21
0.5 = MAC 21 to 22
1.0 = MAC 22 or greater ☐.☐

R Calf circumference (CC) in cm
0 = CC less than 31   1 = CC 31 or greater ☐

Assessment (max. 16 points) ☐☐.☐

Screening score ☐☐

Total Assessment (max. 30 points) ☐☐.☐

Malnutrition Indicator Score

17 to 23.5 points	at risk of malnutrition	☐
Less than 17 points	malnourished	☐

Ref.: Guigoz Y, Vellas B and Garry PJ. 1994. Mini Nutritional Assessment: A practical assessment tool for grading the nutritional state of elderly patients. *Facts and Research in Gerontology.* Supplement #2:15-59.
Rubenstein LZ, Harker J, Guigoz Y and Vellas B. Comprehensive Geriatric Assessment (CGA) and the MNA: An Overview of CGA, Nutritional Assessment, and Development of a Shortened Version of the MNA. In: "Mini Nutritional Assessment (MNA): Research and Practice in the Elderly". Vellas B, Garry PJ and Guigoz Y, editors. Nestlé Nutrition Workshop Series. Clinical & Performance Programme, vol. 1. Karger, Bâle, in press.
® Société des Produits Nestlé S.A., Vevey, Switzerland, Trademark Owners

08.98 USA

Figure 10.14 The Mini Nutritional Assessment.
This is designed to identify elderly persons at nutritional risk who would benefit from a more intensive assessment of nutritional status.

Source: Reprinted courtesy of Société des Produits Nestlé S.A.

Box 10.6 **Eating Disorder Not Otherwise Specified**

1. For females, all of the criteria for anorexia nervosa are met except that the individual has regular menses.
2. All of the criteria for anorexia nervosa are met except that, despite significant weight loss, the individual's current weight is in the normal range.
3. All of the criteria for bulimia nervosa are met except that the binge eating and inappropriate compensatory mechanisms occur at a frequency of less than twice a week or for a duration of less than 3 months.
4. The regular use of inappropriate compensatory behavior by an individual of normal body weight after eating small amounts of food (e.g., self-induced vomiting after the consumption of two cookies)
5. Repeatedly chewing and spitting out, but not swallowing, large amounts of food
6. Binge-eating disorder: recurrent episodes of binge eating in the absence of the regular use of inappropriate compensatory behaviors characteristic of bulimia nervosa

From American Psychiatric Association. 2000. *Diagnostic and Statistical Manual of Mental Disorders,* 4th ed., text revision. Washington, DC: American Psychiatric Association.

SUMMARY

1. The first step in the clinical assessment of nutritional status is obtaining a patient's history. This includes pertinent facts about past and current health and use of medications, as well as personal and household information. Sources include the patient's medical record and data obtained directly from the patient or those familiar with the patient.

2. A diet history is valuable in understanding a patient's nutritional status. This includes information about a patient's usual eating pattern, food likes and dislikes, and intolerances and allergies, as well as money available for purchasing food, ability to obtain and prepare food, eligibility for and access to food assistance programs, and use of vitamin, mineral, and other supplements.

3. Subjective Global Assessment is a clinical technique for assessing the nutritional status of a patient based on features of the patient's history and physical examination, rather than relying on more objective measures of nutritional status, such as anthropometric and biochemical data.

4. In severe PEM, the conditions known as kwashiorkor and marasmus are seen. Kwashiorkor is predominantly a protein deficiency characterized by a relatively normal weight, generally intact skeletal musculature, decreased concentrations of serum proteins, and edema. Marasmus is mainly an energy deficiency characterized by significant loss of body weight, skeletal muscle, and adipose tissue mass, but with serum protein concentrations relatively intact and no edema.

5. Severe cases of PEM and wasting can result from AIDS, certain cancers, some gastrointestinal diseases, and alcoholism and other drug abuse. The emaciation and general ill health seen in these diseases is sometimes called cachexia.

6. Growth failure and flag sign are two conditions seen in severe PEM. The flag sign is characterized by alternating bands of depigmented and normal-colored hair produced by alternating periods of poor and relatively good protein intake. Growth failure, a failure to gain weight and height at the expected rate, is the most common sign of malnutrition in children.

7. The severity of PEM in children and adolescents can be assessed by calculating weight as a percentage of reference median weight for height and by calculating height as a percentage of reference height for age. These two values can then be compared with published guidelines. The severity of PEM in an adult can be assessed by comparing body mass index (kg/m^2) with the reference values.

8. Prior to the development of protease inhibitors for treating HIV infection, HIV wasting was a common feature of patients with AIDS. Although advances in HIV/AIDS drug treatment have led to decreased incidence of HIV wasting syndrome, altered metabolism and body fat distribution remain common in HIV patients, particularly those treated with protease inhibitors. Metabolic alterations include hyperlipidemia, insulin resistance, and diabetes mellitus. Changes in body fat distribution include fat accumulation in the abdominal region (truncal and visceral obesity) and in the dorsocervical pads of the neck ("buffalo hump" or

"bull neck") and loss of fat in the arms, legs, and nasolabial and cheek pads (peripheral lipodystrophy).

9. Anorexia nervosa is characterized by a refusal to maintain a minimally normal body weight, an intense fear of gaining weight, and a distorted perception of body shape or size. Bulimia nervosa is characterized by episodes of bingeing, followed by some behavior to prevent weight gain, such as purging, fasting, or exercising excessively.

10. The Mini Nutritional Assessment is an 18-item questionnaire designed to identify elderly patients at nutritional risk who may subsequently need a more extensive nutritional assessment. Although some anthropometric data are required to complete the instrument, most of the necessary information is obtained from the physical examination and a brief patient interview. Completing the MNA yields a "malnutrition indicator score," used to classify the patient's nutritional status and to decide whether a more detailed evaluation of the patient's nutritional status is warranted.

REFERENCES

1. Corish CA, Kennedy NP. 2000. Protein-energy undernutrition in hospital in-patients. *British Journal of Nutrition* 83:575–591.

2. Hopkins B. 1993. Assessment of nutritional status. In Gottschlich MM, Matarese LE, Shronts EP, eds. *Nutrition support dietetics core curriculum,* 2nd ed. Silver Spring, MD: American Society for Parenteral and Enteral Nutrition.

3. Jeejeebhoy KN. 1994. Clinical and functional assessments. In Shils ME, Olson JA, Shike M, eds. *Modern nutrition in health and disease,* 8th ed. Philadelphia: Lea & Febiger.

4. Detsky AS, McLaughlin JR, Baker JP, Johnston N, Whittaker S, Mendelson RA, Jeejeebhoy KN. 1987. What is subjective global assessment of nutritional status? *Journal of Parenteral and Enteral Nutrition* 11:8–13.

5. Detsky AS, Smalley PS, Change J. 1994. Is this patient malnourished? *Journal of the American Medical Association* 271:54–58.

6. Torun B, Chew F. 1999. Protein-energy malnutrition. In Shils ME, Olson JA, Shike M, Ross AC, eds. *Modern nutrition in health and disease,* 9th ed. Baltimore, MD: Williams & Wilkins.

7. Phinney SD. 1981. The assessment of protein nutrition in the hospitalized patient. *Clinics in Laboratory Medicine* 1:767–774.

8. McLaren DS. 1992. *A colour atlas and text of diet-related disorders,* 2nd ed. London: Mosby Europe.

9. James WPT, Ferro-Luzzi A, Waterlow JC. 1988. Definition of chronic energy deficiency in adults. Report of a working party of the International Dietary Energy Consultative Group. *European Journal of Clinical Nutrition* 42:969–981.

10. Kotler DP. 2000. Nutritional alterations associated with HIV infection. *Journal of Acquired Immune Deficiency Syndromes* 25(suppl 1):S81–S87.

11. Corcoran C, Grinspoon S. 1999. Treatments for wasting in patients with the acquired immunodeficiency syndrome. *New England Journal of Medicine* 340:1740–1750.

12. Scevola D, DiMatteo A, Uberti F, Minoia G, Poletti F, Faga A. 2000. Reversal of cachexia in patients treated with potent antiretroviral therapy. *The AIDS Reader* 10:365–369.

13. Nemecheck PM, Polsky B, Gottlieb MS. 2000. Treatment guidelines for HIV-associated wasting. *Mayo Clinic Proceedings* 75:386–394.

14. Engleson ES, Kotler DP, Tan YX, Agin D, Wang J, Pierson RN, Heymsfield SB. 1999. Fat distribution in HIV-infected patients reporting truncal enlargement quantified by whole-body magnetic resonance imaging. *American Journal of Clinical Nutrition* 69:1162–1169.

15. Peters W, Phillips A. 1999. Buffalo hump and HIV-1 infection: Current concepts and treatment of a patient with the use of suction-assisted lipectomy. *Canadian Journal of Plastic Surgery* 7:129–131.

16. American Psychiatric Association. 2000. *Diagnostic and Statistical Manual of Mental Disorders,* 4th ed., text revision. Washington, DC: American Psychiatric Association.

17. American Psychiatric Association. 2000. *Practice guideline for the treatment of patients with eating disorders,* 2nd ed. Washington, DC: American Psychiatric Association.

18. Vellas B, Guigoz Y, Garry PJ, Nourhashemi F, Bennahum D, Lauque S, Albarede JL. 1999. The mini nutritional assessment (MNA) and its use in grading the nutritional state of elderly patients. *Nutrition* 15:116–122.

19. Guigoz Y, Vellas B, Garry PJ. 1996. Assessing the nutritional status of the elderly: The mini nutritional assessment as part of the geriatric evaluation. *Nutrition Reviews* 54(suppl):S59–S65.

20. Vellas B, Guigoz Y, Baumgartner M, Garry PJ, Lauque S, Albarede JL. 2000. Relationships between nutritional markers and the mini-nutritional assessment in 155 older persons. *Journal of the American Geriatrics Society* 48:1300–1309.

21. Rubenstein LZ, Harker JO, Salva A, Guigoz Y, Vellas B. 2001. Screening for undernutrition in geriatric practice: Developing the short-form mini-nutritional assessment (MNA-SF). *The Journals of Gerontology. Series A, Biological Sciences and Medical Sciences* 56:M366–M372.

ASSESSMENT ACTIVITY 10.1

Using Subjective Global Assessment

This assessment activity gives you an opportunity to practice using Subjective Global Assessment (SGA), a clinical technique for assessing nutritional status using data from a patient's history and physical examination, both of which can be found in a patient's medical record. Begin by making two photocopies of the SGA rating form found in Figure 10.1. Then, using the information from each of the following two cases, complete the chart and arrive at an SGA rating of each patient's nutritional status. You may find it helpful to review the section "Subjective Global Assessment," which explains SGA.

The following cases are straightforward; you and your classmates should arrive at the same rating for each case. However, because of the subjective nature of this approach, there may be an occasional instance when two or more health professionals do not arrive at the same rating of one patient's nutritional status. This should not detract from the usefulness of SGA because clinicians generally arrive at decisions by carefully evaluating the available evidence in light of professional knowledge and past experiences. Thus, health care is not only a science but also an art.

Case 1

A 73-year-old female is admitted to the hospital complaining of loss of appetite and rapid onset of satiety for 6 weeks. For the past 3 days, she has vomited practically all food and beverages consumed. She is ambulatory but has felt weak and has been unable to carry out her activities of daily living for the past 2 weeks. On physical examination, the woman looks somewhat wasted with moderate loss of subcutaneous tissue in the upper arms, shoulders, and thoracic regions. There is moderate edema in the ankles but no ascites present. For the past 10 years or so, her body weight has been stable at approximately 147 lb (66.8 kg). However, in the past 4 months or so, she has steadily lost weight. Her current weight is 123 lb (55.9 kg). Using SGA, how would you rate her nutritional status?

Case 2

A 61-year-old male is admitted to the hospital for resection of his sigmoid colon and rectum, following discovery of a mass in the sigmoid colon by his physician during a flexible sigmoidoscopy. The patient originally complained of bright red blood in his bowel movements. He reported no significant gastrointestinal symptoms other than the bleeding. He denies any change in his functional capacity. His maximum weight was 167 lb (75.9 kg) at age 46 years. In his late 40s, he lost about 15 lb (6.8 kg) and for the past 12 years has maintained his weight at about 152 lb (69.1 kg). Between 2 and 6 months before admission, his appetite was less than normal and he gradually lost 13 lb (5.9 kg). In the past 2 months before admission, his appetite improved and he gained 5 lb (2.3 kg). On physical examination, there is no evidence of subcutaneous tissue loss, muscle wasting, edema, or ascites.

11

COUNSELING THEORY AND TECHNIQUE

INTRODUCTION

Awareness of nutritional status and dietary practices obtained through nutritional assessment often is followed by attempts to change dietary practices. This chapter provides a brief introduction to several counseling theories that provide a variety of useful techniques for initiating and maintaining dietary change.

The purpose of this chapter is *not* to teach you how to be a therapist. It is intended to briefly introduce you to those theories that are most pertinent to nutritional counseling and to acquaint you with some fundamental approaches to counseling your clients. The most effective counselors are those who adapt techniques from several counseling theories to suit their needs and those of their individual clients. As you study this chapter, note the different counseling theories and techniques. Then, based on your professional judgment, use those techniques you feel are best suited to you and the needs of your clients.

Because communication lies at the foundation of interviewing and counseling, the first part of this chapter deals with fundamentals of communication theory and basic skills necessary for effective listening and interviewing. The chapter ends with a practical plan for initiating and maintaining dietary change.

Finally, as important as good nutrition is to health, do not lose sight of the fact that other practices, such as smoking and excessive alcohol use, have a profound impact on health. Cigarette smoking, for example, has been called the "leading cause of preventable death in the United States."[1] You should be a model of good health habits, not only those relating to diet but in all areas. By so doing, you will be most effective in helping your clients achieve better health.

COMMUNICATION

Communication is the process of sending and receiving messages. It lies at the foundation of all efforts to interview, counsel, educate, and change behavior. Although we all communicate (or at least attempt to) and have a basic idea of what it involves, communication is a complex process and is not easily defined. The simplified communication model in Figure 11.1 shows the major components of human communication: sender, receiver, message, and feedback.

The *sender* is the one initiating the communication, the first person to speak. The *message* is the communication. It contains components that are both verbal (what is spoken) and nonverbal (what is implied by the emotional tone of the sender's voice, facial expression, posture, diction, pronunciation, choice of words, dress, and the environment in which the communication occurs).[2] Verbal and nonverbal communication occur simultaneously. The *receiver* is the listener, the one to whom the message is sent. *Feedback* is the response the receiver gives to mes-

sages after interpreting them. Feedback distinguishes one-way communication from two-way communication.[2] The absence of feedback or making no provision for it will likely result in distorted communication because the sender is unable to determine how the message was received. As with the message, feedback is both verbal and nonverbal.

Interference is anything adversely affecting transmission or interpretation of the message. It can arise from the environment or the emotional or physiologic state of either the sender or the receiver. Noise, lack of privacy, interruptions, an office that is too hot or too cold, and uncomfortable seating are examples of environmental factors that may cause interference. Emotional factors leading to interference include fear of disease or death, loneliness, grief, prejudice, and bias. Physiologic factors such as pain, deficits of hearing or vision, and difficulty in speaking can often be sources of interference.

Verbal Communication

Dietary counseling generally involves some type of behavioral change on the receiver's part. The receiver may perceive attempts to change lifelong habits or practices he or she enjoys as a potential threat. Thus, the receiver may become defensive, which interferes with good communication. The receiver's defensive reactions can be prevented or minimized through the use of the guidelines to supportive communication outlined in Box 11.1 and the following paragraphs. The more supportive communication is, the less the receiver perceives it as a threat and the more he or she is able to concentrate on the structure, content, and meaning of the message.[2,3]

Describe behavior rather than evaluate it. Discussing a client's behavior in a judgmental or evaluative way will likely cause the client to become defensive. The client will then be thinking of ways to defend himself or herself rather than concentrating on the counselor's message. Evaluating or judging behavior can lead to an argument. Instead, the counselor can present the facts or seek information in objective, nonjudgmental ways that do not imply guilt or ask the client to change his or her behavior.

For example, in an attempt to raise awareness of the seriousness of the problem at hand, a counselor may accuse a client with poorly controlled diabetes of being

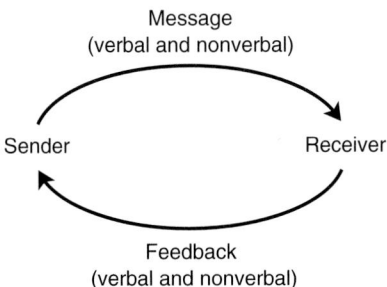

Message
(verbal and nonverbal)

Sender   Receiver

Feedback
(verbal and nonverbal)

Figure 11.1
A communication model.

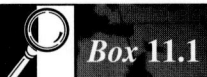

Box 11.1   Guidelines to More Supportive Communication

Description rather than evaluation   Empathy rather than neutrality
Problem orientation rather than manipulation   Provisionalism rather than certainty
Equality rather than superiority

From Gibb JR. 1982. Defensive communication. *Journal of Nursing Administration* 12:14–17.

"irresponsible" or "committing suicide." A better approach would be to objectively discuss the client's blood sugar levels and nonjudgmentally discuss factors that may be affecting them.

Use problem orientation rather than manipulation. Much of our speech is an attempt to persuade others to alter their behavior, attitudes, or activities. Often, when we want people to see things our way, we lead them through a series of questions until they arrive at the "correct conclusion." This is a form of manipulation and implies that the person being directed is inadequate or inferior. This is likely to result in a defensive response that interferes with communication. Problem orientation, on the other hand, is the antithesis of persuasion. The sender communicates a desire to work with the receiver in defining a mutual problem and seeking a workable solution. The sender implies that he or she has no prearranged answer or viewpoint and no hidden agenda to exert control over the receiver. Thus, the receiver arrives at his or her own conclusions and establishes goals and objectives to which there will be greater adherence.

Communicate equality rather than superiority. A sender can promote supportive communication by considering himself or herself a collaborator with or an equal to the receiver. When treated with respect and trust and involved in participative problem solving, the receiver will feel more obligated to the success of any agreed-on solution. If the sender communicates superiority, the receiver will likely become defensive. Although clients often need and appreciate the reassurance of a dietitian's nutritional expertise, dietitians should avoid urging a particular plan of action based primarily on their superior knowledge or ability.

Empathize rather than remain neutral. Communication conveying compassion and respect for others is supportive and defense-reducing. Particularly reassuring is a sender who identifies with the problems and shares in the feelings of the receiver. Communication conveying neutrality may indicate a lack of concern for the receiver's welfare. Attempts to reassure the receiver that he or she is overly anxious or need not feel rejected or bad deny the legitimacy of the receiver's emotions and suggest a lack of acceptance.

Be receptive rather than dogmatic. A willingness to hold one's own attitudes as provisional, to examine other ideas rather than take sides, and to solve problems rather than debate issues gives listeners a sense of participation in and control over the problem-solving process. On the other hand, persons who seem to know all the answers or who regard themselves as teachers rather than team players tend to put others on guard and stifle supportive communication.

Nonverbal Communication

As was shown in Figure 11.1, communication occurs simultaneously on two levels—verbal and nonverbal.

Sometimes referred to as *body language,* nonverbal communication in the form of gestures, posture, facial expressions, and tone of voice is sometimes a more reliable indicator of the client's feelings and attitudes than are his or her words.[4] Verbal communication is generally under conscious control and is subject to censorship. It can be used to persuade, mislead, or cover facts a client wishes to hide. Nonverbal communication, on the other hand, is not as easily controlled by conscious thought and often can be a more reliable indicator of a person's dominant emotions than are his or her words.[2,4] Lack of congruence, or agreement, between verbal and nonverbal communication can be an important indicator that a client is consciously or unconsciously omitting something.

Facial expressions are an important source of nonverbal communication. Sadness often can be seen in the face of a distressed client through a downturned mouth or quivering lip. Unusually prolonged and intense eye contact may indicate anger. Guilt, insecurity, or fear may be indicated by failure to maintain eye contact, especially when this occurs during discussion of a particularly sensitive topic.[4,5]

Posture may indicate a person's feelings. A client seated with arms relaxed at the sides and slightly slouched in the chair can communicate openness, whereas a client may communicate a distrustful, defensive attitude by sitting up very straight with arms tightly crossed over the chest. A client who leans away from the counselor or moves her chair to distance herself may indicate defensiveness or distrust. One leaning closer to the counselor may express a desire for greater intimacy.[4,6] Cultural differences exist in what is considered to be a comfortable distance between two communicating persons. In general, people from Latin cultures prefer being closer, whereas those from North America and parts of Europe favor a somewhat greater distance.[6]

The tone of voice is an important indicator, as well. A client asked about his diet may warmly and pleasantly respond, "It's going well," and mean just that. The same words uttered in a mechanistic and toneless way may indicate a problem with the diet.

Nonverbal communication also facilitates the dietitian's communication to clients. Appropriate eye contact, gestures, facial expressions, and posture assure the client of the dietitian's attention, interest, acceptance, and support. The astute dietitian should carefully note the client's nonverbal cues and their possible significance and use nonverbal communication to respond to the client in a supportive way.[2]

Effective Communication

Effective communication requires consideration of several factors. It is important that messages and feedback be transmitted in ways that are understandable to both sender and receiver. When talking with clients or providing instruction, health professionals should use understandable language and minimize use of medical terminology. Feedback should be encouraged, and the receiver should be given ample opportunity to ask questions and clarify any potential misunderstandings. Both sender and receiver should be aware of their nonverbal communication, so that it supports, rather than interferes with, effective communication.

The environment in which communication takes place should be comfortable, conducive to good communication, and as free as possible of interferences that can adversely affect communication. Adequate time for counseling and client instruction is necessary before clients can even begin to change lifelong habits and adopt new ones. Awareness of the client's abilities, concerns, and fears is also important to effective communication. The dietitian also should be aware of his or her own concerns and limitations and should avoid allowing these to interfere with the communication process.

Consider a dietitian seated at the bedside of a patient in whom diabetes has been recently diagnosed. The dietitian is giving the patient some last-minute instructions on the diabetic exchange system before the patient is discharged. Environmental interference can come from the roommate's television, interruptions from a nurse or physician, a phone call, or the arrival of a visitor. The patient's fear about having diabetes, concerns about being able to manage a new diet, worries about hospitalization costs, and thoughts about what the future holds may preoccupy her mind and interfere with the instruction. The dietitian also may be preoccupied with concerns of his own, such as other patients needing assessment and instruction, and these can interfere with the communication process. This is obviously not an ideal situation for communication or instruction, but, unfortunately, it is one commonly encountered in real life. Awareness of these and other impediments to good communication, however, is necessary before they can be addressed and effectively dealt with.

Listening

Communication is a two-way process. It involves not only *sending* messages but *receiving* them as well. Listening, therefore, is essential to the interviewing and counseling process. In some instances, the best help a counselor can give a client is to simply listen attentively and nonjudgmentally. It is also an excellent way to establish good rapport with a client.[5] As important as listening is, most of us are not very good at it.[6] Listening is a highly active process demanding concentration and attention. It involves six steps (Table 11.1).[6]

A number of misconceptions exist about listening.[6] For example, some people believe that *hearing* and *listening* are the same activity. Listening is a process involving much more than simply hearing sounds, such as

TABLE 11.1	The Six Steps of Listening

1. Hearing: Receiving sound waves by the ear
2. Attending: Mentally focusing on a specific sound
3. Understanding: Interpreting the message and assignment of meaning by the brain
4. Remembering: Storing the message for later use
5. Evaluating: Making an evaluative judgment about the message
6. Responding: Making a verbal and/or nonverbal response to the message

Samovar LA. 2000. *Oral communication: Speaking across cultures*, 11th ed. Los Angeles: Roxbury.

music or voices. It is mistakenly assumed that, when several people hear the same sound (for example, a person talking), they all receive the same message. Quite the opposite is true. Listening is a highly subjective experience, and the interpretations placed on what is heard can vary widely from person to person.

Some people believe that listening is a passive activity, when in reality it is an active process requiring concentration and specific skills that can be learned if one wants to be a better listener.[6–8] Listening skills can be grouped under four categories: openness, concentration, attention, and comprehension.[7]

Openness, or objectivity, involves a willingness to investigate new ideas and to interact with others with minimal internal distortion from personal prejudices. Openness does not necessarily mean acceptance or approval of another's ideas but simply a willingness to "hear a person out." It requires the listener to set aside his or her personal biases, which may interfere with effective listening.[5–7]

Concentration entails focusing the mind on what the speaker is saying. It is made easier when environmental distractions and interferences are minimized. Counseling should take place in a room that is quiet, comfortable, and private.

It is estimated that people with normal intelligence think about five times faster than they talk.[2] Thus, while listening to another person talk, our minds can simultaneously be thinking other things. Unfortunately, many people have allowed this to become a major barrier to effective listening. Rather than focusing the mind on critical and careful listening, we often take mental excursions ranging from thinking about the speaker's hair style to daydreaming.[6] A good listener uses this extra mental capacity to analyze and understand the speaker's verbal and nonverbal messages.

The counselor should indicate that the client has his or her full attention and acceptance by maintaining good eye contact with the client and having an empathic facial expression and relaxed posture. The counselor should give the client ample opportunity for expression without interruption while providing occasional, brief verbal and nonverbal responses indicating reception of the message. Appropriately timed nods or verbal responses such as "I understand" or "I see" will help assure the client of the counselor's attentive listening.

Comprehension involves not only attaching meaning to information but also correctly interpreting the meaning of the client's communication. The counselor's comprehension of the client's message can be enhanced through use of such techniques as reflection, paraphrasing, clarification, and probing.[7] Reflection is restating the affective, or emotional, part of the client's words. This gives the client an opportunity to hear what she has just said and to elaborate on her emotions. A client may say, "I feel depressed about my lack of progress." The affective part of this message is the statement "I feel depressed." In reflection, the counselor simply restates the client's words: "You say you feel depressed." This gives the client an opportunity to elaborate on her feelings.[7,9] In paraphrasing, the client's message is restated, or rephrased, in the counselor's own words. This helps ensure that the counselor has correctly interpreted the client's message. Clarification is simply asking the client to repeat or restate what was just said. Probing is asking the client to provide greater detail on some specific point. It is often used when collecting a 24-hour dietary recall.

INTERVIEWING

Interviewing can be defined as a guided communication process between two persons or parties with the predetermined purpose of obtaining or exchanging specific information through the asking and answering of questions.[2,8] The goal of the interview is obtaining specific information from the client while maintaining an interpersonal environment conducive to disclosure by the client.[2] Of the several types of interviews that exist, the nutrition counselor is primarily concerned with interviews to gather information from clients, give information to clients, and deal with client problems.[8]

Interviewing Skills

As in communication, there are several basic conditions or skills that increase a person's effectiveness as an interviewer. Among these are physical surroundings, freedom from interruption and interference, privacy, good rapport, attentiveness, openness, and the client's context.[2] Factors to consider in the physical surroundings are the comfort of both the client and the interviewer, the seating arrangement, the distance between the interviewer and client, and the presence of physical barriers separating them.

It is best to conduct an interview in a location free of interruptions and interferences. In an office setting, the counselor should arrange to have phone calls held. In a hospital, interviews should not be scheduled during the time of physicians' rounds, nursing or other care, or visiting hours. A convenient time should be arranged with nursing and other staff. When held in the patient's room, arrangements can be made with nursing staff to avoid unnecessary interruptions, the patient's door can be closed, televisions and radios can be turned down or off, and visitors can be kindly asked to step outside.[2,4,8] However, parents, spouses, partners, and siblings can be important sources of information about the patient. The counselor may want to have them present during the interview or available for questions later.

Early establishment of good rapport is essential to an effective interview. Establishing good client rapport will place the client at ease and make him or her more willing to share important information.[2] A counselor should begin the interview with a pleasant greeting. She should introduce herself and briefly give the reason for the interview. If the counselor is late, she should apologize for any inconvenience and explain why.[8]

Attentiveness, as in the context of listening, is also an important interviewing skill. Nonverbal and verbal expressions of attention, such as appropriate eye contact, posture, facial expressions, well-timed nods, or relevant verbal responses, will help assure the client of the counselor's interest and attention. Openness, or interviewer objectivity, as in listening, is an important interviewing skill.

The client's emotional context—his or her beliefs, attitudes, feelings, and values—is also an important consideration when interviewing. Fears about health, concerns about death, feelings of loneliness, or grief may preoccupy a client's thoughts and interfere with his or her ability to participate in the interview. Putting apprehensive clients at ease and allowing them to express their feelings can help alleviate their fears and facilitate the interviewing process.

Obtaining Information

Before the interview, the counselor should review the client's medical record for pertinent information. This provides the counselor with considerable background information on the client and allows the interview to be more directed and concise. Using the "funnel sequence" is suggested. This begins with more general, open questions and gradually narrows to more specific inquiries using closed questions.[8]

Open questions invite rather than demand answers and provide clients substantial freedom in determining the amount and type of information to give.[2,8] Open questions let the client talk and offer information that he or she feels is important. They are generally easy to answer and pose little threat to the client. They give the counselor the opportunity to listen and observe. However, they have the disadvantage of consuming large amounts of time if clients dwell on irrelevant information.[8] Examples of open questions are given in Box 11.2.

Closed questions, on the other hand, are restrictive; they allow the counselor to control answers and to ask for

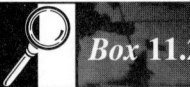

Box 11.2   Examples of Different Types of Questions

OPEN QUESTIONS

"Tell me about yourself."

"Tell me about your eating habits."

"What have you been doing to lower your blood cholesterol level?"

CLOSED QUESTIONS

"Do you smoke?"

"Do you salt your food at the table?"

"Do you eat chicken with or without the skin?"

NEUTRAL QUESTIONS

"What is the first thing you have to eat or drink after waking up in the morning?"

"What kind of milk do you drink?"

"How many times a week do you eat ice cream?"

LEADING QUESTIONS

"What do you eat for breakfast?"

"You don't use whole milk, do you?"

"Do you eat ice cream *every* evening?"

---

specific information. They often provide too little information and fail to reveal why a client has a particular attitude.[8] Examples of closed questions are given in Box 11.2.

Questions also can be classified as neutral or leading (Box 11.2).[8] *Neutral questions* allow the client to answer without pressure or direction from the counselor. In *leading questions,* the counselor makes implicit or explicit suggestions about the expected or desired answer. In answering leading questions, the client merely agrees with what the counselor is apparently suggesting. Counselors should avoid leading clients either by verbal or nonverbal means. When clients respond to their questions, counselors must avoid such expressions as surprise, agreement, disagreement, or disgust, which can suggest expected or desired answers.[2]

When information is sought from or provided to clients, counselors should use understandable language. Health care professionals often make the mistake of assuming that clients understand the technical language used daily in hospitals and other health care organizations. Or they assume that if a client does not understand something, he or she will simply ask what a word means. Many clients are so overwhelmed by the unfamiliar or intimidated by the authority of health care professionals that they fail to seek answers to their questions. Thus, a counselor should avoid using technical language with clients and should not assume that clients will understand medical terminology even if it is explained to them.

COUNSELING THEORIES

Several counseling theories and techniques have been developed and are currently in use today. The purpose of this section is not to teach you how to be a therapist; that takes considerable professional training and practice. Rather, the purpose is to briefly introduce you to those theories that are most pertinent to nutritional counseling and to acquaint you with some fundamental approaches to counseling your clients.

Each counseling theory discussed in the following pages has something of value to offer the dietetic practitioner. Each also has certain limitations or drawbacks. An awareness of these theories and an ability to adapt their more fundamental and benign counseling techniques to suit each unique counseling situation will greatly enhance your ability as a helping professional.

Person-Centered Approach

The person-centered approach to counseling is based primarily on the work of psychologist Carl Rogers.[10–12] Rogers taught that, if people could experience human relationships characterized by respect and trust, they would develop in a positive and constructive manner. He objected to the idea that people need to be instructed, punished, rewarded, and managed by others who are in a superior and "expert" position. He believed that people possess an innate ability to move away from maladjustment to psychologic health. The primary responsibility for this rests with the client, rather than with an authority who directs a passive client.[13]

Rogers advocated three qualities of counselors that create a growth-promoting climate in which persons advance to become what they are capable of becoming. These counselor qualities are genuineness, or realness; unconditional positive regard and acceptance of the client; and deep understanding of the client's feelings. According to Rogers, if a counselor communicates these attitudes, clients will become less defensive, more open to experiences within themselves and the world, and able to relate to others in social and constructive ways.[13] Rogers wrote, "If I can provide a certain type of relationship, the other person will discover within himself the capacity to use that relationship for growth and change, and personal development will occur."[10]

The client's personality change is brought about by the counselor's attitudes instead of by certain techniques, theories, or knowledge. The counselor's primary task is providing a therapeutic climate in which the client feels free to explore areas of his or her life that are currently distorted or denied to awareness. Within this climate, the client is then able to lose his or her "defenses and rigid perceptions and move to a higher level of personal functioning."[13]

The counselor's genuineness, or realness, is the congruence between what is expressed to the client and what is experienced within the counselor's mind. Through genuineness, the counselor serves as a model of a human struggling toward greater awareness and personal functioning.[13]

Unconditional positive regard and acceptance allow the client to be accepted as he or she is and to express feelings and attitudes without risk of losing the counselor's acceptance. Although the client's *feelings* are accepted, not all *overt behavior* is approved or accepted. According to Rogers, the greater the counselor's degree of positive regard and acceptance of the client, the greater will be the success of therapy.[13]

As the counselor develops a deep understanding of the client's feelings and experiences, he or she is able to sense the client's feelings as if they were his or her own. This permits the counselor to expand the client's awareness and understanding of these feelings and to help the client resolve internal conflicts and become more the person the client wishes to become.[13]

The person-centered approach has the advantage of being a safer approach to counseling than other models that place the counselor in a directive position of making interpretations, forming diagnoses, and attempting more drastic personality changes. Its core skills of listening, understanding, caring, and acceptance are needed by all counselors. No matter what counseling approach they use, counselors lacking in these core skills will not be effective in carrying out their treatment. These skills are also valuable for others in the helping professions. Although people in crisis do not necessarily need answers, they do need someone willing to really listen, care, and understand and on whom they can unload their feelings and experiences without fear of rejection. The presence of a caring, listening, understanding person can do much to promote healing.[13]

Counselors using the person-centered approach have been criticized for merely giving support to clients without challenging them. Rogers has suggested, therefore, that counselors include more "caring confrontations." Counselors using caring confrontation are more active in suggesting topics for exploration, interpreting behavior, helping clients set goals, and giving advice.[13]

Behavior Modification

Behavior modification (also known as behavior therapy) attempts to alter previously learned human behavior or to encourage the development of new behavior through a variety of action-oriented methods, as opposed to changing feelings or thoughts.[2,13–15] A major premise of behavior modification is that "all behavior, normal or abnor-

mal, is acquired and maintained according to certain definable principles."[16] Behaviors resulting in positive consequences tend to be repeated, and those behaviors not followed by favorable consequences tend not to be repeated.[15]

Early, or "radical," behaviorists viewed human behavior as almost totally the result of positive reinforcements (the addition of something, such as praise or money, as a consequence of behavior) or negative reinforcements (the removal of unpleasant stimuli once a certain behavior is performed). Currently, behaviorists view humans as both the *product* of environmental influences and the *producer* of their environment. Early behaviorists viewed humans as lacking freedom and self-determination. Modern behaviorists, on the other hand, acknowledge the presence of freedom and self-determination. They attempt to increase clients' freedom and control by assisting them in overcoming crippling behaviors and becoming freer to choose from options that were previously not available to them.[13]

Antecedents and Consequences

Behaviorists view actions as being preceded by antecedents and followed by consequences.[14,17] For example, eating is generally preceded by some antecedent or stimulus, such as smelling or seeing food, coming home from work or school, sitting down to study or watch television, seeing an advertisement for food on television or in a magazine, or experiencing anxiety, boredom, or loneliness. Behavior modification holds that, when antecedents to behaviors are recognized, they can be modified or controlled to decrease the occurrence of negative behaviors and increase the occurrence of positive behaviors. This is referred to as stimulus control. Examples of stimulus control include eating before grocery shopping, preparing a shopping list and purchasing only the items on the list, storing food out of sight, and avoiding the purchase of ready-to-eat foods.

Consequences reinforce the behavior they follow. They may be positive, negative, or neutral. When consequences are positive, behavior is more likely to be repeated. Behavior followed by negative consequences is less likely to be repeated. The delicious tastes and feelings of satiety accompanying a meal are examples of positive consequences that reinforce, or reward, the practice of eating. Behaviorists also believe that positive consequences are more effective in promoting behavioral change than are negative consequences.[14]

Self-monitoring

A valuable behavior modification technique is self-monitoring, or recordkeeping—the careful observation and accurate recording of the behavior to be controlled.[13,16,18] If the behavior is eating, for example, clients carefully observe their eating and record its occurrence, along with comments about relevant antecedents and consequences related to their eating. Self-monitoring has several functions:[18]

- It provides information about eating habits and the factors influencing them.
- It involves clients in observing and analyzing their dietary habits.
- It increases clients' awareness of their diets and behavior as it happens.
- It gives the counselor and client something to review objectively and impartially. For example, they focus on specific problem behaviors in the record, not in the client.
- It increases the clients' skills in manipulating their diets to achieve desired results (for example, finding suitable low-fat entrees to replace others that are high in total fat and saturated fat or finding acceptable low-calorie snack foods to replace high-calorie snacks).
- It increases counselor-client interaction.
- It allows client and counselor to monitor behavior over time and track client progress.

Various forms have been developed for self-monitoring.[18] One example is shown in Appendix U. In general, forms for self-monitoring eating behavior should allow the recording of such information as the food eaten, how food was prepared, the amount eaten, where and when the food was eaten, what happened or how the client felt before eating, what happened or how the client felt after eating, and whether the food was eaten alone or with someone else and with whom.

For monitoring behaviors related to a specific goal (for example, substitution of high-calorie snacks with low-calorie snacks), the client can record the day, time, type of snack eaten, and amount eaten on a pocket-sized card, which he or she can carry.

To be successful, the self-monitoring method ought to be easy to use, convenient, and readily available when the behavior occurs; be clearly understood by the client; be relevant to the dietary problem; and be used for observational purposes rather than to judge the problem.

Goals and Self-contracts

Behaviorists believe that feelings result from behavior.[13,15] Consequently, the focus of attention in counseling is changing behavior, not altering feelings or delving into past experiences. Goals are of central importance in behavior modification and are expressed in terms of altering overt behavior in ways that are both specific and measurable. Therefore, the goals of therapy must be clear, specific, measurable, attainable, and agreed on by both the client and the counselor. The client selects counseling goals at the beginning of the counseling process.

For example, a client may want to decrease his elevated total cholesterol level to less than 200 mg/dL. Having been taught by the counselor that total cholesterol

levels are related to saturated fat intake, the client, with the counselor's assistance, may decide to use soft tub margarine instead of butter at home and to remove the skin from chicken before eating it. The client's progress then can be evaluated objectively in terms of goal attainment and other measurable ways. For example, the client's self-monitoring records can demonstrate adherence to the goals, and measurements of total serum cholesterol may indicate overall progress in lowering serum cholesterol.

Once goals are identified, the counselor can help the client write a self-contract. This is an agreement the client enters into with himself or herself to help build commitment to the goal for change.[15,17,18] The contract should clearly state the goal in terms of a specific time frame and detail the reward for successfully achieving the goal. As an option, it may state the punishment, if any, for not reaching the goal. An example of a self-contract is shown in Figure 11.2.

Modeling

In addition to believing that learning occurs through positive or negative reinforcements, behaviorists hold that people learn through the process of modeling.[13,14,17,18] Also known as observational learning or imitation, modeling is "the process by which the behavior of an individual or a group (the model) acts as a stimulus for similar thoughts, attitudes, and behaviors on the part of observers."[13] Through modeling, clients develop new behaviors without trial-and-error learning. Clients, for

Figure 11.2 **A self-contract.**

example, can learn new behaviors by observing the success of other group members or through others' success stories shared by the counselor.[14]

Modeling can take place by observing a live model (for example, counselors demonstrate the behavior they hope clients will acquire), symbolic models (the client observes the desired behavior performed on videotape or film), or multiple models (new skills are learned as successful peers within the group demonstrate the desired behavior).[13] Modeling is more likely to be successful when the model is similar to the client in age, sex, race, and attitudes than when the model is unlike the client. The likelihood that behaviors will be imitated by clients is increased when models are competent in performing the behavior, exhibit warmth, and possess a realistic degree of prestige and status.

Reinforcers

According to behavior modification, behavior is maintained and strengthened when followed by positive reinforcers.[13,16,17] Thus, a positive reinforcer is any consequence that maintains and strengthens behavior by its presence; in other words, the positive reinforcer makes the behavior more likely to recur.[17] A negative reinforcer is an unpleasant consequence that maintains and strengthens behavior by its being removed from the situation.[17] Reinforcers are often referred to as rewards. Rewards that are effective in reinforcing behavior can take many forms and vary from client to client.

If rewards are used, the counselor must identify rewards likely to effectively reinforce desired behaviors and set up a reinforcement system. As an example, consider a client on a weight control program. The counselor and client can set up a system that allows the client to receive a reward for having lost a certain amount of weight. The weight loss goal may be set rather low to make it easily attainable at the beginning of counseling. As counseling progresses and the client develops skill in managing his behavior, successive goals can be somewhat more difficult to attain. Rewards can include money or material items (an amount of money or a certain purchase for each goal reached), activities (doing something the client especially enjoys each time a goal is reached), or social interaction (visiting someone special or making a phone call when a goal is attained).[14,17] Examples of rewards are shown in Box 11.3.

Behavior Modification Techniques Summarized

Behavior modification uses a number of techniques. The major ones employed in weight management are outlined in Table 11.2.[16] Some of these techniques were not originally developed by behaviorists but were adapted from other approaches or disciplines and incorporated into behavior modification programs to increase the success of behavioral change. Among these are nutrition education, physical activity, and cognitive restructuring. Cognitive restructuring will be discussed in the section "Rational-Emotive Therapy."

Behavior modification has contributed a variety of specific behavioral techniques to nutritional counseling and the treatment of diet-related problems. Its emphasis on changing problem behaviors rather than merely talking about problems and gathering insights allows counselors to focus on assisting clients in formulating a specific plan of action. However, in its attempt to deal with problem solving and the changing of certain behaviors, it has been criticized for deemphasizing the role of feelings and emotions in counseling.[13]

Rational-Emotive Therapy

Unlike behavior modification, which primarily focuses on the relationship between our environment and behavior, rational-emotive therapy (RET) deals with the effects that our thoughts have on our behavior.[2] The major premise of RET is that emotional disturbances are largely the product of irrational thinking.[13] RET holds that our emotions are mainly the product of our beliefs, evaluations, interpretations, and reactions to life situations.[13]

RET views humans as having the potential for both rational thinking and irrational thinking. It views humans as engaging in considerable self-talk and self-evaluation, much of which is irrational and self-denigrating and can result in emotional disturbances. Rather than factors outside of ourselves being the main determinants of behavior, RET holds that our irrational beliefs about ourselves primarily determine our behavior, emotions, and the resulting consequences. In other words, people "are disturbed not by things, but by the view which they take of them."[13] Thus, RET focuses on disputing irrational beliefs and helping people change the irrational beliefs that directly result in disturbed emotions and dysfunctional behavior.[13]

| **Box 11.3** | **Examples of Rewards Used in Behavior Modification** |

Spending money on appropriate things
Reading a book
Watching television
Making a long-distance call

Taking an afternoon or day off
Visiting a friend
Spending time at a favorite hobby
Relaxing or taking a nap

TABLE 11.2 | Examples of Behavior Modification Techniques Used in Weight Control Programs

Stimulus Control

Shopping

Shop for food after eating.
Shop from a list.
Avoid ready-to-eat foods.
Do not carry more cash than needed for shopping.

Plans

Plan to limit food intake.
Substitute exercise for snacking.
Eat meals and snacks at scheduled times.
Do not accept food offered by others.

Activities

Store food out of sight.
Eat all food in the same place.
Remove food from inappropriate storage areas in the house.
Keep serving dishes off the table.
Use smaller dishes and utensils.
Avoid being the food server.
Leave the table immediately after eating.
Do not save leftovers.

Holidays and Parties

Drink fewer alcoholic beverages.
Plan eating habits before parties.
Eat a low-calorie snack before parties.
Practice polite ways to decline food.
Do not get discouraged by an occasional setback.

Eating Behavior

Put the fork down between mouthfuls.
Chew thoroughly before swallowing.
Prepare foods one portion at a time.
Leave some food on the plate.
Pause in the middle of the meal.
Do nothing else while eating (read, watch television).
Solicit help from family and friends.
Have family and friends provide help in the form of praise and material reward.
Use self-monitoring records as basis for rewards.
Plan specific rewards for specific behaviors (behavioral contracts).

Self-monitoring

Keep diet diary that includes time and place of eating, type and amount of food, who is present, and how you feel.

Nutrition Education

Use diet diary to identify problem areas.
Make small changes that you can continue.
Learn nutritional values of foods.
Decrease fat intake; increase intake of complex carbohydrates.

Physical Activity

Routine activity: increase routine activity, increase use of stairs, and keep record of distance walked daily.
Exercise: begin a very mild exercise program, keep a record of daily exercise, and increase the exercise very gradually.

Cognitive Restructuring

Avoid setting unreasonable goals.
Think about progress, not shortcomings.
Avoid imperatives, such as "always" and "never."
Counter negative thoughts with rational statements.
Set weight goals.

From Stunkard AJ, Berthold HC. 1985. What is behavior therapy? A very short description of behavioral weight control. *American Journal of Clinical Nutrition* 41:821–823.

A client's self-talk can be viewed as positive, neutral, or negative. Positive self-talk supports behavioral change, whereas negative self-talk opposes change. Consider a client beginning a weight management program. An example of positive self-talk is the client's silently observing, "I'm going to like this program." Negative self-talk is the thought "I don't think I can handle this" or "I'm no good at dieting; I'll never succeed at this program." According to RET, the likelihood of successful behavioral change is considerably less when people view themselves as failing, as compared with when they see themselves succeeding. In addition, persons viewing themselves as failing at weight management are less likely to begin addressing their behavioral problems, and, when faced with difficult challenges (for example, the urging of friends to eat fattening food at a party), they are more likely to slip from their program and to give it up altogether.[13,14]

Although our irrational beliefs may have begun through early indoctrination by our parents or significant others ("You're never going to amount to anything!"), it is primarily our own repetition of these irrational thoughts that keeps these dysfunctional attitudes alive and operative within us. Thus, RET teaches that we are largely responsible for creating our own problems, that we have the ability to change, that we must identify our irrational beliefs, and that we must dispute these irrational beliefs using the process of cognitive restructuring.[13]

The first step in cognitive restructuring is becoming aware of negative self-talk.[2,13,19,20] One approach is asking the client to record his or her irrational and destructive internal messages on a form similar to the one shown in Table 11.3.[20] Once an irrational internal message is identified, it can be disputed by substituting it with a rational, self-defensive statement. This can also be recorded on the form shown in Table 10.6.

Clients can be led to dispute their irrational self-talk and beliefs by encouraging them to ask such questions as "What is the factual evidence in support of my thoughts?" "Why do I assume I am a rotten person because of the way I behave?" "Would it really be catastrophic if my worst fears were to come true?" and "What can I say in defense of myself?"[13,19] As clients learn to recognize and dispute their irrational self-criticisms, they then can be encouraged to substitute negative self-talk with positive, self-affirming statements.

Other RET techniques include the changing of one's language, cognitive rehearsal, and thought stopping.[2,13,17,19,20] An example of changing one's language is avoiding negative self-fulfilling statements ("I will fail, I will look like a pig, and no one will like me"). People telling themselves that they will fail may actually increase the probability of failure. Cognitive rehearsal (also known as rational-emotive imagery) involves clients' thinking, feeling, and behaving the way they would like to in real life. As clients see themselves overcoming in their thoughts, the likelihood of them overcoming in real life is increased. Thought stopping is a two-step process. First, whenever a negative thought enters the client's mind, he or she says, "Stop!" either out loud or very clearly within the mind. This is followed by substituting a positive, rational thought for the negative, irrational thought. Again, the basis of these exercises is that our language (either audible or silent) influences our thoughts, which in turn influence our emotions and behavior.

Reality Therapy

The central premises of reality therapy are that individuals are responsible for their behavior and that, if a person's current behavior is not meeting his or her needs, steps can be taken to change behavior so that personal needs are met.[13,21] Reality therapy is based primarily on the work of psychiatrist William Glasser, who abandoned traditional psychoanalysis early in his career and went on to develop his own counseling approach. According to Glasser, every person's behavior is an attempt to fulfill his or her basic human needs. "It is always what we want at the time that causes our behavior."[22] According to

TABLE 11.3	Identifying and Disputing Irrational and Destructive Thoughts
Irrational Thought	**Rational, Self-defensive Statement**
"I can't believe I ate six of those cookies! I've blown it. Oh well, I may as well go ahead and finish the rest of the bag."	"I *did* slip by eating those six cookies, but I *did not* blow my program. The best thing for me to do now is to stop eating them. I *can* do better."
"I ate half a bag of potato chips! I'm an absolute failure."	"My success or failure at anything is not based on one incident. I'm human. It's okay to make mistakes once in awhile. I don't have to be perfect."
"The way she's looking at me, she must think my idea is stupid."	"I can't read other people's minds. The way to find out what she thinks is to just ask. Besides, not everyone has to like my idea."

Glasser, rather than being determined by outside forces (as is taught by behaviorists), behavior is completely driven from within the person by the necessity to fulfill five innate needs: survival, love, power, fun, and freedom.[22] "All of our lives we must attempt to live in a way that will best satisfy one or more of these needs."[22]

Glasser teaches that each of us creates our own inner world from which we view the world outside of ourselves. Each person is responsible for the kind of inner world he or she creates. Instead of external factors depressing or angering us, we anger or depress ourselves. "Neurotic" and "psychotic" behavior does not just happen to us; it is something we choose in an attempt to control our world. If a client complains of anxiety, the counselor may ask what behavior is causing the anxiety. The focus is not on the anxiety but on whatever behavior is causing the anxiety. According to Glasser, once people acknowledge and act on the reality that their behavior is the result of their choices, change occurs.[13]

Reality therapy begins by the counselor's establishing an accepting and supportive relationship with the client. The client is then led to examine and evaluate his own behavior to determine if it is contributing to his problems. Once the client acknowledges he is not getting what he wants from his behavior, the counselor helps the client develop an action plan for changing his behavior so that it contributes to his success. The plan should have goals that are simple, specific, clear, and attainable and that involve something the client will do soon and on a daily basis. The counselor then helps the client make a commitment to follow through with the plan and to refuse to give up. The counselor makes it clear to the client that he will neither accept excuses nor use punishment to coerce the client.

Many people tend to blame other individuals or circumstances for their problems. Reality therapy asserts that people are responsible for their own behavior and attacks the excuses many people make for their actions in an attempt to evade responsibility.[23] A client who runs to the refrigerator every time she feels anxious, for example, may benefit from acknowledging that her behavior does not depend on an outside stimulus (in this case, the "anxiety") but on her own conscious choice. The client should be helped to recognize that she has a variety of options for dealing with her anxiety. Then, under the guidance of a counselor, the client can select from her options and develop a plan to deal with her problematic behavior in positive ways.[23]

INITIATING AND MAINTAINING DIETARY CHANGE: A PRACTICAL PLAN

A number of counselor characteristics and behavioral change techniques can be identified. These characteristics and techniques are effective in initiating and maintaining nutrition behavior, but their use does not guarantee success. Each nutrition counselor will want to integrate them into a total program with which he or she feels comfortable. The counselor will also want to consider clients' needs, resources, and social support, as well as the skill level of support staff.

No single counseling approach can be recommended for all clients. Rather, counselors are encouraged to use an eclectic approach—that is, one composed of elements drawn from a variety of approaches. An effective behavioral change program would selectively incorporate several techniques into a multicomponent program that is suitable to both the counselor and the client. However, it is neither necessary nor wise to use all the counseling techniques at one's disposal.

Motivation

No counselor can motivate a client. Motivation comes only from within the client. A counselor can only create a climate that will help clients motivate themselves. People tend to be motivated by challenge, growth, achievement, promotion, and recognition. Emphasis should be placed on providing a proper environment for self-growth by challenging clients, giving them responsibility and encouragement, and giving full range to individual strength.

Characteristics of Effective Counselors

From this discussion of counseling theories, it is possible to identify several characteristics of effective counselors. By practicing good communication, listening, and counseling skills, one of the first steps in initiating behavioral change can take place—establishing good rapport with the client. The following are characteristics of effective counselors:

- Empathy—the ability to climb into the world of the client and communicate back feelings of understanding
- Respect—a deep and genuine appreciation for the worth of a client, separate and apart from his or her behavior; the strength and ability of the client to overcome and adjust is appreciated
- Warmth—communication of concern and appropriate affection
- Genuineness—being freely and deeply oneself; one is congruent and not just playing a role
- Concreteness—essential ideas and elements are ferreted out
- Self-disclosure—information about self is revealed for the benefit of the client at the appropriate time
- Potency and self-actualization—one is dynamic, is in command, conveys feelings of trust and warmth, is competent, is inner-directed, is creative, is

sensitive, is nonjudgmental, is productive, is serene, and is satisfied; this comes across to the client in a helpful way.[24]

Initial Assessment

The initial assessment of the client serves several important functions:

- It makes the counselor and client aware of the client's dietary habits and health history, as well as related factors.
- It provides baseline information from which to gauge progress.
- It alerts the counselor and client to the various demands being placed on the client, so that realistic priorities can be set.
- It gives the counselor and client ideas for making dietary changes.
- It gives the counselor an opportunity to develop rapport and a sense of partnership with the client.
- It enables the counselor to develop a plan of gradual change suitable to the client's way of living.[18]

As discussed in Chapters 3 and 8, a variety of techniques can be used for obtaining dietary information. In addition to these data, however, information should be collected on the client's current health status, health history, and past and present health habits.

Initiating Dietary Change

Counselors and clients should have reasonable expectations about what changes should be undertaken, the extent of change, and the rate at which change is made. Clients should be carefully guided in what benefits they can reasonably expect from dietary change and the amount of change necessary to realize those benefits.[18,25,26]

Goals can be set by the client under the guidance of the counselor. Goals should be specific, measurable, reasonable, and attainable. Whatever the final behavioral goal is, most people will not be able to master it at the first effort or in one step. Behavioral change should be approached gradually, with a number of small, easily attained goals that collectively lead to the final goal. A client can never begin too low and the steps upward can never be too small.[17] Short-term goals spanning 1 to 2 weeks are more effective than long-term goals covering months.[25] Because obstacles and setbacks will be encountered, goals should have some flexibility. One approach to building a client's commitment to attaining goals can be through a written self-contract.

Reinforcers, or rewards, can help promote maintenance of behavioral change, especially at the beginning of a program. If they are used, counselors will need to work with each client (and possibly with a key individual providing social support for the client) to identify rein-

forcers providing ample incentive to goal attainment. At this time, the use of other behavior modification strategies (review Table 10.5) can be discussed with the client. Serious consideration should be given to using stimulus control, self-monitoring, and cognitive restructuring in ways suitable to both counselor and client.

Maintaining Dietary Change

Although counselors can assist clients in making dietary changes (for example, in learning about nutrition, setting realistic goals, and managing the antecedents to behaviors), it is ultimately the client's responsibility to change dietary habits. To be permanently successful, clients will need to be guided toward self-sufficiency.[18]

A key element in self-sufficiency is the client's involvement in the change process.[18] The client should be asked, "What changes can *you* make?" "What can *you* say when someone offers you another serving of dessert?" "What steps can *you* take to avoid overeating at a party?" The more the client "owns" the program, the more successful he or she will be at maintaining dietary change.

Four areas where counselors can help clients increase self-control over eating habits are maintenance of commitment, recordkeeping, environmental restructuring, and use of rewards.[18] At first, most clients are enthusiastic about behavioral change. After several days or weeks, however, this enthusiasm begins to wane. Some suggestions for strengthening commitment to dietary change include the following:

- Praise the client for his or her successful experiences and attribute success to the client's abilities.
- Encourage the client to tell family members and friends about his or her dietary goals. After making a public commitment to dietary change, adherence to the program is more likely.
- Ask the client to state the kinds of problems he or she will likely encounter. Problems will occur, but they will be less likely to derail the client's progress when they are anticipated and planned for.
- Concentrate on foods the client can eat, rather than those to be avoided. Help clients realize that healthy eating is not synonymous with deprivation.[18]

Recordkeeping provides information on the client's performance, aids the client in observing and analyzing his or her environment, and helps in recognizing the antecedents to eating behavior. Recordkeeping can range from marking a 3×5-inch card every time a between-meal snack is declined to keeping elaborate food records.[18]

Some researchers think that restructuring the environment is the most important technique in maintaining change. Counselors can ask clients to identify specific changes that can be made in their physical, social, and cognitive (mental) environments to promote long-term dietary change.

A client may associate an event—such as sitting in a favorite chair, reading the newspaper or watching television—with eating high-calorie foods. The presence of inappropriate foods at home also can be a deterrent to successful change. Altering the arrangement of furniture in the room where television is watched or the newspaper is read can help promote and maintain change. Purchasing healthful foods to substitute for inappropriate items can be helpful as well.

The counselor should ask the client to identify social situations that promote poor eating habits. How is the client's eating behavior affected by various social functions or what family and friends say to the client? The counselor should explore with the client ways that social interactions can be supportive of dietary change. What could family and friends say to promote the client's success? Through role playing, the client can develop skill in asking for support from others.[18] In dealing with the mental environment, the client should be encouraged to use some of the cognitive restructuring techniques discussed in the "Rational-Emotive Therapy" section.

Relapse Prevention

For the purposes of behavioral change, a relapse can be defined as the resumption of an unwanted habit or behavior that one has, for a period of time, overcome or turned from.[17,27] Consider a man with the habit of eating a half-pint of premium butter-pecan ice cream every evening. For several weeks he has limited himself to only 1 cup of nonfat frozen dessert four evenings a week. When he returns to 2 cups of butter-pecan ice cream every evening for several weeks, he has relapsed. However, if he merely indulges once or twice in butter-pecan ice cream while spending a weekend with relatives and then returns to 1 cup of the nonfat variety four evenings a week, he has only experienced a lapse. A lapse can be defined as "a single event, a reemergence of a previous habit, which may or may not lead to a state of relapse."[26] Thus, a lapse is a temporary fall, a slip, or a mistake. When a lapse occurs, corrective action can be taken to prevent a relapse—a total loss of control—from occurring.[26]

A key to relapse prevention is to prepare clients for the occurrence of lapses and to help them cope in ways that prevent a relapse.[25] If counselors and clients have previously discussed the likelihood of lapses' occurring, clients will be better prepared when they do occur, and the risk of lapses' leading to full-blown relapses will be minimized. Clients should be taught to anticipate situa-

tions likely to produce lapses, such as illness, travel, live-in visitors, overwork, emotional distress, and schedule changes.[25]

Counselors should help clients view lapses for what they really are—merely a temporary fall. A counselor and client can discuss what corrective actions the client can take to recover from the lapse and to prevent a relapse from occurring. Techniques such as modeling, role playing, cognitive rehearsal, and direct instruction can help in this.[2] A client needs to be assured that, if a relapse does occur, it is not the end of the world. The client has suffered a setback, but prompt action can limit the lapse to a temporary setback.

KNOWING ONE'S LIMITS

When working with clients, it is important that counselors know the limits of their abilities to help people and when they need to refer a client to more experienced help. Emotional problems are common, and from time to time nutrition counselors encounter individuals needing psychologic counseling. If a client indicates that she is having emotional problems, a nutrition counselor may very gently and tactfully ask if she would like assistance in getting psychologic counseling from a local mental health clinic or professional. The counselor may help her in calling and making an appointment with an appropriate agency or person.[13,25]

Some individuals may not be ready or willing to change certain habits. Circumstances in a person's life may not be conducive to change at the particular time he is seeing a counselor. It may be necessary to suggest that a client postpone weight loss or control of mildly elevated serum cholesterol until *after* he deals with a more pressing problem, such as separation, divorce, bankruptcy, or substance abuse.

This chapter has offered a very brief overview of dietary counseling. It is meant to be only an introduction to the topic. Readers interested in developing the skill of nutritional counseling are encouraged to take coursework and to study other sources for further information. Other excellent resources include the following:

Bauer KD, Sokolik CA. 2002. *Basic nutrition counseling skill development.* Belmont, CA: Wadsworth/Thomson Learning.

Holli BB, Calabrese RJ. 1998. *Communication and education skills for dietetics professionals,* 3rd ed. Baltimore, MD: Williams & Wilkins.

Watson DL, Tharp RG. 2002. *Self-directed behavior: Self-modification for personal adjustment,* 8th ed. Belmont, CA: Wadsworth/Thomson Learning.

SUMMARY

1. Communication, the process of sending and receiving messages, lies at the foundation of all efforts to interview, counsel, educate, and change diet. The basic components of human communication are the sender, receiver, message, feedback, and interference.

2. A counselor's attempts to help bring about dietary change may elicit a defensive reaction from the receiver or client. When this occurs, the receiver fails to concentrate on the structure, content, and meaning of the message. This is one source of interference to communication. When communication is supportive of the receiver, this defensive reaction can be prevented, and the interference to communication can be minimized.

3. Communication occurs simultaneously at both the verbal and nonverbal levels. Nonverbal communication involves gestures, posture, facial expressions, and tone of voice. It is sometimes a more reliable indicator of a person's true feelings than are words. Unlike verbal communication, which is generally under conscious control and subject to censorship, nonverbal communication is not as easily controlled by conscious thought. It is also an effective way for the counselor to communicate to the client.

4. Effective communication is promoted by proper use of feedback, language that is understandable to both counselor and client, an environment that is conducive to good communication, and awareness of the physical and psychologic barriers to communication.

5. Listening is an important part of interviewing and counseling and an excellent way to establish rapport. Despite its importance, most people are not good listeners. Listening involves six steps: hearing, attending, understanding, remembering, evaluating, and responding.

6. Rather than being a passive activity, listening is a highly active process demanding concentration and attention. It is also a skill that can be learned. Listening skills can be grouped under four categories: openness, concentration, attention, and comprehension.

7. Interviewing is a guided communication process between two persons for the purpose of obtaining or exchanging specific information through the asking and answering of questions. The goal of the interview is obtaining specific information from the client while maintaining an interpersonal environment conducive to disclosure by the client. Conditions that increase interviewing effectiveness include comfortable physical surroundings, freedom from interruption and interference, and privacy. Counselor qualities that contribute to a successful interview include the ability to establish good rapport, attentiveness, openness, and an understanding of the client's situation.

8. Several types of questions can be used in the interview. Open questions invite rather than demand answers and give the client substantial freedom in determining the amount and type of information to give. Closed questions are restrictive and allow the counselor to control answers and ask for specific information. Neutral questions allow the client to answer without pressure or direction from the counselor. Leading questions contain implicit or explicit suggestions about the expected or desired answer.

9. The person-centered approach to counseling is largely based on the idea that, if people experience human relationships characterized by respect and trust, they will develop in a positive and constructive manner. Three counselor qualities that create a growth-promoting climate for the client are genuineness, or realness; unconditional positive regard and acceptance of the client; and deep understanding of the client's feelings. Within this climate, the client is then able to lose his or her "defenses and rigid perceptions and move to a higher level of personal functioning."[10]

10. The main contribution of person-centered therapy is its core skills: listening, understanding, caring, and acceptance. Regardless of the approach used, counselors deficient in these skills will lack efficiency in carrying out their treatment. The presence of a caring, listening, understanding person can do much to promote healing in a person experiencing a crisis.

11. Behavior modification attempts to alter previously learned human behavior or encourage the learning of new behavior through a variety of action-oriented methods, as opposed to changing feelings or thoughts. Although early behaviorists viewed human behavior as almost totally the result of reinforcements, modern behaviorists view humans as both the product of environmental influences and the producer of their environment.

12. Behaviorists view actions as being preceded by antecedents and followed by consequences. The modification or control of antecedents to decrease the occurrence of negative behaviors and increase the occurrence of positive behaviors is referred to as stimulus control. Other techniques of behavior modification include self-monitoring, or recordkeeping; modeling; cognitive restructuring;

education; physical activity; and the use of goals, self-contracts, and reinforcers.

13. The major premise of rational-emotive therapy (RET) is that emotional disturbances are largely the product of irrational thinking. RET holds that our emotions are mainly the product of our beliefs, evaluations, interpretations, and reactions to life situations. Rather than factors outside of ourselves being the main determinants of behavior, RET holds that our irrational beliefs about ourselves primarily determine our behavior, emotions, and the resulting consequences.

14. A major technique of RET is cognitive restructuring, which focuses on helping people dispute their irrational beliefs and change the thoughts that directly result in disturbed emotions and dysfunctional behavior. RET also uses such techniques as cognitive rehearsal and thought stopping.

15. Reality therapy views every person's behavior as an attempt to fulfill his or her basic human needs. Reality therapy views behavior as being driven not by outside forces but from within the person by the necessity to fulfill the need for survival, love, power, fun, and freedom. Each individual is responsible for his or her behavior, and, if current behavior is not meeting a person's needs, he or she can take steps to change behavior so that personal needs are met.

16. In reality therapy, the counselor begins by establishing an accepting and supportive relationship with a client. The client is then led to examine and evaluate his behavior to determine if it is contributing to his problems. Once the client acknowledges he is not getting what he wants from his behavior, the counselor helps the client develop an action plan for changing his behavior, so that it contributes to his success.

17. No single counseling approach can be recommended for all clients. Counselors are encouraged to use an eclectic approach—one composed of elements drawn from a variety of methods. An effective behavioral change program would selectively incorporate several techniques into a multicomponent program that is suitable to both the counselor and the client.

18. In addition to having good communication and listening skills, effective counselors convey empathy, respect, warmth, genuineness, concreteness, openness, potency, and self-actualization.

19. It is important for counselors and clients to have reasonable expectations about what changes should be undertaken, the extent of change, and the rate at which change is made. Goals set by the client under the guidance of the counselor should be specific, measurable, reasonable, and attainable. Behavioral change will be more successful when achieved through a number of small steps. Short-term goals spanning 1 to 2 weeks are more effective than long-term goals covering months.

20. If rewards are used, counselors will need to work with each client to identify those providing ample incentive to goal attainment. Serious consideration also should be given to using stimulus control, self-monitoring, and cognitive restructuring in ways suitable to both counselor and client.

21. It is ultimately the client's responsibility to change dietary habits. To be permanently successful, clients need to be guided toward self-sufficiency. Four areas where counselors can help clients develop self-sufficiency in dietary change are maintenance of commitment, recordkeeping, environmental restructuring, and use of reinforcers.

22. A relapse can be defined as the resumption of an unwanted habit or behavior that one has, for a period of time, overcome or turned from. A lapse can be defined as a temporary fall, or a reemergence of a previous habit, which may or may not lead to a state of relapse. Counselors should prepare clients for the occurrence of lapses and help them cope in ways that will prevent a relapse. Clients should be taught to anticipate situations likely to produce lapses, such as illness, travel, live-in visitors, overwork, emotional distress, and schedule changes.

23. Counselors should know the limits of their abilities and when they need to refer clients needing psychologic counseling to more experienced help. Some individuals may not be ready or willing to change certain habits. It may be necessary to suggest that a client postpone dietary change until after his or her more pressing problems have been resolved.

REFERENCES

1. Office on Smoking and Health. 2001. *Women and smoking: A report of the surgeon general—2001.* Rockville, MD: U.S. Centers for Disease Control and Prevention, U.S. Department of Health and Human Services.

2. Holli BB, Calabrese RJ. 1998. *Communication and education skills for dietetics professionals,* 3rd ed.

Baltimore, MD: Williams & Wilkins.

3. Gibb JR. 1982. Defensive communication. *Journal of Nursing Administration* 12:14–17.

4. Bauer KD, Sokolik CA. 2002. *Basic nutrition counseling skill development.* Belmont, CA: Wadsworth/Thomson Learning.

5. Curry KR, Jaffe A. 1998. *Nutrition counseling and communication skills.* Philadelphia: Saunders.

6. Samovar LA. 2000. *Oral communication: Speaking across cultures,* 11th ed. Los Angeles: Roxbury.

7. Curry-Bartley KR. 1986. The art and science of listening. *Topics in Clinical Nutrition* 1:14–24.

8. Stewart CJ, Cash WB. 1999. *Interviewing: Principles and practices,* 9th ed. Boston: McGraw-Hill College.

9. Snetselaar LG. 1997. *Nutrition counseling skills for medical nutrition therapy.* Gaithersburg, MD: Aspen.

10. Rogers C. 1961. *On becoming a person.* Boston: Houghton Mifflin.

11. Rogers C. 1970. *Carl Rogers on encounter groups.* New York: Harper & Row.

12. Rogers C. 1977. *Carl Rogers on personal power: Inner strength and its revolutionary impact.* New York: Delacorte.

13. Corey G. 2000. *Theory and practice of counseling and psychotherapy,* 6th ed. Pacific Grove, CA: Brooks/Cole.

14. Elder JA, Ayala GX, Harris S. 1999. Theories and intervention approaches to health-behavior change in primary care. *American Journal of Preventive Medicine* 17:275–284.

15. Hodges PAM, Vickery CE. 1989. *Effective counseling: Strategies for dietary management.* Rockville, MD: Aspen.

16. Stunkard AJ, Berthold HC. 1985. What is behavior therapy? A very short description of behavioral weight control. *American Journal of Clinical Nutrition* 41:821–823.

17. Watson DL, Tharp RG. 2002. *Self-directed behavior: Self-modification for personal adjustment,* 8th ed. Belmont, CA: Wadsworth/Thomson Learning.

18. Raab C, Tillotson JL. 1985. *Heart to heart: A manual on nutrition counseling for the reduction of cardiovascular disease risk factors.* Bethesda, MD: U.S. Department of Health and Human Services,

Public Health Service; National Institutes of Health.

19. Bandura A. 1997. *Self-efficacy: The exercise of control.* New York: W.H. Freeman.

20. Burns DD. 2000. *Feeling good: The new mood therapy.* New York: Quill.

21. Burns DD. 1999. *The feeling good handbook.* New York: Plume.

22. Glasser W. 2001. *Reality therapy in action.* New York: HarperCollins.

23. Glasser W. 1998. *The quality school: Managing students without coercion.* New York: HarperPerennial.

24. Hoeltzel KE. 1986. Counseling methods for dietitians. *Topics in Clinical Nutrition* 1:33–42.

25. Nieman DC. 1999. *Exercise testing and prescription: A health-related approach,* 4th ed. Mountain View, CA: Mayfield.

26. Baladay GJ. 2000. *ASCM's guidelines for exercise testing and prescription,* 6th ed. Philadelphia: Williams & Wilkins.

27. Brownell KD, Marlatt GA, Lichtenstein E, Wilson GT. 1986. Understanding and preventing relapse. *American Psychologist* 41:765–782.

ASSESSMENT ACTIVITY 11.1

Counseling Practice

Becoming an effective counselor requires considerable skill and practice. This assessment activity is designed to help you get your feet wet.

Members of your class should divide into groups of two students each. You should take the 3-day food record that you completed in Assessment Activity 3.2 and the result of the computerized analysis of that food record and give these to your partner.

Review your partner's food record and computerized analysis. Study the Competency Checklist for Nutrition Counselors shown in Appendix U. Use this as a guide for your counseling session and to evaluate yourself after you have counseled your partner.

Using techniques discussed in this chapter, assist your partner in identifying one specific, measurable, and attainable goal that will improve his or her diet. Guide your partner in developing a simple action plan for attaining the goal he or she has decided on.

Videotape (or audiotape) the counseling session and view (or listen to) it alone later to see how you did. Look for what you did right and note improvements you can make next time. Use the Competency Checklist for Nutrition Counselors in Appendix U to evaluate your counseling skills.

If time allows, repeat this exercise.

APPENDIX A

Dietary Reference Values for Food Energy and Nutrients for the United Kingdom

From Department of Health. 1991. Report on Health and Social Subjects No. 41: *Dietary reference values for food energy and nutrients for the United Kingdom.* London: Her Majesty's Stationery Office. Reproduced with permission of the Controller of Her Brittanic Majesty's Stationery Office.

Dietary Reference Values for Fat and Carbohydrate for Adults as a Percentage of Daily Total Energy Intake (Percentage of Food Energy)

	Individual Minimum	Population Average	Individual Maximum
Saturated fatty acids		10 (11)	
Cis-polyunsaturated fatty acids		6 (6.5)	10
	n–3 0.2		
	n–6 1.0		
Cis-monounsaturated fatty acids		12 (13)	
Trans fatty acids		2 (2)	
Total fatty acids		30 (32.5)	
Total fat		33 (35)	
Nonmilk extrinsic sugars	0	10 (11)	
Intrinsic and milk sugars and starch		37 (39)	
Total carbohydrate		47 (50)	
Nonstarch polysaccharide (g/d)	12	18	24

The average percentage contribution to total energy does not total 100% because figures for protein and alcohol are excluded. Protein intakes average 15% of total energy which is above the RNI. It is recognized that many individuals will derive some energy from alcohol, and this has been assumed to average 5% approximating to current intakes. However, the panel allowed that some groups might not drink alcohol and that for some purposes nutrient intakes as a proportion of food energy (without alcohol) might be useful. Therefore, average figures are given as percentages both of total energy and, in parentheses, of food energy.

Reference Nutrient Intakes for Protein

Age	Reference Nutrient Intake[*] (g/day)
0–3 months	12.5[†]
4–6 months	12.7
7–9 months	13.7
10–12 months	14.9
1–3 years	14.5
4–6 years	19.7
7–10 years	28.3
Males	
11–14 years	42.1
15–18 years	55.2
19–50 years	55.5
50+ years	53.3
Females	
11–14 years	41.2
15–18 years	45.0
19–50 years	45.0
50+ years	46.5
Pregnancy[‡]	+ 6
Lactation[‡]	
0–4 months	+11
4 + months	+ 8

[*]These figures, based on egg and milk protein, assume complete digestibility.
[†]No values for infants 0–3 months are given by WHO. The RNI is calculated from the recommendations of COMA.
[‡]To be added to adult requirement through all stages of pregnancy and lactation.

Reference Nutrient Intakes for Minerals (SI Units)

Age	Calcium mmol/d	Phosphorus[1] mmol/d	Magnesium mmol/d	Sodium mmol/d	Potassium mmol/d	Chloride[4] mmol/d	Iron μmol/d	Zinc μmol/d	Copper μmol/d	Selenium μmol/d	Iodine μmol/d
0–3 months	13.1	13.1	2.2	9	20	9	30	60	5	0.1	0.4
4–6 months	13.1	13.1	2.5	12	22	12	80	60	5	0.2	0.5
7–9 months	13.1	13.1	3.2	14	18	14	140	75	5	0.1	0.5
10–12 months	13.1	13.1	3.3	15	18	15	140	75	5	0.1	0.5
1–3 years	8.8	8.8	3.5	22	20	22	120	75	6	0.2	0.6
4–6 years	11.3	11.3	4.8	30	28	30	110	100	9	0.3	0.8
7–10 years	13.8	13.8	8.0	50	50	50	160	110	11	0.4	0.9
Males											
11–14 years	25.0	25.0	11.5	70	80	70	200	140	13	0.6	1.0
15–18 years	25.0	25.0	12.3	70	90	70	200	145	16	0.9	1.0
19–50 years	17.5	17.5	12.3	70	90	70	160	145	19	0.9	1.0
50+ years	17.5	17.5	12.3	70	90	70	160	145	19	0.9	1.0
Females											
11–14 years	20.0	20.0	11.5	70	80	70	260[5]	140	13	0.6	1.0
15–18 years	20.0	20.0	12.3	70	90	70	260[5]	110	16	0.8	1.1
19–50 years	17.5	17.5	10.9	70	90	70	260[5]	110	19	0.8	1.1
50+ years	17.5	17.5	10.9	70	90	70	160	110	19	0.8	1.1
Pregnancy	*	*	*	*	*	*	*	*	*	*	*
Lactation											
0–4 months	+14.3	+14.3	+2.1	*	*	*	*	+90	+5	+0.2	*
4+ months	+14.3	+14.3	+2.1	*	*	*	*	+40	+5	+0.2	*

Age	Calcium mg/d	Phosphorus[1] mg/d	Magnesium mg/d	Sodium mg/d[2]	Potassium mg/d[3]	Chloride[4] mg/d	Iron mg/d	Zinc mg/d	Copper mg/d	Selenium μg/d	Iodine μg/d
0–3 months	525	400	55	210	800	320	1.7	4.0	0.2	10	50
4–6 months	525	400	60	280	850	400	4.3	4.0	0.3	13	60
7–9 months	525	400	75	320	700	500	7.8	5.0	0.3	10	60
10–12 months	525	400	80	350	700	500	7.8	5.0	0.3	10	60
1–3 years	350	270	85	500	800	800	6.9	5.0	0.4	15	70
4–6 years	450	350	120	700	1100	1100	6.1	6.5	0.6	20	100
7–10 years	550	450	200	1200	2000	1800	8.7	7.0	0.7	30	110
Males											
11–14 years	1000	775	280	1600	3100	2500	11.3	9.0	0.8	45	130
15–18 years	1000	775	300	1600	3500	2500	11.3	9.5	1.0	70	140
19–50 years	700	550	300	1600	3500	2500	8.7	9.5	1.2	75	140
50+ years	700	550	300	1600	3500	2500	8.7	9.5	1.2	75	140
Females											
11–14 years	800	625	280	1600	3100	2500	14.8[5]	9.0	0.8	45	130
15–18 years	800	625	300	1600	3500	2500	14.8[5]	7.0	1.0	60	140
19–50 years	700	550	270	1600	3500	2500	14.8[5]	7.0	1.2	60	140
50+ years	700	550	270	1600	3500	2500	8.7	7.0	1.2	60	140
Pregnancy	*	*	*	*	*	*	*	*	*	*	*
Lactation											
0–4 months	+550	+440	+50	*	*	*	*	+6.0	+0.3	+15	*
4 + months	+550	+440	+50	*	*	*	*	+2.5	+0.3	+15	*

*No increment. [1]Phosphorus RNI is set equal to calcium in molar terms. [2]1 mmol sodium = 23 mg. [3]1 mmol potassium = 39 mg.
[4]Corresponds to sodium 1 mmol = 35.5 mg. [5]Insufficient for women with high menstrual losses where the most practical way of meeting iron requirements is to take iron supplements.

Reference Nutrient Intakes for Vitamins

Age	Thiamin mg/d	Riboflavin mg/d	Niacin (Nicotinic Acid Equivalent) mg/d	Vitamin B_6 mg/d[§]	Vitamin B_{12} µg/d	Folate µg/d	Vitamin C mg/d	Vitamin A µg/d	Vitamin D µg/d
0–3 months	0.2	0.4	3	0.2	0.3	50	25	350	8.5
4–6 months	0.2	0.4	3	0.2	0.3	50	25	350	8.5
7–9 months	0.2	0.4	4	0.3	0.4	50	25	350	7
10–12 months	0.3	0.4	5	0.4	0.4	50	25	350	7
1–3 years	0.5	0.6	8	0.7	0.5	70	30	400	7
4–6 years	0.7	0.8	11	0.9	0.8	100	30	500	—
7–10 years	0.7	1.0	12	1.0	1.0	150	30	500	—
Males									
11–14 years	0.9	1.2	15	1.2	1.2	200	35	600	—
15–18 years	1.1	1.3	18	1.5	1.5	200	40	700	—
19–50 years	1.0	1.3	17	1.4	1.5	200	40	700	—
50+ years	0.9	1.3	16	1.4	1.5	200	40	700	†
Females									
11–14 years	0.7	1.1	12	1.0	1.2	200	35	600	—
15–18 years	0.8	1.1	14	1.2	1.5	200	40	600	—
19–50 years	0.8	1.1	13	1.2	1.5	200	40	600	—
50+ years	0.8	1.1	12	1.2	1.5	200	40	600	†
Pregnancy	+0.1‡	+0.3	*	*	*	+100	+10	+100	10
Lactation									
0–4 months	+0.2	+0.5	+2	*	+0.5	+60	+30	+350	10
4+ months	+0.2	+0.5	+2	*	+0.5	+60	+30	+350	10

*No increment. †After age 65 the RNI is 10 µg/d for men and women. ‡For last trimester only. §Based on protein providing 14.7% of EAR for energy.

Safe Intakes

Nutrient	Safe Intake
Vitamins	
Pantothenic Acid	
Adults	3–7 mg/day
Infants	1.7 mg/day
Biotin	10–200 µg/day
Vitamin E	
Men	Above 4 mg/day
Women	Above 3 mg/day
Infants	0.4 mg/g polyunsaturated fatty acids
Vitamin K	
Adults	1 µg/kg/day
Infants	10 µg/day
Minerals	
Manganese	
Adults	1.4 mg (26 µmol)/day
Infants and children	16 µg (0.3 µmol)/day
Molybdenum	
Adults	50–400 µg/day
Infants, children and adolescents	0.5–1.5 µg/kg/day
Chromium	
Adults	25 µg (0.5 µmol)/day
Children and adolescents	0.1–1.0 µg (2–20 µmol)/kg/day
Fluoride (for infants only)	0.05 mg (3 µmol)/kg/day

APPENDIX B

The U.S. Recommended Daily Allowances (U.S. RDAs)

From *Federal Register,* 19 July 1990, page 29477.

Vitamins and Minerals	Unit of Measurement	Infants	Children Under 4 Years of Age	Adults and Children 4 or More Years of Age	Pregnant or Lactating Women
Vitamin A	International units	1500	2500	5000	8000
Vitamin D	International units	400	400	400	400
Vitamin E	International units	5	10	30	30
Vitamin C	Milligrams	35	40	60	60
Folic acid	Milligrams	.1	.2	.4	.8
Thiamin	Milligrams	.5	.7	1.5	1.7
Riboflavin	Milligrams	.6	.8	1.7	2
Niacin	Milligrams	8	9	20	20
Vitamin B_6	Milligrams	.4	.7	2	2.5
Vitamin B_{12}	Micrograms	2	3	6	8
Biotin	Milligrams	.05	.15	.30	.30
Pantothenic acid	Milligrams	3	5	10	10
Calcium	Grams	.6	.8	1	1
Phosphorus	Grams	.6	.8	1	1
Iodine	Micrograms	45	70	150	150
Iron	Milligrams	15	10	18	18
Magnesium	Milligrams	70	200	400	450
Copper	Milligrams	.6	1	2	2
Zinc	Milligrams	5	8	15	15

*1998 Continuing Survey of Food Intakes by Individuals 24-Hour Recall Form**

*This appendix contains the major portions of the 24-hour recall form. For the complete form, visit the *Nutritional Assessment* website at www.mhhe.com/hper/nutrition. From the Food Surveys Research Group, USDA.

WHAT WE EAT IN AMERICA

Day One Intake Questionnaire

PLACE CASE LABEL HERE

SAMPLE PERSON #: |__|__|

INTERVIEWER NAME: _____

INTERVIEWER ID: |__|__|__|

DATE OF INTERVIEW: |__|__|–|__|__|–19 |__|__|
                       MO   DA   YR

DAY OF INTERVIEW: _____

FIRST NAME OF
   SAMPLE PERSON: _____

DATE OF BIRTH: |__|__|–|__|__|–|__|__|__|__|
               MO   DA   YEAR

OR
AGE: |__|__|__| YRS 1
                 MOS 2

SEX: M 1   F 2

|__|__|:|__|__| AM 1
TIME STARTED PM 2

|__|__|:|__|__| AM 1
TIME ENDED PM 2

INTERVIEW CONDUCTED:
     IN PERSON 1
     BY TELEPHONE 2

FOR HOME OFFICE USE ONLY
DATE RECEIVED: _____
DATE REVIEWED: _____
START TIME: _____ AM PM
END TIME: _____ AM PM
BATCH #: _____

TIME STARTED _____

Day 1

1. | HAND CARD I1 | I'd like you to give me the list of everything (you/NAME) had to eat and drink all day yesterday, (DAY), from midnight to midnight. I'll ask you for the detailed descriptions and amounts later. Please include everything (you/NAME) ate and drank at home and away—even snacks. [DO NOT INTERRUPT RESPONDENT. USE HANDCARD I1 IF NECESSARY.]

[IF INFANT OR CHILD SP UNDER 6:] I'd like you to give me the list of everything (NAME) had to eat and drink all day yesterday, (DAY), from midnight to midnight. I'll ask you for the detailed descriptions and amounts later. Please include everything (he/she) ate and drank at home and away, including snacks and drinks (and bottles or breast milk).

[WHEN RESPONDENT STOPS, ASK: Anything else?]

Now I'm going to ask you the specific questions about the foods and beverages you just listed. When you remember anything else (you/NAME) ate or drank as we go along, please tell me.

Use these measuring guides to help estimate amounts or any of your own cups, mugs, bowls, or package labels.

> WHEN ASKING ABOUT FIRST FOOD RECORDED ON QUICK LIST, GO TO 2b.

2a. Did (you/NAME) have (NEXT QUICK LIST ITEM) at (TIME) with (your/his/her) (OCCASION) or was that at another time? [CONFIRM IF OBVIOUS OR IF RECORDED ON QUICK LIST. IF SAME TIME AND OCCASION, SKIP TO BOX 1; IF AT ANOTHER TIME, ASK Q2b.]

2b. About what time did (you/NAME) begin to (eat/drink) the (FOOD)? [OR CONFIRM IF RECORDED ON QUICK LIST]

3. Looking at this card, please tell me what (you/NAME) would call this occasion. [OR CONFIRM IF RECORDED ON QUICK LIST]

HAND CARD I2		

01	BREAKFAST	06	FOOD AND/OR BEVERAGE BREAK
02	BRUNCH		SNACK
03	LUNCH		OTHER BEVERAGE
04	DINNER	07	FEEDING (INFANT ONLY)
05	SUPPER	08	OTHER (SPECIFY)

BOX 1

STEP 1:   TRANSFER QUICK LIST FOOD TO THE FOOD/DRINK COLUMN. CHECK OFF FOOD IN QUICK LIST AS IT IS TRANSFERRED.

STEP 2 (Q4):   GO TO FIB COLUMN Q4 FOR FOOD PROBES. BE SURE TO REQUEST FOOD LABELS IF RESPONDENT CANNOT ANSWER PROBES IN COLUMN Q4.

STEP 3 (Q5):   GO TO FIB COLUMN Q5 HEADING FOR AMOUNT QUESTION.

STEP 4:   RETURN TO Q2a FOR NEXT FOOD RECORDED IN QUICK LIST.

Individual Intake Form (Continued)

Q2 Time	Q3 Occ. (Hand Card I2)	Food/Drink and Additions	Q4 Description of Food/Drink and Ingredient Amount
a p		33.	
a p		34.	
a p		35.	
a p		36.	
a p		37.	
a p		38.	
a p		39.	
a p		40.	
a p		41.	
a p		42.	
a p		43.	
a p		44.	
a p		45.	
a p		46.	
a p		47.	
a p		48.	

Q5 How Much of This (Food) Did You Actually (Eat/Drink)?	Q7 Where Obtained (Hand Card I3)	Q8 Eaten at Home	Q9 Ever at Home
		YES ....1 (Q7) NO 2	YES ....1 NO 2
		YES ....1 (Q7) NO 2	YES ....1 NO 2
		YES ....1 (Q7) NO 2	YES ....1 NO 2
		YES ....1 (Q7) NO 2	YES ....1 NO 2
		YES ....1 (Q7) NO 2	YES ....1 NO 2
		YES ....1 (Q7) NO 2	YES ....1 NO 2
		YES ....1 (Q7) NO 2	YES ....1 NO 2
		YES ....1 (Q7) NO 2	YES ....1 NO 2
		YES ....1 (Q7) NO 2	YES ....1 NO 2
		YES ....1 (Q7) NO 2	YES ....1 NO 2
		YES ....1 (Q7) NO 2	YES ....1 NO 2
		YES ....1 (Q7) NO 2	YES ....1 NO 2
		YES ....1 (Q7) NO 2	YES ....1 NO 2
		YES ....1 (Q7) NO 2	YES ....1 NO 2
		YES ....1 (Q7) NO 2	YES ....1 NO 2
		YES ....1 (Q7) NO 2	YES ....1 NO 2

Review

6. Now let's see if I have everything. I'd like you to try to remember anything else (you/NAME) ate or drank yesterday that you haven't already told me about, including anything (you/NAME) ate or drank while preparing a meal or while waiting to eat.

   6a. Did (you/NAME) have anything to eat or drink between midnight yesterday and (your/NAME'S) (TIME) (FIRST OCCASION)?

   6b. Now at (TIME) for (THIS OCCASION) (you/NAME) had (FOODS), did (you/NAME) have anything else?

   6c. Did (you/NAME) have anything to eat or drink between (your/NAME's) (TIME) (THIS OCCASION) and (TIME) when (you/NAME) had (NEXT OCCASION)?

   > REPEAT 6b AND 6c FOR EACH OCCASION EXCEPT LAST OCCASION.
   > FOR LAST OCCASION, GO TO 6d.

   6d. Now at (TIME) for (LAST OCCASION) (you/NAME) had (FOODS), did (you/NAME) have anything else?

   6e. Did (you/NAME) have anything to eat or drink after (your/NAME's) (TIME) (LAST OCCASION) but before midnight last night?

Now let's go back to the beginning of the day and find out where (you/NAME), or other people who live here, obtained the food (you/NAME) ate and where (you/NAME) ate it.

7. (Looking at this card) Where did (you/NAME) obtain (THIS FOOD/MOST OF THE INGREDIENTS FOR THIS FOOD)?

> HAND
> CARD
> I3

01 STORE, SUCH AS SUPERMARKET, GROCERY STORE, OR WAREHOUSE, CONVENIENCE STORE, DRUG STORE, OR GAS STATION
SPECIALTY STORE, SUCH AS BAKERY, DELI, SEAFOOD, ETHNIC FOOD, HEALTH FOOD
COMMISSARY
PRODUCE STAND OR FARMER'S MARKET

02 RESTAURANT WITH WAITER/ WAITRESS SERVICE

03 FAST FOOD PLACE, PIZZA PLACE

04 BAR, TAVERN, LOUNGE

05 SCHOOL CAFETERIA

06 OTHER CAFETERIA

07 VENDING MACHINE

08 CHILD CARE CENTER, FAMILY DAY CARE HOME, ADULT DAY CARE

09 SOUP KITCHEN, SHELTER, FOOD PANTRY

10 MEALS ON WHEELS

11 OTHER COMMUNITY FOOD PROGRAM

12 GROWN OR CAUGHT BY YOU OR SOMEONE YOU KNOW

   IF FISH OR SEAFOOD, ASK: Did it come from a
   71 Freshwater lake, pond, or river
   72 The ocean, or
   73 A bay, sound, or estuary?
   74 DON'T KNOW BODY OF WATER

13 SOMEONE ELSE/GIFT

SOME OTHER PLACE (PLEASE DESCRIBE)
   14 MAIL ORDER PURCHASE
   15 COMMON COFFEE POT OR SNACK TRAY
   16 RESIDENTIAL DINING FACILITY
   17 OTHER (SPECIFY)
   98 DON'T KNOW

8. Did (you/NAME) (eat/drink) this (FOOD) at your home?

> IF YES, GO BACK TO Q7 FOR NEXT FOOD.
> IF NO, GO TO Q9.

9. Before (you/NAME) (ate/drank) this particular (FOOD), was it ever at your home?

> REPEAT Q7–9 FOR EACH FOOD.

10. Was the amount of food that (you/NAME) ate yesterday about usual, less than usual, or more than usual?

      USUAL 1   (Q13)
      LESS THAN USUAL 2   (Q11)
      MORE THAN USUAL 3   (Q12)

11. What is the main reason the amount (you/NAME) ate yesterday was less than usual?

      SICKNESS 01
      SHORT OF MONEY 02
      TRAVELING 03
      AT A SOCIAL OCCASION OR ON A 04
        SPECIAL DAY
      ON VACATION 05
      TOO BUSY 06   (Q13)
      NOT HUNGRY 07
      DIETING 08
      FASTING 09
      BORED OR STRESSED 10
      SOME OTHER REASON (SPECIFY) 11

      _____ |_|_|

12. What is the main reason the amount (you/NAME) ate yesterday was more than usual?

      TRAVELING 1
      AT A SOCIAL OCCASION OR ON A SPECIAL DAY . .2
      ON VACATION 3
      VERY HUNGRY 4
      BORED OR STRESSED 5
      SOME OTHER REASON 6
        (SPECIFY) _____ |_|_|

13. | HAND CARD I4 | What type of salt, if any, (do you/does NAME) add to (you/his/her) food <u>at the table</u>? Would you say it is ordinary salt, seasoned salt, lite salt, or a salt substitute?

      ORDINARY SALT/SEA SALT .1
      SEASONED SALT OR OTHER FLAVORED SALT 2
      LITE SALT 3
      SALT SUBSTITUTE 4
      NONE 5   (Q15)
      DON'T KNOW 8   (Q15)

14. How often (do you/does NAME) add (ANSWER IN Q13) to (your/his/her) food <u>at the table</u>? Is it always, frequently, sometimes, or rarely?

      ALWAYS 1
      FREQUENTLY 2
      SOMETIMES 3
      RARELY 4

HAND	Now I'd like you to think about all of the <u>plain drinking water</u> that (you/NAME) had yesterday,
CARD	regardless of where (you/he/she) drank it. By <u>plain drinking water</u>, I mean tap water or any bottled water
I5	that is not carbonated, with nothing added to it, not even lemon.

15. How many fluid ounces of <u>plain drinking water</u> did (you/he/she) drink yesterday?

       |__|__|__|

       FLUID OUNCES

       NONE 000 (Q18)

16. How much of this plain drinking water came from your home? Would you say all, most, some, or none?

       ALL 1   (Q18)

       MOST 2

       SOME 3

       NONE 4

17. What was the main source of plain drinking water that did *not* come from your home? Was it tap water, water from a drinking fountain, bottled water, or something else?

       TAP WATER AND/OR DRINKING FOUNTAIN 1

       BOTTLED WATER 2

       OTHER SOURCE 3

         (SPECIFY) _____ |__|__|

       DON'T KNOW 8

18. (Are you/is NAME) on any kind of diet either to lose weight or for some other health-related reason?

       YES 1

       NO 2   (Q22)

CIRCLE ALL THAT APPLY AND ASK Q20 AND Q21 IN SEQUENCE FOR EACH DIET CIRCLED.	WEIGHT LOSS OR LOW-CALORIE DIET		LOW-FAT OR CHOLESTEROL DIET		LOW-SALT OR SODIUM DIET	
19. HAND CARD I6 Looking at this card, please tell me which of these diets (you are/NAME is) on.	01		02		03	
20. (Are you/is NAME) on this (ANSWER IN Q19) because . . .	YES	NO	YES	NO	YES	NO
A doctor or dietitian suggested or prescribed it?	1	2	1	2	1	2
A medical condition runs in your family?	1	2	1	2	1	2
You joined another person on his/her diet?	1	2	1	2	1	2
You want to maintain or improve your health?	1	2	1	2	1	2
You want to lose weight?	1	2	1	2	1	2
Some other reason? . . . . (IF YES, SPECIFY)	1	2	1	2	1	2
	(SPECIFY) ⌊_⌊_⌋		(SPECIFY) ⌊_⌊_⌋		(SPECIFY) ⌊_⌊_⌋	
21. HAND CARD I7 Looking at this card, please tell me which of these *best* describes the source of (your/his/her) (ANSWER IN Q19). (CODE ONLY ONE)						
AN ORGANIZED WEIGHT LOSS PROGRAM	1		1		1	
A DOCTOR OR DIETITIAN	2		2		2	
SOMETHING YOU READ OR HEARD ABOUT	3		3		3	
SOMETHING YOU MADE UP	4		4		4	
SOMETHING ELSE . . . . (SPECIFY UNDER CODE 5)	5		5		5	
	(SPECIFY) ⌊_⌊_⌋		(SPECIFY) ⌊_⌊_⌋		(SPECIFY) ⌊_⌊_⌋	

SUGAR-FREE OR LOW-SUGAR DIET	LOW-FIBER DIET	HIGH-FIBER DIET	DIABETIC DIET	OTHER DIET
				(SPECIFY)
04	05	06	07	08
				└─┴─┘
YES NO	YES NO	YES NO	YES NO	YES NO
.....1 2	.......1 2	........1 2	.....1 2	.......1 2
.....1 2	.......1 2	........1 2	.....1 2	.......1 2
.....1 2	.......1 2	........1 2	.....1 2	.......1 2
.....1 2	.......1 2	........1 2	.....1 2	.......1 2
.....1 2	.......1 2	........1 2	.....1 2	.......1 2
.....1 2	.......1 2	........1 2	.....1 2	.......1 2
(SPECIFY)	(SPECIFY)	(SPECIFY)	(SPECIFY)	(SPECIFY)
└─┴─┘	└─┴─┘	└─┴─┘	└─┴─┘	└─┴─┘
.......1	1	1	1	1
........2	2	2	2	2
.......3	3	3	3	3
.......4	4	4	4	4
.......5	5	5	5	5
(SPECIFY)	(SPECIFY)	(SPECIFY)	(SPECIFY)	(SPECIFY)
└─┴─┘	└─┴─┘	└─┴─┘	└─┴─┘	└─┴─┘

22. Do you consider (yourself/NAME) to be a vegetarian?

> YES 1
> NO 2

23. How often, if at all, (do you/does NAME) take any vitamin or mineral supplement in pill or liquid form? Would you say every day or almost every day, every so often, or not at all?

> EVERY DAY OR ALMOST EVERY DAY 1
> EVERY SO OFTEN 2
> NOT AT ALL 3   (Q26)

24. | HAND CARD I8 | Looking at this card, which of these types of supplements (do you/does NAME) usually take: a multivitamin; multivitamin with iron or other minerals; combination of vitamin C and iron; or single vitamins or minerals? (CIRCLE ALL THAT APPLY)

> MULTIVITAMIN 1
> MULTIVITAMIN WITH IRON OR 2
>   OTHER MINERALS
> COMBINATION OF VITAMIN C AND IRON 3
> SINGLE VITAMINS/MINERALS 4

```
+--------------------------------------------+
|                   BOX 2                    |
|                                            |
|  IS "4" CIRCLED IN Q24?                    |
|     YES . . . . . . . . . . . . . .1   (Q25)  |
|     NO . . . . . . . . . . . . . . .2   (Q26)  |
+--------------------------------------------+
```

25. | HAND CARD I9 | Looking at this card, which of these single vitamins and minerals (do you/does he/she) usually take? (CIRCLE ALL THAT APPLY)

> VITAMIN A 01
> VITAMIN B/B COMPLEX 02
> VITAMIN C 03
> VITAMIN D 04
> VITAMIN E 05
> CALCIUM 06
> FOLACIN 07
> FLUORIDE 08
> IRON 09
> ZINC 10
> SELENIUM 11
> CHROMIUM 12
> SOMETHING ELSE (SPECIFY) 13
> _____

26. (Do you/Does NAME) take a fish oil supplement?

> YES 1
> NO 2

27. (Do you/Does he/she) take a fiber supplement?

> YES 1
> NO 2

28. (Have you/Has NAME) ever had (your/his/her) blood cholesterol checked?

> YES 1
> NO 2
> DON'T KNOW 8

29. How tall (are you/is he/she) <u>without</u> shoes?

|__|__| |__|__|
FEET   INCHES

30. About how much (do you/does NAME) weigh <u>without</u> shoes?

|__|__|__|
POUNDS

31. In general, would you say (your/his/her) health is excellent, very good, good, fair, or poor?

EXCELLENT 1
VERY GOOD 2
GOOD 3
FAIR 4
POOR 5

32. (Do you/Does NAME) have any food allergies that make it necessary to avoid certain foods?

YES 1
NO 2   (Q34)

33. What food allergies (do you/does NAME) have? (CIRCLE ALL THAT APPLY)

WHEAT 01
COW'S MILK 02
EGGS 03
FISH OR SHELLFISH 04
CORN 05
PEANUTS 06
OTHER NUTS 07
SOY PRODUCTS 08
OTHER (SPECIFY) 09

__	__
__	__
__	__

_____

34. Has a doctor ever told (you/NAME) that (you have/he/she has): (CIRCLE A NUMBER FOR EACH)

	YES	NO
Diabetes?	1	2
High blood pressure (hypertension)?	1	2
Heart disease?	1	2
Cancer?	1	2
Osteoporosis?	1	2
High blood cholesterol?	1	2
Stroke?	1	2

35. How many hours did (you/NAME) watch television or videotapes yesterday?

|__|__|
#OF HOURS

| THANK RESPONDENT |

CODER USE ONLY.
QLIST: |__|__|

TIME ENDED _____ AM
                                             PM

Interviewer Observation Form
[Do Not Read These Questions to the Respondent.]

A. WHO WAS THE MAIN RESPONDENT FOR THIS INTERVIEW?

SAMPLE PERSON 01
MOTHER OF SAMPLE PERSON 02
FATHER OF SAMPLE PERSON 03
WIFE OF SAMPLE PERSON 04
HUSBAND OF SAMPLE PERSON 05
DAUGHTER OF SAMPLE PERSON 06
SON OF SAMPLE PERSON 07
SISTER OF SAMPLE PERSON 08
BROTHER OF SAMPLE PERSON 09
GRANDPARENT OF SAMPLE PERSON 10
AUNT OF SAMPLE PERSON 11
UNCLE OF SAMPLE PERSON 12
SOMEONE ELSE (SPECIFY) 13   ⌊_⌋_⌋

_____

B. WHO ELSE HELPED IN RESPONDING FOR THIS INTERVIEW? (CIRCLE ALL THAT APPLY)

NO ONE 00
SAMPLE PERSON 01
MOTHER OF SAMPLE PERSON 02
FATHER OF SAMPLE PERSON 03
WIFE OF SAMPLE PERSON 04
HUSBAND OF SAMPLE PERSON 05
DAUGHTER OF SAMPLE PERSON 06
SON OF SAMPLE PERSON 07
SISTER OF SAMPLE PERSON 08
BROTHER OF SAMPLE PERSON 09
GRANDPARENT OF SAMPLE PERSON 10
AUNT OF SAMPLE PERSON 11
UNCLE OF SAMPLE PERSON 12   ⌊_⌋_⌋
SOMEONE ELSE (SPECIFY)—OTHER
    THAN INTERVIEWER 13   ⌊_⌋_⌋
                                               ⌊_⌋_⌋

_____

C. DID YOU OR THE RESPONDENT HAVE DIFFICULTY WITH THIS INTAKE INTERVIEW?

YES 1
NO 2   (E)

D. WHAT WAS THE REASON FOR THIS DIFFICULTY?

_____

_____

_____

_____

_____

7 - Day Food Diary

Name _____ Age _____

Address _____ City _____

State _____ Zip _____ Phone _____

Height _____ Weight _____ Sex _____

Physician/Dietitian _____ Phone _____

For Females Only: Are you pregnant? _____

Are you breast-feeding? _____

Directions for Using the Food Diary

1. Keep your food diary current. List foods immediately after they are eaten. **Please print all entries.**
2. Record only one food item per line in this record booklet.
3. Be as specific as possible when describing the food item eaten: the way it was cooked (if it was cooked) and the amount that was eaten.
4. Include brand names whenever possible.
5. Report only the food portion that was actually eaten — for example: **T-bone steak, 4-oz broiled.** (Do not include the bones.)
6. Record amounts in household measures — for example: **ounces, tablespoons, cups, slices** or **units**, as in 1 cup nonfat milk, two slices of wheat toast, or one raw apple.
7. Include method that was used to prepare food item — for example: **fresh, frozen, stewed, fried, baked, canned, broiled, raw,** or **braised.**
8. For canned foods, include the liquid in which it was canned — for example: **sliced peaches in heavy syrup, fruit cocktail in light syrup,** or **tuna in water.**
9. Food items listed without specific amounts eaten will be analyzed using portion sizes.
10. Do not alter your normal diet during the period you keep this diary.
11. Remember to record the amounts of visible fats (oils, butter, salad dressings, margarine, and so on) you eat or use in cooking.

* The following are examples of the way to list food items and amounts.

Time	Food Item and Method of Preparation	Amount Eaten
7 am	Apple, raw, fresh	1 medium
12 pm	Beef Stew	10 oz portion
12 pm	Bread, whole wheat, fresh	2 Slices
3 pm	Cereal, Corn Flakes	2 Cups
	with sugar	2 Tbs.
	with milk, non fat	½ cup
7 pm	Chicken, fried	2 legs
7 pm	Coleslaw, with mayo	1 cup
7 pm	Eggs, Chicken (fried in butter)	2 large
7 pm	Fish, salmon, baked	10 oz

Name _____		Date _____
Time	**Food Item and Method of Preparation**	**Amount Eaten**

Third National Health and Nutrition Examination Survey Food Frequency Questionnarie

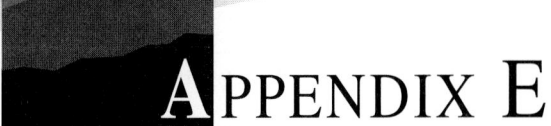

APPENDIX E

From National Center for Health Statistics.

DIET (AGES 17+ YEARS)	
M1. CHECK ITEM. REFER TO AGE OF SP.	1 ☐ UNDER 60 YEARS (M4) 2 ☐ 60+ YEARS (M2)
Now I'm going to ask you some general questions about your eating habits. **M2.** Some cities, churches, and other organizations provide meals for senior citizens. Do you receive meals from any such programs?	1 ☐ Y 2 ☐ N (M4)
M3. Are these meals ever delivered to your home, such as Meals on Wheels?	1 ☐ Y 2 ☐ N
M4. How often do you eat <u>breakfast</u> - every day, on some days, rarely, never, on weekends only?	1 ☐ every day 2 ☐ some days 3 ☐ rarely 4 ☐ never 5 ☐ weekends only
M5. How tall are you without shoes?	_____ feet/ _____ inches or _____ centimeters 999 ☐ DK
M6. How much do you weigh without clothes or shoes? FEMALES: IF CURRENTLY PREGNANT, ASK: About how much did you weigh <u>before</u> your pregnancy?	_____ pounds or _____ kilograms 999 ☐ DK
M7. CHECK ITEM. REFER TO AGE OF SP.	1 ☐ 25 YEARS OR LESS (M10) 2 ☐ 26 YEARS THROUGH 35 YEARS (M9) 3 ☐ 36 YEARS AND OLDER
M8. How much did you weigh <u>10 years ago</u>?	_____ pounds or _____ kilograms 999 ☐ DK
M9. How much did you weigh when you were <u>25 years old</u>?	_____ pounds or _____ kilograms 999 ☐ DK
M10. Up to the present time, what is the most you have ever weighed? (FEMALES): Do not include any times when you were pregnant.	_____ pounds or _____ kilograms 999 ☐ DK

M11. Do you consider yourself <u>now</u> to be overweight, underweight, or about the right weight?	1 ☐ overweight 2 ☐ underweight 3 ☐ about the right weight
M12. Would you like to weigh more, less, or stay about the same?	1 ☐ more 2 ☐ less 3 ☐ stay about the same
M13. During the <u>past 12 months</u>, have you tried to lose weight?	1 ☐ Y 2 ☐ N
M14. During the <u>past 12 months</u>, have you changed what you eat because of any medical reason or health condition?	1 ☐ Y 2 ☐ N (N1)
M15. What was the medical reason or health condition that caused you to change what you eat? MARK ALL THAT APPLY.	01 ☐ OVERWEIGHT/OBESITY 02 ☐ HIGH BLOOD PRESSURE/HYPERTENSION 03 ☐ HIGH BLOOD CHOLESTEROL 04 ☐ DIABETES 05 ☐ HEART DISEASE 06 ☐ ALLERGY 07 ☐ ULCER 08 ☐ OTHER 10 _____ SPECIFY 99 ☐ DK

FOOD FREQUENCY (AGES 17+ YEARS)

HAND CARD HAQ-5.

Now I'm going to ask you how often you usually eat certain foods. When answering think about your <u>usual</u> diet over the <u>past month</u>. Tell me how often you usually ate or drank these foods per day, per week, per month, or not at all.

Times	Day	Week	Month	Never	DK
_ _ per	1 ☐ D	2 ☐ W	3 ☐ M or	4 ☐ N	9 ☐ DK

N1. <u>MILK AND MILK PRODUCTS</u>

First are milk and milk products. Do not include their use in cooking.

a. How often did you have chocolate milk and hot cocoa?

_ _ per 1 ☐ D 2 ☐ W 3 ☐ M or 4 ☐ N 9 ☐ DK

b. How often did you have milk to drink or on cereal? Do not count <u>small</u> amounts of milk added to coffee or tea.

_ _ per 1 ☐ D 2 ☐ W 3 ☐ M or 4 ☐ N 9 ☐ DK

c. CHECK ITEM. REFER TO RESPONSES IN N1a AND N1b.

1 ☐ "NEVER" IN BOTH N1a AND N1b (N1e)

2 ☐ OTHER

d. What type of milk was it? Was it <u>usually</u> whole, 2%, 1%, skim, nonfat, or some other type?

IF SP CANNOT PROVIDE USUAL TYPE, MARK ALL THAT APPLY.

01 ☐ whole/regular

02 ☐ 2%/low fat

03 ☐ 1%

04 ☐ skim/nonfat

05 ☐ buttermilk

06 ☐ evaporated

07 ☐ other 08 _____
                              specify

99 ☐ DK

e. Yogurt and frozen yogurt

_ _ per 1 ☐ D 2 ☐ W 3 ☐ M or 4 ☐ N 9 ☐ DK

f. Ice cream, ice milk, and milkshakes

_ _ per 1 ☐ D 2 ☐ W 3 ☐ M or 4 ☐ N 9 ☐ DK

g. Cheese, all types including American, Swiss, cheddar, and cottage cheese

_ _ per 1 ☐ D 2 ☐ W 3 ☐ M or 4 ☐ N 9 ☐ DK

h. Pizza, calzone, and lasagna

_ _ per 1 ☐ D 2 ☐ W 3 ☐ M or 4 ☐ N 9 ☐ DK

i. Cheese dishes such as macaroni and cheese, cheese nachos, cheese enchiladas, and quesadillas

_ _ per 1 ☐ D 2 ☐ W 3 ☐ M or 4 ☐ N 9 ☐ DK

N2. MAIN DISHES, MEAT, FISH, CHICKEN, AND EGGS

Next are main dishes, meat, fish, chicken, and eggs.

	Times	Day	Week	Month		Never	DK
	__ __ per	1 ☐ D	2 ☐ W	3 ☐ M	or	4 ☐ N	9 ☐ DK
a. How often did you eat any type of stew, or soup containing <u>vegetables</u>, including minestrone, tomato, and split pea?	__ __ per	1 ☐ D	2 ☐ W	3 ☐ M	or	4 ☐ N	9 ☐ DK
b. Spaghetti and pasta with tomato sauce	__ __ per	1 ☐ D	2 ☐ W	3 ☐ M	or	4 ☐ N	9 ☐ DK
c. Bacon, sausage (chorizo) and luncheon meats such as hot dogs, salami, and bologna	__ __ per	1 ☐ D	2 ☐ W	3 ☐ M	or	4 ☐ N	9 ☐ DK
d. Liver and other organ meats such as heart, kidney, tongue, and tripe (menudo)	__ __ per	1 ☐ D	2 ☐ W	3 ☐ M	or	4 ☐ N	9 ☐ DK
e. Beef, including hamburger, steaks, roast beef, and meatloaf	__ __ per	1 ☐ D	2 ☐ W	3 ☐ M	or	4 ☐ N	9 ☐ DK
f. Pork and ham, including roast pork, pork chops, and spare ribs	__ __ per	1 ☐ D	2 ☐ W	3 ☐ M	or	4 ☐ N	9 ☐ DK
g. Shrimp, clams, oysters, crab, and lobster	__ __ per	1 ☐ D	2 ☐ W	3 ☐ M	or	4 ☐ N	9 ☐ DK
h. Fish including fillets, fish sticks, fish sandwiches, and tuna fish	__ __ per	1 ☐ D	2 ☐ W	3 ☐ M	or	4 ☐ N	9 ☐ DK
i. Chicken, all types, including baked, fried, chicken nuggets, and chicken salad. Include turkey.	__ __ per	1 ☐ D	2 ☐ W	3 ☐ M	or	4 ☐ N	9 ☐ DK
j. How often did you have eggs including scrambled, fried, omelettes, hard-boiled eggs, and egg salad?	__ __ per	1 ☐ D	2 ☐ W	3 ☐ M	or	4 ☐ N	9 ☐ DK

N3. FRUIT AND FRUIT JUICES

Next are fruit juices and fruit. Include all forms - fresh, frozen, canned, and dried.

	Times	Day	Week	Month		Never	DK
a. How often did you have orange juice, grapefruit juice, and tangerine juice?	__ __ per	1 ☐ D	2 ☐ W	3 ☐ M	or	4 ☐ N	9 ☐ DK
b. Other fruit juices such as grape juice, apple juice, cranberry juice, and fruit nectars	__ __ per	1 ☐ D	2 ☐ W	3 ☐ M	or	4 ☐ N	9 ☐ DK
c. Citrus fruits including oranges, grapefruits, and tangerines	__ __ per	1 ☐ D	2 ☐ W	3 ☐ M	or	4 ☐ N	9 ☐ DK
d. Melons including cantaloupe, honeydew, and watermelon	__ __ per	1 ☐ D	2 ☐ W	3 ☐ M	or	4 ☐ N	9 ☐ DK
e. Peaches, nectarines, apricots, guava, mango, and papaya	__ __ per	1 ☐ D	2 ☐ W	3 ☐ M	or	4 ☐ N	9 ☐ DK
f. How often did you have any other fruits such as apples, bananas, pears, berries, cherries, grapes, plums, and strawberries? (Include plantains.)	__ __ per	1 ☐ D	2 ☐ W	3 ☐ M	or	4 ☐ N	9 ☐ DK

N4. VEGETABLES

These next questions are about vegetables. Please remember to include fresh, raw, frozen, canned, and cooked vegetables.

	Times	Day	Week	Month	Never	DK
	_ _ per	1 ☐ D	2 ☐ W	3 ☐ M or	4 ☐ N	9 ☐ DK

		Times	Day	Week	Month	Never	DK
a.	How often did you have carrots and vegetable mixtures containing carrots?	_ _ per	1 ☐ D	2 ☐ W	3 ☐ M or	4 ☐ N	9 ☐ DK
b.	Broccoli	_ _ per	1 ☐ D	2 ☐ W	3 ☐ M or	4 ☐ N	9 ☐ DK
c.	Brussels sprouts and cauliflower	_ _ per	1 ☐ D	2 ☐ W	3 ☐ M or	4 ☐ N	9 ☐ DK
d.	White potatoes, including baked, mashed, boiled, french-fries, and potato salad	_ _ per	1 ☐ D	2 ☐ W	3 ☐ M or	4 ☐ N	9 ☐ DK
e.	Sweet potatoes, yams, and orange squash including acorn, butternut, hubbard, and pumpkin	_ _ per	1 ☐ D	2 ☐ W	3 ☐ M or	4 ☐ N	9 ☐ DK
f.	Tomatoes including fresh and stewed tomatoes, tomato juice, and salsa	_ _ per	1 ☐ D	2 ☐ W	3 ☐ M or	4 ☐ N	9 ☐ DK
g.	Spinach, greens, collards, and kale	_ _ per	1 ☐ D	2 ☐ W	3 ☐ M or	4 ☐ N	9 ☐ DK
h.	Tossed salad	_ _ per	1 ☐ D	2 ☐ W	3 ☐ M or	4 ☐ N	9 ☐ DK
i.	Cabbage, cole slaw, and sauerkraut	_ _ per	1 ☐ D	2 ☐ W	3 ☐ M or	4 ☐ N	9 ☐ DK
j.	Hot red chili peppers. Do not count ground red chili peppers.	_ _ per	1 ☐ D	2 ☐ W	3 ☐ M or	4 ☐ N	9 ☐ DK
k.	Peppers including green, red, and yellow peppers	_ _ per	1 ☐ D	2 ☐ W	3 ☐ M or	4 ☐ N	9 ☐ DK
l.	Any other vegetables such as green beans, corn, peas, mushrooms, and zucchini	_ _ per	1 ☐ D	2 ☐ W	3 ☐ M or	4 ☐ N	9 ☐ DK

N5. BEANS, NUTS, CEREALS, AND GRAIN PRODUCTS

		Times	Day	Week	Month	Never	DK
a.	How often did you have beans, lentils, and (chickpeas/garbanzos)? Include kidney, pinto, refried, black, and baked beans.	_ _ per	1 ☐ D	2 ☐ W	3 ☐ M or	4 ☐ N	9 ☐ DK
b.	Peanuts, peanut butter, other types of nuts, and seeds	_ _ per	1 ☐ D	2 ☐ W	3 ☐ M or	4 ☐ N	9 ☐ DK

Now I'm going to ask how often you ate certain cereals.

		Times	Day	Week	Month	Never	DK
c.	How about All-Bran, All-Bran Extra Fiber, 100% Bran, and Fiber One?	_ _ per	1 ☐ D	2 ☐ W	3 ☐ M or	4 ☐ N	9 ☐ DK
d.	Total, Product 19, Most, and Just Right	_ _ per	1 ☐ D	2 ☐ W	3 ☐ M or	4 ☐ N	9 ☐ DK

	Times	Day	Week	Month	Never	DK
N5. **BEANS, NUTS, CEREALS, AND GRAIN PRODUCTS** (cont.)	_ _ per	1 ☐ D	2 ☐ W	3 ☐ M or	4 ☐ N	9 ☐ DK

e. All other cold-cereals like corn flakes, Cheerios, Rice Krispies, and presweetened cereals
_ _ per 1 ☐ D 2 ☐ W 3 ☐ M or 4 ☐ N 9 ☐ DK

f. Cooked, hot cereals like oatmeal, cream of wheat, cream of rice, and grits
_ _ per 1 ☐ D 2 ☐ W 3 ☐ M or 4 ☐ N 9 ☐ DK

Now let's talk about white bread products only. I'll ask about dark breads next.

g. How often did you have white bread, rolls, bagels, biscuits, English muffins, and crackers? Include those used for sandwiches.
_ _ per 1 ☐ D 2 ☐ W 3 ☐ M or 4 ☐ N 9 ☐ DK

h. Dark breads and rolls, including whole wheat, rye, and pumpernickel
_ _ per 1 ☐ D 2 ☐ W 3 ☐ M or 4 ☐ N 9 ☐ DK

i. Corn bread, corn muffins, and corn tortillas
_ _ per 1 ☐ D 2 ☐ W 3 ☐ M or 4 ☐ N 9 ☐ DK

j. Flour tortillas
_ _ per 1 ☐ D 2 ☐ W 3 ☐ M or 4 ☐ N 9 ☐ DK

k. Rice
_ _ per 1 ☐ D 2 ☐ W 3 ☐ M or 4 ☐ N 9 ☐ DK

l. Salted snacks such as potato chips, taco chips, corn chips, and salted pretzels and popcorn
_ _ per 1 ☐ D 2 ☐ W 3 ☐ M or 4 ☐ N 9 ☐ DK

N6. **DESSERTS, SWEETS, AND BEVERAGES**

a. How often did you have cakes, cookies, brownies, pies, doughnuts, and pastries?
_ _ per 1 ☐ D 2 ☐ W 3 ☐ M or 4 ☐ N 9 ☐ DK

b. Chocolate candy and fudge
_ _ per 1 ☐ D 2 ☐ W 3 ☐ M or 4 ☐ N 9 ☐ DK

Next are hot and iced beverages.

c. How often did you have Hi-C, Tang, Hawaiian Punch, Koolaid, and other drinks with added vitamin C?
_ _ per 1 ☐ D 2 ☐ W 3 ☐ M or 4 ☐ N 9 ☐ DK

d. Diet colas, diet sodas, and diet drinks such as Crystal Light
_ _ per 1 ☐ D 2 ☐ W 3 ☐ M or 4 ☐ N 9 ☐ DK

e. Regular colas and sodas, not diet
_ _ per 1 ☐ D 2 ☐ W 3 ☐ M or 4 ☐ N 9 ☐ DK

f. Regular coffee with caffeine
_ _ per 1 ☐ D 2 ☐ W 3 ☐ M or 4 ☐ N 9 ☐ DK

g. Regular tea with caffeine
_ _ per 1 ☐ D 2 ☐ W 3 ☐ M or 4 ☐ N 9 ☐ DK

h. Beer and lite beer
_ _ per 1 ☐ D 2 ☐ W 3 ☐ M or 4 ☐ N 9 ☐ DK

i. Wine, wine coolers, sangria, and champagne
_ _ per 1 ☐ D 2 ☐ W 3 ☐ M or 4 ☐ N 9 ☐ DK

j. Hard liquor such as tequila, gin, vodka, scotch, rum, whiskey and liqueurs, either alone or mixed
_ _ per 1 ☐ D 2 ☐ W 3 ☐ M or 4 ☐ N 9 ☐ DK

N7. **FATS**

How often were these items added to your foods <u>after preparation</u>? For example, this would include on top of vegetables or baked potatoes, or as a spread on bread.

Times	Day	Week	Month	Never	DK
_ _ per	1 ☐ D	2 ☐ W	3 ☐ M or	4 ☐ N	9 ☐ DK

a. Margarine

_ _ per 1 ☐ D 2 ☐ W 3 ☐ M or 4 ☐ N 9 ☐ DK

b. Butter

_ _ per 1 ☐ D 2 ☐ W 3 ☐ M or 4 ☐ N 9 ☐ DK

c. Oil and vinegar, mayonnaise and salad dressings such as Italian and Thousand Island, including those added to salads and sandwiches

_ _ per 1 ☐ D 2 ☐ W 3 ☐ M or 4 ☐ N 9 ☐ DK

N8. Have I missed any other foods or beverages that you had <u>at least once per week</u> in the <u>past month</u>?

1. ☐ Y (specify) ⟶↓   2. ☐ N (N9)

PROBE: How often did you eat . . . in the past month?

a. 1 _____

_ _ per 1 ☐ D 2 ☐ W 3 ☐ M or 4 ☐ N 9 ☐ DK

b. 1 _____

_ _ per 1 ☐ D 2 ☐ W 3 ☐ M or 4 ☐ N 9 ☐ DK

c. 1 _____

_ _ per 1 ☐ D 2 ☐ W 3 ☐ M or 4 ☐ N 9 ☐ DK

d. 1 _____

_ _ per 1 ☐ D 2 ☐ W 3 ☐ M or 4 ☐ N 9 ☐ DK

e. 1 _____

_ _ per 1 ☐ D 2 ☐ W 3 ☐ M or 4 ☐ N 9 ☐ DK

f. 1 _____

_ _ per 1 ☐ D 2 ☐ W 3 ☐ M or 4 ☐ N 9 ☐ DK

N9. CHECK ITEM. REFER TO AGE OF SP.

1 ☐   UNDER 20 YEARS (P1)

2 ☐   20 + YEARS

N10. REFER TO AGE OF SP. HAND CARD HAQ-6.
READ RESPONSE CATEGORIES TO SP IF NECESSARY.

Now I am going to ask how often you drank milk over your <u>lifetime</u>. Try to remember whether you were a milk drinker or a non-milk drinker during different times in your life. Then think of certain events that might have occurred during each time period, for example, were you in school, at home with children, on a farm, or in the service.

How often did you drink any type of milk, including milk added to cereal, when you were a _____? Do <u>not</u> count small amounts of milk added to coffee or tea.

Time period (age)	more than once per day	once per day	less than once per day but more than once per week	once per week	less than once per week	never	don't know
a. Child (5–12)	1 ☐	2 ☐	3 ☐	4 ☐	5 ☐	0 ☐	9 ☐
b. Teenager (13–17)	1 ☐	2 ☐	3 ☐	4 ☐	5 ☐	0 ☐	9 ☐
c. Young adult (18–35)	1 ☐	2 ☐	3 ☐	4 ☐	5 ☐	0 ☐	9 ☐
d. Middle-aged adult (36–65)	1 ☐	2 ☐	3 ☐	4 ☐	5 ☐	0 ☐	9 ☐
e. Older adult (over 65)	1 ☐	2 ☐	3 ☐	4 ☐	5 ☐	0 ☐	9 ☐

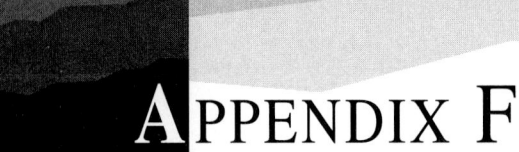

APPENDIX F

Database and Age- and Sex-Specific Portion Sizes for Food Items on Screening Questionnaire for Fat Intake Shown in Chapter 3

From National Cancer Institute, Division of Cancer Prevention and Control, National Institutes of Health.

Age- and Sex-Specific Portion Sizes* for Food Items on Screening Questionnaire

		Age- and Sex-Specific Portion Sizes (g)					
		Females			Males		
		Small	Medium	Large	Small	Medium	Large
Hamburgers, cheeseburgers							
Age	19–29	56.0	84.0	134.0	70.0	100.0	168.0
	30–60	56.0	84.0	111.0	67.0	100.0	168.0
	61+	50.0	70.0	84.0	53.0	84.0	126.0
Beef steaks, roasts							
Age	19–29	63.0	108.0	168.0	84.0	126.0	210.0
	30–60	60.0	85.0	157.0	84.0	126.0	168.0
	61+	50.0	84.0	126.0	70.0	112.0	168.0
Pork, incl. chops, roasts							
Age	19–29	53.0	84.0	126.0	70.0	112.0	168.0
	30–60	54.0	84.0	126.0	67.0	100.0	168.0
	61+	42.0	84.0	105.0	56.0	84.0	126.0
Hot dogs							
Age	19–29	44.0	88.0	132.0	45.0	90.0	135.0
	30–60	44.0	88.0	132.0	44.0	88.0	132.0
	61+	44.0	88.0	132.0	45.0	90.0	135.0
Ham, lunch meats							
Age	19–29	28.0	56.0	84.0	28.0	56.0	112.0
	30–60	28.0	56.0	84.0	28.0	56.0	84.0
	61+	28.0	56.0	84.0	28.0	56.0	84.0
Whole milk							
Age	19–29	150.0	270.0	330.0	226.0	270.0	330.0
	30–60	150.0	270.0	330.0	150.0	270.0	330.0
	61+	150.0	270.0	330.0	150.0	270.0	330.0
Doughnuts, cookies, cake							
Age	19–29	21.0	42.0	64.0	36.0	49.0	84.0
	30–60	28.0	42.0	63.0	31.0	48.0	84.0
	61+	24.0	42.0	53.0	23.0	42.0	64.0

continued

Age- and Sex-Specific Portion Sizes* for Food Items on Screening Questionnaire—*continued*

		Age- and Sex-Specific Portion Sizes (g)					
		Females			**Males**		
		Small	**Medium**	**Large**	**Small**	**Medium**	**Large**
White bread, rolls, etc.							
Age	19–29	28.0	46.0	56.0	40.0	56.0	92.0
	30–60	28.0	46.0	56.0	40.0	56.0	92.0
	61+	23.0	46.0	69.0	28.0	46.0	69.0
Eggs							
Age	19–29	50.0	100.0	150.0	50.0	100.0	128.0
	30–60	50.0	100.0	150.0	50.0	100.0	150.0
	61+	50.0	100.0	150.0	50.0	100.0	150.0
Cheese, excluding cottage							
Age	19–29	28.0	56.0	84.0	28.0	56.0	84.0
	30–60	28.0	56.0	84.0	28.0	56.0	84.0
	61+	28.0	56.0	69.0	28.0	56.0	84.0
Margarine, butter							
Age	19–29	5.5	11.0	16.0	5.5	11.0	16.0
	30–60	5.5	11.0	16.0	5.5	11.0	16.0
	61+	5.5	11.0	16.0	5.5	11.0	16.0
Mayonnaise, salad dressing							
Age	19–29	9.0	15.0	24.0	9.0	15.0	28.0
	30–60	9.0	18.0	28.0	9.0	15.0	28.0
	61+	9.0	18.0	28.0	9.0	18.0	28.0
French fries							
Age	19–29	52.0	115.0	126.0	52.0	126.0	252.0
	30–60	52.0	126.0	144.0	52.0	126.0	178.0
	61+	52.0	60.0	126.0	52.0	126.0	157.0

*Portion sizes are those used in the database developed by Gladys Block of the National Cancer Institute. They derive ultimately from portion sizes actually reported by respondents, using three-dimensional abstract models, in the NHANES II data. However, many of the items on this screener are unitary (e.g., one or two eggs, one or two pats of butter), and the portion sizes for unitary items were modified in some instances to correspond to those units.

Food List and Database for Screening Questionnaire for Fat Intake[*†]

	Portion Sizes (g)			Nutrient Content			
	Small	Medium	Large	Total Fat (g) per 100 g	Saturated Fat (g) per 100 g[‡]	Oleic Acid (g) per 100 g[‡]	Linoleic Acid (g) per 100 g[‡]
Hamburgers, cheeseburgers	43	85	128	20.3	9.7	8.9	0.4
Beef steaks, roasts	56	112	168	10.2	4.9	4.5	0.2
Pork, incl. chops, roast	44	88	132	15.4	5.5	6.5	1.4
Hot dogs	44	88	132	29.0	12.9	13.0	0.9
Ham, lunch meats	28	56	84	25.0	9.0	10.0	1.5
Whole milk (as a beverage)	122	244	366	3.5	1.9	1.2	0.1
Doughnuts, cookies, cake, pastry	24	42	63	16.8	4.5	8.0	2.2
White bread, rolls, bagels, etc., including sandwiches	25	50	75	4.0	0.7	1.5	0.8
Eggs	50	100	150	12.9	4.4	5.1	0.8
Cheese, excluding cottage	28	56	84	25.0	15.4	7.8	0.6
Margarine or butter	5	10	15	80.7	17.2[§]	35.0[§]	26.0[§]
Salad dressing, mayonnaise	8	16	24	60.0	10.7	13.6	31.2
French fries	51	102	153	8.4	2.1	1.8	4.2

Do you eat these every day?[‖]

  Dark bread, such as whole-wheat, rye, pumpernickel? Yes/No

  Breakfast cereal? Yes/No

---

[*]Foods are listed in the order in which they might be used in an actual questionnaire with a respondent, *not* in order of their importance as nutrient sources. The two categorical variables are not important sources of fat at all, but are to be used only as behavioral markers.

[†]Fat scores would be calculated as follows:
Algorithm for 13-item list: Use foods 1–13. "Times" = No. of times, in the "How often" column; "Factor" indicates the time unit: Day = 7; Week = 1; Month = 0.2333; Year = 0.01923. Calculate sum of (Times × Factor × Reported portion size/100 × fat per 100 g). After adding all the foods, divide by 7 for daily estimate. Divide resulting distribution at midpoint, for above and below median. (Midpoint of the screener distribution among this population of mostly white, health-conscious women aged 45–69 years was 21.3 g.) Quintile cutpoints were 1–11.9, 12–19.5, 19.6–23.9, 24–36.9, 37 or higher.
Algorithm for 13-item augmented list: for the sum, use foods 1–13; calculate as in Algorithm 1. Include in the questionnaire, but not in the sum, food 14 ("Dark bread such as whole-wheat, rye, pumpernickel") and food 15 ("Breakfast cereal"). Then the algorithm for categorizing as "high" or "low" on percent of calories from fat is as follows: If below screener median (calculated from foods 1–13), then categorize as "low"; if above screener median, categorize as "high"; if above screener median *and* eats dark bread every day *and* eats breakfast cereal every day, then move from "high" to "low."

[‡]Saturated fat and oleic acid (monounsaturated fat) are not used in calculating the screener estimate used to identify respondents with a high (or low) mean percent of calories from fat. They are provided here for investigators who may wish to use the instrument to rank respondents on gram intake of these nutrients. Linoleic acid is provided for the same reason, but it should be noted that the questionnaire was not designed to assess this nutrient. Since its correlation with reference data was tolerable, some investigators may wish to calculate linoleic in studies in which the main purpose is to assess one of the other fats.

[§]Values are for margarine. Butter has 44.6 g saturated fat, 26.7 g oleic acid, 2.4 g linoleic acid. If linoleic and oleic acids are of central importance to a proposed study, rather than total fat, consider asking butter and margarine separately.

[‖]Included as a categorical variable, but not included in the grams-of-fat calculation.

MEDFICTS* Dietary Assessment Questionnaire

APPENDIX G

In each food category for both Group 1 and Group 2 foods check one box from the "Weekly Consumption" column (number of servings eaten per week) and then check one box from the "Serving Size" column. If you check Rarely/Never, do not check a serving size box. See next page for score.

Food Category	Weekly Consumption			Serving Size			Score
	Rarely/ never	3 or less	4 or more	Small <5 oz/d 1 pt	Average 5 oz/d 2 pts	Large >5 oz/d 3 pts	

Meats

- Recommended amount per day: ≤5 oz (equal in size to 2 decks of playing cards)
- Base your estimate on the food you consume most often.
- Beef and lamb selections are trimmed to 1/8" fat.

Food Category	Rarely/never	3 or less	4 or more	Small	Average	Large	Score
Group 1. 10 gm or more total fat in 3 oz cooked portion **Beef** – Ground beef, Ribs, Steak (T-bone, Flank, Porterhouse, Tenderloin), Chuck blade roast, Brisket, Meatloaf (w/ground beef), Corned beef **Processed meats** – ¼ lb burger or lg. sandwich, Bacon, Lunch meat, Sausage/knockwurst, Hot dogs, Ham (bone-end), Ground turkey **Other meats, Poultry, Seafood**—Pork chops (center loin), Pork roast (Blade, Boston, Sirloin), Pork spareribs, Ground pork, Lamb chops, Lamb (ribs), Organ meats†, Chicken w/skin, Eel, Mackerel, Pompano	☐	☐ 3 pts	☐ 7pts	x ☐ 1 pt	☐ 2 pts	☐ 3 pts	_____
Group 2. Less than 10 gm total fat in 3 oz cooked portion **Lean beef** – Round steak (Eye of round, Top round), Sirloin‡, Tip & bottom round‡, Chuck arm pot roast‡, Top Loin‡ **Low-fat processed meats** – Low-fat lunch meat, Canadian bacon, "Lean" fast food sandwich, Boneless ham **Other meats, Poultry, Seafood** – Chicken, Turkey (w/o skin)§, most Seafood†, Lamb leg shank, Pork tenderloin, Sirloin top loin, Veal cutlets, Sirloin, Shoulder, Ground veal, Venison, Veal chops and ribs‡, Lamb (whole leg, loin, fore-shank, sirloin)‡	☐	☐	☐	☐	☐	☐¥ 6 pts	_____

Eggs – Weekly consumption is the number of times you eat eggs each week   Check the number of eggs eaten each time

Food Category	Rarely/never	3 or less	4 or more	≤1 1 pt	2 2 pts	≥3 3 pts	Score
Group 1. Whole eggs, Yolks	☐	☐ 3 pts	☐ 7 pts	x ☐	☐	☐	_____
Group 2. Egg whites, Egg substitutes (½ cup)	☐	☐	☐	☐	☐	☐	_____

Dairy

Food Category	Rarely/never	3 or less	4 or more	Small 1 pt	Average 2 pts	Large 3 pts	Score
Milk – Average serving 1 cup **Group 1.** Whole milk, 2% milk, 2% buttermilk, Yogurt (whole milk)	☐	☐ 3 pts	☐ 7 pts	x ☐ 1 pt	☐ 2 pts	☐ 3 pts	_____
Group 2. Fat-free milk, 1% milk, Fat-free buttermilk, Yogurt (Fat-free, 1% low fat)	☐	☐	☐	☐	☐	☐	_____
Cheese – Average serving 1 oz **Group 1.** Cream cheese, Cheddar, Monterey Jack, Colby, Swiss, American processed, Blue cheese, Regular cottage cheese (½ cup), and Ricotta (¼ cup)	☐	☐ 3 pts	☐ 7 pts	x ☐ 1 pt	☐ 2 pts	☐ 3 pts	_____
Group 2. Low-fat & fat-free cheeses, Fat-free milk mozzarella, String cheese, Low-fat, Fat-free milk & Fat-free cottage cheese (½ cup) and Ricotta (¼ cup)	☐	☐	☐	☐	☐	☐	_____
Frozen Desserts – Average serving ½ cup **Group 1.** Ice cream, Milk shakes	☐	☐ 3 pts	☐ 7 pts	x ☐ 1 pt	☐ 2 pts	☐ 3 pts	_____
Group 2. Low-fat ice cream, Frozen yogurt	☐	☐	☐	☐	☐	☐	_____

Food Category	Weekly Consumption			Serving Size			Score
	Rarely/ never	3 or less	4 or more	Small <5 oz/d 1 pt	Average 5 oz/d 2 pts	Large >5 oz/d 3 pts	

Frying Foods – Average servings: see below. This section refers to method of prepartion for vegetables and meat.

Group 1. French fries, Fried vegetables (½ cup), Fried chicken, fish, meat (3 oz)	☐	☐ 3 pts	☐ 7 pts	x ☐ 1 pt	☐ 2 pts	☐ 3 pts	_____
Group 2. Vegetables, not deep fried (½ cup), Meat, poultry, or fish—prepared by baking, broiling, grilling, poaching, roasting, stewing: (3 oz)	☐	☐	☐	☐	☐	☐	_____

In Baked Goods – 1 Average serving

Group 1. Doughnuts, Biscuits, Butter rolls, Muffins, Croissants, Sweet rolls, Danish, Cakes, Pies, Coffee cakes, Cookies	☐	☐ 3 pts	☐ 7 pts	x ☐ 1 pt	☐ 2 pts	☐ 3 pts	_____
Group 2. Fruit bars, Low-fat cookies/cakes/pastries, Angel food cake, Homemade baked goods with vegetable oils, breads, bagels	☐	☐	☐	☐	☐	☐	_____

Convenience Foods

Group 1. Canned, Packaged, or Frozen dinners: e.g., Pizza (1 slice), Macaroni & cheese (1 cup), Pot pie (1), Cream soups (1 cup), Potato, rice & pasta dishes with cream/cheese sauces (½ cup)	☐	☐ 3 pts	☐ 7 pts	x ☐ 1 pt	☐ 2 pts	☐ 3 pts	_____
Group 2. Diet/Reduced calorie or reduced fat dinners (1), Potato, rice & pasta dishes without cream/cheese sauces (½ cup)	☐	☐	☐	☐	☐	☐	_____

Table Fats – Average serving: 1 Tbsp

Group 1. Butter, Stick margarine, Regular salad dressing, Mayonnaise, Sour cream (2 Tbsp)	☐	☐ 3 pts	☐ 7 pts	x ☐ 1 pt	☐ 2 pts	☐ 3 pts	_____
Group 2. Diet and tub margarine, Low-fat & fat-free salad dressing, Low-fat & fat-free mayonnaise	☐	☐	☐	☐	☐	☐	_____

Snacks

Group 1. Chips (potato, corn, taco), Cheese puffs, Snack mix, Nuts (1 oz), Regular crackers (½ oz), Candy (milk chocolate, caramel, coconut) (about 1½ oz), Regular popcorn (3 cups)	☐	☐ 3 pts	☐ 7 pts	x ☐ 1 pt	☐ 2 pts	☐ 3 pts	_____
Group 2. Pretzels, Fat-free chips (1 oz), Low-fat crackers (1/2 oz), Fruit, Fruit rolls, Licorice, Hard candy (1 med piece), Bread sticks (1–2 pcs), Air-popped or low-fat popcorn (3 cups)	☐	☐	☐	☐	☐	☐	_____

†   Organ meats, shrimp, abalone, and squid are low in fat but high in cholesterol.

‡   Only lean cuts with all visible fat trimmed. If not trimmed of all visible fat, score as if in Group 1.

¥   Score 6 pts if this box is checked.

§   All parts not listed in group 1 have <10 gm total fat.

Total from page 1 _____

Total from page 2 _____

FINAL SCORE _____

To Score: For each food category, multiply points in weekly consumption box by points in serving size box and record total in score column. If Group 2 foods checked, no points are scored (except for Group 2 meats, large serving = 6 pts).

Example:

☐	☐ 3 pts	☑ 7 pts	x ☐ 1 pt	☐ 2 pts	☑ 3 pts	21

Add score on page 1 and page 2 to get final score.

Key:

≥70   Need to make some dietary changes
40–70 Heart-Healthy Diet
<40   TLC Diet

From National Cholesterol Education Program. 2001. *Third report of the Expert Panel on Detection, Evaluation, and Treatment of High Blood Cholesterol in Adults.* Bethesda, MD: U.S. Department of Health and Human Services.

*MEDFICTS = **M**eats, **E**ggs, **D**airy, **F**rying Foods, **I**n baked goods, **C**onvenience foods, **T**able fats, **S**nacks.

Harvard University School of Public Health Food Frequency Questionnaire

APPENDIX H

DIETARY ASSESSMENT

ID NUMBER: _____

DATE: _____

USE NO. 2 PENCIL ONLY 2

- **Darken one circle per question that corresponds to your answer**

- **Follow arrows**

VITAMINS

1. Have you ever regularly taken **multi-vitamins**?

⊢ ○ **Never** have
  ○ Have in the **Past only** →

 a) For how many years did you take them in the past?

  ○ 1 year or less   ○ 2–4 years   ○ 5–9 years   ○ 10 or more years

○ **Currently** take them →

 a) If you currently take multi-vitamins, how many do you take per week?

  ○ 2 or less   ○ 3–5   ○ 6–9   ○ 10 or more

 b) If you are currently taking multi-vitamins, for how many years have you been taking them?

  ○ 1 year or less   ○ 2–4 years   ○ 5–9 years   ○ 10 or more years

 c) If you currently take them, what <u>brand</u> do you usually use?
 (Specify exact brand and type)

 [   ]

2. <u>**Not counting multi-vitamins,**</u> have you <u>ever</u> taken any of the following specific vitamins or minerals?

Vitamin A　　　　　　　　→ **Dose per day?** →　　　**How long?**

⊢ ○ **Never** taken
  ○ Taken in the **past only** ⇒
  ○ Yes, **currently** take it

Dose per day?
○ Less than 8,000 IU
○ 8,000 to 12,000 IU
○ 13,000 to 22,000 IU
○ 23,000 IU or more
○ Don't know

How long?
○ 0–1 year
○ 2–4 years
○ 5–9 years
○ 10 years or more

PLEASE DO NOT WRITE IN THIS AREA

20158

2. (Continued) **Not counting multi-vitamins,** have you <u>ever</u> taken any of the following specific vitamins or minerals?

Beta Carotene

○ Never taken
○ Taken in the past only
○ Yes, currently take it

Dose per day?
○ Less than 8,000 IU
○ 8,000 to 12,000 IU
○ 13,000 to 22,000 IU
○ 23,000 IU or more
○ Don't know

How long?
○ 0–1 year
○ 2–4 years
○ 5–9 years
○ 10 years or more

Vitamin B₆

○ Never taken
○ Taken in the past only
○ Yes, currently take it

Dose per day?
○ Less than 10 mg
○ 10 to 39 mg
○ 40 to 79 mg
○ 80 mg or more
○ Don't know

How long?
○ 0–1 year
○ 2–4 years
○ 5–9 years
○ 10 years or more

Vitamin C

○ Never taken
○ Taken in the past only
○ Yes, currently take it

Dose per day?
○ Less than 400 mg
○ 400 to 700 mg
○ 750 to 1,250 mg
○ 1,300 mg or more
○ Don't know

How long?
○ 0–1 year
○ 2–4 years
○ 5–9 years
○ 10 years or more

Vitamin E

○ Never taken
○ Taken in the past only
○ Yes, currently take it

Dose per day?
○ Less than 100 IU
○ 100 to 250 IU
○ 300 to 500 IU
○ 600 IU or more
○ Don't know

How long?
○ 0–1 year
○ 2–4 years
○ 5–9 years
○ 10 years or more

Selenium

○ Never taken
○ Taken in the past only
○ Yes, currently take it

Dose per day?
○ Less than 80 mcg
○ 80 to 130 mcg
○ 140 to 250 mcg
○ 260 mcg or more
○ Don't know

How long?
○ 0–1 year
○ 2–4 years
○ 5–9 years
○ 10 years or more

Iron

○ Never taken
○ Taken in the past only
○ Yes, currently take it

Dose per day?
mg of elemental iron (325 mg Ferrous Sulfate = 65 mg elemental iron)
○ Less than 41 mg
○ 41 to 80 mg
○ 81 to 150 mg
○ 151 mg or more
○ Don't know

How long?
○ 0–1 year
○ 2–4 years
○ 5–9 years
○ 10 years or more

Zinc

○ Never taken
○ Taken in the past only
○ Yes, currently take it

Dose per day?
○ Less than 25 mg
○ 25 to 74 mg
○ 75 to 100 mg
○ 101 mg or more
○ Don't know

How long?
○ 0–1 year
○ 2–4 years
○ 5–9 years
○ 10 years or more

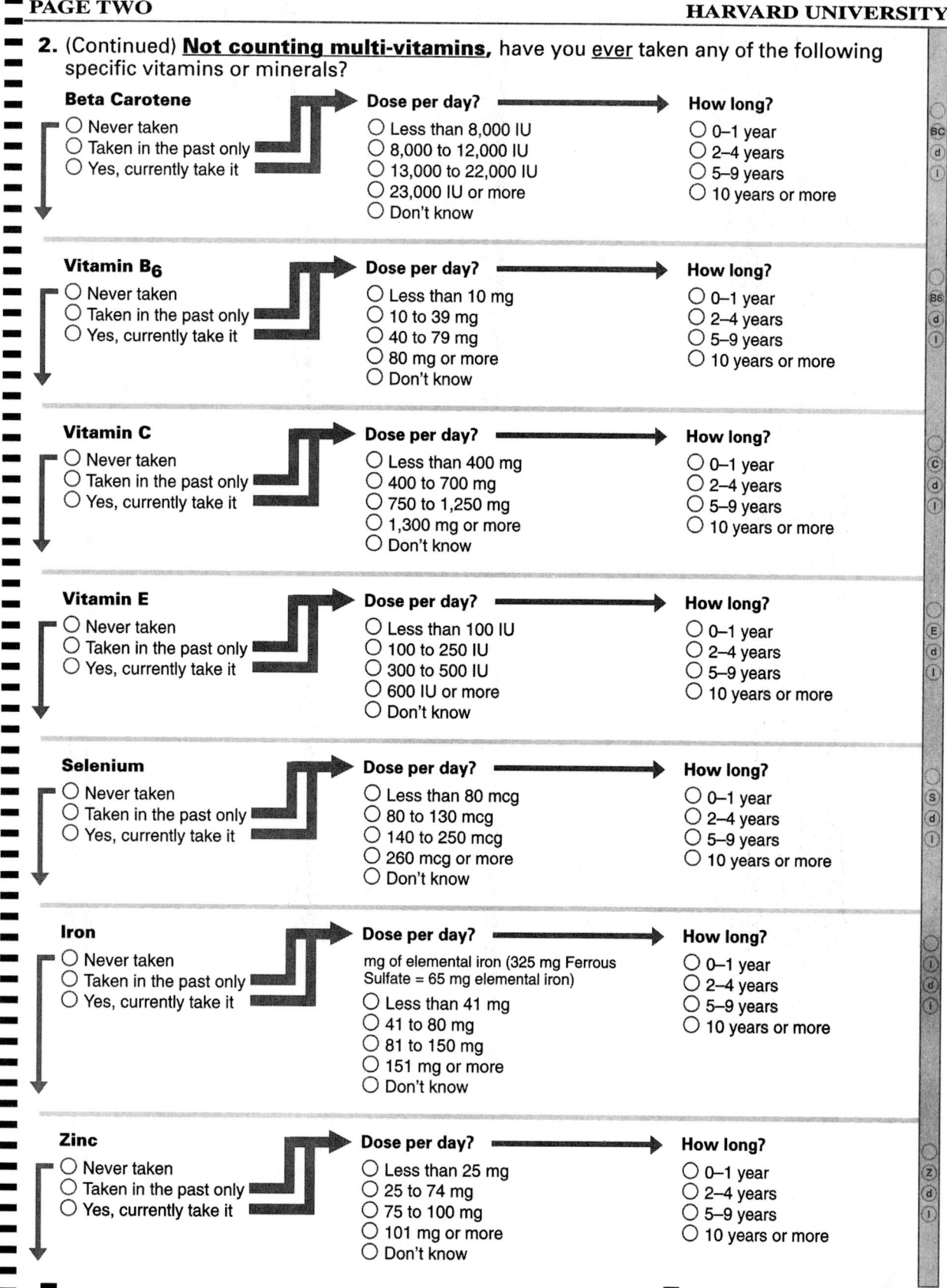

405

2. (Continued) **Not counting multi-vitamins,** have you <u>ever</u> taken any of the following specific vitamins or minerals?

Calcium or Dolomite (Include Tums)

○ Never taken
○ Taken in the past only
○ Yes, currently take it

Dose per day? ➡

mg of elemental Calcium (1 Tums = 500 mg Calcium Carbonate = 200 mg elemental.)

○ Less than 400 mg
○ 400 to 900 mg
○ 901 to 1,300 mg
○ 1,301 mg or more
○ Don't know

How long?

○ 0–1 year
○ 2–4 years
○ 5–9 years
○ 10 years or more

Fish Oil (Omega 3 fatty acids)

○ Never taken
○ Taken in the past only
○ Yes, currently take it

Dose per day? ➡

○ Less than 2500 mg
○ 2500 to 4999 mg
○ 5000 to 9999 mg
○ 10,000 mg or more
○ Don't know

How long?

○ 0–1 year
○ 2–4 years
○ 5–9 years
○ 10 years or more

Which <u>other</u> supplements are you taking <u>currently</u> on a regular basis (at least once per week)?

○ None
○ Metamucil
○ Cod liver oil
○ Brewer's yeast
○ Vitamin D
○ Folic acid or folate (B_9)
○ Potassium
○ Magnesium
○ Niacin
○ Other Supplements (specify) _____

DAIRY FOODS

In the following section, please describe how often <u>on average</u> you have used the amount specified in the past year. Please indicate your average <u>total</u> use, taking the portion size into account. For example, if you use 1/2 a glass of milk twice a week, mark 1 glass per week to represent your average total intake.

3. For each food listed, fill in the circle indicating your <u>average total</u> use of the amount specified <u>during the past year</u>.

Skim milk (8 oz. glass)	1% or 2% milk (8 oz. glass)	Whole milk (8 oz. glass)
○ Never	○ Never	○ Never
○ Less than once per month	○ Less than once per month	○ Less than once per month
○ 1–3 glasses per month	○ 1–3 glasses per month	○ 1–3 glasses per month
○ 1 glass per week	○ 1 glass per week	○ 1 glass per week
○ 2–4 glasses per week	○ 2–4 glasses per week	○ 2–4 glasses per week
○ 5–6 glasses per week	○ 5–6 glasses per week	○ 5–6 glasses per week
○ 1 glass per day	○ 1 glass per day	○ 1 glass per day
○ 2–3 glasses per day	○ 2–3 glasses per day	○ 2–3 glasses per day
○ 4 or more glasses per day	○ 4 or more glasses per day	○ 4 or more glasses per day

3. (Continued) Please fill in your <u>average</u> total use, <u>during the past year</u>, of each specified food.

Cream, e.g., in coffee, whipped or sour cream (1 tbs.)
- ○ Never
- ○ Less than once per month
- ○ 1–3 tbs. per month
- ○ 1 tbs. per week
- ○ 2–4 tbs. per week
- ○ 5–6 tbs. per week
- ○ 1 tbs. per day
- ○ 2 or more tbs. per day

Non-dairy coffee whitener (tsp.)
- ○ Never
- ○ Less than once per month
- ○ 1–3 tsp. per month
- ○ 1 tsp. per week
- ○ 2–4 tsp. per week
- ○ 5–6 tsp. per week
- ○ 1 tsp. per day
- ○ 2 or more tsp. per day

Frozen yogurt, sherbet or non-fat ice cream (1/2 cup)
- ○ Never
- ○ Less than once per month
- ○ 1–3 times per month
- ○ Once per week
- ○ 2–4 times per week
- ○ 5–6 times per week
- ○ Once per day
- ○ 2 or more servings per day

Ice cream (1/2 cup)
- ○ Never
- ○ Less than once per month
- ○ 1–3 times per month
- ○ Once per week
- ○ 2–4 times per week
- ○ 5–6 times per week
- ○ Once per day
- ○ 2 or more servings per day

Flavored yogurt, <u>without</u> Nutrasweet (1 cup)
- ○ Never
- ○ Less than once per month
- ○ 1–3 cups per month
- ○ 1 cup per week
- ○ 2–4 cups per week
- ○ 5–6 cups per week
- ○ 1 cup per day
- ○ 2 or more servings per day

Yogurt, plain or with Nutrasweet (1 cup)
- ○ Never
- ○ Less than once per month
- ○ 1–3 cups per month
- ○ 1 cup per week
- ○ 2–4 cups per week
- ○ 5–6 cups per week
- ○ 1 cup per day
- ○ 2 or more servings per day

What type of yogurt do you usually eat?
- ○ None
- ○ Regular
- ○ Low fat
- ○ Nonfat

Cottage or ricotta cheese (1/2 cup)
- ○ Never
- ○ Less than once per month
- ○ 1–3 times per month
- ○ Once per week
- ○ 2–4 times per week
- ○ 5–6 times per week
- ○ Once per day
- ○ 2 or more servings per day

Cream cheese (1 oz.)
- ○ Never
- ○ Less than once per month
- ○ 1–3 times per month
- ○ Once per week
- ○ 2–4 times per week
- ○ 5–6 times per week
- ○ Once per day
- ○ 2 or more servings per day

Other cheese, e.g., American, cheddar, etc., plain or as part of a dish (1 slice or 1 oz. serving)
- ○ Never
- ○ Less than once per month
- ○ 1–3 slices per month
- ○ 1 slice per week
- ○ 2–4 slices per week
- ○ 5–6 slices per week
- ○ 1 slice per day
- ○ 2 or more slices per day

What type of cheese do you usually eat?
- ○ None
- ○ Regular
- ○ Low fat or lite
- ○ Nonfat

Butter (small pat or tsp.), added to food or bread; exclude use in cooking
- ○ Never
- ○ Less than once per month
- ○ 1–3 pats per month
- ○ 1 pat per week
- ○ 2–4 pats per week
- ○ 5–6 pats per week
- ○ 1 pat per day
- ○ 2–3 pats per day
- ○ 4 or more pats per day

3. (Continued) Please fill in your <u>average</u> total use, <u>during the past year</u>, of each specified food.

Margarine (small pat or tsp.), added to food or bread; exclude use in cooking

○ Never
○ Less than once per month
○ 1–3 pats per month
○ 1 pat per week
○ 2–4 pats per week
○ 5–6 pats per week
○ 1 pat per day
○ 2–3 pats per day
○ 4 or more pats per day

What form of margarine do you usually use? (Do not include "spray" type margarine)

○ None

Form?
○ Stick
○ Tub
○ Squeeze (liquid)

Type?
○ Regular
○ Light spread
○ Extra light spread
○ Nonfat

What specific **brand** and **type** (e.g., Land O' Lakes Country Morning Blend Light)?

FRUITS

4. Please fill in your <u>average</u> total use, <u>during the past year</u>, of each specified food.

Please try to average your seasonal use of foods over the entire year. For example, if a food such as cantaloupe is eaten 4 times a week during the 3 months that it is in season, then the <u>average</u> total use would be once per week over the year.

Raisins (1 oz. or small pack) or grapes

○ Never
○ Less than once per month
○ 1–3 times per month
○ Once per week
○ 2–4 times per week
○ 5–6 times per week
○ Once per day
○ 2 or more servings per day

Prunes (7 prunes or 1/2 cup)

○ Never
○ Less than once per month
○ 1–3 times per month
○ Once per week
○ 2–4 times per week
○ 5–6 times per week
○ Once per day

Bananas (1)

○ Never
○ Less than once per month
○ 1–3 per month
○ 1 per week
○ 2–4 per week
○ 5–6 per week
○ 1 per day
○ 2 or more per day

Cantaloupe (1/4 melon)

○ Never
○ Less than once per month
○ 1–3 times per month
○ Once per week
○ 2–4 times per week
○ 5–6 times per week
○ Once per day
○ 2–3 times per day
○ 4 or more servings per day

Avocado (1/2 fruit or 1/2 cup)

○ Never
○ Less than once per month
○ 1–3 times per month
○ Once per week
○ 2–4 times per week
○ 5–6 times per week
○ One per day
○ Two or more per day

Applesauce (1/2 cup)

○ Never
○ Less than once per month
○ 1–3 times per month
○ Once per week
○ 2–4 times per week
○ 5–6 times per week
○ One or more per day

Fresh apples or pears (1)

○ Never
○ Less than once per month
○ 1–3 per month
○ 1 per week
○ 2–4 per week
○ 5–6 per week
○ 1 per day
○ 2–3 per day
○ 4 or more per day

Apple juice or cider (small glass)

○ Never
○ Less than once per month
○ 1–3 glasses per month
○ 1 glass per week
○ 2–4 glasses per week
○ 5–6 glasses per week
○ 1 glass per day
○ 2 or more glasses per day

Oranges (1)

○ Never
○ Less than once per month
○ 1–3 per month
○ 1 per week
○ 2–4 per week
○ 5–6 per week
○ 1 per day
○ 2–3 per day
○ 4 or more per day

4. (Continued) Please fill in your <u>average</u> total use, <u>during the past year</u>, of each specified food.

Orange juice (small glass)
- ○ Never
- ○ Less than once per month
- ○ 1–3 glasses per month
- ○ 1 glass per week
- ○ 2–4 glasses per week
- ○ 5–6 glasses per week
- ○ 1 glass per day
- ○ 2 or more glasses per day

Grapefruit (1/2)
- ○ Never
- ○ Less than once per month
- ○ 1–3 times per month
- ○ Once per week
- ○ 2–4 times per week
- ○ 5–6 times per week
- ○ Once per day
- ○ 2–3 times per day
- ○ 4 or more times per day

Grapefruit juice (small glass)
- ○ Never
- ○ Less than once per month
- ○ 1–3 glasses per month
- ○ 1 glass per week
- ○ 2–4 glasses per week
- ○ 5–6 glasses per week
- ○ 1 glass per day
- ○ 2 or more glasses per day

Other fruit juices (small glass)
- ○ Never
- ○ Less than once per month
- ○ 1–3 glasses per month
- ○ 1 glass per week
- ○ 2–4 glasses per week
- ○ 5–6 glasses per week
- ○ 1 glass per day
- ○ 2 or more glasses per day

Strawberries, fresh, frozen or canned (1/2 cup)
- ○ Never
- ○ Less than once per month
- ○ 1–3 times per month
- ○ Once per week
- ○ 2–4 times per week
- ○ 5–6 times per week
- ○ Once or more per day

Blueberries, fresh, frozen or canned (1/2 cup)
- ○ Never
- ○ Less than once per month
- ○ 1–3 times per month
- ○ Once per week
- ○ 2–4 times per week
- ○ 5 or more servings per week

Peaches, apricots or plums (1 fresh, or 1/2 cup canned)
- ○ Never
- ○ Less than once per month
- ○ 1–3 per month
- ○ Once per week
- ○ 2–4 per week
- ○ 5–6 per week
- ○ 1 or more per day

In summary, how many servings of fruit do you usually eat, <u>not counting juices</u>?
- ○ None
- ○ Less than one per month
- ○ 1–3 per month
- ○ 1 per week
- ○ 2–4 per week
- ○ 5–6 per week
- ○ 1 per day
- ○ 2–3 per day
- ○ 4–5 per day
- ○ 6+ per day

VEGETABLES

5. Please fill in your <u>average</u> total use, <u>during the past year</u>, of each specified food.

Tomatoes (1)
- ○ Never
- ○ Less than once per month
- ○ 1–3 per month
- ○ 1 per week
- ○ 2–4 per week
- ○ 5–6 per week
- ○ 1 or more per day

Tomato juice (small glass)
- ○ Never
- ○ Less than once per month
- ○ 1–3 glasses per month
- ○ 1 glass per week
- ○ 2–4 glasses per week
- ○ 5–6 glasses per week
- ○ 1 glass per day
- ○ 2 or more glasses per day

Tomato sauce (1/2 cup) e.g., spaghetti sauce
- ○ Never
- ○ Less than once per month
- ○ 1–3 times per month
- ○ Once per week
- ○ 2–4 times per week
- ○ 5 or more servings per week

Salsa, picante or taco sauce (1/4 cup)
- ○ Never
- ○ Less than once per month
- ○ 1–3 times per month
- ○ Once per week
- ○ 2–4 times per week
- ○ 5–6 times per week
- ○ Once per day
- ○ 2 or more servings per day

Tofu or soybeans (3–4 oz.)
- ○ Never
- ○ Less than once per month
- ○ 1–3 times per month
- ○ Once per week
- ○ 2–4 times per week
- ○ 5–6 times per week
- ○ Once per day
- ○ 2 or more servings per day

String beans (1/2 cup)
- ○ Never
- ○ Less than once per month
- ○ 1–3 times per month
- ○ Once per week
- ○ 2–4 times per week
- ○ 5 or more servings per week

5. (Continued) Please fill in your <u>average</u> total use, <u>during the past year</u>, of each specified food.

Broccoli (1/2 cup)
○ Never
○ Less than once per month
○ 1–3 times per month
○ Once per week
○ 2–4 times per week
○ 5–6 times per week
○ 1 or more servings per day

Cabbage or cole slaw (1/2 cup)
○ Never
○ Less than once per month
○ 1–3 times per month
○ Once per week
○ 2–4 times per week
○ 5–6 times per week
○ 1 or more servings per day

Cauliflower (1/2 cup)
○ Never
○ Less than once per month
○ 1–3 times per month
○ Once per week
○ 2–4 times per week
○ 5–6 times per week
○ 1 or more servings per day

Brussels sprouts (1/2 cup)
○ Never
○ Less than once per month
○ 1–3 times per month
○ Once per week
○ 2–4 times per week
○ 5–6 times per week
○ 1 or more servings per day

Carrots, raw (1/2 carrot or 2–4 sticks)
○ Never
○ Less than once per month
○ 1–3 times per month
○ Once per week
○ 2–4 times per week
○ 5–6 times per week
○ Once per day
○ 2 or more servings per day

Carrots, cooked (1/2 cup) or carrot juice (2–3 oz.)
○ Never
○ Less than once per month
○ 1–3 times per month
○ Once per week
○ 2–4 times per week
○ 5–6 times per week
○ Once per day
○ 2 or more servings per day

Corn (1 ear or 1/2 cup frozen or canned)
○ Never
○ Less than once per month
○ 1–3 per month
○ 1 per week
○ 2–4 per week
○ 5–6 per week
○ 1 or more servings per day

Peas or lima beans (1/2 cup fresh, frozen or canned)
○ Never
○ Less than once per month
○ 1–3 times per month
○ Once per week
○ 2–4 times per week
○ 5–6 times per week
○ 1 or more servings per day

Mixed vegetables (1/2 cup)
○ Never
○ Less than once per month
○ 1–3 times per month
○ Once per week
○ 2–4 times per week
○ 5–6 times per week
○ 1 or more servings per day

Beans or lentils, baked or dried (1/2 cup)
○ Never
○ Less than once per month
○ 1–3 times per month
○ Once per week
○ 2–4 times per week
○ 5–6 times per week
○ 1 or more servings per day

Dark orange (winter) squash (1/2 cup)
○ Never
○ Less than once per month
○ 1–3 times per month
○ Once per week
○ 2–4 times per week
○ 5–6 times per week
○ 1 or more servings per day

Eggplant, zucchini or other summer squash (1/2 cup)
○ Never
○ Less than once per month
○ 1–3 times per month
○ Once per week
○ 2–4 times per week
○ 5–6 times per week
○ 1 or more servings per day

Yams or sweet potatoes (1/2 cup)
○ Never
○ Less than once per month
○ 1–3 times per month
○ Once per week
○ 2–4 times per week
○ 5–6 times per week
○ 1 or more servings per day

Spinach, cooked (1/2 cup)
○ Never
○ Less than once per month
○ 1–3 times per month
○ Once per week
○ 2–4 times per week
○ 5–6 times per week
○ 1 or more servings per day

Spinach, raw as in salad
○ Never
○ Less than once per month
○ 1–3 times per month
○ Once per week
○ 2–4 times per week
○ 5–6 times per week
○ 1 or more servings per day

5. (Continued) Please fill in your <u>average</u> total use, <u>during the past year</u>, of each specified food.

Kale, mustard, or chard greens (1/2 cup)

- ○ Never
- ○ Less than once per month
- ○ 1–3 times per month
- ○ Once per week
- ○ 2–4 times per week
- ○ 5–6 times per week
- ○ 1 or more servings per day

Iceberg or head lettuce (serving)

- ○ Never
- ○ Less than once per month
- ○ 1–3 times per month
- ○ Once per week
- ○ 2–4 times per week
- ○ 5–6 times per week
- ○ Once per day
- ○ 2 or more servings per day

Romaine or leaf lettuce (serving)

- ○ Never
- ○ Less than once per month
- ○ 1–3 times per month
- ○ Once per week
- ○ 2–4 times per week
- ○ 5–6 times per week
- ○ Once per day
- ○ 2 or more servings per day

Celery (4" stick)

- ○ Never
- ○ Less than once per month
- ○ 1–3 per month
- ○ Once per week
- ○ 2–4 per week
- ○ 5–6 per week
- ○ Once per day
- ○ 2 or more servings per day

Green peppers (3 slices or 1/4 pepper)

- ○ Never
- ○ Less than once per month
- ○ 1–3 times per month
- ○ Once per week
- ○ 2–4 times per week
- ○ 5–6 times per week
- ○ 1 or more servings per day

Onions as a garnish or in a salad (1 slice)

- ○ Never
- ○ Less than once per month
- ○ 1–3 slices per month
- ○ 1 slice per week
- ○ 2–4 slices per week
- ○ 5–6 slices per week
- ○ 1 or more slices per day

Onions as a vegetable, rings or soup (1 onion)

- ○ Never
- ○ Less than once per month
- ○ 1–3 per month
- ○ 1 per week
- ○ 2–4 per week
- ○ 5–6 per week
- ○ 1 or more per day

In summary, how many servings of vegetables do you usually eat, <u>not counting salad or potatoes</u>?

- ○ None
- ○ Less than one per month
- ○ 1–3 per month
- ○ 1 per week
- ○ 2–4 per week
- ○ 5–6 per week
- ○ 1 per day
- ○ 2–3 per day
- ○ 4–5 per day
- ○ 6+ per day

EGGS, MEAT & FISH

6. Please fill in your <u>average</u> total use, <u>during the past year</u>, of each specified food.

Egg Beaters or egg whites only (1/4 cup or 1 egg)
- ○ Never
- ○ Less than once per month
- ○ 1–3 eggs per month
- ○ 1 egg per week
- ○ 2–4 eggs per week
- ○ 5–6 eggs per week
- ○ 1 egg per day
- ○ 2 or more eggs per day

Eggs whole, with yolk (1)
- ○ Never
- ○ Less than once per month
- ○ 1–3 eggs per month
- ○ 1 egg per week
- ○ 2–4 eggs per week
- ○ 5–6 eggs per week
- ○ 1 egg per day
- ○ 2 or more eggs per day

Bacon (2 slices)
- ○ Never
- ○ Less than once per month
- ○ 1–3 times per month
- ○ Once per week
- ○ 2–4 times per week
- ○ 5–6 times per week
- ○ 1 or more servings per day

Chicken or turkey sandwich
- ○ Never
- ○ Less than once per month
- ○ 1–3 times per month
- ○ Once per week
- ○ 2–4 times per week
- ○ 5 or more per week

Other chicken or turkey, with skin (4–6 oz.)
- ○ Never
- ○ Less than once per month
- ○ 1–3 times per month
- ○ Once per week
- ○ 2–4 times per week
- ○ 5–6 times per week
- ○ Once per day
- ○ 2 or more servings per day

Other chicken or turkey, without skin (4–6 oz.)
- ○ Never
- ○ Less than once per month
- ○ 1–3 times per month
- ○ Once per week
- ○ 2–4 times per week
- ○ 5–6 times per week
- ○ Once per day
- ○ 2 or more servings per day

Beef or pork hot dogs (1)
- ○ Never
- ○ Less than once per month
- ○ 1–3 per month
- ○ 1 per week
- ○ 2–4 per week
- ○ 5–6 per week
- ○ 1 per day
- ○ 2 or more per day

Chicken or turkey hot dogs (1)
- ○ Never
- ○ Less than once per month
- ○ 1–3 per month
- ○ 1 per week
- ○ 2–4 per week
- ○ 5–6 per week
- ○ 1 per day
- ○ 2 or more per day

Salami, bologna, or other processed meat sandwiches
- ○ Never
- ○ Less than once per month
- ○ 1–3 times per month
- ○ Once per week
- ○ 2–4 times per week
- ○ 5 or more per week

Processed meats, e.g., sausage, kielbasa, etc. (2 oz. or 2 small links)
- ○ Never
- ○ Less than once per month
- ○ 1–3 times per month
- ○ Once per week
- ○ 2–4 times per week
- ○ 5–6 times per week
- ○ Once per day
- ○ 2 or more servings per day

Hamburger, <u>lean or extra lean</u> (1 patty)
- ○ Never
- ○ Less than once per month
- ○ 1–3 per month
- ○ 1 per week
- ○ 2–4 per week
- ○ 5–6 per week
- ○ 1 or more per day

Hamburger, <u>regular</u> (1 patty)
- ○ Never
- ○ Less than once per month
- ○ 1–3 per month
- ○ 1 per week
- ○ 2–4 per week
- ○ 5–6 per week
- ○ 1 or more per day

6. (Continued) Please fill in your <u>average</u> total use, <u>during the past year</u>, of each specified food.

Beef, pork, or lamb as a sandwich or mixed dish, e.g., stew, casserole, lasagna, etc.

○ Never
○ Less than once per month
○ 1–3 times per month
○ Once per week
○ 2–4 times per week
○ 5–6 times per week
○ 1 or more times per day

Pork as a main dish, e.g., ham or chops (4–6 oz.)

○ Never
○ Less than once per month
○ 1–3 times per month
○ Once per week
○ 2–4 times per week
○ 5–6 times per week
○ 1 or more times per day

Beef or lamb as a main dish, e.g., steak, roast (4–6 oz.)

○ Never
○ Less than once per month
○ 1–3 times per month
○ Once per week
○ 2–4 times per week
○ 5–6 times per week
○ 1 or more times per day

Liver: beef, calf or pork (4 oz.)

○ Never
○ Less than once per month
○ 1–3 times per month
○ Once per week
○ 2 or more servings per week

Liver: chicken or turkey (1 oz.)

○ Never
○ Less than once per month
○ 1–3 times per month
○ Once per week
○ 2 or more servings per week

Canned tuna fish (3–4 oz.)

○ Never
○ Less than once per month
○ 1–3 times per month
○ Once per week
○ 2–4 times per week
○ 5–6 times per week
○ Once per day
○ 2 or more servings per day

Breaded fish cakes, pieces, or fish sticks (1 serving, store bought)

○ Never
○ Less than once per month
○ 1–3 times per month
○ Once per week
○ 2–4 times per week
○ 5–6 times per week
○ 1 or more per day

Shrimp, lobster, scallops, clams as a main dish (1 serving)

○ Never
○ Less than once per month
○ 1–3 times per month
○ Once per week
○ 2–4 times per week
○ 5–6 times per week
○ 1 or more times per day

Dark meat fish, e.g., mackerel, salmon, sardines, bluefish, swordfish (3–5 oz.)

○ Never
○ Less than once per month
○ 1–3 times per month
○ Once per week
○ 2–4 times per week
○ 5–6 times per week
○ 1 or more servings per day

Other fish, e.g., cod, haddock, halibut (3–5 oz.)

○ Never
○ Less than once per month
○ 1–3 times per month
○ Once per week
○ 2–4 times per week
○ 5–6 times per week
○ 1 or more servings per day

CEREALS, BREADS & STARCHES

7. Please fill in your <u>average</u> total use, <u>during the past year</u>, of each specified food.

Cold breakfast cereal (1 cup)
○ Never
○ Less than once per month
○ 1–3 cups per month
○ 1 cup per week
○ 2–4 cups per week
○ 5–6 cups per week
○ 1 cup per day
○ 2–3 cups per day
○ 4 or more cups per day

Cooked oatmeal/cooked oat bran (1 cup)
○ Never
○ Less than once per month
○ 1–3 cups per month
○ 1 cup per week
○ 2–4 cups per week
○ 5–6 cups per week
○ 1 cup per day
○ 2–3 cups per day
○ 4 or more cups per day

Other cooked breakfast cereal (1 cup)
○ Never
○ Less than once per month
○ 1–3 cups per month
○ 1 cup per week
○ 2–4 cups per week
○ 5–6 cups per week
○ 1 cup per day
○ 2–3 cups per day
○ 4 or more cups per day

What brand and type of <u>cold</u> breakfast cereal do you usually eat? ➡ Specify brand & type (e.g., "Ralston Rice Chex")
○ Don't eat cold breakfast cereal

White bread (slice), including pita bread
○ Never
○ Less than once per month
○ 1–3 slices per month
○ 1 slice per week
○ 2–4 slices per week
○ 5–6 slices per week
○ 1 slice per day
○ 2–3 slices per day
○ 4–5 slices per day
○ 6+ slices per day

Dark bread (slice), including wheat pita bread
○ Never
○ Less than once per month
○ 1–3 slices per month
○ 1 slice per week
○ 2–4 slices per week
○ 5–6 slices per week
○ 1 slice per day
○ 2–3 slices per day
○ 4–5 slices per day
○ 6+ slices per day

Bagels, English muffins, or rolls (1 whole)
○ Never
○ Less than once per month
○ 1–3 times per month
○ Once per week
○ 2–4 times per week
○ 5–6 times per week
○ Once per day
○ 2 or more per day

Muffins (regular) or biscuits (1)
○ Never
○ Less than once per month
○ 1–3 per month
○ 1 per week
○ 2–4 per week
○ 5–6 per week
○ 1 per day
○ 2 or more per day

Brown rice (1 cup)
○ Never
○ Less than once per month
○ 1–3 cups per month
○ 1 cup per week
○ 2–4 cups per week
○ 5–6 cups per week
○ 1 cup per day
○ 2 or more cups per day

White rice (1 cup)
○ Never
○ Less than once per month
○ 1–3 cups per month
○ 1 cup per week
○ 2–4 cups per week
○ 5–6 cups per week
○ 1 cup per day
○ 2 or more cups per day

7. (Continued) Please fill in your <u>average</u> total use, <u>during the past year</u>, of each specified food.

Pasta, e.g., spaghetti, noodles, etc. (1 cup)

- ○ Never
- ○ Less than once per month
- ○ 1–3 cups per month
- ○ 1 cup per week
- ○ 2–4 cups per week
- ○ 5–6 cups per week
- ○ 1 cup per day
- ○ 2 or more cups per day

Tortillas (1)

- ○ Never
- ○ Less than once per month
- ○ 1–3 per month
- ○ 1 per week
- ○ 2–4 per week
- ○ 5–6 per week
- ○ 1 per day
- ○ 2–3 per day
- ○ 4 or more per day

Other grains, e.g., bulgar, kasha, couscous, etc. (1 cup)

- ○ Never
- ○ Less than once per month
- ○ 1–3 cups per month
- ○ 1 cup per week
- ○ 2–4 cups per week
- ○ 5–6 cups per week
- ○ 1 cup per day
- ○ 2 or more cups per day

Pancakes or waffles (3 pieces)

- ○ Never
- ○ Less than once per month
- ○ 1–3 servings per month
- ○ 1 serving per week
- ○ 2–4 servings per week
- ○ 5–6 servings per week
- ○ 1 serving per day
- ○ 2 or more servings per day

French fried potatoes (small order or 1/2 cup)

- ○ Never
- ○ Less than once per month
- ○ 1–3 times per month
- ○ Once per week
- ○ 2–4 times per week
- ○ 5–6 times per week
- ○ 1 or more servings per day

Potatoes, baked, boiled (1) or mashed (1 cup)

- ○ Never
- ○ Less than once per month
- ○ 1–3 per month
- ○ 1 per week
- ○ 2–4 per week
- ○ 5–6 per week
- ○ 1 per day
- ○ 2 or more servings per day

Potato chips or corn chips (small bag or 1 oz.)

- ○ Never
- ○ Less than once per month
- ○ 1–3 per month
- ○ 1 per week
- ○ 2–4 per week
- ○ 5–6 per week
- ○ 1 per day
- ○ 2 or more servings per day

Crackers, Triscuits, Wheat Thins (5)

- ○ Never
- ○ Less than once per month
- ○ 1–3 times per month
- ○ Once per week
- ○ 2–4 times per week
- ○ 5–6 times per week
- ○ Once per day
- ○ 2–3 times per day
- ○ 4 or more servings per day

Pizza (2 slices)

- ○ Never
- ○ Less than once per month
- ○ 1–3 times per month
- ○ Once per week
- ○ 2–4 times per week
- ○ 5–6 times per week
- ○ Once per day
- ○ 2 or more servings per day

BEVERAGES

CARBONATED BEVERAGES—Consider the serving size as one 12 oz. glass, bottle or can for these carbonated beverages.

8. Please fill in your <u>average</u> total use, <u>during the past year</u>, of each specified food.

LOW-CALORIE (Sugar-free types)

Low-calorie cola, e.g., Diet Coke <u>with caffeine</u> (1 glass, bottle, can)

- ○ Never
- ○ Less than once per month
- ○ 1–3 cans per month
- ○ 1 can per week
- ○ 2–4 cans per week
- ○ 5–6 cans per week
- ○ 1 can per day
- ○ 2–3 cans per day
- ○ 4 or more cans per day

Low-calorie <u>caffeine-free</u> soda (1 glass, bottle, can)

- ○ Never
- ○ Less than once per month
- ○ 1–3 cans per month
- ○ 1 can per week
- ○ 2–4 cans per week
- ○ 5–6 cans per week
- ○ 1 can per day
- ○ 2–3 cans per day
- ○ 4 or more cans per day

Other low-calorie carbonated beverage, e.g., Diet 7-Up, Fresca, diet ginger ale (1 glass, bottle, can)

- ○ Never
- ○ Less than once per month
- ○ 1–3 cans per month
- ○ 1 can per week
- ○ 2–4 cans per week
- ○ 5–6 cans per week
- ○ 1 can per day
- ○ 2–3 cans per day
- ○ 4 or more cans per day

8. (Continued) Please fill in your <u>average</u> total use, <u>during the past year</u>, of each specified food.

REGULAR TYPES (not sugar-free)

Coke, Pepsi, or other cola <u>with sugar</u> (1 glass, bottle, can)

- ○ Never
- ○ Less than once per month
- ○ 1–3 cans per month
- ○ 1 can per week
- ○ 2–4 cans per week
- ○ 5–6 cans per week
- ○ 1 can per day
- ○ 2–3 cans per day
- ○ 4 or more cans per day

Caffeine-Free Coke, Pepsi, or other cola <u>with sugar</u> (1 glass, bottle, can)

- ○ Never
- ○ Less than once per month
- ○ 1–3 cans per month
- ○ 1 can per week
- ○ 2–4 cans per week
- ○ 5–6 cans per week
- ○ 1 can per day
- ○ 2–3 cans per day
- ○ 4 or more cans per day

Other carbonated beverage <u>with sugar</u>, e.g., 7-Up (1 glass, bottle, can)

- ○ Never
- ○ Less than once per month
- ○ 1–3 cans per month
- ○ 1 can per week
- ○ 2–4 cans per week
- ○ 5–6 cans per week
- ○ 1 can per day
- ○ 2–3 cans per day
- ○ 4 or more cans per day

OTHER BEVERAGES

Hawaiian Punch, lemonade, or other non-carbonated fruit drinks (1 glass, bottle, can)

- ○ Never
- ○ Less than once per month
- ○ 1–3 glasses per month
- ○ 1 glass per week
- ○ 2–4 glasses per week
- ○ 5–6 glasses per week
- ○ 1 glass per day
- ○ 2–3 glasses per day
- ○ 4 or more glasses per day

Beer, regular (1 glass, bottle, can)

- ○ Never
- ○ Less than once per month
- ○ 1–3 cans per month
- ○ 1 can per week
- ○ 2–4 cans per week
- ○ 5–6 cans per week
- ○ 1 can per day
- ○ 2–3 cans per day
- ○ 4–5 cans per day
- ○ 6+ cans per day

Light beer, e.g., Bud Light (1 glass, bottle, can)

- ○ Never
- ○ Less than once per month
- ○ 1–3 cans per month
- ○ 1 can per week
- ○ 2–4 cans per week
- ○ 5–6 cans per week
- ○ 1 can per day
- ○ 2–3 cans per day
- ○ 4–5 cans per day
- ○ 6+ cans per day

Red wine (4 oz. glass)

- ○ Never
- ○ Less than once per month
- ○ 1–3 glasses per month
- ○ 1 glass per week
- ○ 2–4 glasses per week
- ○ 5–6 glasses per week
- ○ 1 glass per day
- ○ 2–3 glasses per day
- ○ 4–5 glasses per day
- ○ 6+ glasses per day

White wine (4 oz. glass)

- ○ Never
- ○ Less than once per month
- ○ 1–3 glasses per month
- ○ 1 glass per week
- ○ 2–4 glasses per week
- ○ 5–6 glasses per week
- ○ 1 glass per day
- ○ 2–3 glasses per day
- ○ 4–5 glasses per day
- ○ 6+ glasses per day

Liquor, e.g., whiskey, gin, etc. (1 drink or shot)

- ○ Never
- ○ Less than once per month
- ○ 1–3 drinks per month
- ○ 1 drink per week
- ○ 2–4 drinks per week
- ○ 5–6 drinks per week
- ○ 1 drink per day
- ○ 2–3 drinks per day
- ○ 4–5 drinks per day
- ○ 6+ drinks per day

8. (Continued) Please fill in your <u>average</u> total use, <u>during the past year</u>, of each specified food.

Plain water, bottled or tap including mineral water and soda water (1 cup or glass)

- ○ Never
- ○ Less than once per month
- ○ 1–3 glasses per month
- ○ 1 glass per week
- ○ 2–4 glasses per week
- ○ 5–6 glasses per week
- ○ 1 glass per day
- ○ 2–3 glasses per day
- ○ 4–5 glasses per day
- ○ 6+ glasses per day

Herbal tea (1 cup)

- ○ Never
- ○ Less than once per month
- ○ 1–3 cups per month
- ○ 1 cup per week
- ○ 2–4 cups per week
- ○ 5–6 cups per week
- ○ 1 cup per day
- ○ 2–3 cups per day
- ○ 4–5 cups per day
- ○ 6+ cups per day

Tea (1 cup), <u>Not</u> <u>herbal</u> teas

- ○ Never
- ○ Less than once per month
- ○ 1–3 cups per month
- ○ 1 cup per week
- ○ 2–4 cups per week
- ○ 5–6 cups per week
- ○ 1 cup per day
- ○ 2–3 cups per day
- ○ 4–5 cups per day
- ○ 6+ cups per day

Decaffeinated coffee (1 cup)

- ○ Never
- ○ Less than once per month
- ○ 1–3 cups per month
- ○ 1 cup per week
- ○ 2–4 cups per week
- ○ 5–6 cups per week
- ○ 1 cup per day
- ○ 2–3 cups per day
- ○ 4–5 cups per day
- ○ 6+ cups per day

Coffee with caffeine (1 cup)

- ○ Never
- ○ Less than once per month
- ○ 1–3 cups per month
- ○ 1 cup per week
- ○ 2–4 cups per week
- ○ 5–6 cups per week
- ○ 1 cup per day
- ○ 2–3 cups per day
- ○ 4–5 cups per day
- ○ 6+ cups per day

SWEETS, BAKED GOODS & MISCELLANEOUS

9. Please fill in your <u>average</u> total use, <u>during the past year</u>, of each specified food.

Pure chocolate candy bar or packet, (e.g., Hershey's, M&M's)

- ○ Never
- ○ Less than once per month
- ○ 1–3 per month
- ○ 1 per week
- ○ 2–4 per week
- ○ 5–6 per week
- ○ 1 per day
- ○ 2–3 per day
- ○ 4 or more per day

Other mixed candy bars, (e.g., Snickers, Milky Way, Reeses)

- ○ Never
- ○ Less than once per month
- ○ 1–3 candy bars per month
- ○ 1 candy bar per week
- ○ 2–4 candy bars per week
- ○ 5–6 candy bars per week
- ○ 1 candy bar per day
- ○ 2–3 candy bars per day
- ○ 4 or more candy bars per day

Candy <u>without</u> chocolate (e.g., 1 pack mints, Lifesavers)

- ○ Never
- ○ Less than once per month
- ○ 1–3 times per month
- ○ Once per week
- ○ 2–4 times per week
- ○ 5–6 times per week
- ○ Once per day
- ○ 2–3 times per day
- ○ 4 or more times per day

Jams, jellies, preserves, syrup, or honey (1 tbs.)

- ○ Never
- ○ Less than once per month
- ○ 1–3 tbs. per month
- ○ 1 tbs. per week
- ○ 2–4 tbs. per week
- ○ 5–6 tbs. per week
- ○ 1 tbs. per day
- ○ 2–3 tbs. per day
- ○ 4 or more tbs. per day

Peanut butter (1 tbs.)

- ○ Never
- ○ Less than once per month
- ○ 1–3 tbs. per month
- ○ 1 tbs. per week
- ○ 2–4 tbs. per week
- ○ 5–6 tbs. per week
- ○ 1 tbs. per day
- ○ 2–3 tbs. per day
- ○ 4 or more tbs. per day

Popcorn (1 cup)

- ○ Never
- ○ Less than once per month
- ○ 1–3 cups per month
- ○ 1 cup per week
- ○ 2–4 cups per week
- ○ 5–6 cups per week
- ○ 1 cup per day
- ○ 2 or more cups per day

9. (Continued) Please fill in your <u>average</u> total use, <u>during the past year</u>, of each specified food.

Pretzels (1 oz., or small bag)
- ○ Never
- ○ Less than once per month
- ○ 1–3 servings per month
- ○ One serving per week
- ○ 2–4 servings per week
- ○ 5–6 servings per week
- ○ One serving per day
- ○ 2 or more servings per day

Cookies, <u>home baked</u> (1)
- ○ Never
- ○ Less than once per month
- ○ 1–3 cookies per month
- ○ 1 cookie per week
- ○ 2–4 cookies per week
- ○ 5–6 cookies per week
- ○ 1 cookie per day
- ○ 2–3 cookies per day
- ○ 4 or more cookies per day

Cookies, <u>ready made</u> (1)
- ○ Never
- ○ Less than once per month
- ○ 1–3 cookies per month
- ○ 1 cookie per week
- ○ 2–4 cookies per week
- ○ 5–6 cookies per week
- ○ 1 cookie per day
- ○ 2–3 cookies per day
- ○ 4 or more cookies per day

Brownies (1)
- ○ Never
- ○ Less than once per month
- ○ 1–3 per month
- ○ 1 per week
- ○ 2–4 per week
- ○ 5–6 per week
- ○ 1 per day
- ○ 2 or more per day

Doughnuts (1)
- ○ Never
- ○ Less than once per month
- ○ 1–3 per month
- ○ 1 per week
- ○ 2–4 per week
- ○ 5–6 per week
- ○ 1 per day
- ○ 2–3 per day
- ○ 4 or more per day

Cake, <u>home baked</u> (slice)
- ○ Never
- ○ Less than once per month
- ○ 1–3 slices per month
- ○ 1 slice per week
- ○ 2–4 slices per week
- ○ 5–6 slices per week
- ○ 1 or more slices per day

Cake, <u>ready made</u> (slice)
- ○ Never
- ○ Less than once per month
- ○ 1–3 slices per month
- ○ 1 slice per week
- ○ 2–4 slices per week
- ○ 5–6 slices per week
- ○ 1 or more slices per day

Pie, <u>homemade</u> (slice)
- ○ Never
- ○ Less than once per month
- ○ 1–3 slices per month
- ○ 1 slice per week
- ○ 2–4 slices per week
- ○ 5–6 slices per week
- ○ 1 or more slices per day

Pie, <u>ready made</u> (slice)
- ○ Never
- ○ Less than once per month
- ○ 1–3 slices per month
- ○ 1 slice per week
- ○ 2–4 slices per week
- ○ 5–6 slices per week
- ○ 1 or more slices per day

Sweet roll, coffee cake or other pastry, <u>home baked</u> (serving)
- ○ Never
- ○ Less than once per month
- ○ 1–3 times per month
- ○ Once per week
- ○ 2–4 times per week
- ○ 5–6 times per week
- ○ Once per day
- ○ 2 or more servings per day

Sweet roll, coffee cake or other pastry, <u>ready made</u> (serving)
- ○ Never
- ○ Less than once per month
- ○ 1–3 times per month
- ○ Once per week
- ○ 2–4 times per week
- ○ 5–6 times per week
- ○ Once per day
- ○ 2 or more servings per day

Peanuts (small packet or 1 oz.)
- ○ Never
- ○ Less than once per month
- ○ 1–3 per month
- ○ 1 per week
- ○ 2–4 per week
- ○ 5–6 per week
- ○ 1 per day
- ○ 2 or more servings per day

Other nuts (small packet or 1 oz.)
- ○ Never
- ○ Less than once per month
- ○ 1–3 per month
- ○ 1 per week
- ○ 2–4 per week
- ○ 5–6 per week
- ○ 1 per day
- ○ 2 or more servings per day

Oat bran, added to food (1 tbs.)
- ○ Never
- ○ Less than once per month
- ○ 1–3 tbs. per month
- ○ 1 tbs. per week
- ○ 2–4 tbs. per week
- ○ 5–6 tbs. per week
- ○ 1 tbs. per day
- ○ 2 or more servings per day

Other bran, added to food (1 tbs.)
- ○ Never
- ○ Less than once per month
- ○ 1–3 tbs. per month
- ○ 1 tbs. per week
- ○ 2–4 tbs. per week
- ○ 5–6 tbs. per week
- ○ 1 tbs. per day
- ○ 2 or more servings per day

9. (Continued) Please fill in your <u>average</u> total use, <u>during the past year</u>, of each specified food.

Wheat germ (1 tbs.)

○ Never
○ Less than once per month
○ 1–3 tbs. per month
○ 1 tbs. per week
○ 2–4 tbs. per week
○ 5–6 tbs. per week
○ 1 tbs. per day
○ 2 or more servings per day

Chowder or cream soup (1 cup)

○ Never
○ Less than once per month
○ 1–3 cups per month
○ 1 cup per week
○ 2–4 cups per week
○ 5–6 cups per week
○ 1 or more cups per day

Ketchup or red chili sauce (1 tbs.)

○ Never
○ Less than once per month
○ 1–3 tbs. per month
○ 1 tbs. per week
○ 2–4 tbs. per week
○ 5–6 tbs. per week
○ 1 tbs. per day
○ 2 or more servings per day

Salt added at table (1 shake)

○ Never
○ Less than once per month
○ 1–3 shakes per month
○ 1 shake per week
○ 2–4 shakes per week
○ 5–6 shakes per week
○ 1 shake per day
○ 2–3 shakes per day
○ 4–5 shakes per day
○ 6+ shakes per day

How many teaspoons of sugar do you add to your beverages or food each day?

Teaspoons

[ ]

Nutrasweet or Equal (1 packet) NOT Sweet 'N Low

○ Never
○ Less than once per month
○ 1–3 per month
○ 1 per week
○ 2–4 per week
○ 5–6 per week
○ 1 per day
○ 2–3 per day
○ 4–5 per day
○ 6+ per day

⓪⓪ ①① ②② ③③ ④④ ⑤⑤ ⑥⑥ ⑦⑦ ⑧⑧ ⑨⑨

Garlic (1 clove or 4 shakes)

○ Never
○ Less than once per month
○ 1–3 per month
○ 1 per week
○ 2–4 per week
○ 5–6 per week
○ 1 per day
○ 2–3 per day
○ 4–5 per day
○ 6+ per day

Low fat mayonnaise/fat free mayonnaise (2 tbs.)

○ Never
○ Less than once per month
○ 1–3 tbs. per month
○ 1 tbs. per week
○ 2–4 tbs. per week
○ 5–6 tbs. per week
○ 1 tbs. per day
○ 2 or more tbs. per day

Regular mayonnaise (2 tbs.)

○ Never
○ Less than once per month
○ 1–3 tbs. per month
○ 1 tbs. per week
○ 2–4 tbs. per week
○ 5–6 tbs. per week
○ 1 tbs. per day
○ 2 or more tbs. per day

Salad dressing (2 tbs.) ⟶

○ Never
○ Less than once per month
○ 1–3 tbs. per month
○ 1 tbs. per week
○ 2–4 tbs. per week
○ 5–6 tbs. per week
○ 1 tbs. per day
○ 2–3 tbs. per day
○ 4 or more tbs. per day

Type of salad dressing:

○ Nonfat
○ Low fat
○ Olive oil dressing
○ Regular

Olive oil added to food or bread (1 tbs.); exclude use in cooking

○ Never
○ Less than once per month
○ 1–3 tbs. per month
○ 1 tbs. per week
○ 2–4 tbs. per week
○ 5–6 tbs. per week
○ 1 tbs. per day
○ 2–3 tbs. per day
○ 4–5 tbs. per day
○ 6+ tbs. per day

10. How much of the visible fat on your beef, pork or lamb do you remove before eating?

- ○ Don't eat meat
- ○ Remove all visible fat
- ○ Remove most
- ○ Remove small part of fat
- ○ Remove none

11. What kind of fat is usually used for frying and sautéing at home?

- ○ Don't fry
- ○ Real butter
- ○ Margarine
- ○ Olive oil
- ○ Vegetable oil
- ○ Vegetable shortening
- ○ Lard/bacon fat
- ○ Pam type spray

12. What kind of fat is usually used for baking at home?

- ○ Don't bake
- ○ Real butter
- ○ Margarine
- ○ Olive oil
- ○ Vegetable oil
- ○ Vegetable shortening
- ○ Lard/bacon fat
- ○ Pam type spray

13. How often do you eat food fried, stir-fried in oil, or sautéed at home?

- ○ Never
- ○ Less than once a week
- ○ Once per week
- ○ 2–4 times per week
- ○ 5–6 times per week
- ○ Daily

14. How often do you eat deep fried food away from home or as take out (e.g., french fries, fried chicken, fish, clams, shrimp, etc.)?

- ○ Never
- ○ Less than once a week
- ○ Once per week
- ○ 2–4 times per week
- ○ 5–6 times per week
- ○ Daily

15. What type of cooking oil is usually used at home (e.g., Wesson Corn Oil)?

(Specify brand and type)

16. Are there any other foods not mentioned above that you usually eat <u>at least once per week</u>?

Include for example: Paté, cream sauce, custard, radishes, fava beans, coconut, mango, horseradish, parsnips, rhubarb, papaya, dried apricots, dates, figs. (Do not include dry spices and do not list something that has been listed in the previous sections.)

Other foods that you usually eat at least once per week	Usual serving size	Servings per week
(a)		
(b)		
(c)		

DIET CHANGES

17. Do you currently follow a special diet?

○ No
○ Yes ⟶ ○ Physician prescribed
         ○ Self prescribed

a) If yes, for how many years?

(Number of years on diet)

b) If yes, what kind of diet do you follow?
(Select more than one if necessary.)
○ Weight reduction (low calorie)
○ Low cholesterol
○ Low sodium
○ Diabetic
○ Low fat
○ Low triglyceride
○ Ulcer
○ High Potassium

(Specify type of diet)

○ Other ⟶

18. How has your use of the following foods and beverages <u>changed</u> over the
PAST TEN YEARS?

Whole milk
○ Use has decreased
○ Use about the same
○ Use has increased

Butter
○ Use has decreased
○ Use about the same
○ Use has increased

Margarine
○ Use has decreased
○ Use about the same
○ Use has increased

Eggs
○ Use has decreased
○ Use about the same
○ Use has increased

Fish
○ Use has decreased
○ Use about the same
○ Use has increased

Red meat
○ Use has decreased
○ Use about the same
○ Use has increased

Fruits
○ Use has decreased
○ Use about the same
○ Use has increased

Vegetables
○ Use has decreased
○ Use about the same
○ Use has increased

Whole wheat bread
○ Use has decreased
○ Use about the same
○ Use has increased

Whole grains
○ Use has decreased
○ Use about the same
○ Use has increased

Sugar
○ Use has decreased
○ Use about the same
○ Use has increased

Alcohol
○ Use has decreased
○ Use about the same
○ Use has increased

APPENDIX I

The Youth/Adolescent Questionnaire, a Food Frequency Questionnaire Designed by Researchers at Brigham and Women's Hospital and Harvard University for Assessing the Dietary Intake of Older Children and Adolescents

From Helaine R. H. Rockett, MS, RD, FADA, Department of Medicine, Channing Laboratory, 180 Longwood Avenue, Boston, MA 02115.

MARKING INSTRUCTIONS

- Use a **NO. 2 PENCIL** only.
- Do not use ink or ballpoint pen.
- Darken in the circle completely.
- Erase cleanly any marks you wish to change.
- Do not make any stray marks on this form.

The **RIGHT** way ● to mark your answer!

The **WRONG** way ⊘ ⊗ ⊖ ⊙ to mark your answers!

USE NO. 2 PENCIL ONLY

1. What is your AGE?

- ○ Less than 9
- ○ 9
- ○ 10
- ○ 11
- ○ 12
- ○ 13
- ○ 14
- ○ 15
- ○ 16
- ○ 17
- ○ 18 or older

2. Are you:

- ○ Male
- ○ Female

3. Your Height

FEET	INCHES

4. Current Weight (lbs)

5. Do you currently take multi-vitamins (like Flintstones, One-A-Day, etc.)?

○ No   ○ Yes ➡ **If yes)**

a) How many tablets do you take per week?
- ○ 2 or less
- ○ 3 - 5
- ○ 6 - 9
- ○ 10 or more

b) For how many years?
- ○ 0 - 1 years
- ○ 2 - 4
- ○ 5 - 9
- ○ 10+ years

6. How many teaspoons of sugar do you ADD to your beverages or food each day?

- ○ None
- ○ 1 - 2 teaspoons per day
- ○ 3 - 4 teaspoons per day
- ○ 5 or more teaspoons per day

7. Which cold breakfast cereal do you usually eat?

○ Never eat cold breakfast cereal

8. Where do you usually eat breakfast?

- ○ At home
- ○ At school
- ○ Don't eat breakfast
- ○ Other

9. How many times each week (including weekdays and weekends) do you eat breakfast <u>prepared away from home</u>?

- ○ Never or almost never
- ○ 1 - 2 times per week
- ○ 3 - 4 times per week
- ○ 5 or more times per week

3531

10. How many times each week (including weekdays and weekends) do you eat lunch <u>prepared away from home</u>?

○ Never or almost never
○ 1 - 2 times per week
○ 3 - 4 times per week
○ 5 or more times per week

11. How many times each week do you eat after-school snacks or foods <u>prepared away from home</u>?

○ Never or almost never
○ 1 - 2 times per week
○ 3 - 4 times per week
○ 5 or more times per week

12. How many times each week (weekdays and weekends) do you eat dinner <u>prepared away from home</u>?

○ Never or almost never
○ 1 - 2 times per week
○ 3 - 4 times per week
○ 5 or more times per week

13. How many times per week do you prepare dinner for yourself (and/or others in your house)?

○ Never or almost never
○ Less than once per week
○ 1 - 2 times per week
○ 3 - 4 times per week
○ 5 or more times per week

14. How often do you have dinner that is ready made, like frozen dinners, Spaghetti-O's, etc.

○ Never
○ 1 - 2 times per week
○ 3 - 4 times per week
○ 5'or more times per week

15. How many times each week (including weekdays and weekends) do you eat late night snacks <u>prepared away from home</u>?

○ Never
○ 1 - 2 times per week
○ 3 - 4 times per week
○ 5 or more times per week

16. How often do you eat food that is fried at home, like fried chicken?

○ Less than once per week
○ 1 - 3 times per week
○ 4 - 6 times per week
○ Daily

17. How often do you eat fried food away from home (like french fries, fried chicken)?

○ Less than once per week
○ 1 - 3 times per week
○ 4 - 6 times per week
○ Daily

DIETARY INTAKE

Estimate how often you eat the following foods:

<u>Example 1</u> If you drink one can of diet soda 2 - 3 times per week, then your answer should look like this:

**E1. Diet soda
(1 can or glass)**

○ Never
○ 1 - 3 cans per month
○ 1 can per week
● 2 - 6 cans per week
○ 1 can per day
○ 2 or more cans per day

BEVERAGES

FILL OUT ONE BUBBLE FOR EACH FOOD ITEM

18. Diet soda (1 can or glass)

- ○ Never
- ○ 1 - 3 cans per month
- ○ 1 can per week
- ○ 2 - 6 cans per week
- ○ 1 can per day
- ○ 2 or more cans per day

19. Soda - not diet (1 can or glass)

- ○ Never
- ○ 1 - 3 cans per month
- ○ 1 can per week
- ○ 2 - 6 cans per week
- ○ 1 can per day
- ○ 2 or more cans per day

20. Hawaiian Punch, lemonade, Koolaid or other non-carbonated fruit drink (1 glass)

- ○ Never
- ○ 1 - 3 glasses per month
- ○ 1 glass per week
- ○ 2 - 4 glasses per week
- ○ 5 - 6 glasses per week
- ○ 1 glass per day
- ○ 2 or more glasses per day

21. Iced Tea - sweetened (1 glass)

- ○ Never
- ○ 1 - 3 glasses per month
- ○ 1 - 4 glasses per week
- ○ 5 or more glasses per week

22. Tea (1 cup)

- ○ Never
- ○ 1 - 3 cups per month
- ○ 1 - 2 cups per week
- ○ 3 - 6 cups per week
- ○ 1 or more cups per day

23. Coffee - not decaf. (1 cup)

- ○ Never
- ○ 1 - 3 cups per month
- ○ 1 - 2 cups per week
- ○ 3 - 6 cups per week
- ○ 1 or more cups per day

24. Beer (1 glass, bottle or can)

- ○ Never
- ○ 1 - 3 cans per month
- ○ 1 can per week
- ○ 2 or more cans per week

25. Wine or wine coolers (1 glass)

- ○ Never
- ○ 1 - 3 glasses per month
- ○ 1 glass per week
- ○ 2 or more glasses per week

26. Liquor, like vodka or rum (1 drink or shot)

- ○ Never
- ○ 1 - 3 drinks per month
- ○ 1 drink per week
- ○ 2 or more drinks per week

Example 2 **If you eat:**

2	pats of margarine on toast
1 - 2	pats of margarine on sandwich
1	pat of margarine on vegetables

5 - 6 **pats total all day**

then answer this way →

E2. Margarine (1 pat) - not butter

- ○ Never
- ○ 1 - 3 pats per month
- ○ 1 pat per week
- ○ 2 - 6 pats per week
- ○ 1 pat per day
- ○ 2 - 4 pats per day
- ● 5 or more pats per day

DAIRY PRODUCTS

27. What TYPE of milk do you usually drink?

- ○ Whole milk
- ○ 2% milk
- ○ 1% milk
- ○ Skim/nonfat milk
- ○ Don't know
- ○ Don't drink milk

28. Milk (glass or with cereal)

- ○ Never
- ○ 1 glass per week or less
- ○ 2 - 6 glasses per week
- ○ 1 glass per day
- ○ 2 - 3 glasses per day
- ○ 4+ glasses per day

29. Chocolate milk (glass)

- ○ Never
- ○ 1 - 3 glasses per month
- ○ 1 glass per week
- ○ 2 - 6 glasses per week
- ○ 1 - 2 glasses per day
- ○ 3 or more glasses per day

3531

30. Instant Breakfast Drink (1 packet)
- ○ Never
- ○ 1 - 3 times per month
- ○ Once per week
- ○ 2 - 4 times per week
- ○ 5 or more times per week

31. Whipped cream
- ○ Never
- ○ 1 - 3 times per month
- ○ Once per week
- ○ 2 - 4 times per week
- ○ 5 or more times per week

32. Yogurt (1 cup) - Not frozen
- ○ Never
- ○ 1 - 3 cups per month
- ○ 1 cup per week
- ○ 2 - 6 cups per week
- ○ 1 cup per day
- ○ 2 or more cups per day

33. Cottage or ricotta cheese
- ○ Never
- ○ 1 - 3 times per month
- ○ Once per week
- ○ 2 or more times per week

34. Cheese (1 slice)
- ○ Never
- ○ 1 - 3 slices per month
- ○ 1 slice per week
- ○ 2 - 6 slices per week
- ○ 1 slice per day
- ○ 2 or more slices per day

35. Cream cheese
- ○ Never
- ○ 1 - 3 times per month
- ○ Once per week
- ○ 2 or more times per week

36. What TYPE of yogurt, cottage cheese & dairy products (besides milk) do you use mostly?
- ○ Nonfat/Skim
- ○ Lowfat
- ○ Regular
- ○ Don't know

37. Butter (1 pat) - NOT margarine
- ○ Never
- ○ 1 - 3 pats per month
- ○ 1 pat per week
- ○ 2 - 6 pats per week
- ○ 1 pat per day
- ○ 2 - 4 pats per day
- ○ 5 or more pats per day

38. Margarine (1 pat) - NOT butter
- ○ Never
- ○ 1 - 3 pats per month
- ○ 1 pat per week
- ○ 2 - 6 pats per week
- ○ 1 pat per day
- ○ 2 - 4 pats per day
- ○ 5 or more pats per day

39. What FORM and BRAND of margarine does your family usually use?
- ○ None
- ○ Stick
- ○ Tub
- ○ Squeeze (liquid)

⓪①②③④⑤⑥⑦⑧⑨
⓪①②③④⑤⑥⑦⑧⑨
⓪①②③④⑤⑥⑦⑧⑨

WHAT SPECIFIC BRAND AND TYPE (LIKE "PARKAY CORN OIL SPREAD")?

Leave blank if you don't know.

40. What TYPE of oil does your family use at home?
- ○ Canola oil
- ○ Corn oil
- ○ Safflower oil
- ○ Olive oil
- ○ Vegetable oil
- ○ Don't know

MAIN DISHES

41. Cheeseburger (1)
- ○ Never
- ○ 1 - 3 per month
- ○ One per week
- ○ 2 - 4 per week
- ○ 5 or more per week

42. Hamburger (1)
- ○ Never
- ○ 1 - 3 per month
- ○ One per week
- ○ 2 - 4 per week
- ○ 5 or more per week

43. Pizza (2 slices)
- ○ Never
- ○ 1 - 3 times per month
- ○ Once per week
- ○ 2 - 4 times per week
- ○ 5 or more times per week

44. Tacos/burritos (1)
- ○ Never
- ○ 1 - 3 per month
- ○ One per week
- ○ 2 - 4 per week
- ○ 5 or more per week

45. Which taco filling do you usually have:
- ○ Beef & beans
- ○ Beef
- ○ Chicken
- ○ Beans

46. Chicken nuggets (6)
- ○ Never
- ○ 1 - 3 times per month
- ○ Once per week
- ○ 2 - 4 times per week
- ○ 5 or more times per week

47. Hot dogs (1)

○ Never
○ 1 - 3 per month
○ One per week
○ 2 - 4 per week
○ 5 or more per week

**48. Peanut butter sandwich (1)
(plain or with jelly, fluff, etc.)**

○ Never
○ 1 - 3 per month
○ One per week
○ 2 - 4 per week
○ 5 or more per week

49. Chicken or turkey sandwich (1)

○ Never
○ 1 - 3 per month
○ One per week
○ 2 or more per week

**50. Roast beef or ham
sandwich (1)**

○ Never
○ 1 - 3 per month
○ One per week
○ 2 or more per week

**51. Salami, bologna, or other
deli meat sandwich (1)**

○ Never
○ 1 - 3 per month
○ One per week
○ 2 or more per week

52. Tuna sandwich (1)

○ Never
○ 1 - 3 per month
○ One per week
○ 2 or more per week

**53. Chicken or turkey as
main dish (1 serving)**

○ Never
○ 1 - 3 times per month
○ Once per week
○ 2 - 4 times per week
○ 5 or more times per week

**54. Fish sticks, fish cakes or fish
sandwich (1 serving)**

○ Never
○ 1 - 3 times per month
○ Once per week
○ 2 or more times per week

55. Fresh fish as main dish (1 serving)

○ Never
○ 1 - 3 times per month
○ Once per week
○ 2 - 4 times per week
○ 5 or more times per week

**56. Beef (steak, roast) or lamb
as main dish (1 serving)**

○ Never
○ 1 - 3 times per month
○ Once per week
○ 2 - 4 times per week
○ 5 or more times per week

**57. Pork or ham as main dish
(1 serving)**

○ Never
○ 1 - 3 times per month
○ Once per week
○ 2 - 4 times per week
○ 5 or more times per week

58. Meatballs or meatloaf (1 serving)

○ Never
○ 1 - 3 times per month
○ Once per week
○ 2 - 4 times per week
○ 5 or more times per week

**59. Lasagna/baked ziti
(1 serving)**

○ Never
○ 1 - 3 times per month
○ Once per week
○ 2 or more times per week

**60. Macaroni and cheese
(1 serving)**

○ Never
○ 1 - 3 times per month
○ Once per week
○ 2 or more times per week

**61. Spaghetti with tomato sauce
(1 serving)**

○ Never
○ 1 - 3 times per month
○ Once per week
○ 2 - 4 times per week
○ 5 or more times per week

62. Eggs (1)

○ Never
○ 1 - 3 eggs per month
○ One egg per week
○ 2 - 4 eggs per week
○ 5 or more eggs per week

**63. Liver: beef, calf,
or pork (1 serving)**

○ Never
○ Less than once per month
○ Once per month
○ 2 - 3 times per month
○ Once per week or more

**64. Shrimp, lobster, scallops
(1 serving)**

○ Never
○ 1 - 3 times per month
○ Once per week
○ 2 or more times per week

3531

427

MISCELLANEOUS FOODS

65. Brown gravy
- ○ Never
- ○ Once per week or less
- ○ 2 - 6 times per week
- ○ Once per day
- ○ 2 or more times per day

66. Ketchup
- ○ Never
- ○ 1 - 3 times per month
- ○ Once per week
- ○ 2 - 4 times per week
- ○ 5 or more times per week

67. Clear soup (with rice, noodles, vegetables) 1 bowl
- ○ Never
- ○ 1 - 3 bowls per month
- ○ 1 bowl per week
- ○ 2 or more bowls per week

68. Cream (milk) soups or chowder (1 bowl)
- ○ Never
- ○ 1 - 3 bowls per month
- ○ 1 bowl per week
- ○ 2 - 6 bowls per week
- ○ 1 or more bowls per day

69. Mayonnaise
- ○ Never
- ○ 1 - 3 times per month
- ○ Once per week
- ○ 2 - 6 times per week
- ○ Once per day

70. Low calorie salad dressing
- ○ Never
- ○ 1 - 3 times per month
- ○ Once per week
- ○ 2 - 6 times per week
- ○ Once or more per day

71. Salad dressing (not low calorie)
- ○ Never
- ○ 1 - 3 times per month
- ○ Once per week
- ○ 2 - 6 times per week
- ○ Once or more per day

72. Salsa
- ○ Never
- ○ 1 - 3 times per month
- ○ Once per week
- ○ 2 - 6 times per week
- ○ Once or more per day

73. How much fat on your beef, pork, or lamb do you eat?
- ○ Eat all
- ○ Eat some
- ○ Eat none
- ○ Don't eat meat

74. Do you eat the skin of the chicken or turkey?
- ○ Yes
- ○ No
- ○ Sometimes

BREADS & CEREALS

75. Cold breakfast cereal (1 bowl)
- ◯ Never
- ◯ 1 - 3 bowls per month
- ◯ 1 bowl per week
- ◯ 2 - 4 bowls per week
- ◯ 5 - 7 bowls per week
- ◯ 2 or more bowls per day

76. Hot breakfast cereal, like oatmeal, grits (1 bowl)
- ◯ Never
- ◯ 1 - 3 bowls per month
- ◯ 1 bowl per week
- ◯ 2 - 4 bowls per week
- ◯ 5 - 7 bowls per week
- ◯ 2 or more bowls per day

77. White bread, pita bread, or toast (1 slice)
- ◯ Never
- ◯ 1 slice per week or less
- ◯ 2 - 4 slices per week
- ◯ 5 - 7 slices per week
- ◯ 2 - 3 slices per day
- ◯ 4+ slices per day

78. Dark bread (1 slice)
- ◯ Never
- ◯ 1 slice per week or less
- ◯ 2 - 4 slices per week
- ◯ 5 - 7 slices per week
- ◯ 2 - 3 slices per day
- ◯ 4+ slices per day

79. English muffins or bagels (1)
- ◯ Never
- ◯ 1 - 3 per month
- ◯ 1 per week
- ◯ 2 - 4 per week
- ◯ 5 or more per week

80. Muffin (1)
- ◯ Never
- ◯ 1 - 3 muffins per month
- ◯ 1 muffin per week
- ◯ 2 - 4 muffins per week
- ◯ 5 or more muffins per week

81. Cornbread (1 square)
- ◯ Never
- ◯ 1 - 3 times per month
- ◯ Once per week
- ◯ 2 - 4 times per week
- ◯ 5 or more per week

82. Biscuit/roll (1)
- ◯ Never
- ◯ 1 - 3 per month
- ◯ 1 per week
- ◯ 2 - 4 per week
- ◯ 5 or more per week

83. Rice
- ◯ Never
- ◯ 1 - 3 times per month
- ◯ Once per week
- ◯ 2 - 4 times per week
- ◯ 5 or more times per week

84. Noodles, pasta
- ◯ Never
- ◯ 1 - 3 times per month
- ◯ Once per week
- ◯ 2 - 4 times per week
- ◯ 5 or more times per week

85. Tortilla - no filling (1)
- ◯ Never
- ◯ 1 - 3 per month
- ◯ 1 per week
- ◯ 2 - 4 per week
- ◯ 5 or more per week

86. Other grains, like kasha, couscous, bulgar
- ◯ Never
- ◯ 1 - 3 times per month
- ◯ Once per week
- ◯ 2 or more times per week

87. Pancakes (2) or waffles (1)
- ◯ Never
- ◯ 1 - 3 times per month
- ◯ Once per week
- ◯ 2 or more times per week

88. French fries (large order)
- ◯ Never
- ◯ 1 - 3 orders per month
- ◯ 1 order per week
- ◯ 2 - 4 orders per week
- ◯ 5 or more orders per week

89. Potatoes - baked, boiled, mashed
- ◯ Never
- ◯ 1 - 3 times per month
- ◯ Once per week
- ◯ 2 - 4 times per week
- ◯ 5 or more times per week

FRUITS & VEGETABLES

90. Raisins (small pack)
- ○ Never
- ○ 1 - 3 times per month
- ○ 1 per week
- ○ 2 - 4 times per week
- ○ 5 or more times per week

91. Grapes (bunch)
- ○ Never
- ○ 1 - 3 times per month
- ○ Once per week
- ○ 2 - 4 times per week
- ○ 5 or more times per week

92. Bananas (1)
- ○ Never
- ○ 1 - 3 per month
- ○ 1 per week
- ○ 2 - 4 per week
- ○ 5 or more per week

93. Cantaloupe, melons (1/4 melon)
- ○ Never
- ○ 1 - 3 times per month
- ○ 1 per week
- ○ 2 or more times per week

94. Apples (1) or applesauce
- ○ Never
- ○ 1 - 3 per month
- ○ 1 per week
- ○ 2 - 6 per week
- ○ 1 or more per day

95. Pears (1)
- ○ Never
- ○ 1 - 3 per month
- ○ 1 per week
- ○ 2 - 6 per week
- ○ 1 or more per day

96. Oranges (1), grapefruit (1/2)
- ○ Never
- ○ 1 - 3 per month
- ○ 1 per week
- ○ 2 - 6 per week
- ○ 1 or more per day

97. Strawberries
- ○ Never
- ○ 1 - 3 times per month
- ○ Once per week
- ○ 2 or more times per week

98. Peaches, plums, apricots (1)
- ○ Never
- ○ 1 - 3 per month
- ○ 1 per week
- ○ 2 or more per week

99. Orange juice (1 glass)
- ○ Never
- ○ 1 - 3 glasses per month
- ○ 1 glass per week
- ○ 2 - 6 glasses per week
- ○ 1 glass per day
- ○ 2 or more glasses per day

100. Apple juice and other fruit juices (1 glass)
- ○ Never
- ○ 1 - 3 glasses per month
- ○ 1 glass per week
- ○ 2 - 6 glasses per week
- ○ 1 glass per day
- ○ 2 or more glasses per day

101. Tomatoes (1)
- ○ Never
- ○ 1 - 3 per month
- ○ 1 per week
- ○ 2 - 6 per week
- ○ 1 or more per day

102. Tomato/spaghetti sauce
- ○ Never
- ○ 1 - 3 times per month
- ○ Once per week
- ○ 2 - 4 times per week
- ○ 5 or more times per week

103. Tofu
- ○ Never
- ○ 1 - 3 times per month
- ○ Once per week
- ○ 2 - 4 times per week
- ○ 5 or more times per week

104. String beans
- ○ Never
- ○ 1 - 3 times per month
- ○ Once per week
- ○ 2 - 4 times per week
- ○ 5 or more times per week

45803-3/3

3531

105. Broccoli
- ○ Never
- ○ 1 - 3 times per month
- ○ Once per week
- ○ 2 - 4 times per week
- ○ 5 or more times per week

106. Beets (not greens)
- ○ Never
- ○ Once per week or less
- ○ 2 or more times per week

107. Corn
- ○ Never
- ○ 1 - 3 times per month
- ○ Once per week
- ○ 2 - 4 times per week
- ○ 5 or more times per week

108. Peas or lima beans
- ○ Never
- ○ 1 - 3 times per month
- ○ Once per week
- ○ 2 - 4 times per week
- ○ 5 or more times per week

109. Mixed vegetables
- ○ Never
- ○ 1 - 3 times per month
- ○ Once per week
- ○ 2 - 4 times per week
- ○ 5 or more times per week

110. Spinach
- ○ Never
- ○ 1 - 3 times per month
- ○ Once a week
- ○ 2 - 4 times per week
- ○ 5 or more times per week

111. Greens/kale
- ○ Never
- ○ 1 - 3 times per month
- ○ Once per week
- ○ 2 - 4 times per week
- ○ 5 or more times per week

112. Green/red peppers
- ○ Never
- ○ 1 - 3 times per month
- ○ Once a week
- ○ 2 - 4 times per week
- ○ 5 or more times per week

113. Yams/sweet potatoes (1)
- ○ Never
- ○ 1 - 3 times per month
- ○ Once a week
- ○ 2 - 4 times per week
- ○ 5 or more times per week

114. Zucchini, summer squash, eggplant
- ○ Never
- ○ 1 - 3 times per month
- ○ Once per week
- ○ 2 - 4 times per week
- ○ 5 or more times per week

115. Carrots, cooked
- ○ Never
- ○ 1 - 3 times per month
- ○ Once per week
- ○ 2 - 4 times per week
- ○ 5 or more times per week

116. Carrots, raw
- ○ Never
- ○ 1 - 3 times per month
- ○ Once per week
- ○ 2 - 4 times per week
- ○ 5 or more times per week

117. Celery
- ○ Never
- ○ 1 - 3 times per month
- ○ Once per week
- ○ 2 - 4 times per week
- ○ 5 or more times per week

118. Lettuce/tossed salad
- ○ Never
- ○ 1 - 3 times per month
- ○ Once per week
- ○ 2 - 6 times per week
- ○ One or more per day

119. Coleslaw
- ○ Never
- ○ 1 - 3 times per month
- ○ Once per week
- ○ 2 or more times per week

120. Potato salad
- ○ Never
- ○ 1 - 3 times per month
- ○ Once per week
- ○ 2 or more times per week

121. Beans/lentils/soybeans
- ○ Never
- ○ Once per week or less
- ○ 2 - 6 times per week
- ○ Once per day

SNACK FOODS/DESSERTS

122. **Fill in the number of snacks (food or drinks) eaten on school days and weekends/vacation days.**

Snacks	School Days					Vacation/Weekend Days				
	NONE	1	2	3	4 OR MORE	NONE	1	2	3	4 OR MORE
Between breakfast and lunch	○	○	○	○	○	○	○	○	○	○
After lunch, before dinner	○	○	○	○	○	○	○	○	○	○
After dinner	○	○	○	○	○	○	○	○	○	○

Think about your usual snacks. Estimate how often you eat each type of snack food.

Example 3 If you eat poptarts rarely (about 6 per year) then your answer should look like this:

E3. Poptarts (1)
- ● Never/less than 1 per month
- ○ 1 - 3 per month
- ○ 1 - 6 per week
- ○ 1 or more per day

123. Potato chips (1 small bag)
- ○ Never/less than 1 per month
- ○ 1 - 3 small bags per month
- ○ One small bag per week
- ○ 2 - 6 small bags per week
- ○ 1 or more small bags per day

124. Corn chips/Doritos (small bag)
- ○ Never/less than 1 per month
- ○ 1 - 3 small bags per month
- ○ One small bag per week
- ○ 2 - 6 small bags per week
- ○ 1 or more small bags per day

125. Nachos with cheese (1 serving)
- ○ Never/less than 1 per month
- ○ 1 - 3 times per month
- ○ Once per week
- ○ 2 or more times per week

126. Popcorn (1 small bag)
- ○ Never/less than 1 per month
- ○ 1 - 3 small bags per month
- ○ 1 - 4 small bags per week
- ○ 5 or more small bags per week

127. Pretzels (1 small bag)
- ○ Never/less than 1 per month
- ○ 1 - 3 small bags per month
- ○ 1 small bags per week
- ○ 2 or more small bags per week

128. Peanuts, nuts (1 small bag)
- ○ Never/less than 1 per month
- ○ 1 - 3 small bags per month
- ○ 1 - 4 small bags per week
- ○ 5 or more small bags per week

129. Fun fruit (1 pack)
- ○ Never/less than 1 per month
- ○ 1 - 3 packs per month
- ○ 1 - 4 packs per week
- ○ 5 or more packs per week

130. Graham crackers
- ○ Never/less than 1 per month
- ○ 1 - 3 times per month
- ○ 1 - 4 times per week
- ○ 5 or more times per week

131. Crackers, like saltines or wheat thins
- ○ Never/less than 1 per month
- ○ 1 - 3 times per month
- ○ 1 - 4 times per week
- ○ 5 or more times per week

3531

132. Poptarts (1)

- ◯ Never/less than 1 per month
- ◯ 1 - 3 poptarts per month
- ◯ 1 - 6 poptarts per week
- ◯ 1 or more poptarts per day

133. Cake (1 slice)

- ◯ Never/less than 1 per month
- ◯ 1 - 3 slices per month
- ◯ 1 slice per week
- ◯ 2 or more slices per week

134. Snack cakes, Twinkies (1 package)

- ◯ Never/less than 1 per month
- ◯ 1 - 3 per month
- ◯ Once per week
- ◯ 2 - 6 per week
- ◯ 1 or more per day

135. Danish, sweetrolls, pastry (1)

- ◯ Never/less than 1 per month
- ◯ 1 - 3 per month
- ◯ 1 per week
- ◯ 2 - 4 per week
- ◯ 5 or more per week

136. Donuts (1)

- ◯ Never/less than 1 per month
- ◯ 1 - 3 donuts per month
- ◯ 1 donut per week
- ◯ 2 - 6 donuts per week
- ◯ 1 or more donuts per day

137. Cookies (1)

- ◯ Never/less than 1 per month
- ◯ 1 - 3 cookies per month
- ◯ 1 cookie per week
- ◯ 2 - 6 cookies per week
- ◯ 1 - 3 cookies per day
- ◯ 4 or more cookies per day

138. Brownies (1)

- ◯ Never/less than 1 per month
- ◯ 1 - 3 per month
- ◯ 1 per week
- ◯ 2 - 4 per week
- ◯ 5 or more per week

139. Pie (1 slice)

- ◯ Never/less than 1 per month
- ◯ 1 - 3 slices per month
- ◯ 1 slice per week
- ◯ 2 or more slices per week

140. Chocolate (1 bar or packet) like Hershey's or M & M's

- ◯ Never/less than 1 per month
- ◯ 1 - 3 per month
- ◯ 1 per week
- ◯ 2 - 6 per week
- ◯ 1 or more per day

141. Other candy bars (Milky Way, Snickers)

- ◯ Never/less than 1 per month
- ◯ 1 - 3 candy bars per month
- ◯ 1 candy bar per week
- ◯ 2 - 4 candy bars per week
- ◯ 5 or more candy bars per week

142. Other candy without chocolate (mints, Lifesavers) (1 pack)

- ◯ Never/less than 1 per month
- ◯ 1 - 3 times per month
- ◯ Once per week
- ◯ 2 - 4 times per week
- ◯ 5 or more times per week

143. Jello

- ◯ Never/less than 1 per month
- ◯ 1 - 3 times per month
- ◯ Once per week
- ◯ 2 - 4 times per week
- ◯ 5 or more times per week

144. Pudding

- ◯ Never/less than 1 per month
- ◯ 1 - 3 times per month
- ◯ Once per week
- ◯ 2 - 4 times per week
- ◯ 5 or more times per week

145. Frozen yogurt

- ◯ Never/less than 1 per month
- ◯ 1 - 3 times per month
- ◯ Once per week
- ◯ 2 - 4 times per week
- ◯ 5 or more times per week

146. Ice cream

- ◯ Never/less than 1 per month
- ◯ 1 - 3 times per month
- ◯ Once per week
- ◯ 2 - 4 times per week
- ◯ 5 or more times per week

147. Milkshake or frappe (1)

- ◯ Never/less than 1 per month
- ◯ 1 - 3 per month
- ◯ 1 per week
- ◯ 2 or more per week

148. Popsicles

- ◯ Never/less than 1 per month
- ◯ 1 - 3 popsicles per month
- ◯ 1 popsicle per week
- ◯ 2 - 4 popsicles per week
- ◯ 5 or more popsicles per week

149. Please list any other important foods that you usually eat <u>at least once per week</u> that are not listed (for example, coconut, hummus, falafel, eggrolls, chili, plantains, mangoes, etc. . .)

FOODS

a) _____

b) _____

c) _____

d) _____

HOW OFTEN?

a) _____

b) _____

c) _____

d) _____

THANK YOU FOR COMPLETING THIS SURVEY!

*The Diet History Questionnaire (DHQ)**

APPENDIX J

From the Risk Factor Monitoring and Methods Branch, Division of Cancer Control and Population Studies, National Cancer Institute, National Institutes of Health, U.S. Department of Health and Human Services.

*This appendix contains the first eight pages of the Diet History Questionnaire. For the complete questionnaire, visit the *Nutritional Assessment* website at www.mhhe.com/hper/nutrition.

Diet History Questionnaire

GENERAL INSTRUCTIONS

- Answer each question as best you can. Estimate if you are not sure. A guess is better than leaving a blank.
- Use only a No. 2 pencil.
- Be certain to completely blacken in each of the answers.
- Erase completely if you make any changes.
- Do not make any stray marks on this form.
- If you blacken **NEVER** or **NO** for a question, please follow any arrows or instructions that direct you to the next question.

BEFORE TURNING THE PAGE, PLEASE COMPLETE THE FOLLOWING QUESTIONS.

Today's date:

MONTH	DAY	YEAR
JAN		1998
FEB		1999
MAR	⓪⓪	2000
APR	①①	2001
MAY	②②	2002
JUN	③③	
JUL	④	
AUG	⑤	
SEP	⑥	
OCT	⑦	
NOV	⑧	
DEC	⑨	

In what month were you born?

- JAN
- FEB
- MAR
- APR
- MAY
- JUN
- JUL
- AUG
- SEP
- OCT
- NOV
- DEC

In what year were you born?

1 9

⓪⓪
①①
②②
③③
④④
⑤⑤
⑥⑥
⑦⑦
⑧⑧
⑨⑨

Are you male or female?

- Male
- Female

SERIAL #

1. Over the past 12 months, how often did you drink **tomato juice** or **vegetable juice**?

○ NEVER (GO TO QUESTION 2)

○ 1 time per month or less ○ 1 time per day
○ 2–3 times per month ○ 2–3 times per day
○ 1–2 times per week ○ 4–5 times per day
○ 3–4 times per week ○ 6 or more times per day
○ 5–6 times per week

1a. Each time you drank **tomato juice** or **vegetable juice**, how much did you usually drink?

○ Less than $^3/_4$ cup (6 ounces)
○ $^3/_4$ to $1^1/_4$ cups (6 to 10 ounces)
○ More than $1^1/_4$ cups (10 ounces)

2. Over the past 12 months, how often did you drink **orange juice** or **grapefruit juice?**

○ NEVER (GO TO QUESTION 3)

○ 1 time per month or less ○ 1 time per day
○ 2–3 times per month ○ 2–3 times per day
○ 1–2 times per week ○ 4–5 times per day
○ 3–4 times per week ○ 6 or more times per day
○ 5–6 times per week

2a. Each time you drank **orange juice** or **grapefruit juice,** how much did you usually drink?

○ Less than $^3/_4$ cup (6 ounces)
○ $^3/_4$ to $1^1/_4$ cups (6 to 10 ounces)
○ More than $1^1/_4$ cups (10 ounces)

3. Over the past 12 months, how often did you drink **other 100% fruit juice** or **100% fruit juice mixtures** (such as apple, grape, pineapple, or others)?

○ NEVER (GO TO QUESTION 4)

○ 1 time per month or less ○ 1 time per day
○ 2–3 times per month ○ 2–3 times per day
○ 1–2 times per week ○ 4–5 times per day
○ 3–4 times per week ○ 6 or more times per day
○ 5–6 times per week

3a. Each time you drank **other fruit juice** or **fruit juice mixtures**, how much did you usually drink?

○ Less than $^3/_4$ cup (6 ounces)
○ $^3/_4$ to $1^1/_2$ cups (6 to 12 ounces)
○ More than $1^1/_2$ cups (12 ounces)

Question 4 appears in the next column.

Over the past 12 months...

4. How often did you drink other **fruit drinks** (such as cranberry cocktail, Hi-C, lemonade, or Kool-Aid, diet or regular)?

○ NEVER (GO TO QUESTION 5)

○ 1 time per month or less ○ 1 time per day
○ 2–3 times per month ○ 2–3 times per day
○ 1–2 times per week ○ 4–5 times per day
○ 3–4 times per week ○ 6 or more times per day
○ 5–6 times per week

4a. Each time you drank **fruit drinks**, how much did you usually drink?

○ Less than 1 cup (8 ounces)
○ 1 to 2 cups (8 to 16 ounces)
○ More than 2 cups (16 ounces)

4b. How often were your fruit drinks **diet** or **sugar-free drinks**?

○ Almost never or never
○ About $^1/_4$ of the time
○ About $^1/_2$ of the time
○ About $^3/_4$ of the time
○ Almost always or always

5. How often did you drink **milk as a beverage** (NOT in coffee, NOT in cereal)? (Please include chocolate milk and hot chocolate.)

○ NEVER (GO TO QUESTION 6)

○ 1 time per month or less ○ 1 time per day
○ 2–3 times per month ○ 2–3 times per day
○ 1–2 times per week ○ 4–5 times per day
○ 3–4 times per week ○ 6 or more times per day
○ 5–6 times per week

5a. Each time you drank **milk as a beverage**, how much did you usually drink?

○ Less than 1 cup (8 ounces)
○ 1 to $1^1/_2$ cups (8 to 12 ounces)
○ More than $1^1/_2$ cups (12 ounces)

5b. What kind of **milk** did you usually drink?

○ Whole milk
○ 2% fat milk
○ 1 % fat milk
○ Skim, nonfat, or $^1/_2$% fat milk
○ Soy milk
○ Rice milk
○ Other

Question 6 appears on the next page.

2

Over the past 12 months...

6. How often did you drink **meal replacement, energy, or high-protein beverages** such as Instant Breakfast, Ensure, Slimfast, Sustacal or others?

○ NEVER (GO TO QUESTION 7)

○ 1 time per month or less   ○ 1 time per day
○ 2–3 times per month   ○ 2–3 times per day
○ 1–2 times per week   ○ 4–5 times per day
○ 3–4 times per week   ○ 6 or more times
○ 5–6 times per week   per day

6a. Each time you drank **meal replacement beverages**, how much did you usually drink?

○ Less than 1 cup (8 ounces)
○ 1 to 1^1/$_2$ cups (8 to 12 ounces)
○ More than 1^1/$_2$ cups (12 ounces)

7. Over the past 12 months, did you drink **soft drinks, soda, or pop**?

○ NO (GO TO QUESTION 8)

○ YES

7a. How often did you drink **soft drinks, soda,** or **pop IN THE SUMMER**?

○ NEVER

○ 1 time per month or less   ○ 1 time per day
○ 2–3 times per month   ○ 2–3 times per day
○ 1–2 times per week   ○ 4–5 times per day
○ 3–4 times per week   ○ 6 or more times
○ 5–6 times per week   per day

7b. How often did you drink **soft drinks, soda,** or **pop DURING THE REST OF THE YEAR**?

○ NEVER

○ 1 time per month or less   ○ 1 time per day
○ 2–3 times per month   ○ 2–3 times per day
○ 1–2 times per week   ○ 4–5 times per day
○ 3–4 times per week   ○ 6 or more times
○ 5–6 times per week   per day

7c. Each time you drank **soft drinks, soda,** or **pop**, how much did you usually drink?

○ Less than 12 ounces or less than 1 can or bottle
○ 12 to 16 ounces or 1 can or bottle
○ More than 16 ounces or more than 1 can or bottle

Question 8 appears in the next column.

7d. How often were these soft drinks, soda, or pop **diet** or **sugar-free**?

○ Almost never or never
○ About ^{1}/$_4$ of the time
○ About ^{1}/$_2$ of the time
○ About ^{3}/$_4$ of the time
○ Almost always or always

7e. How often were these soft drinks, soda, or pop **caffeine-free**?

○ Almost never or never
○ About ^{1}/$_4$ of the time
○ About ^{1}/$_2$ of the time
○ About ^{3}/$_4$ of the time
○ Almost always or always

8. Over the past 12 months, did you drink **beer**?

○ NO (GO TO QUESTION 9)

○ YES

8a. How often did you drink **beer IN THE SUMMER**?

○ NEVER

○ 1 time per month or less   ○ 1 time per day
○ 2–3 times per month   ○ 2–3 times per day
○ 1–2 times per week   ○ 4–5 times per day
○ 3–4 times per week   ○ 6 or more times
○ 5–6 times per week   per day

8b. How often did you drink **beer DURING THE REST OF THE YEAR**?

○ NEVER

○ 1 time per month or less   ○ 1 time per day
○ 2–3 times per month   ○ 2–3 times per day
○ 1–2 times per week   ○ 4–5 times per day
○ 3–4 times per week   ○ 6 or more times
○ 5–6 times per week   per day

8c. Each time you drank **beer**, how much did you usually drink?

○ Less than a 12-ounce can or bottle
○ 1 to 3 12-ounce cans or bottles
○ More than 3 12-ounce cans or bottles

Question 9 appears on the next page.

3

9. How often did you drink **wine** or **wine coolers**?

○ NEVER (GO TO QUESTION 10)

○ 1 time per month or less ○ 1 time per day
○ 2–3 times per month ○ 2–3 times per day
○ 1–2 times per week ○ 4–5 times per day
○ 3–4 times per week ○ 6 or more times
○ 5–6 times per week   per day

9a. Each time you drank **wine** or **wine coolers**, how much did you usually drink?

○ Less than 5 ounces or less than 1 glass
○ 5 to 12 ounces or 1 to 2 glasses
○ More than 12 ounces or more than 2 glasses

10. How often did you drink **liquor** or **mixed drinks**?

○ NEVER (GO TO QUESTION 11)

○ 1 time per month or less ○ 1 time per day
○ 2–3 times per month ○ 2–3 times per day
○ 1–2 times per week ○ 4–5 times per day
○ 3–4 times per week ○ 6 or more times per day
○ 5–6 times per week

10a. Each time you drank **liquor** or **mixed drinks**, how much did you usually drink?

○ Less than 1 shot of liquor
○ 1 to 3 shots of liquor
○ More than 3 shots of liquor

11. Over the <u>past 12 months</u>, did you eat **oatmeal, grits,** or **other cooked cereal?**

○ NO (GO TO QUESTION 12)

○ YES

11a. How often did you eat **oatmeal, grits,** or **other cooked cereal IN THE WINTER?**

○ NEVER

○ 1–6 times per winter ○ 2 times per week
○ 7–11 times per winter ○ 3–4 times per week
○ 1 time per month ○ 5–6 times per week
○ 2–3 times per month ○ 1 time per day
○ 1 time per week ○ 2 or more times
   per day

Question 12 appears in the next column.

11b. How often did you eat **oatmeal, grits,** or **other cooked cereal DURING THE REST OF THE YEAR?**

○ NEVER

○ 1–6 times per year ○ 2 times per week
○ 7–11 times per year ○ 3–4 times per week
○ 1 time per month ○ 5–6 times per week
○ 2–3 times per month ○ 1 time per day
○ 1 time per week ○ 2 or more times
   per day

11c. Each time you ate **oatmeal, grits,** or **other cooked cereal,** how much did you usually eat?

○ Less than $^3/_4$ cup
○ $^3/_4$ to $1^1/_4$ cups
○ More than $1^1/_4$ cups

12. How often did you eat **cold cereal**?

○ NEVER (GO TO QUESTION 13)

○ 1–6 times per year ○ 2 times per week
○ 7–11 times per year ○ 3–4 times per week
○ 1 time per month ○ 5–6 times per week
○ 2–3 times per month ○ 1 time per day
○ 1 time per week ○ 2 or more times per day

12a. Each time you ate **cold cereal,** how much did you usually eat?

○ Less than 1 cup
○ 1 to $2^1/_2$ cups
○ More than $2^1/_2$ cups

12b. How often was the cold cereal you ate **Total, Product 19,** or **Right Start**?

○ Almost never or never
○ About $^1/_4$ of the time
○ About $^1/_2$ of the time
○ About $^3/_4$ of the time
○ Almost always or always

12c. How often was the cold cereal you ate **All Bran, Fiber One, 100% Bran,** or **Bran Buds?**

○ Almost never or never
○ About $^1/_4$ of the time
○ About $^1/_2$ of the time
○ About $^3/_4$ of the time
○ Almost always or always

Question 13 appears on the next page.

4

213950 · 2/9

439

Over the past 12 months...

12d. How often was the cold cereal you ate **some other bran** or **fiber cereal** (such as Cheerios, Shredded Wheat, Raisin Bran, Bran Flakes, Grape-Nuts, Granola, Wheaties, or Healthy Choice)?

○ Almost never or never
○ About $^1/_4$ of the time
○ About $^1/_2$ of the time
○ About $^3/_4$ of the time
○ Almost always or always

12e. How often was the cold cereal you ate any **other type of cold cereal** (such as Corn Flakes, Rice Krispies, Frosted Flakes, Special K, Froot Loops, Cap'n Crunch, or others)?

○ Almost never or never
○ About $^1/_4$ of the time
○ About $^1/_2$ of the time
○ About $^3/_4$ of the time
○ Almost always or always

12f. Was **milk** added to your cold cereal?

○ NO (GO TO QUESTION 13)

○ YES

12g. What kind of **milk** was usually added?

○ Whole milk
○ 2% fat milk
○ 1% fat milk
○ Skim, nonfat, or $^1/_2$% fat milk
○ Soy milk
○ Rice milk
○ Other

12h. Each time **milk was added to your cold cereal**, how much was usually added?

○ Less than $^1/_2$ cup
○ $^1/_2$ to 1 cup
○ More than 1 cup

13. How often did you eat **applesauce**?

○ NEVER (GO TO QUESTION 14)

○ 1–6 times per year	○ 2 times per week
○ 7–11 times per year	○ 3–4 times per week
○ 1 time per month	○ 5–6 times per week
○ 2–3 times per month	○ 1 time per day
○ 1 time per week	○ 2 or more times per day

Question 14 appears in the next column.

13a. Each time you ate **applesauce**, how much did you usually eat?

○ Less than $^1/_2$ cup
○ $^1/_2$ to 1 cup
○ More than 1 cup

14. How often did you eat **apples**?

○ NEVER (GO TO QUESTION 15)

○ 1–6 times per year	○ 2 times per week
○ 7–11 times per year	○ 3–4 times per week
○ 1 time per month	○ 5–6 times per week
○ 2–3 times per month	○ 1 time per day
○ 1 time per week	○ 2 or more times per day

14a. Each time you ate **apples**, how many did you usually eat?

○ Less than 1 apple
○ 1 apple
○ More than 1 apple

15. How often did you eat **pears** (fresh, canned, or frozen)?

○ NEVER (GO TO QUESTION 16)

○ 1–6 times per year	○ 2 times per week
○ 7–11 times per year	○ 3–4 times per week
○ 1 time per month	○ 5–6 times per week
○ 2–3 times per month	○ 1 time per day
○ 1 time per week	○ 2 or more times per day

15a. Each time you ate **pears**, how much did you usually eat?

○ Less than 1 pear
○ 1 pear
○ More than 1 pear

16. How often did you eat **bananas**?

○ NEVER (GO TO QUESTION 17)

○ 1–6 times per year	○ 2 times per week
○ 7–11 times per year	○ 3–4 times per week
○ 1 time per month	○ 5–6 times per week
○ 2–3 times per month	○ 1 time per day
○ 1 time per week	○ 2 or more times per day

Question 17 appears on the next page.

Perf

16a. Each time you ate **bananas**, how many did you usually eat?

- ○ Less than 1 banana
- ○ 1 banana
- ○ More than 1 banana

17. How often did you eat **dried fruit**, such as prunes or raisins (not including dried apricots)?

├─ ○ NEVER (GO TO QUESTION 18)

- ○ 1–6 times per year
- ○ 7–11 times per year
- ○ 1 time per month
- ○ 2–3 times per month
- ○ 1 time per week
- ○ 2 times per week
- ○ 3–4 times per week
- ○ 5–6 times per week
- ○ 1 time per day
- ○ 2 or more times per day

17a. Each time you ate **dried fruit**, how much did you usually eat (not including dried apricots)?

- ○ Less than 2 tablespoons
- ○ 2 to 5 tablespoons
- ○ More than 5 tablespoons

18. Over the past 12 months, did you eat **peaches, nectarines,** or **plums**?

├─ ○ NO (GO TO QUESTION 19)

○ YES

18a. How often did you eat **fresh peaches, nectarines,** or **plums** WHEN IN SEASON?

- ○ NEVER

- ○ 1–6 times per season
- ○ 7–11 times per season
- ○ 1 time per month
- ○ 2–3 times per month
- ○ 1 time per week
- ○ 2 times per week
- ○ 3–4 times per week
- ○ 5–6 times per week
- ○ 1 time per day
- ○ 2 or more times per day

18b. How often did you eat **peaches, nectarines,** or **plums** (fresh, canned, or frozen) **DURING THE REST OF THE YEAR**?

- ○ NEVER

- ○ 1–6 times per year
- ○ 7–11 times per year
- ○ 1 time per month
- ○ 2–3 times per month
- ○ 1 time per week
- ○ 2 times per week
- ○ 3–4 times per week
- ○ 5–6 times per week
- ○ 1 time per day
- ○ 2 or more times per day

Question 19 appears in the next column.

18c. Each time you ate **peaches, nectarines,** or **plums,** how much did you usually eat?

- ○ Less than 1 fruit or less than $1/2$ cup
- ○ 1 to 2 fruits or $1/2$ to $3/4$ cup
- ○ More than 2 fruits or more than $3/4$ cup

19. How often did you eat **grapes**?

├─ ○ NEVER (GO TO QUESTION 20)

- ○ 1–6 times per year
- ○ 7–11 times per year
- ○ 1 time per month
- ○ 2–3 times per month
- ○ 1 time per week
- ○ 2 times per week
- ○ 3–4 times per week
- ○ 5–6 times per week
- ○ 1 time per day
- ○ 2 or more times per day

19a. Each time you ate **grapes**, how much did you usually eat?

- ○ Less than $1/2$ cup or less than 10 grapes
- ○ $1/2$ to 1 cup or 10 to 30 grapes
- ○ More than 1 cup or more than 30 grapes

20. Over the past 12 months, did you eat **cantaloupe**?

├─ ○ NO (GO TO QUESTION 21)

○ YES

20a. How often did you eat **fresh cantaloupe WHEN IN SEASON**?

- ○ NEVER

- ○ 1–6 times per season
- ○ 7–11 times per season
- ○ 1 time per month
- ○ 2–3 times per month
- ○ 1 time per week
- ○ 2 times per week
- ○ 3–4 times per week
- ○ 5–6 times per week
- ○ 1 time per day
- ○ 2 or more times per day

20b. How often did you eat **fresh or frozen cantaloupe DURING THE REST OF THE YEAR**?

- ○ NEVER

- ○ 1–6 times per year
- ○ 7–11 times per year
- ○ 1 time per month
- ○ 2–3 times per month
- ○ 1 time per week
- ○ 2 times per week
- ○ 3–4 times per week
- ○ 5–6 times per week
- ○ 1 time per day
- ○ 2 or more times per day

Question 21 appears on the next page.

213950 - 3/9

Over the past 12 months...

20c. Each time you ate **cantaloupe**, how much did you usually eat?

○ Less than $^1/_4$ melon or less than $^1/_2$ cup
○ $^1/_4$ melon or $^1/_2$ to 1 cup
○ More than $^1/_4$ melon or more than 1 cup

21. Over the past 12 months, did you eat **melon, other than cantaloupe** (such as watermelon or honeydew)?

○ NO (GO TO QUESTION 22)

○ YES

21a. How often did you eat **fresh melon, other than cantaloupe,** (such as watermelon or honeydew) **WHEN IN SEASON?**

○ NEVER

○ 1–6 times per season   ○ 2 times per week
○ 7–11 times per season   ○ 3–4 times per week
○ 1 time per month   ○ 5–6 times per week
○ 2–3 times per month   ○ 1 time per day
○ 1 time per week   ○ 2 or more times
                              per day

21b. How often did you eat **fresh** or **frozen melon, other than cantaloupe** (such as watermelon or honeydew) **DURING THE REST OF THE YEAR?**

○ NEVER

○ 1–6 times per year   ○ 2 times per week
○ 7–11 times per year   ○ 3–4 times per week
○ 1 time per month   ○ 5–6 times per week
○ 2–3 times per month   ○ 1 time per day
○ 1 time per week   ○ 2 or more times
                              per day

21c. Each time you ate **melon other than cantaloupe**, how much did you usually eat?

○ Less than $^1/_2$ cup or 1 small wedge
○ $^1/_2$ to 2 cups or 1 medium wedge
○ More than 2 cups or 1 large wedge

Question 22 appears in the next column.

Perf

22. Over the past 12 months, did you eat **strawberries?**

○ NO (GO TO QUESTION 23)

○ YES

22a. How often did you eat **fresh strawberries WHEN IN SEASON?**

○ NEVER

○ 1–6 times per season   ○ 2 times per week
○ 7–11 times per season   ○ 3–4 times per week
○ 1 time per month   ○ 5–6 times per week
○ 2–3 times per month   ○ 1 time per day
○ 1 time per week   ○ 2 or more times
                              per day

22b. How often did you eat **fresh** or **frozen strawberries DURING THE REST OF THE YEAR?**

○ NEVER

○ 1–6 times per year   ○ 2 times per week
○ 7–11 times per year   ○ 3–4 times per week
○ 1 time per month   ○ 5–6 times per week
○ 2–3 times per month   ○ 1 time per day
○ 1 time per week   ○ 2 or more times
                              per day

22c. Each time you ate **strawberries**, how much did you usually eat?

○ Less than $^1/_4$ cup or less than 3 berries
○ $^1/_4$ to $^3/_4$ cup or 3 to 8 berries
○ More than $^3/_4$ cup or more than 8 berries

23. Over the past 12 months, did you eat **oranges, tangerines, or tangelos?**

○ NO (GO TO QUESTION 24)

○ YES

23a. How often did you eat **fresh oranges, tangerines, or tangelos WHEN IN SEASON?**

○ NEVER

○ 1–6 times per season   ○ 2 times per week
○ 7–11 times per season   ○ 3–4 times per week
○ 1 time per month   ○ 5–6 times per week
○ 2–3 times per month   ○ 1 time per day
○ 1 time per week   ○ 2 or more times
                              per day

Question 24 appears on the next page.

7

■ **Over the past 12 months...**

23b. How often did you eat **oranges, tangerines, or tangelos** (fresh or canned) **DURING THE REST OF THE YEAR?**

○ NEVER

○ 1–6 times per year	○ 2 times per week
○ 7–11 times per year	○ 3–4 times per week
○ 1 time per month	○ 5–6 times per week
○ 2–3 times per month	○ 1 time per day
○ 1 time per week	○ 2 or more times per day

23c. Each time you ate **oranges, tangerines,** or **tangelos,** how many did you usually eat?

○ Less than 1 fruit
○ 1 fruit
○ More than 1 fruit

24. Over the past 12 months, did you eat **grapefruit?**

○ NO (GO TO QUESTION 25)

○ YES

24a. How often did you eat **fresh grapefruit WHEN IN SEASON?**

○ NEVER

○ 1–6 times per season	○ 2 times per week
○ 7–11 times per season	○ 3–4 times per week
○ 1 time per month	○ 5–6 times per week
○ 2–3 times per month	○ 1 time per day
○ 1 time per week	○ 2 or more times per day

24b. How often did you eat **grapefruit** (fresh or canned) **DURING THE REST OF THE YEAR?**

○ NEVER

○ 1–6 times per year	○ 2 times per week
○ 7–11 times per year	○ 3–4 times per week
○ 1 time per month	○ 5–6 times per week
○ 2–3 times per month	○ 1 time per day
○ 1 time per week	○ 2 or more times per day

24c. Each time you ate **grapefruit,** how much did you usually eat?

○ Less than $^1/_2$ grapefruit
○ $^1/_2$ grapefruit
○ More than $^1/_2$ grapefruit

Question 25 appears in the next column.

25. How often did you eat **other kinds of fruit?**

○ NEVER (GO TO QUESTION 26)

○ 1–6 times per year	○ 2 times per week
○ 7–11 times per year	○ 3–4 times per week
○ 1 time per month	○ 5–6 times per week
○ 2–3 times per month	○ 1 time per day
○ 1 time per week	○ 2 or more times per day

25a. Each time you ate **other kinds of fruit,** how much did you usually eat?

○ Less than $^1/_4$ cup
○ $^1/_4$ to $^3/_4$ cup
○ More than $^3/_4$ cup

26. How often did you eat **COOKED greens** (such as spinach, turnip, collard, mustard, chard, or kale)?

○ NEVER (GO TO QUESTION 27)

○ 1–6 times per year	○ 2 times per week
○ 7–11 times per year	○ 3–4 times per week
○ 1 time per month	○ 5–6 times per week
○ 2–3 times per month	○ 1 time per day
○ 1 time per week	○ 2 or more times per day

26a. Each time you ate **COOKED greens,** how much did you usually eat?

○ Less than $^1/_2$ cup
○ $^1/_2$ to 1 cup
○ More than 1 cup

27. How often did you eat **RAW greens** (such as spinach, turnip, collard, mustard, chard, or kale)? (*We will ask about lettuce later.*)

○ NEVER (GO TO QUESTION 28)

○ 1–6 times per year	○ 2 times per week
○ 7–11 times per year	○ 3–4 times per week
○ 1 time per month	○ 5–6 times per week
○ 2–3 times per month	○ 1 time per day
○ 1 time per week	○ 2 or more times per day

27a. Each time you ate **RAW greens,** how much did you usually eat?

○ Less than $^1/_2$ cup
○ $^1/_2$ to 1 cup
○ More than 1 cup

Question 28 appears on the next page.

8

213950 · 4/9

443

APPENDIX K

Code	Food Name	Unit Amount	Kilocalories (kcal)	Protein (g)	Carbohydrate (g)
2047	Salt, table (sodium Chloride)	1 tsp.	0.0	0.0	0.0
16104	Bacon, vegetarian, meatless	1 strip	15.5	0.5	0.3
18005	Bagel, cinnamon-raisin	1 mini bagel 2.5" diam	126.0	4.5	25.4
18003	Bagel, egg	1 bagel 3.5" diam	177.9	6.8	33.9
18007	Bagel, oatbran	1 bagel 3.5" diam	163.2	6.8	34.1
918008	Bagel, oatbran, toasted, mini/small sizes	1 mini bagel 2.5" diam	126.0	5.3	26.4
18001	Bagel, plain/onion/poppy/sesame, enriched	1 bagel 3.5" diam	176.0	6.7	34.2
924037	Bean burrito	8.0 oz	463.7	20.0	64.0
16112	Bean sauce, fermented soy product, miso	1/2 cup	284.3	16.3	38.6
16008	Beans, baked w/franks, canned	1 cup	363.5	17.3	39.4
16011	Beans, baked w/pork & tomato sauce, canned	1 cup	222.5	11.7	44.0
16006	Beans, baked, plain or vegetarian, canned	1 cup	236.2	12.2	52.1
16018	Beans, black turtle soup, mature seeds, canned	1 cup	230.2	15.3	41.9
16054	Beans, broadbeans (fava) mature seeds, canned	1/2 cup	66.7	5.1	11.7
16026	Beans, great northern, mature seeds, canned	1/2 cup	149.3	9.7	27.5
16029	Beans, kidney, mature seeds, canned	1/2 cup	103.7	6.7	19.0
16070	Beans, lentils, mature seeds, boiled w/o salt	1/2 cup	114.8	8.9	19.9
16081	Beans, mung, mature seeds, boiled w/o salt	1/2 cup	54.6	3.7	10.0
16039	Beans, navy, mature seeds, canned	1/2 cup	102.8	6.9	18.6
16044	Beans, pinto, mature seeds, canned	1/2 cup	97.2	5.5	17.2
16103	Beans, refried, canned (includes USDA Commodity)	1/2 cup	118.4	6.9	19.6
16111	Beans, soy, mature seeds, dry-roasted	1/2 cup	648.0	57.0	47.1
16162	Beans, soy, tofu, Mori-Nu, silken, firm	1/4 block	52.1	5.8	2.0
913524	Beef brisket, all grades, lean (1/2" trim) braised	3.5 oz	241.0	29.4	0.0
913522	Beef brisket, all grades, lean & fat (1/2" trim) braised	3.5 oz	391.0	23.0	0.0
924246	Beef chop suey	1 cup	300.0	26.0	12.5
924222	Beef chow mein/LaChoy	3/4 cup	60.0	6.0	5.0
924002	Beef pot pie, frz (Banquet)	7.0 oz	485.1	19.8	36.8
924034	Beef stroganoff, frz (Stouffer's)	4.0 oz	200.2	15.6	5.8
913512	Beef, all cuts, all grades, lean (1/2" trim) ckd	3.5 oz	222.0	30.4	0.0
13012	Beef, all cuts, all grades, lean (1/4" trim) ckd	3.5 oz	216.0	29.6	0.0
913504	Beef, all cuts, all grades, lean & fat (1/2" trim) ckd	3.5 oz	349.0	25.0	0.0
13004	Beef, all cuts, all grades, lean & fat (1/4" trim) ckd	3.5 oz	305.0	25.9	0.0
13366	Beef, all cuts, select, lean (0" trim) ckd	3.5 oz	201.0	29.9	0.0
924108	Beef, corned beef hash	3.5 oz	184.0	8.5	8.5
924325	Beef, creamed chipped	4.0 oz	174.0	9.3	8.0
13347	Beef, cured corned beef brisket, cooked	3.5 oz	251.0	18.2	0.5
13418	Beef, eye of round, all grades, lean (0" trim) roasted		166.0	29.0	0.0
13300	Beef, ground, extra lean, pan-fried, medium	4.0 oz	303.5	29.7	0.0
13305	Beef, ground, lean, broiled, medium	3.5 oz	272.0	24.7	0.0
13307	Beef, ground, lean, pan-fried, medium	3.5 oz	275.0	24.2	0.0
13312	Beef, ground, regular, broiled, medium	3.5 oz	289.0	24.1	0.0
13314	Beef, ground, regular, pan-fried, medium	4.0 oz	364.1	28.5	0.0
13315	Beef, ground, regular, pan-fried, well-done	4.0 oz	340.3	32.1	0.0
14006	Beverage, alcoholic, beer, light	12.0 oz	100.8	0.7	4.7

Dietary Fiber (g)	Total Fat (g)	Cholesterol (mg)	Calcium (mg)	Iron (mg)	Magnesium (mg)	Sodium (mg)	Zinc (mg)	Vitamin A (μgRE)	Vitamin C (mg)	Vitamin E (mgαT)	Thiamin (mg)	Riboflavin (mg)	Niacin (mg)	Vitamin B₆ (mg)	Folate (μg)
0.0	0.0	0.0	1.4	0.0	0.1	2325.5	0.0	0.0	0.0	0.0	0.0	0.0	0.0	0.0	0.0
0.1	1.5	0.0	1.2	0.1	1.0	73.3	0.0	0.5	0.0	0.3	0.2	0.0	0.4	0.0	2.1
1.1	0.8	0.0	8.7	1.7	12.9	148.1	0.5	0.0	0.3	0.1	0.2	0.1	1.4	0.0	41.4
1.5	1.3	15.4	8.3	2.5	16.0	323.2	0.5	21.1	0.4	0.0	0.3	0.2	2.2	0.1	56.3
2.3	0.8	0.0	7.7	2.0	19.8	324.5	0.6	0.0	0.1	0.1	0.2	0.2	1.9	0.0	51.8
1.7	0.6	0.1	6.0	1.5	28.5	250.7	1.0	0.0	0.0	0.1	0.1	0.2	1.3	0.1	16.1
1.5	1.0	0.0	47.4	2.3	18.6	341.8	0.6	0.0	0.0	0.0	0.3	0.2	2.9	0.0	56.3
1.5	14.3	0.0	275.7	1.6	103.4	1387.7	0.0	0.0	0.0	0.0	0.0	0.0	0.0	0.0	0.0
7.5	8.4	0.0	91.1	3.8	58.0	5032.9	4.6	12.4	0.0	0.0	0.1	0.3	1.2	0.3	45.5
17.7	16.8	15.4	122.9	4.4	71.7	1100.8	4.8	38.4	5.9	1.2	0.1	0.1	2.3	0.1	76.8
10.9	2.3	15.9	127.1	7.4	79.5	998.8	13.3	27.2	7.0	1.2	0.1	0.1	1.1	0.2	51.1
12.7	1.1	0.0	127.0	0.7	81.3	1008.4	3.6	43.2	7.9	1.3	0.4	0.2	1.1	0.3	60.7
17.5	0.7	0.0	88.6	4.8	88.6	971.5	1.4	0.0	6.8	0.0	0.4	0.3	1.6	0.1	153.8
3.5	0.2	0.0	24.4	0.9	30.1	425.8	0.6	0.9	1.7	0.0	0.0	0.0	0.9	0.0	30.7
6.4	0.5	0.0	69.4	2.1	66.8	5.2	0.9	0.0	1.7	0.0	0.2	0.1	0.6	0.1	106.5
4.5	0.4	0.0	34.6	1.6	39.7	444.2	0.7	0.0	1.5	0.0	0.1	0.1	0.6	0.1	63.0
7.8	0.4	0.0	18.8	3.3	35.6	2.0	1.3	1.0	1.5	0.1	0.2	0.1	1.0	0.2	179.0
4.0	0.2	0.0	14.0	0.7	25.0	1.0	0.4	1.0	0.5	0.3	0.1	0.0	0.3	0.0	82.6
4.6	0.4	0.0	42.8	1.7	42.8	407.7	0.7	0.0	0.6	0.3	0.1	0.1	0.4	0.1	56.7
5.2	0.9	0.0	48.6	1.6	30.5	332.2	0.8	2.3	1.0	1.1	0.1	0.1	0.3	0.1	68.0
6.7	1.6	10.1	44.1	2.1	41.6	376.7	1.5	0.0	7.6	0.0	0.0	0.0	0.4	0.2	13.9
11.7	31.1	0.0	201.6	5.7	328.3	2.9	6.9	2.9	6.6	0.0	0.6	1.1	1.5	0.3	294.6
0.1	2.3	0.0	26.9	0.9	22.7	30.2	0.5	0.0	0.0	0.2	0.1	0.0	0.2	0.0	0.0
0.0	12.8	5.8	6.0	2.8	23.0	72.0	6.9	0.0	0.0	0.0	0.1	0.2	3.8	0.3	8.0
0.0	32.4	14.7	9.0	2.2	18.0	61.0	5.0	0.0	0.0	0.0	0.1	0.2	3.0	0.3	6.0
1.3	17.0	0.0	60.0	4.8	0.0	1053.0	0.0	120.0	33.0	0.0	0.3	0.4	5.0	0.0	0.0
2.0	1.0	16.0	80.0	1.4	0.0	890.0	0.0	150.0	2.0	0.0	0.1	0.1	1.2	0.0	0.0
1.7	28.3	39.6	27.3	3.6	0.0	561.9	3.0	795.8	5.7	0.0	0.3	0.3	4.5	0.2	27.3
0.0	12.8	56.5	33.9	1.4	0.0	795.5	0.0	8.5	0.0	0.0	0.1	0.3	2.6	0.0	0.0
0.0	10.2	4.5	8.0	3.2	27.0	65.0	7.1	0.0	0.0	0.0	0.1	0.3	4.2	0.4	9.0
0.0	9.9	86.0	9.0	3.0	26.0	67.0	6.9	0.0	0.0	0.1	0.1	0.2	4.1	0.4	8.0
0.0	26.9	12.0	10.0	2.6	21.0	59.0	5.5	0.0	0.0	0.0	0.1	0.2	3.5	0.3	7.0
0.0	21.5	88.0	10.0	2.6	22.0	62.0	5.9	0.0	0.0	0.2	0.1	0.2	3.6	0.3	7.0
0.0	8.1	86.0	8.0	3.0	26.0	66.0	6.8	0.0	0.0	0.0	0.1	0.2	4.0	0.4	8.0
1.2	12.7	155.3	34.1	5.2	0.0	672.9	5.2	0.0	9.4	0.0	0.1	0.5	5.3	0.5	17.6
0.0	11.6	29.5	118.5	0.9	0.0	809.0	0.0	81.2	0.5	0.0	0.1	0.2	0.7	0.0	0.0
0.0	19.0	98.0	8.0	1.9	12.0	1134.0	4.6	0.0	0.0	0.2	0.0	0.2	3.0	0.2	6.0
0.0	4.7	69.0	5.0	2.0	27.0	62.0	4.7	0.0	0.0	0.1	0.1	0.2	3.8	0.4	7.0
0.0	19.5	96.4	8.3	2.8	25.0	83.3	6.4	0.0	0.0	0.2	0.1	0.3	5.6	0.3	10.7
0.0	18.5	87.0	11.0	2.1	21.0	77.0	5.4	0.0	0.0	0.2	0.1	0.2	5.2	0.3	9.0
0.0	19.1	84.0	10.0	2.2	20.0	77.0	5.2	0.0	0.0	0.2	0.1	0.2	4.8	0.3	9.0
0.0	20.7	90.0	11.0	2.4	20.0	83.0	5.2	0.0	0.0	0.2	0.0	0.2	5.8	0.3	9.0
0.0	26.8	105.9	13.1	2.9	23.8	100.0	6.0	0.0	0.0	0.3	0.0	0.2	6.9	0.3	10.7
0.0	22.5	116.6	15.5	3.2	26.2	110.7	6.7	0.0	0.0	0.0	0.0	0.2	7.7	0.3	11.9
0.0	0.0	0.0	18.0	0.1	18.0	10.8	0.1	0.0	0.0	0.0	0.0	0.1	1.4	0.1	14.8

Code	Food Name	Unit Amount	Kilocalories (kcal)	Protein (g)	Carbohydrate (g)
14003	Beverage, alcoholic, beer, regular	12.0 oz	147.6	1.1	13.3
914008	Beverage, alcoholic, bloody mary, prep from recipe	5.0 oz	115.4	0.7	4.9
914870	Beverage, alcoholic, champagne	3.5 oz	72.1	0.2	2.6
14414	Beverage, alcoholic, coffee liqueur 53-proof	1.5 oz	174.7	0.1	24.3
14009	Beverage, alcoholic, daiquiri, canned	6.8 oz	261.3	0.0	32.8
14037	Beverage, alcoholic, distilled spirits (gin, rum, vodka, or whisky) 80-proof	1.5 oz	97.0	0.0	0.0
914011	Beverage, alcoholic, gin and tonic, prep from recipe	7.5 oz	171.0	0.0	15.8
914014	Beverage, alcoholic, martini, prep from recipe	2.5 oz	156.1	0.0	0.2
14015	Beverage, alcoholic, pina colada, canned	6.8 oz	495.3	1.3	57.7
14027	Beverage, alcoholic, whiskey sour, canned	6.8 oz	248.7	0.0	28.0
14084	Beverage, alcoholic, wine (all table)	3.5 oz	72.1	0.2	1.4
14115	Beverage, alpine spiced cider, instant apple flavor drink mix, powder	2 Tbsp.	31.6	0.0	7.9
14181	Beverage, chocolate syrup w/o added nutrients	2 Tbsp.	82.8	0.7	22.4
14186	Beverage, chocolate syrup, fortified, mixed w/milk	8.0 oz	168.0	7.2	20.2
14390	Beverage, cocoa mix w/aspartame, dry, low kcal, prep w/H$_2$O	8.0 oz	56.0	4.5	9.9
14194	Beverage, cocoa mix, dry, w/o added nutrients, prep w/H$_2$O	8.0 oz	112.0	3.4	24.4
14417	Beverage, cocoa mix, fortified, dry, prep w/H$_2$O	8.0 oz	127.7	2.0	25.8
14195	Beverage, cocoa, hot cocoa mix w/marshmallows/Carnation	2 Tbsp.	87.8	1.1	19.1
14418	Beverage, coffee mix w/sugar (cappuccino) dry, prep w/H$_2$O	8.0 oz	71.7	0.4	12.5
14209	Beverage, coffee, brewed	6.0 oz	3.4	0.2	0.7
14219	Beverage, coffee, instant powder, decaffeinated, prep	1 rd tsp.	0.0	0.0	0.0
14215	Beverage, coffee, instant, prep	6.0 oz	3.4	0.2	0.7
14400	Beverage, cola w/caffeine	12.0 oz	137.8	0.0	34.9
1057	Beverage, eggnog	8.0 oz	341.9	9.7	34.4
914840	Beverage, fruit tea punch	6.0 oz	107.5	0.0	27.0
14123	Beverage, kiwi strawberry cocktail/Snapple	6.0 oz	80.0	0.2	19.8
14305	Beverage, malt beverage	6.0 oz	100.8	0.5	22.6
14137	Beverage, Nestea Ice Tea, Lemon Flavor	6.0 oz	61.7	0.0	14.3
914814	Beverage, soft drink, chocolate carbonated	12.0 oz	163.3	0.0	41.5
14121	Beverage, soft drink, club soda	12.0 oz	0.0	0.0	0.0
14166	Beverage, soft drink, cola or pepper-type, low kcal w/saccharin & caffeine	12.0 oz	0.0	0.0	0.4
14535	Beverage, soft drink, cola, low kcal w/saccharin & aspartame, w/caffeine	12.0 oz	3.6	0.4	0.4
14416	Beverage, soft drink, cola, w/aspartame, low kcal	12.0 oz	3.6	0.4	0.4
14130	Beverage, soft drink, cream soda	12.0 oz	181.1	0.0	47.2
914818	Beverage, soft drink, diet fruit flavor	12.0 oz	3.6	0.0	0.0
914819	Beverage, soft drink, diet ginger ale	12.0 oz	3.6	0.0	1.5
914820	Beverage, soft drink, diet lemon-lime	12.0 oz	0.0	0.0	0.0
914887	Beverage, soft drink, diet root beer	12.0 oz	0.0	0.0	0.4
14136	Beverage, soft drink, ginger ale	12.0 oz	120.7	0.0	30.9
14142	Beverage, soft drink, grape	12.0 oz	152.7	0.0	39.8
14145	Beverage, soft drink, lemon-lime	12.0 oz	142.0	0.0	36.9
914888	Beverage, soft drink, mineral H$_2$O	12.0 oz	0.0	0.0	0.0
14537	Beverage, soft drink, not cola or pepper-type, w/saccharin, low kcal	12.0 oz	0.0	0.0	0.4
14150	Beverage, soft drink, orange	12.0 oz	170.4	0.0	43.7
14153	Beverage, soft drink, pepper-type	12.0 oz	145.6	0.0	36.9
14157	Beverage, soft drink, root beer	12.0 oz	145.6	0.0	37.6
14376	Beverage, tea mix, instant w/lemon flavor, w/saccharin, dry, prep	2 tsp.	0.0	0.0	0.0
14369	Beverage, tea mix, instant w/lemon, unsweetened, dry, prep	2 tsp.	0.0	0.0	0.0
14367	Beverage, tea mix, instant, unsweetened, dry, prep	2 tsp.	0.0	0.0	0.0
14355	Beverage, tea, brewed	6.0 oz	2.4	0.0	0.7
14545	Beverage, tea, chamomile, brewed	6.0 oz	2.4	0.0	0.5
14381	Beverage, tea, herbal (not chamomile) brewed	6.0 oz	2.4	0.0	0.5
14549	Beverage, tea, instant, w/sugar, lemon-flavored, w/added vit C, dry, prep	6.0 oz	81.6	0.2	20.4
914906	Beverage, tea, sweetened, canned	12.0 oz	196.8	0.0	48.7
14133	Beverage, tomato cocktail/bloody Mary mix, mild/tabasco	6.0 oz	55.7	2.2	11.8
14429	Beverage, water	1.0 fl oz	0.3	0.0	0.0
14155	Beverage, water, carbonated, tonic (quinine)	12.0-oz can or bottle	124.4	0.0	32.2
14384	Beverage, water, Perrier	6.5 fl oz bottle	0.0	0.0	0.0
18615	Biscuit, buttermilk biscuit mix, dry/Martha White	1 biscuit	171.4	3.0	26.4
18009	Biscuit, plain or buttermilk, commercially baked	1 small (2.5″ diam)	127.4	2.2	17.0
918011	Biscuit, plain or buttermilk, dry mix, prep	1 biscuit (3″ diam)	191.0	4.2	27.6
18016	Biscuit, plain or buttermilk, homemade	1 medium biscuit (2.5″ diam)	212.4	4.2	26.8
20015	Bran, corn, crude	1 Tbsp.	10.8	0.4	4.1
20034	Bran, oat, ckd	1 Tbsp.	5.5	0.4	1.6
20060	Bran, rice, crude	1 Tbsp.	23.4	1.0	3.7

446

Dietary Fiber (g)	Total Fat (g)	Cholesterol (mg)	Calcium (mg)	Iron (mg)	Magnesium (mg)	Sodium (mg)	Zinc (mg)	Vitamin A (μgRE)	Vitamin C (mg)	Vitamin E (mgαT)	Thiamin (mg)	Riboflavin (mg)	Niacin (mg)	Vitamin B$_6$ (mg)	Folate (μg)
0.7	0.0	0.0	18.0	0.1	21.6	18.0	0.1	0.0	0.0	0.0	0.0	0.1	1.6	0.2	21.6
0.4	0.1	0.0	10.4	0.5	11.8	331.5	0.1	50.3	20.4	0.0	0.1	0.0	0.6	0.1	19.7
0.0	0.0	0.0	0.0	0.0	0.0	0.0	0.0	0.0	0.0	0.0	0.0	0.0	0.0	0.0	0.0
0.0	0.2	0.0	0.5	0.0	1.6	4.2	0.0	0.0	0.0	0.0	0.0	0.0	0.1	0.0	0.0
0.0	0.0	0.0	0.0	0.0	2.1	83.6	0.1	0.0	2.7	0.0	0.0	0.0	0.0	0.0	1.7
0.0	0.0	0.0	0.0	0.0	0.0	0.4	0.0	0.0	0.0	0.0	0.0	0.0	0.0	0.0	0.0
0.0	0.0	0.0	4.5	0.0	2.3	9.0	0.2	0.0	0.9	0.0	0.0	0.0	0.0	0.0	1.1
0.0	0.0	0.0	1.4	0.1	1.4	2.1	0.0	0.0	0.0	0.0	0.0	0.0	0.0	0.0	0.1
0.2	15.9	0.0	2.1	0.1	12.5	148.4	0.4	4.2	3.1	0.0	0.0	0.0	0.2	0.0	12.5
0.2	0.0	0.0	0.0	0.0	2.1	92.0	0.1	2.1	3.3	0.0	0.0	0.0	0.0	0.0	0.0
0.0	0.0	0.0	8.2	0.4	10.3	8.2	0.1	0.0	0.0	0.0	0.0	0.0	0.1	0.0	1.1
0.0	0.0	0.0	0.0	0.0	0.0	0.1	0.0	0.0	29.0	0.0	0.0	0.0	0.0	0.0	0.0
0.7	0.3	0.0	5.3	0.8	24.7	36.5	0.3	1.1	0.1	0.0	0.0	0.0	0.1	0.0	1.5
0.2	7.2	29.1	248.6	2.3	26.9	125.4	0.8	273.3	2.0	0.0	0.1	0.5	5.6	0.1	10.3
0.4	0.4	2.2	105.3	0.9	38.1	201.6	0.6	0.0	0.0	0.0	0.0	0.2	0.2	0.1	2.7
2.7	1.3	2.2	105.3	0.4	26.9	161.3	0.5	0.0	0.4	0.0	0.0	0.2	0.2	0.0	0.0
0.9	3.1	0.0	112.0	1.9	24.6	221.8	0.3	161.3	6.5	0.0	0.2	0.2	2.1	0.0	0.0
0.4	0.8	1.3	32.3	0.2	12.8	75.5	0.2	0.0	0.0	0.0	0.0	0.1	0.1	0.0	0.9
0.0	2.5	0.0	9.0	0.2	11.2	121.0	0.1	0.0	0.0	0.0	0.0	0.0	0.4	0.0	0.0
0.0	0.0	0.0	3.4	0.1	8.4	3.4	0.0	0.0	0.0	0.0	0.0	0.0	0.4	0.0	0.2
0.0	0.0	0.0	0.1	0.0	0.1	0.1	0.0	0.0	0.0	0.0	0.0	0.0	0.0	0.0	0.0
0.0	0.0	0.0	5.0	0.1	6.7	5.0	0.1	0.0	0.0	0.0	0.0	0.0	0.5	0.0	0.0
0.0	0.0	0.0	10.1	0.1	3.4	13.4	0.0	0.0	0.0	0.0	0.0	0.0	0.0	0.0	0.0
0.0	19.0	149.1	330.2	0.5	47.0	138.2	1.2	203.2	3.8	0.6	0.1	0.5	0.3	0.1	2.3
0.0	0.0	0.0	0.0	0.0	0.0	9.1	0.0	0.0	0.0	0.0	0.0	0.0	0.0	0.0	0.0
0.0	0.0	0.0	0.0	0.0	0.0	4.2	0.0	0.0	0.0	0.0	0.0	0.0	0.0	0.0	0.0
0.0	0.2	0.0	8.4	0.1	11.8	21.8	0.0	0.0	0.8	0.0	0.0	0.1	1.9	0.0	23.5
0.0	0.5	0.0	0.0	0.0	0.0	0.0	0.0	0.0	0.0	0.0	0.0	0.0	0.0	0.0	0.0
0.0	0.0	0.0	0.0	0.0	0.0	26.6	0.0	0.0	0.0	0.0	0.0	0.0	0.0	0.0	0.0
0.0	0.0	0.0	17.8	0.0	3.6	74.6	0.4	0.0	0.0	0.0	0.0	0.0	0.0	0.0	0.0
0.0	0.0	0.0	14.2	0.1	3.6	56.8	0.2	0.0	0.0	0.0	0.0	0.0	0.0	0.0	0.0
0.0	0.0	0.0	14.2	0.1	3.6	32.0	0.3	0.0	0.0	0.0	0.0	0.1	0.0	0.0	0.0
0.0	0.0	0.0	14.2	0.1	3.6	21.3	0.3	0.0	0.0	0.0	0.0	0.1	0.0	0.0	0.0
0.0	0.0	0.0	17.8	0.2	3.6	42.6	0.2	0.0	0.0	0.0	0.0	0.0	0.0	0.0	0.0
0.0	0.0	0.0	35.5	0.0	0.0	21.7	0.0	0.0	0.0	0.0	0.0	0.0	0.0	0.0	0.0
0.0	0.0	0.0	17.8	0.0	0.0	31.6	0.0	0.0	0.0	0.0	0.0	0.0	0.0	0.0	0.0
0.0	0.0	0.0	34.5	0.0	0.0	48.3	0.0	0.0	0.0	0.0	0.0	0.0	0.0	0.0	0.0
0.0	0.0	0.0	0.0	0.0	0.0	56.6	0.0	0.0	0.0	0.0	0.0	0.0	0.0	0.0	0.0
0.0	0.0	0.0	10.7	0.6	3.6	24.9	0.2	0.0	0.0	0.0	0.0	0.0	0.0	0.0	0.0
0.0	0.0	0.0	10.7	0.3	3.6	53.3	0.2	0.0	0.0	0.0	0.0	0.0	0.0	0.0	0.0
0.0	0.0	0.0	7.1	0.2	3.6	39.1	0.2	0.0	0.0	0.0	0.0	0.0	0.1	0.0	0.0
0.0	0.0	0.0	48.1	0.0	1.8	5.5	0.0	0.0	0.0	0.0	0.0	0.0	0.0	0.0	0.0
0.0	0.0	0.0	14.2	0.1	3.6	56.8	0.2	0.0	0.0	0.0	0.0	0.0	0.0	0.0	0.0
0.0	0.0	0.0	17.8	0.2	3.6	42.6	0.4	0.0	0.0	0.0	0.0	0.0	0.0	0.0	0.0
0.0	0.4	0.0	10.7	0.1	0.0	35.5	0.1	0.0	0.0	0.0	0.0	0.0	0.0	0.0	0.0
0.0	0.0	0.0	17.8	0.2	3.6	46.2	0.2	0.0	0.0	0.0	0.0	0.0	0.0	0.0	0.0
0.0	0.0	0.0	0.0	0.0	0.0	0.1	0.0	0.0	0.0	0.0	0.0	0.0	0.0	0.0	0.0
0.0	0.0	0.0	0.0	0.0	0.0	0.1	0.0	0.0	0.0	0.0	0.0	0.0	0.0	0.0	0.0
0.0	0.0	0.0	0.0	0.0	0.0	0.0	0.0	0.0	0.0	0.0	0.0	0.0	0.0	0.0	0.0
0.0	0.0	0.0	0.0	0.0	7.2	7.2	0.0	0.0	0.0	0.0	0.0	0.0	0.0	0.0	12.5
0.0	0.0	0.0	4.8	0.2	2.4	2.4	0.1	4.8	0.0	0.2	0.0	0.0	0.0	0.0	1.4
0.0	0.0	0.0	4.8	0.2	2.4	2.4	0.1	0.0	0.0	0.0	0.0	0.0	0.0	0.0	1.4
0.0	0.0	0.0	4.8	0.0	4.8	7.2	0.1	0.0	21.6	0.0	0.0	0.0	0.1	0.0	8.9
0.0	0.0	0.0	0.0	0.0	0.0	17.3	0.0	0.0	0.0	0.0	0.0	0.0	0.0	0.0	0.0
0.0	0.0	0.0	0.0	1.7	0.0	1164.0	0.0	0.0	0.0	0.0	0.0	0.0	0.0	0.0	0.0
0.0	0.0	0.0	0.6	0.0	0.3	0.9	0.0	0.0	0.0	0.0	0.0	0.0	0.0	0.0	0.0
0.0	0.0	0.0	3.7	0.0	0.0	14.6	0.4	0.0	0.0	0.0	0.0	0.0	0.0	0.0	0.0
0.0	0.0	0.0	26.9	0.0	0.0	1.9	0.0	0.0	0.0	0.0	0.0	0.0	0.0	0.0	0.0
0.0	5.9	0.0	60.7	0.0	0.0	504.3	0.0	0.0	0.0	0.0	0.0	0.0	0.0	0.0	0.0
0.5	5.8	0.4	17.2	1.2	6.0	368.2	0.2	0.4	0.0	1.0	0.1	0.1	1.2	0.0	20.7
1.0	6.9	2.4	105.5	1.2	14.3	544.4	0.3	14.8	0.2	0.0	0.2	0.2	1.7	0.0	3.4
0.9	9.8	1.8	141.0	1.7	10.8	348.0	0.3	13.8	0.1	0.8	0.2	0.2	1.8	0.0	36.6
4.1	0.0	0.0	2.0	0.1	3.1	0.3	0.1	0.3	0.0	0.1	0.0	0.0	0.1	0.0	0.2
0.4	0.1	0.0	1.4	0.1	5.5	0.1	0.1	0.0	0.0	0.0	0.0	0.0	0.0	0.0	0.8
1.6	1.5	0.0	4.2	1.4	57.8	0.4	0.4	0.0	0.0	0.4	0.2	0.0	2.5	0.3	4.7

Code	Food Name	Unit Amount	Kilocalories (kcal)	Protein (g)	Carbohydrate (g)
20077	Bran, wheat, crude	1 Tbsp.	7.6	0.5	2.3
18376	Bread crumbs, dry, grated, seasoned	1.0 oz	102.8	4.0	19.7
18079	Bread crumbs, plain, grated, dry	1/4 cup	106.7	3.4	19.6
18080	Bread sticks, plain	1 small stick (4.25″ long)	20.6	0.6	3.4
18085	Bread stuffing, corn, dry mix, prep	1/2 cup	179.0	2.9	21.9
18082	Bread stuffing, plain, dry mix, prep	1/2 cup	178.0	3.2	21.7
918083	Bread stuffing, plain, homemade	1/2 cup	168.0	3.8	22.2
918020	Bread, banana, homemade w/vegetable shortening	1/2 cup	392.1	5.0	63.9
18021	Bread, Boston brown, canned	1 slice	87.8	2.3	19.5
918023	Bread, corn, dry mix, prep	1 piece	188.4	4.3	28.9
918026	Bread, cracked wheat, toasted	1 thin slice	50.9	1.7	9.7
18027	Bread, egg	1 slice (5″ x 3″ x 0.5″)	114.8	3.8	19.1
18029	Bread, French/Vienna/sourdough	1 medium slice (4.75″ x 4″ x 0.5″)	68.5	2.2	13.0
18604	Bread, garlic, frozen/Campione	1 slice	181.2	4.3	22.2
18641	Bread, hamburger rolls/Wonder	1 roll	115.5	4.3	21.2
18033	Bread, Italian	1 medium slice	54.2	1.8	10.0
18035	Bread, mixed-grain/7-grain/whole-grain	1 large slice	80.0	3.2	14.8
18037	Bread, oatbran	1 slice	70.8	3.1	11.9
18049	Bread, oatbran, reduced kcal	1.0 oz	57.0	2.3	11.7
18039	Bread, oatmeal	1.0 oz	76.3	2.4	13.7
18041	Bread, pita, white, enriched	1 small pita (4″ diam)	77.0	2.5	15.6
18042	Bread, pita, whole-wheat	1 small pita (4″ diam)	74.5	2.7	15.4
18044	Bread, pumpernickel	1 thin slice	50.0	1.7	9.5
918046	Bread, pumpkin, homemade	1 slice (3.75″ x 3″ x 0.5″)	198.6	2.4	30.7
18047	Bread, raisin, enriched	1 slice	71.2	2.1	13.6
18059	Bread, rice bran	1 slice	65.6	2.4	11.7
18060	Bread, rye	1 slice	82.9	2.7	15.5
18064	Bread, wheat (includes wheat berry)	1 slice	65.0	2.3	11.8
18066	Bread, wheat bran	1 slice	89.3	3.2	17.2
18055	Bread, wheat, reduced kcal	1 slice	45.5	2.1	10.0
18069	Bread, white, commercially prep, crumbs/cubes/slices	1/4 cup of crumbs	32.0	1.0	5.9
18057	Bread, white, reduced kcal	1 slice	47.6	2.0	10.2
18075	Bread, whole-wheat, commercially prep	1 slice	71.3	2.8	13.4
18022	Bread/muffins, corn, dry mix, enriched	1/4 cup of crumbs	50.2	0.8	8.3
1001	Butter, regular (with salt)	1 pat (1″ sq, 1/3″ high)	35.9	0.0	0.0
1145	Butter, unsalted	1 Tbsp.	100.4	0.1	0.0
1002	Butter, whipped (with salt)	1 pat (1″ sq, 1/3″ high)	28.7	0.0	0.0
18086	Cake, angelfood, commercially prep	1 piece (1/12 of 12 oz-cake)	74.8	1.7	16.8
18088	Cake, angelfood, dry mix, prep	1 piece (1/12 of 10″ diam)	128.5	3.1	29.4
918823	Cake, apple streusel crumb	1 piece	240.2	2.0	33.0
918824	Cake, banana	1/12 cake	249.8	3.0	36.0
18090	Cake, Boston cream pie, commercially prep	1 piece (1/6 of pie)	231.8	2.2	39.5
918093	Cake, carrot, dry mix, prep, w/o icing	1 piece (1/12 of 9″ diam)	239.4	3.6	32.7
918828	Cake, chocolate fudge	1/6 cake	310.2	30.0	40.0
918858	Cake, chocolate Suzy Q's/Hostess	2 cakes	480.0	4.0	74.0
18099	Cake, chocolate, dry mix, regular	1 package (18.5 oz)	2242.7	30.9	382.5
918129	Cake, chocolate, dry mix, special dietary	1 package (8 oz)	874.0	7.5	176.2
18101	Cake, chocolate, homemade, w/o icing	1 piece (1/12 of 9″ diam)	340.1	5.0	50.7
918846	Cake, cinnamon streusel, frozen	1/8 cake	145.9	2.2	19.4
918851	Cake, devil square/LittleDeb	2 squares	295.1	1.9	32.9
918831	Cake, german chocolate, frozen	1/8 cake	198.0	2.5	22.1
918115	Cake, gingerbread, dry mix, prep	1.0 oz	86.5	1.1	14.2
918853	Cake, Ho Ho's/Hostess	2 cakes	240.2	2.0	34.0
918838	Cake, pineapple upside down mix	1/9 cake	250.2	2.0	39.0
18120	Cake, pound, commercially prep w/butter	1 piece (1/10 of cake)	116.4	1.7	14.6
918855	Cake, Snoballs/Hostess	2 cakes	300.1	2.0	56.0
18133	Cake, sponge, commercially prep	1 piece (1/12 of 16-oz cake)	109.8	2.1	23.2
918859	Cake, Twinkies/Hostess	2 cakes	319.9	2.0	52.0
918811	Cake, white w/chocolate icing, slice	1/16 cake	250.4	3.0	45.0
18137	Cake, white, dry mix, regular	1.0 oz	123.5	1.3	22.6
18140	Cake, yellow w/chocolate icing, commercially prep	1 piece (1/8 of 18-oz cake)	242.6	2.4	35.5
18141	Cake, yellow w/vanilla icing, commercially prep	1 piece (1/8 of 18-oz cake)	238.7	2.2	37.6
19159	Candy bar, 3 Musketeers/M&M Mars	1 bar (.8 oz)	95.7	0.7	17.7
19065	Candy bar, Almond Joy/Hershey	1.76 oz	233.5	2.1	29.2
19111	Candy bar, Baby Ruth/Nestle	2.1 oz	288.6	4.5	39.1

Dietary Fiber (g)	Total Fat (g)	Cholesterol (mg)	Calcium (mg)	Iron (mg)	Magnesium (mg)	Sodium (mg)	Zinc (mg)	Vitamin A (µgRE)	Vitamin C (mg)	Vitamin E (mgαT)	Thiamin (mg)	Riboflavin (mg)	Niacin (mg)	Vitamin B6 (mg)	Folate (µg)
1.5	0.1	0.0	2.6	0.4	21.4	0.1	0.3	0.0	0.0	0.1	0.0	0.0	0.5	0.0	2.8
1.2	0.7	0.3	27.7	0.9	10.6	742.0	0.3	0.8	0.1	0.0	0.0	0.0	0.8	0.0	30.5
0.6	1.5	0.0	61.3	1.7	12.4	232.7	0.3	0.0	0.0	0.2	0.2	0.1	1.8	0.0	29.4
0.2	0.5	0.0	1.1	0.2	1.6	32.9	0.0	0.0	0.0	0.1	0.0	0.0	0.3	0.0	6.1
2.9	8.8	0.0	26.0	0.9	13.0	455.0	0.2	85.0	0.8	1.4	0.1	0.1	1.2	0.0	97.0
2.9	8.6	0.0	32.0	1.1	12.0	543.0	0.3	81.0	0.0	1.4	0.1	0.1	1.5	0.0	101.0
0.0	7.2	3.2	64.0	1.6	15.0	461.0	0.3	69.0	1.7	0.0	0.2	0.1	1.6	0.1	17.0
0.0	13.7	5.8	20.9	1.6	16.2	229.7	0.4	27.8	2.0	0.0	0.2	0.2	1.7	0.2	12.8
2.1	0.7	0.5	31.5	0.9	28.4	284.0	0.2	5.0	0.0	0.3	0.0	0.1	0.5	0.0	5.0
1.4	6.0	3.1	43.8	1.1	12.0	466.8	0.4	26.4	0.1	0.0	0.1	0.2	1.2	0.1	6.6
1.1	0.8	0.4	8.5	0.5	10.3	105.3	0.2	0.0	0.0	0.1	0.1	0.0	0.6	0.1	5.4
0.9	2.4	20.4	37.2	1.2	7.6	196.8	0.3	9.2	0.0	0.2	0.2	0.2	1.9	0.0	42.0
0.8	0.8	0.0	18.8	0.6	6.8	152.3	0.2	0.0	0.0	0.1	0.1	0.1	1.2	0.0	23.8
2.4	8.4	0.0	0.0	0.5	0.0	275.0	0.0	0.0	0.0	0.0	0.0	0.0	0.0	0.0	0.0
0.0	1.5	0.0	74.8	1.0	0.0	256.3	0.0	0.0	0.0	0.0	0.0	0.0	0.0	0.0	0.0
0.5	0.7	0.0	15.6	0.6	5.4	116.8	0.2	0.0	0.0	0.1	0.1	0.1	0.9	0.0	19.0
2.0	1.2	0.0	29.1	1.1	17.0	155.8	0.4	0.0	0.1	0.2	0.1	0.1	1.4	0.1	25.6
1.4	1.3	0.0	19.5	0.9	10.5	122.1	0.3	0.0	0.0	0.2	0.2	0.1	1.4	0.0	24.3
3.4	0.9	0.0	16.2	0.9	15.6	99.5	0.3	0.0	0.0	0.1	0.1	0.1	1.1	0.0	18.7
1.1	1.2	0.0	18.7	0.8	10.5	169.8	0.3	0.6	0.0	0.2	0.1	0.1	0.9	0.0	17.6
0.6	0.3	0.0	24.1	0.7	7.3	150.1	0.2	0.0	0.0	0.0	0.2	0.1	1.3	0.0	26.6
2.1	0.7	0.0	4.2	0.9	19.3	149.0	0.4	0.0	0.0	0.3	0.1	0.0	0.8	0.1	14.0
1.3	0.6	0.0	13.6	0.6	10.8	134.2	0.3	0.0	0.0	0.1	0.1	0.1	0.6	0.0	16.0
0.0	7.7	1.9	10.8	1.0	7.8	187.8	0.2	334.2	0.6	0.0	0.1	0.1	0.8	0.0	6.6
1.1	1.1	0.0	17.2	0.8	6.8	101.4	0.2	0.0	0.0	0.1	0.1	0.1	0.9	0.0	22.6
1.3	1.2	0.0	18.6	1.0	21.6	118.8	0.4	0.0	0.0	0.2	0.2	0.1	1.8	0.1	17.6
1.9	1.1	0.0	23.4	0.9	12.8	211.2	0.4	0.3	0.1	0.1	0.1	0.1	1.2	0.0	27.5
1.1	1.0	0.0	26.3	0.8	11.5	132.5	0.3	0.0	0.0	0.1	0.1	0.1	1.0	0.0	19.3
1.4	1.2	0.0	26.6	1.1	29.2	175.0	0.5	0.0	0.0	0.2	0.1	0.1	1.6	0.1	24.8
2.8	0.5	0.0	18.4	0.7	9.0	117.5	0.3	0.0	0.0	0.0	0.1	0.1	0.9	0.0	16.3
0.3	0.4	0.1	13.0	0.4	2.9	64.6	0.1	0.0	0.0	0.1	0.0	0.0	0.5	0.0	11.4
2.2	0.6	0.0	21.6	0.7	5.3	104.2	0.3	0.2	0.1	0.0	0.1	0.1	0.8	0.0	21.9
2.0	1.2	0.0	20.9	1.0	24.9	152.8	0.6	0.0	0.0	0.2	0.1	0.1	1.1	0.1	14.5
0.8	1.5	0.2	6.8	0.3	2.9	133.3	0.1	1.4	0.0	0.2	0.1	0.0	0.4	0.0	12.6
0.0	4.1	10.9	1.2	0.0	0.1	41.3	0.0	37.7	0.0	0.1	0.0	0.0	0.0	0.0	0.2
0.0	11.4	30.6	3.3	0.0	0.3	1.5	0.0	105.6	0.0	0.2	0.0	0.0	0.0	0.0	0.4
0.0	3.2	8.8	0.9	0.0	0.1	33.1	0.0	30.2	0.0	0.1	0.0	0.0	0.0	0.0	0.1
0.4	0.2	0.0	40.6	0.2	3.5	217.2	0.0	0.0	0.0	0.0	0.0	0.1	0.3	0.0	10.2
0.1	0.2	0.0	42.0	0.1	4.0	254.5	0.1	0.0	0.0	0.0	0.0	0.1	0.1	0.0	15.0
0.3	11.0	45.0	11.0	0.8	0.0	190.0	0.0	13.0	15.0	0.0	0.1	0.1	0.9	0.0	0.0
0.3	11.0	0.0	0.0	0.0	0.0	290.0	0.0	0.0	0.0	0.0	0.0	0.0	0.0	0.0	0.0
1.3	7.8	34.0	21.2	0.3	5.5	132.5	0.1	21.2	0.2	1.0	0.4	0.2	0.2	0.0	13.8
1.4	11.0	3.4	77.0	0.9	4.9	249.2	0.2	172.9	1.7	0.0	0.1	0.1	0.8	0.1	8.4
0.0	15.0	35.0	0.0	0.0	0.0	300.0	0.0	0.0	0.0	0.0	0.0	0.0	0.0	0.0	0.0
0.5	20.0	32.0	42.0	1.6	0.0	600.0	0.0	0.0	0.0	0.0	0.0	0.1	1.0	0.0	5.0
12.6	81.7	0.0	786.0	23.6	246.3	4323.0	4.2	0.0	0.0	12.6	0.9	0.8	8.4	0.2	283.0
0.0	22.2	9.0	81.7	5.8	104.4	935.2	1.9	0.0	0.0	0.0	0.5	0.4	4.4	0.0	22.7
1.5	14.3	55.1	57.0	1.5	30.4	299.3	0.7	38.0	0.2	1.5	0.1	0.2	1.1	0.0	25.7
0.3	7.1	0.0	12.0	0.7	6.0	134.0	0.0	51.2	0.0	0.0	0.1	0.1	0.8	0.0	0.0
0.5	17.3	0.0	0.0	1.0	0.0	136.0	0.0	0.0	0.0	0.0	0.1	0.1	0.7	0.0	5.0
0.9	11.4	0.0	28.0	0.9	14.0	153.0	0.0	37.8	0.0	0.0	0.0	0.1	0.3	0.0	5.0
0.3	2.9	1.6	19.3	0.9	4.5	128.2	0.1	4.5	0.0	0.4	0.1	0.1	0.4	0.0	2.8
0.5	12.0	26.0	24.0	0.6	0.0	180.0	0.0	0.0	0.0	0.0	0.0	0.0	0.0	0.0	4.0
0.7	10.0	40.0	0.0	0.0	0.0	210.0	0.0	0.0	0.0	0.0	0.0	0.0	0.0	0.0	0.0
0.1	6.0	66.3	10.5	0.4	3.3	119.4	0.1	46.8	0.0	0.0	0.0	0.1	0.4	0.0	12.3
0.5	8.0	4.0	24.0	1.0	0.0	340.0	0.0	0.0	0.0	0.0	0.0	0.1	0.0	0.0	0.0
0.2	1.0	38.8	26.6	1.0	4.2	92.7	0.2	17.5	0.0	0.1	0.1	0.1	0.7	0.0	14.8
0.5	10.0	40.0	38.0	1.1	0.0	300.0	0.0	0.0	0.0	0.0	0.1	0.1	1.0	0.0	5.0
0.5	8.0	1.0	70.0	0.7	15.0	238.0	0.2	8.0	0.0	0.0	0.1	0.1	0.8	0.0	4.0
0.3	3.2	0.0	55.7	0.4	3.2	192.6	0.1	0.0	0.1	0.6	0.1	0.1	0.3	0.0	13.9
1.2	11.1	35.2	23.7	1.3	19.2	215.7	0.4	21.1	0.0	1.5	0.1	0.1	0.8	0.0	14.1
0.2	9.3	35.2	39.7	0.7	3.8	220.2	0.2	12.2	0.0	0.0	0.1	0.0	0.3	0.0	17.3
0.4	3.0	2.5	19.3	0.2	6.7	44.6	0.1	5.5	0.1	0.1	0.0	0.0	0.1	0.0	0.0
2.4	13.4	2.0	30.5	0.7	0.0	73.0	0.0	0.0	0.0	0.0	0.0	0.0	0.0	0.0	0.0
1.7	12.7	2.4	24.6	0.1	48.0	135.6	0.8	0.0	0.0	1.1	0.1	0.1	1.7	0.0	18.6

Code	Food Name	Unit Amount	Kilocalories (kcal)	Protein (g)	Carbohydrate (g)
19075	Candy bar, Caramello/Hershey	1.6 oz	213.3	2.7	28.5
919944	Candy bar, Chocolate Almond/Hershey	1.0 oz	157.1	3.2	13.9
19119	Candy bar, Chunky	1.0 oz	138.6	2.5	16.0
19130	Candy bar, Golden Almond Chocolate Bar/Hershey	3.2 oz	522.3	11.2	41.6
19109	Candy bar, Kit Kat Wafer/Hershey	1.62 oz	236.4	3.3	29.4
19115	Candy bar, Mars Almond/M&M Mars	1.76 oz (69 pieces)	224.2	3.9	30.1
19135	Candy bar, Mars Milky Way/M&M Mars	2.1 oz	253.8	2.7	43.0
19142	Candy bar, Mounds/Hershey	1.55 oz	209.9	1.7	25.9
19143	Candy bar, Mr. Goodbar/Hershey	1.75 oz	272.5	5.4	25.9
19136	Candy bar, Skor Toffee Candy/Hershey	1.4 oz	222.4	1.8	23.1
19155	Candy bar, Snickers/M&M Mars	2.16 oz	292.2	4.9	36.1
19164	Candy bar, Special Dark Sweet Chocolate/Hershey	1.45-oz bar	226.3	2.0	24.8
919967	Candy bar, Summit Bar	0.75-oz bar	100.1	1.0	11.0
19093	Candy bar, Symphony Milk Chocolate/Hershey	1.4 oz	221.2	2.9	23.2
919951	Candy bar, Tiger Milk Bar	2.0 oz	249.8	9.0	35.0
19160	Candy bar, Twix Caramel Cookie/M&M Mars	2.0 oz	284.4	2.6	37.4
919912	Candy, candy corn	1/4 cup	182.0	0.1	44.8
19074	Candy, caramel	1 piece (0.75" cube)	38.2	0.5	7.7
19071	Candy, carob	3.0 oz	469.8	7.1	49.0
919901	Candy, chocolate caramel turtle	0.6 oz	81.9	1.1	9.9
19080	Candy, chocolate chips, semisweet	1 cup, large chips	871.8	7.6	114.8
919921	Candy, chocolate chips/Bakers	1/4 cup	200.6	1.7	32.0
919956	Candy, chocolate w/cream center	1.0 oz	122.9	1.1	19.9
919946	Candy, chocolate, dietetic	1 bar	333.8	7.2	14.0
19014	Candy, fruit leather, roll	1 small roll	49.0	0.1	11.8
919970	Candy, fruit roll snack	1 large roll	73.1	0.2	17.7
19100	Candy, fudge, chocolate, homemade	1 piece	64.8	0.3	13.5
19103	Candy, fudge, vanilla, homemade	1 piece	59.0	0.2	13.2
19105	Candy, Goobers Chocolate Covered Peanuts/Nestle	10 pieces	51.3	1.4	4.9
19106	Candy, Gumdrops/Gummy Bears/Fish/Worm/Dinosaur	1 small gumdrop (0.5" diam)	11.6	0.0	3.0
19117	Candy, halvah, plain	1 bar (8 oz)	1064.6	28.4	137.3
19107	Candy, hard candy	1 lollipop (0.75" diam)	23.6	0.0	5.9
19108	Candy, jellybeans	10 small	40.4	0.0	10.2
19140	Candy, M&M's Peanut Chocolate	1 piece	10.3	0.2	1.2
19141	Candy, M&M's Plain Chocolate	1 piece	3.4	0.0	0.5
19148	Candy, peanut brittle, homemade	1.0 oz	126.8	2.1	19.4
19150	Candy, Peanut Butter Cups, Reese's/Hershey	1 miniature cup	37.9	0.7	3.8
19126	Candy, peanuts, milk chocolate–coated	10 pieces	207.6	5.2	19.8
919072	Candy, pudding pops, chocolate, frozen	1 pop	71.9	1.9	11.9
919073	Candy, pudding pops, vanilla, frozen	1 pop	74.7	1.9	12.6
19149	Candy, Raisinets/Nestle	10 pieces	41.2	0.5	7.1
19127	Candy, raisins, milk chocolate–coated	10 pieces	39.0	0.4	6.8
19152	Candy, Rolo Caramel, milk chocolate/Hershey	1.94 oz (8 pieces)	226.6	2.7	29.4
919923	Candy, semisweet chocolate chips/Nestle	1.0 oz	148.1	1.0	17.8
919947	Candy, semisweet chocolate/Baker	1.0 oz	135.0	2.0	16.3
919948	Candy, semisweet chocolate/Hershey	1.0 oz	147.0	1.2	17.5
19370	Candy, Skittles, Original Bite Size Candy/M&M Mars	2.3 oz (59 pieces)	263.3	0.1	58.9
919958	Candy, Sno Caps	1.0 oz	131.9	1.5	20.6
19156	Candy, Starburst Fruit Chews/M&M Mars	2.07 oz	233.6	0.2	49.9
919966	Candy, taffy	0.5 oz piece	56.0	0.0	13.7
19112	Candy, Twizzlers Strawberry/Hershey	1 package (2.5 oz)	237.1	2.4	55.0
19091	Candy, York Peppermint Patty	0.39 oz, 1 sm patty	43.2	0.2	8.8
8053	Cereal, 100% bran (wheat bran & barley)	1 cup	177.5	8.3	48.1
908912	Cereal, 100% Natural/Quaker	1/4 cup	127.1	3.3	18.0
8153	Cereal, 40% Bran Flakes/Ralston Purina	1.0 oz, @ 3/4 cup	94.0	3.3	23.1
8001	Cereal, All-Bran/Kellogg	1/2 cup	79.2	3.7	22.8
8006	Cereal, Bran Chex (wheat & corn)	1 cup	156.3	5.0	39.1
8010	Cereal, Cap'n Crunch/Quaker	3/4 cup	107.2	1.4	23.0
8013	Cereal, Cheerios/Gen Mills	1 cup	109.5	3.1	22.9
8014	Cereal, Cocoa Krispies/Kellogg	3/4 cup	120.3	1.6	27.2
8017	Cereal, Cookie Crisp, Chocolate Chip & Vanilla	1 cup	120.0	1.5	26.3
8019	Cereal, Corn Chex	1 single serving box (.75 oz)	83.5	1.5	18.7
8022	Cereal, corn flakes, low sodium	1.0 oz	113.1	2.2	25.2
8020	Cereal, Corn Flakes/Kellogg	1 cup	102.2	1.8	24.2
8023	Cereal, Cracklin' Oat Bran/Kellogg	3/4 cup	225.0	4.6	40.1

Dietary Fiber (g)	Total Fat (g)	Cholesterol (mg)	Calcium (mg)	Iron (mg)	Magnesium (mg)	Sodium (mg)	Zinc (mg)	Vitamin A (μgRE)	Vitamin C (mg)	Vitamin E (mgαT)	Thiamin (mg)	Riboflavin (mg)	Niacin (mg)	Vitamin B6 (mg)	Folate (μg)
0.7	9.8	12.2	82.8	0.3	0.0	61.7	0.0	0.0	0.0	0.0	0.0	0.0	0.0	0.0	0.0
0.4	9.8	7.5	73.8	0.5	25.3	34.8	0.5	5.1	0.0	0.0	0.0	0.1	0.1	0.0	0.0
1.3	8.2	3.1	40.0	0.4	20.4	14.8	0.5	3.1	0.1	0.0	0.0	0.1	0.5	0.0	6.2
4.4	34.7	13.7	203.8	1.6	0.0	61.0	0.0	0.0	0.0	0.0	0.0	0.0	0.0	0.0	0.0
0.9	11.7	2.8	75.9	0.4	17.9	34.5	0.6	22.1	0.3	0.4	0.1	0.2	1.2	0.1	65.3
1.0	11.0	8.2	80.6	0.5	34.6	81.6	0.5	24.0	0.3	2.2	0.0	0.1	0.5	0.0	9.1
1.0	9.7	8.4	78.0	0.5	20.4	144.0	0.4	19.2	0.6	0.4	0.0	0.1	0.2	0.0	6.0
2.6	11.0	0.9	6.6	0.9	24.6	65.6	0.4	0.4	0.2	0.3	0.0	0.0	0.1	0.0	1.3
1.8	17.5	4.0	54.0	0.7	43.0	74.5	0.9	18.5	0.2	1.4	0.1	0.1	1.7	0.0	19.5
0.6	13.6	20.4	52.0	0.2	0.0	110.4	0.0	0.0	0.0	0.0	0.0	0.0	0.0	0.0	0.0
1.5	15.0	7.9	57.3	0.5	43.9	162.3	1.4	23.8	0.4	0.9	0.1	0.1	2.6	0.1	24.4
2.1	13.3	0.4	11.1	1.0	45.5	2.9	0.6	1.6	0.0	0.2	0.0	0.0	0.2	0.0	0.8
0.4	6.0	0.0	0.0	0.0	0.0	0.0	0.0	0.0	0.0	0.0	0.0	0.0	0.0	0.0	0.0
0.8	13.1	8.8	86.0	0.5	0.0	36.8	0.0	0.0	0.0	0.0	0.0	0.0	0.0	0.0	0.0
29.1	8.0	0.0	0.0	6.3	0.0	0.0	0.0	0.0	0.0	0.0	0.5	0.7	0.6	0.0	0.0
0.6	13.9	2.9	51.3	0.5	18.2	110.0	0.4	14.3	0.2	0.7	0.1	0.1	0.7	0.0	13.7
0.0	1.0	0.0	7.0	0.6	0.0	106.0	0.0	0.0	0.0	0.0	0.0	0.0	0.0	0.0	0.5
0.1	0.8	0.7	13.8	0.0	1.7	24.5	0.0	0.8	0.1	0.0	0.0	0.0	0.0	0.0	0.5
3.3	27.3	2.6	263.6	1.1	31.3	93.1	3.1	7.0	0.4	1.4	0.1	0.2	0.9	0.1	24.4
0.0	4.7	4.0	27.0	0.2	0.0	16.0	0.0	6.0	0.0	0.0	0.0	0.0	0.1	0.0	0.0
10.7	54.6	0.0	58.2	5.7	209.3	20.0	2.9	3.6	0.0	2.2	0.1	0.2	0.8	0.1	5.5
0.7	9.0	0.0	66.5	0.9	35.8	26.6	0.5	0.8	0.0	0.0	0.0	0.1	0.1	0.0	2.0
0.4	4.8	0.0	36.0	0.2	0.0	52.0	0.0	0.0	0.0	0.0	0.0	0.0	0.0	0.0	0.0
0.0	27.8	0.0	0.0	0.0	0.0	0.0	0.0	0.0	0.0	0.0	0.0	0.0	0.0	0.0	0.0
0.5	0.4	0.0	4.5	0.1	2.8	8.5	0.0	1.7	0.9	0.0	0.0	0.0	0.0	0.0	1.1
0.5	0.6	0.0	7.0	0.2	4.0	13.0	0.0	2.0	1.0	0.0	0.0	0.0	0.0	0.1	0.0
0.1	1.4	2.4	7.1	0.1	4.3	10.5	0.1	7.8	0.0	0.0	0.0	0.0	0.0	0.0	0.3
0.0	0.9	2.6	6.2	0.0	0.8	10.7	0.0	8.0	0.0	0.0	0.0	0.0	0.0	0.0	0.2
0.6	3.4	0.9	12.7	0.1	11.9	4.1	0.2	0.0	0.0	0.0	0.0	0.0	0.5	0.0	0.8
0.0	0.0	0.0	0.1	0.0	0.0	1.3	0.0	0.0	0.0	0.0	0.0	0.0	0.0	0.0	0.0
10.2	48.9	0.0	74.9	10.3	494.9	442.7	9.8	0.0	0.2	6.4	1.0	0.2	6.5	0.8	147.6
0.0	0.0	0.0	0.2	0.2	0.2	2.3	0.0	0.0	0.0	0.0	0.0	0.0	0.0	0.0	0.0
0.0	0.1	0.0	0.3	0.1	0.2	2.8	0.0	0.0	0.0	0.0	0.0	0.0	0.0	0.0	0.0
0.1	0.5	0.2	2.0	0.0	1.5	1.0	0.0	0.5	0.0	0.0	0.0	0.0	0.1	0.0	0.7
0.0	0.1	0.1	0.7	0.0	0.3	0.4	0.0	0.4	0.0	0.0	0.0	0.0	0.0	0.0	0.0
0.6	5.3	3.6	8.4	0.4	14.0	126.6	0.3	13.2	0.0	0.5	0.1	0.0	1.0	0.0	19.6
0.2	2.2	0.4	5.5	0.1	6.2	22.2	0.1	1.3	0.0	0.3	0.0	0.0	0.3	0.0	3.9
1.9	13.4	3.6	41.6	0.5	37.6	16.4	0.8	0.0	0.0	1.0	0.0	0.1	1.7	0.1	3.2
0.2	2.2	0.9	66.3	0.2	9.9	77.6	0.2	15.5	0.2	0.0	0.0	0.1	0.1	0.0	1.4
0.0	2.1	0.9	60.6	0.0	5.2	49.8	0.2	24.4	0.1	0.0	0.0	0.1	0.0	0.0	2.4
0.5	1.6	0.4	10.8	0.1	4.5	3.6	0.1	0.9	0.0	0.0	0.0	0.0	0.0	0.0	0.5
0.4	1.5	0.3	8.6	0.2	4.5	3.6	0.1	0.7	0.0	0.1	0.0	0.0	0.0	0.0	0.5
0.4	11.0	9.9	84.2	0.3	21.5	96.8	0.5	20.4	0.2	0.5	0.0	0.1	0.1	0.0	2.8
1.0	7.9	0.0	10.0	1.0	0.0	4.0	0.4	0.1	0.0	0.0	0.0	0.0	0.2	0.0	3.6
0.5	9.0	0.0	11.0	1.0	41.0	1.0	1.0	1.6	0.0	0.0	0.0	0.0	0.2	0.0	1.0
0.5	9.2	0.0	9.0	0.9	0.0	5.0	0.0	2.0	0.0	0.0	0.0	0.1	0.1	0.0	1.0
0.0	2.8	0.0	0.0	0.0	0.7	10.4	0.0	0.0	43.5	0.2	0.0	0.0	0.0	0.0	0.0
0.2	5.6	0.0	38.0	0.4	0.0	20.0	0.5	6.0	0.0	0.0	0.0	0.1	0.1	0.0	0.0
0.0	4.9	0.0	2.4	0.1	0.6	33.0	0.0	0.0	31.2	0.9	0.0	0.0	0.0	0.0	0.0
0.0	0.4	1.0	0.0	0.0	0.0	13.0	0.0	5.0	0.0	0.0	0.0	0.0	0.0	0.0	0.0
1.0	1.1	0.0	5.0	0.2	0.0	175.4	0.0	0.0	0.0	0.0	0.0	0.0	0.0	0.0	0.0
0.2	0.8	0.1	1.7	0.1	0.0	2.6	0.0	0.0	0.0	0.0	0.0	0.0	0.0	0.0	0.0
19.5	3.3	0.0	46.2	8.1	312.2	457.4	5.7	0.0	62.7	1.5	1.6	1.8	20.9	2.1	46.9
2.0	5.5	0.0	43.0	0.8	31.0	14.0	0.6	0.0	0.0	0.0	0.1	0.1	0.4	0.1	12.0
4.1	0.4	0.0	13.3	4.6	69.6	270.0	1.2	384.0	15.4	0.0	0.4	0.4	5.1	0.5	102.4
9.7	0.9	0.0	105.9	4.5	128.7	60.9	3.8	225.3	15.0	0.6	0.4	0.4	5.0	0.5	90.0
7.9	1.4	0.0	29.4	14.0	69.1	345.5	6.5	10.8	26.0	0.6	0.6	0.3	8.6	0.9	173.0
0.9	1.4	0.0	5.4	4.5	9.5	208.4	3.8	3.5	0.0	0.1	0.4	0.4	5.0	0.5	100.2
2.6	1.8	0.0	55.2	8.1	32.7	284.1	3.8	375.3	15.0	0.2	0.4	0.4	5.0	0.5	99.9
0.4	0.8	0.0	4.0	1.8	11.5	210.2	1.5	225.1	15.0	0.1	0.4	0.4	5.0	0.5	93.0
0.4	1.1	0.0	5.7	4.8	8.4	206.7	3.2	0.0	0.0	0.1	0.4	0.3	5.3	0.5	105.9
0.4	0.1	0.0	2.3	6.1	3.0	232.8	0.1	10.7	11.3	0.1	0.3	0.1	3.7	0.4	75.2
0.3	0.1	0.0	12.2	0.6	3.7	2.8	0.1	10.8	0.0	0.0	0.0	0.1	0.1	0.0	2.0
0.8	0.2	0.0	1.1	8.7	3.4	297.9	0.2	210.3	14.0	0.0	0.4	0.4	4.7	0.5	98.8
6.5	7.0	0.0	24.8	2.0	76.5	195.3	1.7	253.0	16.8	0.4	0.4	0.5	5.6	0.6	152.9

Code	Food Name	Unit Amount	Kilocalories (kcal)	Protein (g)	Carbohydrate (g)
8101	Cereal, cream of rice, prep w/o salt	1 Tbsp.	7.9	0.1	1.7
8109	Cereal, cream of wheat, plain, mix 'n eat, prep	1 packet, prep	102.2	2.7	21.4
8103	Cereal, cream of wheat, regular, prep w/o salt	1 cup	133.0	3.8	27.6
8259	Cereal, Crispix/Kellogg	1 cup	108.5	2.1	25.0
8018	Cereal, Crunchy Bran/Quaker	3/4 cup	89.9	1.9	22.7
8244	Cereal, Fiber One/Gen Mills	1 cup	123.0	5.6	48.0
8030	Cereal, Froot Loops/Kellogg	1 cup	117.3	1.5	26.5
8319	Cereal, Frosted Mini-Wheats, bite size/Kellogg	1 cup, bite size	187.0	5.2	44.8
8035	Cereal, Golden Grahams/Gen Mills	3/4 cup	115.5	1.6	25.7
8037	Cereal, granola (oats & wheat germ) homemade	1.0 oz	135.4	4.3	15.4
908038	Cereal, Grape-Nuts	1½-oz box	135.7	4.4	31.2
8040	Cereal, Heartland natural, plain (oats & wheat germ)	1 cup	499.1	11.6	78.5
8211	Cereal, Honey Graham Ohs/Quaker	3/4 cup	111.8	1.4	22.7
908046	Cereal, Honeycomb	1.0 oz	109.5	1.6	24.9
8242	Cereal, Just Right w/crunchy nuggets/Kellogg	1 cup	404.4	8.4	91.2
8048	Cereal, Kix/Gen Mills	1 cup	400.1	6.8	90.7
8049	Cereal, Life, Plain/Quaker	1 cup	416.9	10.8	86.6
8050	Cereal, Lucky Charms/Gen Mills	1 cup	445.1	8.3	96.5
8117	Cereal, malt-o-meal, plain & chocolate, prep w/o salt	1 cup	15.3	0.5	3.2
8277	Cereal, Nature Valley Low Fat Fruit Granola/Gen Mills	1 cup	84.9	1.8	17.5
8043	Cereal, Nut & Honey Crunch/Kellogg	3/4 cup	109.4	2.0	22.6
8291	Cereal, Nutri-Grain Almond and Raisin/Kellogg	1-1/3 cup	110.1	2.4	23.3
8292	Cereal, Nutri-Grain Wheat/Kellogg	3/4 cup	107.2	3.2	25.6
8202	Cereal, Oatmeal Crisp w/almonds/Gen Mills	1 cup	218.9	5.8	42.0
8190	Cereal, Oatmeal Crisp w/apples/Gen Mills	1 cup	205.2	4.3	46.2
8227	Cereal, oatmeal, instant w/fruit & cream, prep/Quaker	3.5 oz @ 1 cup	118.0	2.5	23.1
8304	Cereal, oatmeal, Quick 'N Hearty Regular Flavor, microwave/Quaker	1 packet	105.9	3.8	19.1
8127	Cereal, oats, instant w/bran & raisins, fortified, prep	1 packet prep	158.0	4.9	30.4
8123	Cereal, oats, instant, plain, fortified, prep	1 cup, cooked	138.1	5.9	23.9
8180	Cereal, oats, regular/quick/instant, ckd w/salt	1 packet, prep	98.0	4.1	17.1
8058	Cereal, Product 19/Kellogg	3/4 cup	640.5	15.6	145.6
8066	Cereal, Puffed Rice/Quaker	1 cup	114.9	2.1	26.3
908911	Cereal, Puffed Wheat/Quaker	1 cup	50.0	2.4	10.5
908061	Cereal, Raisin Bran, Post	1 single-serving box (1.25 oz)	107.5	3.3	26.5
8261	Cereal, Raisin Nut Bran/Gen Mills	1 cup	209.0	5.2	41.5
8287	Cereal, Raisin Squares Mini-Wheats/Kellogg	3/4 cup	187.0	4.4	42.9
8185	Cereal, Ralston, ckd w/salt	1 cup	134.1	5.6	28.3
8064	Cereal, Rice Chex	1 cup	130.4	1.7	29.4
8065	Cereal, Rice Krispies/Kellogg	5/8-oz box	67.9	1.1	15.6
8156	Cereal, rice, puffed, fortified	0.5 oz	57.1	0.9	12.8
8067	Cereal, Special K/Kellogg	0.63-oz box	66.6	3.7	13.0
8070	Cereal, Sugar Frosted Flakes/Ralston Purina	1 cup	148.6	2.0	34.2
8074	Cereal, Tasteeos	10 pieces	3.9	0.1	0.8
908075	Cereal, Team	1 cup	164.2	2.7	36.0
8077	Cereal, Total/Gen Mills	3/4 cup	105.3	3.0	23.9
8082	Cereal, Wheat Chex	1 cup	168.8	4.6	37.8
8157	Cereal, wheat, puffed, fortified	1 cup	43.7	1.8	9.6
8148	Cereal, wheat, shredded, small biscuit	1 single-serving box (.875 oz)	88.5	2.7	19.9
8089	Cereal, Wheaties/Gen Mills	1 cup	110.1	3.2	23.8
924035	Cheese blintzes	8.0 oz	431.3	19.2	31.2
1163	Cheese fondue	1.0 oz	64.1	4.0	1.1
1150	Cheese spread, pasteurized process, American w/disodium phosphate	1.0 oz	81.3	4.6	2.4
1161	Cheese substitute, mozzarella	1.0 oz	69.4	3.2	6.6
1004	Cheese, blue	1.0 oz	98.9	6.0	0.7
1005	Cheese, brick	1.0 oz	103.9	6.5	0.8
1006	Cheese, Brie	1.0 oz	93.4	5.8	0.1
1007	Cheese, camembert	1.0 oz	83.9	5.5	0.1
1008	Cheese, caraway	1.0 oz	105.3	7.1	0.9
1009	Cheese, cheddar	1.0 oz	112.7	7.0	0.4
1169	Cheese, cheddar or colby, low-sodium	1.0 oz	111.4	6.8	0.5
1168	Cheese, cheddar or colby, low fat	1.0 oz	48.4	6.8	0.5
1011	Cheese, colby	1.0 oz	110.2	6.7	0.7
1012	Cheese, cottage, creamed, large or small curd	1.0 oz or 1 Tbsp.	28.9	3.5	0.8
1013	Cheese, cottage, creamed, w/fruit	1.0 oz or 1 Tbsp.	34.6	2.8	3.7
1016	Cheese, cottage, low-fat, 1% fat	1.0 oz or 1 Tbsp.	20.3	3.5	0.8

Dietary Fiber (g)	Total Fat (g)	Cholesterol (mg)	Calcium (mg)	Iron (mg)	Magnesium (mg)	Sodium (mg)	Zinc (mg)	Vitamin A (μgRE)	Vitamin C (mg)	Vitamin E (mgαT)	Thiamin (mg)	Riboflavin (mg)	Niacin (mg)	Vitamin B_6 (mg)	Folate (μg)
0.0	0.0	0.0	0.5	0.0	0.5	0.2	0.0	0.0	0.0	0.0	0.0	0.0	0.1	0.0	0.5
0.4	0.3	0.0	19.9	8.1	7.1	241.4	0.2	376.3	0.0	0.0	0.4	0.3	5.0	0.6	100.8
1.8	0.5	0.0	50.2	10.3	10.0	2.5	0.3	0.0	0.0	0.0	0.3	0.0	1.5	0.5	45.2
0.6	0.3	0.0	3.5	1.8	7.0	240.1	1.5	225.3	15.0	0.1	0.4	0.4	5.0	0.5	87.0
4.8	0.9	0.0	20.5	7.6	14.3	253.3	3.8	3.8	0.0	0.1	0.1	0.4	5.0	0.5	100.2
28.5	1.7	0.0	117.0	9.0	136.2	285.0	2.5	0.0	18.0	0.7	0.8	0.9	10.0	1.0	199.8
0.6	0.9	0.0	3.3	4.2	8.7	140.7	3.8	211.2	14.1	0.1	0.4	0.4	5.0	0.5	90.0
5.9	0.9	0.0	0.0	15.4	55.6	1.7	1.4	0.0	0.0	0.0	0.3	0.4	4.7	0.4	110.0
0.9	1.1	0.0	14.4	4.5	9.3	274.5	3.8	225.3	15.0	0.2	0.4	0.4	5.0	0.5	99.9
3.0	7.1	0.0	23.5	1.2	51.6	7.0	1.2	1.2	0.4	3.7	0.2	0.1	0.6	0.1	24.9
3.8	0.2	0.0	3.6	10.9	25.5	264.1	0.8	503.1	0.0	0.1	0.5	0.6	6.7	0.7	134.1
7.0	17.7	0.0	74.8	4.3	147.2	293.3	3.0	6.9	1.2	0.8	0.4	0.2	1.6	0.2	64.4
0.7	1.9	0.0	12.4	4.5	12.7	177.9	3.8	301.3	12.0	0.1	0.4	0.4	5.0	0.5	100.4
0.8	0.5	0.1	4.8	2.7	9.5	157.6	1.5	370.7	0.0	0.1	0.4	0.4	4.9	0.5	98.8
5.6	2.9	0.0	28.3	32.2	67.6	669.3	1.7	744.5	0.0	4.4	0.8	0.9	9.9	1.0	202.7
2.8	2.2	0.0	152.3	28.4	32.6	920.9	13.1	1313.6	52.5	0.3	1.3	1.5	17.5	1.8	349.7
7.0	4.4	0.0	335.5	30.8	106.7	599.5	13.8	4.4	0.0	0.6	1.4	1.6	18.3	1.8	367.4
4.6	4.2	0.0	124.2	17.3	74.8	778.6	14.4	863.7	57.5	0.5	1.4	1.6	19.2	1.9	383.0
0.1	0.0	0.0	0.6	1.2	0.6	0.3	0.0	0.0	0.0	0.0	0.1	0.0	0.7	0.0	0.6
1.4	1.2	0.0	15.8	0.6	7.5	82.1	0.3	0.0	0.0	0.3	0.0	0.0	0.4	0.0	2.9
0.4	1.2	0.0	2.7	2.2	2.4	181.7	0.2	110.7	7.4	0.1	0.2	0.2	2.5	0.2	54.0
2.4	1.7	0.0	91.5	0.8	6.9	106.5	2.0	0.0	0.0	3.0	0.2	0.2	2.7	0.3	60.0
4.0	1.1	0.0	10.2	1.1	25.9	235.5	4.0	0.0	16.0	5.8	0.4	0.4	5.3	0.5	96.0
4.3	4.6	0.0	35.8	4.5	57.2	250.3	3.8	0.0	9.0	3.1	0.4	0.4	5.0	0.5	99.6
4.5	1.8	0.0	23.1	4.5	45.1	281.6	3.8	0.0	9.0	0.4	0.4	0.4	5.0	0.5	99.6
1.9	2.2	0.0	94.0	3.5	25.0	150.0	0.6	277.0	0.1	0.1	0.3	0.3	3.7	0.4	74.0
2.4	2.1	0.0	107.9	8.5	38.6	152.5	0.9	315.2	0.0	0.0	0.3	0.4	4.2	0.4	84.1
5.5	2.0	0.0	173.6	7.6	56.6	247.7	1.3	479.7	0.0	0.0	0.6	0.6	8.1	0.8	156.0
4.0	2.3	0.0	215.3	8.3	56.2	376.7	1.1	599.0	0.0	0.3	0.7	0.4	7.2	1.0	198.9
2.7	1.6	0.0	12.6	1.1	37.9	252.8	0.8	3.2	0.0	0.0	0.2	0.0	0.2	0.0	6.3
5.8	2.3	0.0	15.8	105.0	71.8	1260.0	87.5	1314.3	350.0	129.5	8.8	10.0	116.7	11.7	2275.0
0.4	0.3	0.0	2.7	0.9	9.0	1.5	0.3	0.0	0.0	0.0	0.1	0.0	1.9	0.0	3.0
1.0	0.2	0.0	3.0	0.6	19.0	1.0	0.4	0.0	0.0	0.0	0.1	0.0	1.6	0.0	4.0
4.9	0.7	0.1	16.5	5.6	59.5	228.2	1.9	463.4	0.0	0.8	0.5	0.5	6.2	0.6	123.6
5.1	4.4	0.0	73.7	4.5	53.9	245.9	1.1	0.0	0.0	2.0	0.4	0.4	5.0	0.5	99.6
5.2	1.5	0.0	18.7	16.8	47.9	3.3	1.5	0.0	0.0	0.3	0.4	0.4	5.2	0.5	110.0
6.1	0.8	0.0	12.7	1.6	58.2	475.6	1.4	0.0	0.0	0.0	0.2	0.2	2.0	0.1	17.7
0.6	0.1	0.0	4.6	9.4	8.3	275.9	0.5	2.0	17.5	0.0	0.4	0.0	5.8	0.6	116.5
0.2	0.2	0.0	1.8	1.1	8.6	193.0	0.3	135.2	9.0	0.0	0.2	0.3	3.0	0.3	63.5
0.2	0.1	0.0	0.9	4.5	3.6	0.4	0.1	0.0	0.0	0.0	0.4	0.3	5.0	0.0	2.7
0.6	0.2	0.0	2.7	5.1	10.3	145.1	2.2	130.7	8.7	0.0	0.3	0.3	4.1	0.4	54.0
0.8	0.5	0.0	4.2	1.0	2.7	246.6	0.8	503.1	20.1	0.1	0.5	0.6	6.7	0.7	2.7
0.1	0.0	0.0	0.5	0.3	1.1	7.6	0.0	13.2	0.5	0.0	0.0	0.0	0.2	0.0	3.5
0.5	0.8	0.2	6.3	12.0	11.8	259.6	0.6	556.1	22.3	0.1	0.5	0.6	7.4	0.8	6.7
2.6	0.7	0.0	258.3	18.0	32.1	198.6	15.0	375.3	60.0	23.5	1.5	1.7	20.1	2.0	399.9
4.1	1.2	0.0	17.9	13.1	58.4	308.2	1.2	0.0	24.4	0.2	0.6	0.2	8.1	0.8	162.4
0.5	0.1	0.0	3.4	3.8	17.4	0.5	0.3	0.0	0.0	0.0	0.3	0.2	4.2	0.0	3.8
2.4	0.4	0.0	9.4	1.0	32.7	2.5	0.8	0.0	0.0	0.1	0.1	0.1	1.3	0.1	12.4
2.1	0.9	0.0	54.6	8.1	31.8	222.3	0.7	225.3	15.0	0.4	0.4	0.4	5.0	0.5	99.9
0.0	25.6	436.0	336.0	4.8	0.0	246.0	0.0	313.6	0.0	0.0	0.0	0.3	2.0	3.9	0.0
0.0	3.8	12.6	133.3	0.1	6.4	37.0	0.5	31.9	0.0	0.0	0.0	0.1	0.1	0.0	2.2
0.0	5.9	15.5	157.3	0.1	8.0	455.0	0.7	52.9	0.0	0.0	0.0	0.1	0.0	0.0	2.0
0.0	3.4	0.0	170.8	0.1	11.5	191.8	0.5	122.4	0.0	0.6	0.0	0.1	0.1	0.0	3.1
0.0	8.0	21.1	147.7	0.1	6.4	390.7	0.7	63.8	0.0	0.2	0.0	0.1	0.3	0.0	10.2
0.0	8.3	26.4	188.6	0.1	6.8	156.7	0.7	84.6	0.0	0.1	0.0	0.1	0.0	0.0	5.7
0.0	7.8	28.0	51.5	0.1	5.6	176.2	0.7	51.0	0.0	0.2	0.0	0.1	0.1	0.1	18.2
0.0	6.8	20.2	108.5	0.1	5.6	235.7	0.7	70.6	0.0	0.2	0.0	0.1	0.2	0.1	17.4
0.0	8.2	26.0	188.5	0.2	6.2	193.2	0.8	80.9	0.0	0.0	0.0	0.1	0.1	0.0	5.1
0.0	9.3	29.4	202.0	0.2	7.8	173.7	0.9	77.8	0.0	0.1	0.0	0.1	0.0	0.0	5.1
0.0	9.1	28.0	196.8	0.2	7.6	5.9	0.9	80.6	0.0	0.1	0.0	0.1	0.0	0.0	5.0
0.0	2.0	5.9	116.2	0.1	4.5	171.4	0.5	17.9	0.0	0.0	0.0	0.1	0.0	0.0	3.1
0.0	9.0	26.6	191.7	0.2	7.2	169.2	0.9	77.0	0.0	0.1	0.0	0.1	0.0	0.0	5.1
0.0	1.3	4.2	16.8	0.0	1.5	113.3	0.1	13.4	0.0	0.0	0.0	0.0	0.0	0.0	3.4
0.0	1.0	3.1	13.3	0.0	1.2	113.3	0.1	10.1	0.0	0.0	0.0	0.0	0.0	0.0	2.7
0.0	0.3	1.2	17.1	0.0	1.5	113.7	0.1	3.1	0.0	0.0	0.0	0.0	0.0	0.0	3.5

Code	Food Name	Unit Amount	Kilocalories (kcal)	Protein (g)	Carbohydrate (g)
1015	Cheese, cottage, low-fat, 2% fat	1.0 oz or 1 Tbsp.	25.1	3.8	1.0
1014	Cheese, cottage, nonfat, uncreamed, dry, large or small curd	1.0 oz or 1 Tbsp.	23.7	4.8	0.5
1017	Cheese, cream	1.0 oz or 1 Tbsp.	97.7	2.1	0.7
1186	Cheese, cream, fat free	1.0 oz or 1 Tbsp.	26.9	4.0	1.6
1018	Cheese, edam	1.0 oz	99.8	7.0	0.4
1019	Cheese, feta	1.0 oz	73.8	4.0	1.1
1020	Cheese, fontina	1.0 oz	108.9	7.2	0.4
1022	Cheese, gouda	1.0 oz	99.8	7.0	0.6
1023	Cheese, gruyere	1.0 oz	115.6	8.3	0.1
1165	Cheese, Mexican, Queso Anejo	1.0 oz	104.4	6.0	1.3
1025	Cheese, monterey	1.0 oz	104.5	6.9	0.2
1028	Cheese, mozzarella, part skim milk	1.0 oz	71.2	6.8	0.8
1026	Cheese, mozzarella, whole milk	1.0 oz	78.8	5.4	0.6
1030	Cheese, muenster	1.0 oz	103.1	6.6	0.3
1031	Cheese, neufchatel	1.0 oz or 1 Tbsp.	72.8	2.8	0.8
1032	Cheese, parmesan, grated	1.0 oz	127.6	11.6	1.0
1033	Cheese, parmesan, hard	1.0 oz	109.8	10.0	0.9
1146	Cheese, parmesan, shredded	1.0 oz	116.2	10.6	1.0
1042	Cheese, pasteurized process, American with disodium phosphate	1 cup, shredded	424.3	25.0	1.8
1043	Cheese, pasteurized process, pimiento	1 cup, shredded	424.2	25.0	2.0
1044	Cheese, pasteurized process, Swiss with disodium phosphate	1 cup, shredded	376.9	27.9	2.4
901903	Cheese, process, Cheez Whiz	1.0 oz	77.0	4.6	1.8
901901	Cheese, process, Velveeta	1.0 oz	84.0	5.2	2.2
1035	Cheese, provolone	1 cup, diced	464.0	33.8	2.8
1037	Cheese, ricotta, part skim milk	1.0 oz or 1 Tbsp.	21.3	1.8	0.8
1036	Cheese, ricotta, whole milk	1.0 oz or 1 Tbsp.	26.8	1.7	0.5
1038	Cheese, romano	1.0 oz	108.3	8.9	1.0
1039	Cheese, roquefort	1.0 oz	103.3	6.0	0.6
1040	Cheese, Swiss	1.0 oz	405.8	30.7	3.7
22703	Chicken & dumplings, canned/Sweet Sue	1 package	619.7	42.9	64.7
924003	Chicken a la king frz (Le Menu 10. 5-oz meal)	1 package	574.1	32.9	14.6
924006	Chicken chow mein	10.0 oz	289.7	35.2	11.4
924005	Chicken chow mein, canned	3/4 cup	76.0	5.6	14.4
924248	Chicken chow mein/Chun King	3/4 cup	200.0	13.6	28.7
924068	Chicken egg roll/LaChoy	3 medium	89.9	3.0	12.0
924043	Chicken Kiev, frozen	1 breast w/filling	604.8	22.3	41.4
924051	Chicken parmigiana	11.5 oz	548.2	38.4	39.3
22527	Chicken pie, frozen/Stouffers	1 slice	468.6	19.0	29.9
924007	Chicken pot pie	7.0 oz	465.3	19.6	35.8
924171	Chicken teriyaki/LaChoy	3/4 cup	85.2	8.0	8.0
924242	Chicken w/vegetables & pasta	9.5 oz	121.1	10.8	13.7
924004	Chicken & Noodles	1 cup	364.8	22.0	26.0
924047	Chicken & Rice	7.0-oz pkg	364.0	22.0	26.0
5060	Chicken, broiler or fryer, breast w/skin, roasted	3.5 oz	197.0	29.8	0.0
5061	Chicken, broiler or fryer, breast w/skin, stewed	3.5 oz	184.0	27.4	0.0
5063	Chicken, broiler or fryer, breast, no skin, fried	3.5 oz	187.0	33.4	0.5
5064	Chicken, broiler or fryer, breast, no skin, roasted	3.5 oz	165.0	31.0	0.0
5065	Chicken, broiler or fryer, breast, no skin, stewed	3.5 oz	151.0	29.0	0.0
5037	Chicken, broiler or fryer, dark meat w/skin, roasted	3.5 oz	253.0	26.0	0.0
5038	Chicken, broiler or fryer, dark meat w/skin, stewed	3.5 oz	233.0	23.5	0.0
5044	Chicken, broiler or fryer, dark meat, no skin, fried	4.0 oz	284.4	34.5	3.1
5045	Chicken, broiler or fryer, dark meat, no skin, roasted	3.5 oz	205.0	27.4	0.0
5046	Chicken, broiler or fryer, dark meat, no skin, stewed	3.5 oz	192.0	26.0	0.0
5078	Chicken, broiler or fryer, leg w/skin, roasted	3.5 oz	232.0	26.0	0.0
5079	Chicken, broiler or fryer, leg w/skin, stewed	3.5 oz	220.0	24.2	0.0
5081	Chicken, broiler or fryer, leg, no skin, fried	4.0 oz	247.5	33.8	0.8
5082	Chicken, broiler or fryer, leg, no skin, roasted	3.5 oz	191.0	27.0	0.0
5083	Chicken, broiler or fryer, leg, no skin, stewed	3.5 oz	185.0	26.3	0.0
5032	Chicken, broiler or fryer, light meat w/skin, roasted	3.5 oz	222.0	29.0	0.0
5033	Chicken, broiler or fryer, light meat w/skin, stewed	3.5 oz	201.0	26.1	0.0
5040	Chicken, broiler or fryer, light meat, no skin, fried	4.0 oz	228.5	39.1	0.5
5041	Chicken, broiler or fryer, light meat, no skin, roasted	3.5 oz	173.0	30.9	0.0
5042	Chicken, broiler or fryer, light meat, no skin, stewed	3.5 oz	159.0	28.9	0.0
5009	Chicken, broiler or fryer, meat & skin, roasted	3.5 oz	239.0	27.3	0.0
5010	Chicken, broiler or fryer, meat & skin, stewed	3.5 oz	219.0	24.7	0.0

Dietary Fiber (g)	Total Fat (g)	Cholesterol (mg)	Calcium (mg)	Iron (mg)	Magnesium (mg)	Sodium (mg)	Zinc (mg)	Vitamin A (μgRE)	Vitamin C (mg)	Vitamin E (mgαT)	Thiamin (mg)	Riboflavin (mg)	Niacin (mg)	Vitamin B$_6$ (mg)	Folate (μg)
0.0	0.5	2.4	19.2	0.0	1.7	113.7	0.1	5.6	0.0	0.0	0.0	0.1	0.0	0.0	3.7
0.0	0.1	1.9	8.9	0.1	1.1	3.6	0.1	2.2	0.0	0.0	0.0	0.0	0.0	0.0	4.1
0.0	9.8	30.7	22.4	0.3	1.8	82.7	0.2	107.0	0.0	0.3	0.0	0.1	0.0	0.0	3.7
0.0	0.4	2.2	51.8	0.1	3.9	152.6	0.2	78.1	0.0	0.0	0.0	0.0	0.0	0.0	10.4
0.0	7.8	25.0	204.7	0.1	8.3	270.2	1.1	70.8	0.0	0.2	0.0	0.1	0.0	0.0	4.5
0.0	6.0	24.9	137.9	0.2	5.4	312.5	0.8	35.8	0.0	0.0	0.0	0.2	0.3	0.1	9.0
0.0	8.7	32.5	154.0	0.1	3.9	224.0	1.0	81.2	0.0	0.1	0.0	0.1	0.0	0.0	1.7
0.0	7.7	31.9	195.9	0.1	8.1	229.4	1.1	48.7	0.0	0.1	0.0	0.1	0.0	0.0	5.9
0.0	9.1	30.8	283.1	0.0	10.1	94.1	1.1	84.3	0.0	0.1	0.0	0.1	0.0	0.0	2.9
0.0	8.4	29.4	190.4	0.1	7.8	316.7	0.8	17.6	0.0	0.0	0.0	0.1	0.0	0.0	0.3
0.0	8.5	24.9	209.0	0.2	7.6	150.2	0.8	70.8	0.0	0.1	0.0	0.1	0.0	0.0	5.1
0.0	4.5	16.2	180.8	0.1	6.5	130.5	0.8	49.6	0.0	0.1	0.0	0.1	0.0	0.0	2.5
0.0	6.0	22.0	144.8	0.1	5.2	104.5	0.6	67.5	0.0	0.1	0.0	0.1	0.0	0.0	2.0
0.0	8.4	26.8	200.8	0.1	7.7	175.8	0.8	88.5	0.0	0.1	0.0	0.1	0.0	0.0	3.4
0.0	6.6	21.3	21.1	0.1	2.1	111.8	0.1	84.0	0.0	0.0	0.0	0.1	0.0	0.0	3.2
0.0	8.4	22.0	385.2	0.3	14.2	521.2	0.9	48.4	0.0	0.2	0.0	0.1	0.1	0.0	2.2
0.0	7.2	19.0	331.4	0.2	12.2	448.4	0.8	41.7	0.0	0.2	0.0	0.1	0.1	0.0	1.9
0.0	7.7	20.2	350.8	0.2	14.2	474.9	0.9	48.4	0.0	0.0	0.0	0.1	0.1	0.0	2.2
0.0	35.3	106.7	695.5	0.4	25.1	1616.4	3.4	327.7	0.0	0.5	0.0	0.4	0.1	0.1	8.8
0.0	35.3	106.4	694.3	0.5	25.1	1613.1	3.4	363.9	2.5	0.5	0.0	0.4	0.1	0.1	8.8
0.0	28.3	95.8	872.2	0.7	32.9	1548.4	4.1	258.8	0.0	0.8	0.0	0.3	0.0	0.0	6.7
0.0	5.7	16.0	147.0	0.1	8.0	370.0	0.7	38.6	0.0	0.0	0.0	0.1	0.1	0.0	4.0
0.0	6.1	21.0	154.0	0.1	8.0	454.0	0.6	68.6	0.0	0.0	0.0	0.1	0.0	0.0	6.0
0.0	35.1	90.9	997.8	0.7	36.4	1155.7	4.3	348.5	0.0	0.5	0.0	0.4	0.2	0.1	13.7
0.0	1.2	4.7	41.9	0.1	2.3	19.2	0.2	17.4	0.0	0.0	0.0	0.0	0.0	0.0	2.0
0.0	2.0	7.8	31.9	0.1	1.7	13.0	0.2	20.6	0.0	0.1	0.0	0.0	0.0	0.0	1.9
0.0	7.5	29.1	297.9	0.2	11.5	336.0	0.7	39.5	0.0	0.2	0.0	0.1	0.0	0.0	1.9
0.0	8.6	25.2	185.3	0.2	8.3	506.5	0.6	83.7	0.0	0.0	0.0	0.2	0.2	0.0	13.7
0.0	29.6	99.0	1037.8	0.2	38.8	280.8	4.2	273.2	0.0	0.5	0.0	0.4	0.1	0.1	6.9
7.5	21.1	102.2	0.0	7.3	0.0	2683.1	0.0	0.0	0.0	0.0	0.0	0.0	0.0	0.0	0.0
0.1	41.5	269.7	155.0	3.0	0.0	927.5	2.2	275.8	14.6	0.0	0.1	0.5	6.6	0.3	13.4
3.4	14.2	85.2	65.9	2.8	0.0	815.6	2.4	63.6	11.4	0.0	0.1	0.3	4.9	0.5	21.6
1.6	0.8	6.4	36.0	1.0	0.0	580.0	1.0	24.0	10.4	0.0	0.0	0.1	0.8	0.1	9.6
0.0	3.3	0.0	14.6	1.1	0.0	845.5	0.0	68.6	2.2	0.0	0.1	0.1	1.6	0.0	0.0
0.0	3.0	3.0	9.0	0.8	0.0	140.0	0.0	5.0	2.0	0.0	0.1	0.1	1.1	0.0	0.0
0.0	39.0	0.0	54.3	1.5	0.0	95.0	0.0	397.4	2.5	0.0	0.2	0.2	9.0	0.0	0.0
0.0	26.3	0.0	309.7	11.2	0.0	637.2	0.0	494.1	28.5	0.0	0.3	0.3	8.5	0.0	0.0
2.6	30.4	62.6	83.5	2.5	0.0	772.6	0.0	0.0	0.0	0.0	0.0	0.0	0.0	0.0	0.0
1.5	27.7	47.8	59.7	2.6	0.0	506.9	1.7	1232.4	4.3	0.0	0.3	0.3	4.2	0.4	24.8
1.0	2.0	20.0	20.0	1.1	0.0	850.0	0.0	200.0	12.0	0.0	0.0	0.1	2.0	0.0	0.0
0.0	2.4	0.0	50.0	1.3	0.0	965.0	0.0	493.4	5.0	0.0	0.1	0.1	2.9	0.0	0.0
0.1	18.0	103.0	26.0	2.2	0.0	600.0	2.1	86.0	0.0	0.0	0.1	0.2	4.3	0.2	9.0
1.0	18.0	103.0	26.0	2.4	0.0	600.0	2.1	26.0	1.0	0.0	0.1	0.2	4.3	0.2	9.0
0.0	7.8	84.0	14.0	1.1	27.0	71.0	1.0	27.0	0.0	0.3	0.1	0.1	12.7	0.6	4.0
0.0	7.4	75.0	13.0	0.9	22.0	62.0	1.0	24.0	0.0	0.3	0.0	0.1	7.8	0.3	3.0
0.0	4.7	91.0	16.0	1.1	31.0	79.0	1.1	7.0	0.0	0.4	0.1	0.1	14.8	0.6	4.0
0.0	3.6	85.0	15.0	1.0	29.0	74.0	1.0	6.0	0.0	0.3	0.1	0.1	13.7	0.6	4.0
0.0	3.0	77.0	13.0	0.9	24.0	63.0	1.0	6.0	0.0	0.3	0.0	0.1	8.5	0.3	3.0
0.0	15.8	91.0	15.0	1.4	22.0	87.0	2.5	58.0	0.0	0.0	0.1	0.2	6.4	0.3	7.0
0.0	14.7	82.0	14.0	1.3	18.0	70.0	2.3	54.0	0.0	0.0	0.1	0.2	4.5	0.2	6.0
0.0	13.8	114.2	21.4	1.8	29.8	115.4	3.5	28.6	0.0	0.0	0.1	0.3	8.4	0.4	10.7
0.0	9.7	93.0	15.0	1.3	23.0	93.0	2.8	22.0	0.0	0.3	0.1	0.2	6.5	0.4	8.0
0.0	9.0	88.0	14.0	1.4	20.0	74.0	2.7	21.0	0.0	0.3	0.1	0.2	4.7	0.2	7.0
0.0	13.5	92.0	12.0	1.3	23.0	87.0	2.6	39.0	0.0	0.3	0.1	0.2	6.2	0.3	7.0
0.0	12.9	84.0	11.0	1.4	20.0	73.0	2.4	36.0	0.0	0.3	0.1	0.2	4.6	0.2	6.0
0.0	11.1	117.8	15.5	1.7	29.8	114.2	3.5	23.8	0.0	0.0	0.1	0.3	8.0	0.5	10.7
0.0	8.4	94.0	12.0	1.3	24.0	91.0	2.9	19.0	0.0	0.3	0.1	0.2	6.3	0.4	8.0
0.0	8.1	89.0	11.0	1.4	21.0	78.0	2.8	18.0	0.0	0.3	0.1	0.2	4.8	0.2	8.0
0.0	10.9	84.0	15.0	1.1	25.0	75.0	1.2	32.0	0.0	0.0	0.1	0.1	11.1	0.5	3.0
0.0	10.0	74.0	13.0	1.0	20.0	63.0	1.1	28.0	0.0	0.3	0.0	0.1	6.9	0.3	3.0
0.0	6.6	107.1	19.0	1.4	34.5	96.4	1.5	10.7	0.0	0.0	0.1	0.1	15.9	0.7	4.8
0.0	4.5	85.0	15.0	1.1	27.0	77.0	1.2	9.0	0.0	0.3	0.1	0.1	12.4	0.6	4.0
0.0	4.0	77.0	13.0	0.9	22.0	65.0	1.2	8.0	0.0	0.3	0.0	0.1	7.8	0.3	3.0
0.0	13.6	88.0	15.0	1.3	23.0	82.0	1.9	47.0	0.0	0.3	0.1	0.2	8.5	0.4	5.0
0.0	12.6	78.0	13.0	1.2	19.0	67.0	1.8	42.0	0.0	0.3	0.0	0.1	5.6	0.2	5.0

Code	Food Name	Unit Amount	Kilocalories (kcal)	Protein (g)	Carbohydrate (g)
5094	Chicken, broiler or fryer, thigh w/skin, roasted	3.5 oz	247.0	25.1	0.0
5095	Chicken, broiler or fryer, thigh w/skin, stewed	3.5 oz	232.0	23.3	0.0
5097	Chicken, broiler or fryer, thigh, no skin, fried	4.0 oz	259.4	33.5	1.4
5098	Chicken, broiler or fryer, thigh, no skin, roasted	3.5 oz	209.0	25.9	0.0
5099	Chicken, broiler or fryer, thigh, no skin, stewed	3.5 oz	195.0	25.0	0.0
5103	Chicken, broiler or fryer, wing w/skin, roasted	3.5 oz	290.0	26.9	0.0
5104	Chicken, broiler or fryer, wing w/skin, stewed	3.5 oz	249.0	22.8	0.0
5106	Chicken, broiler or fryer, wing, no skin, fried	4.0 oz	251.1	35.9	0.0
5107	Chicken, broiler or fryer, wing, no skin, roasted	3.5 oz	203.0	30.5	0.0
5108	Chicken, broiler or fryer, wing, no skin, stewed	3.5 oz	181.0	27.2	0.0
22697	Chicken, chicken salad ready to serve sandwich salad/Libby Spreadable	1 package	329.2	11.1	22.9
5277	Chicken, meat only w/broth, canned	2.5 oz	117.2	15.5	0.0
51608	Chicken, nugget, breaded/Pierre product #1879	3.5 oz	329.0	16.8	13.3
924008	Chili con carne	3/4 cup	159.6	8.9	14.6
22904	Chili con carne w/beans, canned entree	1 cup	293.3	23.2	28.1
924243	Chili w/beans	1 package	909.5	30.9	90.8
16059	Chili w/beans, canned	1 cup	246.4	12.6	26.2
924059	Chili w/beans, homemade	1 cup	328.5	18.5	30.1
924056	Chili w/o beans, homemade	1 cup	472.0	24.3	13.7
22720	Chili, vegetarian chili w/beans, canned entree/Hormel	1 cup	205.0	11.9	38.0
18606	Chocolate cake, snack cake, chocolate creme filling–Ding Dongs/Hostess	1 cup	1015.5	6.8	130.2
918804	Chocolate, baking, Choco-Bake/Nestle	1 serving	480.0	4.0	34.0
918805	Chocolate, baking, Hershey	1.0 oz	185.1	4.0	6.7
19146	Chocolate, baking, M&M's Milk Chocolate Mini Baking Bits	1.0 oz	139.4	1.3	18.8
19139	Chocolate, baking, M&M's Semisweet Chocolate Mini Baking Bits	1 serving	73.6	0.6	9.4
19124	Chocolate, baking, Mexican, squares	1 Tbsp.	59.6	0.5	10.8
918806	Chocolate, baking, unsweetened liquid	1 tablet	95.8	2.4	6.9
918870	Cobbler, peach	1.0 oz	44.8	0.3	7.1
14198	Cocoa mix, No Sugar Added Hot Cocoa Mix/Carnation	1/3 cup	365.0	28.7	56.2
14197	Cocoa mix, Rich Chocolate Hot Cocoa Mix/Carnation	1 envelope	60.0	0.7	13.0
1105	Cocoa, hot, homemade w/whole milk	1 envelope	21.6	1.1	3.3
18104	Coffee cake, cinnamon w/crumb topping, enriched, commercially prep	1.0 oz	121.2	2.0	13.5
14210	Coffee, brewed, espresso, restaurant-prep	2.0 oz	5.1	0.0	0.9
902912	Condiment, A-1 sauce	6 fl oz	118.6	0.0	29.5
902922	Condiment, enchilada sauce	1/4 cup	21.0	0.0	2.8
2055	Condiment, horseradish, prep	1 Tbsp.	7.2	0.2	1.7
902916	Condiment, mustard, brown	1 tsp.	5.0	0.3	0.3
902917	Condiment, mustard, yellow	1 tsp.	4.0	0.2	0.3
902925	Condiment, picante sauce	3 Tbsp.	16.0	0.0	4.0
902918	Condiment, pickle, sour relish	1 Tbsp.	16.1	0.0	3.8
902926	Condiment, salsa	3 Tbsp.	24.9	1.0	6.0
902927	Condiment, taco sauce, chunky	3 Tbsp.	24.9	1.0	6.0
902928	Condiment, taco sauce, hot/mild	3 Tbsp.	15.1	0.0	4.0
11935	Condiment, vege, tomato catsup	1 Tbsp.	15.6	0.2	4.1
11949	Condiment, vege, tomato catsup, low-sodium	1 Tbsp.	15.6	0.2	4.1
902919	Condiment, Worcestershire sauce	1 Tbsp.	11.0	0.3	2.7
18150	Cookie, animal crackers/arrowroot/tea biscuits	1 cracker	8.9	0.1	1.5
918153	Cookie, brownies, dry mix, prep	1 brownie (2" square)	139.6	1.4	20.4
18197	Cookie, brownies, dry mix, prep, special dietary	1 brownie (2" square)	84.5	0.8	15.7
18154	Cookie, brownies, homemade	1 brownie (2" square)	111.8	1.5	12.0
18155	Cookie, butter, enriched, commercially prep	1 cookie	23.4	0.3	3.4
918861	Cookie, Capri/PepFarm	1 cookie	81.9	0.8	9.7
18614	Cookie, Chewy Fudge Brownie Mix, dry/Martha White	1 serving	114.1	1.3	23.2
18159	Cookie, chocolate chip, enriched, commercially prep	1 large Keebler RichnChip/PecanChipDelux	67.3	0.8	9.4
18378	Cookie, chocolate chip, homemade w/butter	1 medium cookie (2.25" diam)	78.1	0.9	9.3
918895	Cookie, Chocolate Coated Graham/Lance	1.8 oz	249.0	3.5	32.7
918854	Cookie, Chocolate Marshmallow Pie/LittleDeb	1.4 oz	170.0	1.5	27.1
18169	Cookie, coconut macaroons, homemade	1 individual pkg (2-oz pkg w/2 3"bars	230.3	2.1	41.2
18170	Cookie, fig bar	1 cookie	55.7	0.6	11.3
18171	Cookie, fortune	1 cookie	30.2	0.3	6.7
918822	Cookie, Fudge Brownie/LittleDeb	1 brownie	236.0	2.7	38.6
18172	Cookie, ginger snaps	1 cookie	29.1	0.4	5.4
18609	Cookie, Golden Vanilla Wafers/Keebler	1 large (3.5" - 4" diam)	152.0	1.7	22.3
18174	Cookie, graham crackers, chocolate-coated	1 cracker (2.5" square)	67.8	0.8	9.3
18173	Cookie, graham crackers, plain/honey/cinnamon	1 large or 4 small rectangular pieces	59.2	1.0	10.8

Dietary Fiber (g)	Total Fat (g)	Cholesterol (mg)	Calcium (mg)	Iron (mg)	Magnesium (mg)	Sodium (mg)	Zinc (mg)	Vitamin A (μgRE)	Vitamin C (mg)	Vitamin E (mgαT)	Thiamin (mg)	Riboflavin (mg)	Niacin (mg)	Vitamin B$_6$ (mg)	Folate (μg)
0.0	15.5	93.0	12.0	1.3	22.0	84.0	2.4	48.0	0.0	0.3	0.1	0.2	6.4	0.3	7.0
0.0	14.7	84.0	11.0	1.4	19.0	71.0	2.3	44.0	0.0	0.3	0.1	0.2	4.9	0.2	6.0
0.0	12.3	121.4	15.5	1.7	30.9	113.1	3.3	25.0	0.0	0.0	0.1	0.3	8.5	0.5	10.7
0.0	10.9	95.0	12.0	1.3	24.0	88.0	2.6	20.0	0.0	0.3	0.1	0.2	6.5	0.4	8.0
0.0	9.8	90.0	11.0	1.4	21.0	75.0	2.6	19.0	0.0	0.3	0.1	0.2	5.2	0.2	7.0
0.0	19.5	84.0	15.0	1.3	19.0	82.0	1.8	47.0	0.0	0.3	0.0	0.1	6.6	0.4	3.0
0.0	16.8	70.0	12.0	1.1	16.0	67.0	1.6	40.0	0.0	0.3	0.0	0.1	4.6	0.2	3.0
0.0	10.9	100.0	17.9	1.4	25.0	108.3	2.5	21.4	0.0	0.0	0.1	0.2	8.6	0.7	4.8
0.0	8.1	85.0	16.0	1.2	21.0	92.0	2.1	18.0	0.0	0.3	0.0	0.1	7.3	0.6	4.0
0.0	7.2	74.0	13.0	1.1	18.0	73.0	2.0	16.0	0.0	0.3	0.0	0.1	5.2	0.3	3.0
0.0	21.3	59.0	0.0	0.0	0.0	1062.4	0.0	0.0	0.0	0.0	0.0	0.0	0.0	0.0	0.0
0.0	5.6	44.0	9.9	1.1	8.5	357.1	1.0	24.1	1.4	0.2	0.0	0.1	4.5	0.2	2.8
1.1	23.4	39.0	36.0	2.2	24.0	697.0	2.5	0.0	0.0	2.7	0.3	0.2	6.3	0.3	29.0
2.8	7.5	13.2	38.6	2.0	0.0	637.2	2.4	14.1	3.8	0.0	0.0	0.1	1.6	0.2	19.3
9.4	9.4	28.1	76.5	3.8	63.8	1185.8	2.8	107.1	1.0	0.3	0.2	0.2	2.4	0.2	66.3
11.6	52.2	125.6	183.5	12.4	0.0	1931.8	3.9	566.0	77.3	0.0	0.8	0.6	8.5	0.5	48.3
9.7	12.1	37.4	103.4	7.5	99.0	1148.4	4.4	74.8	3.7	1.6	0.1	0.2	0.8	0.3	49.9
1.5	15.1	0.0	79.0	4.2	0.0	1311.6	0.0	29.6	0.0	0.0	0.1	0.2	3.2	0.0	0.0
0.5	34.9	101.5	89.7	3.3	0.0	3138.8	11.8	70.8	4.7	0.0	0.0	0.3	5.2	0.6	0.0
9.9	0.7	0.0	96.3	3.5	81.5	778.1	1.7	0.0	1.2	0.0	0.0	0.0	0.0	0.0	0.0
4.6	51.9	30.1	0.0	5.1	0.0	547.8	0.0	0.0	0.0	0.0	0.0	0.0	0.0	0.0	0.0
0.0	39.4	0.0	0.0	0.0	0.0	8.6	0.0	0.0	0.0	0.0	0.0	0.0	0.0	0.0	0.0
0.7	15.8	0.0	20.0	2.0	84.0	3.0	1.1	1.2	0.0	0.0	0.0	0.1	0.3	0.0	3.0
0.8	6.5	4.2	32.5	0.3	12.9	19.0	0.3	12.6	0.2	0.3	0.0	0.1	0.1	0.0	1.4
1.0	3.7	0.4	4.8	0.4	15.1	0.4	0.2	1.0	0.0	0.1	0.0	0.0	0.1	0.0	4.0
0.5	2.2	0.0	4.8	0.3	13.3	0.4	0.2	0.3	0.0	0.1	0.0	0.0	0.3	0.0	0.3
0.0	9.6	0.0	10.7	0.8	53.6	2.1	0.7	2.4	0.0	0.0	0.0	0.1	0.4	0.0	0.0
0.3	1.8	0.0	2.0	0.1	0.0	44.2	0.0	26.8	7.3	0.0	0.0	0.0	0.3	0.0	0.0
5.0	2.8	19.0	823.0	2.6	180.0	947.0	4.0	0.0	2.7	0.1	0.4	1.5	1.2	0.4	39.0
0.4	0.6	0.9	21.5	0.2	14.7	54.5	0.2	0.0	0.0	0.0	0.0	0.1	0.1	0.0	1.1
0.2	0.7	2.2	35.3	0.1	7.8	14.3	0.2	15.4	0.3	0.0	0.0	0.0	0.0	0.0	1.7
0.6	6.8	9.3	15.7	0.6	6.4	101.8	0.2	9.6	0.1	1.0	0.1	0.1	0.5	0.0	17.7
0.0	0.1	0.0	1.1	0.1	45.6	8.0	0.0	0.0	0.1	0.0	0.0	0.1	3.0	0.0	0.6
0.0	0.0	0.0	9.8	1.0	0.0	2625.5	0.0	0.0	0.0	0.0	0.0	0.0	0.0	0.0	0.0
0.0	0.0	0.0	9.8	0.6	0.0	209.3	0.0	99.1	7.0	0.0	0.0	0.0	0.4	0.0	0.0
0.5	0.1	0.0	8.4	0.1	4.1	47.1	0.1	0.0	3.7	0.0	0.0	0.0	0.1	0.0	8.6
0.1	0.3	0.0	6.0	0.1	0.0	65.0	0.0	0.0	0.0	0.0	0.0	0.0	0.0	0.0	0.0
0.1	0.2	0.0	4.0	0.1	0.0	63.0	0.0	0.0	0.0	0.0	0.0	0.0	0.0	0.0	0.0
0.0	0.0	0.0	12.0	0.2	0.0	650.0	0.0	45.0	10.0	0.0	0.0	0.1	0.5	0.0	0.0
0.2	0.0	0.0	4.3	0.2	0.0	75.0	0.0	4.7	0.0	0.0	0.0	0.0	0.1	0.0	0.0
0.0	0.0	0.0	35.0	0.2	0.0	350.0	0.0	94.0	17.0	0.0	0.0	0.3	0.7	0.0	0.0
0.0	0.0	0.0	20.0	0.7	0.0	310.0	0.0	87.0	16.0	0.0	0.0	0.2	0.7	0.0	0.0
0.0	0.0	0.0	25.0	0.2	0.0	310.0	0.0	46.0	7.0	0.0	0.0	0.0	0.5	0.0	0.0
0.2	0.1	0.0	2.9	0.1	3.3	177.9	0.0	15.3	2.3	0.2	0.0	0.0	0.2	0.0	2.3
0.2	0.1	0.0	2.9	0.1	3.3	3.0	0.0	15.3	2.3	0.2	0.0	0.0	0.2	0.0	2.3
0.0	0.0	0.0	15.0	0.9	0.0	234.0	0.0	10.2	27.0	0.0	0.0	0.0	0.0	0.0	0.0
0.0	0.3	0.0	0.9	0.1	0.4	7.9	0.0	0.0	0.0	0.0	0.0	0.0	0.1	0.0	1.7
0.9	6.6	2.0	6.3	0.6	10.9	83.2	0.2	4.3	0.0	0.0	0.0	0.0	0.5	0.0	2.6
0.8	2.4	0.0	2.6	0.3	1.3	20.7	0.0	0.0	0.0	0.4	0.0	0.0	0.2	0.0	7.5
0.0	7.0	17.5	13.7	0.4	12.7	82.3	0.2	47.8	0.1	0.0	0.0	0.0	0.2	0.0	7.0
0.0	0.9	5.9	1.5	0.1	0.6	17.6	0.0	8.4	0.0	0.0	0.0	0.0	0.2	0.0	2.0
0.1	4.6	0.0	6.0	0.3	0.0	39.0	0.0	0.0	0.0	0.0	0.0	0.0	0.2	0.0	0.0
0.0	1.8	0.0	0.0	1.1	0.0	138.3	0.0	0.0	0.0	0.0	0.0	0.0	0.0	0.0	0.0
0.4	3.2	0.0	3.5	0.4	4.3	44.1	0.1	0.0	0.0	0.4	0.0	0.0	0.4	0.0	5.9
0.0	4.5	11.2	6.1	0.4	8.8	54.6	0.2	23.5	0.0	0.0	0.0	0.0	0.2	0.0	5.3
0.0	13.5	0.0	120.0	0.1	0.0	79.0	0.0	0.0	0.0	0.0	0.1	0.1	0.6	0.0	0.0
0.0	6.2	0.0	0.0	0.7	0.0	77.0	0.0	0.0	0.0	0.0	0.1	0.0	0.0	0.0	0.0
1.0	7.2	0.0	4.0	0.4	12.0	140.8	0.4	0.0	0.0	0.2	0.0	0.1	0.1	0.1	2.3
0.7	1.2	0.0	10.2	0.5	4.3	56.0	0.1	0.6	0.0	0.2	0.0	0.0	0.3	0.0	4.3
0.1	0.2	0.2	1.0	0.1	0.6	21.9	0.0	0.1	0.0	0.0	0.0	0.0	0.1	0.0	4.4
0.0	8.0	1.0	0.0	1.7	0.0	121.0	0.0	0.0	0.0	0.0	0.1	0.1	0.1	0.0	0.0
0.2	0.7	0.0	5.4	0.4	3.4	45.8	0.0	0.0	0.0	0.1	0.0	0.0	0.2	0.0	5.0
0.0	6.2	0.0	0.0	0.0	0.0	123.5	0.0	0.0	0.0	0.0	0.0	0.0	0.0	0.0	0.0
0.4	3.2	0.0	8.1	0.5	8.1	40.7	0.1	0.1	0.0	0.2	0.0	0.0	0.3	0.0	2.4
0.4	1.4	0.0	3.4	0.5	4.2	84.7	0.1	0.0	0.0	0.3	0.0	0.0	0.6	0.0	8.4

Code	Food Name	Unit Amount	Kilocalories (kcal)	Protein (g)	Carbohydrate (g)
918812	Cookie, iced brownies w/nuts	1 ladyfinger	44.6	0.5	7.0
18423	Cookie, ladyfinger/egg jumbo/breakfast treat/anisette sponge w/o lemon	1 ladyfinger	40.2	1.2	6.6
918863	Cookie, Lemon Nut/PepFarm	2 large	336.0	3.8	40.3
18612	Cookie, Little Debbie Nutty Bars, Chocolate Covered Wafers w/Peanut Butter	1 bar	312.4	4.6	31.5
18176	Cookie, marshmallow, chocolate coated/marshmallow pie	1 marshmallow pie (3" diam x 0.75")	164.2	1.6	26.4
18177	Cookie, molasses	1 large (3.5"–4" diam/Archway Brand)	137.6	1.8	23.6
18178	Cookie, oatmeal, commercially prep	1 cookie	81.0	1.1	12.4
918809	Cookie, Oreos	3 cookies	100.0	2.0	16.0
918821	Cookie, peanut butter brownie	1 brownie	120.0	3.0	16.0
18185	Cookie, peanut butter, commercially prep	1 cookie	71.6	1.4	8.8
18191	Cookie, raisin, soft	1 cookie	60.2	0.6	10.2
18166	Cookie, sandwich, chocolate, cream-filled	1.0 oz	47.2	0.5	7.0
18199	Cookie, sandwich, chocolate, cream-filled, special dietary	1 cookie	46.1	0.5	6.8
18190	Cookie, sandwich, peanut butter, regular	1 cookie	66.9	1.2	9.2
18201	Cookie, sandwich, peanut butter, special dietary	1 cookie	53.5	1.0	5.1
18210	Cookie, sandwich, vanilla, cream-filled	1 oval cookie (3-1/8" x 1.25" x 3/8")	72.5	0.7	10.8
918194	Cookie, shortbread, homemade w/butter	1 medium cookie (1.5" diam)	60.1	0.7	6.2
18193	Cookie, shortbread, pecan, commercially prep	1 cookie (2" diam)	75.9	0.7	8.2
18192	Cookie, shortbread, plain, commercially prep	1 cookie (1.6" square)	40.2	0.5	5.2
18209	Cookie, sugar wafer, cream-filled	1 large wafer (3.5" x 1" x 0.5")	46.0	0.4	6.3
18202	Cookie, sugar wafer, cream-filled, special dietary	1 wafer	20.1	0.1	2.6
918207	Cookie, sugar, homemade w/butter	1 cookie (3" diam)	65.9	0.8	8.4
18206	Cookie, sugar, refrig dough, baked	1 cookie	58.1	0.6	7.9
18204	Cookie, sugar/vanilla, commercially prep	1 cookie	71.7	0.8	10.2
18213	Cookie, vanilla wafer	1 wafer	28.4	0.3	4.3
18212	Cookie, vanilla wafer, lower-fat	1 large wafer	26.5	0.3	4.4
20018	Corn flour, degermed, unenriched, yellow	1 Tbsp.	29.6	0.4	6.5
924077	Corn fritter	1 fritter	132.0	2.7	13.9
13348	Corned beef brisket, canned	1.0 oz	70.9	7.7	0.0
20027	Cornstarch	1 Tbsp.	30.5	0.0	7.3
18214	Cracker, cheese	1 cracker (1" square)	5.0	0.1	0.6
18216	Cracker, crispbread, rye	1 crispbread, wafer or cracker	36.6	0.8	8.2
919977	Cracker, Goldfish/PepFarm	12 crackers	30.0	0.0	4.0
18218	Cracker, matzo, egg	1 matzo	110.8	3.5	22.3
18219	Cracker, matzo, whole-wheat	1 matzo	99.5	3.7	22.4
18220	Cracker, Melba Toast Rounds, plain	1 melba round	11.7	0.4	2.3
18221	Cracker, Melba Toast, rye or pumpernickel	1 toast	19.5	0.6	3.9
18223	Cracker, milk	1 cracker	50.1	0.8	7.7
18620	Cracker, Original Premium Saltine Crackers/Nabisco	1 serving	58.8	1.5	10.0
18621	Cracker, Ritz/Nabisco	1 serving	78.7	1.2	10.3
18224	Cracker, Rusk Toast	1 rusk	40.7	1.4	7.2
918808	Cracker, Rye Krisps	1/4 large square	40.0	1.5	13.0
18425	Cracker, saltine/oyster/soda/soup, low-salt	1 oyster cracker	4.3	0.1	0.7
18426	Cracker, saltines/oyster/soda/soup, unsalted	1 saltine	13.0	0.3	2.1
18230	Cracker, sandwich, cheese-filled	1 sandwich cracker	33.4	0.7	4.3
18215	Cracker, sandwich, cheese w/peanut butter filling	1 sandwich cracker	33.7	0.9	4.0
18231	Cracker, sandwich, peanut butter–filled	1 sandwich cracker	34.2	0.8	4.1
18234	Cracker, sandwich, wheat w/peanut butter filling	1 sandwich cracker	34.7	0.9	3.8
18622	Cracker, Snackwell Zesty Cheese, Reduced Fat/Nabisco	1 serving	124.1	2.9	23.1
18229	Cracker, standard snack, regular	1 rectangular cracker	20.1	0.3	2.4
18624	Cracker, Wheat Thins, baked/Nabisco	1 serving	136.2	2.4	20.0
18235	Cracker, whole-wheat	1 cracker	17.7	0.4	2.7
18429	Cracker, whole-wheat, low-sodium	1 cracker	17.7	0.4	2.7
18434	Crackers, cheese, Cheez-its/Goldfish, low sodium	1 goldfish	3.0	0.1	0.3
18457	Crackers, saltines, fat-free, low-sodium	3 saltines	59.0	1.6	12.3
1067	Cream substitute, nondairy, liquid w/hydrogenated vege oil and soy protein	1 Tbsp.	20.3	0.2	1.7
1069	Cream substitute, nondairy, powder	1 tsp.	10.9	0.1	1.1
1058	Cream, filled cream, nonbutterfat sour dressing, cultured	1 cup	417.5	7.6	11.0
1049	Cream, half and half	1 Tbsp.	19.6	0.4	0.6
1053	Cream, heavy whipping	1 Tbsp.	51.7	0.3	0.4
1052	Cream, light whipping	1 Tbsp.	43.9	0.3	0.4
1056	Cream, sour, cultured	1 Tbsp.	25.7	0.4	0.5
1074	Cream, sour, imitation, cultured	1.0 oz	60.5	0.7	1.9
1055	Cream, sour, reduced-fat (half and half) cultured	2 Tbsp.	40.4	0.9	1.3
1054	Cream, whipped cream topping, pressurized	1 Tbsp.	7.7	0.1	0.4

Dietary Fiber (g)	Total Fat (g)	Cholesterol (mg)	Calcium (mg)	Iron (mg)	Magnesium (mg)	Sodium (mg)	Zinc (mg)	Vitamin A (μgRE)	Vitamin C (mg)	Vitamin E (mgαT)	Thiamin (mg)	Riboflavin (mg)	Niacin (mg)	Vitamin B$_6$ (mg)	Folate (μg)
0.0	1.9	0.0	5.5	0.3	4.4	25.9	0.2	6.5	0.0	0.0	0.0	0.0	0.2	0.0	1.1
0.1	1.0	40.2	5.2	0.4	1.3	16.2	0.1	18.4	0.0	0.1	0.0	0.0	0.2	0.0	8.5
0.0	17.9	0.0	22.0	0.4	0.0	189.0	0.0	0.0	0.0	0.0	0.0	0.1	0.3	0.0	0.0
0.0	18.7	0.0	0.0	0.0	0.0	127.1	0.0	0.0	1.1	0.0	0.0	0.0	0.0	0.0	0.0
0.8	6.6	0.0	17.9	1.0	14.0	65.5	0.3	0.4	0.0	0.8	0.0	0.1	0.3	0.0	7.4
0.3	4.1	0.0	23.7	2.1	16.6	146.9	0.1	0.0	0.0	0.5	0.1	0.1	1.0	0.0	23.7
0.5	3.3	0.0	6.7	0.5	5.9	68.9	0.1	0.4	0.1	0.5	0.0	0.0	0.4	0.0	8.1
0.6	4.0	0.0	0.0	0.0	0.0	150.0	0.0	0.0	0.0	0.0	0.0	0.0	0.0	0.0	0.0
0.2	5.0	0.0	6.0	0.9	15.0	100.0	0.2	10.0	0.0	0.0	0.0	0.0	1.1	0.0	2.0
0.3	3.5	0.2	5.3	0.4	6.8	62.3	0.1	0.5	0.0	0.5	0.0	0.0	0.6	0.0	9.3
0.2	2.0	0.3	6.9	0.3	3.2	50.7	0.0	0.2	0.1	0.3	0.0	0.0	0.3	0.0	6.6
0.3	2.1	0.0	2.6	0.4	4.5	60.4	0.1	0.0	0.0	0.3	0.0	0.0	0.2	0.0	4.3
0.4	2.2	0.0	9.8	0.5	2.6	24.3	0.1	0.0	0.0	0.4	0.1	0.0	0.4	0.0	6.2
0.3	3.0	0.0	7.4	0.4	6.9	51.5	0.1	0.1	0.0	0.5	0.0	0.0	0.5	0.0	6.2
0.0	3.4	0.0	4.3	0.3	5.1	41.2	0.1	0.0	0.0	0.6	0.0	0.0	0.5	0.0	5.4
0.2	3.0	0.0	4.1	0.3	2.1	52.4	0.1	0.0	0.0	0.5	0.0	0.0	0.4	0.0	8.9
0.0	3.7	1.0	2.0	0.3	1.4	51.2	0.0	33.6	0.0	0.0	0.0	0.0	0.3	0.0	1.2
0.3	4.6	4.6	4.2	0.3	2.5	39.3	0.1	0.1	0.0	0.0	0.0	0.0	0.3	0.0	8.8
0.1	1.9	1.6	2.8	0.2	1.4	36.4	0.0	1.0	0.0	0.3	0.0	0.0	0.3	0.0	4.7
0.1	2.2	0.0	1.6	0.2	1.0	13.2	0.0	0.0	0.0	0.4	0.0	0.0	0.2	0.0	3.9
0.0	1.0	0.0	2.1	0.1	0.2	0.4	0.0	0.0	0.0	0.0	0.0	0.0	0.1	0.0	1.7
0.0	3.3	0.9	9.9	0.3	1.7	64.3	0.1	31.2	0.0	0.0	0.0	0.0	0.3	0.0	1.7
0.1	2.8	3.8	10.8	0.2	1.0	56.2	0.0	1.3	0.0	0.4	0.0	0.0	0.3	0.0	6.4
0.1	3.2	7.7	3.2	0.3	1.8	53.6	0.1	4.1	0.0	0.4	0.0	0.0	0.4	0.0	6.8
0.1	1.2	0.0	1.5	0.1	0.7	18.4	0.0	0.0	0.0	0.0	0.0	0.0	0.2	0.0	2.6
0.1	0.9	3.1	2.9	0.1	0.8	18.7	0.0	0.5	0.0	0.1	0.0	0.0	0.2	0.0	3.0
0.2	0.1	0.0	0.2	0.1	1.4	0.1	0.0	0.4	0.0	0.0	0.0	0.0	0.2	0.0	3.8
1.0	7.5	0.0	22.0	0.6	0.0	167.0	0.0	28.0	1.0	0.0	0.1	0.1	0.6	0.0	0.0
0.0	4.2	24.4	3.4	0.6	4.0	285.2	1.0	0.0	0.0	0.0	0.0	0.0	0.7	0.0	2.6
0.1	0.0	0.0	0.2	0.0	0.2	0.7	0.0	0.0	0.0	0.0	0.0	0.0	0.0	0.0	0.0
0.0	0.3	0.1	1.5	0.0	0.4	10.0	0.0	0.3	0.0	0.0	0.0	0.0	0.0	0.0	0.8
1.7	0.1	0.0	3.1	0.2	7.8	26.4	0.2	0.0	0.0	0.1	0.0	0.0	0.1	0.0	4.7
0.5	2.0	0.0	4.0	0.2	0.0	50.0	0.0	0.2	0.0	0.0	0.0	0.0	0.2	0.0	0.0
0.8	0.6	23.5	11.3	0.8	6.8	6.0	0.2	3.7	0.0	0.0	0.2	0.2	1.4	0.0	33.2
3.3	0.4	0.0	6.5	1.3	38.0	0.6	0.7	0.0	0.0	0.4	0.1	0.1	1.5	0.0	13.6
0.2	0.1	0.0	2.8	0.1	1.8	24.9	0.1	0.0	0.0	0.0	0.0	0.0	0.1	0.0	3.7
0.4	0.2	0.0	3.9	0.2	2.0	45.0	0.1	0.0	0.0	0.0	0.0	0.0	0.2	0.0	4.3
0.2	1.7	1.2	18.9	0.4	2.4	65.1	0.1	0.8	0.0	0.3	0.1	0.0	0.5	0.0	9.0
0.4	1.4	0.0	27.0	0.7	2.9	177.8	0.0	0.0	0.0	0.0	0.0	0.1	0.6	0.0	11.8
0.3	3.7	0.0	23.5	0.6	3.2	124.2	0.2	0.0	0.0	0.0	0.0	0.0	0.6	0.0	9.6
0.0	0.7	7.8	2.7	0.3	3.6	25.3	0.1	1.2	0.0	0.0	0.0	0.0	0.5	0.0	8.7
2.5	0.2	0.0	12.0	0.4	34.0	112.0	0.8	0.0	0.0	0.0	0.0	0.1	0.3	0.1	7.0
0.0	0.1	0.0	1.2	0.1	0.3	6.4	0.0	0.0	0.0	0.0	0.0	0.0	0.1	0.0	1.2
0.1	0.4	0.0	3.6	0.2	0.8	23.0	0.0	0.0	0.0	0.0	0.0	0.0	0.2	0.0	3.7
0.1	1.5	0.1	18.0	0.2	2.5	98.1	0.0	1.3	0.0	0.0	0.0	0.0	0.3	0.0	5.9
0.2	1.6	0.4	5.5	0.2	4.1	69.4	0.1	2.4	0.0	0.3	0.0	0.0	0.5	0.1	6.2
0.2	1.7	0.0	6.8	0.2	3.7	65.9	0.1	0.0	0.0	0.3	0.0	0.0	0.4	0.0	5.9
0.3	1.9	0.0	11.9	0.2	2.7	56.5	0.1	0.0	0.0	0.0	0.0	0.0	0.4	0.0	4.9
0.7	2.2	1.5	40.5	1.0	9.6	275.1	0.5	0.0	0.1	0.0	0.1	0.1	1.3	0.1	17.4
0.1	1.0	0.0	4.8	0.1	1.1	33.9	0.0	0.0	0.0	0.2	0.0	0.0	0.2	0.0	3.1
1.7	5.2	0.0	25.8	1.0	15.1	167.6	0.0	0.0	0.0	0.0	0.1	0.1	1.2	0.0	12.2
0.4	0.7	0.0	2.0	0.1	4.0	26.4	0.1	0.0	0.0	0.0	0.0	0.0	0.2	0.0	1.6
0.4	0.7	0.0	2.0	0.1	4.0	9.9	0.1	0.0	0.0	0.0	0.0	0.0	0.2	0.0	1.6
0.0	0.2	0.1	0.9	0.0	0.2	2.7	0.0	0.2	0.0	0.0	0.0	0.0	0.0	0.0	0.5
0.4	0.2	0.0	3.3	1.2	3.9	95.4	0.1	0.0	0.0	0.0	0.1	0.1	0.9	0.0	18.6
0.0	1.5	0.0	1.4	0.0	0.0	11.9	0.0	1.4	0.0	0.2	0.0	0.0	0.0	0.0	0.0
0.0	0.7	0.0	0.4	0.0	0.1	3.6	0.0	0.4	0.0	0.0	0.0	0.0	0.0	0.0	0.0
0.0	38.9	12.7	265.8	0.1	23.3	113.3	0.9	4.7	2.2	0.3	0.1	0.4	0.2	0.0	27.7
0.0	1.7	5.5	15.7	0.0	1.5	6.1	0.1	16.1	0.1	0.0	0.0	0.0	0.0	0.0	0.4
0.0	5.6	20.6	9.7	0.0	1.1	5.6	0.0	63.2	0.1	0.1	0.0	0.0	0.0	0.0	0.6
0.0	4.6	16.7	10.4	0.0	1.1	5.1	0.0	44.3	0.1	0.1	0.0	0.0	0.0	0.0	0.6
0.0	2.5	5.3	14.0	0.0	1.3	6.4	0.0	23.4	0.1	0.1	0.0	0.0	0.0	0.0	1.3
0.0	5.7	0.0	0.7	0.1	1.9	29.6	0.3	0.0	0.0	0.0	0.0	0.0	0.0	0.0	0.0
0.0	3.6	11.6	31.3	0.0	3.0	12.2	0.2	33.6	0.3	0.1	0.0	0.0	0.0	0.0	3.2
0.0	0.7	2.3	3.0	0.0	0.3	3.9	0.0	6.2	0.0	0.0	0.0	0.0	0.0	0.0	0.1

Code	Food Name	Unit Amount	Kilocalories (kcal)	Protein (g)	Carbohydrate (g)
18242	Croutons, plain	1 cup	122.1	3.6	22.1
18243	Croutons, seasoned	4 cubes	4.7	0.1	0.6
919168	Custard, egg, baked, homemade	1/2 cup	148.1	7.2	15.1
19205	Custard, egg, dry mix prep w/reduced-fat (2%) milk	1 cup	297.9	11.2	47.1
919186	Dessert, apple crisp, homemade	1/2 cup	229.8	2.5	45.5
919094	Dessert, flan (caramel custard) homemade	1/2 cup	220.3	6.9	34.9
902923	Dip, jalapeno bean	1.0 oz	33.0	1.5	2.9
18251	Donut, cake, chocolate w/sugar or glaze	1 small donut (3″ diam)	175.1	1.9	24.1
18249	Donut, cake, plain w/chocolate icing	1 small donut (2″ diam)	132.7	1.4	13.4
18250	Donut, cake, plain w/sugar or glaze	1.0 oz	120.8	1.5	14.4
918865	Donut, cake/Hostess	1 donut	110.0	1.0	12.0
918866	Donut, chocolate/Hostess	1 donut	129.9	1.0	14.0
918867	Donut, cinnamon/Hostess	1 donut	110.0	1.0	15.0
18253	Donut, French cruller, glazed	1 cruller (3″ diam)	168.9	1.3	24.4
918868	Donut, powdered sugar/Hostess	1 mini donut	110.0	1.0	15.0
18254	Donut, yeast-leavened, cream-filled	1 donut (3.5″ x 2.5″ oval)	306.9	5.4	25.5
18256	Donut, yeast-leavened, jelly	1 donut (3.5″ x 2.5″ oval)	289.0	5.0	33.2
18255	Donut/honey bun, yeast-leavened, glazed	1 extra large (~ 5″ diam)	491.7	7.8	54.0
924066	Egg Foo Young/LaChoy	2 patties	159.6	8.0	19.0
924181	Egg souffle w/cheese	1 cup	207.1	9.4	5.9
924182	Egg souffle w/spinach, frozen/Stouffer	4.0 oz	141.3	6.7	9.4
901910	Egg substitute, Country Morning	1/2 cup	173.0	14.6	1.3
1142	Egg substitute, frozen	1/4 cup	95.9	6.8	1.9
1143	Egg substitute, liquid	1 Tbsp.	13.2	1.9	0.1
901912	Egg substitute, scramblend	1/2 cup	142.8	12.1	3.0
924272	Egg & cheese bagel, frozen/Swanson	3.6 oz	256.0	12.7	29.0
924323	Egg, omelet w/bacon & onion	6.5 oz	364.6	17.4	12.7
924322	Egg, omelet w/cheese	4.0 oz	313.0	15.9	1.3
924012	Egg, quiche lorraine	1 slice	600.2	13.0	29.0
1128	Egg, whole, fried	1 large egg	91.5	6.2	0.6
1129	Egg, whole, hard-cooked	1 large egg	77.5	6.3	0.6
1130	Egg, whole, omelet	1 Tbsp.	23.1	1.6	0.2
1131	Egg, whole, poached	1 large egg	74.5	6.2	0.6
1123	Egg, whole, raw	1 large egg	74.5	6.2	0.6
1132	Egg, whole, scrambled	1 large egg	101.3	6.8	1.3
1125	Egg, yolk, raw, fresh	1 large egg yolk	59.4	2.8	0.3
18260	English muffin, mixed-grain/granola	1 muffin	155.1	6.0	30.6
18258	English muffin, plain/sourdough, enriched	1 muffin	134.0	4.4	26.2
18262	English muffin, raisin-cinn/apple cinnamon	1 muffin	138.5	4.3	27.8
18264	English muffin, wheat	1 muffin	127.1	5.0	25.5
18266	English muffin, whole-wheat	1 muffin	134.0	5.8	26.7
921897	Fast food, apple pie/McD	1 pie	259.8	2.2	30.0
921915	Fast food, bean burrito/TB	1 burrito	447.0	15.0	63.0
921916	Fast food, beef burrito/TB	1 burrito	492.3	25.0	48.0
921805	Fast food, biscuit/MCD	1 biscuit	260.3	4.6	31.9
921919	Fast Food, burrito supreme/TB	1 burrito	502.4	20.0	55.0
21069	Fast food, burrito w/apples or cherries	1 small burrito	230.9	2.5	35.0
21060	Fast food, burrito w/beans	2 burritos	447.0	14.1	71.4
21061	Fast food, burrito w/beans & cheese	2 burritos	377.6	15.1	55.0
21063	Fast food, burrito w/beans & meat	2 burritos	508.2	22.5	66.0
21064	Fast food, burrito w/beans, cheese, & beef	2 burritos	330.9	14.6	39.7
21066	Fast food, burrito w/beef	2 burritos	523.6	26.6	58.5
21068	Fast food, burrito w/beef, cheese, & chili peppers	2 burritos	632.3	40.9	63.7
921813	Fast food, chicken center breast, extra crispy/KFC	1 piece	341.6	33.0	11.7
921867	Fast food, chicken center breast, original recipe/KFC	1 piece	282.9	27.5	8.8
921812	Fast food, chicken drumstick, extra crispy/KFC	1 piece	204.2	13.6	6.1
921866	Fast food, chicken drumstick, original recipe/KFC	1 piece	145.9	13.1	4.2
921946	Fast food, Chicken McNuggets/McD	1 serving	290.4	19.0	16.5
921884	Fast food, Chicken Peg Legs/Long John	5 pieces	350.0	22.0	26.0
921876	Fast food, Chicken Planks/Long John	4 pieces	456.5	27.0	35.0
921963	Fast food, Chicken Strips/JB	4 pieces	348.8	29.0	28.0
921800	Fast food, Chicken Tenders/BK	6 pieces	235.8	16.0	14.0
921815	Fast food, chicken thigh, extra crispy/KFC	1 piece	405.8	20.0	14.4
921869	Fast food, chicken thigh, original recipe/KFC	1 piece	294.3	17.9	11.1
921816	Fast food, chicken wing, extra crispy/KFC	1 piece	254.2	12.4	9.3

Dietary Fiber (g)	Total Fat (g)	Cholesterol (mg)	Calcium (mg)	Iron (mg)	Magnesium (mg)	Sodium (mg)	Zinc (mg)	Vitamin A (μgRE)	Vitamin C (mg)	Vitamin E (mgαT)	Thiamin (mg)	Riboflavin (mg)	Niacin (mg)	Vitamin B₆ (mg)	Folate (μg)
1.5	2.0	0.0	22.8	1.2	9.3	209.4	0.3	0.0	0.0	0.0	0.2	0.1	1.6	0.0	39.6
0.1	0.2	0.1	1.0	0.0	0.4	12.4	0.0	0.1	0.0	0.0	0.0	0.0	0.0	0.0	0.9
0.0	6.6	2.1	157.9	0.4	19.7	108.6	0.7	84.6	0.7	0.0	0.0	0.3	0.1	0.1	14.1
0.0	7.4	149.0	393.7	0.7	53.2	399.0	1.4	149.0	2.1	0.0	0.1	0.6	0.3	0.2	21.3
2.4	5.1	2.2	39.5	1.1	9.9	256.6	0.2	43.7	3.2	0.0	0.1	0.1	1.1	0.1	7.1
0.0	6.3	2.1	131.6	0.5	16.8	85.7	0.7	87.2	0.8	0.0	0.0	0.3	0.1	0.1	13.8
0.3	1.1	1.0	7.0	0.4	0.0	163.0	0.1	8.4	0.0	0.0	0.0	0.0	1.1	0.0	0.0
0.9	8.4	23.9	89.5	1.0	14.3	142.8	0.2	4.6	0.0	1.1	0.0	0.0	0.2	0.0	16.0
0.6	8.7	17.1	9.8	0.7	11.2	120.1	0.2	3.1	0.1	1.2	0.0	0.0	0.4	0.0	8.1
0.4	6.5	9.1	17.0	0.3	4.8	114.0	0.1	0.9	0.0	0.0	0.1	0.1	0.4	0.0	13.0
0.5	7.0	7.0	12.0	0.4	0.0	135.0	0.0	0.0	0.0	0.0	0.1	0.0	0.5	0.0	0.0
0.5	8.0	4.0	10.0	0.4	0.0	150.0	0.0	0.0	0.0	0.0	0.0	0.0	0.3	0.0	0.0
0.5	6.0	6.0	10.0	0.3	0.0	140.0	0.0	0.0	0.0	0.0	0.0	0.0	0.4	0.0	0.0
0.5	7.5	4.5	10.7	1.0	4.9	141.5	0.1	1.2	0.0	1.0	0.1	0.1	0.9	0.0	14.4
0.5	5.0	6.0	9.0	0.3	0.0	140.0	0.0	0.0	0.0	0.0	0.0	0.0	0.4	0.0	0.0
0.7	20.8	20.4	21.3	1.6	17.0	262.7	0.7	16.2	0.0	2.3	0.3	0.1	1.9	0.1	54.4
0.7	15.9	22.1	21.3	1.5	17.0	249.1	0.6	13.6	0.0	2.1	0.3	0.1	1.8	0.1	52.7
1.5	27.8	7.3	52.5	2.5	26.8	417.2	0.9	4.9	0.1	3.7	0.4	0.3	3.5	0.1	52.5
1.0	7.0	275.0	60.0	1.8	0.0	1250.0	0.0	50.0	0.0	0.0	1.2	0.1	0.0	0.0	0.0
0.0	16.2	184.0	191.0	1.0	0.0	346.0	1.2	152.0	0.0	0.0	0.1	0.2	0.2	0.0	0.0
0.0	8.6	88.0	107.0	1.5	0.0	599.0	0.0	316.4	4.0	0.0	0.1	0.3	0.5	0.0	0.0
0.0	12.1	594.0	52.0	2.1	0.0	180.0	0.0	227.6	0.0	0.0	0.1	0.5	0.0	0.0	0.0
0.0	6.7	1.2	43.7	1.2	9.0	119.6	0.6	81.0	0.3	1.3	0.1	0.2	0.1	0.1	9.8
0.0	0.5	0.2	8.3	0.3	1.4	27.8	0.2	33.9	0.0	0.1	0.0	0.0	0.0	0.0	2.3
0.0	9.1	466.0	77.0	1.7	0.0	173.0	0.0	214.2	0.0	0.0	0.1	0.4	0.0	0.0	0.0
0.0	9.9	0.0	137.0	2.1	0.0	621.0	0.0	55.8	0.0	0.0	0.2	0.4	1.6	0.0	0.0
0.1	27.1	365.0	267.0	2.2	0.0	1148.0	0.0	141.8	2.0	0.0	0.2	0.5	1.2	0.0	0.0
0.0	27.1	328.0	245.0	1.6	0.0	398.0	0.0	0.0	0.0	0.0	0.1	0.0	0.0	0.0	0.0
1.0	48.0	285.0	211.0	1.0	0.0	653.0	2.0	328.0	0.0	0.0	0.1	0.3	0.0	0.1	17.0
0.0	6.9	211.1	25.3	0.7	5.1	162.4	0.5	114.1	0.0	0.8	0.0	0.2	0.0	0.1	17.5
0.0	5.3	212.0	25.0	0.6	5.0	62.0	0.5	84.0	0.0	0.5	0.0	0.3	0.0	0.1	22.0
0.0	1.7	53.2	6.4	0.2	1.4	41.0	0.1	28.4	0.0	0.2	0.0	0.1	0.0	0.0	4.4
0.0	5.0	211.5	24.5	0.7	5.0	140.0	0.6	95.0	0.0	0.5	0.0	0.2	0.0	0.1	17.5
0.0	5.0	212.5	24.5	0.7	5.0	63.0	0.6	95.5	0.0	0.5	0.0	0.3	0.0	0.1	23.5
0.0	7.4	214.7	43.3	0.7	7.3	170.8	0.6	119.0	0.1	0.8	0.0	0.3	0.0	0.1	18.3
0.0	5.1	212.6	22.7	0.6	1.5	7.1	0.5	96.9	0.0	0.5	0.0	0.1	0.0	0.1	24.2
1.8	1.2	0.0	129.4	2.0	27.1	274.6	0.9	0.0	0.0	0.2	0.3	0.2	2.4	0.0	52.8
1.5	1.0	0.0	99.2	1.4	12.0	264.5	0.4	0.0	0.0	0.1	0.3	0.2	2.2	0.0	46.2
1.7	1.5	0.0	83.8	1.4	8.6	254.8	0.6	0.0	0.2	0.2	0.2	0.2	2.0	0.0	46.2
2.6	1.1	0.0	101.5	1.6	21.1	217.7	0.6	0.0	0.0	0.3	0.2	0.2	1.9	0.0	31.4
4.4	1.4	0.0	174.9	1.6	46.9	420.4	1.1	0.0	0.0	0.5	0.2	0.1	2.3	0.1	27.7
0.5	14.8	6.0	11.0	0.7	0.0	240.0	0.2	0.0	11.0	0.0	0.1	0.0	0.3	0.0	5.0
9.6	14.0	9.0	144.0	2.6	0.0	1148.0	2.4	156.0	2.4	0.0	0.8	0.5	3.3	1.2	66.0
2.2	21.0	57.0	113.0	2.4	0.0	1311.0	4.4	22.0	2.2	0.0	0.3	0.5	3.7	0.2	30.0
0.5	12.7	1.0	75.0	1.3	0.0	730.0	0.3	0.0	0.0	0.0	0.2	0.1	1.7	0.0	9.0
5.8	22.0	33.0	163.0	2.5	0.0	1181.0	3.5	212.8	10.4	0.0	0.5	0.5	3.6	0.6	46.0
0.0	9.5	3.7	15.5	1.1	7.4	211.6	0.4	37.0	0.7	0.0	0.2	0.2	1.9	0.1	24.4
0.0	13.5	4.3	112.8	4.5	86.8	985.2	1.5	32.6	2.0	0.0	0.6	0.6	4.1	0.3	86.8
0.0	11.7	27.9	213.9	2.3	80.0	1166.2	1.6	238.1	1.7	0.0	0.2	0.7	3.6	0.2	74.4
0.0	17.8	48.5	106.3	4.9	83.2	1335.2	3.8	64.7	1.8	0.0	0.5	0.8	5.4	0.4	115.5
0.0	13.3	123.8	129.9	3.7	50.8	990.6	2.4	150.2	5.1	0.0	0.3	0.7	3.9	0.2	75.1
0.0	20.8	63.8	83.6	6.1	81.4	1491.6	4.7	28.6	1.1	0.0	0.2	0.9	6.4	0.3	129.8
0.0	24.8	170.2	221.9	7.8	69.9	2091.5	7.9	112.5	3.6	0.0	0.6	1.2	8.3	0.4	139.8
0.5	19.7	114.0	33.0	0.9	0.0	790.0	0.7	12.0	0.0	0.0	0.1	0.1	13.1	0.3	8.0
0.1	15.3	93.0	36.0	1.0	0.0	672.0	0.7	12.0	0.0	0.0	0.1	0.2	11.5	0.3	8.0
0.5	13.9	71.0	13.0	0.7	0.0	324.0	1.3	8.0	0.0	0.0	0.1	0.1	3.7	0.2	6.0
0.1	8.5	67.0	21.0	1.1	0.0	275.0	1.3	6.0	1.0	0.0	0.1	0.1	3.2	0.1	4.0
0.5	16.3	65.0	13.0	1.0	0.0	520.0	0.9	0.0	0.0	0.0	0.1	0.1	9.0	0.4	11.0
0.5	28.0	0.0	0.0	0.0	0.0	0.0	0.0	0.0	0.0	0.0	0.0	0.0	0.0	0.0	0.0
1.0	23.0	0.0	0.0	0.0	0.0	0.0	0.0	0.0	0.0	0.0	0.0	0.0	0.0	0.0	0.0
0.0	14.0	68.0	0.0	0.0	0.0	748.0	0.0	0.0	0.0	0.0	0.0	0.0	0.0	0.0	0.0
0.0	13.0	46.0	18.0	0.7	24.0	541.0	0.6	19.0	0.0	0.0	0.1	0.1	7.3	0.3	10.0
0.5	29.9	129.0	49.0	1.2	0.0	688.0	1.7	26.2	0.0	0.0	0.1	0.2	6.5	0.2	9.0
0.1	19.7	123.0	65.0	1.3	0.0	619.0	1.7	20.8	0.0	0.0	0.1	0.3	5.5	0.2	9.0
0.5	18.6	67.0	18.0	0.6	0.0	422.0	0.6	6.0	0.0	0.0	0.0	0.1	3.3	0.1	5.0

Code	Food Name	Unit Amount	Kilocalories (kcal)	Protein (g)	Carbohydrate (g)
921870	Fast food, chicken wing, original recipe/KFC	1 piece	178.2	12.2	6.0
921807	Fast food, chicken, Hot Wings/KFC	6 pieces	376.0	22.4	17.3
21042	Fast food, chili con carne	8 fl oz cup	255.5	24.6	21.9
921927	Fast food, chili/Wendy	1 serving	219.3	21.0	23.0
21070	Fast food, chimichanga w/beef	1 chimichanga	424.6	19.6	42.8
21071	Fast food, chimichanga w/beef & cheese	1 chimichanga	442.9	20.1	39.3
921951	Fast food, chocolate chip cookies/McD	1 box	329.8	4.2	41.9
21043	Fast food, clams (shellfish) breaded, fried	1 Tbsp.	37.6	1.1	3.2
921896	Fast food, cookies, McDonaldland	1 box	290.1	4.2	47.1
21128	Fast food, corn on the cob w/butter	1 ear	154.8	4.5	31.9
921044	Fast food, crab (shellfish) baked	1 crab	160.2	28.5	4.2
921045	Fast food, crab (shellfish) soft shell, fried	1 crab	333.8	11.0	31.2
21046	Fast food, crab cake (shellfish)	1 cake	159.6	11.3	5.1
21015	Fast food, Danish pastry, cheese	1 pastry	353.1	5.8	28.7
21016	Fast food, Danish pastry, cinnamon	1 pastry	349.4	4.8	46.9
21017	Fast food, Danish pastry, fruit	1 pastry	334.6	4.8	45.1
21074	Fast food, enchilada w/cheese	1 enchilada	319.5	9.6	28.5
21075	Fast food, enchilada w/cheese & beef	1 enchilada	322.6	11.9	30.5
21076	Fast food, enchirito w/cheese, beef & beans	1 enchirito	343.5	17.9	33.8
921933	Fast food, Fish Tenders/BK	1 serving	267.3	12.0	18.0
921879	Fast food, fish, 2 pieces/Long John	2 pieces	651.4	30.0	53.0
921986	Fast food, French fries, large/Hardee	1 large	360.5	4.0	48.0
921984	Fast food, French fries, regular/Hardee	1 regular	230.0	3.0	30.0
921837	Fast food, French fries, small/DQ	1 small	200.2	2.0	25.0
21024	Fast food, French toast sticks	5 sticks	513.2	8.3	57.9
21077	Fast food, frijoles (beans) w/cheese	8.0 oz	225.5	11.4	28.7
921834	Fast food, frozen dessert, Freeze/DQ	1 serving, 14.0 oz	500.2	9.0	89.0
921835	Fast food, frozen dessert, Mr Misty Freeze/DQ	1 serving, 15.0 oz	501.4	9.0	91.0
921841	Fast food, frozen dessert, Mr Misty Kiss/DQ	1 serving 3.0 oz	70.3	0.0	17.0
921842	Fast food, frozen dessert/DQ	1 serving 4.0 oz	179.7	5.0	27.0
921802	Fast food, ham & cheese sandwich	1 sandwich	471.5	24.0	44.0
21202	Fast food, hamburger, large, one meat patty w/condiments	1 sandwich	425.3	23.0	36.7
921895	Fast food, hot cakes w/butter & syrup/McD	1 serving	410.1	8.2	74.4
21119	Fast food, hot dog w/chili, plain	1 hot dog	296.4	13.5	31.3
21120	Fast food, hot dog w/corn-flour coating, corn dog	1 hot dog	460.3	16.8	55.8
21118	Fast food, hot dog, plain	1 hot dog	242.1	10.4	18.0
21129	Fast food, hush puppies	5 hush puppies	256.6	4.9	34.9
921850	Fast food, ice cream cone, dipped, regular/DQ	1 regular	340.1	6.0	42.0
921849	Fast food, ice cream cone, dipped, small/DQ	1 small	190.3	3.0	25.0
921847	Fast food, ice cream cone, regular/DQ	1 regular	240.0	6.0	38.0
921846	Fast food, ice cream cone, small/DQ	1 small	139.9	3.0	22.0
921852	Fast food, ice cream parfait/DQ	1 serving	428.8	8.0	76.0
921853	Fast food, ice cream sandwich/DQ	1 sandwich	139.8	3.0	24.0
921859	Fast food, ice cream sundae, regular/DQ	1 regular	309.8	5.0	56.0
921858	Fast food, ice cream sundae, small/DQ	1 small	189.7	3.0	33.0
921823	Fast food, ice cream, banana split/DQ	1 split	540.0	9.0	103.0
921824	Fast food, ice cream, Buster Bar/DQ	1 bar	460.6	10.0	41.0
921829	Fast food, ice cream, Dilly Bar/DQ	1 bar	210.0	3.0	21.0
921832	Fast food, ice cream, float/DQ	1 serving	408.9	5.0	82.0
921839	Fast food, ice cream, malt, regular/DQ	1 regular	760.8	14.0	134.0
921838	Fast food, ice cream, malt, small/DQ	1 small	520.9	10.0	91.0
21028	Fast food, ice milk cone, soft, vanilla	1 cone	163.8	3.9	24.1
14346	Fast food, milk beverage, chocolate shake/McD	1 fl oz	26.4	0.7	4.3
14428	Fast food, milk beverage, strawberry shake	10 fl oz	319.8	9.6	53.5
14347	Fast food, shake, vanilla/McD	1 fl oz	23.1	0.7	3.7
21078	Fast food, nachos w/cheese	6–8 nachos	345.8	9.1	36.3
21079	Fast food, nachos w/cheese & jalapeno peppers	6–8 nachos	607.9	16.8	60.1
21080	Fast food, nachos w/cheese, beans, ground beef, & peppers	6–8 nachos	568.7	19.8	55.8
21081	Fast food, nachos w/cinnamon & sugar	6–8 nachos	591.9	7.2	63.4
21130	Fast food, onion rings, breaded, fried	8–9 onion rings	275.6	3.7	31.3
21048	Fast food, oysters (shellfish) battered/breaded, fried	6 oysters	368.4	12.5	39.9
21025	Fast food, pancakes w/butter & syrup	3 cakes	519.7	8.3	90.9
21049	Fast food, pizza w/cheese	1 slice (1/8 12"-pizza)	140.5	7.7	20.5
21050	Fast food, pizza w/cheese, meat, & veges	1 slice (1/8 12"-pizza)	184.1	13.0	21.3
21051	Fast food, pizza w/pepperoni	1 slice (1/8 12"-pizza)	181.1	10.1	19.9

Dietary Fiber (g)	Total Fat (g)	Cholesterol (mg)	Calcium (mg)	Iron (mg)	Magnesium (mg)	Sodium (mg)	Zinc (mg)	Vitamin A (μgRE)	Vitamin C (mg)	Vitamin E (mgαT)	Thiamin (mg)	Riboflavin (mg)	Niacin (mg)	Vitamin B₆ (mg)	Folate (μg)
0.2	11.7	64.0	48.0	1.2	0.0	372.0	0.6	11.2	0.0	0.0	0.0	0.1	3.7	0.1	4.0
0.5	24.1	148.0	0.0	0.0	0.0	677.0	0.0	0.0	0.0	0.0	0.0	0.0	0.0	0.0	0.0
0.0	8.3	134.1	68.3	5.2	45.5	1006.9	3.6	167.0	1.5	0.0	0.1	1.1	2.5	0.3	45.5
6.0	7.0	45.0	64.0	4.5	0.0	750.0	3.8	237.6	6.0	0.0	0.2	0.2	3.0	0.3	40.0
0.0	19.7	8.7	62.6	4.5	62.6	910.0	5.0	15.7	4.7	0.0	0.5	0.6	5.8	0.3	83.5
0.0	23.4	51.2	237.9	3.8	60.4	957.1	3.4	126.3	2.7	0.0	0.4	0.9	4.7	0.2	91.5
1.0	15.6	4.0	24.0	2.2	0.0	280.0	0.5	0.0	0.0	0.0	0.2	0.2	2.5	0.0	6.0
0.0	2.2	7.3	1.7	0.3	2.6	69.6	0.1	3.1	0.0	0.0	0.0	0.0	0.2	0.0	3.6
1.0	9.2	10.0	9.0	2.1	0.0	300.0	0.3	0.0	0.0	0.0	0.2	0.2	2.5	0.0	6.0
0.0	3.4	5.8	4.4	0.9	40.9	29.2	0.9	96.4	6.9	0.0	0.2	0.1	2.2	0.3	43.8
0.0	2.3	0.6	415.3	1.4	81.8	549.4	7.0	22.9	2.6	0.0	0.3	0.2	4.5	0.5	20.7
0.0	17.9	7.7	55.0	1.8	25.0	1117.5	1.1	3.8	0.8	0.0	0.1	0.1	1.8	0.2	20.0
0.2	10.4	82.2	202.2	1.1	25.2	491.4	2.1	82.2	0.2	0.0	0.1	0.1	1.2	0.1	24.6
0.0	24.6	20.0	70.1	1.8	15.5	319.4	0.6	42.8	2.6	0.0	0.3	0.2	2.5	0.1	54.6
0.0	16.7	27.3	37.0	1.8	14.1	326.5	0.5	5.3	2.6	0.0	0.3	0.2	2.2	0.1	54.6
0.0	15.9	18.8	21.6	1.4	14.1	332.8	0.5	24.4	1.6	0.0	0.3	0.2	1.8	0.1	31.0
0.0	18.8	44.0	324.4	1.3	50.5	784.0	2.5	185.8	1.0	0.0	0.1	0.4	1.9	0.4	65.2
0.0	17.6	40.3	228.5	3.1	82.6	1319.0	2.7	142.1	1.3	0.0	0.1	0.4	2.5	0.3	67.2
0.0	16.1	50.2	218.1	2.4	71.4	1250.6	2.8	133.2	4.6	0.0	0.2	0.7	3.0	0.2	59.8
0.0	16.0	28.0	0.0	0.0	0.0	870.0	0.0	0.0	0.0	0.0	0.0	0.0	0.0	0.0	0.0
1.0	36.0	27.0	0.0	0.0	0.0	1543.0	0.0	0.0	0.0	0.0	0.0	0.0	0.0	0.0	0.0
1.8	17.0	0.0	19.0	1.0	0.0	135.0	0.1	0.0	16.0	0.0	0.1	0.0	0.6	0.0	0.0
1.2	11.0	0.0	12.0	1.0	0.0	85.0	0.1	0.0	10.0	0.0	0.1	0.0	1.0	0.0	0.0
1.0	10.0	10.0	0.0	0.3	16.0	115.0	0.0	0.0	9.0	0.0	0.1	0.0	0.8	0.2	15.0
2.7	29.0	74.7	77.6	3.0	26.8	499.1	0.9	12.7	0.0	4.0	0.2	0.3	3.0	0.3	81.8
0.0	7.8	36.7	188.7	2.2	85.2	881.8	1.7	70.1	1.5	0.0	0.1	0.3	1.5	0.2	111.9
0.0	12.0	30.0	300.0	1.8	0.0	180.0	0.0	80.0	0.0	0.0	0.2	0.5	0.0	0.0	0.0
0.0	12.0	30.0	300.0	1.4	0.0	140.0	0.0	80.0	0.0	0.0	0.1	0.5	0.0	0.0	0.0
0.0	0.0	0.0	0.0	0.0	0.0	10.0	0.0	0.0	0.0	0.0	0.0	0.0	0.0	0.0	0.0
0.0	6.0	20.0	150.0	0.0	0.0	0.0	0.0	20.0	0.0	0.0	0.1	0.2	0.0	0.0	0.0
0.5	23.0	70.0	195.0	3.2	42.0	1534.0	2.4	170.0	7.0	0.0	0.9	0.4	6.0	0.3	25.0
2.1	20.9	70.3	133.8	4.1	34.3	728.9	4.8	0.0	2.6	0.0	0.3	0.3	6.5	0.2	61.7
1.0	9.3	21.0	114.0	2.1	0.0	640.0	0.7	34.6	0.0	0.0	0.3	0.3	2.8	0.1	9.0
0.0	13.4	51.3	19.4	3.3	10.3	479.9	0.8	5.7	2.7	0.0	0.2	0.4	3.7	0.0	73.0
0.0	18.9	78.8	101.5	6.2	17.5	973.0	1.3	36.8	0.0	0.0	0.3	0.7	4.2	0.1	103.3
0.0	14.5	44.1	23.5	2.3	12.7	670.3	2.0	0.0	0.1	0.0	0.2	0.3	3.6	0.0	48.0
0.0	11.6	134.9	68.6	1.4	16.4	964.9	0.4	26.5	0.0	0.0	0.0	0.0	2.0	0.1	13.3
0.0	16.0	20.0	150.0	0.7	0.0	100.0	0.7	40.0	0.0	0.0	0.1	0.3	0.0	0.1	3.0
0.0	9.0	10.0	100.0	0.4	0.0	55.0	0.5	40.0	0.0	0.0	0.1	0.3	0.0	0.0	2.0
0.0	7.0	15.0	150.0	0.7	0.0	80.0	0.7	40.0	0.0	0.0	0.1	0.3	0.0	0.1	3.0
0.0	4.0	10.0	100.0	0.4	0.0	45.0	0.5	20.0	0.0	0.0	0.0	0.2	0.0	0.0	2.0
0.5	8.0	30.0	250.0	1.4	0.0	140.0	0.0	80.0	0.0	0.0	0.1	0.4	0.4	0.0	0.0
0.5	4.0	5.0	60.0	0.0	0.0	40.0	0.0	20.0	0.0	0.0	0.0	0.1	0.4	0.0	0.0
0.5	8.0	20.0	200.0	1.1	0.0	120.0	0.9	40.0	0.0	0.0	0.1	0.3	0.3	0.1	4.0
0.5	4.0	10.0	100.0	0.4	0.0	75.0	0.5	20.0	0.0	0.0	0.0	0.2	0.2	0.0	2.0
1.0	11.0	30.0	250.0	1.8	0.0	150.0	2.1	150.0	15.0	0.0	0.1	0.5	0.4	0.8	9.0
0.5	29.0	10.0	100.0	1.1	0.0	175.0	0.0	20.0	0.0	0.0	0.1	0.2	2.0	0.0	0.0
0.5	13.0	10.0	100.0	0.4	0.0	50.0	0.0	20.0	0.0	0.0	0.0	0.2	0.0	0.0	0.0
0.0	7.0	20.0	200.0	1.1	0.0	85.0	0.0	40.0	0.0	0.0	0.1	0.3	0.0	0.0	0.0
0.5	18.0	50.0	450.0	4.5	0.0	260.0	0.1	150.0	0.0	0.0	0.3	0.8	0.8	0.2	4.0
0.5	13.0	35.0	350.0	2.7	0.0	180.0	0.1	100.0	0.0	0.0	0.2	0.6	0.4	0.1	3.0
0.1	6.1	27.8	153.5	0.2	15.5	91.7	0.6	51.5	1.1	0.4	0.1	0.3	0.3	0.1	12.4
0.2	0.8	2.7	23.5	0.1	3.5	20.2	0.1	4.8	0.1	0.0	0.0	0.1	0.0	0.0	0.7
1.1	7.9	31.1	319.8	0.3	36.8	234.9	1.0	82.1	2.3	0.0	0.1	0.6	0.5	0.1	8.5
0.1	0.6	2.3	25.4	0.0	2.5	17.1	0.1	6.7	0.2	0.0	0.0	0.0	0.0	0.0	0.7
0.0	19.0	18.1	272.3	1.3	55.4	815.9	1.8	91.5	1.2	0.0	0.2	0.4	1.5	0.2	10.2
0.0	34.1	83.6	620.2	2.4	108.1	1736.0	2.9	471.2	1.0	0.0	0.1	0.5	2.8	0.4	18.4
0.0	30.7	20.4	385.1	2.8	96.9	1800.3	3.6	469.2	4.8	0.0	0.2	0.7	3.3	0.4	38.3
0.0	36.0	39.2	85.0	2.9	19.6	439.3	0.6	10.9	8.0	0.0	0.2	0.4	3.9	0.2	7.6
0.0	15.5	14.1	73.0	0.8	15.8	429.9	0.3	0.8	0.6	0.3	0.1	0.1	0.9	0.1	54.8
0.0	17.9	108.4	27.8	4.5	23.6	676.9	15.6	108.4	4.2	0.0	0.3	0.3	4.4	0.0	30.6
0.0	14.0	58.0	127.6	2.6	48.7	1104.3	1.0	69.6	3.5	1.4	0.4	0.6	3.4	0.1	30.2
0.0	3.2	9.5	116.6	0.6	15.8	335.8	0.8	73.7	1.3	0.0	0.2	0.2	2.5	0.0	34.7
0.0	5.4	20.5	101.1	1.5	18.2	382.4	1.1	101.1	1.6	0.0	0.2	0.2	2.0	0.1	32.4
0.0	7.0	14.2	64.6	0.9	8.5	267.0	0.5	54.7	1.6	0.0	0.1	0.2	3.0	0.1	36.9

Code	Food Name	Unit Amount	Kilocalories (kcal)	Protein (g)	Carbohydrate (g)
921911	Fast food, pizza, cheese pan/PH	2 slices	492.0	30.0	57.0
921906	Fast food, pizza, cheese, thin/PH	2 slices	398.1	28.0	37.0
921912	Fast food, pizza, pepperoni Pan/PH	2 slices	540.2	29.0	62.0
921905	Fast food, pizza, pepperoni, personal/PH	1 pizza	675.8	37.0	76.0
921907	Fast food, pizza, pepperoni, thin/PH	2 slices	413.2	26.0	36.0
921913	Fast food, pizza, super supreme pan/PH	2 slices	562.8	33.0	53.0
921908	Fast food, pizza, super supreme, thin/PH	2 slices	462.8	29.0	44.0
921914	Fast food, pizza, supreme pan/PH	2 slices	589.1	32.0	53.0
921910	Fast food, pizza, supreme personal/PH	1 pizza	646.8	33.0	76.0
921909	Fast food, pizza, supreme, thin/PH	2 slices	460.0	28.0	41.0
21132	Fast food, potato, baked, topped w/cheese & bacon	1 potato	451.5	18.4	44.4
21133	Fast food, potato, baked, topped w/cheese & broccoli	1 potato	403.4	13.7	46.6
21134	Fast food, potato, baked, topped w/cheese & chili	1 potato	481.9	23.2	55.9
21131	Fast food, potato, baked, topped w/cheese sauce	1 potato	473.6	14.6	46.5
21135	Fast food, potato, baked, topped w/sour cream & chives	1 potato	392.6	6.7	50.0
21139	Fast food, potato, mashed	1 Tbsp.	12.5	0.3	2.4
21026	Fast food, potatoes, hash brown	1 Tbsp.	18.9	0.2	2.0
21122	Fast food, roast beef sandwich w/cheese	1 sandwich	473.4	32.2	45.4
21121	Fast food, roast beef sandwich, plain	1 sandwich	346.1	21.5	33.4
4021	Fast food, salad dressing, Italian, w/salt, diet (2 kcal/tsp.)	1 Tbsp.	15.8	0.0	0.7
4025	Fast food, salad dressing, mayonnaise, soybean oil, w/salt	1 cup	1577.0	2.4	5.9
921983	Fast food, salad, chef/Hardee	1 salad	241.1	22.0	5.0
921864	Fast food, salad, chunky chicken/BK	1 salad	141.9	20.0	8.0
21127	Fast food, salad, cole slaw	1 Tbsp.	12.3	0.1	1.1
921871	Fast food, salad, cole slaw/KFC	1 serving	119.2	1.5	13.2
921803	Fast food, salad, garden/BK	1 salad	95.9	6.0	8.0
21140	Fast food, salad, potato	1 Tbsp.	20.3	0.3	2.4
21083	Fast food, salad, taco	1 Tbsp.	11.4	0.5	1.0
21084	Fast food, salad, taco w/chili con carne	1 Tbsp.	12.1	0.7	1.1
921974	Fast food, sandwich, beef & cheddar/Arby	1 sandwich	490.6	24.0	51.0
921981	Fast food, sandwich, Big Deluxe Hamburger/Hardee	1 burger	499.0	27.0	32.0
921971	Fast food, sandwich, Big Roast Beef/Hardee	1 sandwich	300.2	18.0	32.0
921989	Fast food, sandwich, Big Twin/Hardee	1 sandwich	449.8	23.0	34.0
21002	Fast food, sandwich, biscuit w/egg	1 biscuit	315.5	11.1	24.2
21003	Fast food, sandwich, biscuit w/egg & bacon	1 biscuit	457.5	17.0	28.6
21004	Fast food, sandwich, biscuit w/egg & ham	1 biscuit	441.6	20.4	30.3
21005	Fast food, sandwich, biscuit w/egg & sausage	1 biscuit	581.4	19.2	41.1
21006	Fast food, sandwich, biscuit w/egg & steak	1 biscuit	410.0	17.9	21.3
21007	Fast food, sandwich, biscuit w/egg, cheese, & bacon	1 biscuit	476.6	16.3	33.4
21093	Fast food, sandwich, cheeseburger (2 patty) condiments & veges	1 burger	416.7	21.2	35.2
21092	Fast food, sandwich, cheeseburger (2 patty) plain	1 burger	457.3	27.7	22.1
921969	Fast food, sandwich, cheeseburger, 1/4 pound/Hardee	1 burger	500.5	29.0	34.0
921952	Fast food, sandwich, cheeseburger, Big Classic/Wendy	1 burger	640.2	30.0	46.0
921926	Fast food, sandwich, cheeseburger, junior/Wendy	1 burger	300.1	17.0	31.0
21100	Fast food, sandwich, cheeseburger, large (2 patty) w/condiments & vege	1 burger	704.3	38.0	39.7
21096	Fast food, sandwich, cheeseburger, large, one meat patty, plain	1 burger	608.7	30.1	47.4
21089	Fast food, sandwich, cheeseburger, one meat patty, plain	1 burger	319.3	14.8	31.8
21090	Fast food, sandwich, cheeseburger, one meat patty, w/condiments	1 burger	294.9	16.0	26.5
21102	Fast food, sandwich, chicken filet, plain	1 sandwich	515.1	24.1	38.7
921934	Fast food, sandwich, chicken/BK	1 sandwich	684.7	26.0	56.0
921979	Fast food, sandwich, club/Arby	1 sandwich	559.4	30.0	43.0
921809	Fast food, sandwich, Colonel's Chicken/KFC	1 sandwich	481.4	20.8	38.6
921801	Fast food, sandwich, croissandwich/BK	1 sandwich	345.6	19.0	19.0
21011	Fast food, sandwich, croissant w/egg & cheese	1 croissant	368.3	12.8	24.3
21012	Fast food, sandwich, croissant w/egg, cheese, & bacon	1 croissant	412.8	16.2	23.6
21013	Fast food, sandwich, croissant w/egg, cheese, & ham	1 croissant	474.2	18.9	24.2
21020	Fast food, sandwich, English muffin w/cheese & sausage	1 muffin	393.3	15.3	29.2
21021	Fast food, sandwich, English muffin w/egg, cheese, & Canadian bacon	1 sandwich	289.1	16.7	26.7
21047	Fast food, sandwich, fish filet, battered/breaded, fried	1 fillet	211.1	13.3	15.4
21105	Fast food, sandwich, fish w/tartar sauce	1 sandwich	431.3	16.9	41.0
21106	Fast food, sandwich, fish w/tartar sauce & cheese	1 sandwich	523.4	20.6	47.6
921977	Fast food, sandwich, ham & cheese/Arby	1 sandwich	352.7	26.0	33.0
21110	Fast food, sandwich, hamburger (2 patties) plain	1 burger	543.8	29.9	42.9
21111	Fast food, sandwich, hamburger (2 patties) w/condiments	1 burger	576.2	31.8	38.7
921929	Fast food, sandwich, hamburger, Big Classic/Wendy	1 burger	570.6	27.0	46.0

Dietary Fiber (g)	Total Fat (g)	Cholesterol (mg)	Calcium (mg)	Iron (mg)	Magnesium (mg)	Sodium (mg)	Zinc (mg)	Vitamin A (μgRE)	Vitamin C (mg)	Vitamin E (mgαT)	Thiamin (mg)	Riboflavin (mg)	Niacin (mg)	Vitamin B₆ (mg)	Folate (μg)
5.0	18.0	34.0	500.0	5.4	0.0	940.0	0.0	200.0	0.0	0.0	0.7	0.7	7.0	0.0	0.0
4.0	17.0	33.0	450.0	4.5	0.0	867.0	0.0	150.0	0.0	0.0	0.3	0.5	5.0	0.0	0.0
5.0	22.0	42.0	400.0	5.4	0.0	1127.0	0.0	250.0	4.0	0.0	0.7	0.7	8.0	0.0	0.0
8.0	29.0	53.0	0.0	0.0	0.0	1335.0	0.0	0.0	0.0	0.0	0.0	0.0	0.0	0.0	0.0
4.0	20.0	46.0	300.0	4.5	0.0	986.0	0.0	200.0	4.0	0.0	0.3	0.5	6.0	0.0	0.0
6.0	26.0	55.0	400.0	7.2	0.0	1447.0	0.0	150.0	1.0	0.0	0.9	0.8	9.0	0.0	0.0
5.0	21.0	56.0	350.0	6.3	0.0	1336.0	0.0	200.0	1.0	0.0	0.4	0.7	7.0	0.0	0.0
7.0	30.0	48.0	400.0	7.2	0.0	1363.0	0.0	200.0	9.0	0.0	0.7	0.8	9.0	0.0	0.0
9.0	28.0	49.0	0.0	0.0	0.0	1313.0	0.0	0.0	0.0	0.0	0.0	0.0	0.0	0.0	0.0
5.0	22.0	42.0	350.0	7.2	0.0	1328.0	0.0	250.0	2.0	0.0	0.4	0.7	7.0	0.0	0.0
0.0	25.9	29.9	308.0	3.1	68.8	971.8	2.2	173.4	28.7	0.0	0.3	0.2	4.0	0.7	29.9
0.0	21.4	20.3	335.6	3.3	78.0	484.8	2.0	278.0	48.5	0.0	0.3	0.3	3.6	0.8	61.0
0.0	21.8	31.6	410.8	6.1	110.6	699.2	3.8	173.8	31.6	0.0	0.3	0.4	4.2	0.9	47.4
0.0	28.7	17.8	310.8	3.0	65.1	381.8	1.9	227.9	26.0	0.0	0.2	0.2	3.3	0.7	26.6
0.0	22.3	24.2	105.7	3.1	69.5	181.2	0.9	277.8	33.8	0.0	0.3	0.2	3.7	0.8	33.2
0.0	0.2	0.3	3.2	0.1	2.7	34.1	0.0	1.5	0.1	0.0	0.0	0.0	0.2	0.0	1.2
0.0	1.2	1.2	0.9	0.1	2.0	36.3	0.0	0.4	0.7	0.0	0.0	0.0	0.1	0.0	1.0
0.0	18.0	77.4	183.0	5.1	40.5	1633.3	5.4	45.8	0.0	0.0	0.4	0.5	5.9	0.3	63.4
0.0	13.8	51.4	54.2	4.2	30.6	792.3	3.4	20.9	2.1	0.0	0.4	0.3	5.9	0.3	57.0
0.0	1.5	0.9	0.3	0.0	0.0	118.1	0.0	0.0	0.0	0.0	0.2	0.0	0.0	0.0	0.0
0.0	174.7	129.8	39.6	1.1	2.2	1250.5	0.4	184.8	0.0	25.9	0.0	0.0	0.0	1.3	16.9
0.0	15.0	115.0	279.0	2.0	0.0	930.0	0.0	0.0	0.0	0.0	0.0	0.0	0.0	0.0	0.0
0.0	4.0	49.0	0.0	0.0	0.0	443.0	0.0	0.0	0.0	0.0	0.0	0.0	0.0	0.0	0.0
0.0	0.9	0.4	2.8	0.1	0.7	22.4	0.0	4.2	0.7	0.0	0.0	0.0	0.0	0.0	3.2
1.0	6.6	5.0	33.0	0.2	0.0	197.0	0.1	62.0	22.0	0.0	0.0	0.0	0.2	0.1	10.0
0.0	5.0	15.0	0.0	0.0	0.0	125.0	0.0	0.0	0.0	0.0	0.0	0.0	0.0	0.0	0.0
0.0	1.1	10.7	2.5	0.1	1.4	58.4	0.0	3.0	0.2	0.0	0.0	0.0	0.0	0.0	4.5
0.0	0.6	1.8	7.9	0.1	2.1	31.2	0.1	3.2	0.1	0.0	0.0	0.0	0.1	0.0	3.4
0.0	0.5	0.2	10.2	0.1	2.2	37.0	0.1	8.9	0.1	0.0	0.0	0.0	0.1	0.0	3.8
0.5	21.0	51.0	80.0	5.4	0.0	1520.0	0.0	14.2	3.0	0.0	0.1	0.3	5.0	0.0	0.0
0.0	30.0	70.0	185.0	5.0	0.0	760.0	0.0	0.0	0.0	0.0	0.0	0.0	0.0	0.0	0.0
0.5	12.0	45.0	106.0	5.0	0.0	880.0	0.0	129.6	8.0	0.0	1.0	0.2	5.2	0.0	0.0
0.0	25.0	55.0	180.0	4.0	0.0	580.0	0.0	0.0	0.0	0.0	0.0	0.0	0.0	0.0	0.0
0.0	20.2	232.6	153.7	3.1	20.4	654.2	1.1	178.2	0.0	0.0	0.3	0.3	0.7	0.1	61.2
0.8	31.1	352.5	189.0	3.7	24.0	999.0	1.6	52.5	2.7	2.1	0.1	0.2	2.4	0.1	60.0
0.8	27.0	299.5	220.8	4.6	30.7	1382.4	2.2	240.0	0.0	2.2	0.7	0.6	2.0	0.3	65.3
0.9	38.7	302.4	154.8	4.0	25.2	1141.2	2.2	163.8	0.0	2.8	0.5	0.5	3.6	0.2	64.8
0.0	28.4	272.3	137.6	5.3	25.2	888.0	2.8	190.9	0.1	0.0	0.4	0.5	3.1	0.2	56.2
0.0	31.4	260.6	164.2	2.5	20.2	1260.0	1.5	165.6	1.6	0.0	0.3	0.4	2.3	0.1	53.3
0.0	21.1	59.8	171.0	3.4	29.9	1050.8	3.5	64.7	1.7	0.0	0.3	0.3	8.1	0.2	61.4
0.0	28.5	110.1	232.5	3.4	32.6	635.5	5.0	79.1	0.0	1.2	0.2	0.4	6.0	0.2	68.2
0.4	29.0	70.0	248.0	5.0	0.0	1060.0	3.6	101.6	33.0	0.0	0.3	0.6	14.0	0.3	0.0
2.0	38.0	100.0	180.0	5.4	0.0	1370.0	9.0	87.8	2.3	0.0	0.5	0.7	11.4	0.5	31.0
0.0	13.0	45.0	0.0	0.0	0.0	745.0	0.0	0.0	0.0	0.0	0.0	0.0	0.0	0.0	0.0
0.0	43.7	141.9	239.9	5.9	51.6	1148.1	6.7	54.2	1.0	0.0	0.4	0.5	7.2	0.4	74.8
0.0	33.0	96.2	90.7	5.5	38.9	1589.2	5.6	148.0	0.0	0.0	0.5	0.6	11.2	0.3	74.0
0.0	15.1	50.0	140.8	2.4	21.4	499.8	2.4	36.7	0.0	0.0	0.4	0.4	3.7	0.1	54.1
0.0	14.1	37.3	110.7	2.4	20.3	615.9	2.1	93.8	1.9	0.5	0.2	0.2	3.7	0.1	54.2
0.0	29.4	60.1	60.1	4.7	34.6	957.3	1.9	30.9	8.9	0.0	0.3	0.2	6.8	0.2	100.1
0.5	40.0	82.0	79.0	3.3	54.0	1417.0	1.1	25.2	0.0	0.0	0.5	0.3	9.6	0.4	18.0
1.0	30.0	100.0	200.0	3.6	0.0	1610.0	0.0	0.0	0.0	0.0	0.7	0.4	7.0	0.0	0.0
1.0	27.3	47.0	46.0	1.3	0.0	1060.0	0.0	0.0	0.0	0.0	0.4	0.3	11.1	0.0	0.0
0.5	21.0	241.0	136.0	2.2	24.0	962.0	1.9	85.2	0.0	0.0	0.5	0.3	3.2	0.0	0.0
0.0	24.7	215.9	243.8	2.2	21.6	551.2	1.8	255.3	0.1	0.0	0.2	0.4	1.5	0.1	47.0
0.0	28.4	215.4	150.9	2.2	23.2	888.8	1.9	120.0	2.2	0.0	0.3	0.3	2.2	0.1	45.2
0.0	33.6	212.8	144.4	2.1	25.8	1080.7	2.2	117.0	11.4	0.0	0.5	0.3	3.2	0.2	45.6
1.5	24.3	58.7	167.9	2.3	24.2	1036.2	1.7	86.3	1.3	0.5	0.7	0.3	4.1	0.1	66.7
1.5	12.6	234.3	150.7	2.4	23.3	728.8	1.6	156.2	1.8	0.9	0.5	0.4	3.3	0.1	43.8
0.5	11.2	30.9	16.4	1.9	21.8	484.1	0.4	10.9	0.0	0.0	0.1	0.1	1.9	0.1	15.5
0.0	22.8	55.3	83.7	2.6	33.2	614.6	1.0	30.0	2.8	0.9	0.3	0.2	3.4	0.1	85.3
0.0	28.6	67.7	184.8	3.5	36.6	938.8	1.2	97.0	2.7	1.8	0.5	0.4	4.2	0.1	91.5
0.5	13.0	50.0	200.0	1.8	0.0	1655.0	2.4	40.0	24.0	0.0	1.0	0.5	6.0	0.3	26.0
0.0	27.9	98.6	86.2	4.6	37.0	554.4	5.7	0.0	0.0	1.3	0.3	0.4	8.3	0.3	77.4
0.0	32.5	103.2	92.5	5.5	45.2	741.8	5.8	4.3	1.1	0.0	0.3	0.4	6.7	0.4	83.9
1.0	33.0	85.0	48.0	6.3	0.0	1075.0	8.4	25.6	0.0	0.0	0.2	0.4	9.0	0.5	29.0

Code	Food Name	Unit Amount	Kilocalories (kcal)	Protein (g)	Carbohydrate (g)
921887	Fast food, sandwich, hamburger, Big Mac/McD	1 burger	559.0	25.2	42.5
921931	Fast food, sandwich, hamburger, junior/Wendy	1 burger	259.7	14.0	30.0
21107	Fast food, sandwich, hamburger, plain	1 burger	274.5	12.3	30.5
921930	Fast food, sandwich, hamburger, single/Wendy	1 burger	340.2	24.0	38.0
921894	Fast food, sandwich, hamburger/McD	1 burger	260.1	12.2	30.6
921825	Fast food, sandwich, hot dog w/cheese/DQ	1 hot dog	330.0	15.0	21.0
921827	Fast food, sandwich, hot dog w/chili/DQ	1 hot dog	320.0	13.0	23.0
921844	Fast food, sandwich, hot dog/DQ	1 hot dog	280.2	11.0	21.0
921976	Fast food, sandwich, Jr. Roast Beef/Arby	1 sandwich	218.3	12.0	22.0
921973	Fast food, sandwich, roast beef/Arby	1 sandwich	350.0	22.0	32.0
921972	Fast food, sandwich, roast beef/Hardee	1 sandwich	259.9	15.0	31.0
921806	Fast food, sandwich, Sausage McMuffin/McD	1 sandwich	369.7	16.5	27.3
921978	Fast food, sandwich, Turkey Deluxe/Arby	1 sandwich	375.2	24.0	32.0
921890	Fast food, scrambled eggs/McD	1 serving	140.0	12.4	1.2
921988	Fast food, shake, chocolate/Hardee	1 shake	460.4	11.0	85.0
921932	Fast food, shake, Frosty/Wendy	1 shake	401.0	8.0	59.0
921903	Fast food, shake, strawberry/McD	1 shake	320.3	10.7	67.0
921821	Fast food, shake, vanilla/BK	1 shake	335.1	9.0	51.0
21059	Fast food, shrimp (shellfish) breaded, fried	6–8 shrimp	454.3	18.9	40.0
21123	Fast food, steak sandwich	1 sandwich	459.0	30.3	52.0
21124	Fast food, submarine sandwich, cold cuts	1 sub	456.0	21.8	51.0
21125	Fast food, submarine sandwich, roast beef	1 sub	410.4	28.6	44.3
21126	Fast food, submarine sandwich, tuna salad	1 sub	583.7	29.7	55.4
21082	Fast food, taco	1 small taco	369.4	20.7	26.7
921958	Fast food, taco/JB	1 taco	191.2	8.0	16.0
21085	Fast food, tostada w/beans & cheese	1 tostada	223.2	9.6	26.5
21086	Fast food, tostada w/beans, beef, & cheese	1 tostada	333.0	16.1	29.7
4002	Fat, animal, lard, pork	1 cup	1849.1	0.0	0.0
924073	Fish cakes, fried	4.0 oz	206.4	17.6	11.2
924074	Fish cakes, frozen	4.0 oz	253.5	11.6	27.3
15187	Fish, bass, freshwater, cooked w/dry heat	3.5 oz	146.0	24.2	0.0
15188	Fish, bass, striped, cooked w/dry heat	1 fillet	153.8	28.2	0.0
15189	Fish, bluefish, cooked w/dry heat	1 fillet	186.0	30.1	0.0
15009	Fish, carp, baked or broiled (dry heat)	1 fillet	275.4	38.9	0.0
15235	Fish, catfish, channel, farmed, cooked w/dry heat	1 fillet	217.4	26.8	0.0
15233	Fish, catfish, channel, wild, cooked w/dry heat	1 fillet	150.2	26.4	0.0
15012	Fish, caviar, black/red, granular	1.0 oz	73.1	7.1	1.2
15016	Fish, cod, Atlantic, baked/broiled (dry heat)	1 fillet	189.0	41.1	0.0
15018	Fish, cod, Atlantic, dried & salted	1 piece (5.5" x 1.5" x 0.5")	232.0	50.3	0.0
15192	Fish, cod, Pacific, cooked w/dry heat	3.0 oz	89.3	19.5	0.0
15027	Fish, fish sticks, frozen & reheated	1 piece (4" x 2" x 0.5")	155.0	8.9	13.5
15032	Fish, grouper, baked or broiled (dry heat)	3.0 oz	100.3	21.1	0.0
15034	Fish, haddock, baked or broiled (dry heat)	3.0 oz	95.2	20.6	0.0
15035	Fish, haddock, smoked	1 cubic inch, boneless	19.7	4.3	0.0
15037	Fish, halibut, Atlantic & Pacific, baked or broiled (dry heat)	3.0 oz	119.0	22.7	0.0
15196	Fish, halibut, Greenland, cooked w/dry heat	3.0 oz	203.2	15.7	0.0
15040	Fish, herring, Atlantic, baked or broiled (dry heat)	3.5 oz	203.0	23.0	0.0
15042	Fish, herring, Atlantic, kippered	1.5 oz (1 piece 4 3/8" x 1 3/4" x 1/4")	95.5	10.8	0.0
15041	Fish, herring, Atlantic, pickled	0.5 oz (1 piece 3/4" x 7/8" x 1/2")	39.3	2.1	1.4
15121	Fish, light tuna, canned in H₂O drained	3.5 oz	116.0	25.5	0.0
15183	Fish, light tuna, canned in oil w/o salt, drained	3.5 oz	198.0	29.1	0.0
15119	Fish, light tuna, canned in oil, drained	3.0 oz, 1 sm can	168.3	24.8	0.0
15047	Fish, mackerel, Atlantic, baked or broiled (dry heat)	3.5 oz	262.0	23.9	0.0
15200	Fish, mackerel, king, cooked w/dry heat	3.5 oz	134.0	26.0	0.0
15058	Fish, ocean perch, Atlantic, baked or broiled (dry heat)	3.5 oz	121.0	23.9	0.0
15061	Fish, perch, baked or broiled (dry heat)	3.5 oz	117.0	24.9	0.0
15063	Fish, Pike, northern, baked or broiled (dry heat)	3.5 oz	113.0	24.7	0.0
15204	Fish, pike, walleye, cooked w/dry heat	3.5 oz	119.0	24.5	0.0
15205	Fish, pollock, Atlantic, cooked w/dry heat	3.5 oz	118.0	24.9	0.0
15067	Fish, pollock, walleye, baked or broiled	3.5 oz	113.0	23.5	0.0
15069	Fish, pompano, Florida, baked or broiled (dry heat)	3.5 oz	211.0	23.7	0.0
915902	Fish, roe, canned	1.0 oz	33.0	6.0	0.1
15232	Fish, roughy, orange, cooked w/dry heat	3.5 oz	89.0	18.9	0.0
15237	Fish, salmon, Atlantic, farmed, cooked w/dry heat	3.5 oz	206.0	22.1	0.0
15209	Fish, salmon, Atlantic, wild, cooked w/dryheat	3.5 oz	182.0	25.4	0.0

Dietary Fiber (g)	Total Fat (g)	Cholesterol (mg)	Calcium (mg)	Iron (mg)	Magnesium (mg)	Sodium (mg)	Zinc (mg)	Vitamin A (μgRE)	Vitamin C (mg)	Vitamin E (mgαT)	Thiamin (mg)	Riboflavin (mg)	Niacin (mg)	Vitamin B_6 (mg)	Folate (μg)
1.0	32.5	103.0	256.0	4.0	0.0	950.0	4.7	70.4	2.0	0.0	0.5	0.4	6.8	0.3	21.0
0.0	9.0	34.0	0.0	0.0	0.0	545.0	0.0	0.0	0.0	0.0	0.0	0.0	0.0	0.0	0.0
0.0	11.8	35.1	63.0	2.4	18.9	387.0	2.0	0.0	0.0	0.5	0.3	0.3	3.7	0.1	53.1
1.0	17.0	65.0	32.0	4.5	0.0	475.0	2.0	18.8	0.0	0.0	0.2	0.2	5.0	0.1	0.5
0.5	9.5	37.0	122.0	2.3	0.0	500.0	2.1	30.4	2.0	0.0	0.3	0.2	3.8	0.1	17.0
0.5	21.0	55.0	150.0	1.4	0.0	990.0	1.9	20.0	0.0	0.0	0.1	0.2	3.0	0.1	25.0
0.5	20.0	55.0	80.0	1.8	0.0	985.0	1.8	30.0	0.0	0.0	0.1	0.3	4.0	0.2	30.0
0.5	16.0	45.0	80.0	1.4	21.0	830.0	1.4	0.0	0.0	0.0	0.1	0.1	3.0	0.1	20.0
0.5	8.0	20.0	40.0	1.8	0.0	345.0	1.2	0.0	0.0	0.0	0.2	0.3	4.0	0.1	7.0
0.5	15.0	39.0	80.0	3.6	0.0	590.0	0.0	17.0	1.0	0.0	0.2	0.4	7.6	0.2	14.0
0.5	10.0	34.0	105.0	4.0	0.0	730.0	0.0	108.4	3.0	0.0	0.9	0.2	3.7	0.0	0.0
0.5	21.9	64.0	235.0	2.3	0.0	820.0	1.3	48.0	0.0	0.0	0.6	0.3	4.8	0.1	12.0
0.5	17.0	39.0	80.0	2.7	0.0	850.0	2.2	60.0	4.8	0.0	0.2	0.4	12.0	0.5	20.0
0.0	9.8	399.0	57.0	2.1	0.0	290.0	1.7	103.6	0.0	0.0	0.1	0.3	0.1	0.2	65.0
0.0	8.0	45.0	480.0	1.0	0.0	340.0	1.6	58.4	0.0	0.0	0.2	0.8	0.4	0.1	0.0
0.0	14.0	50.0	45.0	0.9	0.0	220.0	0.9	71.0	0.0	0.0	0.2	0.6	0.5	0.1	17.0
0.0	1.3	10.0	327.0	0.1	0.0	170.0	1.0	61.2	0.0	0.0	0.1	0.5	0.3	0.1	11.0
0.0	10.0	33.0	295.0	0.0	32.0	213.0	1.0	0.0	0.0	0.0	0.1	0.6	0.0	0.0	0.0
0.0	24.9	200.1	83.6	3.0	39.4	1446.5	1.2	36.1	0.0	0.0	0.2	0.9	0.0	0.1	36.1
0.0	14.1	73.4	91.8	5.2	49.0	797.6	4.5	44.9	5.5	0.0	0.4	0.4	7.3	0.4	89.8
0.0	18.6	36.5	189.2	2.5	68.4	1650.7	2.6	79.8	12.3	0.0	1.0	0.8	5.5	0.1	86.6
0.0	13.0	73.4	41.0	2.8	67.0	844.6	4.4	49.7	5.6	0.0	0.4	0.4	6.0	0.3	71.3
0.0	28.0	48.6	74.2	2.6	79.4	1292.8	1.9	41.0	3.6	0.0	0.5	0.3	11.3	0.2	102.4
0.0	20.6	56.4	220.6	2.4	70.1	802.0	3.9	147.1	2.2	0.0	0.2	0.4	3.2	0.2	68.4
1.2	11.0	21.0	100.0	1.1	0.0	406.0	1.2	80.0	2.8	0.0	0.1	0.2	1.0	0.1	0.0
0.0	9.9	30.2	210.2	1.9	59.0	542.9	1.9	85.0	1.3	0.0	0.1	0.3	1.3	0.2	43.2
0.0	16.9	74.3	189.0	2.5	67.5	870.8	3.2	173.3	4.1	0.0	0.1	0.5	2.9	0.2	85.5
0.0	205.0	194.8	0.1	0.0	0.0	0.0	0.2	0.0	0.0	2.5	0.0	0.0	0.0	0.0	0.0
0.0	9.6	0.0	56.0	0.9	0.0	0.0	12.8	0.0	0.0	0.0	0.0	0.0	0.0	0.0	0.0
0.0	10.8	0.0	79.0	1.6	0.0	824.6	0.0	0.0	0.0	0.0	0.2	0.3	1.6	0.0	0.0
0.0	4.7	87.0	103.0	1.9	38.0	90.0	0.8	35.0	2.1	0.0	0.1	0.1	1.5	0.1	17.0
0.0	3.7	127.7	23.6	1.3	63.2	109.1	0.6	38.4	0.0	0.0	0.1	0.0	3.2	0.4	12.4
0.0	6.4	88.9	10.5	0.7	49.1	90.1	1.2	161.5	0.0	0.0	0.1	0.1	8.5	0.5	2.3
0.0	12.2	142.8	88.4	2.7	64.6	107.1	3.2	15.3	2.7	0.0	0.2	0.1	3.6	0.4	29.4
0.0	11.5	91.5	12.9	1.2	37.2	114.4	1.5	21.5	1.1	0.0	0.6	0.1	3.6	0.2	10.0
0.0	4.1	103.0	15.7	0.5	40.0	71.5	0.9	21.5	1.1	0.0	0.3	0.1	3.4	0.2	14.3
0.0	5.2	170.5	79.8	3.4	87.0	435.0	0.3	162.4	0.0	2.0	0.1	0.2	0.0	0.1	14.5
0.0	1.5	99.0	25.2	0.9	75.6	140.4	1.0	25.2	1.8	0.5	0.2	0.1	4.5	0.5	14.6
0.0	1.9	121.6	128.0	2.0	106.4	5621.6	1.3	33.6	2.8	0.5	0.2	0.2	6.0	0.7	19.8
0.0	0.7	40.0	7.7	0.3	26.4	77.4	0.4	8.5	2.6	0.0	0.0	0.0	2.1	0.4	6.8
0.0	7.0	63.8	11.4	0.4	14.3	331.7	0.4	17.7	0.0	0.8	0.1	0.1	1.2	0.0	10.4
0.0	1.1	40.0	17.9	1.0	31.5	45.1	0.4	42.5	0.0	0.0	0.1	0.0	0.3	0.3	8.7
0.0	0.8	62.9	35.7	1.1	42.5	74.0	0.4	16.2	0.0	0.0	0.0	0.0	3.9	0.3	11.3
0.0	0.2	13.1	8.3	0.2	9.2	129.7	0.1	3.7	0.0	0.1	0.0	0.0	0.9	0.1	2.6
0.0	2.5	34.9	51.0	0.9	91.0	58.7	0.5	45.9	0.0	0.9	0.1	0.1	6.1	0.3	11.7
0.0	15.1	50.2	3.4	0.7	28.1	87.6	0.4	15.3	0.0	0.0	0.1	0.1	1.6	0.4	0.9
0.0	11.6	77.0	74.0	1.4	41.0	115.0	1.3	31.0	0.7	1.3	0.1	0.3	4.1	0.3	11.5
0.0	5.4	36.1	37.0	0.7	20.2	403.9	0.6	17.2	0.4	0.4	0.1	0.1	1.9	0.2	6.0
0.0	2.7	2.0	11.6	0.2	1.2	130.5	0.1	38.7	0.0	0.2	0.0	0.0	0.5	0.0	0.4
0.0	0.8	30.0	11.0	1.5	27.0	338.0	0.8	17.0	0.0	0.5	0.0	0.1	13.3	0.4	4.0
0.0	8.2	18.0	13.0	1.4	31.0	50.0	0.9	23.0	0.0	0.0	0.0	0.1	12.4	0.1	5.3
0.0	7.0	15.3	11.1	1.2	26.4	300.9	0.8	19.6	0.0	1.0	0.0	0.1	10.5	0.1	4.5
0.0	17.8	75.0	15.0	1.6	97.0	83.0	0.9	54.0	0.4	0.0	0.2	0.4	6.9	0.5	1.5
0.0	2.6	68.0	40.0	2.3	41.0	203.0	0.7	252.0	1.6	0.0	0.1	0.6	10.5	0.5	9.0
0.0	2.1	54.0	137.0	1.2	39.0	96.0	0.6	14.0	0.8	0.0	0.1	0.1	2.4	0.3	10.4
0.0	1.2	115.0	102.0	1.2	38.0	79.0	1.4	10.0	1.7	0.0	0.1	0.1	1.9	0.1	5.8
0.0	0.9	50.0	73.0	0.7	40.0	49.0	0.9	24.0	3.8	0.0	0.1	0.1	2.8	0.1	17.3
0.0	1.6	110.0	141.0	1.7	38.0	65.0	0.8	24.0	0.0	0.0	0.3	0.2	2.8	0.1	17.0
0.0	1.3	91.0	77.0	0.6	86.0	110.0	0.6	12.0	0.0	0.0	0.1	0.2	4.0	0.3	3.0
0.0	1.1	96.0	6.0	0.3	73.0	116.0	0.6	23.0	0.0	0.2	0.1	0.1	1.7	0.1	3.6
0.0	12.1	64.0	43.0	0.7	31.0	76.0	0.7	36.0	0.0	0.0	0.7	0.2	3.8	0.2	17.3
0.0	0.8	0.0	4.2	0.3	0.0	0.0	0.0	0.0	0.0	0.0	0.0	0.0	0.0	0.0	0.0
0.0	0.9	26.0	38.0	0.2	38.0	81.0	1.0	24.0	0.0	0.0	0.1	0.2	3.7	0.3	8.0
0.0	12.4	63.0	15.0	0.3	30.0	61.0	0.4	15.0	3.7	0.0	0.3	0.1	8.0	0.6	34.0
0.0	8.1	71.0	15.0	1.0	37.0	56.0	0.8	13.0	0.0	0.0	0.3	0.5	10.1	0.9	29.0

Code	Food Name	Unit Amount	Kilocalories (kcal)	Protein (g)	Carbohydrate (g)
15210	Fish, salmon, chinook, cooked w/dry heat	3.5 oz	231.0	25.7	0.0
15077	Fish, salmon, chinook, smoked	3.5 oz	117.0	18.3	0.0
15179	Fish, salmon, chinook, smoked, lox, regular	1.0 oz	32.8	5.1	0.0
15239	Fish, salmon, coho, farmed, cooked w/dry heat	3.5 oz	178.0	24.3	0.0
15247	Fish, salmon, coho, wild, cooked w/dry heat	3.5 oz	139.0	23.5	0.0
15082	Fish, salmon, coho, wild, cooked w/moist heat	3.5 oz	184.0	27.4	0.0
15084	Fish, salmon, pink, canned, solids & liquid	3.5 oz	139.0	19.8	0.0
15212	Fish, salmon, pink, cooked w/dry heat	3.5 oz	149.0	25.6	0.0
15088	Fish, sardine, Atlantic, w/bone, canned in oil, drained	1 small fish (2.66" x 0.5" x 0.25")	25.0	3.0	0.0
15089	Fish, sardine, Pacific, w/bone, canned in tom sauce, drained	1 sardine	67.6	6.2	0.0
15092	Fish, sea bass, baked or broiled (dry heat)	3.5 oz	124.0	23.6	0.0
15214	Fish, sea trout, cooked w/dry heat	3.5 oz	133.0	21.5	0.0
15215	Fish, shad, American, cooked w/dry heat	3.5 oz	252.0	21.7	0.0
15096	Fish, shark, battered, fried	4.0 oz	273.6	22.3	7.7
15102	Fish, snapper, baked or broiled (dry heat)	3.5 oz	128.0	26.3	0.0
15218	Fish, sunfish/pumpkin seed, cooked w/dry heat	3.5 oz	114.0	24.9	0.0
15109	Fish, surimi	3.0 oz	84.2	12.9	5.8
15111	Fish, swordfish, baked or broiled (dry heat)	3.5 oz	155.0	25.4	0.0
15219	Fish, trout, cooked w/dry heat	3.5 oz	190.0	26.6	0.0
15241	Fish, trout, rainbow, farmed, cooked w/dry heat	3.5 oz	169.0	24.3	0.0
15116	Fish, trout, rainbow, wild, cooked w/dry heat	3.5 oz	150.0	22.9	0.0
924207	Fish, tuna noodle casserole	6.0 oz	193.8	11.4	15.8
924208	Fish, tuna pot pie, frozen/Banquet	7.0 oz	540.5	17.0	44.0
15128	Fish, tuna salad	3.0 oz	159.0	13.6	8.0
15118	Fish, tuna, bluefin, baked or broiled (dry heat)	3.0 oz	156.4	25.4	0.0
915905	Fish, tuna, canned, low-sodium	2.0 oz	70.2	15.0	0.0
15221	Fish, tuna, yellowfin, fresh, cooked w/dry heat	3.5 oz	139.0	30.0	0.0
15222	Fish, turbot, European, cooked w/dry heat	3.5 oz	122.0	20.6	0.0
15126	Fish, white tuna, canned in H_2O, drained	3.0 oz	108.8	20.1	0.0
15124	Fish, white tuna, canned in oil, drained	3.0 oz	158.1	22.6	0.0
15223	Fish, whitefish, cooked w/dry heat	3.0 oz	146.2	20.8	0.0
15133	Fish, whiting, baked or broiled (dry heat)	1 fillet	83.5	16.9	0.0
15225	Fish, yellowtail, cooked w/dry heat	3.5 oz	159.0	25.2	0.0
2050	Flavoring, vanilla extract	1 tsp.	12.1	0.0	0.5
920904	Flour, Bisquick Mix	1/2 cup	240.0	4.0	37.0
20090	Flour, brown rice	1 cup	573.5	11.4	120.8
20316	Flour, corn, white, whole-grain	1 cup	422.4	8.1	89.9
20016	Flour, corn, yellow, whole-grain	1 cup	422.4	8.1	89.9
924291	Flour, potato	1/2 cup	315.9	7.2	71.9
20061	Flour, rice, white	1 cup	596.6	9.7	130.6
920906	Flour, rye & wheat	1 cup	457.0	14.1	96.5
20063	Flour, rye, dark	1 cup	414.7	18.0	88.0
20065	Flour, rye, light	1 cup	469.8	10.7	102.7
20064	Flour, rye, medium	1 cup	453.1	12.0	99.2
20070	Flour, triticale, whole-grain	1 cup	432.6	16.9	93.6
20081	Flour, wheat, white, all purpose, bleached, enriched	1 cup	455.0	12.9	95.4
20082	Flour, wheat, white, all purpose, self-rise, enriched	1 cup	442.5	12.4	92.8
20083	Flour, wheat, white, bread, enriched	1 cup	451.3	15.0	90.7
20084	Flour, wheat, white, cake, enriched	1 cup	452.5	10.3	97.5
20086	Flour, wheat, white, tortilla mix, enriched	1 cup	506.3	12.1	83.9
20080	Flour, whole-wheat, whole-grain	1 cup	423.8	17.1	90.7
18268	French toast, frozen	1 piece	125.7	4.4	18.9
18269	French toast, homemade w/reduced-fat (2%) milk	1 slice	148.9	5.0	16.3
918381	French toast, homemade w/whole milk	1 slice	150.8	5.0	16.2
924287	Frozen meal, beef chop suey	12.0 oz	282.2	13.6	38.8
924062	Frozen meal, beef chop suey/Banquet	8.0 oz	104.4	9.8	9.8
924255	Frozen meal, beef enchilada/Banquet	7.0 oz	269.3	10.0	28.0
22402	Frozen meal, beef macaroni/Healthy Choice	1 serving	211.2	14.1	33.5
924026	Frozen meal, beef oriental/LeMenuLite	10.0 oz	221.5	18.8	24.5
924080	Frozen meal, beef pepper steak, diet/Armour	11.25 oz	220.1	17.0	29.0
22578	Frozen meal, beef pot roast w/whipped potatoes/Stouffer's Lean Cuisine Homestyle	1 package	206.6	17.3	22.4
22616	Frozen meal, beef sirloin salisbury steak w/red skinned pots & vege/Budget Gourmet	1 package	261.2	18.3	33.9
924032	Frozen meal, beef stew/Stouffer's	5.0 oz	129.2	9.7	7.2
924229	Frozen meal, beef stroganoff, diet/Armour	11.25 oz	248.8	18.0	33.0
924230	Frozen meal, beef stroganoff/LeMenu	10.0 oz	383.4	26.5	23.8

Dietary Fiber (g)	Total Fat (g)	Cholesterol (mg)	Calcium (mg)	Iron (mg)	Magnesium (mg)	Sodium (mg)	Zinc (mg)	Vitamin A (μgRE)	Vitamin C (mg)	Vitamin E (mgαT)	Thiamin (mg)	Riboflavin (mg)	Niacin (mg)	Vitamin B6 (mg)	Folate (μg)
0.0	13.4	85.0	28.0	0.9	122.0	60.0	0.6	149.0	4.1	0.0	0.0	0.2	10.0	0.5	35.0
0.0	4.3	23.0	11.0	0.9	18.0	784.0	0.3	26.0	0.0	1.4	0.0	0.1	4.7	0.3	1.9
0.0	1.2	6.4	3.1	0.2	5.0	560.0	0.1	7.3	0.0	0.0	0.0	0.0	1.3	0.1	0.5
0.0	8.2	63.0	12.0	0.4	34.0	52.0	0.5	59.0	1.5	0.0	0.1	0.1	7.4	0.6	14.0
0.0	4.3	55.0	45.0	0.6	33.0	58.0	0.6	39.0	1.4	0.8	0.1	0.1	8.0	0.6	13.0
0.0	7.5	57.0	46.0	0.7	35.0	53.0	0.5	32.0	1.0	0.0	0.1	0.2	7.8	0.6	9.0
0.0	6.1	55.0	213.0	0.8	34.0	554.0	0.9	17.0	0.0	1.4	0.0	0.2	6.5	0.3	15.4
0.0	4.4	67.0	17.0	1.0	33.0	86.0	0.7	41.0	0.0	0.0	0.2	0.1	8.5	0.2	5.0
0.0	1.4	17.0	45.8	0.4	4.7	60.6	0.2	8.0	0.0	0.0	0.0	0.0	0.6	0.2	1.4
0.0	4.6	23.2	91.2	0.9	12.9	157.3	0.5	26.6	0.4	1.4	0.0	0.1	1.6	0.0	9.2
0.0	2.6	53.0	13.0	0.4	53.0	87.0	0.5	64.0	0.0	0.0	0.1	0.2	1.9	0.5	5.8
0.0	4.6	106.0	22.0	0.4	40.0	74.0	0.6	35.0	0.0	0.0	0.1	0.2	2.9	0.5	6.0
0.0	17.7	96.0	60.0	1.2	38.0	65.0	0.5	36.0	0.0	0.0	0.2	0.3	10.8	0.5	17.0
0.0	16.6	70.8	60.0	1.3	51.6	146.4	0.6	64.8	0.0	0.0	0.1	0.1	3.3	0.4	18.0
0.0	1.7	47.0	40.0	0.2	37.0	57.0	0.4	35.0	1.6	0.0	0.1	0.0	0.3	0.5	5.8
0.0	0.9	86.0	103.0	1.5	38.0	103.0	2.0	17.0	1.0	0.0	0.1	0.1	1.5	0.1	17.0
0.0	0.8	25.5	7.7	0.2	36.6	121.6	0.3	17.0	0.0	0.0	0.0	0.0	0.2	0.0	1.4
0.0	5.1	50.0	6.0	1.0	34.0	115.0	1.5	41.0	1.1	0.0	0.0	0.1	11.8	0.4	2.3
0.0	8.5	74.0	55.0	1.9	28.0	67.0	0.9	19.0	0.5	0.0	0.4	0.4	5.8	0.2	15.0
0.0	7.2	68.0	86.0	0.3	32.0	42.0	0.5	86.0	3.3	0.0	0.2	0.1	8.8	0.4	24.0
0.0	5.8	69.0	86.0	0.4	31.0	56.0	0.5	15.0	2.0	0.0	0.2	0.1	5.8	0.3	19.0
1.0	9.4	27.0	102.0	1.0	0.0	731.0	0.0	13.6	0.0	0.0	0.1	0.3	3.4	0.0	0.0
0.0	33.0	30.0	146.0	2.0	0.0	810.0	0.0	116.0	2.0	0.0	0.4	0.4	6.3	0.0	0.0
0.0	7.9	11.1	14.5	0.9	16.2	341.7	0.5	23.0	1.9	0.0	0.0	0.1	5.7	0.1	6.8
0.0	5.3	41.7	8.5	1.1	54.4	42.5	0.7	642.6	0.0	0.0	0.2	0.3	9.0	0.4	1.9
0.0	1.0	20.0	3.0	0.7	54.0	120.0	0.3	0.0	0.0	0.0	0.0	0.0	7.5	0.2	2.0
0.0	1.2	58.0	21.0	0.9	64.0	47.0	0.7	20.0	1.0	0.0	0.5	0.1	11.9	1.0	2.0
0.0	3.8	62.0	23.0	0.5	65.0	192.0	0.3	12.0	1.7	0.0	0.1	0.1	2.7	0.2	9.0
0.0	2.5	35.7	11.9	0.8	28.1	320.5	0.4	5.1	0.0	1.4	0.0	0.0	4.9	0.2	1.7
0.0	6.9	26.4	3.4	0.6	28.9	336.6	0.4	20.4	0.0	0.0	0.0	0.1	9.9	0.4	3.9
0.0	6.4	65.5	28.1	0.4	35.7	55.3	1.1	33.2	0.0	0.0	0.1	0.1	3.3	0.3	14.5
0.0	1.2	60.5	44.6	0.3	19.4	95.0	0.4	24.5	0.0	0.2	0.0	0.1	1.2	0.1	10.8
0.0	5.7	60.4	24.7	0.5	32.3	42.5	0.6	26.4	2.5	0.0	0.1	0.0	7.4	0.2	3.4
0.0	0.0	0.0	0.5	0.0	0.5	0.4	0.0	0.0	0.0	0.0	0.0	0.0	0.0	0.0	0.0
0.0	8.0	0.0	0.0	0.0	0.0	700.0	0.0	0.0	0.0	0.0	0.0	0.0	0.0	0.0	0.0
7.3	4.4	0.0	17.4	3.1	177.0	12.6	3.9	0.0	0.0	1.1	0.7	0.1	10.0	1.2	25.3
11.2	4.5	0.0	8.2	2.8	108.8	5.9	2.0	0.0	0.0	0.3	0.3	0.1	2.2	0.4	29.3
15.7	4.5	0.0	8.2	2.8	108.8	5.9	2.0	55.0	0.0	0.3	0.3	0.1	2.2	0.4	29.3
0.0	0.7	0.0	30.0	15.5	0.0	31.0	0.0	0.0	17.0	0.0	0.4	0.1	3.1	0.0	0.0
3.9	2.3	0.0	16.3	0.6	57.1	0.0	1.3	0.0	0.0	0.2	0.2	0.0	4.2	0.7	6.5
0.0	1.7	0.0	27.4	4.6	0.0	2.3	0.0	0.0	0.0	0.0	0.6	0.3	5.0	0.0	0.0
28.9	3.4	0.0	71.7	8.3	317.4	1.3	7.2	0.0	0.0	3.3	0.4	0.3	5.5	0.6	76.8
18.7	1.7	0.0	26.9	2.3	89.6	2.6	2.2	0.0	0.0	0.7	0.4	0.1	1.0	0.3	28.2
18.7	2.3	0.0	30.7	2.7	96.0	3.8	2.5	0.0	0.0	1.7	0.4	0.1	2.2	0.3	24.3
18.7	2.3	0.0	44.8	3.3	195.8	2.6	3.4	0.0	0.0	2.4	0.5	0.2	3.7	0.5	94.7
3.4	1.2	0.0	18.8	5.8	27.5	2.5	0.9	0.0	0.0	0.1	1.0	0.6	7.4	0.1	192.5
3.4	1.2	0.0	422.5	5.8	23.8	1587.5	0.8	0.0	0.0	0.1	0.8	0.5	7.3	0.1	192.5
3.0	2.1	0.0	18.8	5.5	31.3	2.5	1.1	0.0	0.0	0.1	1.0	0.6	9.4	0.0	192.5
2.1	1.1	0.0	17.5	9.2	20.0	2.5	0.8	0.0	0.0	0.1	1.1	0.5	8.5	0.0	192.5
0.0	13.3	0.0	256.3	8.8	26.3	846.3	0.8	0.0	0.0	0.0	0.9	0.6	7.3	0.1	170.0
15.3	2.3	0.0	42.5	4.9	172.5	6.3	3.7	0.0	0.0	1.5	0.6	0.3	8.0	0.4	55.0
0.7	3.6	48.4	63.1	1.3	10.0	292.1	0.5	31.9	0.2	0.4	0.2	0.2	1.6	0.3	30.7
0.0	7.0	75.4	65.0	1.1	11.1	311.4	0.4	85.8	0.2	0.0	0.1	0.2	1.1	0.0	28.0
0.0	7.3	3.0	64.4	1.1	11.1	310.7	0.4	80.6	0.2	0.0	0.1	0.2	1.1	0.0	15.0
0.0	8.2	0.0	44.0	2.4	0.0	1802.0	0.0	68.0	4.0	0.0	0.1	0.1	3.0	0.0	0.0
0.0	3.0	0.0	32.0	2.1	0.0	1334.0	0.0	32.2	2.0	0.0	0.0	0.1	1.1	0.0	0.0
0.0	13.0	0.0	52.0	1.0	0.0	1477.0	0.0	35.8	0.0	0.0	0.2	0.1	1.9	0.0	0.0
4.6	2.2	14.4	45.6	2.7	36.0	444.0	1.2	50.4	58.1	1.5	0.3	0.2	3.1	0.2	105.6
0.0	5.4	39.0	39.0	3.4	0.0	560.0	0.0	289.8	9.0	0.0	0.1	0.5	3.4	0.0	0.0
0.0	4.0	35.0	50.0	2.0	0.0	970.0	0.0	105.4	15.0	0.0	0.2	0.3	1.6	0.0	0.0
3.6	5.4	38.3	0.0	0.0	0.0	494.7	0.0	0.0	0.0	0.0	0.0	0.0	0.0	0.0	0.0
7.2	5.9	43.5	0.0	3.0	0.0	494.5	0.0	0.0	51.0	0.0	0.0	0.0	0.0	0.0	0.0
0.0	6.8	28.0	14.0	1.3	0.0	540.0	0.0	213.0	3.0	0.0	0.1	0.1	1.4	0.0	0.0
0.0	6.0	55.0	56.0	2.0	0.0	510.0	0.0	580.8	43.0	0.0	0.3	0.2	1.6	0.0	0.0
0.0	20.3	0.0	107.0	4.3	0.0	867.0	0.0	220.6	1.0	0.0	0.1	0.3	5.1	0.0	0.0

Code	Food Name	Unit Amount	Kilocalories (kcal)	Protein (g)	Carbohydrate (g)
924137	Frozen meal, beef szechuan/LeanCuisine	9.2 oz	280.3	20.0	25.0
924231	Frozen meal, beef teriyaki	9.0 oz	270.3	20.0	36.0
924025	Frozen meal, beef w/gravy/Banquet	4.0 oz	99.4	8.0	5.0
924268	Frozen meal, Belgian waffles & berries/Swanson	3.5 oz	201.0	3.2	30.8
22679	Frozen meal, breakfast burrito, ham & cheese flavor	1 package	211.9	9.6	27.8
924031	Frozen meal, cannelloni/LeanCuisine	9.6 oz	270.3	19.0	25.0
924232	Frozen meal, cheese cannelloni/Stouffer's	5.5 oz	171.6	10.1	13.7
924292	Frozen meal, cheese enchilada/Banquet	12.0 oz	550.8	22.0	71.0
924122	Frozen meal, cheese lasagna/DiningLite	9.0 oz	261.0	14.0	36.0
924233	Frozen meal, cheese tomato cannelloni/LeanCuisine	9.1 oz	270.9	22.0	24.0
22577	Frozen meal, chicken & vegetables w/vermicelli/Stouffer's Lean Cuisine	1 package	252.5	18.7	32.1
22581	Frozen meal, chicken a l'orange in sauce w/broccoli & rice/Stouffer's Lean Cuisine	1 package	267.8	24.5	38.5
924040	Frozen meal, chicken ala king & rice/Swanson	9.0 oz	275.4	14.4	32.1
22610	Frozen meal, chicken Alfredo w/fettucini & vege/Stouffer's Lunch Express	1 package	372.6	19.0	32.6
924048	Frozen meal, chicken cacciatore/LeanCuisine	10.9 oz	280.3	23.0	25.0
924234	Frozen meal, chicken cannelloni, diet/LeMenu	10.3 oz	261.9	14.9	39.2
924254	Frozen meal, chicken chow mein/LeanCuisine	11.3 oz	248.8	14.0	36.0
22588	Frozen meal, chicken enchilada suprema w/green chili sauce, rice, corn, & apple	1 package	297.6	13.0	46.0
924257	Frozen meal, chicken enchilada/LeMenuLite	8.25 oz	269.1	19.1	33.2
924084	Frozen meal, chicken fettucini/Armour	11.0 oz	259.0	17.0	28.0
924326	Frozen meal, chicken fried steak/Worthington	6.2 oz	580.8	28.0	25.0
924244	Frozen meal, chicken parmesan/LeanCuisine	10.0 oz	249.0	25.0	19.0
924240	Frozen meal, chicken piccata	11.0 oz	343.2	21.0	22.9
22906	Frozen meal, chicken pot pie, frozen entree	1 serving	483.9	13.0	42.7
22587	Frozen meal, chicken teriyaki w/rice, mixed vege w/butter sauce & apple cherry	1 package	268.3	17.1	37.1
924283	Frozen meal, chicken & noodle/Armour	11.0 oz	230.9	19.0	23.0
924091	Frozen meal, chicken, sweet & sour dinner/LeMenu	10.5 oz	381.4	18.8	41.0
924289	Frozen meal, corned beef hash	10.0 oz	372.0	19.9	42.6
924180	Frozen meal, egg souffle w/broccoli & cheese/Stouffer's	4.0 oz	151.4	8.4	7.7
22614	Frozen meal, escalloped chicken & noodles/Stouffer's	1 package	365.1	17.0	3.7
924294	Frozen meal, filet of sole/LeMenu	10.0 oz	355.0	17.9	43.5
924216	Frozen meal, fried chicken/Banquet	10.0 oz	400.4	15.0	45.0
924046	Frozen meal, glazed chicken/LeanCuisine	8.5 oz	269.9	26.0	23.0
924261	Frozen meal, green pepper steak/Stouffer's	3.0 oz	85.9	7.7	3.8
22673	Frozen meal, Italian sausage lasagna/Budget Gourmet	1 package	455.9	20.6	39.9
924296	Frozen meal, lasagna	13.0 oz	391.1	13.0	54.0
22570	Frozen meal, lasagna w/meat & sauce/Stouffer's	1 package	767.6	51.8	73.2
924117	Frozen meal, lasagna/LeanCuisine	10.3 oz	279.4	27.0	24.0
924267	Frozen meal, linguini w/clam sauce/LeanCuisine	9.6 oz	261.1	16.0	32.0
22576	Frozen meal, macaroni & beef in tomato sauce/Stouffer's Lean Cuisine	1 package	249.0	13.9	36.5
22680	Frozen meal, macaroni & beef in tomato sauce/WW	1 package	282.5	15.6	44.7
924092	Frozen meal, macaroni & cheese dinner/Banquet	10.0 oz	420.3	14.0	46.0
924280	Frozen meal, manicotti w/tomato sauce/LeMenu	11.7 oz	392.9	20.0	44.3
22675	Frozen meal, meat loaf w/tomato sauce, mashed potatoes, & carrots in seasoned sauce	1 package	611.6	29.1	33.6
924114	Frozen meal, meatballs Italian style/Stouffer's	13.0 oz	483.4	24.5	60.4
924093	Frozen meal, meat loaf/LeMenu	10.0 oz	301.0	17.8	27.3
924302	Frozen meal, Mexican combo dinner/Banquet	12.0 oz	520.2	20.0	72.0
924305	Frozen meal, noodles & chicken/Banquet	10.0 oz	349.3	10.0	42.0
22571	Frozen meal, original fried chicken meal w/mashed pots & corn in seasoned sauce	1 package	469.7	21.5	35.1
924238	Frozen meal, pasta primavera/Campbell	10.0 oz	14.2	22.2	39.9
924177	Frozen meal, pasta, cheese tortellini/Stouffer's	4.5 oz	267.5	15.4	26.9
924308	Frozen meal, pasta, ravioli dinner/Swanson	16.0 oz	486.7	16.1	68.3
924193	Frozen meal, pasta, spaghetti w/meat sauce/Banquet	8.0 oz	270.1	14.0	35.0
924191	Frozen meal, pasta, spaghetti w/meat sauce/LeMenuLite	9.5 oz	285.1	12.6	44.6
924311	Frozen meal, pasta, spaghetti & meatballs/Swanson	12.5 oz	375.2	13.5	46.0
22569	Frozen meal, pepper, stuffed w/beef in tomato sauce/Stouffer's	1 package	377.5	15.8	41.7
924090	Frozen meal, pork ham/LeMenu	10.0 oz	286.8	18.3	31.0
22609	Frozen meal, rice & chicken stir-fry w/vegetables/Stouffer's Lean Cuisine Lunch	1 package	270.3	11.7	39.5
924156	Frozen meal, rigatoni pasta/Stouffer's	6.0 oz	180.2	11.7	17.0
22712	Frozen meal, roasted chicken w/garlic sauce, pasta, & vegetable medley/Tyson	1 package	214.2	16.9	21.5
22583	Frozen meal, salisbury steak in gravy & macaroni & cheese/Stouffer's Homestyle	1 package	386.2	22.6	26.4
924157	Frozen meal, salisbury steak/Banquet	5.0 oz	190.3	9.0	8.0
924204	Frozen meal, sliced beef/Swanson	15.2 oz	453.6	37.8	50.0
22580	Frozen meal, spaghetti w/meat sauce/Stouffer's Lean Cuisine	1 package	313.0	14.3	50.5
924260	Frozen meal, stuffed shells/LeMenuLite	10.0 oz	269.8	17.3	33.5

Dietary Fiber (g)	Total Fat (g)	Cholesterol (mg)	Calcium (mg)	Iron (mg)	Magnesium (mg)	Sodium (mg)	Zinc (mg)	Vitamin A (μgRE)	Vitamin C (mg)	Vitamin E (mgαT)	Thiamin (mg)	Riboflavin (mg)	Niacin (mg)	Vitamin B$_6$ (mg)	Folate (μg)
0.0	11.0	95.0	40.0	1.8	0.0	720.0	0.0	250.0	12.0	0.0	0.1	0.3	4.0	0.0	0.0
0.0	5.0	45.0	29.0	2.0	0.0	850.0	0.0	146.4	2.0	0.0	0.2	0.2	3.4	0.0	0.0
0.0	5.0	40.0	10.0	2.0	0.0	426.0	0.0	5.8	0.0	0.0	0.0	0.1	1.2	0.0	0.0
0.0	7.1	0.0	45.0	1.1	0.0	235.0	0.0	3.8	3.0	0.0	0.1	0.1	0.7	0.0	0.0
1.4	6.9	192.1	0.0	3.2	0.0	404.9	0.0	0.0	0.0	0.0	0.0	0.0	0.0	0.0	0.0
0.0	10.0	45.0	200.0	1.4	0.0	940.0	0.0	400.0	0.0	0.0	0.2	0.3	2.0	0.0	0.0
0.0	8.7	20.0	218.0	0.6	0.0	608.0	0.0	156.0	17.0	0.0	0.1	0.2	0.9	0.0	0.0
0.0	19.0	0.0	281.0	3.0	0.0	2170.0	0.0	142.2	7.0	0.0	0.4	0.3	2.4	0.0	0.0
0.0	6.0	0.0	307.0	2.0	0.0	800.0	0.0	397.6	7.0	0.0	0.2	0.3	1.9	0.0	0.0
0.0	10.0	30.0	300.0	0.7	0.0	900.0	0.0	150.0	6.0	0.0	0.1	0.3	1.2	0.0	0.0
5.0	5.6	23.8	104.0	1.3	0.0	582.1	0.0	0.0	14.6	0.0	0.0	0.0	0.0	0.0	0.0
0.0	1.8	45.9	0.0	0.0	0.0	359.6	0.0	0.0	18.1	0.0	0.0	0.0	0.0	0.0	0.0
1.0	9.9	0.0	64.0	0.9	0.0	859.0	0.0	116.6	2.0	0.0	0.1	0.3	5.0	0.0	0.0
3.8	18.5	57.1	146.9	0.0	0.0	587.5	0.0	0.0	24.2	0.0	0.0	0.0	0.0	0.0	0.0
0.0	10.0	45.0	40.0	1.8	0.0	950.0	0.0	100.0	12.0	0.0	0.1	0.2	5.0	0.0	0.0
0.0	5.0	38.0	93.0	3.1	0.0	621.0	0.0	350.6	9.0	0.0	0.6	0.4	3.2	0.0	0.0
0.0	5.0	30.0	40.0	1.1	0.0	1030.0	0.0	20.0	15.0	0.0	0.1	0.2	4.0	0.0	0.0
4.2	6.7	38.4	134.4	0.8	0.0	563.2	0.0	0.0	18.2	0.0	0.1	0.4	3.2	0.0	0.0
0.0	6.6	33.0	215.0	1.8	0.0	537.0	0.0	68.8	11.0	0.0	0.1	0.4	3.2	0.0	0.0
0.0	9.0	50.0	146.0	2.0	0.0	660.0	0.0	329.8	61.0	0.0	0.2	0.2	3.8	0.0	0.0
1.0	41.0	95.0	20.0	4.1	0.0	1040.0	0.0	9.4	0.0	0.0	0.2	0.2	4.9	0.0	0.0
0.0	8.0	70.0	150.0	1.4	0.0	850.0	0.0	100.0	6.0	0.0	0.2	0.3	7.0	0.0	0.0
0.0	18.5	0.0	96.0	2.9	0.0	1148.0	0.0	178.6	6.0	0.0	0.2	0.1	8.0	0.0	0.0
1.7	29.1	41.2	32.6	2.1	23.9	857.2	1.0	342.9	1.5	3.8	0.3	0.4	4.1	0.2	52.1
2.8	5.6	43.7	37.4	1.1	0.0	602.2	0.0	0.0	12.2	0.0	0.0	0.0	0.0	0.0	0.0
0.0	7.0	50.0	87.0	2.0	0.0	660.0	0.0	895.6	57.0	0.0	0.2	0.2	4.7	0.0	0.0
0.0	15.7	0.0	80.0	2.1	0.0	1020.0	0.0	329.6	5.0	0.0	0.1	0.2	5.5	0.0	0.0
0.0	13.3	0.4	65.0	4.0	0.0	1752.0	0.0	70.4	13.0	0.0	0.2	0.1	3.1	0.0	0.0
0.0	9.6	141.0	130.0	0.9	0.0	509.0	0.0	65.6	9.0	0.0	0.1	0.3	0.5	0.0	0.0
0.0	31.4	76.4	116.0	1.1	0.0	1211.2	0.0	0.0	0.0	0.0	0.0	0.0	0.0	0.0	0.0
3.7	12.1	0.0	105.0	2.0	0.0	956.0	0.0	415.8	2.0	0.0	0.2	0.3	2.4	0.0	0.0
0.0	22.0	0.0	46.0	1.0	0.0	1100.0	0.0	112.8	8.0	0.0	0.1	0.1	4.9	0.0	0.0
0.0	8.0	60.0	20.0	0.7	0.0	710.0	0.0	20.0	2.0	0.0	0.1	0.1	8.0	0.0	0.0
0.0	4.4	19.0	14.0	0.9	0.0	527.0	0.0	27.2	7.0	0.0	0.0	0.1	1.5	0.0	0.0
3.0	23.8	47.7	315.9	2.7	0.0	902.9	0.0	0.0	0.0	0.0	0.0	0.0	0.0	0.0	0.0
0.0	14.0	0.0	0.0	0.0	0.0	825.0	0.0	0.0	0.0	0.0	0.0	0.0	0.0	0.0	0.0
8.9	29.8	113.1	636.7	0.0	0.0	2034.9	0.0	0.0	0.0	0.0	0.0	0.0	0.0	0.0	0.0
0.0	8.0	70.0	250.0	1.4	0.0	1000.0	0.0	400.0	5.0	0.0	0.9	0.4	4.0	0.0	0.0
0.0	7.0	30.0	20.0	1.8	0.0	800.0	0.0	0.0	0.0	0.0	0.1	0.1	1.2	0.0	0.0
3.4	5.4	22.6	0.0	2.2	0.0	563.2	0.0	0.0	157.3	0.0	0.0	0.0	0.0	0.0	0.0
6.7	4.6	13.5	0.0	5.7	0.0	492.3	0.0	0.0	27.4	0.0	0.0	0.0	0.0	0.0	0.0
0.0	20.0	30.0	272.0	3.0	0.0	450.0	0.0	1517.6	7.0	0.0	0.3	0.4	2.4	0.0	0.0
0.0	15.2	0.0	493.0	3.1	0.0	871.0	0.0	22.0	17.0	0.0	0.3	0.4	4.0	0.0	0.0
6.3	40.0	113.3	77.0	3.9	0.0	1943.4	0.0	0.0	7.7	0.0	0.0	0.0	0.0	0.0	0.0
0.2	15.9	0.0	148.0	5.7	0.0	935.0	0.0	335.8	16.0	0.0	0.3	0.4	4.9	0.0	0.0
0.0	13.3	0.0	97.0	4.0	0.0	860.0	0.0	934.4	5.0	0.0	0.2	0.3	4.3	0.0	0.0
0.0	17.0	0.0	194.0	3.0	0.0	1980.0	0.0	107.8	7.0	0.0	0.4	0.2	2.7	0.0	0.0
0.0	15.0	45.0	29.0	2.0	0.0	460.0	0.0	1378.0	2.0	0.0	0.2	0.2	3.8	0.0	0.0
2.1	27.0	88.9	38.8	1.4	0.0	1500.2	0.0	0.0	1.4	0.0	0.0	0.0	0.0	0.0	0.0
0.0	0.0	0.0	265.0	2.4	0.0	882.0	0.0	204.4	2.0	0.0	0.1	0.3	2.1	0.0	0.0
0.0	10.9	77.0	243.0	1.0	0.0	326.0	0.0	7.6	1.0	0.0	0.1	0.2	1.2	0.0	0.0
0.0	16.8	0.0	162.0	4.4	0.0	975.0	0.0	196.6	25.0	0.0	0.3	0.3	4.2	0.0	0.0
1.0	8.0	0.0	29.0	3.0	0.0	1250.0	0.0	179.6	14.0	0.0	0.1	0.1	3.2	0.0	0.0
0.0	6.1	14.0	45.0	3.9	0.0	406.0	0.0	146.4	32.0	0.0	0.2	0.3	3.0	0.0	0.0
0.0	15.1	0.0	113.0	3.1	0.0	1097.0	2.4	242.4	14.0	0.0	0.2	0.2	3.4	0.2	0.0
10.5	16.2	43.9	0.0	0.0	0.0	1154.6	0.0	0.0	173.0	0.0	0.0	0.0	0.0	0.0	0.0
0.0	10.1	0.0	67.0	2.2	0.0	1486.0	0.0	1479.4	31.0	0.0	0.6	0.3	4.5	0.0	0.0
5.9	7.4	25.5	0.0	0.0	0.0	632.4	0.0	0.0	23.7	0.0	0.0	0.0	0.0	0.0	0.0
0.0	7.1	22.0	170.0	1.7	0.0	510.0	0.0	85.0	9.0	0.0	0.1	0.2	2.2	0.0	0.0
3.6	6.7	28.1	0.0	1.6	0.0	466.7	0.0	0.0	0.0	0.0	0.0	0.0	0.0	0.0	0.0
0.0	21.2	62.6	195.8	2.3	0.0	1014.6	0.0	0.0	0.0	0.0	0.0	0.0	0.0	0.0	0.0
0.5	14.0	35.0	49.0	1.9	0.0	766.0	0.0	5.8	0.0	0.0	0.1	0.1	1.1	0.2	0.0
0.0	11.3	0.0	43.0	5.9	0.0	1003.0	0.0	105.2	7.0	0.0	0.2	0.4	7.7	0.0	0.0
5.5	5.9	13.0	0.0	2.1	0.0	609.6	0.0	0.0	34.9	0.0	0.0	0.0	0.0	0.0	0.0
0.0	7.3	20.0	241.0	2.7	0.0	686.0	0.0	268.2	34.0	0.0	0.1	0.1	2.0	0.0	0.0

Code	Food Name	Unit Amount	Kilocalories (kcal)	Protein (g)	Carbohydrate (g)
22573	Frozen meal, swedish meatballs w/pasta/Stouffer's Lean Cuisine	1 package	276.1	21.7	31.2
924101	Frozen meal, swiss steak/Swanson	10.0 oz	346.5	26.2	37.0
22683	Frozen meal, teriyaki chicken breast w/Oriental veges/Budget Gourmet Light & Healthy	1 package	317.2	18.7	52.2
924176	Frozen meal, turkey w/gravy	5.0 oz	95.1	8.4	6.6
924215	Frozen meal, turkey w/gravy/Banquet	5.0 oz	99.4	7.0	5.0
924175	Frozen meal, turkey & dressing/Armour	11.5 oz	319.5	19.0	34.0
924103	Frozen meal, turkey/Banquet	10.5 oz	390.4	18.0	35.0
924304	Frozen meal, veal marsala/LeMenuLite	10.0 oz	249.9	25.3	25.4
924314	Frozen meal, veal parmigiana dinner/Armour	11.25 oz	398.8	18.0	34.0
924061	Frozen meal, vegetable chow mein/LeanCuisine	3/4 cup	34.6	2.0	6.0
924115	Frozen meal, vegetable lasagna/LeMenuLite	10.5 oz	253.3	12.4	34.0
924121	Frozen meal, vegetarian lasagna	7.8 oz	316.0	20.0	30.0
924301	Frozen meal, ziti w/meat sauce/Swanson	17.6 oz	557.5	28.4	58.4
914896	Fruit beverage mix, fruit punch drink, dry, prep	8 fl oz	96.9	0.0	24.8
914847	Fruit beverage mix, grape/Crystal Light	8 fl oz	2.4	0.1	0.3
914844	Fruit beverage mix, Kool-Aid	8 fl oz	98.4	0.0	25.1
14127	Fruit beverage mix, Kool-Aid, sugar free w/aspartame & vit C, dry mix, cherry flavor	1/8 envelope	3.5	0.1	1.0
14290	Fruit beverage mix, lemonade w/aspartame, low kcal, dry, prep	1 fl oz	0.6	0.0	0.1
14288	Fruit beverage mix, lemonade, dry, prep w/H$_2$O	1 cup H$_2$O & 2 Tbsp. mix	103.0	0.0	26.9
914845	Fruit beverage mix, lemonade/CountryTime	8 fl oz	81.6	0.0	20.5
14408	Fruit beverage mix, orange flavor drink, dry, prep w/H$_2$O	1 fl oz	14.3	0.0	3.7
914807	Fruit beverage mix, w/sugar/Kool-Aid	8 fl oz	81.6	0.0	21.0
914897	Fruit beverage, cherry juice drink	6 fl oz	96.5	0.2	23.6
14263	Fruit beverage, citrus drink, frozen concentrate, prep w/H$_2$O	1 cup (8 fl oz)	112.7	0.7	28.2
14238	Fruit beverage, cranberry-apple drink, bottled	1 cup (8 fl oz)	164.2	0.2	41.9
14242	Fruit beverage, cranberry cocktail, bottled	12 fl oz can	248.0	0.0	62.6
14431	Fruit beverage, cranberry juice cocktail, frozen concentrate, prep w/H$_2$O	1 cup (8 fl oz)	144.1	0.0	36.7
14267	Fruit beverage, fruit punch, canned	1 cup	116.1	0.0	29.4
14269	Fruit beverage, fruit punch, frozen concentrate, prep w/H$_2$O	1 cup	113.6	0.0	28.9
14282	Fruit beverage, grape juice drink, canned	6 fl oz glass	94.0	0.2	24.3
914848	Fruit beverage, grapefruit juice cocktail	6 fl oz	79.2	0.0	20.0
914842	Fruit beverage, Hawaiian punch	8 fl oz	121.0	0.0	29.0
14406	Fruit beverage, juice drink, frozen concentrate, prep	1 fl oz	15.5	0.0	3.8
914898	Fruit beverage, lemonade, canned	6 fl oz	64.4	0.0	16.5
14543	Fruit beverage, lemonade, pink, frozen conc, prep w/H$_2$O	6 fl oz	74.4	0.2	19.5
14293	Fruit beverage, lemonade, white, frozen, prep w/H$_2$O	6 fl oz	74.4	0.2	19.5
14303	Fruit beverage, limeade, frozen concentrate, prep w/H$_2$O	6 fl oz	76.3	0.0	20.5
914843	Fruit beverage, low kcal/Hawaiian punch	8 fl oz	34.6	0.1	8.0
14323	Fruit beverage, orange drink, canned	6 fl oz	94.9	0.0	24.0
914900	Fruit beverage, orange-pineapple juice drink	6 fl oz	93.6	0.6	23.0
14334	Fruit beverage, pineapple & grapefruit juice drink, canned	6 fl oz	87.4	0.4	21.6
14341	Fruit beverage, pineapple & orange juice drink, canned	6 fl oz	93.0	2.4	21.9
914808	Fruit beverage, sugar free/Kool-Aid	8 fl oz	2.4	0.1	0.3
914903	Fruit beverage, wild berry juice drink	6 fl oz	90.7	0.0	23.0
9101	Fruit cocktail (peach, pineapple, pear, grape, & cherry) canned in ex-heavy syrup	1/2 cup	114.4	0.5	29.8
9098	Fruit cocktail (peach, pineapple, pear, grape, & cherry) canned in extralite syrup	1/2 cup	54.9	0.5	14.2
914839	Fruit juice, apple, Juice Works/Campbells	6 fl oz	97.2	0.3	23.7
9400	Fruit juice, apple, canned or bottled, unsweetened w/added vit C	6 fl oz	84.6	0.1	21.0
9411	Fruit juice, apple, frozen concentrate, unsweetened w/added vit C, prep	6 fl oz container	99.2	0.3	24.3
9403	Fruit juice, apricot nectar, canned, w/added vit C	6 fl oz container	118.2	0.8	30.4
914910	Fruit juice, cranberry apple juice	6 fl oz container	192.0	1.1	48.8
914907	Fruit juice, cranberry apple juice, low kcal	6 fl oz container	35.9	0.2	8.4
9137	Fruit juice, grape, frozen concentrate, sweetened w/added vit C, prep	6 fl oz container	110.2	0.4	27.5
9124	Fruit juice, grapefruit, canned, sweetened	6 fl oz container	99.4	1.3	24.0
9123	Fruit juice, grapefruit, canned, unsweetened	6 fl oz container	82.1	1.1	19.4
9126	Fruit juice, grapefruit, frozen concentrate, unsweetened, prep	1 fl oz	12.7	0.2	3.0
9404	Fruit juice, grapefruit, pink or red, fresh	1 cup	96.3	1.2	22.7
9128	Fruit juice, grapefruit, white, fresh	juice from 1 fruit	76.4	1.0	18.0
9153	Fruit juice, lemon, canned or bottled	1 Tbsp.	3.2	0.1	1.0
9152	Fruit juice, lemon, fresh	1 Tbsp.	3.8	0.1	1.3
9161	Fruit juice, lime, canned or bottled unsweetened	1 Tbsp.	3.2	0.0	1.0
9160	Fruit juice, lime, fresh	1 Tbsp.	4.1	0.1	1.4
9207	Fruit juice, orange, canned, unsweetened	1 fl oz	13.1	0.2	3.1
9206	Fruit juice, orange, fresh	juice from 1 fruit (2.6" diam)	38.7	0.6	8.9
9215	Fruit juice, orange, frozen concentrate, unsweetened, prep	1 fl oz	14.0	0.2	3.4

Dietary Fiber (g)	Total Fat (g)	Cholesterol (mg)	Calcium (mg)	Iron (mg)	Magnesium (mg)	Sodium (mg)	Zinc (mg)	Vitamin A (µgRE)	Vitamin C (mg)	Vitamin E (mgαT)	Thiamin (mg)	Riboflavin (mg)	Niacin (mg)	Vitamin B_6 (mg)	Folate (µg)
2.6	7.2	46.4	0.0	2.1	0.0	562.4	0.0	0.0	0.0	0.0	0.0	0.0	0.0	0.0	0.0
0.0	10.5	0.0	49.0	4.4	0.0	701.0	0.0	112.6	11.0	0.0	0.2	0.2	4.6	0.0	0.0
4.0	3.7	24.9	0.0	0.0	0.0	674.9	0.0	0.0	44.5	0.0	0.0	0.0	0.0	0.0	0.0
0.1	3.7	45.0	20.0	1.3	12.0	786.0	1.0	11.8	0.0	0.0	0.0	0.2	2.6	0.1	0.0
0.1	6.0	45.0	19.0	0.7	0.0	586.0	0.0	1.6	0.0	0.0	0.0	0.1	1.7	0.0	0.0
0.0	12.0	50.0	95.0	2.0	0.0	1280.0	0.0	601.2	8.0	0.0	0.3	0.2	5.5	0.0	0.0
0.0	20.0	40.0	49.0	1.0	0.0	1110.0	0.0	109.2	6.0	0.0	0.1	0.2	5.8	0.0	0.0
0.0	5.2	112.0	33.0	1.8	0.0	728.0	0.0	243.2	3.0	0.0	0.2	0.5	7.4	0.0	0.0
0.0	22.0	55.0	164.0	3.0	0.0	1320.0	0.0	220.4	27.0	0.0	0.3	0.3	3.6	0.0	0.0
2.0	0.0	0.0	80.0	0.7	0.0	780.0	0.0	200.0	15.0	0.0	0.0	0.0	0.4	0.0	0.0
0.0	7.4	24.0	174.0	2.8	0.0	462.0	0.0	367.6	44.0	0.0	0.2	0.4	2.8	0.0	0.0
2.0	14.0	30.0	457.0	2.4	0.0	760.0	2.0	33.6	7.0	0.0	0.2	0.3	2.0	0.2	14.0
0.0	23.5	0.0	255.0	7.5	0.0	1689.0	0.0	476.2	38.0	0.0	0.4	0.4	6.6	0.0	0.0
0.0	23.6	0.0	41.0	0.1	3.0	38.0	0.1	0.0	31.0	0.0	0.0	0.0	0.0	0.0	0.0
0.0	0.0	0.0	0.0	0.0	14.0	0.0	0.0	0.0	6.0	0.0	0.0	0.0	0.0	0.0	0.0
0.0	0.0	0.0	15.0	0.0	0.0	14.0	0.0	0.0	6.0	0.0	0.0	0.0	0.0	0.0	0.0
0.0	0.0	0.0	0.0	0.0	0.0	5.1	0.0	0.0	6.7	0.0	0.0	0.0	0.0	0.0	0.0
0.0	0.0	0.0	6.2	0.0	0.3	0.9	0.0	0.0	0.7	0.0	0.0	0.0	0.0	0.0	0.0
0.0	0.0	0.0	71.3	0.2	2.6	13.2	0.1	0.0	8.4	0.0	0.0	0.0	0.0	0.0	3.4
0.0	0.0	0.0	1.0	0.0	16.0	21.0	0.0	0.0	6.0	0.0	0.0	0.0	0.0	0.0	0.0
0.0	0.0	0.0	7.8	0.0	0.3	1.6	0.0	68.8	15.1	0.0	0.0	0.0	0.0	0.0	17.9
0.0	0.0	0.0	26.0	0.0	0.0	19.0	0.0	0.0	6.0	0.0	0.0	0.0	0.0	0.0	0.0
0.0	0.1	0.0	20.0	0.9	0.0	18.0	0.0	0.0	7.0	0.0	0.0	0.0	0.4	0.0	0.0
0.0	0.0	0.0	22.1	2.7	14.7	7.4	0.1	9.8	66.4	0.0	0.0	0.0	0.4	0.1	4.9
0.2	0.0	0.0	17.2	0.1	4.9	4.9	0.1	0.0	78.4	0.0	0.0	0.0	0.1	0.1	0.5
0.4	0.4	0.0	13.1	0.7	8.7	8.7	0.3	0.0	154.0	0.0	0.0	0.0	0.2	0.1	0.9
0.3	0.0	0.0	13.1	0.2	5.2	7.9	0.1	2.6	25.9	0.0	0.0	0.0	0.0	0.0	0.0
0.2	0.0	0.0	19.8	0.5	4.9	54.3	0.3	2.5	73.1	0.0	0.1	0.1	0.1	0.0	3.2
0.2	0.0	0.0	9.9	0.2	4.9	9.9	0.1	2.5	108.4	0.0	0.0	0.0	0.1	0.0	2.2
0.2	0.0	0.0	5.6	0.2	7.5	1.9	0.1	0.0	30.1	0.0	0.0	0.0	0.2	0.0	1.5
0.1	0.0	0.0	14.0	0.2	8.0	15.0	0.1	0.0	100.0	0.0	0.0	0.0	0.0	0.0	0.0
0.0	0.0	0.0	4.0	0.4	0.0	23.0	0.0	2.6	80.0	0.0	0.0	0.0	0.0	0.0	0.0
0.0	0.1	0.0	2.2	0.1	1.2	1.6	0.1	0.3	1.7	0.0	0.0	0.0	0.0	0.0	0.0
0.0	0.0	0.0	0.0	0.0	0.0	33.0	0.0	0.0	22.0	0.0	0.0	0.0	0.0	0.0	0.0
0.0	0.0	0.0	5.6	0.3	3.7	5.6	0.1	0.0	7.3	0.0	0.0	0.0	0.0	0.0	4.1
0.2	0.0	0.0	5.6	0.3	3.7	5.6	0.1	3.7	7.3	0.0	0.0	0.0	0.0	0.0	4.1
0.2	0.0	0.0	5.6	0.1	1.9	3.7	0.0	0.0	5.0	0.0	0.0	0.0	0.0	0.0	1.9
0.0	0.0	0.0	0.0	0.0	0.0	0.0	0.0	0.0	0.0	0.0	0.0	0.0	0.0	0.0	0.0
0.2	0.0	0.0	11.2	0.5	3.7	29.8	0.2	3.7	63.4	0.0	0.0	0.0	0.1	0.0	4.1
1.0	0.0	0.0	0.0	0.0	0.0	1.0	0.0	115.2	60.0	0.0	0.0	0.0	0.0	0.0	0.0
0.2	0.2	0.0	13.0	0.6	11.2	26.0	0.1	7.4	85.6	0.0	0.1	0.0	0.5	0.1	19.5
0.2	0.0	0.0	9.3	0.5	11.2	5.6	0.1	98.6	41.9	0.0	0.1	0.0	0.4	0.1	20.3
0.0	0.0	0.0	24.0	0.0	0.0	13.0	0.0	0.0	6.0	0.0	0.0	0.0	0.0	0.0	0.0
0.0	0.0	0.0	2.0	0.4	0.0	19.0	0.0	2.8	60.0	0.0	0.0	0.0	0.0	0.0	0.0
1.4	0.1	0.0	7.8	0.4	6.5	7.8	0.1	26.0	2.5	0.0	0.0	0.0	0.5	0.1	3.4
1.3	0.1	0.0	9.8	0.4	7.3	4.9	0.1	28.1	3.7	0.0	0.0	0.0	0.6	0.1	3.3
0.0	0.1	0.0	19.0	0.9	0.0	30.0	0.0	0.0	5.0	0.0	0.0	0.0	0.3	0.0	0.0
0.2	0.2	0.0	12.6	0.7	5.4	5.4	0.1	0.0	74.9	0.0	0.0	0.0	0.0	0.1	0.2
0.2	0.2	0.0	12.7	0.5	10.6	14.8	0.1	0.0	52.8	0.0	0.0	0.0	0.1	0.1	0.6
1.3	0.2	0.0	14.8	0.8	10.6	6.3	0.2	278.5	114.8	0.0	0.0	0.0	0.5	0.0	2.7
1.1	10.2	0.0	20.4	0.2	0.0	5.7	0.1	0.2	90.8	0.0	0.0	0.1	0.2	0.1	1.1
0.0	0.2	0.0	19.3	0.1	0.0	9.1	0.0	0.0	68.1	0.0	0.0	0.0	0.0	0.0	0.0
0.2	0.2	0.0	8.6	0.2	8.6	4.3	0.1	2.2	51.6	0.1	0.0	0.1	0.3	0.1	2.8
0.2	0.2	0.0	17.3	0.8	21.6	4.3	0.1	0.0	58.1	0.1	0.1	0.0	0.7	0.0	22.5
0.2	0.2	0.0	15.1	0.4	21.6	2.2	0.2	2.2	63.1	0.1	0.1	0.0	0.5	0.0	22.5
0.0	0.0	0.0	2.5	0.0	3.4	0.3	0.0	0.3	10.4	0.0	0.0	0.0	0.1	0.0	1.1
0.0	0.2	0.0	22.2	0.5	29.6	2.5	0.1	108.7	93.9	0.0	0.1	0.0	0.5	0.1	25.2
0.2	0.2	0.0	17.6	0.4	23.5	2.0	0.1	2.0	74.5	0.1	0.1	0.0	0.4	0.1	20.0
0.1	0.0	0.0	1.7	0.0	1.2	3.2	0.0	0.3	3.8	0.0	0.0	0.0	0.0	0.0	1.5
0.1	0.0	0.0	1.1	0.0	0.9	0.2	0.0	0.3	6.9	0.0	0.0	0.0	0.0	0.0	1.9
0.1	0.0	0.0	1.8	0.0	1.1	2.4	0.0	0.3	1.0	0.0	0.0	0.0	0.0	0.0	1.2
0.1	0.0	0.0	1.4	0.0	0.9	0.2	0.0	0.2	4.4	0.0	0.0	0.0	0.0	0.0	1.2
0.1	0.0	0.0	2.5	0.1	3.4	0.6	0.0	5.6	10.7	0.0	0.0	0.0	0.1	0.0	5.6
0.2	0.2	0.0	9.5	0.2	9.5	0.9	0.0	17.2	43.0	0.1	0.1	0.0	0.3	0.0	26.1
0.1	0.0	0.0	2.8	0.0	3.1	0.3	0.0	2.5	12.1	0.1	0.0	0.0	0.1	0.0	13.6

Code	Food Name	Unit Amount	Kilocalories (kcal)	Protein (g)	Carbohydrate (g)
914889	Fruit juice, orange-grapefruit juice	1 cup	110.3	1.6	25.5
9229	Fruit juice, papaya nectar, canned	6 fl oz	121.4	0.4	30.9
9232	Fruit juice, passion fruit, purple, fresh	6 fl oz	111.2	0.9	29.6
9407	Fruit juice, peach nectar, canned, w/added vit C	6 fl oz	115.0	0.6	29.6
9408	Fruit juice, pear nectar, canned, w/added vit C	6 fl oz	127.8	0.2	33.6
9409	Fruit juice, pineapple, canned, unsweetened w/added vit C	6 fl oz	119.3	0.7	29.4
9294	Fruit juice, prune, canned	6 fl oz	151.2	1.3	37.2
9223	Fruit juice, tangerine, canned, sweetened	6 fl oz	106.5	1.1	25.6
9105	Fruit salad (peach, pineapple, pear, apricot, & cherry) canned in heavy syrup	1/2 cup	92.7	0.4	24.3
9103	Fruit salad (peach, pineapple, pear, apricot, & cherry) canned in juice	1/2 cup	62.0	0.6	16.2
9104	Fruit salad (peach, pineapple, pear, apricot, & cherry) canned in lite syrup	1/2 cup	73.1	0.4	19.1
9003	Fruit, apple w/skin, raw	1 medium (2.75" diam) (3/lb)	81.4	0.3	21.0
9009	Fruit, apple, dehydrated, sulfured	1 cup	207.6	0.8	56.1
9014	Fruit, apple, frozen, unsweetened	1 cup slices	83.0	0.5	21.3
9004	Fruit, apple, peeled, raw, medium	1 fruit (2.75" diam) (3/lb)	73.0	0.2	19.0
9007	Fruit, apple, slices, sweetened, canned, drained	1/2 cup slices	68.3	0.2	17.0
9402	Fruit, applesauce, canned, sweetened w/added vit C	1/2 cup	96.5	0.2	25.3
9401	Fruit, applesauce, canned, unsweetened w/added vit C	1/2 cup	52.5	0.2	13.8
9024	Fruit, apricot w/skin, canned in juice	1/2 cup of halves	59.0	0.8	15.2
9026	Fruit, apricot w/skin, canned in lite syrup	1/2 cup of halves	77.5	0.7	20.3
9032	Fruit, apricot, dried, sulfured	1/2 cup of halves	8.3	0.1	2.2
9035	Fruit, apricot, frozen, sweetened	1 cup	118.6	0.8	30.4
9023	Fruit, apricot, peeled, canned in H$_2$O	4 halves & 2 Tbsp. liquid	19.8	0.6	4.9
9028	Fruit, apricot, peeled, canned in heavy syrup	4 halves & 2 Tbsp. liquid	74.7	0.5	19.3
9021	Fruit, apricot, raw	1 apricot	16.8	0.5	3.9
9037	Fruit, avocado, all varieties, peeled, raw	1 fruit w/o pit	185.2	2.3	8.5
9041	Fruit, banana, dried or powder	1 Tbsp.	173.0	1.9	44.1
9046	Fruit, blackberries, canned in heavy syrup	1/2 cup	112.2	1.6	28.2
9048	Fruit, blackberries, frozen, unsweetened	1 cup	163.2	3.0	40.0
9042	Fruit, blackberries, raw	1 cup	74.9	1.0	18.4
9052	Fruit, blueberries, canned in heavy syrup	1/2 cup	113.5	0.8	28.5
9054	Fruit, blueberries, frozen, unsweetened	1/2 cup	72.4	0.6	17.3
9050	Fruit, blueberries, raw	1 cup	81.2	1.0	20.5
9056	Fruit, boysenberries, canned in heavy syrup	1/2 cup	125.0	1.4	31.7
9057	Fruit, boysenberries, frozen, unsweetened	1/2 cup	71.0	1.6	17.3
9059	Fruit, breadfruit, peeled, raw	1/4 small fruit w/o seeds	98.9	1.0	26.0
9060	Fruit, crambola (starfruit) raw	1 small (3" long)	23.1	0.4	5.5
9061	Fruit, carissa (natal-plum) peeled, raw	1 fruit w/o seeds	12.4	0.1	2.7
9062	Fruit, cherimoya, peeled, raw	1 fruit w/o seeds	514.2	7.1	131.3
9065	Fruit, cherries, sour, red, canned in lite syrup	1/2 cup	94.5	0.9	24.3
9068	Fruit, cherries, sour, red, frozen, unsweetened	1/2 cup	57.5	1.2	13.8
9063	Fruit, cherries, sour, red, raw	1 cup w/pits	51.5	1.0	12.5
9064	Fruit, cherries, sour/tart, red, canned in H$_2$O	1/2 cup	43.9	0.9	10.9
9072	Fruit, cherries, sweet, canned in juice	1/2 cup w/o pits	67.5	1.1	17.3
9073	Fruit, cherries, sweet, canned in lite syrup	1/2 cup w/o pits	84.4	0.8	21.8
9076	Fruit, cherries, sweet, frozen, sweetened	10 oz package	126.4	1.6	31.8
9070	Fruit, cherries, sweet, raw	1 cup w/pits, edible part	84.2	1.4	19.4
9078	Fruit, cranberries, raw	1 cup whole	46.6	0.4	12.0
9082	Fruit, cranberry-orange relish, canned	1/2 cup	245.6	0.4	63.8
9081	Fruit, cranberry sauce, canned, sweetened	1 slice (0.5" thick, ~8 slices/can)	86.1	0.1	22.2
9083	Fruit, currant, European, black, raw	1 cup	70.6	1.6	17.2
9084	Fruit, currant, red or white, raw	1 cup	62.7	1.6	15.5
9087	Fruit, dates, domestic, natural, dried	1 date	22.8	0.2	6.1
9091	Fruit, figs, canned in lite syrup	1 fig w/liquid	19.3	0.1	5.0
9094	Fruit, figs, dried, raw	1 fig	48.5	0.6	12.4
9095	Fruit, figs, dried, stewed	1/2 cup	140.4	1.7	35.8
9089	Fruit, figs, raw	1 small (1.5" diam)	29.6	0.3	7.7
9107	Fruit, gooseberries, raw	1/2 cup	33.0	0.7	7.6
9120	Fruit, grapefruit, canned in juice	1/2 cup	46.3	0.9	11.5
9121	Fruit, grapefruit, canned in lite syrup	1/2 cup	94.8	0.9	24.4
9111	Fruit, grapefruit, red, white or pink, peeled, raw	1/2 cup sections w/juice	43.2	0.9	10.9
9131	Fruit, grapes, American-type (slip skin) raw	1 cup	61.6	0.6	15.8
9139	Fruit, guava, common, raw	1/2 cup	43.4	0.7	10.1
9148	Fruit, kiwifruit (Chinese gooseberry) peeled, raw	1 medium fruit	46.4	0.8	11.3
9149	Fruit, kumquat, raw	1 fruit	12.0	0.2	3.1

Dietary Fiber (g)	Total Fat (g)	Cholesterol (mg)	Calcium (mg)	Iron (mg)	Magnesium (mg)	Sodium (mg)	Zinc (mg)	Vitamin A (μgRE)	Vitamin C (mg)	Vitamin E (mg αT)	Thiamin (mg)	Riboflavin (mg)	Niacin (mg)	Vitamin B6 (mg)	Folate (μg)
0.1	0.1	0.0	24.0	0.3	25.0	1.0	0.2	56.2	107.0	0.0	0.2	0.0	0.7	0.1	7.0
1.3	0.3	0.0	21.3	0.7	6.4	10.7	0.3	23.4	6.4	0.0	0.0	0.0	0.3	0.1	4.5
0.4	0.1	0.0	8.7	0.5	37.1	13.1	0.1	157.0	65.0	0.1	0.0	0.3	3.2	0.1	15.3
1.3	0.0	0.0	10.7	0.4	8.5	14.9	0.2	55.4	57.1	0.0	0.0	0.0	0.6	0.0	3.0
1.3	0.0	0.0	10.7	0.6	6.4	8.5	0.1	0.0	57.5	0.0	0.0	0.0	0.3	0.0	2.6
0.4	0.2	0.0	36.2	0.6	27.7	2.1	0.2	0.0	51.1	0.0	0.1	0.0	0.5	0.2	49.2
2.1	0.1	0.0	25.6	2.5	29.8	8.5	0.4	0.0	8.7	0.0	0.0	0.1	1.7	0.5	0.9
0.4	0.4	0.0	38.3	0.4	17.0	2.1	0.1	89.5	46.9	0.2	0.1	0.0	0.2	0.1	9.8
1.3	0.1	0.0	7.6	0.4	6.4	7.6	0.1	63.5	3.0	0.6	0.0	0.0	0.4	0.0	3.2
1.2	0.0	0.0	13.6	0.3	9.9	6.2	0.2	74.4	4.1	0.0	0.0	0.0	0.4	0.0	3.2
1.3	0.1	0.0	8.8	0.4	6.3	7.6	0.1	54.2	3.2	0.0	0.0	0.0	0.5	0.0	3.3
3.7	0.5	0.0	9.7	0.2	6.9	0.0	0.1	6.9	7.9	0.4	0.0	0.0	0.1	0.1	3.9
7.4	0.3	0.0	11.4	1.2	13.2	74.4	0.2	4.8	1.3	2.1	0.0	0.1	0.4	0.2	0.6
3.3	0.6	0.0	6.9	0.3	5.2	5.2	0.1	5.2	0.2	0.0	0.0	0.0	0.1	0.1	1.2
2.4	0.4	0.0	5.1	0.1	3.8	0.0	0.1	5.1	5.1	0.1	0.0	0.0	0.1	0.1	0.5
1.7	0.5	0.0	4.1	0.2	2.0	3.1	0.0	5.1	0.4	0.0	0.0	0.0	0.1	0.0	0.3
1.5	0.2	0.0	5.1	0.4	3.8	35.6	0.1	1.3	2.2	0.0	0.0	0.0	0.2	0.0	0.8
1.5	0.1	0.0	3.7	0.1	3.7	2.4	0.0	3.7	25.9	0.0	0.0	0.0	0.2	0.0	0.7
2.0	0.0	0.0	14.8	0.4	12.3	4.9	0.1	207.9	6.0	1.1	0.0	0.0	0.4	0.1	2.1
2.0	0.1	0.0	13.5	0.5	9.8	4.9	0.1	162.4	3.3	1.1	0.0	0.0	0.4	0.1	2.1
0.3	0.0	0.0	1.6	0.2	1.6	0.4	0.0	25.3	0.1	0.1	0.0	0.0	0.1	0.0	0.4
2.7	0.1	0.0	12.1	1.1	10.9	4.8	0.1	203.3	10.9	1.1	0.0	0.0	1.0	0.1	2.1
1.0	0.0	0.0	7.2	0.5	8.1	9.9	0.1	162.9	1.6	0.0	0.0	0.0	0.4	0.0	1.5
1.4	0.1	0.0	8.1	0.4	7.2	9.9	0.1	111.6	2.5	0.0	0.0	0.0	0.4	0.0	1.5
0.8	0.1	0.0	4.9	0.2	2.8	0.4	0.1	91.4	3.5	0.3	0.0	0.0	0.2	0.0	3.0
5.8	17.6	0.0	12.7	1.2	44.9	11.5	0.5	70.2	9.1	1.5	0.1	0.1	2.2	0.3	71.2
3.8	0.9	0.0	11.0	0.6	54.0	1.5	0.3	15.5	3.5	0.0	0.1	0.1	1.4	0.2	7.0
4.1	0.2	0.0	25.6	0.8	20.7	3.7	0.2	26.8	3.4	0.9	0.0	0.0	0.4	0.0	32.3
12.8	1.1	0.0	74.0	2.0	56.1	2.6	0.6	28.1	7.9	1.8	0.1	0.1	3.1	0.2	86.7
7.6	0.6	0.0	46.1	0.8	28.8	0.0	0.4	23.0	30.2	1.0	0.0	0.1	0.6	0.1	49.0
1.9	0.4	0.0	6.5	0.4	5.2	3.9	0.1	7.7	1.4	1.3	0.0	0.1	0.1	0.0	2.1
3.8	0.9	0.0	11.4	0.3	7.1	1.4	0.1	11.4	3.6	1.4	0.0	0.1	0.7	0.1	9.5
3.9	0.6	0.0	8.7	0.2	7.3	8.7	0.2	14.5	18.9	1.5	0.1	0.1	0.5	0.1	9.3
3.7	0.2	0.0	25.6	0.6	15.6	4.3	0.3	5.7	8.8	1.0	0.0	0.0	0.3	0.1	48.8
5.5	0.4	0.0	38.3	1.2	22.7	1.4	0.3	9.9	4.4	0.6	0.1	0.1	1.1	0.1	89.9
4.7	0.2	0.0	16.3	0.5	24.0	1.9	0.1	3.8	27.8	1.1	0.1	0.0	0.9	0.1	13.4
1.9	0.2	0.0	2.8	0.2	6.3	1.4	0.1	34.3	14.8	0.3	0.0	0.0	0.3	0.1	9.8
0.0	0.3	0.0	2.2	0.3	3.2	0.6	0.0	0.8	7.6	0.0	0.0	0.0	0.0	0.0	0.0
13.1	2.2	0.0	125.8	2.7	0.0	0.0	0.0	5.5	49.2	0.0	0.5	0.6	7.1	0.0	0.0
1.0	0.1	0.0	12.6	1.7	7.6	8.8	0.1	92.0	2.5	0.0	0.0	0.0	0.2	0.1	9.7
2.0	0.6	0.0	16.3	0.7	11.3	1.3	0.1	108.8	2.1	0.2	0.1	0.0	0.2	0.1	5.6
1.6	0.3	0.0	16.5	0.3	9.3	3.1	0.1	131.8	10.3	0.1	0.0	0.0	0.4	0.0	7.7
1.3	0.1	0.0	13.4	1.7	7.3	8.5	0.1	91.5	2.6	0.2	0.0	0.1	0.2	0.1	9.8
1.9	0.0	0.0	17.5	0.7	15.0	3.8	0.1	16.3	3.1	0.1	0.0	0.0	0.5	0.0	5.3
1.9	0.2	0.0	11.3	0.5	11.3	3.8	0.1	20.2	4.7	0.2	0.0	0.1	0.5	0.0	5.3
3.0	0.2	0.0	17.0	0.5	14.2	1.4	0.1	27.0	1.4	0.2	0.0	0.1	0.3	0.1	6.0
2.7	1.1	0.0	17.6	0.5	12.9	0.0	0.1	24.6	8.2	0.2	0.1	0.1	0.5	0.0	4.9
4.0	0.2	0.0	6.7	0.2	4.8	1.0	0.1	4.8	12.8	0.1	0.0	0.0	0.1	0.1	1.6
0.0	0.1	0.0	15.2	0.3	5.5	44.2	0.0	9.7	24.8	0.0	0.0	0.0	0.1	0.0	0.6
0.6	0.1	0.0	2.3	0.1	1.7	16.5	0.0	1.1	1.1	0.1	0.0	0.0	0.1	0.0	0.6
0.0	0.5	0.0	61.6	1.7	26.9	2.2	0.3	25.8	202.7	0.1	0.1	0.1	0.3	0.1	0.0
4.8	0.2	0.0	37.0	1.1	14.6	1.1	0.3	13.4	45.9	0.1	0.0	0.1	0.1	0.1	9.0
0.6	0.0	0.0	2.7	0.1	2.9	0.2	0.0	0.4	0.0	0.0	0.0	0.0	0.2	0.0	1.0
0.5	0.0	0.0	7.6	0.1	2.8	0.3	0.0	1.1	0.3	0.2	0.0	0.0	0.1	0.0	0.6
2.3	0.2	0.0	27.4	0.4	11.2	2.1	0.1	2.5	0.2	0.0	0.0	0.0	0.1	0.0	1.4
6.6	0.6	0.0	79.3	1.2	32.5	6.5	0.3	20.8	5.7	0.0	0.0	0.1	0.8	0.2	1.3
1.3	0.1	0.0	14.0	0.1	6.8	0.4	0.1	5.6	0.8	0.4	0.0	0.0	0.2	0.0	2.4
3.2	0.4	0.0	18.8	0.2	7.5	0.8	0.1	21.8	20.8	0.3	0.0	0.0	0.2	0.1	4.5
0.5	0.1	0.0	18.8	0.3	13.8	8.8	0.1	0.0	42.4	0.3	0.0	0.0	0.3	0.0	11.0
0.6	0.2	0.0	22.1	0.6	15.8	3.2	0.1	0.0	33.7	0.4	0.1	0.0	0.4	0.0	13.4
1.5	0.1	0.0	16.2	0.1	10.8	0.0	0.1	16.2	46.4	0.3	0.0	0.0	0.3	0.1	13.8
0.9	0.3	0.0	12.9	0.3	4.6	1.8	0.0	9.2	3.7	0.3	0.1	0.1	0.3	0.1	3.6
4.6	0.5	0.0	17.0	0.3	8.5	2.6	0.2	67.2	156.0	1.0	0.0	0.0	1.0	0.1	11.9
2.6	0.3	0.0	19.8	0.3	22.8	3.8	0.1	13.7	74.5	0.9	0.0	0.0	0.4	0.1	28.9
1.3	0.0	0.0	8.4	0.1	2.5	1.1	0.0	5.7	7.1	0.0	0.0	0.0	0.1	0.0	3.0

Code	Food Name	Unit Amount	Kilocalories (kcal)	Protein (g)	Carbohydrate (g)
9150	Fruit, lemon, peeled, raw	1 medium fruit (2.1″ diam)	16.8	0.6	5.4
9165	Fruit, lychee (litchi) shelled, dried	1 fruit	6.9	0.1	1.8
9176	Fruit, mango, peeled, raw	1 fruit w/o seed	134.6	1.1	35.2
9185	Fruit, melon balls (cantaloupe & honeydew) frozen	1 cup thawed	57.1	1.5	13.7
9183	Fruit, melon, casaba, peeled, raw	1 cup cubes	44.2	1.5	10.5
9184	Fruit, melon, honeydew, peeled, wedges, raw	10 honeydew balls	48.3	0.6	12.7
9188	Fruit, mixed (prune, apricot, & pear) dried	3.5 w/o pits	243.0	2.5	64.1
9187	Fruit, mixed (peach, pear, & pineapple) canned in heavy syrup	1 Tbsp.	11.4	0.1	3.0
9191	Fruit, nectarine, raw	1 fruit w/o pit (2.5″ diam)	66.6	1.3	16.0
9193	Fruit, olives, ripe, pitted, canned	1 tsp.	3.2	0.0	0.2
9216	Fruit, orange peel, raw	1 tsp.	1.9	0.0	0.5
9200	Fruit, orange, all varieties, peeled, raw	1 cup sections w/o membrane	84.6	1.7	21.2
9226	Fruit, papayas, peeled, cubed/mashed, raw	1 cup cubes	54.6	0.9	13.7
9231	Fruit, passion fruit/granadilla, purple, peeled, raw	1 fruit	17.5	0.4	4.2
9241	Fruit, peach, canned in heavy syrup	1 half w/liquid	72.5	0.4	19.5
9238	Fruit, peach, canned in juice	1 half w/liquid	43.1	0.6	11.3
9240	Fruit, peach, canned in lite syrup	1 half w/liquid	52.9	0.4	14.3
9246	Fruit, peach, dried, sulfured	1 half	31.1	0.5	8.0
9250	Fruit, peach, frozen, sweetened	10 slices	145.7	1.0	37.2
9236	Fruit, peach, peeled, raw	1 large (2.75″ diam) (2.5/lb)	67.5	1.1	17.4
9254	Fruit, pear, canned in juice	1/2 cup halves	62.0	0.4	16.0
9256	Fruit, pear, canned in lite syrup	1/2 cup halves	71.8	0.2	19.1
9259	Fruit, pear, dried, sulfured	10 halves	458.5	3.3	122.0
9252	Fruit, pear, raw	1 large pear (2/lb)	123.3	0.8	31.6
9265	Fruit, persimmon, native, raw	1 fruit w/o seeds	31.8	0.2	8.4
9268	Fruit, pineapple, canned in juice	1/2 cup crushed, sliced or chunks	75.0	0.5	19.6
9269	Fruit, pineapple, canned in lite syrup	1/2 cup crushed, sliced or chunks	65.5	0.5	16.9
9272	Fruit, pineapple, frozen, chunks, sweetened	1/2 cup of chunks, frz sweetened	104.6	0.5	27.3
9266	Fruit, pineapple, peeled, raw	1 fruit	231.3	1.8	58.5
9276	Fruit, pitanga (surinam cherry) peeled, raw	1 fruit w/o seeds	2.3	0.1	0.5
9277	Fruit, plantain, peeled, raw	1 medium fruit	218.4	2.3	57.1
9282	Fruit, plum, purple, canned in juice	1/2 cup w/o pits	73.1	0.6	19.1
9283	Fruit, plum, purple, canned in lite syrup	1/2 cup w/o pits	79.4	0.5	20.5
9279	Fruit, plum, raw	1 fruit (2.1″ diam) w/o pit	36.3	0.5	8.6
9286	Fruit, pomegranates, peeled, raw	1 fruit: 3.35″ diam	104.7	1.5	26.4
9287	Fruit, prickly pear, peeled, raw	1 fruit	42.2	0.8	9.9
9292	Fruit, prune, dried, stewed w/o added sugar	1 Tbsp. w/o pits	16.6	0.2	4.4
9290	Fruit, prunes, dehydrated, stewed	1/2 cup	158.2	1.7	41.6
9291	Fruit, prunes, dried	1 prune	20.1	0.2	5.3
9295	Fruit, pummelo, peeled, raw	1 fruit w/o seeds & membrane	231.4	4.6	58.6
9296	Fruit, quinces, peeled, raw	1 fruit w/o seeds	52.4	0.4	14.1
9297	Fruit, raisins, golden, seedless	1/2 cup packed	250.7	2.8	66.0
9298	Fruit, raisins, seedless	1/2 cup packed	249.0	2.7	65.7
9302	Fruit, raspberries, raw	10 raspberries	9.3	0.2	2.2
9304	Fruit, raspberries, red, canned in heavy syrup	1/2 cup	116.5	1.1	29.9
9306	Fruit, raspberries, red, frozen, sweetened	10 oz package	292.5	2.0	74.3
9310	Fruit, rhubarb, frozen, cooked w/sugar	1/2 cup	139.2	0.5	37.4
9307	Fruit, rhubarb, raw	1/2 cup diced	12.8	0.5	2.8
9317	Fruit, strawberries, canned in heavy syrup	1/2 cup	70.8	0.4	18.1
9320	Fruit, strawberries, frozen, sliced, sweetened	1 cup thawed	244.8	1.4	66.1
9318	Fruit, strawberries, unsweetened, frozen	1 cup	52.2	0.6	13.6
9322	Fruit, tamarind, raw	1 fruit w/o pods & seeds: 3″ x 1″	4.8	0.1	1.3
9326	Fruit, watermelon, balls, raw	1 cup balls	49.3	1.0	11.1
20005	Grain, barley	1 Tbsp.	40.7	1.4	8.5
20008	Grain, barley, pearled, ckd	1 Tbsp.	12.1	0.2	2.8
20009	Grain, buckwheat groats, roasted, ckd	1 Tbsp.	9.7	0.4	2.1
20012	Grain, bulgar, ckd	1 Tbsp.	7.0	0.3	1.6
20014	Grain, corn, shite	1 Tbsp.	38.0	1.0	7.7
20029	Grain, corn, yellow	1 Tbsp.	38.0	1.0	7.7
20030	Grain, couscous, dry	1 Tbsp.	40.6	1.4	8.4
20330	Grain, hominy, yellow	1 cup	128.3	2.7	27.9
20031	Grain, millet, ckd	1 Tbsp.	13.0	0.4	2.6
20035	Grain, oats	1 Tbsp.	38.1	1.7	6.5
20036	Grain, rice, brown, long-grain, ckd	1 Tbsp.	13.5	0.3	2.8
20040	Grain, rice, brown, medium-grain, ckd	1 Tbsp.	13.7	0.3	2.9

Dietary Fiber (g)	Total Fat (g)	Cholesterol (mg)	Calcium (mg)	Iron (mg)	Magnesium (mg)	Sodium (mg)	Zinc (mg)	Vitamin A (μgRE)	Vitamin C (mg)	Vitamin E (mgαT)	Thiamin (mg)	Riboflavin (mg)	Niacin (mg)	Vitamin B_6 (mg)	Folate (μg)
1.6	0.2	0.0	15.1	0.3	4.6	1.2	0.0	1.7	30.7	0.1	0.0	0.0	0.1	0.0	6.1
0.1	0.0	0.0	0.8	0.0	1.1	0.1	0.0	0.0	4.6	0.0	0.0	0.0	0.1	0.0	0.3
3.7	0.6	0.0	20.7	0.3	18.6	4.1	0.1	805.2	57.3	2.3	0.1	0.1	1.2	0.3	29.0
1.2	0.4	0.0	17.3	0.5	24.2	53.6	0.3	306.2	10.7	0.3	0.3	0.0	1.1	0.2	44.5
1.4	0.2	0.0	8.5	0.7	13.6	20.4	0.3	5.1	27.2	0.3	0.1	0.0	0.7	0.2	28.9
0.8	0.1	0.0	8.3	0.1	9.7	13.8	0.1	5.5	34.2	0.2	0.1	0.0	0.8	0.1	8.3
7.8	0.5	0.0	38.0	2.7	39.0	18.0	0.5	244.0	3.8	0.0	0.0	0.2	1.9	0.2	3.9
0.2	0.0	0.0	0.2	0.1	0.8	0.6	0.0	3.0	11.0	0.0	0.0	0.0	0.1	0.0	0.5
2.2	0.6	0.0	6.8	0.2	10.9	0.0	0.1	100.6	7.3	1.2	0.0	0.1	1.3	0.0	5.0
0.1	0.3	0.0	2.5	0.1	0.1	24.4	0.0	1.1	0.0	0.1	0.0	0.0	0.0	0.0	0.0
0.2	0.0	0.0	3.2	0.0	0.4	0.1	0.0	0.8	2.7	0.0	0.0	0.0	0.0	0.0	0.6
4.3	0.2	0.0	72.0	0.2	18.0	0.0	0.1	37.8	95.8	0.4	0.2	0.1	0.5	0.1	54.5
2.5	0.2	0.0	33.6	0.1	14.0	4.2	0.1	39.2	86.5	1.6	0.0	0.0	0.5	0.0	53.2
1.9	0.1	0.0	2.2	0.3	5.2	5.0	0.0	12.6	5.4	0.2	0.0	0.0	0.3	0.0	2.5
1.3	0.1	0.0	2.9	0.3	4.9	5.9	0.1	32.3	2.7	0.9	0.0	0.0	0.6	0.0	3.1
1.3	0.0	0.0	5.9	0.3	6.9	3.9	0.1	37.2	3.5	1.5	0.0	0.0	0.6	0.0	3.3
1.3	0.0	0.0	2.9	0.4	4.9	4.9	0.1	34.3	2.4	0.9	0.0	0.0	0.6	0.0	3.2
1.1	0.1	0.0	3.6	0.5	5.5	0.9	0.1	28.1	0.6	0.0	0.0	0.0	0.6	0.0	0.0
2.8	0.2	0.0	4.7	0.6	7.8	9.3	0.1	43.4	146.0	1.4	0.0	0.1	1.0	0.0	5.0
3.1	0.1	0.0	7.9	0.2	11.0	0.0	0.2	84.8	10.4	1.1	0.0	0.1	1.6	0.0	5.3
2.0	0.1	0.0	11.2	0.4	8.7	5.0	0.1	1.2	2.0	0.6	0.0	0.0	0.2	0.0	1.5
2.0	0.0	0.0	6.3	0.4	5.0	6.3	0.1	0.0	0.9	0.6	0.0	0.0	0.2	0.0	1.5
13.1	1.1	0.0	59.5	3.7	57.8	10.5	0.7	0.0	12.3	0.0	0.0	0.3	2.4	0.1	0.0
5.0	0.8	0.0	23.0	0.5	12.5	0.0	0.3	4.2	8.4	1.0	0.0	0.1	0.2	0.0	15.3
0.0	0.1	0.0	6.8	0.6	0.0	0.3	0.0	0.0	16.5	0.0	0.0	0.0	0.0	0.0	0.0
1.0	0.1	0.0	17.5	0.4	17.5	1.3	0.1	5.0	11.9	0.1	0.1	0.0	0.4	0.1	6.0
1.0	0.2	0.0	17.6	0.5	20.2	1.3	0.2	1.3	9.5	0.1	0.1	0.0	0.4	0.1	5.9
1.4	0.1	0.0	11.1	0.5	12.3	2.5	0.1	3.7	9.8	0.1	0.1	0.0	0.4	0.1	13.0
5.7	2.0	0.0	33.0	1.7	66.1	4.7	0.4	9.4	72.7	0.5	0.4	0.2	2.0	0.4	50.0
0.0	0.0	0.0	0.6	0.0	0.8	0.2	0.0	10.5	1.8	0.0	0.0	0.0	0.0	0.0	0.0
4.1	0.7	0.0	5.4	1.1	66.2	7.2	0.3	202.3	32.9	0.5	0.1	0.1	1.2	0.5	39.4
1.3	0.0	0.0	12.6	0.4	10.1	1.3	0.1	127.3	3.5	0.9	0.0	0.1	0.6	0.0	3.3
1.3	0.1	0.0	11.3	1.1	6.3	25.2	0.1	32.8	0.5	0.9	0.0	0.1	0.4	0.0	3.3
1.0	0.4	0.0	2.6	0.1	4.6	0.0	0.1	21.1	6.3	0.4	0.0	0.1	0.3	0.1	1.5
0.9	0.5	0.0	4.6	0.5	4.6	4.6	0.2	0.0	9.4	0.8	0.0	0.0	0.5	0.2	9.2
3.7	0.5	0.0	57.7	0.3	87.6	5.2	0.1	5.2	14.4	0.0	0.0	0.1	0.5	0.1	6.2
1.0	0.0	0.0	3.6	0.2	3.1	0.3	0.0	4.8	0.4	0.0	0.0	0.0	0.1	0.0	0.0
0.0	0.3	0.0	33.6	1.6	29.4	2.8	0.4	72.8	0.0	0.0	0.1	0.0	1.4	0.3	0.3
0.6	0.0	0.0	4.3	0.2	3.8	0.3	0.0	16.7	0.3	0.1	0.0	0.0	0.2	0.0	0.3
6.1	0.2	0.0	24.4	0.7	36.5	6.1	0.5	0.0	371.5	0.0	0.2	0.2	1.3	0.2	0.0
1.7	0.1	0.0	10.1	0.6	7.4	3.7	0.0	3.7	13.8	0.5	0.0	0.0	0.2	0.0	2.8
3.3	0.4	0.0	44.0	1.5	29.1	10.0	0.3	3.3	2.7	0.6	0.0	0.2	0.9	0.3	2.7
3.3	0.4	0.0	40.7	1.7	27.4	10.0	0.2	0.8	2.7	0.6	0.1	0.1	0.7	0.2	2.7
1.3	0.1	0.0	4.2	0.1	3.4	0.0	0.1	2.5	4.8	0.1	0.0	0.0	0.2	0.0	4.9
4.2	0.2	0.0	14.1	0.5	15.4	3.8	0.2	3.8	11.1	0.6	0.0	0.0	0.6	0.1	13.4
12.5	0.5	0.0	42.6	1.8	36.9	2.8	0.5	17.0	46.9	1.3	0.1	0.1	0.7	0.1	73.8
2.4	0.1	0.0	174.0	0.3	14.4	1.2	0.1	8.4	4.0	0.2	0.0	0.0	0.2	0.0	6.4
1.1	0.1	0.0	52.5	0.1	7.3	2.4	0.1	6.1	4.9	0.1	0.0	0.0	0.2	0.0	4.3
1.3	0.2	0.0	10.0	0.4	6.2	3.1	0.1	2.3	24.4	0.1	0.0	0.0	0.0	0.0	21.6
4.8	0.3	0.0	28.1	1.5	17.9	7.7	0.2	5.1	105.6	0.4	0.0	0.1	1.0	0.1	38.0
3.1	0.2	0.0	23.8	1.1	16.4	3.0	0.2	6.0	61.4	0.4	0.0	0.1	0.7	0.0	25.0
0.1	0.0	0.0	1.5	0.1	1.8	0.6	0.0	0.1	0.1	0.0	0.0	0.0	0.0	0.0	0.3
0.8	0.7	0.0	12.3	0.3	16.9	3.1	0.1	57.0	14.8	0.2	0.1	0.0	0.3	0.2	3.4
2.0	0.3	0.0	3.8	0.4	15.3	1.4	0.3	0.2	0.0	0.1	0.1	0.0	0.5	0.0	2.2
0.4	0.0	0.0	1.1	0.1	2.2	0.3	0.1	0.1	0.0	0.0	0.0	0.0	0.2	0.0	1.6
0.3	0.1	0.0	0.7	0.1	5.4	0.4	0.1	0.0	0.0	0.0	0.0	0.0	0.1	0.0	1.5
0.4	0.0	0.0	0.8	0.1	2.7	0.4	0.0	0.0	0.0	0.0	0.0	0.0	0.1	0.0	1.5
0.0	0.5	0.0	0.7	0.3	13.2	3.6	0.2	0.0	0.0	0.0	0.0	0.0	0.4	0.1	0.0
0.0	0.5	0.0	0.7	0.3	13.2	3.6	0.2	4.9	0.0	0.1	0.0	0.0	0.4	0.1	2.0
0.5	0.1	0.0	2.6	0.1	4.8	1.1	0.1	0.0	0.0	0.0	0.0	0.0	0.4	0.0	2.2
1.6	0.6	0.0	9.0	2.3	0.0	701.0	0.0	55.4	0.0	0.0	0.0	0.1	0.1	0.0	0.0
0.1	0.1	0.0	0.3	0.1	4.8	0.2	0.1	0.0	0.0	0.0	0.0	0.0	0.1	0.0	2.1
1.0	0.7	0.0	5.3	0.5	17.3	0.2	0.4	0.0	0.0	0.1	0.1	0.0	0.1	0.0	5.5
0.2	0.1	0.0	1.2	0.1	5.2	0.6	0.1	0.0	0.0	0.1	0.0	0.0	0.2	0.0	0.5
0.2	0.1	0.0	1.2	0.1	5.4	0.1	0.1	0.0	0.0	0.0	0.0	0.0	0.2	0.0	0.5

Code	Food Name	Unit Amount	Kilocalories (Kcal)	Protein (g)	Carbohydrate (g)
20054	Grain, rice, white, glutinous, ckd	1 Tbsp., cooked	10.6	0.2	2.3
20047	Grain, rice, white, long-grain, enriched, ckd w/salt	1 Tbsp.	12.9	0.3	2.8
20048	Grain, rice, white, long-grain, precooked/instant, enriched, ckd	1 Tbsp.	10.1	0.2	2.2
20044	Grain, rice, white, long-grain, regular, enriched, ckd	1 Tbsp.	12.9	0.3	2.8
20444	Grain, rice, white, long-grain, regular, unenriched, ckd w/o salt	1 Tbsp.	12.7	0.3	2.8
20051	Grain, rice, white, long-grain, unenriched, ckd w/salt	1 Tbsp.	12.9	0.3	2.8
20050	Grain, rice, white, medium-grain, ckd	1 Tbsp.	15.1	0.3	3.3
20450	Grain, rice, white, medium-grain, unenriched, ckd	1 Tbsp.	15.1	0.3	3.3
20056	Grain, rice, white, w/pasta, ckd	1 Tbsp.	15.4	0.3	2.7
20066	Grain, rye	1 Tbsp.	35.5	1.6	7.4
20466	Grain, semolina, enriched	1 Tbsp.	37.4	1.3	7.6
20068	Grain, sorghum	1 Tbsp.	40.7	1.4	9.0
20069	Grain, tapioca, pearl, dry	1 Tbsp.	34.0	0.0	8.4
20076	Grain, wheat germ, crude	1 Tbsp.	34.6	2.2	5.0
20071	Grain, wheat, durum	1 Tbsp.	40.7	1.6	8.5
6115	Gravy, au jus, canned	1 cup	38.1	2.9	6.0
6116	Gravy, au jus, dry, made w/H_2O	1 cup (8 fl oz)	32.0	1.2	4.0
6561	Gravy, beef, canned	1 cup	123.5	8.7	11.2
6118	Gravy, brown gravy, dry mix/Nestle Trio	1 Tbsp.	24.4	0.6	3.5
6119	Gravy, brown, dry, made w/H_2O	1 cup (8 fl oz)	74.8	2.4	13.0
6120	Gravy, chicken, canned	1 cup	188.0	4.6	12.9
6572	Gravy, chicken, dry, made w/H_2O	1 cup (8 fl oz)	83.2	2.6	14.4
6746	Gravy, dry, made w/H_2O	1/4 cup	21.8	0.8	3.6
6579	Gravy, hearty beef gravy, glass jar/PepFarm	1 package	146.2	10.2	21.1
6122	Gravy, mushroom, canned	1/4 cup	30.0	0.8	3.3
6124	Gravy, onion, dry, made w/H_2O	1/4 cup	18.0	0.5	3.7
6563	Gravy, pork, dry, made w/H_2O	1/4 cup	18.0	0.4	3.1
6126	Gravy, turkey, canned	1 Tbsp.	7.7	0.4	0.8
5151	Gravy, turkey, dry, made w/H_2O	1 Tbsp.	5.0	0.2	0.9
22700	Hamburger Helper	1 serving	341.3	20.3	30.0
2023	Herb, ginger root, peeled, sliced, raw	5 slices (1″ diam x 0.12″ thick)	7.6	0.2	1.7
17170	Hopping John (rice & blackeyed peas)	1/3 cup	118.0	5.0	17.8
901932	Ice cream bar, vanilla	1 bar	162.1	2.1	14.5
18272	Ice cream cone, cake or wafer	1 cone	16.7	0.3	3.2
901920	Ice cream cone, sugar, rolled	1 cone	40.2	0.8	8.4
19270	Ice cream sandwich	1 bar	166.8	3.1	26.1
901917	Ice cream, chocolate	1 individual container (3.5 fl oz)	125.3	2.2	16.4
901918	Ice cream, creamsicle	1 bar	103.2	1.2	17.6
19264	Ice cream, drumstick	1 stick	186.3	2.6	21.5
19090	Ice cream, Eskimo Pie Vanilla Ice Cream Bar w/dark chocolate coating	1 bar	165.7	2.1	12.3
901919	Ice cream, French vanilla custard, soft serve	1 cup (8 fl oz)	369.8	7.1	38.2
19262	Ice cream, fudgsicle	1 bar	91.3	3.8	18.6
901922	Ice cream, Klondike Vanilla Ice Cream Bar w/chocolate coating	1 bar (5 fl oz)	488.5	6.2	35.7
901923	Ice cream, light, chocolate (ice milk)	2/3 cup	136.8	4.3	20.2
19088	Ice cream, light, strawberry (ice milk)	2/3 cup	133.2	4.3	22.1
19096	Ice cream, light, vanilla	1 cup (8 fl oz)	183.5	5.0	30.0
19260	Ice cream, light, vanilla, soft serve	1 cup (8 fl oz)	221.8	8.6	38.4
19271	Ice cream, light, w/aspartame, no sugar, vanilla	1 Tbsp.	12.3	0.4	1.5
19095	Ice cream, strawberry	1 individual container (3.5 fl oz)	111.4	1.9	16.0
19089	Ice cream, vanilla	1 individual container (3.5 fl oz)	116.6	2.0	13.7
17003	Lamb, domestic, choice, composite, lean (1/4″ trim) ckd	3.0 oz	175.1	24.0	0.0
7001	Lobster (shellfish) egg roll/LaChoy	1 medium	26.4	0.7	4.2
7274	Lunch meat, barbecue loaf (pork & beef)	1.0 oz, 1 slice	48.4	4.4	1.8
7042	Lunch meat, beef pastrami, cooked, smoked, chopped, pressed/Carl Buddig	2.5 oz, 1 pkg	100.1	13.9	0.7
7043	Lunch meat, beef, smoked, sliced/Carl Buddig	2.5 oz, 1 pkg	98.7	13.7	0.4
7008	Lunch meat, beef, thin slices	1.0 oz, 6 paper-thin slices	49.6	7.9	1.6
7202	Lunch meat, bologna (beef & pork)	1.0 oz, 1 slice	88.5	3.3	0.8
7007	Lunch meat, bologna (beef light)/Oscar Mayer	1.0 oz, 2 slices	55.4	3.3	1.7
7201	Lunch meat, bologna (beef)	1.0 oz, 1 slice	87.4	3.4	0.2
7010	Lunch meat, bologna (chicken, pork, & beef)/Oscar Mayer	1.0 oz, 1 slice	89.0	3.1	0.7
7011	Lunch meat, bologna (pork)	1.0 oz, 1 slice	69.2	4.3	0.2
7206	Lunch meat, bologna (turkey)	1.0 oz, 1 slice	55.7	3.8	0.3
7039	Lunch meat, bologna, fat-free/Oscar Mayer	1.0 oz, 1 slice	22.1	3.5	1.7
7249	Lunch meat, braunschweiger liver sausage, sliced/Oscar Mayer	1.0 oz, 1 slice	94.1	3.9	0.6
7209	Lunch meat, chicken breast classic baked/grill, Carving Board/Louis Rich	1.0 oz, 1 slice	27.4	5.5	1.0

Dietary Fiber (g)	Total Fat (g)	Cholesterol (mg)	Calcium (mg)	Iron (mg)	Magnesium (mg)	Sodium (mg)	Zinc (mg)	Vitamin A (μgRE)	Vitamin C (mg)	Vitamin E (mgαT)	Thiamin (mg)	Riboflavin (mg)	Niacin (mg)	Vitamin B₆ (mg)	Folate (μg)
0.1	0.0	0.0	0.2	0.0	0.5	0.5	0.0	0.0	0.0	0.0	0.0	0.0	0.0	0.0	0.1
0.0	0.0	0.0	1.0	0.1	1.2	37.8	0.0	0.0	0.0	0.0	0.0	0.0	0.1	0.0	5.7
0.1	0.0	0.0	0.8	0.1	0.5	0.3	0.0	0.0	0.0	0.0	0.0	0.0	0.1	0.0	4.2
0.0	0.0	0.0	1.0	0.1	1.2	0.1	0.0	0.0	0.0	0.0	0.0	0.0	0.1	0.0	5.7
0.0	0.0	0.0	1.0	0.0	1.2	0.1	0.0	0.0	0.0	0.0	0.0	0.0	0.0	0.0	0.3
0.0	0.0	0.0	1.0	0.0	1.2	37.8	0.0	0.0	0.0	0.0	0.0	0.0	0.0	0.0	0.3
0.0	0.0	0.0	0.3	0.2	1.5	0.0	0.0	0.0	0.0	0.0	0.0	0.0	0.2	0.0	6.7
0.0	0.0	0.0	0.3	0.0	1.5	0.0	0.0	0.0	0.0	0.0	0.0	0.0	0.0	0.0	0.2
0.3	0.4	0.1	1.0	0.1	1.5	71.6	0.0	0.0	0.0	0.0	0.0	0.0	0.2	0.0	5.5
1.5	0.3	0.0	3.5	0.3	12.8	0.6	0.4	0.0	0.0	0.2	0.0	0.0	0.5	0.0	6.4
0.4	0.1	0.0	1.8	0.5	4.9	0.1	0.1	0.0	0.0	0.0	0.1	0.1	0.6	0.0	16.0
0.0	0.4	0.0	3.4	0.5	0.0	0.7	0.0	0.0	0.0	0.0	0.0	0.0	0.4	0.0	0.0
0.1	0.0	0.0	1.9	0.2	0.1	0.1	0.0	0.0	0.0	0.0	0.0	0.0	0.0	0.0	0.4
1.3	0.9	0.0	3.7	0.6	22.9	1.2	1.2	0.0	0.0	0.0	0.2	0.0	0.7	0.1	27.0
0.0	0.3	0.0	4.1	0.4	17.3	0.2	0.5	0.0	0.0	0.0	0.1	0.0	0.8	0.1	5.2
0.0	0.5	0.0	9.5	1.4	4.8	119.2	2.4	0.0	2.4	0.0	0.0	0.1	2.1	0.0	4.8
0.0	1.3	2.5	22.1	0.0	7.4	964.3	0.1	0.0	0.0	0.0	0.0	0.0	0.0	0.0	0.0
0.9	5.5	7.0	14.0	1.6	4.7	1304.8	2.3	0.0	0.0	0.1	0.1	0.1	1.5	0.0	4.7
0.2	0.9	0.0	2.2	0.1	0.5	261.8	0.0	0.0	0.0	0.0	0.0	0.0	0.0	0.0	1.6
0.0	1.7	2.6	67.1	0.2	10.3	1075.9	0.3	0.0	0.0	0.0	0.0	0.1	0.8	0.0	0.0
1.0	13.6	4.8	47.6	1.1	4.8	1373.3	1.9	264.2	0.0	0.4	0.0	0.1	1.1	0.0	4.8
0.0	1.9	2.6	39.0	0.3	10.4	1133.6	0.3	0.0	2.6	0.0	0.1	0.1	0.8	0.0	2.6
0.0	0.5	0.0	9.2	0.1	2.6	359.0	0.1	0.0	0.5	0.0	0.0	0.0	0.2	0.0	0.9
0.0	2.4	17.0	0.0	0.0	0.0	2145.4	0.0	0.0	0.0	0.0	0.0	0.0	0.0	0.0	0.0
0.2	1.6	0.0	4.2	0.4	1.2	342.0	0.4	0.0	0.0	0.0	0.0	0.0	0.4	0.0	7.2
0.0	0.2	0.0	16.8	0.0	0.6	232.8	0.1	0.0	0.0	0.0	0.0	0.0	0.0	0.0	0.0
0.2	0.4	0.6	7.2	0.1	2.4	287.4	0.1	0.0	0.4	0.0	0.0	0.0	0.2	0.0	0.7
0.1	0.3	0.3	0.6	0.1	0.3	86.6	0.1	0.0	0.0	0.0	0.0	0.0	0.2	0.0	0.3
0.1	0.1	0.2	2.9	0.0	0.6	86.0	0.0	0.0	0.1	0.0	0.0	0.0	0.1	0.0	0.2
0.0	15.7	0.0	0.0	0.0	0.0	1043.0	0.0	0.0	0.0	0.0	0.0	0.0	0.0	0.0	0.0
0.2	0.1	0.0	2.0	0.1	4.7	1.4	0.0	0.0	0.6	0.0	0.0	0.0	0.1	0.0	1.2
0.5	3.6	0.0	22.0	1.0	1.0	447.0	0.0	4.2	2.0	0.0	0.5	0.0	0.3	0.0	0.0
0.0	10.6	0.0	70.0	0.0	8.0	28.0	0.0	41.8	0.0	0.0	0.0	0.1	0.1	0.0	0.0
0.1	0.3	0.0	1.0	0.1	1.0	5.7	0.0	0.0	0.0	0.1	0.0	0.0	0.2	0.0	4.1
0.2	0.4	0.0	4.4	0.4	3.1	32.0	0.1	0.0	0.0	0.0	0.1	0.0	0.5	0.0	8.3
0.1	6.2	0.0	73.0	0.1	8.0	92.0	0.0	38.6	0.0	0.0	0.0	0.1	0.5	0.0	0.0
0.7	6.4	19.7	63.2	0.5	16.8	44.1	0.3	69.0	0.4	0.2	0.0	0.1	0.1	0.0	9.3
0.0	3.1	0.0	46.0	0.0	5.0	27.0	0.0	25.0	0.0	0.0	0.0	0.1	0.3	0.0	0.0
0.2	9.9	0.0	67.0	0.1	7.0	57.0	0.0	37.0	0.0	0.0	0.0	0.1	0.5	0.0	0.0
0.0	12.1	14.2	59.5	0.0	0.0	34.2	0.0	0.0	0.0	0.0	0.0	0.0	0.0	0.0	0.0
0.0	22.4	156.5	225.3	0.4	20.6	104.9	0.9	264.9	1.4	0.6	0.1	0.3	0.2	0.1	15.5
0.0	0.2	0.0	129.0	0.1	14.0	55.0	0.0	0.0	0.0	0.0	0.0	0.2	0.7	0.0	0.0
0.0	35.7	39.8	211.6	0.0	0.0	107.9	0.0	0.0	0.0	0.0	0.0	0.0	0.0	0.0	0.0
0.0	4.6	13.0	140.0	0.1	12.0	61.0	0.8	38.0	1.0	0.0	0.0	0.2	0.1	0.1	5.0
0.1	3.1	13.0	161.0	0.3	12.0	64.0	0.9	25.8	0.0	0.0	0.1	0.2	0.1	0.1	5.0
0.0	5.7	18.5	183.5	0.1	19.8	112.2	0.6	62.0	1.1	0.0	0.1	0.3	0.1	0.1	7.9
0.0	4.6	21.1	276.3	0.1	24.6	123.2	0.9	51.0	1.6	0.0	0.1	0.3	0.2	0.1	10.6
0.0	0.5	1.3	15.9	0.0	0.0	7.2	0.0	0.0	0.0	0.0	0.0	0.0	0.0	0.0	0.0
0.2	4.9	16.8	69.6	0.1	8.1	34.8	0.2	45.2	4.5	0.0	0.0	0.1	0.1	0.0	7.0
0.0	6.4	25.5	74.2	0.1	8.1	46.4	0.4	67.9	0.3	0.0	0.0	0.1	0.1	0.0	2.9
0.0	8.1	78.2	12.8	1.7	22.1	64.6	4.5	0.0	0.0	0.2	0.1	0.2	5.4	0.1	19.6
0.0	0.7	0.0	3.9	0.2	0.0	52.7	0.0	1.8	1.1	0.0	0.0	0.0	0.3	0.0	0.0
0.0	2.5	10.4	15.4	0.3	4.8	373.5	0.7	2.0	0.0	0.0	0.1	0.1	0.6	0.1	2.5
0.0	4.6	46.2	12.1	1.7	0.0	749.8	0.0	0.0	0.0	0.0	0.1	0.2	2.9	0.0	0.0
0.0	4.6	47.6	9.9	1.6	0.0	1016.0	0.0	0.0	0.0	0.0	0.1	0.2	2.7	0.0	0.0
0.0	1.1	11.5	3.1	0.8	5.3	402.9	1.1	0.0	0.0	0.1	0.0	0.1	1.5	0.1	3.1
0.0	7.9	15.4	3.4	0.4	3.1	285.3	0.5	0.0	0.0	0.1	0.0	0.0	0.7	0.1	1.4
0.0	4.0	12.6	3.6	0.3	3.9	313.9	0.5	0.0	0.0	0.0	0.0	0.0	0.0	0.0	1.4
0.0	8.0	16.2	3.4	0.5	3.4	274.7	0.6	0.0	0.0	0.1	0.0	0.0	0.7	0.0	1.4
0.0	8.2	28.8	19.3	0.5	5.9	289.2	0.4	0.0	0.0	0.0	0.0	0.0	0.0	0.0	0.0
0.0	5.6	16.5	3.1	0.2	3.9	331.5	0.6	0.0	0.0	0.1	0.1	0.0	1.1	0.1	1.4
0.0	4.3	27.7	23.5	0.4	3.9	245.8	0.5	0.0	0.0	0.1	0.0	0.0	1.0	0.1	2.0
0.0	0.2	7.0	4.2	0.3	6.2	273.6	0.3	0.0	0.0	0.0	0.0	0.0	0.0	0.0	0.0
0.1	8.5	49.0	2.5	2.7	3.9	324.0	1.0	0.0	2.5	0.0	0.1	0.4	2.6	0.1	13.2
0.0	0.1	14.6	2.2	0.4	9.0	319.8	0.2	0.0	0.0	0.0	0.0	0.0	0.0	0.0	0.0

Code	Food Name	Unit Amount	Kilocalories (Kcal)	Protein (g)	Carbohydrate (g)
7250	Lunch meat, chicken breast, honey-glazed/Oscar Mayer	1.0 oz, 1 slice	30.5	5.5	1.2
7210	Lunch meat, chicken breast, oven-roasted deluxe/Louis Rich	1.0 oz, 1 slice	28.3	5.1	0.7
7053	Lunch meat, chicken breast, oven-roasted, fat free/Oscar Mayer	1.0 oz, 1 slice	23.8	5.1	0.5
7018	Lunch meat, chicken roll, light meat	2.0 oz, 2 slices	90.6	11.1	1.4
7271	Lunch meat, chicken spread, canned	1.5 oz.	82.6	6.6	2.3
7251	Lunch meat, chicken, light and dark meat, sliced, smoked/Carl Buddig	2.5 oz, 1 pkg	117.2	12.7	0.5
7021	Lunch meat, Corned Beef, cooked, chopped, pressed/Carl Buddig	2.5 oz, 1 pkg	100.8	13.7	0.7
7252	Lunch meat, Dutch brand (old fashion) loaf (pork & beef)	1.0 oz, 1 slice	67.2	3.8	1.6
7253	Lunch meat, franks (turkey & chicken cheese)/Louis Rich	1.6 oz, 1 frank	90.5	5.7	2.3
7054	Lunch meat, franks (turkey & chicken)/Louis Rich	1.6 oz, 1 frank	84.6	5.0	2.4
7033	Lunch meat, ham & cheese loaf or roll	1.0 oz, 1 slice	72.5	4.7	0.4
7211	Lunch meat, ham & cheese spread	3 Tbsp.	105.4	7.0	1.0
7031	Lunch meat, ham and cheese loaf/Oscar Mayer	1.0 oz, 1 slice	64.4	3.9	1.0
7212	Lunch meat, ham salad spread	1.0 oz, 1 Tbsp.	60.5	2.4	3.0
7030	Lunch meat, ham, honey, water-added/Oscar Mayer	1 slice	23.3	3.5	0.7
7028	Lunch meat, ham, minced	1 slice	55.2	3.4	0.4
7029	Lunch meat, ham, slices, extra lean (5% fat)	1 slice : 6.25" x 4" x 0.06"	37.1	5.5	0.3
7217	Lunch meat, ham, slices, regular (11% fat)	1 slice : 6.25" x 4" x 4" x 0.06"	51.6	5.0	0.9
7216	Lunch meat, ham, smoked, sliced/Carl Buddig	2.5 oz, 1 pkg	115.7	13.1	0.8
7214	Lunch meat, ham, water-added, baked, 96% fat-free/Oscar Mayer	2.25 oz	64.9	10.4	0.6
7035	Lunch meat, head cheese/Oscar Mayer	1.0 oz, 1 slice	51.8	4.4	0.0
7219	Lunch meat, honey loaf (pork & beef)	2 slices: 4" x 4" x 0.09"	73.0	9.0	3.0
7220	Lunch meat, jellied, beef	1 slice (4" x 4" x 0.9" thick)	32.2	5.5	0.0
7055	Lunch meat, liver cheese (pork)	1.0 oz slice	85.1	4.3	0.6
7041	Lunch meat, liver pate, canned	1.0 oz, 2 Tbsp.	89.3	4.0	0.4
7221	Lunch meat, liver sausage (liverwurst)	1 slice: 2.5" diam x 0.25" thick	58.7	2.5	0.4
7060	Lunch meat, luncheon loaf, spiced/Oscar Mayer	1.0 oz, 1 slice	65.5	3.8	2.0
7223	Lunch meat, old fashioned loaf/Oscar Mayer	1.0 oz, 1 slice	64.7	3.7	2.2
7051	Lunch meat, olive loaf (chicken, pork, & turkey)/Oscar Mayer	1.0 oz, 1 slice	73.6	2.8	1.9
13355	Lunch meat, olive loaf (pork)	1.0 oz, 1 slice	65.8	3.3	2.6
7052	Lunch meat, pastrami (beef)	1.0 oz, 1 slice	97.7	4.8	0.9
7056	Lunch meat, pastrami (turkey)	1.0 oz, 1 slice	39.5	5.1	0.5
7058	Lunch meat, peppered loaf (pork & beef)	1.0 oz, 1 slice	41.4	4.8	1.3
7224	Lunch meat, pickle & pimento loaf	1.0 oz, 1 slice	73.4	3.2	1.7
7045	Lunch meat, pork sausage links, cooked/Oscar Mayer	1 link	82.3	3.9	0.2
7067	Lunch meat, pork, canned	0.75 oz, 1 slice	70.1	2.6	0.4
7227	Lunch meat, salami beef cotto/Oscar Mayer	0.75 oz, 1 slice	43.3	3.0	0.4
7230	Lunch meat, salami cotto (beef, pork, & chicken)/Oscar Mayer	0.75 oz, 1 slice	51.5	2.8	0.5
7073	Lunch meat, salami, hard/Oscar Mayer	0.33 oz, 1 slice	35.8	2.5	0.3
7231	Lunch meat, sandwich spread (pork & beef)	1.0 oz, 2 Tbsp.	65.8	2.1	3.3
7232	Lunch meat, sandwich spread (pork, chicken, & beef)/Oscar Mayer	1.0 oz, 2 Tbsp.	66.4	1.8	4.3
7233	Lunch meat, smokie links sausage/Oscar Mayer	1.5 oz, 1 link	129.9	5.3	0.7
7236	Lunch meat, smokies sausage little (pork & turkey)/Oscar Mayer	0.33 oz, 1 sm link	27.1	1.1	0.2
7237	Lunch meat, smokies sausage little cheese (pork & turkey)/Oscar Mayer	0.33 oz, 1 sm link	28.4	1.2	0.2
7254	Lunch meat, summer sausage thuringer cervalat/Oscar Mayer	1.0 oz, 1 slice	85.1	4.2	0.3
7255	Lunch meat, turkey bacon/Louis Rich	0.5 oz, 1 slice	34.2	2.2	0.3
7256	Lunch meat, turkey bologna/Louis Rich	1.0 oz, 1 slice	51.5	3.2	1.3
7259	Lunch meat, turkey breast meat	1.5 oz, 2 slices	46.2	9.5	0.0
7260	Lunch meat, turkey breast, oven-roasted, fat-free/Louis Rich	1.0 oz, 1 slice	23.5	4.2	1.3
7239	Lunch meat, turkey breast, smoked, Carving Board/Louis Rich	2.0 oz, 1.0 oz slices	42.3	8.9	0.7
7080	Lunch meat, turkey ham, 10% water-added/Louis Rich	1.0 oz slice	31.6	5.1	0.3
7265	Lunch meat, turkey ham, cured	2 slices	73.0	10.8	0.2
7081	Lunch meat, turkey roll, light & dark meat	2.0 oz slice	83.4	10.2	1.2
7267	Lunch meat, turkey roll, light meat	2.0 oz slice	82.3	10.5	0.3
7266	Lunch meat, turkey salami cotto/Louis Rich	1.0 oz, 1 slice	41.7	4.2	0.3
5300	Lunch meat, turkey smoked sausage/Louis Rich	2.0 oz slice	89.6	8.1	2.2
7273	Lunch meat, turkey, honey-roasted, fat-free/Louis Rich	2.0 oz slice	57.1	10.8	2.5
7243	Lunch meat, wieners (beef franks) bun length/Oscar Mayer	1 frank	183.5	6.4	1.6
7241	Lunch meat, wieners (beef franks) light/Oscar Mayer	1 frank	110.0	6.1	2.3
7246	Lunch meat, wieners (cheese hot dogs w/turkey)/Oscar Mayer	1 frank	143.1	5.4	1.3
7247	Lunch meat, wieners (hot dogs) fat-free/Oscar Mayer	1 frank	36.5	6.3	2.2
7248	Lunch meat, wieners (pork & turkey)/Oscar Mayer	1 frank	144.9	5.0	1.3
924132	Macaroni & beef/FrancoAm	7.5 oz	191.7	9.0	30.1
924274	Macaroni & cheese mix/Kraft	3/4 cup	254.3	10.8	36.3
924275	Macaroni & cheese, frozen	6.0 oz	195.5	11.0	21.8

Dietary Fiber (g)	Total Fat (g)	Cholesterol (mg)	Calcium (mg)	Iron (mg)	Magnesium (mg)	Sodium (mg)	Zinc (mg)	Vitamin A (μgRE)	Vitamin C (mg)	Vitamin E (mgαT)	Thiamin (mg)	Riboflavin (mg)	Niacin (mg)	Vitamin B6 (mg)	Folate (μg)
0.0	0.4	15.1	2.8	0.3	10.1	388.1	0.2	0.0	0.0	0.0	0.0	0.0	0.0	0.0	0.0
0.0	0.6	13.7	2.0	0.3	6.7	332.6	0.2	0.0	0.0	0.0	0.0	0.0	0.0	0.0	0.0
0.0	0.2	12.3	3.4	0.4	10.1	347.8	0.2	0.0	0.0	0.0	0.0	0.0	0.0	0.0	0.0
0.0	4.2	28.5	24.5	0.6	10.8	332.9	0.4	13.7	0.0	0.2	0.0	0.1	3.0	0.1	1.1
0.0	5.0	22.4	53.8	1.0	5.2	166.0	0.5	10.8	0.0	0.0	0.0	0.0	1.2	0.1	1.3
0.0	7.2	37.6	88.0	1.1	0.0	677.3	0.0	0.0	0.0	0.0	0.0	0.2	4.8	0.0	0.0
0.0	4.8	46.2	12.1	1.7	0.0	952.8	0.0	0.0	0.0	0.0	0.1	0.2	3.0	0.0	0.0
0.0	5.0	13.2	23.5	0.3	5.9	350.0	0.5	0.0	0.0	0.1	0.1	0.1	0.7	0.1	0.6
0.0	6.5	42.3	109.4	0.9	9.9	481.5	0.8	0.0	0.0	0.0	0.0	0.0	0.0	0.0	0.0
0.0	6.1	41.4	59.0	1.0	10.4	511.2	0.8	0.0	0.0	0.0	0.0	0.0	0.0	0.0	0.0
0.0	5.7	16.0	16.2	0.3	4.5	376.0	0.6	6.4	0.0	0.1	0.2	0.1	1.0	0.1	0.8
0.0	8.0	26.2	93.3	0.3	7.7	514.7	1.0	39.1	0.0	0.0	0.1	0.1	0.9	0.1	1.3
0.0	5.0	18.5	18.8	0.2	5.3	350.8	0.5	0.0	0.0	0.0	0.2	0.1	1.0	0.1	0.8
0.0	4.3	10.4	2.2	0.2	2.8	255.4	0.3	0.0	0.0	0.5	0.1	0.0	0.6	0.0	0.3
0.0	0.7	9.5	2.1	0.3	6.5	262.1	0.4	0.0	0.0	0.0	0.0	0.0	0.0	0.0	0.0
0.0	4.3	14.7	2.1	0.2	3.4	261.5	0.4	0.0	0.0	0.1	0.1	0.0	0.9	0.1	0.2
0.0	1.4	13.3	2.0	0.2	4.8	405.1	0.5	0.0	0.0	0.1	0.3	0.1	1.4	0.1	1.1
0.0	3.0	16.2	2.0	0.3	5.4	373.4	0.6	0.0	0.0	0.1	0.2	0.1	1.5	0.1	0.9
0.0	6.6	39.1	11.4	1.4	0.0	980.5	0.0	0.0	0.0	0.0	0.5	0.2	3.7	0.0	0.0
0.0	2.3	30.2	6.3	0.8	19.5	764.8	1.1	0.0	0.0	0.0	0.0	0.0	0.0	0.0	0.0
0.0	3.8	25.5	5.9	0.5	3.1	300.4	0.3	0.0	0.0	0.0	0.0	0.0	0.3	0.0	0.3
0.0	2.5	19.4	9.7	0.8	9.7	752.4	1.4	0.0	0.0	0.1	0.3	0.1	1.8	0.2	4.6
0.0	1.0	9.9	2.9	1.0	5.2	383.4	1.0	0.0	0.0	0.0	0.0	0.1	1.4	0.1	2.0
0.0	7.2	48.7	2.2	3.0	3.4	343.0	1.0	1470.6	0.8	0.0	0.1	0.6	3.3	0.1	29.1
0.0	7.8	71.4	19.6	1.5	3.6	195.2	0.8	279.7	0.6	0.0	0.0	0.0	0.9	0.0	16.8
0.0	5.1	28.4	4.7	1.2	2.2	154.8	0.4	1494.0	0.0	0.0	0.0	0.2	0.8	0.0	5.4
0.0	4.7	18.8	30.5	0.4	6.7	343.3	0.5	0.0	0.0	0.0	0.0	0.0	0.0	0.0	0.0
0.0	4.6	17.1	31.6	0.4	6.4	331.5	0.5	0.0	0.0	0.0	0.0	0.0	0.0	0.0	0.0
0.0	6.1	19.9	31.1	0.5	7.6	369.0	0.3	0.0	0.0	0.0	0.0	0.0	0.0	0.0	0.0
0.0	4.6	10.6	30.5	0.2	5.3	415.5	0.4	5.6	0.0	0.1	0.1	0.1	0.5	0.1	0.6
0.0	8.2	26.0	2.5	0.5	5.0	343.6	1.2	0.0	0.0	0.1	0.0	0.0	1.4	0.1	2.0
0.0	1.7	15.1	2.5	0.5	3.9	292.6	0.6	0.0	0.0	0.1	0.0	0.1	1.0	0.1	1.4
0.0	1.8	12.9	15.1	0.3	5.6	426.4	0.9	0.0	0.0	0.1	0.1	0.1	0.9	0.1	0.6
0.0	5.9	10.4	26.6	0.3	5.0	388.9	0.4	2.0	0.0	0.1	0.1	0.1	0.6	0.1	1.4
0.0	7.3	18.5	3.8	0.4	4.3	200.6	0.6	0.0	0.0	0.0	0.0	0.0	0.0	0.0	0.0
0.0	6.4	13.0	1.3	0.2	2.1	270.7	0.3	0.0	0.2	0.1	0.1	0.0	0.7	0.0	1.3
0.0	3.3	17.4	1.5	0.6	3.6	274.9	0.4	0.0	0.0	0.0	0.0	0.0	0.0	0.0	0.0
0.0	4.3	16.8	15.8	0.6	6.1	230.0	0.4	0.0	0.0	0.0	0.0	0.0	0.0	0.0	0.0
0.0	2.8	8.6	1.1	0.2	1.9	169.4	0.3	0.0	0.0	0.0	0.1	0.0	0.5	0.0	0.3
0.1	4.9	10.6	3.4	0.2	2.2	283.6	0.3	2.5	0.0	0.5	0.0	0.0	0.5	0.0	0.6
0.1	4.6	12.6	7.6	0.2	3.4	229.9	0.2	0.0	0.0	0.0	0.0	0.0	0.0	0.0	0.0
0.0	11.7	27.1	4.3	0.5	7.3	433.0	0.9	0.0	0.0	0.0	0.0	0.0	0.0	0.0	0.0
0.0	2.4	5.8	1.0	0.1	1.5	92.0	0.2	0.0	0.0	0.0	0.0	0.0	0.0	0.0	0.0
0.0	2.5	6.0	6.0	0.1	1.9	93.2	0.2	0.0	0.0	0.0	0.0	0.0	0.0	0.0	0.0
0.0	7.5	23.5	2.5	0.6	4.2	400.4	0.6	0.0	0.0	0.0	0.1	0.1	1.2	0.1	1.4
0.0	2.7	12.5	5.6	0.2	2.7	184.2	0.4	0.0	0.0	0.0	0.0	0.0	0.0	0.0	0.0
0.0	3.7	19.0	34.7	0.5	6.2	269.9	0.5	0.0	0.0	0.0	0.0	0.0	0.0	0.0	0.0
0.0	0.7	17.2	2.9	0.2	8.4	601.0	0.5	0.0	0.0	0.0	0.0	0.0	3.5	0.2	1.7
0.0	0.2	9.0	3.1	0.3	7.6	333.8	0.2	0.0	0.0	0.0	0.0	0.0	0.0	0.0	0.0
0.0	0.5	19.4	6.8	0.7	14.0	540.5	0.4	0.0	0.0	0.0	0.0	0.0	0.0	0.0	0.0
0.0	1.1	18.8	1.4	0.4	6.2	315.6	0.7	0.0	0.0	0.0	0.0	0.0	0.0	0.0	0.0
0.0	2.9	31.9	5.7	1.6	9.1	567.7	1.7	0.0	0.0	0.4	0.0	0.1	2.0	0.1	3.4
0.0	3.9	30.8	17.9	0.8	10.1	328.2	1.1	0.0	0.0	0.2	0.1	0.2	2.7	0.2	2.8
0.0	4.0	24.1	22.4	0.7	9.0	273.8	0.9	0.0	0.0	0.1	0.0	0.1	3.9	0.2	2.2
0.0	2.7	21.6	8.7	0.5	5.9	285.0	0.7	0.0	0.0	0.0	0.0	0.0	0.0	0.0	0.0
0.0	5.4	35.8	14.6	0.8	11.8	515.2	1.2	0.0	0.0	0.0	0.0	0.0	0.0	0.0	0.0
0.0	0.4	22.4	8.4	0.6	15.7	660.8	0.6	0.0	0.0	0.0	0.0	0.0	0.0	0.0	0.0
0.0	16.9	32.5	7.4	0.9	8.6	575.7	1.3	0.0	0.0	0.0	0.0	0.0	0.0	0.0	0.0
0.0	8.5	27.9	12.0	0.9	10.3	615.0	1.2	0.0	0.0	0.0	0.0	0.0	0.0	0.0	0.0
0.0	12.9	33.3	73.8	0.7	11.3	514.4	0.8	0.0	0.0	0.0	0.0	0.0	0.0	0.0	0.0
0.0	0.3	14.5	7.5	0.5	10.5	487.0	0.6	0.0	0.0	0.0	0.0	0.0	0.0	0.0	0.0
0.0	13.3	32.4	27.0	0.5	7.7	434.7	0.8	0.0	0.0	0.0	0.0	0.0	0.0	0.0	0.0
0.0	3.8	0.0	43.0	2.2	0.0	792.0	0.0	192.6	7.0	0.0	0.2	0.2	3.2	0.0	0.0
1.0	7.5	18.0	123.0	1.9	29.0	652.0	1.3	77.6	0.0	0.0	0.3	0.2	1.7	0.0	12.0
1.0	7.1	17.0	269.0	0.7	0.0	358.0	0.0	17.6	4.0	0.0	0.2	0.2	0.9	0.0	0.0

Code	Food Name	Unit Amount	Kilocalories (Kcal)	Protein (g)	Carbohydrate (g)
924276	Macaroni & cheese/FrancoAm	7.5 oz	166.1	6.5	23.1
20099	Macaroni, enriched, ckd	1 cup elbow-shaped	197.4	6.7	39.7
20499	Macaroni, unenriched, ckd	1 cup	162.2	5.5	32.6
20105	Macaroni, vegetable, enriched, ckd	1 cup elbow-shaped	179.2	6.3	37.3
20107	Macaroni, whole-wheat, ckd	1 cup	166.2	7.1	35.6
4585	Margarine (about 40% fat) imitation	1 Tbsp.	483.3	0.7	0.6
4132	Margarine, blend: 60% corn oil & 40% butter	1 Tbsp.	753.9	0.9	0.7
4522	Margarine, hard w/salt	1 Tbsp.	107.8	0.1	0.1
4067	Margarine, hard, corn, corn-hydrogenated	1 Tbsp.	107.8	0.1	0.1
4068	Margarine, hard, corn, soybean-hydrogenated & cottonseed-hydrogenated w/salt	1 Tbsp.	107.8	0.1	0.1
4071	Margarine, hard, corn, soybean-hydrogenated & cottonseed-hydrogenated, no salt	1 Tbsp.	107.1	0.1	0.1
4091	Margarine, hard, corn-hydrogenated	1 Tbsp.	107.8	0.1	0.1
4131	Margarine, hard, lard-hydrogenated	1 Tbsp.	110.0	0.1	0.1
4089	Margarine, hard, no salt	1 Tbsp.	107.1	0.1	0.1
4079	Margarine, hard, safflower, soybean-hydrogenated	1 Tbsp.	107.8	0.1	0.1
4081	Margarine, hard, soybean, soybean-hydrogenated	1 Tbsp.	107.8	0.1	0.1
4076	Margarine, hard, soybean-hydrogenated	1 Tbsp.	107.8	0.1	0.1
4082	Margarine, hard, soybean-hydrogenated & palm-hydrogenated	1 Tbsp.	107.8	0.1	0.1
4521	Margarine, hard, soybean-hydrogenated, cottonseed	1 Tbsp.	107.8	0.1	0.1
4109	Margarine, imitation (about 40% fat) corn, corn-hydrogenated	1 Tbsp.	51.8	0.1	0.1
4112	Margarine, imitation (about 40% fat) soybean-hydrogenated	1 Tbsp.	51.8	0.1	0.1
4130	Margarine, liquid, soybean-hydrogenated, soybean, cottonseed	1 Tbsp.	108.2	0.3	0.0
4092	Margarine, soft w/salt	1 Tbsp.	107.5	0.1	0.1
4129	Margarine, soft, corn, corn-hydrogenated	1 Tbsp.	107.5	0.1	0.1
4101	Margarine, soft, no salt	1 Tbsp.	107.5	0.1	0.1
4094	Margarine, soft, safflower, safflower-hydrogenated	1 Tbsp.	107.5	0.1	0.1
4093	Margarine, soft, soybean, soybean-hydrogenated w/salt	1 Tbsp.	107.5	0.1	0.1
4103	Margarine, soft, soybean, soybean-hydrogenated, no salt	1 Tbsp.	107.5	0.1	0.1
4099	Margarine, soft, soybean, soybean & cottonseed-hydrogenated	1 Tbsp.	107.5	0.1	0.1
4095	Margarine, soft, soybean-hydrogenated & safflower	1 Tbsp.	107.5	0.1	0.1
4523	Margarine, soft, soybean-hydrogenated, cottonseed	1 Tbsp.	107.5	0.1	0.1
4525	Margarine, soft, soybean-hydrogenated, palm-hydrogenated, & palm	1 Tbsp.	107.5	0.1	0.1
4527	Margarine-like spread (about 60% fat) tub	1 Tbsp.	80.9	0.1	0.0
920900	Mayonnaise dressing, low kcal	2 Tbsp.	42.9	0.0	4.3
902934	Meat extender, vegetarian, meatless	1 cup	275.4	33.5	33.7
902935	Meat tenderizer	1 tsp.	2.0	0.0	0.0
924327	Meat & shrimp (shellfish) egg roll/LaChoy	3 medium	79.9	3.0	11.0
14422	Meat loaf	3.5 oz	159.7	17.0	4.6
1111	Milk shake, thick, chocolate	1 container (10.6 oz net wt)	355.8	9.2	63.5
1094	Milk shake, thick, vanilla	1 container (11 oz net wt)	350.0	12.1	55.6
1088	Milk, buttermilk, dry	1 Tbsp.	25.1	2.2	3.2
1059	Milk, buttermilk, low-fat, cultured	1 cup	99.0	8.1	11.7
1082	Milk, human, mature breast	1 fl oz	21.4	0.3	2.1
1083	Milk, lowfat, 1% fat w/added vitamin A	1 cup	102.1	8.0	11.7
1104	Milk, low-fat, 1% fat w/NFDM & vit A added	1 cup	104.4	8.5	12.2
1084	Milk, low-fat, 1% fat, chocolate	1 cup	157.6	8.1	26.1
1154	Milk, low-fat, 1% fat, protein-fortified, vit A added	1 cup	119.1	9.7	13.6
1093	Milk, nonfat, dry w/added vit A	1/4 cup	108.7	10.8	15.6
1092	Milk, nonfat, dry, calcium-reduced	1.0 oz	100.3	10.1	14.7
1155	Milk, nonfat, dry, instant w/added vit A	1 cup	243.6	23.9	35.5
1091	Milk, nonfat, dry, instant w/o vit A added	1 cup	243.4	23.9	35.5
1097	Milk, nonfat, dry, regular w/o vit A added	1 Tbsp.	27.2	2.7	3.9
1085	Milk, nonfat, skim, evaporated, canned	1 Tbsp.	12.5	1.2	1.8
1086	Milk, nonfat/fat-free, skim w/added vit A	1 cup	85.5	8.4	11.9
1151	Milk, nonfat/fat-free, skim w/NFDM & vit A added	1 cup	90.3	8.7	12.3
1087	Milk, nonfat/fat-free, skim w/o added vit A	1 cup	85.8	8.4	11.9
1079	Milk, nonfat/fat-free, skim, protein-fortified, vit A added	1 cup	99.9	9.7	13.7
1080	Milk, reduced-fat, 2% fat w/added vitamin A	1 cup	121.2	8.1	11.7
1152	Milk, reduced-fat, 2% fat w/NFDM & vit A added	1 cup	124.9	8.5	12.2
1103	Milk, reduced-fat, 2% fat w/NFDM, w/o added vit A	1 cup	136.0	9.7	13.5
1081	Milk, reduced-fat, 2% fat, chocolate	1 fl oz	22.3	1.0	3.2
16120	Milk, reduced-fat, 2% fat, protein-fortified, vit A added	1 cup	136.6	9.7	13.5
1075	Milk, soy, fluid	1 cup	79.2	6.6	4.3
1077	Milk, sweetened condensed, canned	1 fl oz	122.5	3.0	20.8
1078	Milk, whole, 3.25% fat	1 Tbsp.	9.3	0.5	0.7

Dietary Fiber (g)	Total Fat (g)	Cholesterol (mg)	Calcium (mg)	Iron (mg)	Magnesium (mg)	Sodium (mg)	Zinc (mg)	Vitamin A (μgRE)	Vitamin C (mg)	Vitamin E (mgαT)	Thiamin (mg)	Riboflavin (mg)	Niacin (mg)	Vitamin B$_6$ (mg)	Folate (μg)
1.0	5.4	0.0	95.0	1.5	0.0	934.0	1.4	173.4	0.0	0.0	0.2	0.2	2.1	0.0	0.0
1.8	0.9	0.0	9.8	2.0	25.2	1.4	0.7	0.0	0.0	0.0	0.3	0.1	2.3	0.0	98.0
1.5	0.8	0.0	8.1	0.6	20.7	1.2	0.6	0.0	0.0	0.0	0.0	0.0	0.5	0.0	8.1
6.0	0.2	0.0	15.4	0.7	26.6	8.4	0.6	7.0	0.0	0.1	0.2	0.1	1.5	0.0	91.0
3.8	0.7	0.0	20.1	1.4	40.2	4.0	1.1	0.0	0.0	0.1	0.1	0.1	0.9	0.1	6.7
0.0	54.3	0.0	24.9	0.0	2.2	1343.4	0.0	1118.6	0.1	3.3	0.0	0.0	0.0	0.0	1.0
0.0	84.7	92.4	29.4	0.1	2.1	941.9	0.0	839.0	0.1	8.0	0.0	0.0	0.0	0.0	2.1
0.0	12.1	0.0	4.5	0.0	0.4	141.5	0.0	119.9	0.0	1.9	0.0	0.0	0.0	0.0	0.2
0.0	12.1	0.0	4.5	0.0	0.4	141.5	0.0	119.9	0.0	2.2	0.0	0.0	0.0	0.0	0.2
0.0	12.1	0.0	4.5	0.0	0.4	141.5	0.0	119.9	0.0	0.0	0.0	0.0	0.0	0.0	0.2
0.0	12.0	0.0	2.6	0.0	0.2	0.3	0.0	119.9	0.0	1.7	0.0	0.0	0.0	0.0	0.1
0.0	12.1	0.0	4.5	0.0	0.4	141.5	0.0	119.9	0.0	0.0	0.0	0.0	0.0	0.0	0.2
0.0	12.1	7.7	0.0	0.0	0.0	141.5	0.0	0.0	0.0	0.0	0.0	0.0	0.0	0.0	0.0
0.0	12.0	0.0	2.6	0.0	0.2	0.3	0.0	119.9	0.0	1.9	0.0	0.0	0.0	0.0	0.1
0.0	12.1	0.0	4.5	0.0	0.4	141.5	0.0	119.9	0.0	0.0	0.0	0.0	0.0	0.0	0.2
0.0	12.1	0.0	4.5	0.0	0.4	141.5	0.0	119.9	0.0	0.0	0.0	0.0	0.0	0.0	0.2
0.0	12.1	0.0	4.5	0.0	0.4	141.5	0.0	119.9	0.0	1.6	0.0	0.0	0.0	0.0	0.2
0.0	12.1	0.0	4.5	0.0	0.4	141.5	0.0	119.9	0.0	0.0	0.0	0.0	0.0	0.0	0.2
0.0	12.1	0.0	4.5	0.0	0.4	141.5	0.0	119.9	0.0	0.0	0.0	0.0	0.0	0.0	0.2
0.0	5.8	0.0	2.7	0.0	0.2	143.9	0.0	119.9	0.0	0.0	0.0	0.0	0.0	0.0	0.1
0.0	5.8	0.0	2.7	0.0	0.2	143.9	0.0	119.9	0.0	0.0	0.0	0.0	0.0	0.0	0.1
0.0	12.1	0.0	9.9	0.0	0.9	117.1	0.0	119.9	0.1	0.8	0.0	0.0	0.0	0.0	0.4
0.0	12.1	0.0	4.0	0.0	0.3	161.8	0.0	119.9	0.0	1.8	0.0	0.0	0.0	0.0	0.2
0.0	12.1	0.0	4.0	0.0	0.3	161.8	0.0	119.9	0.0	0.0	0.0	0.0	0.0	0.0	0.2
0.0	12.0	0.0	4.0	0.0	0.3	4.1	0.0	119.9	0.0	1.3	0.0	0.0	0.0	0.0	0.2
0.0	12.1	0.0	4.0	0.0	0.3	161.8	0.0	119.9	0.0	0.0	0.0	0.0	0.0	0.0	0.2
0.0	12.1	0.0	4.0	0.0	0.3	161.8	0.0	119.9	0.0	0.0	0.0	0.0	0.0	0.0	0.2
0.0	12.0	0.0	4.0	0.0	0.3	4.1	0.0	119.9	0.0	0.0	0.0	0.0	0.0	0.0	0.2
0.0	12.1	0.0	4.0	0.0	0.3	161.8	0.0	119.9	0.0	0.0	0.0	0.0	0.0	0.0	0.2
0.0	12.1	0.0	4.0	0.0	0.3	161.8	0.0	119.9	0.0	0.0	0.0	0.0	0.0	0.0	0.2
0.0	12.1	0.0	4.0	0.0	0.3	161.8	0.0	119.9	0.0	0.0	0.0	0.0	0.0	0.0	0.2
0.0	12.1	0.0	4.0	0.0	0.3	161.8	0.0	119.9	0.0	0.0	0.0	0.0	0.0	0.0	0.2
0.0	9.1	0.0	3.1	0.0	0.3	149.1	0.0	119.9	0.0	1.4	0.0	0.0	0.0	0.0	0.1
0.0	4.3	4.3	6.4	0.0	0.0	40.7	0.0	17.1	0.0	0.0	0.0	0.0	0.0	0.0	0.0
15.4	2.6	0.0	179.5	10.6	190.1	8.8	1.9	2.6	0.0	0.0	0.6	0.8	19.4	1.2	174.2
0.0	0.0	0.0	11.0	0.1	2.0	1695.0	0.0	1.0	0.0	0.0	0.0	0.0	0.0	0.0	0.0
0.0	3.0	4.0	9.0	0.8	0.0	115.0	0.0	2.0	3.0	0.0	0.1	0.1	1.0	0.0	0.0
0.2	7.6	92.0	38.0	2.3	0.0	653.0	0.0	35.8	2.0	0.0	0.1	0.2	8.0	0.0	0.0
0.9	8.1	31.5	396.0	0.9	48.0	333.0	1.4	63.0	0.0	0.3	0.1	0.7	0.4	0.1	14.7
0.0	9.5	36.9	457.3	0.3	36.8	298.6	1.2	87.6	0.0	0.3	0.1	0.6	0.5	0.1	20.7
0.0	0.4	4.5	77.0	0.0	7.1	33.6	0.3	3.5	0.4	0.0	0.0	0.1	0.1	0.0	3.1
0.0	2.2	8.6	285.2	0.1	26.8	257.0	1.0	19.6	2.4	0.1	0.1	0.4	0.1	0.1	12.3
0.0	1.3	4.3	9.9	0.0	1.0	5.2	0.1	19.7	1.5	0.3	0.0	0.0	0.1	0.0	1.6
0.0	2.6	9.8	300.1	0.1	33.7	123.2	1.0	144.0	2.4	0.1	0.1	0.4	0.2	0.1	12.4
0.0	2.4	9.8	312.9	0.1	35.2	128.4	1.0	144.6	2.5	0.1	0.1	0.4	0.2	0.1	13.0
1.3	2.5	7.3	286.8	0.6	33.3	151.8	1.0	147.5	2.3	0.1	0.1	0.4	0.3	0.1	12.0
0.0	2.9	9.8	349.3	0.1	39.3	143.4	1.1	145.1	2.8	0.0	0.1	0.5	0.2	0.1	14.5
0.0	0.2	5.9	377.1	0.1	33.0	160.6	1.2	198.0	2.0	0.0	0.1	0.5	0.3	0.1	15.0
0.0	0.1	0.6	79.4	0.1	17.0	646.4	1.1	0.6	1.9	0.0	0.0	0.5	0.2	0.1	14.0
0.0	0.5	12.4	836.9	0.2	79.6	373.1	3.0	482.8	3.8	0.0	0.3	1.2	0.6	0.2	33.9
0.0	0.5	12.2	837.1	0.2	79.6	373.3	3.0	3.4	3.8	0.0	0.3	1.2	0.6	0.2	34.0
0.0	0.1	1.5	94.3	0.0	8.3	40.1	0.3	0.6	0.5	0.0	0.0	0.1	0.1	0.0	3.8
0.0	0.0	0.6	46.3	0.0	4.3	18.4	0.1	18.7	0.2	0.0	0.0	0.0	0.0	0.0	1.4
0.0	0.4	4.4	302.3	0.1	27.8	126.2	1.0	149.5	2.4	0.1	0.1	0.3	0.2	0.1	12.7
0.0	0.6	4.9	316.3	0.1	35.5	129.9	1.0	149.5	2.5	0.1	0.1	0.4	0.2	0.1	13.2
0.0	0.4	4.9	301.4	0.1	27.0	127.4	1.0	2.5	2.4	0.1	0.1	0.3	0.2	0.1	12.3
0.0	0.6	4.9	351.8	0.1	39.5	144.4	1.1	150.1	2.8	0.0	0.1	0.5	0.2	0.1	14.8
0.0	4.7	18.3	296.7	0.1	33.4	121.8	1.0	139.1	2.3	0.2	0.1	0.4	0.2	0.1	12.4
0.0	4.7	18.4	312.9	0.1	35.2	128.4	1.0	139.7	2.5	0.2	0.1	0.4	0.2	0.1	13.0
0.0	4.9	18.9	350.6	0.1	35.5	144.1	1.0	149.5	2.7	0.0	0.1	0.5	0.2	0.1	13.2
0.2	0.6	2.1	35.4	0.1	4.1	18.8	0.1	17.8	0.3	0.0	0.0	0.1	0.0	0.0	1.5
0.0	4.9	18.9	352.0	0.1	39.6	144.6	1.1	140.2	2.8	0.0	0.1	0.5	0.2	0.1	14.8
3.1	4.6	0.0	9.6	1.4	45.6	28.8	0.6	7.2	0.0	0.0	0.4	0.2	0.4	0.1	3.6
0.0	3.3	12.9	108.3	0.1	9.8	48.5	0.4	30.9	1.0	0.1	0.0	0.2	0.2	0.0	4.3
0.0	0.5	2.1	18.1	0.0	2.0	7.4	0.1	4.7	0.1	0.0	0.0	0.0	0.0	0.0	0.8

Code	Food Name	Unit Amount	Kilocalories (kcal)	Protein (g)	Carbohydrate (g)
1102	Milk, whole, 3.7% fat	1 cup	156.6	8.0	11.3
1090	Milk, whole, chocolate	8 fl oz	221.7	8.4	27.5
1153	Milk, whole, dry	1 Tbsp.	39.7	2.1	3.1
1096	Milk, whole, evaporated, canned, w/added vit A	1 fl oz	42.3	2.1	3.2
1106	Milk, whole, evaporated, canned, w/o vit A added	1 Tbsp.	21.2	1.1	1.6
1108	Milk, whole, goat	1 fl oz	21.0	1.1	1.4
1089	Milk, whole, Indian buffalo	8 fl oz	235.8	9.2	12.6
1109	Milk, whole, low-sodium	1 cup	148.6	7.6	10.9
18613	Muffin, almond poppyseed mix, dry/Krusteaz	1 piece	8.4	0.1	1.5
18274	Muffin, blueberry mix/Martha White	1 small muffin	161.6	2.0	30.4
18275	Muffin, blueberry, commercially prep	1 serving	110.8	2.2	19.2
18278	Muffin, blueberry, dry mix, prep	1 muffin (2.25″ diam x 1.75″)	149.5	2.6	24.4
918391	Muffin, blueberry, homemade w/reduced-fat (2%) milk	1 muffin	162.5	3.7	23.2
18279	Muffin, blueberry, homemade w/whole milk	1 muffin (2.75″ diam x 2″)	165.3	3.7	23.1
918280	Muffin, corn, commercially prep	1 muffin (2.5″ diam x 2.25″)	173.9	3.4	29.0
918393	Muffin, corn, homemade w/reduced-fat (2%) milk	1 muffin (2.75″ diam x 2″)	180.1	4.0	25.2
18605	Muffin, corn, homemade w/whole milk	1 muffin (2.75″ diam x 2″)	183.0	4.0	25.2
18273	Muffin, oatbran	1 muffin (2.5″ diam x 2.25″)	153.9	4.0	27.5
918389	Muffin, plain, homemade w/reduced-fat (2%) milk	1 muffin	168.7	3.9	23.6
18639	Muffin, plain, homemade w/whole milk	1 muffin (2.75″ diam x 2″)	171.6	3.9	23.6
18284	Muffin, Thomas' English muffins, plain/Best Foods	1.0 oz	66.9	2.5	13.2
918287	Muffin, wheat bran, dry mix, prep	1 muffin (2.25″ diam x 1.75″)	138.0	3.3	23.3
918394	Muffin, wheat bran, homemade w/reduced-fat (2%) milk	1 muffin (2.75″ diam x 2″)	161.3	4.0	23.9
18601	Muffin, wheat bran, homemade w/whole milk	1 muffin (2.75″ diam x 2″)	164.2	4.0	23.8
20134	Muffin, wild blueberry, dry mix/General Mills-Betty Crocker	1 serving	128.4	2.1	26.0
22702	Noodle Weenee/VanCamp	1 cup	244.2	9.3	32.9
16082	Noodles, alfredo egg noodles in a creamy sauce, dry mix/Lipton	1 cup	388.6	14.4	58.0
20113	Noodles, beans, mung, long rice or cellophane, dry	1 Tbsp.	30.9	0.0	7.6
20110	Noodles, Chinese, chow mein	1 Tbsp.	14.8	0.2	1.6
20310	Noodles, egg, enriched, ckd w/salt	1 Tbsp.	13.3	0.5	2.5
20111	Noodles, egg, spinach, enriched, ckd	1 cup	211.2	8.1	38.8
20510	Noodles, egg, unenriched, ckd w/o salt	1 cup	212.8	7.6	39.7
20409	Noodles, egg, unenriched, ckd w/salt	1 cup	212.8	7.6	39.7
20114	Noodles, Japanese, soba, ckd	1 cup	112.9	5.8	24.4
20116	Noodles, Japanese, somen, ckd	1 cup	230.6	7.0	48.5
20133	Noodles, ramen	1 cup	231.5	6.2	34.1
925074	Nutrient/vitamin supplement, 1-A-Day Essential	1 tablet	0.0	0.0	0.0
925042	Nutrient/vitamin supplement, 1-A-Day Maximum	1 tablet	0.0	0.0	0.0
925045	Nutrient/vitamin supplement, Centrum Jr.	1 tablet	0.0	0.0	0.0
925024	Nutrient/vitamin supplement, Geritol Complete	1 tablet	0.0	0.0	0.0
925100	Nutrient/vitamin supplement, Theragran	1 tablet	0.0	0.0	0.0
12072	Nuts, acorns, raw	1.0 oz	108.4	1.7	11.4
12061	Nuts, almonds, dried, blanched	1 Tbsp.	53.3	1.9	1.7
12066	Nuts, almonds, oil roast, blanched w/salt	1 whole kernel	6.1	0.2	0.2
12563	Nuts, almonds, toasted, unblanched	1.0 oz	164.9	5.7	6.4
12565	Nuts, almonds, unblanched, dry-roasted w/salt	1 kernel	5.9	0.2	0.2
12078	Nuts, beechnuts, dried	1.0 oz	161.3	1.7	9.4
12084	Nuts, brazil nuts, dried, unblanched	1.0 oz, 6–8 kernels	183.7	4.0	3.6
12585	Nuts, butternuts, dried	1 cup	734.4	29.9	14.5
12085	Nuts, cashews, dry-roasted w/salt	1 nut	11.5	0.3	0.7
912903	Nuts, cashews, dry-roasted, w/o salt	1 cup, halves and whole	786.4	21.0	44.8
12586	Nuts, cashews, honey roasted	1.0 oz	150.1	4.0	7.0
12086	Nuts, cashews, oil-roasted w/salt	1 nut	11.5	0.3	0.6
12095	Nuts, cashews, oil-roasted, w/o salt	1.0 oz, 18 kernels	161.3	4.5	8.0
12203	Nuts, chestnuts, European, roasted	1 kernel	19.6	0.3	4.2
12118	Nuts, coconut meat, raw	1 cup shredded or grated	283.2	2.7	12.2
12176	Nuts, coconut milk, canned (liquid expressed from grated meat & water)	1 Tbsp.	29.6	0.3	0.4
12177	Nuts, coconut water (liquid from coconuts)	1 Tbsp.	2.9	0.1	0.6
12114	Nuts, coconut, creamed, dried, creamed	1.0 oz	191.5	1.5	6.0
12109	Nuts, coconut, dried, toasted	1.0 oz	165.8	1.5	12.4
12108	Nuts, coconut, sweetened, shredded, dried	7-oz pkg	997.0	5.7	94.9
12121	Nuts, coconut, unsweetened, dried	1.0 oz	184.8	1.9	6.8
12120	Nuts, filberts/hazelnuts, dried, blanched	1.0 oz	188.2	3.6	4.5
12633	Nuts, macadamia, dried	1 kernel	14.0	0.2	0.3
12138	Nuts, mixed (no peanuts) oil-roasted w/salt	1.0 oz	172.2	4.3	6.2

Dietary Fiber (g)	Total Fat (g)	Cholesterol (mg)	Calcium (mg)	Iron (mg)	Magnesium (mg)	Sodium (mg)	Zinc (mg)	Vitamin A (μgRE)	Vitamin C (mg)	Vitamin E (mgαT)	Thiamin (mg)	Riboflavin (mg)	Niacin (mg)	Vitamin B6 (mg)	Folate (μg)
0.0	8.9	34.9	290.4	0.1	32.7	119.1	0.9	83.0	3.6	0.2	0.1	0.4	0.2	0.1	12.2
2.1	9.0	32.5	298.2	0.6	34.7	158.5	1.1	77.1	2.4	0.2	0.1	0.4	0.3	0.1	12.5
0.0	2.1	7.8	73.0	0.0	6.8	29.7	0.3	22.4	0.7	0.1	0.0	0.1	0.1	0.0	3.0
0.0	2.4	9.3	82.2	0.1	7.6	33.3	0.2	17.0	0.6	0.0	0.0	0.1	0.1	0.0	2.5
0.0	1.2	4.6	41.1	0.0	3.8	16.7	0.1	8.5	0.3	0.0	0.0	0.0	0.0	0.0	1.2
0.0	1.3	3.5	40.7	0.0	4.3	15.2	0.1	17.1	0.4	0.0	0.0	0.0	0.1	0.0	0.2
0.0	16.8	46.4	412.4	0.3	75.9	127.4	0.5	129.3	5.5	0.0	0.1	0.3	0.2	0.1	13.7
0.0	8.4	33.2	246.0	0.1	12.2	6.1	0.9	78.1	2.3	0.2	0.0	0.3	0.1	0.1	12.2
0.0	0.2	0.0	0.0	0.0	0.0	12.1	0.0	0.0	0.0	0.0	0.0	0.0	0.0	0.0	0.0
0.0	3.5	0.0	0.0	0.0	0.0	343.2	0.0	0.0	0.0	0.0	0.0	0.0	0.0	0.0	0.0
1.0	2.6	12.0	22.8	0.6	6.4	178.8	0.2	3.6	0.4	0.4	0.1	0.0	0.4	0.0	18.0
0.6	4.4	1.8	12.5	0.6	5.5	218.5	0.2	11.0	0.5	0.0	0.1	0.2	1.1	0.0	5.5
0.0	6.2	21.1	107.7	1.3	9.1	251.4	0.3	22.2	0.9	0.0	0.2	0.2	1.3	0.0	27.4
0.0	6.4	1.6	107.2	1.3	9.1	250.8	0.3	16.0	0.9	0.0	0.2	0.2	1.3	0.0	6.8
1.9	4.8	14.8	42.2	1.6	18.2	297.0	0.3	20.5	0.0	1.0	0.2	0.2	1.2	0.0	35.3
0.0	7.0	23.9	147.6	1.5	13.1	333.5	0.3	29.1	0.2	0.0	0.2	0.2	1.4	0.1	35.3
0.0	7.4	1.8	147.1	1.5	13.1	333.5	0.3	22.8	0.2	0.0	0.2	0.2	1.4	0.1	9.7
2.6	4.2	0.0	35.9	2.4	89.5	224.0	1.0	0.0	0.0	0.7	0.1	0.1	0.2	0.1	29.6
1.5	6.5	22.2	114.0	1.4	9.7	266.2	0.3	22.8	0.2	0.0	0.2	0.2	1.3	0.0	29.1
1.5	6.8	1.7	113.4	1.4	9.1	266.2	0.3	16.5	0.2	0.0	0.2	0.2	1.3	0.0	6.8
0.0	0.4	0.0	38.9	0.9	0.0	107.0	0.0	0.0	0.0	0.5	0.0	0.0	0.0	0.0	42.1
2.1	4.6	2.3	16.0	1.3	28.5	233.5	0.6	15.5	0.0	0.0	0.1	0.1	1.4	0.1	8.0
0.0	7.0	1.7	106.6	2.4	44.5	335.2	1.6	142.5	4.4	0.0	0.2	0.3	2.3	0.2	29.6
0.0	7.3	1.8	106.0	2.4	44.5	335.2	1.6	136.2	4.4	0.0	0.2	0.3	2.3	0.2	29.6
0.0	1.8	0.0	0.0	0.0	0.0	186.0	0.0	0.0	0.0	0.0	0.0	0.0	0.0	0.0	0.0
0.0	8.5	0.0	47.0	6.0	0.0	1245.0	0.0	134.4	0.0	0.0	0.1	0.2	2.1	0.0	0.0
0.0	11.0	104.2	118.1	2.8	0.0	1646.1	0.0	0.0	0.0	0.0	0.0	0.0	0.0	0.0	0.2
0.0	0.0	0.0	2.2	0.2	0.3	0.9	0.0	0.0	0.0	0.0	0.0	0.0	0.2	0.0	2.5
0.1	0.9	0.0	0.6	0.1	1.5	12.3	0.0	0.3	0.0	0.0	0.0	0.0	0.2	0.0	2.5
0.1	0.1	3.3	1.2	0.2	1.9	0.7	0.1	0.6	0.0	0.0	0.0	0.0	0.1	0.0	6.4
3.7	2.5	52.8	30.4	1.7	38.4	19.2	1.0	22.4	0.0	0.1	0.4	0.2	2.4	0.2	102.4
1.8	2.4	52.8	19.2	1.0	30.4	11.2	1.0	9.6	0.0	0.1	0.0	0.0	0.6	0.1	11.2
0.0	2.4	52.8	19.2	1.0	30.4	264.0	1.0	9.6	0.0	0.0	0.0	0.0	0.6	0.1	11.2
0.0	0.1	0.0	4.6	0.5	10.3	68.4	0.1	0.0	0.0	0.0	0.1	0.0	0.6	0.0	8.0
0.0	0.3	0.0	14.1	0.9	3.5	283.4	0.4	0.0	0.0	0.0	0.0	0.1	0.2	0.0	3.5
4.1	8.4	0.0	7.2	2.1	0.0	892.5	0.0	0.0	0.0	0.0	0.2	0.2	2.4	0.0	0.0
0.0	0.0	0.0	0.0	0.0	0.0	0.0	0.0	1000.0	60.0	0.0	1.5	1.7	20.0	2.0	0.4
0.0	0.0	0.0	0.0	18.0	0.0	0.0	15.0	1000.0	60.0	0.0	1.5	1.7	20.0	2.0	0.4
0.0	0.0	0.0	0.0	18.0	0.0	0.0	0.0	1000.0	300.0	0.0	1.5	1.7	20.0	2.0	0.4
0.0	0.0	0.0	0.0	50.0	0.0	0.0	0.0	1000.0	60.0	0.0	1.5	1.7	20.0	2.0	0.4
0.0	0.0	0.0	0.0	0.0	0.0	0.0	0.0	1100.0	120.0	0.0	3.0	3.4	30.0	3.0	0.4
0.0	6.7	0.0	11.5	0.2	17.4	0.0	0.1	1.1	0.0	0.0	0.0	0.0	0.5	0.1	24.4
0.6	4.8	0.0	22.5	0.3	26.0	0.9	0.3	0.0	0.1	1.8	0.0	0.1	0.3	0.0	3.5
0.1	0.6	0.0	1.9	0.1	2.9	7.8	0.0	0.0	0.0	0.1	0.0	0.0	0.0	0.0	0.6
3.1	14.2	0.0	79.2	1.4	85.4	3.1	1.4	0.0	0.2	4.5	0.0	0.2	0.8	0.0	17.9
0.1	0.5	0.0	2.8	0.0	3.0	7.8	0.0	0.0	0.0	0.1	0.0	0.0	0.0	0.0	0.6
0.0	14.0	0.0	0.3	0.7	0.0	10.6	0.1	0.0	4.3	0.0	0.1	0.1	0.2	0.2	31.6
1.5	18.5	0.0	49.3	1.0	63.0	0.6	1.3	0.0	0.2	2.1	0.3	0.0	0.5	0.1	1.1
5.6	68.4	0.0	63.6	4.8	284.4	1.2	3.8	14.4	3.8	4.2	0.5	0.2	1.3	0.7	79.4
0.1	0.9	0.0	0.9	0.1	5.2	12.8	0.1	0.0	0.0	0.0	0.0	0.0	0.0	0.0	1.4
4.1	63.5	0.0	61.7	8.2	356.2	21.9	7.7	0.0	0.0	0.8	0.3	0.3	1.9	0.4	94.8
2.0	13.0	0.0	12.0	1.2	0.0	90.0	1.4	0.0	0.0	0.0	0.1	0.1	0.4	0.1	20.0
0.1	1.0	0.0	0.8	0.1	5.1	12.5	0.1	0.0	0.0	0.0	0.0	0.0	0.0	0.0	1.4
1.1	13.5	0.0	11.5	1.1	71.4	4.8	1.3	0.0	0.0	0.4	0.1	0.0	0.5	0.1	19.0
0.4	0.2	0.0	2.3	0.1	2.6	0.2	0.0	0.2	2.1	0.1	0.0	0.0	0.1	0.0	5.6
7.2	26.8	0.0	11.2	1.9	25.6	16.0	0.9	0.0	2.6	0.6	0.1	0.0	0.4	0.0	21.1
0.0	3.2	0.0	2.7	0.5	6.9	2.0	0.1	0.0	0.2	0.0	0.0	0.0	0.1	0.0	2.0
0.2	0.0	0.0	3.6	0.0	3.8	15.8	0.0	0.0	0.4	0.0	0.0	0.0	0.0	0.0	0.4
0.0	19.3	0.0	7.3	0.9	25.8	10.4	0.6	0.0	0.4	0.0	0.0	0.0	0.2	0.1	2.5
0.0	13.2	0.0	7.6	0.9	25.8	10.4	0.6	0.0	0.4	0.0	0.0	0.0	0.2	0.1	2.6
9.0	70.6	0.0	29.9	3.8	99.5	521.4	3.6	0.0	1.4	2.7	0.1	0.0	0.9	0.5	16.1
4.6	18.1	0.0	7.3	0.9	25.2	10.4	0.6	0.0	0.4	0.4	0.0	0.0	0.2	0.1	2.5
1.8	18.8	0.0	54.6	0.9	82.9	0.8	0.7	2.0	0.3	7.2	0.1	0.0	0.3	0.2	20.9
0.2	1.5	0.0	1.4	0.0	2.3	0.1	0.1	0.0	0.0	0.0	0.0	0.0	0.0	0.0	0.3
1.5	15.7	0.0	29.7	0.7	70.3	196.0	1.3	0.6	0.1	1.7	0.1	0.1	0.5	0.1	15.8

Code	Food Name	Unit Amount	Kilocalories (kcal)	Protein (g)	Carbohydrate (g)
12135	Nuts, mixed w/o peanuts, oil-roasted, w/o salt	1.0 oz	172.2	4.3	6.2
12635	Nuts, mixed w/peanuts, dry-roasted, w/o salt	1.0 oz	166.3	4.8	7.1
12137	Nuts, mixed w/peanuts, dry-roasted w/salt	1.0 oz	166.3	4.8	7.1
12637	Nuts, mixed w/peanuts, oil-roasted, w/o salt	1 Tbsp.	54.9	1.5	1.9
12142	Nuts, mixed w/peanuts, oil-roasted w/salt	1 nut	6.2	0.2	0.2
12143	Nuts, pecans, dried	2 halves	20.0	0.2	0.5
12643	Nuts, pecans, dry-roasted w/o salt	1.0 oz	184.5	2.2	6.3
12144	Nuts, pecans, dry-roasted w/salt	1.0 oz	184.5	2.2	6.3
12644	Nuts, pecans, oil-roasted w/o salt	2 halves	27.4	0.3	0.6
12145	Nuts, pecans, oil-roasted w/salt	2 halves	27.4	0.3	0.6
12149	Nuts, pine nut, Pignolias, dried	1 cup	769.8	32.6	19.3
12152	Nuts, pistachios, dried	2 kernels	5.8	0.2	0.2
12652	Nuts, pistachios, dry-roasted w/o salt	1.0 oz	169.7	4.2	7.7
12154	Nuts, pistachios, dry-roasted w/salt	1.0 oz	169.7	4.2	7.7
12155	Nuts, walnut, black, dried	1 Tbsp.	47.3	1.9	0.9
4501	Oil, vegetable, canola	1 Tbsp.	120.2	0.0	0.0
4047	Oil, vegetable, cocoa butter	1 Tbsp.	120.2	0.0	0.0
904902	Oil, vegetable, coconut	1 Tbsp.	117.2	0.0	0.0
4541	Oil, vegetable, Crisco	1 Tbsp.	120.5	0.0	0.0
4055	Oil, vegetable, oat	1 Tbsp.	120.2	0.0	0.0
4513	Oil, vegetable, palm	1 Tbsp.	120.2	0.0	0.0
4514	Oil, vegetable, palm kernel	1 Tbsp.	117.2	0.0	0.0
4536	Oil, vegetable, rice bran	1 Tbsp.	120.2	0.0	0.0
4060	Oil, vegetable, soybean lecithin	1 Tbsp.	103.8	0.0	0.0
4506	Oil, vegetable, sunflower, linoleic < 60%	1 Tbsp.	120.2	0.0	0.0
4584	Oil, vegetable, sunflower, linoleic > 60%	1 Tbsp.	120.2	0.0	0.0
4545	Oil, vegetable, sunflower, oleic > 70%	1 Tbsp.	120.2	0.0	0.0
4516	Oil, vegetable, sunflower-hydrogenated, linoleic	1 Tbsp.	120.2	0.0	0.0
4502	Oil, vegetable/salad/cooking, corn	1 Tbsp.	120.2	0.0	0.0
4053	Oil, vegetable/salad/cooking, cottonseed	1 Tbsp.	120.2	0.0	0.0
4042	Oil, vegetable/salad/cooking, olive	1 Tbsp.	119.3	0.0	0.0
4510	Oil, vegetable/salad/cooking, peanut	1 Tbsp.	119.3	0.0	0.0
4511	Oil, vegetable/salad/cooking, safflower, linoleic > 70%	1 Tbsp.	120.2	0.0	0.0
4058	Oil, vegetable/salad/cooking, safflower, oleic > 70%	1 Tbsp.	120.2	0.0	0.0
4044	Oil, vegetable/salad/cooking, sesame	1 Tbsp.	120.2	0.0	0.0
4034	Oil, vegetable/salad/cooking, soybean	1 Tbsp.	120.2	0.0	0.0
4543	Oil, vegetable/salad/cooking, soybean, hydrogenated	1 Tbsp.	120.2	0.0	0.0
18294	Pancake/waffle, buttermilk, Eggo/Kellogg	1 serving (2 waffles)	181.7	4.7	29.7
18295	Pancakes, blueberry, homemade	1 pancake (4″ diam)	84.4	2.3	11.0
18611	Pancakes, buckwheat, incomplete dry mix, prep	1 pancake (4″ diam)	62.4	2.4	8.5
918298	Pancakes, buttermilk, homemade	1 pancake (4″ diam)	86.3	2.6	10.9
18297	Pancakes, dry mix, prep, special dietary	1 pancake (4″ diam)	75.6	1.9	16.0
918292	Pancakes, plain, homemade	1.0 oz	63.6	1.8	7.9
18289	Pancakes, plain, incomplete dry mix, prep	1 pancake (4″ diam)	82.8	3.0	11.0
18288	Pancakes, plain/buttermilk, complete dry mix, prep	1 pancake (4″ diam)	73.7	2.0	13.9
18291	Pancakes, plain/buttermilk, frozen	1 pancake (4″ diam)	82.4	1.9	15.7
20097	Pancakes, whole-wheat, incomplete dry mix, prep	1 pancake (4″ diam)	79.0	3.2	11.2
22907	Pasta w/egg, homemade, ckd	2.0 oz, ckd	74.1	3.0	13.4
20098	Pasta w/meatballs in tomato sauce, canned entree	1 can	437.8	18.4	52.2
22522	Pasta w/o egg, homemade, ckd	2.0 oz	70.7	2.5	14.3
22515	Pasta w/sliced franks in tomato sauce, canned entree	1 can	434.7	15.5	49.7
924169	Pasta, beef ravioli w/meat sauce, canned	1 can, 7.8-oz serving	268.4	9.8	34.8
924206	Pasta, Beefaroni, macaroni w/beef in tomato sauce, canned entree/Chef Boyardee	1 package	184.4	8.2	31.1
20092	Pasta, cheese ravioli/Contadina	4.5 oz	369.9	18.0	39.0
20094	Pasta, fettucini alfredo	2.0 oz dry, 1 cup cooked	30.7	1.3	46.0
20093	Pasta, fresh-refrigerated, plain, ckd	2.0 oz dry, 1 cup cooked	74.7	2.9	14.2
20095	Pasta, fresh-refrigerated, spinach, ckd	2.0 oz	74.1	2.9	14.3
924170	Pasta, mini beef ravioli in tomato & meat sauce, canned entree/Chef Boyardee	1 package	403.8	14.8	68.5
924270	Pasta, ravioli, frozen	1.0 oz	59.9	2.0	7.0
924014	Pasta, spaghetti w/meat sauce	1 cup	332.3	18.6	30.7
924126	Pasta, spaghetti w/tomato sauce & cheese	1 cup	260.0	9.0	37.0
924189	Pasta, spaghetti & meatballs	1 cup	329.8	19.0	39.0
20121	Pasta, spaghetti, canned	1 cup	190.0	6.0	39.0
20321	Pasta, spaghetti, enriched, ckd w/o salt	1 cup	197.4	6.7	39.7
20120	Pasta, spaghetti, enriched, ckd w/salt	1 cup	197.4	6.7	39.7

Dietary Fiber (g)	Total Fat (g)	Cholesterol (mg)	Calcium (mg)	Iron (mg)	Magnesium (mg)	Sodium (mg)	Zinc (mg)	Vitamin A (μgRE)	Vitamin C (mg)	Vitamin E (mgαT)	Thiamin (mg)	Riboflavin (mg)	Niacin (mg)	Vitamin B6 (mg)	Folate (μg)
1.5	15.7	0.0	29.7	0.7	70.3	3.1	1.3	0.6	0.1	1.7	0.1	0.1	0.5	0.1	15.8
2.5	14.4	0.0	19.6	1.0	63.0	3.4	1.1	0.3	0.1	1.7	0.1	0.1	1.3	0.1	14.1
2.5	14.4	0.0	19.6	1.0	63.0	187.3	1.1	0.3	0.1	1.7	0.1	0.1	1.3	0.1	14.1
0.9	5.0	0.0	9.6	0.3	20.9	1.0	0.5	0.2	0.0	0.5	0.0	0.0	0.5	0.0	7.4
0.1	0.6	0.0	1.1	0.0	2.4	6.5	0.1	0.0	0.0	0.1	0.0	0.0	0.1	0.0	0.8
0.2	2.0	0.0	1.1	0.1	3.8	0.0	0.2	0.4	0.1	0.1	0.0	0.0	0.0	0.0	1.2
2.6	18.1	0.0	9.8	0.6	37.2	0.3	1.6	3.6	0.6	0.9	0.1	0.0	0.3	0.1	11.4
2.6	18.1	0.0	9.8	0.6	37.2	218.4	1.6	3.6	0.6	0.0	0.1	0.0	0.3	0.1	11.4
0.3	2.8	0.0	1.4	0.1	5.2	0.0	0.2	0.5	0.1	0.0	0.0	0.0	0.0	0.0	1.6
0.3	2.8	0.0	1.4	0.1	5.2	30.2	0.2	0.5	0.1	0.0	0.0	0.0	0.0	0.0	1.6
6.1	69.0	0.0	35.4	12.5	316.9	5.4	5.8	4.1	2.6	4.8	1.1	0.3	4.9	0.1	77.9
0.1	0.5	0.0	1.4	0.1	1.6	0.1	0.0	0.2	0.1	0.1	0.0	0.0	0.0	0.0	0.6
3.0	14.8	0.0	19.6	0.9	36.4	1.7	0.4	6.7	2.0	1.5	0.1	0.1	0.4	0.1	16.5
3.0	14.8	0.0	19.6	0.9	36.4	218.4	0.4	6.7	2.0	1.8	0.1	0.1	0.4	0.1	16.5
0.4	4.4	0.0	4.5	0.2	15.8	0.1	0.3	2.3	0.2	0.2	0.0	0.0	0.1	0.0	5.1
0.0	13.6	0.0	0.0	0.0	0.0	0.0	0.0	0.0	0.0	2.8	0.0	0.0	0.0	0.0	0.0
0.0	13.6	0.0	0.0	0.0	0.0	0.0	0.0	0.0	0.0	0.0	0.0	0.0	0.0	0.0	0.0
0.0	13.6	0.0	0.0	0.0	0.0	0.0	0.0	0.0	0.0	0.0	0.0	0.0	0.0	0.0	0.0
0.0	13.6	0.0	0.0	0.0	0.0	0.0	0.0	0.0	0.0	0.0	0.0	0.0	0.0	0.0	0.0
0.0	13.6	0.0	0.0	0.0	0.0	0.0	0.0	0.0	0.0	2.0	0.0	0.0	0.0	0.0	0.0
0.0	13.6	0.0	0.0	0.0	0.0	0.0	0.0	0.0	0.0	3.0	0.0	0.0	0.0	0.0	0.0
0.0	13.6	0.0	0.0	0.0	0.0	0.0	0.0	0.0	0.0	0.5	0.0	0.0	0.0	0.0	0.0
0.0	13.6	0.0	0.0	0.0	0.0	0.0	0.0	0.0	0.0	0.0	0.0	0.0	0.0	0.0	0.0
0.0	13.6	0.0	0.0	0.0	0.0	0.0	0.0	0.0	0.0	0.7	0.0	0.0	0.0	0.0	0.0
0.0	13.6	0.0	0.0	0.0	0.0	0.0	0.0	0.0	0.0	0.0	0.0	0.0	0.0	0.0	0.0
0.0	13.6	0.0	0.0	0.0	0.0	0.0	0.0	0.0	0.0	6.9	0.0	0.0	0.0	0.0	0.0
0.0	13.6	0.0	0.0	0.0	0.0	0.0	0.0	0.0	0.0	0.0	0.0	0.0	0.0	0.0	0.0
0.0	13.6	0.0	0.0	0.0	0.0	0.0	0.0	0.0	0.0	6.9	0.0	0.0	0.0	0.0	0.0
0.0	13.6	0.0	0.0	0.0	0.0	0.0	0.0	0.0	0.0	2.9	0.0	0.0	0.0	0.0	0.0
0.0	13.6	0.0	0.0	0.0	0.0	0.0	0.0	0.0	0.0	5.2	0.0	0.0	0.0	0.0	0.0
0.0	13.5	0.0	0.0	0.1	0.0	0.0	0.0	0.0	0.0	1.7	0.0	0.0	0.0	0.0	0.0
0.0	13.5	0.0	0.0	0.0	0.0	0.0	0.0	0.0	0.0	1.7	0.0	0.0	0.0	0.0	0.0
0.0	13.6	0.0	0.0	0.0	0.0	0.0	0.0	0.0	0.0	5.9	0.0	0.0	0.0	0.0	0.0
0.0	13.6	0.0	0.0	0.0	0.0	0.0	0.0	0.0	0.0	4.7	0.0	0.0	0.0	0.0	0.0
0.0	13.6	0.0	0.0	0.0	0.0	0.0	0.0	0.0	0.0	0.6	0.0	0.0	0.0	0.0	0.0
0.0	13.6	0.0	0.0	0.0	0.0	0.0	0.0	0.0	0.0	2.5	0.0	0.0	0.0	0.0	0.0
0.0	13.6	0.0	0.0	0.0	0.0	0.0	0.0	0.0	0.0	2.5	0.0	0.0	0.0	0.0	0.0
0.9	5.2	8.6	27.3	2.4	14.0	413.4	0.5	0.0	1.1	0.0	0.2	0.2	2.7	0.3	40.6
0.0	3.5	21.3	78.3	0.7	6.1	156.6	0.2	19.4	0.8	0.0	0.1	0.1	0.6	0.0	13.7
0.7	2.3	0.6	76.8	0.6	16.8	159.9	0.4	20.1	0.2	0.0	0.1	0.1	0.4	0.0	5.1
0.0	3.5	22.0	59.7	0.6	5.7	198.4	0.2	11.4	0.2	0.0	0.1	0.1	0.6	0.0	14.4
0.0	0.3	0.1	22.0	0.7	10.3	99.6	0.3	3.8	0.0	0.0	0.1	0.0	0.6	0.0	1.9
0.0	2.7	16.5	61.3	0.5	4.5	122.9	0.2	15.1	0.1	0.0	0.1	0.1	0.4	0.0	10.6
0.7	2.9	0.8	81.7	0.5	8.4	191.9	0.3	27.4	0.2	0.0	0.1	0.1	0.5	0.0	4.2
0.5	1.0	0.3	47.9	0.6	7.6	238.6	0.1	3.4	0.1	0.0	0.1	0.1	0.7	0.0	3.4
0.6	1.2	3.2	22.3	1.3	5.0	183.2	0.2	10.4	0.1	0.1	0.1	0.2	1.4	0.0	18.0
1.1	2.5	0.7	95.0	1.2	17.5	217.4	0.4	24.3	0.2	0.0	0.1	0.2	0.9	0.0	8.0
0.0	1.0	23.4	5.7	0.7	8.0	47.3	0.3	9.7	0.0	0.0	0.1	0.1	0.7	0.0	24.5
11.5	17.3	34.0	46.8	4.0	59.5	1776.5	3.1	157.3	12.8	2.1	0.3	0.3	5.6	0.3	89.3
0.0	0.6	0.0	3.4	0.6	8.0	42.2	0.2	0.0	0.0	0.0	0.1	0.1	0.8	0.0	24.5
3.8	19.2	37.6	0.0	3.8	0.0	2014.8	0.0	0.0	0.0	0.0	0.0	0.0	0.0	0.0	0.0
0.0	10.1	0.0	51.0	2.2	0.0	814.0	0.0	196.0	7.0	0.0	0.2	0.2	3.3	0.0	0.0
3.0	2.9	17.0	17.0	1.5	0.0	799.2	0.0	0.0	0.4	0.0	0.0	0.0	0.0	0.0	0.0
0.0	15.0	110.0	340.0	1.4	34.0	540.0	1.1	103.0	0.0	0.0	0.2	0.3	1.2	0.1	13.0
0.0	0.9	5.7	13.2	0.3	0.0	47.3	0.0	0.0	0.0	0.0	0.0	0.0	0.2	0.0	0.0
0.0	0.6	18.8	3.4	0.6	10.3	3.4	0.3	3.4	0.0	0.0	0.1	0.1	0.6	0.0	36.5
0.0	0.5	18.8	10.3	0.6	13.7	3.4	0.4	8.0	0.0	0.0	0.1	0.1	0.6	0.1	36.5
5.5	8.0	29.8	38.3	4.1	0.0	2018.8	0.0	0.0	0.4	0.0	0.0	0.0	0.0	0.0	0.0
0.0	2.0	0.0	12.0	0.7	0.0	80.0	0.0	0.0	0.0	0.0	0.1	0.1	0.8	0.0	0.0
0.0	11.7	0.0	124.0	3.7	0.0	1009.0	0.0	318.0	22.0	0.0	0.3	0.3	4.0	0.0	0.0
2.0	9.0	8.0	80.0	2.3	0.0	955.0	1.3	216.0	13.0	0.0	0.3	0.2	2.3	0.2	8.0
1.0	12.0	89.0	124.0	3.7	0.0	1009.0	2.5	318.0	22.0	0.0	0.3	0.3	4.0	0.2	10.0
2.0	2.0	3.0	40.0	2.8	0.0	955.0	1.1	186.0	10.0	0.0	0.4	0.3	4.5	0.1	6.0
2.4	0.9	0.0	9.8	2.0	25.2	1.4	0.7	0.0	0.0	0.1	0.3	0.1	2.3	0.0	98.0
2.4	0.9	0.0	9.8	2.0	25.2	140.0	0.7	0.0	0.0	0.0	0.3	0.1	2.3	0.0	98.0

Code	Food Name	Unit Amount	Kilocalories (kcal)	Protein (g)	Carbohydrate (g)
20126	Pasta, spaghetti, spinach, ckd	1 cup	182.0	6.4	36.6
20521	Pasta, spaghetti, unenriched, ckd w/o salt	1 cup	197.4	6.7	39.7
20420	Pasta, spaghetti, unenriched, ckd w/salt	1 cup	197.4	6.7	39.7
20124	Pasta, spaghetti, whole-wheat, ckd	1 cup	173.6	7.5	37.2
924172	Pasta, Spaghettios & Franks/FrancoAm	8.0 oz	227.0	8.3	28.3
924194	Pasta, Spaghettios & Meatballs/FrancoAm	8.0 oz	222.5	9.9	27.3
22520	Pasta, spinach tortellini/Contadina	8.0 oz	656.0	31.9	97.5
18640	Pasta, whole-wheat macaroni and cheese dinner, dry mix/Hodgson Mill	8.0 oz	852.4	32.0	157.1
18635	Pastry, chocolate eclairs, frozen/WW	1 eclair, frozen	140.5	2.4	23.5
18238	Pastry, cinnamon rolls w/icing, refrigerated dough/Pillsbury	1 serving	150.2	2.4	23.9
18237	Pastry, cream puff/eclair shell, homemade w/custard	1 miniature cream puff	59.3	1.5	5.3
18240	Pastry, cream puff/eclair shell, homemade	1 cream puff shell	238.9	5.9	15.0
18241	Pastry, croissant, butter	1 mini croissant	117.7	2.4	13.3
918816	Pastry, croissant, cheese	1 small croissant	173.9	3.9	19.7
18244	Pastry, Danish, cheese	1 pastry	265.5	5.7	26.4
18431	Pastry, Danish, fruit (apple/cinn/raisin/lemon/raspberry/strawberry) enriched	1 large (7" diam)	526.8	7.7	67.9
18435	Pastry, Danish, nut (almond/raisin nut/cinnamon nut)	1 piece (1/8 of 15-oz ring)	227.9	3.8	24.2
18338	Pastry, eclair/cream puff, homemade, custard filled w/chocolate icing	1 eclair (5" x 2" x 1.75")	262.0	6.4	24.2
18337	Pastry, phyllo dough	1.0 oz	83.7	2.0	14.7
18354	Pastry, puff, frozen, baked	1 shell	223.2	3.0	18.3
18368	Pastry, strudel, apple	1 piece	194.5	2.3	29.2
16398	Peanut butter, chunky w/salt	2 Tbsp.	188.5	7.7	6.9
16099	Peanut butter, smooth w/salt	2 Tbsp.	189.8	8.1	6.2
16090	Peanuts, all types, dry-roasted w/o salt	1 peanut	5.9	0.2	0.2
16389	Peanuts, all types, dry-roasted w/salt	1.0 oz	163.8	6.6	6.0
16089	Peanuts, all types, oil-roasted w/o salt	1 peanut	5.8	0.3	0.2
16087	Peanuts, all types, oil-roasted w/salt	1 peanut	5.2	0.2	0.2
912901	Peanuts, all types, raw	1.0 oz	158.8	7.2	4.5
16392	Peanuts, honey-roasted	1.0 oz	150.1	7.0	4.0
16394	Peanuts, Spanish, raw	1/4 cup (@ 1 handful)	210.9	9.7	5.9
16158	Peas, chickpea/garbanzo, falafel, homemade	1 (2.25" diam) patty	56.6	2.3	5.4
16357	Peas, chickpea/garbanzo, hummus, commercial	1/2 cup	207.5	9.9	17.9
16056	Peas, chickpea/garbanzo/Bengal gram, mature seeds, canned	1/2 cup	142.8	5.9	27.1
18628	Pie, apple snack pie/Hostess	1 pie	390.4	5.0	45.0
18443	Pie, apple turnover, frozen, ready to bake/PepFarm	1 serving	284.1	3.7	31.2
18302	Pie, apple, frozen/Banquet	1 serving	292.3	2.9	41.4
918871	Pie, apple, homemade	1.0 oz	75.1	0.7	10.5
18304	Pie, banana cream, frozen	1/6 pie	180.2	2.0	21.0
18303	Pie, banana cream, homemade	1 piece (1/8 of 9" diam)	387.4	6.3	47.4
918872	Pie, banana cream, no bake mix	1 piece (1/8 of 9" diam)	230.9	3.1	29.1
918873	Pie, banana custard	1/8 pie	251.9	5.1	35.0
918889	Pie, blackberry	1/8 pie	286.7	3.1	40.6
18305	Pie, blueberry snack pie/Hostess	1 pie	390.4	3.0	49.0
18306	Pie, blueberry, commercially prep	1 piece (1/8 of 9" diam)	290.0	2.3	43.6
918307	Pie, blueberry, homemade	1 piece (1/8 of 9" diam)	360.2	4.0	49.2
918890	Pie, butterscotch pudding, homemade	1 piece (1/8 of 9" diam)	354.3	6.0	42.3
18308	Pie, cherry snack pie/Hostess	1 pie	390.4	5.0	55.0
18444	Pie, cherry, commercially prep	1 piece (1/8 of 9" diam)	325.0	2.5	49.8
18309	Pie, cherry, fried	1.0 oz	88.5	0.8	11.9
918874	Pie, cherry, homemade	1.0 oz	78.3	0.8	11.2
18310	Pie, chocolate cream, frozen/Banquet	1/6 pie	190.1	2.0	24.0
918311	Pie, chocolate cream, commercially prep	1 piece (1/6 of 8" pie)	343.5	2.9	38.0
18312	Pie, chocolate cream, homemade	1 piece (1/8 of 9" diam)	400.4	6.8	44.3
918875	Pie, chocolate mousse, no bake mix	1 piece (1/8 of 9" diam)	247.0	3.3	28.1
18313	Pie, coconut cream, frozen	1 piece (1/6 of 8" pie)	288.0	3.0	33.3
918315	Pie, coconut cream, commercially prep	1 piece (1/8 of 7" pie)	143.0	1.0	17.9
18314	Pie, coconut cream, homemade	1 piece (1/8 of 9" diam)	396.3	6.4	45.5
918318	Pie, egg custard, commercially prep	1 piece (1/8 of 8" pie)	220.5	5.8	21.8
18319	Pie, egg custard, homemade	1 piece (1/8 of 9" diam)	261.6	6.5	34.0
918876	Pie, fruit pie, fried	1 fried pie (5" x 3.75")	404.5	3.8	54.5
918877	Pie, lemon chiffon	1 piece (1/8 of 8" pie)	254.3	5.7	35.5
18320	Pie, lemon cream, frozen/Banquet	1 piece (1/6 of 8" pie)	170.3	2.0	23.0
18321	Pie, lemon meringue, commercially prep	1 piece (1/6 of 8" pie)	302.8	1.7	53.3
18445	Pie, lemon meringue, homemade	1 piece (1/8 of 9" diam)	362.0	4.8	49.7
18322	Pie, lemon, fried	1 fried pie (5" x 3.75")	404.5	3.8	54.5

Dietary Fiber (g)	Total Fat (g)	Cholesterol (mg)	Calcium (mg)	Iron (mg)	Magnesium (mg)	Sodium (mg)	Zinc (mg)	Vitamin A (μgRE)	Vitamin C (mg)	Vitamin E (mgαT)	Thiamin (mg)	Riboflavin (mg)	Niacin (mg)	Vitamin B₆ (mg)	Folate (μg)
0.0	0.9	0.0	42.0	1.5	86.8	19.6	1.5	21.0	0.0	0.0	0.1	0.1	2.1	0.1	16.8
2.4	0.9	0.0	9.8	0.7	25.2	1.4	0.7	0.0	0.0	0.1	0.0	0.0	0.6	0.0	9.8
0.0	0.9	0.0	9.8	0.7	25.2	140.0	0.7	0.0	0.0	0.0	0.0	0.0	0.6	0.0	9.8
6.3	0.8	0.0	21.0	1.5	42.0	4.2	1.1	0.0	0.0	0.1	0.2	0.1	1.0	0.1	7.0
1.1	9.1	0.0	34.8	2.4	0.0	1074.2	1.7	111.0	4.3	0.0	0.2	0.2	3.5	0.1	0.0
0.9	8.2	0.0	32.0	2.4	0.0	1024.8	2.2	112.8	4.4	0.0	0.2	0.2	3.3	0.1	0.0
0.0	14.2	115.3	540.9	6.4	16.0	1064.1	0.6	94.0	0.0	0.0	1.3	1.0	11.4	0.0	12.4
17.3	10.7	17.9	258.8	5.9	0.0	1387.0	0.0	0.0	0.0	0.0	0.0	0.0	0.0	0.0	0.0
0.9	4.1	30.1	0.0	0.0	0.0	185.9	0.0	0.0	0.0	0.0	0.0	0.0	0.0	0.0	0.0
0.0	5.0	0.0	0.0	0.0	0.0	334.4	0.0	0.0	0.0	0.0	0.0	0.0	0.0	0.0	0.0
0.1	3.6	30.8	15.2	0.3	2.8	78.4	0.1	45.8	0.1	0.5	0.0	0.1	0.2	0.0	6.4
0.5	17.1	129.4	23.8	1.3	7.9	367.6	0.5	203.3	0.0	2.5	0.1	0.2	1.0	0.0	31.7
0.8	6.1	19.4	10.7	0.6	4.6	215.8	0.2	53.9	0.1	0.1	0.1	0.1	0.6	0.0	18.0
1.1	8.8	23.9	22.3	0.9	10.1	233.1	0.4	82.7	0.1	0.4	0.2	0.1	0.9	0.0	31.1
0.7	15.5	11.4	24.9	1.1	10.7	319.5	0.5	32.0	0.1	1.8	0.1	0.2	1.4	0.0	42.6
2.7	26.3	161.9	65.3	2.5	21.3	502.7	0.8	31.2	5.5	3.5	0.4	0.3	2.8	0.1	46.9
1.1	13.4	24.4	49.8	1.0	17.0	192.4	0.5	7.4	0.9	1.9	0.1	0.1	1.2	0.1	44.0
0.6	15.7	127.0	63.0	1.2	15.0	337.0	0.6	191.0	0.3	2.1	0.1	0.3	0.8	0.1	28.0
0.5	1.7	0.0	3.1	0.9	4.2	135.2	0.1	0.0	0.0	0.3	0.2	0.1	1.1	0.0	20.7
0.6	15.4	0.0	4.0	1.0	6.4	101.2	0.2	0.0	0.0	1.0	0.1	0.1	1.5	0.0	18.8
1.6	8.0	4.3	10.7	0.3	6.4	191.0	0.1	6.4	1.2	2.2	0.0	0.0	0.2	0.0	9.9
2.1	16.0	0.0	13.1	0.6	50.9	155.5	0.9	0.0	0.0	0.0	0.0	0.0	4.4	0.1	29.4
1.9	16.3	0.0	12.2	0.6	50.9	149.4	0.9	0.0	0.0	3.2	0.0	0.0	4.3	0.1	23.7
0.1	0.5	0.0	0.5	0.0	1.8	0.1	0.0	0.0	0.0	0.1	0.0	0.0	0.1	0.0	1.5
2.2	13.9	0.0	15.1	0.6	49.3	227.6	0.9	0.0	0.0	2.1	0.1	0.0	3.8	0.1	40.7
0.1	0.5	0.0	0.9	0.0	1.9	0.1	0.1	0.0	0.0	0.1	0.0	0.0	0.1	0.0	1.3
0.1	0.4	0.0	0.8	0.0	1.7	3.9	0.1	0.0	0.0	0.1	0.0	0.0	0.1	0.0	1.1
2.4	13.8	0.0	25.8	1.3	47.0	5.0	0.9	0.0	0.0	2.6	0.2	0.0	3.4	0.1	67.1
3.0	13.0	0.0	15.0	0.6	0.0	110.0	0.9	0.0	0.0	0.0	0.1	0.0	3.8	0.1	41.0
3.5	18.4	0.0	39.2	1.4	69.6	8.1	0.8	0.0	0.0	0.0	0.2	0.0	5.9	0.1	88.8
0.0	3.0	0.0	9.2	0.6	13.9	50.0	0.3	0.2	0.3	0.0	0.0	0.0	0.2	0.0	15.8
7.5	12.0	0.0	47.5	3.1	88.8	473.8	2.3	3.8	0.0	0.0	0.2	0.1	0.7	0.3	103.8
5.3	1.4	0.0	38.4	1.6	34.8	358.8	1.3	2.4	4.6	0.0	0.0	0.0	0.2	0.6	80.2
0.0	20.0	18.0	26.0	1.4	0.0	540.0	0.0	0.0	1.0	0.0	0.1	0.1	1.6	0.0	0.0
1.6	16.0	0.0	0.0	1.2	0.0	176.2	0.0	0.0	0.0	0.0	0.0	0.0	0.0	0.0	0.0
1.0	13.2	8.7	10.1	0.3	0.0	360.6	0.0	0.0	0.0	0.0	0.0	0.0	0.0	0.0	0.0
0.0	3.5	0.0	2.0	0.3	2.0	59.8	0.1	3.4	0.5	0.0	0.0	0.0	0.3	0.0	6.8
2.0	10.0	0.0	32.0	1.0	0.0	150.0	0.0	1.4	1.0	0.0	0.0	0.1	2.0	0.3	15.0
1.0	19.6	73.4	108.0	1.5	23.0	345.6	0.7	100.8	2.3	2.1	0.2	0.3	1.5	0.2	38.9
0.6	11.9	26.7	67.2	0.4	11.0	266.8	0.3	92.0	0.5	0.0	0.1	0.1	0.7	0.0	19.3
1.0	10.6	0.0	75.0	0.6	0.0	221.0	0.0	58.0	1.0	0.0	0.1	0.2	0.3	0.0	0.0
5.0	13.0	0.0	22.0	0.6	0.0	316.0	0.0	22.0	5.0	0.0	0.0	0.0	0.4	0.0	0.0
0.0	20.0	18.0	28.0	1.5	0.0	450.0	0.0	0.0	2.0	0.0	0.2	0.1	1.8	0.0	0.0
1.3	12.5	0.0	10.0	0.4	6.3	406.3	0.2	42.5	3.4	2.5	0.0	0.0	0.4	0.0	27.5
0.0	17.5	0.0	10.3	1.8	11.8	272.0	0.3	5.9	1.0	0.0	0.2	0.2	1.8	0.0	33.8
0.0	18.2	7.6	128.3	1.6	21.6	335.3	0.7	106.7	0.6	0.0	0.2	0.3	1.3	0.1	14.0
0.0	20.0	18.0	29.0	1.4	0.0	530.0	0.0	0.0	2.0	0.0	0.2	0.1	1.6	0.0	0.0
1.0	13.8	0.0	15.0	0.6	10.0	307.5	0.2	67.5	1.1	1.9	0.0	0.0	0.3	0.1	27.5
0.7	4.5	0.0	6.2	0.3	2.8	104.7	0.1	4.8	0.4	0.0	0.0	0.0	0.4	0.0	5.0
0.0	3.5	0.0	2.9	0.5	2.6	55.4	0.1	13.9	0.3	0.0	0.0	0.0	0.4	0.0	7.8
1.0	10.0	0.0	38.0	1.0	0.0	110.0	0.0	1.4	0.0	0.0	0.0	0.1	0.2	0.0	0.0
2.3	21.9	5.7	40.7	1.2	23.7	153.7	0.3	0.0	0.0	3.1	0.0	0.1	0.8	0.0	14.7
0.0	22.9	9.4	115.0	1.8	36.9	347.9	0.9	103.7	0.7	0.0	0.2	0.3	1.5	0.1	14.2
0.0	14.6	33.3	73.2	1.0	30.4	437.0	0.6	96.0	0.5	0.0	0.0	0.1	0.6	0.0	24.7
0.0	16.7	0.0	45.5	1.5	0.0	181.8	0.0	0.3	0.0	0.0	0.0	0.1	0.3	0.0	0.0
0.6	8.0	0.0	13.9	0.4	9.6	122.4	0.2	0.0	0.0	0.9	0.0	0.0	0.1	0.0	3.4
0.0	21.3	8.0	113.1	1.5	21.3	356.4	0.8	105.1	0.7	0.0	0.2	0.3	1.3	0.1	14.6
1.7	12.2	34.7	84.0	0.6	11.6	252.0	0.5	70.4	0.6	2.0	0.0	0.2	0.3	0.1	21.0
0.0	11.3	4.6	106.7	1.0	16.5	256.5	0.6	81.3	0.5	0.0	0.1	0.3	0.8	0.1	12.7
3.3	20.6	0.0	28.2	1.6	12.8	478.7	0.3	3.8	1.7	3.8	0.2	0.1	1.8	0.0	23.0
1.0	10.2	0.0	19.0	0.7	0.0	211.0	0.0	28.0	2.0	0.0	0.0	0.1	0.2	0.0	0.0
1.0	9.0	0.0	30.0	1.0	0.0	120.0	0.0	0.4	2.0	0.0	0.0	0.0	0.2	0.0	0.0
1.4	9.8	50.9	63.3	0.7	17.0	165.0	0.6	58.8	3.6	2.5	0.1	0.2	0.7	0.0	14.7
0.0	16.4	67.3	15.2	1.3	7.6	307.3	0.4	55.9	4.2	0.0	0.1	0.2	1.2	0.0	31.8
3.3	20.6	0.0	28.2	1.6	12.8	478.7	0.3	3.8	0.0	0.0	0.2	0.1	1.8	0.0	23.0

Code	Food Name	Unit Amount	Kilocalories (kcal)	Protein (g)	Carbohydrate (g)
918878	Pie, mince, homemade	1 piece (1/8 of 9″ diam)	476.9	4.3	79.2
18323	Pie, mincemeat, frozen/Banquet	1 piece (1/6 of 8″ pie)	260.4	3.0	38.0
918891	Pie, peach	1.0 oz	63.6	0.5	9.4
918892	Pie, peach snack pie/Hostess	1 pie	399.4	4.0	53.0
18324	Pie, pecan snack pie/LittleDeb	1 pie	201.8	1.8	33.1
18325	Pie, pecan, commercially prep	1 piece (1/6 of 8″ pie)	452.0	4.5	64.6
918879	Pie, pecan, homemade	1 piece (1/8 of 9″ diam)	502.6	6.0	63.7
918880	Pie, pineapple	1 piece (1/8 of 9″ diam)	298.5	2.6	45.0
918881	Pie, pineapple chiffon	1 piece (1/8 of 9″ diam)	233.3	5.3	31.7
18326	Pie, pineapple custard	1 piece (1/8 of 9″ diam)	250.8	4.6	36.6
18327	Pie, pumpkin, commercially prep	1 piece (1/6 of 8″ pie)	378.0	7.0	49.1
918882	Pie, pumpkin, homemade	1 piece (1/8 of 9″ diam)	232.6	5.1	30.1
918883	Pie, raisin	1 piece (1/8 of 9″ diam)	318.6	3.1	50.7
918885	Pie, rhubarb	1 piece (1/8 of 9″ diam)	298.5	3.0	45.1
18328	Pie, strawberry	1 piece (1/8 of 9″ diam)	184.1	1.8	28.7
22531	Pie, vanilla creme, homemade	1 piece (1/8 of 9″ diam)	258.5	4.5	30.3
22533	Pizza Rolls Pizza Snacks, hamburger, frozen/Totino's	1 serving (1/3 pkg)	231.2	9.4	26.4
22532	Pizza Rolls Pizza Snacks, pepperoni, frozen/Totino's	1 serving	384.9	14.4	39.5
924142	Pizza Rolls Pizza Snacks, sausage, frozen/Totino's	1 serving	351.1	14.1	40.2
924146	Pizza, cheese, meat, vegetable	1/8 of a large pizza	184.1	13.0	21.3
924141	Pizza, cheese, frozen/Celeste	1/4 of a medium pizza	317.5	14.2	27.8
22545	Pizza, cheese, homemade	1 slice	152.8	7.8	18.4
924262	Pizza, combination, sausage & pepperoni, frozen/Jeno's Crisp'n Tasty	1 package	491.0	16.8	51.7
22548	Pizza, combo, frozen/Totino's	1/6 pizza	234.8	11.3	20.0
22554	Pizza, deep dish sausage, frozen/Tony's D'Primo	1 package	1576.1	50.1	163.9
22542	Pizza, deluxe French bread w/sausage, pepperoni, & mushroom, frozen/Stouffer's	1 package	857.5	32.2	88.9
924148	Pizza, deluxe w/sausage, green & red pepper, & mushrooms, frozen/Celeste	1 package	1538.5	66.6	132.5
924133	Pizza, deluxe, frozen/Celeste	1/4 pizza	377.6	15.5	29.3
22553	Pizza, French bread pizza/Pillsbury	5.7 oz	389.6	18.5	43.0
924149	Pizza, French bread w/sausage & pepperoni, frozen/Stouffer's	1 package	895.6	35.4	87.1
924264	Pizza, ground beef/Totino's	3.5 oz	240.0	10.5	24.4
22560	Pizza, Mexican, frozen/Totino's	1/2 pizza	381.4	13.1	35.5
22555	Pizza, original pepperoni, frozen, 12″/Tombstone	1 serving	311.9	14.5	28.3
22557	Pizza, original pepperoni, frozen, 9″/Tombstone	1 serving	413.4	17.8	38.6
22559	Pizza, original sausage & mushroom, frozen/Tombstone	1 serving	306.2	14.4	31.2
22566	Pizza, original sausage & pepperoni, frozen/Tombstone	1 serving	327.5	14.4	30.6
22562	Pizza, pepperoni	1/8 pizza	181.1	10.1	19.9
22903	Pizza, pepperoni w/Italian pastry crust, frozen/Tony's	1 serving	411.6	15.1	36.8
924151	Pizza, pepperoni, frozen	1 serving	378.1	15.3	34.2
22546	Pizza, pepperoni, frozen/Jack's Original	1 serving	323.3	15.0	29.5
22551	Pizza, pepperoni/Pillsbury	1/2 pizza	302.4	13.4	29.0
22563	Pizza, Premium Deep Dish Singles, pepperoni, frozen/Red Baron	1 serving	480.5	16.0	47.9
22543	Pizza, sausage & pepperoni, frozen	1 serving	385.4	15.8	36.2
924158	Pizza, sausage & pepperoni, frozen/Jack's Great Combination	1 serving	348.0	17.4	30.1
924155	Pizza, sausage mushroom, frozen/Celentano	8.5 oz	592.9	23.9	51.3
924153	Pizza, sausage, frozen/LeanCuisine	6.0 oz	329.8	21.0	40.0
924139	Pizza, sausage, homemade	1 slice	156.8	5.2	19.8
924140	Pizza, Sicilian cheese, frozen	1/4 pizza	329.0	15.4	42.5
924145	Pizza, Sicilian deluxe	1/4 pizza	425.9	18.6	43.8
22550	Pizza, Sicilian sausage	1/4 pizza	399.8	18.2	44.5
22598	Pizza, supreme Italian pastry crust w/sausage, pepperoni, mushroom, green & red peppers	1 serving	399.9	15.8	39.1
22564	Pizza, supreme, sausage, mushrooms, pepperoni, frozen/Red Baron	1 serving	344.1	13.6	31.8
924263	Pizza, taco/Mexican sausage & tangy taco sauce on a corn crust, frozen/Tony's	1 serving	437.4	14.3	42.8
18339	Pizza, vegetable, frozen/Totino's	1/2 pizza	304.0	10.6	36.0
18447	Popover, dry mix, prep	1 popover	66.7	2.6	10.4
918395	Popover, homemade w/reduced-fat (2%) milk	1 popover	87.6	3.5	11.2
10131	Pork back rib, fresh, lean & fat, roasted	3.5 oz	370.0	24.3	0.0
10130	Pork bacon, Canadian, cured, grilled	3.5 oz	185.0	24.2	1.4
10123	Pork bacon, cured, broiled, pan-fried, or roasted	3.5 oz	576.0	30.5	0.6
10041	Pork centerloin/chop, fresh, lean & fat w/bone, broiled	3.5 oz	240.0	28.7	0.0
10039	Pork centerloin/roast, fresh, lean w/bone, roasted	3.5 oz	199.0	27.6	0.0
10098	Pork centerloin/roast, fresh, lean & fat w/bone, roasted	3.5 oz	234.0	26.3	0.0
10093	Pork chow mein, canned/LaChoy	3/4 cup	45.6	5.0	4.0
10137	Pork ham, cured, boneless, extra lean (4% fat) canned, roasted	3.5 oz	136.0	21.2	0.5
10140	Pork ham, cured, boneless, regular fat (11% fat) roasted	3.5 oz	178.0	22.6	0.0

Dietary Fiber (g)	Total Fat (g)	Cholesterol (mg)	Calcium (mg)	Iron (mg)	Magnesium (mg)	Sodium (mg)	Zinc (mg)	Vitamin A (μgRE)	Vitamin C (mg)	Vitamin E (mgαT)	Thiamin (mg)	Riboflavin (mg)	Niacin (mg)	Vitamin B$_6$ (mg)	Folate (μg)
4.3	17.8	0.0	36.3	2.5	23.1	419.1	0.4	3.3	9.7	3.1	0.2	0.2	2.0	0.1	38.0
0.0	11.0	0.0	19.0	1.0	0.0	370.0	0.0	0.4	1.0	0.0	0.0	0.0	0.3	0.0	0.0
0.2	2.9	0.0	2.3	0.1	1.7	77.0	0.0	6.3	0.3	0.6	0.0	0.0	0.1	0.0	6.8
0.0	20.0	18.0	37.0	2.0	0.0	445.0	0.0	0.0	1.0	0.0	0.2	0.2	2.3	0.0	0.0
1.0	6.9	1.0	8.0	0.6	0.0	184.0	0.5	0.0	0.0	0.0	0.1	0.1	0.5	0.0	5.0
4.0	20.9	36.2	19.2	1.2	20.3	479.1	0.6	53.1	1.2	2.1	0.1	0.1	0.3	0.0	30.5
0.0	27.1	106.1	39.0	1.8	31.7	319.6	1.2	108.6	0.2	0.0	0.2	0.2	1.0	0.1	31.7
0.6	12.6	0.0	15.0	0.6	0.0	320.0	0.0	4.0	1.0	0.0	0.0	0.0	0.5	0.0	0.0
0.3	9.8	0.0	19.0	0.7	0.0	207.0	0.0	56.0	1.0	0.0	0.0	0.1	0.3	0.0	0.0
0.5	9.9	0.0	27.0	0.5	0.0	212.0	0.0	42.0	1.0	0.0	0.1	0.1	0.5	0.0	0.0
4.9	17.1	36.0	108.0	1.4	27.0	507.6	0.8	669.6	1.8	3.1	0.1	0.3	0.3	0.1	36.0
0.0	10.6	47.9	107.2	1.4	21.7	256.5	0.5	891.5	1.9	0.0	0.1	0.2	0.9	0.1	23.9
0.8	12.6	0.0	21.0	1.1	0.0	336.0	0.0	2.0	1.0	0.0	0.0	0.0	0.4	0.0	0.0
2.0	12.6	0.0	76.0	0.8	0.0	319.0	0.0	12.0	4.0	0.0	0.0	0.0	0.4	0.0	0.0
1.8	7.3	0.0	15.0	0.7	0.0	180.0	0.0	8.0	23.0	0.0	0.0	0.0	0.4	0.0	0.0
0.6	13.4	57.7	83.7	0.9	12.1	241.8	0.5	79.1	0.5	1.3	0.1	0.2	0.9	0.0	24.2
0.0	9.8	0.0	0.0	0.0	0.0	417.4	0.0	0.0	0.0	0.0	0.0	0.0	0.0	0.0	0.0
2.3	18.9	31.0	102.9	0.0	0.0	865.7	0.0	0.0	0.0	0.0	0.0	0.0	0.0	0.0	0.0
2.8	14.9	24.0	101.5	0.0	0.0	631.7	0.0	0.0	0.0	0.0	0.0	0.0	0.0	0.0	0.0
0.0	5.4	21.0	101.0	1.5	18.0	382.0	1.1	101.0	2.0	0.0	0.2	0.2	2.0	0.1	27.0
2.2	16.6	20.0	204.0	1.0	30.0	770.0	3.0	155.8	0.0	0.0	0.1	0.4	1.1	0.1	14.0
1.0	5.4	0.0	144.0	0.7	0.0	456.0	3.0	82.0	5.0	0.0	0.0	0.1	0.7	0.2	100.0
2.8	24.2	25.7	166.3	0.0	0.0	1239.5	0.0	0.0	0.0	0.0	0.0	0.0	0.0	0.0	0.0
0.0	12.2	0.0	177.0	1.5	0.0	539.0	0.0	65.8	3.0	0.0	0.3	0.2	2.0	0.0	0.0
0.0	80.2	62.6	574.7	11.7	0.0	3351.4	0.0	0.0	0.0	0.0	0.0	0.0	0.0	0.0	0.0
7.0	41.3	66.5	462.0	5.4	0.0	1680.0	0.0	0.0	59.9	0.0	0.0	0.0	0.0	0.0	0.0
0.0	82.6	146.5	1118.9	0.0	0.0	3050.3	0.0	0.0	0.0	0.0	0.0	0.0	0.0	0.0	0.0
3.1	22.1	20.0	267.0	1.9	38.0	903.0	3.0	190.0	0.0	0.0	0.2	0.5	2.7	0.2	57.0
0.0	15.8	0.0	309.0	2.2	0.0	708.0	0.0	33.4	1.0	0.0	0.4	0.2	2.7	0.0	0.0
5.0	45.0	74.3	308.0	6.0	0.0	1720.4	0.0	0.0	0.0	0.0	0.0	0.0	0.0	0.0	0.0
0.0	11.0	0.0	134.0	1.7	0.0	712.0	0.0	53.2	3.0	0.0	0.1	0.2	2.4	0.0	0.0
0.0	20.3	0.0	213.0	3.3	0.0	973.0	0.0	84.2	10.0	0.0	0.4	0.3	3.3	0.0	0.0
0.0	15.7	31.6	202.3	0.0	0.0	551.4	0.0	0.0	0.0	0.0	0.0	0.0	0.0	0.0	0.0
0.0	20.8	41.0	272.1	0.0	0.0	869.4	0.0	0.0	0.0	0.0	0.0	0.0	0.0	0.0	0.0
0.0	13.7	26.4	200.6	0.0	0.0	718.1	0.0	0.0	0.0	0.0	0.0	0.0	0.0	0.0	0.0
2.1	16.4	31.3	178.8	0.0	0.0	790.0	0.0	0.0	0.0	0.0	0.0	0.0	0.0	0.0	0.0
0.0	7.0	14.0	65.0	0.9	8.0	267.0	0.5	54.0	2.0	0.0	0.1	0.2	3.1	0.0	53.0
0.0	22.7	32.2	218.4	2.8	0.0	845.6	0.0	0.0	0.0	0.0	0.0	0.0	0.0	0.0	0.0
2.2	20.0	31.7	0.0	2.5	23.5	830.8	1.7	62.1	1.7	1.6	0.4	0.3	3.4	0.1	51.1
0.0	16.1	40.3	220.8	0.0	0.0	612.4	0.0	0.0	0.0	0.0	0.0	0.0	0.0	0.0	0.0
2.0	14.4	0.0	194.0	1.6	0.0	790.0	4.0	87.8	9.0	0.0	0.2	0.2	2.3	0.0	0.0
0.0	25.0	28.6	152.9	3.5	0.0	888.7	0.0	0.0	0.0	0.0	0.0	0.0	0.0	0.0	0.0
2.3	19.7	30.7	191.3	2.8	26.3	854.1	1.6	62.8	3.2	1.4	0.4	0.3	3.6	0.1	51.1
0.0	17.5	43.8	224.7	0.0	0.0	708.3	0.0	0.0	0.0	0.0	0.0	0.0	0.0	0.0	0.0
4.5	32.3	20.0	362.0	2.4	60.0	1179.0	5.0	240.0	0.0	0.0	0.3	0.9	3.9	0.3	82.0
0.0	10.0	30.0	300.0	3.6	0.0	1040.0	0.0	60.0	6.0	0.0	0.5	0.4	5.0	0.0	0.0
1.0	6.2	0.0	11.0	0.8	0.0	488.0	3.0	76.0	6.0	0.0	0.1	0.1	1.0	0.2	100.0
1.5	10.6	0.0	269.0	2.1	0.0	0.0	0.0	123.6	6.0	0.0	0.4	0.3	2.0	0.0	0.0
1.5	19.5	0.0	267.0	2.0	0.0	1000.0	4.0	200.0	6.0	0.0	0.3	0.7	3.0	0.2	65.0
1.2	16.5	0.0	267.0	1.6	0.0	1000.0	3.0	213.2	2.0	0.0	0.3	0.5	2.1	0.2	90.0
0.0	20.0	27.9	212.4	2.9	0.0	771.9	0.0	0.0	0.0	0.0	0.0	0.0	0.0	0.0	0.0
0.0	18.1	23.1	223.0	2.3	0.0	738.5	0.0	0.0	0.0	0.0	0.0	0.0	0.0	0.0	0.0
0.0	23.3	27.7	187.9	2.5	0.0	756.1	0.0	0.0	0.0	0.0	0.0	0.0	0.0	0.0	0.0
0.0	13.4	0.0	210.0	2.6	0.0	909.0	0.0	104.6	13.0	0.0	0.3	0.3	2.9	0.0	0.0
0.0	1.5	0.6	9.2	0.6	4.6	143.2	0.2	16.5	0.0	0.0	0.1	0.1	0.4	0.0	5.6
0.4	3.0	0.9	37.6	0.8	7.2	82.0	0.3	34.0	0.2	0.4	0.1	0.1	0.7	0.0	7.2
0.0	29.6	118.0	45.0	1.4	21.0	101.0	3.4	3.0	0.3	0.0	0.4	0.2	3.6	0.3	3.0
0.0	8.4	58.0	10.0	0.8	21.0	1546.0	1.7	0.0	0.0	0.3	0.8	0.2	6.9	0.5	4.0
0.0	49.2	85.0	12.0	1.6	24.0	1596.0	3.3	0.0	0.0	0.5	0.7	0.3	7.3	0.4	5.0
0.0	13.1	82.0	33.0	0.8	25.0	58.0	2.3	3.0	0.4	0.0	1.1	0.3	5.2	0.4	6.0
0.0	9.0	79.0	25.0	1.0	22.0	66.0	2.1	2.0	1.0	0.0	0.9	0.3	5.5	0.4	4.0
0.0	13.5	80.0	27.0	1.0	20.0	63.0	2.0	2.0	0.9	0.0	0.9	0.3	5.2	0.4	4.0
2.0	1.0	50.0	80.0	0.7	0.0	820.0	0.0	150.0	10.0	0.0	0.0	0.0	0.4	0.0	0.0
0.0	4.9	30.0	6.0	0.9	21.0	1135.0	2.2	0.0	0.0	0.3	1.0	0.2	4.9	0.5	5.0
0.0	9.0	59.0	8.0	1.3	22.0	1500.0	2.5	0.0	0.0	0.3	0.7	0.3	6.2	0.3	3.0

Code	Food Name	Unit Amount	Kilocalories (kcal)	Protein (g)	Carbohydrate (g)
10151	Pork ham, smoked	3.5 oz	122.0	18.9	0.0
10032	Pork loin, blade/chops, fresh, lean & fat w/bone, broiled	3.5 oz	320.0	22.5	0.0
10048	Pork loin, blade/roasts, fresh, lean & fat w/bone, roasted	3.5 oz	323.0	23.7	0.0
10045	Pork loin, center rib chop, fresh, lean w/bone, broiled	3.5 oz	219.0	30.8	0.0
10200	Pork loin, center rib chop, fresh, lean & fat, boneless, pan-fried	4.0 oz	266.6	32.9	0.0
10203	Pork loin, center rib roast, fresh, lean & fat, boneless, roasted	3.5 oz	252.0	27.0	0.0
10215	Pork sirloin chop, fresh, lean & fat, boneless, broiled	3.5 oz	208.0	30.5	0.0
10213	Pork sirloin chop, fresh, lean, boneless, broiled	3.5 oz	193.0	31.1	0.0
10056	Pork sirloin roast, fresh, lean & fat, boneless, roasted	3.5 oz	207.0	28.5	0.0
10053	Pork sirloin, chop, fresh, lean w/bone, broiled	3.5 oz	213.0	28.5	0.0
10059	Pork sirloin, fresh, lean, boneless, roasted	3.5 oz	198.0	28.9	0.0
10218	Pork tenderloin, fresh, lean & fat, broiled	3.5 oz	201.0	29.9	0.0
10223	Pork tenderloin, fresh, lean & fat, roasted	3.5 oz	173.0	27.8	0.0
51612	Pork, bacon bits	1/4 oz	21.0	2.6	0.2
10219	Pork, ground, fresh, ckd	3.5 oz	297.0	25.7	0.0
10088	Pork, spareribs, fresh, lean & fat, braised	3.5 oz	397.0	29.1	0.0
924165	Pork, sweet & sour, canned/LaChoy	3/4 cup	249.6	6.0	48.0
19318	Pudding Pop, chocolate/vanilla swirl	1 pop	78.0	1.9	13.0
919167	Pudding, banana, RTE	1.0 oz	36.0	0.7	6.0
901924	Pudding, bread pudding, homemade	1/2 cup	211.7	6.6	31.0
901927	Pudding, chocolate, RTE	4.0 oz (1 snack-sized can)	150.3	3.1	25.8
19191	Pudding, chocolate, sugar-free	1/2 cup	91.8	4.5	13.0
901928	Pudding, flan (caramel custard) dry mix prep w/whole milk	1 cup	300.6	8.0	50.8
19330	Pudding, Indian	2/3 cup	161.2	5.4	22.6
919182	Pudding, lemon, RTE	1 oz	35.4	0.0	7.1
901929	Pudding, mousse, chocolate, homemade	1/2 cup	446.4	8.7	33.1
19194	Pudding, pistachio	1/2 cup	170.5	4.2	28.2
19198	Pudding, rice, RTE	1.0 oz	46.2	0.6	6.2
919210	Pudding, tapioca, RTE	1 can (5 oz)	169.0	2.8	27.5
901930	Pudding, vanilla, RTE	1 cup (8 oz)	293.8	5.2	49.5
14342	Pudding, vanilla, sugar-free	1/2 cup	82.5	4.2	11.0
924152	Rice beverage, Rice Dream, canned/Imagine Foods	1 cup	120.1	0.4	24.8
924042	Rice, chicken fried rice/Chun King	8 oz	261.1	14.0	41.0
924197	Rice, pork fried rice/Chun King	8 oz	270.1	10.0	44.0
918814	Rice, Spanish	1 cup	213.2	4.4	40.7
918815	Roll, brown & serve	1 roll	80.1	2.0	13.0
18344	Roll, buttermilk	1 roll	80.1	2.0	13.0
918343	Roll, dinner, egg	1 roll (2.5" diam)	107.5	3.3	18.2
18396	Roll, dinner, oat bran	1 roll	77.9	3.1	13.3
18347	Roll, dinner, rye	1 large (3.5"–4" diam)	123.0	4.4	22.8
18342	Roll, dinner, wheat	1 roll (3 oz)	232.1	7.3	39.1
18351	Roll, French	1 roll	105.3	3.3	19.1
18350	Roll, hamburger/hot dog, mixed grain	1 roll	113.1	4.1	19.2
18352	Roll, hamburger/hot dog, plain	1 roll	123.0	3.7	21.6
18353	Roll, hamburger/hot dog, whole-wheat	1 frankfurter roll	114.4	3.7	22.0
918817	Roll, hard/kaiser	1 roll (3.5" diam)	167.0	5.6	30.0
4023	Salad dressing, 1000 island, regular, w/salt	2.0 Tbsp.	113.2	0.3	4.6
902921	Salad dressing, 1000 island, w/salt, low kcal (10 kcal/tsp.)	2.0 Tbsp.	47.6	0.2	4.9
4539	Salad dressing, blue cheese, low kcal	2.0 Tbsp.	80.1	0.6	3.0
4140	Salad dressing, blue/roquefort cheese, regular w/salt	2.0 Tbsp.	151.2	1.4	2.2
4120	Salad dressing, French, low-fat, w/salt, diet (5 kcal/tsp.)	2.0 Tbsp.	40.3	0.1	6.5
4141	Salad dressing, French, regular w/salt	2.0 Tbsp.	128.9	0.2	5.3
4114	Salad dressing, Italian, no salt, diet (2 kcal/tsp.)	2.0 Tbsp.	31.6	0.0	1.5
4143	Salad dressing, Italian, regular w/salt	2.0 Tbsp.	140.2	0.2	3.1
4145	Salad dressing, mayonnaise, safflower & soybean oil, w/salt	2.0 Tbsp.	215.0	0.3	0.8
18625	Salad dressing, mayonnaise-type, regular, w/salt	2.0 Tbsp.	116.9	0.3	7.2
4022	Salad dressing, Russian w/salt	2.0 Tbsp.	148.2	0.5	3.1
4030	Salad dressing, Russian, w/salt, low kcal	2.0 Tbsp.	42.4	0.2	8.3
4016	Salad dressing, sandwich spread w/chopped pickle, regular	2.0 Tbsp.	116.7	0.3	6.7
902932	Salad dressing, sesame seed	2.0 Tbsp.	132.9	0.9	2.6
902933	Salad dressing, sweet & sour	2.0 Tbsp.	57.9	0.4	13.8
4135	Salad dressing, vinaigrette	2.0 Tbsp.	99.9	0.0	8.0
902910	Salad dressing, vinegar & oil, homemade	2.0 Tbsp.	134.6	0.0	0.8
902909	Salt substitute, lite/Morton	1 tsp.	0.0	0.0	0.0
22539	Salt substitute/Morton	1 tsp.	0.0	0.0	0.1

Dietary Fiber (g)	Total Fat (g)	Cholesterol (mg)	Calcium (mg)	Iron (mg)	Magnesium (mg)	Sodium (mg)	Zinc (mg)	Vitamin A (μgRE)	Vitamin C (mg)	Vitamin E (mgαT)	Thiamin (mg)	Riboflavin (mg)	Niacin (mg)	Vitamin B_6 (mg)	Folate (μg)
0.0	4.7	38.8	6.1	1.0	17.3	1280.6	2.0	0.0	27.6	0.0	0.9	0.2	5.4	0.5	6.1
0.0	24.9	86.0	29.0	0.9	22.0	70.0	3.4	2.0	0.7	0.0	0.7	0.3	4.1	0.4	4.0
0.0	24.6	93.0	34.0	1.1	20.0	30.0	3.3	3.0	0.2	0.0	0.5	0.3	4.2	0.4	4.0
0.0	9.7	81.0	31.0	0.8	28.0	65.0	2.4	2.0	0.3	0.3	1.1	0.3	6.2	0.5	3.0
0.0	14.0	83.3	6.0	0.9	32.1	61.9	2.5	2.4	0.4	0.3	0.9	0.4	6.1	0.5	9.5
0.0	15.2	81.0	6.0	0.9	22.0	48.0	2.6	3.0	0.4	0.0	0.6	0.3	5.0	0.4	8.0
0.0	8.6	91.0	18.0	1.2	27.0	56.0	2.6	2.0	0.4	0.3	1.0	0.4	4.7	0.5	6.0
0.0	6.7	92.0	18.0	1.2	27.0	56.0	2.7	2.0	0.4	0.3	1.0	0.4	4.8	0.5	6.0
0.0	9.4	86.0	16.0	1.2	26.0	56.0	2.5	2.0	1.0	0.3	0.9	0.4	5.1	0.5	5.0
0.0	10.1	85.0	13.0	1.1	31.0	72.0	2.7	2.0	1.0	0.3	1.0	0.4	4.8	0.6	5.0
0.0	8.3	86.0	17.0	1.2	27.0	56.0	2.5	2.0	1.0	0.3	0.9	0.4	5.1	0.5	5.0
0.0	8.1	94.0	5.0	1.4	35.0	64.0	2.9	2.0	1.0	0.0	1.0	0.4	5.1	0.5	6.0
0.0	6.1	79.0	6.0	1.5	27.0	55.0	2.6	2.0	0.4	0.3	0.9	0.4	4.7	0.4	6.0
0.0	1.1	6.0	1.0	0.1	2.0	181.0	0.3	0.0	1.0	0.0	0.0	0.0	0.7	0.0	1.0
0.0	20.8	94.0	22.0	1.3	24.0	73.0	3.2	2.0	0.7	0.3	0.7	0.2	4.2	0.4	6.0
0.0	30.3	121.0	47.0	1.9	24.0	93.0	4.6	3.0	0.3	0.4	0.4	0.4	5.5	0.4	4.0
3.0	4.0	18.0	20.0	1.4	0.0	1540.0	0.0	125.0	4.0	0.0	0.1	0.1	1.2	0.0	0.0
0.0	1.9	1.0	71.0	0.2	7.0	66.0	0.1	13.4	0.0	0.0	0.0	0.1	0.1	0.0	2.0
0.0	1.0	0.0	24.1	0.0	2.3	55.6	0.1	8.5	0.1	0.0	0.0	0.0	0.0	0.0	0.6
1.3	7.4	2.7	143.6	1.4	23.9	291.1	0.7	81.9	1.0	0.0	0.1	0.3	0.8	0.1	16.4
1.1	4.5	3.4	101.7	0.6	23.7	145.8	0.5	12.4	2.0	0.1	0.0	0.2	0.4	0.0	3.4
0.0	2.7	9.0	152.0	0.3	25.0	381.0	0.6	50.2	1.0	0.0	0.1	0.2	0.1	0.1	6.0
0.3	8.2	31.9	300.6	0.2	31.9	130.3	0.9	69.2	1.9	0.0	0.1	0.4	0.2	0.1	10.6
0.0	5.6	0.0	221.0	1.4	0.0	0.0	0.0	79.0	0.0	0.0	0.1	0.3	0.4	0.0	0.0
0.0	0.9	0.0	0.6	0.0	0.3	39.7	0.0	0.0	0.0	0.0	0.0	0.0	0.0	0.0	0.0
1.2	32.9	10.3	202.0	1.3	44.4	86.9	1.4	323.2	1.2	0.0	0.1	0.4	0.3	0.1	32.3
0.0	4.8	17.0	149.0	0.1	19.0	408.0	0.5	30.8	1.0	0.0	0.0	0.2	0.1	0.0	7.0
0.0	2.1	0.3	14.7	0.1	2.3	24.1	0.1	9.9	0.1	0.4	0.0	0.0	0.0	0.0	0.9
0.1	5.3	1.4	119.3	0.3	11.4	225.8	0.4	0.0	1.0	0.1	0.0	0.1	0.4	0.0	4.3
0.2	8.1	15.8	198.9	0.3	18.1	305.1	0.6	13.6	0.0	0.3	0.0	0.3	0.6	0.0	0.0
0.0	2.4	9.0	152.0	0.1	18.0	199.0	0.5	50.0	1.0	0.0	0.0	0.2	0.1	0.0	6.0
0.0	2.0	0.0	19.6	0.2	9.8	85.8	0.2	0.0	1.2	1.8	0.1	0.0	1.9	0.0	90.7
0.0	4.0	0.0	38.0	2.0	0.0	1460.0	0.0	136.0	7.0	0.0	0.7	0.2	1.5	0.0	0.0
0.0	6.0	0.0	26.0	1.0	0.0	1210.0	0.0	170.0	4.0	0.0	0.3	0.2	1.5	0.0	0.0
1.6	4.2	0.0	34.0	1.5	0.0	774.0	0.0	324.0	37.0	0.0	0.1	0.1	1.7	0.0	0.0
0.5	2.0	5.0	14.0	0.6	0.0	140.0	0.0	0.0	1.0	0.0	0.1	0.1	0.6	0.0	0.0
0.5	2.0	5.0	0.0	0.0	0.0	140.0	0.0	0.0	0.0	0.0	0.0	0.0	0.0	0.0	0.0
1.3	2.2	17.5	20.7	1.2	8.8	190.8	0.4	2.8	0.0	0.3	0.2	0.2	1.2	0.0	36.8
1.4	1.5	0.0	28.1	1.4	10.9	136.3	0.3	0.0	0.0	0.2	0.1	0.1	1.6	0.0	31.4
2.1	1.5	0.0	12.9	1.2	23.2	383.6	0.4	0.4	0.0	0.2	0.2	0.1	1.7	0.0	37.0
3.2	5.4	0.0	149.6	3.0	30.6	289.0	0.8	0.0	0.0	0.8	0.4	0.2	3.5	0.1	43.4
1.2	1.6	0.0	34.6	1.0	7.6	231.4	0.3	0.0	0.0	0.2	0.2	0.1	1.7	0.0	36.1
1.6	2.6	0.0	40.9	1.7	18.9	196.9	0.5	0.0	0.0	0.2	0.2	0.1	1.9	0.0	40.9
1.2	2.2	0.0	59.8	1.4	8.6	240.8	0.3	0.0	0.0	0.7	0.2	0.1	1.7	0.0	40.9
3.2	2.0	0.0	45.6	1.0	36.6	205.5	0.9	0.0	0.0	0.6	0.1	0.1	1.6	0.1	13.3
1.3	2.5	0.0	54.2	1.9	15.4	310.1	0.5	0.0	0.0	0.2	0.3	0.2	2.4	0.0	54.2
0.0	10.7	7.8	3.3	0.2	0.6	210.0	0.0	28.8	0.0	0.3	0.0	0.0	0.0	0.0	1.9
0.4	3.2	4.5	3.3	0.2	0.2	300.0	0.0	28.8	0.0	0.4	0.0	0.0	0.0	0.0	1.7
0.0	7.4	2.0	0.0	0.0	0.0	394.0	0.0	0.0	0.0	0.0	0.0	0.0	0.0	0.0	0.0
0.0	15.7	5.1	24.3	0.1	0.0	328.2	0.1	19.8	0.6	2.8	0.0	0.0	0.0	0.0	2.4
0.0	1.7	0.0	3.3	0.1	0.0	236.1	0.1	39.0	0.0	0.4	0.0	0.0	0.0	0.0	0.0
0.0	12.3	0.0	3.3	0.1	0.0	411.0	0.0	39.0	0.0	2.5	0.0	0.0	0.0	0.0	1.3
0.0	2.9	1.8	0.6	0.1	0.0	9.0	0.0	0.0	0.0	0.0	0.0	0.0	0.0	0.0	0.0
0.0	14.5	0.0	3.0	0.1	0.2	236.1	0.0	7.2	0.0	3.1	0.0	0.0	0.0	0.0	1.5
0.0	23.8	17.7	5.4	0.2	0.3	170.5	0.0	25.2	0.0	0.0	0.0	0.0	0.0	0.2	2.3
0.0	10.0	7.8	4.2	0.1	0.6	213.2	0.1	25.2	0.0	1.2	0.0	0.0	0.0	0.0	1.9
0.0	15.2	5.4	5.7	0.2	0.5	260.4	0.1	62.1	1.8	3.1	0.0	0.0	0.2	0.0	3.1
0.1	1.2	1.8	5.7	0.2	0.1	260.4	0.0	4.8	1.8	0.2	0.0	0.0	0.0	0.0	1.0
0.1	10.2	22.8	4.2	0.1	0.6	300.0	0.2	25.2	0.0	2.1	0.0	0.0	0.0	0.0	1.8
0.3	13.6	0.0	5.7	0.2	0.0	300.0	0.0	62.1	0.0	0.0	0.0	0.0	0.0	0.0	0.0
0.2	0.6	0.0	2.0	0.0	0.0	136.0	0.0	0.0	0.0	0.0	0.0	0.0	0.0	0.0	0.0
0.0	7.6	0.0	0.0	0.0	0.0	432.0	0.0	0.0	0.0	0.0	0.0	0.0	0.0	0.0	0.0
0.0	15.0	0.0	0.0	0.0	0.0	0.2	0.0	0.0	0.0	2.6	0.0	0.0	0.0	0.0	0.0
0.0	0.0	0.0	0.0	0.0	4.0	1100.0	0.0	0.0	0.0	0.0	0.0	0.0	0.0	0.0	0.0
0.0	0.0	0.0	30.0	0.0	0.0	0.0	0.0	0.0	0.0	0.0	0.0	0.0	0.0	0.0	0.0

Code	Food Name	Unit Amount	Kilocalories (kcal)	Protein (g)	Carbohydrate (g)
22535	Sandwich, hot pockets, beef & cheddar stuffed, frozen	1 package	403.3	16.3	39.2
22537	Sandwich, hot pockets, croissant pocket w/chicken, broccoli, & cheddar, frozen	1 package	601.6	22.8	77.8
22002	Sandwich, lean pockets, glazed chicken supreme stuffed, frozen	1 package	464.1	19.6	68.1
22540	Sandwich, pizza burger	1 burger	243.8	18.2	2.3
6931	Sandwich, sausage biscuits, breakfast sandwich, frozen/Jimmy Dean	1 package	384.6	9.5	23.1
6932	Sauce, pasta, spaghetti/marinara, RTE	1/2 cup	71.3	1.8	10.3
906961	Sauce, 100% natural spaghetti sauce, traditional, jar/Prego	1/2 cup	130.9	2.1	20.0
6721	Sauce, alfredo	1 Tbsp.	42.6	1.6	0.4
6921	Sauce, barbecue, RTE	1 Tbsp.	13.5	0.3	2.3
6140	Sauce, bearnaise, dry, made w/milk & butter	1 cup (8 fl oz)	687.5	8.2	17.2
906978	Sauce, cheddar cheese sauce/LaVictoria	1 Tbsp.	26.2	0.3	1.5
6713	Sauce, cheese	2.0 oz	59.9	2.3	3.5
6139	Sauce, chili	1 Tbsp.	17.0	0.2	3.8
6923	Sauce, chunky chili dip, salsa, canned/LaVictoria	1 Tbsp.	4.7	0.1	1.0
6135	Sauce, con queso sauce, RTE/Nestle Que Bueno	1 cup	335.2	15.4	14.3
6903	Sauce, Coney Island style hot dog sauce, RTE/Nestle Chef-Mate	1/4 cup	75.6	2.2	5.6
6104	Sauce, creole sauce, RTE/Nestle Chef-Mate	1/4 cup	24.8	0.9	3.7
6901	Sauce, curry, dry, made w/milk	1/4 cup	67.3	2.7	6.4
6152	Sauce, deluxe marinara sauce, RTE/Contadina	1/4 cup	37.1	0.8	4.4
6153	Sauce, deluxe pizza sauce, RTE/Contadina	1/4 cup	34.0	1.4	5.5
6179	Sauce, enchilada sauce/LaVictoria	1 Tbsp.	5.0	0.0	0.7
6273	Sauce, green chile salsa, mild/LaVictoria	1 Tbsp.	3.8	0.2	0.7
6259	Sauce, green taco sauce, medium/LaVictoria	1 Tbsp.	4.5	0.1	0.9
906965	Sauce, hoisin, RTE	1 Tbsp.	35.2	0.5	7.1
6155	Sauce, Hollandaise	1/4 cup	264.0	3.1	6.7
6181	Sauce, hot dog chili sauce, RTE/Nestle Chef-Mate	2.25 oz, 1/4 cup	69.3	2.7	9.2
6922	Sauce, Italian sauce, RTE/Nestle Chef-Mate	2.25 oz, 1/4 cup	61.7	1.1	11.6
6905	Sauce, jalapeno cheese sauce, RTE/Nestle Que Bueno	1 package	3876.5	95.9	369.6
906970	Sauce, lemon sauce, RTE/Nestle Chef-Mate	1 package	2848.8	4.7	678.6
906960	Sauce, marinara/Contadina	7.5 oz	100.1	4.0	12.0
906966	Sauce, medium white	1 cup	395.0	10.0	24.0
6136	Sauce, mole poblano, dry mix	1 Tbsp.	94.2	1.2	6.9
6714	Sauce, mushroom, dry, made w/milk	1 cup (8 fl oz)	227.0	11.3	23.8
6910	Sauce, nacho cheese sauce, mild, RTE/Nestle Que Bueno	1 cup	476.3	18.1	10.1
6168	Sauce, oyster, RTE	1 Tbsp.	2.0	0.1	0.4
6169	Sauce, pepper or hot, RTE	1/4 tsp.	0.1	0.0	0.0
924173	Sauce, pepperoni pizza/Contadina	1/4 cup	40.2	1.0	5.0
6157	Sauce, pesto	1.0 oz	155.1	2.8	3.0
906968	Sauce, picante sauce, RTE/Que Bueno Nestle	1 serving	10.2	0.4	2.0
6151	Sauce, pizza/Contadina	1/4 cup	30.0	1.0	5.0
6153	Sauce, plum, RTE	1 Tbsp.	35.0	0.2	8.1
6274	Sauce, red clam (shellfish)	4.0 oz	80.6	3.6	9.3
6907	Sauce, salsa, RTE	1 packet	2.5	0.1	0.6
906969	Sauce, sofrito, homemade	1 Tbsp.	35.3	1.9	0.8
6148	Sauce, sour cream	1/4 cup	123.8	2.8	1.9
906134	Sauce, sour cream, dry, made w/milk	1 cup (8 fl oz)	508.7	19.1	45.3
924192	Sauce, soy sauce, RTE	1 Tbsp.	9.5	0.9	1.5
924195	Sauce, spaghetti sauce w/meat	4.0 oz	70.1	2.0	12.0
6904	Sauce, spaghetti sauce w/mushrooms	4.0 oz	107.4	1.6	14.5
924162	Sauce, spaghetti w/mushrooms, dry	2 tsp.	30.4	1.0	4.9
6107	Sauce, spaghetti & meat/FrancoAm	7.5 oz	212.0	8.5	26.2
906972	Sauce, steak	1 Tbsp.	18.0	0.0	2.5
6109	Sauce, steak & mushrooms	1 fl oz	9.0	0.3	1.9
6716	Sauce, stroganoff, dry, made w/H$_2$O	1 cup (8 fl oz)	272.3	11.7	33.9
6110	Sauce, sweet & sour	1/4 cup	54.9	0.2	13.6
906975	Sauce, Szechuan, RTE/Nestle Chef-Mate	1 Tbsp.	20.8	0.2	2.9
906974	Sauce, tabasco	1 tsp.	0.8	0.1	0.1
6111	Sauce, tartar	1 Tbsp.	70.0	0.0	0.1
6129	Sauce, teriyaki, RTE	1 Tbsp.	15.1	1.1	2.9
906977	Sauce, thick white	1/4 cup	130.7	2.6	7.3
924111	Sauce, thin white	1/4 cup	73.8	2.4	4.6
6113	Sauce, white clam (shellfish)	4.0 oz	121.0	4.5	4.2
7006	Sausage, blood	1 slice: 5" x 4.6" x 0.06"	94.5	3.7	0.3
7014	Sausage, bratwurst (pork) ckd	1 link (4/12 oz)	255.9	12.0	1.8
7022	Sausage, frankfurter (weiner) (beef & pork)	1 frank: 0.85" diam x 5" long—8/lb	182.4	6.4	1.5

Dietary Fiber (g)	Total Fat (g)	Cholesterol (mg)	Calcium (mg)	Iron (mg)	Magnesium (mg)	Sodium (mg)	Zinc (mg)	Vitamin A (μgRE)	Vitamin C (mg)	Vitamin E (mgαT)	Thiamin (mg)	Riboflavin (mg)	Niacin (mg)	Vitamin B$_6$ (mg)	Folate (μg)
0.0	20.2	52.5	336.5	2.9	0.0	906.0	0.0	0.0	0.0	0.0	0.0	0.0	0.0	0.0	0.0
2.8	22.0	74.2	0.0	7.6	0.0	1303.0	0.0	0.0	12.5	0.0	0.0	0.0	0.0	0.0	0.0
0.0	12.5	45.9	242.3	0.0	0.0	1119.5	0.0	0.0	0.0	0.0	0.0	0.0	0.0	0.0	0.0
0.5	18.0	62.0	109.0	2.3	16.0	615.0	3.3	72.6	4.0	0.0	0.1	0.2	6.5	0.0	0.0
1.4	28.2	31.4	75.5	1.6	0.0	881.3	0.0	0.0	0.0	0.0	0.0	0.0	0.0	0.0	0.0
2.0	2.6	0.0	27.5	0.9	21.3	515.0	0.2	47.5	10.0	1.6	0.1	0.1	1.3	0.1	12.5
3.9	4.9	0.0	0.0	0.0	0.0	537.5	0.0	0.0	13.0	0.0	0.0	0.0	0.0	0.0	0.0
0.0	3.8	0.0	28.9	0.2	0.0	104.4	0.0	4.2	0.1	0.0	0.0	0.0	0.0	0.0	0.0
0.2	0.3	0.0	3.4	0.2	3.2	146.7	0.0	15.7	1.3	0.2	0.0	0.0	0.2	0.0	0.7
0.0	67.0	185.0	225.0	0.3	25.0	1240.0	0.8	742.5	1.8	0.0	0.1	0.3	0.3	0.1	10.0
0.0	2.1	0.5	15.0	0.1	0.0	158.2	0.0	0.0	0.0	0.0	0.0	0.0	0.0	0.0	0.0
0.0	4.1	0.0	63.0	0.2	0.0	288.0	3.5	32.2	0.0	0.0	0.0	0.0	0.1	0.0	0.0
0.0	0.0	0.0	3.0	0.1	0.0	191.0	0.0	42.0	2.0	0.0	0.0	0.0	0.2	0.0	9.0
0.1	0.0	0.0	2.1	0.0	0.0	74.0	0.0	0.0	1.6	0.0	0.0	0.0	0.0	0.0	0.0
0.0	24.1	63.0	471.2	0.0	15.1	2220.1	1.3	148.7	0.0	1.3	0.0	0.2	0.2	0.0	7.6
1.4	4.9	1.9	19.8	1.1	11.8	383.2	0.3	63.2	0.1	1.1	0.0	0.0	0.8	0.1	8.1
0.8	0.7	0.0	34.7	0.3	8.7	339.1	0.1	23.6	0.6	0.0	0.0	0.0	0.5	0.1	8.7
0.0	3.7	8.8	121.0	0.3	11.6	318.9	0.3	10.2	0.7	0.0	0.0	0.1	0.1	0.0	4.1
0.8	1.8	0.0	12.2	0.4	7.7	240.0	0.1	22.4	4.5	0.0	0.0	0.0	0.4	0.1	5.8
1.3	0.7	1.9	34.0	0.6	13.2	116.6	0.2	42.2	7.1	1.6	0.0	0.0	0.9	0.1	6.3
0.1	0.2	0.0	1.8	0.0	0.0	99.2	0.0	0.0	0.7	0.0	0.0	0.0	0.0	0.0	0.0
0.1	0.0	0.0	2.3	0.1	0.0	87.4	0.0	0.0	2.0	0.0	0.0	0.0	0.0	0.0	0.0
0.1	0.1	0.0	1.2	0.0	0.0	95.7	0.0	0.0	0.7	0.0	0.0	0.0	0.0	0.0	0.0
0.4	0.5	0.5	5.1	0.2	3.8	258.4	0.1	0.2	0.1	0.0	0.0	0.0	0.2	0.0	3.7
0.0	25.6	71.0	23.0	0.9	0.0	425.0	0.0	205.4	0.0	0.0	0.0	0.0	0.0	0.0	0.0
1.7	2.4	4.4	19.5	1.0	12.6	398.8	0.5	42.2	0.1	0.3	0.0	0.0	0.7	0.1	22.1
0.9	1.2	0.0	34.7	0.4	20.2	308.7	0.3	24.6	4.2	1.2	0.1	0.0	1.1	0.2	16.4
0.0	224.2	300.5	2554.3	5.7	180.3	27255.4	16.2	811.4	24.0	15.7	0.1	2.0	2.0	0.4	90.2
0.0	12.5	0.0	85.0	8.1	42.5	170.1	0.9	0.0	182.8	0.9	0.1	0.1	0.7	0.2	21.3
0.0	4.0	0.0	73.0	2.6	0.0	700.0	0.0	413.2	20.0	0.0	0.2	0.4	2.2	0.0	0.0
0.5	30.0	32.0	292.0	0.9	0.0	888.0	0.5	238.0	2.0	0.0	0.2	0.4	0.8	0.1	12.0
1.7	6.9	0.0	49.8	0.9	21.0	192.1	0.4	0.0	0.0	0.0	0.0	0.1	0.4	0.1	12.2
0.0	10.3	34.7	293.7	0.5	37.4	1535.3	1.3	93.5	1.9	0.0	0.2	0.8	4.8	0.2	40.1
2.0	40.5	80.6	471.2	0.8	25.2	1968.1	2.6	126.0	0.3	1.0	0.0	0.3	0.1	0.0	12.6
0.0	0.0	0.0	1.3	0.0	0.2	109.3	0.0	0.3	0.0	0.0	0.0	0.0	0.1	0.0	0.6
0.0	0.0	0.0	0.1	0.0	0.1	31.7	0.0	0.4	0.9	0.0	0.0	0.0	0.0	0.0	0.1
0.0	2.2	0.0	13.0	0.7	8.0	390.0	0.0	131.8	13.0	0.0	0.0	0.0	0.1	0.0	0.0
0.7	14.6	0.0	98.0	0.3	0.0	244.0	0.0	98.8	0.0	0.0	0.0	0.1	0.2	0.0	0.0
0.0	0.1	0.0	12.6	0.2	4.5	252.0	0.1	8.4	0.6	0.4	0.0	0.0	0.3	0.0	3.0
0.0	1.0	0.0	13.0	0.7	8.0	330.0	0.0	133.8	14.0	0.0	0.0	0.0	0.6	0.0	0.0
0.1	0.2	0.0	2.3	0.3	2.3	102.2	0.0	0.8	0.1	0.0	0.0	0.0	0.2	0.0	1.1
1.0	3.2	0.0	32.0	1.2	0.0	556.0	0.0	128.2	9.0	0.0	0.1	0.1	0.9	0.0	0.0
0.1	0.0	0.0	2.7	0.1	1.2	38.6	0.0	5.3	1.2	0.1	0.0	0.0	0.1	0.0	1.4
0.3	2.7	0.0	3.0	0.1	3.7	170.6	0.2	0.0	3.0	0.0	0.0	0.0	0.4	0.1	6.4
0.0	11.9	1966.0	23.0	0.3	3.0	7.0	0.5	82.0	0.0	0.0	0.0	0.1	0.0	0.0	23.0
3.5	30.2	91.1	546.4	0.6	44.0	1004.8	1.4	144.4	2.5	0.0	0.1	0.7	0.6	0.1	15.7
0.0	0.0	0.0	3.1	0.4	6.1	1028.7	0.1	0.0	0.0	0.0	0.0	0.0	0.6	0.0	2.8
2.0	2.0	2.0	18.0	1.8	0.0	570.0	0.0	156.0	18.0	0.0	0.1	0.1	1.8	0.0	0.0
0.6	4.7	0.0	21.0	1.1	0.0	499.0	0.0	129.8	12.0	0.0	0.1	0.1	1.3	0.0	0.0
0.0	0.9	2.8	39.9	0.2	3.6	942.0	0.2	4.9	0.2	0.0	0.0	0.0	0.2	0.0	2.8
1.0	8.1	0.0	28.0	2.2	0.0	1101.0	0.0	185.6	5.0	0.0	0.2	0.2	3.5	0.0	0.0
0.1	0.0	0.0	6.0	0.4	0.0	149.0	0.0	10.2	11.0	0.0	0.0	0.1	0.0	0.0	0.0
0.2	0.1	0.0	2.0	0.2	0.0	157.0	0.0	0.8	2.0	0.0	0.0	0.0	0.1	0.0	0.0
0.0	10.7	38.5	521.0	1.3	38.5	1829.3	1.1	127.3	1.5	0.0	0.9	0.8	0.8	0.1	8.9
0.0	0.0	0.0	8.0	0.3	0.0	146.0	0.0	0.0	0.0	0.0	0.0	0.0	0.0	0.0	0.0
0.0	0.9	0.0	1.8	0.1	1.6	218.1	0.0	9.9	0.3	0.1	0.0	0.0	0.1	0.0	0.6
0.0	0.0	0.0	0.0	0.0	0.0	22.0	0.0	0.0	0.0	0.0	0.0	0.0	0.0	0.0	0.0
0.1	8.1	5.0	2.0	0.0	0.0	190.0	0.0	30.0	0.0	0.0	0.0	0.0	0.0	0.0	0.0
0.0	0.0	0.0	4.5	0.3	11.0	689.9	0.0	0.0	0.0	0.0	0.0	0.0	0.2	0.0	3.6
0.3	10.3	24.0	71.0	0.2	0.0	263.0	0.0	75.2	0.0	0.0	0.0	0.1	0.2	0.0	0.0
0.1	5.2	18.0	73.0	0.1	0.0	214.0	0.3	42.6	0.0	0.0	0.0	0.1	0.1	0.0	0.0
0.5	9.6	0.0	28.0	1.3	0.0	639.0	0.0	22.4	2.0	0.0	0.0	0.0	0.4	0.0	0.0
0.0	8.6	30.0	1.5	1.6	2.0	170.0	0.3	0.0	0.0	0.1	0.0	0.0	0.3	0.0	1.3
0.0	22.0	51.0	37.4	1.1	12.8	473.5	2.0	0.0	0.9	0.2	0.4	0.2	2.7	0.2	1.7
0.0	16.6	28.5	6.3	0.7	5.7	638.4	1.0	0.0	0.0	0.1	0.1	0.1	1.5	0.1	2.3

Code	Food Name	Unit Amount	Kilocalories (kcal)	Protein (g)	Carbohydrate (g)
7024	Sausage, frankfurter (weiner) (beef)	1 frank: 0.75" diam x 5" long—10/lb	141.8	5.4	0.8
7025	Sausage, frankfurter (weiner) (chicken)	1 frank	115.7	5.8	3.1
7016	Sausage, frankfurter (weiner) (turkey)	1 frank	101.7	6.4	0.7
7089	Sausage, Italian (pork & beef)	1 slice: 4" diam x 0.12" thick	59.8	3.5	0.4
7038	Sausage, kielbasa (kolbassy) (pork, beef, & NFD milk)	1 slice: 6" x 3.75" x 0.06"	80.6	3.4	0.6
7091	Sausage, mortadella (beef & pork)	1 slice (1⅝ oz)	46.7	2.5	0.5
7059	Sausage, pepperoni (pork & beef)	1 sausage @ 9.0 oz	1247.5	52.6	7.1
7064	Sausage, pork, bulk/links/patties, frozen, raw/USDA Commodity	3.5 oz	231.0	15.0	0.0
7068	Sausage, salami (cotto) (beef & pork) ckd	1 slice: 4" diam x 0.12" thick (10/8 oz)	57.5	3.2	0.5
7072	Sausage, salami, (turkey) ckd	2 slices	111.7	9.3	0.3
7074	Sausage, smoked link (pork & beef)	2.4 oz	228.5	9.1	1.0
7077	Sausage, smoked link (pork)	2.4 oz	264.5	15.1	1.4
7076	Sausage, smoked link (pork, beef, & NFD milk)	2.4 oz	212.8	9.0	1.3
7083	Sausage, vegetarian, meatless	2.4 oz	174.1	12.6	6.7
924160	Sausage, Vienna, canned (beef & pork)	1 sm sausage	44.6	1.6	0.3
12037	Seeds, sunflower kernels, dried	1 cup w/hulls (edible part)	262.2	10.5	8.6
12537	Seeds, sunflower kernels, dry-roasted w/o salt	1.0 oz	165.0	5.5	6.8
12538	Seeds, sunflower kernels, oil-roasted w/o salt	1.0 oz	174.4	6.1	4.2
15155	Shellfish, abalone, fried	3.0 oz	160.7	16.7	9.4
15158	Shellfish, clams, boiled/steamed (moist heat)	3.0 oz	125.8	21.7	4.4
15162	Shellfish, clams, breaded & fried	3.0 oz	171.7	12.1	8.8
15160	Shellfish, clams, canned with liquid	3.0 oz	1.7	0.3	0.1
15157	Shellfish, clams, canned, drained	3.0 oz	125.8	21.7	4.4
15138	Shellfish, crab, Alaskan king, boiled/steamed	3.0 oz	82.5	16.4	0.0
15136	Shellfish, crab, Alaskan king, imitation surimi	3.0 oz	86.7	10.2	8.7
15139	Shellfish, crab, blue, crab cakes	1 cake	93.0	12.1	0.3
15143	Shellfish, crab, dungeness, cooked w/moist heat	3.0 oz	93.5	19.0	0.8
15147	Shellfish, lobster, northern, boiled/steamed (moist heat)	3.0 oz	83.3	17.4	1.1
15154	Shellfish, lobster, spiny, cooked w/moist heat	3.0 oz	121.6	22.4	2.7
15164	Shellfish, mussel, blue, boiled/steamed	3.0 oz	146.2	20.2	6.3
15246	Shellfish, oyster, eastern, breaded & fried	3.0 oz	167.5	7.5	9.9
15245	Shellfish, oyster, eastern, farmed, cooked w/dry heat	6 medium oysters	46.6	4.1	4.3
15244	Shellfish, oyster, eastern, farmed, raw	6 medium oysters	49.6	4.4	4.6
15174	Shellfish, scallops, breaded, fried	2 large scallops	66.7	5.6	3.1
15172	Shellfish, scallops, imitation surimi	3.0 oz	84.2	10.9	9.0
924252	Shellfish, shrimp chow mein, frozen	1 cup	72.6	5.9	10.9
15151	Shellfish, shrimp egg roll/LaChoy	3 medium	75.1	2.0	12.0
15150	Shellfish, shrimp, boiled/steamed (moist heat)	1 large shrimp	5.9	1.3	0.0
15152	Shellfish, shrimp, breaded & fried	1 large shrimp	16.9	1.5	0.8
15153	Shellfish, shrimp, canned	1 cup	153.6	29.5	1.3
15149	Shellfish, shrimp, imitation surimi	3.0 oz	85.9	10.5	7.8
4550	Sherbet, orange	1 sherbet bar	91.1	0.7	20.1
4546	Shortening, animal & vegetable fat, lard & vege oil	1 cup	1845.0	0.0	0.0
4556	Shortening, vegetable fat, Crisco	1 Tbsp.	106.0	0.0	0.0
19002	Snack, banana chips	1.0 oz	147.1	0.7	16.6
919972	Snack, beef jerky	1.0 oz	116.2	9.4	3.1
18501	Snack, Bugles	1.0 oz	150.1	2.0	18.0
19419	Snack, Chex Party Mix	1.0 oz (2/3 cup)	119.0	3.1	18.2
19800	Snack, corn cakes	1 cake	34.8	0.7	7.5
919973	Snack, corn chips, BBQ flavor	1.0 oz	148.3	2.0	15.9
19003	Snack, corn chips, light/Fritos	1.0 oz	155.1	1.9	15.9
19803	Snack, corn chips, plain	1.0 oz	152.8	1.9	16.1
19401	Snack, corn cones, plain	1.0 oz	144.6	1.6	17.8
19402	Snack, corn nuts, BBQ flavor	1.0 oz	123.6	2.6	20.3
19008	Snack, corn nuts, plain	1.0 oz	124.5	2.4	20.8
19016	Snack, Doo Dads Party Mix, original flavor	1 Tbsp.	16.0	0.4	2.3
19015	Snack, granola bar, hard, peanut butter	1.0 oz	136.9	2.8	17.7
19017	Snack, granola bar, hard, plain	1.0-oz bar	133.5	2.9	18.3
19405	Snack, granola bar, hard, w/chocolate chips	1.0 oz	124.2	2.1	20.4
19024	Snack, granola bar, soft, chocolate chip, graham & marshmallow	1.0-oz bar	121.1	1.7	20.1
19406	Snack, granola bar, soft, chocolate chip, milk chocolate cover	1.0-oz bar	132.1	1.6	18.1
19027	Snack, granola bar, soft, peanut butter	1.0-oz bar	120.8	3.0	18.3
19022	Snack, granola bar, soft, plain	1.0-oz bar	125.6	2.1	19.1
19404	Snack, granola bar, soft, raisin	1.0-oz bar	127.0	2.2	18.8
19440	Snack, granola bar, soft, w/chocolate chips	1.0-oz bar	119.1	2.1	19.6

Dietary Fiber (g)	Total Fat (g)	Cholesterol (mg)	Calcium (mg)	Iron (mg)	Magnesium (mg)	Sodium (mg)	Zinc (mg)	Vitamin A (μgRE)	Vitamin C (mg)	Vitamin E (mgαT)	Thiamin (mg)	Riboflavin (mg)	Niacin (mg)	Vitamin B6 (mg)	Folate (μg)
0.0	12.8	27.5	9.0	0.6	1.4	461.7	1.0	0.0	0.0	0.1	0.0	0.0	1.1	0.1	1.8
0.0	8.8	45.5	42.8	0.9	4.5	616.5	0.5	17.1	0.0	0.1	0.0	0.1	1.4	0.1	1.8
0.0	8.0	48.2	47.7	0.8	6.3	641.7	1.4	0.0	0.0	0.3	0.0	0.1	1.9	0.1	3.6
0.0	4.8	14.7	3.0	0.3	3.2	271.9	0.6	0.0	0.0	0.0	0.0	0.0	0.8	0.0	0.7
0.0	7.1	17.4	11.4	0.4	4.2	279.8	0.5	0.0	0.0	0.1	0.1	0.1	0.7	0.0	1.3
0.0	3.8	8.4	2.7	0.2	1.7	186.9	0.3	0.0	0.0	0.0	0.0	0.0	0.4	0.0	0.5
0.0	110.4	198.3	25.1	3.5	40.2	5120.4	6.3	0.0	0.0	0.6	0.8	0.6	12.4	0.6	10.0
0.0	18.6	73.0	9.0	1.0	17.0	507.0	2.4	8.0	0.0	0.6	0.7	0.2	2.6	0.2	3.0
0.0	4.6	15.0	3.0	0.6	3.5	245.0	0.5	0.0	0.0	0.1	0.1	0.1	0.8	0.0	0.5
0.0	7.9	46.7	11.4	0.9	8.6	572.3	1.0	0.0	0.0	0.3	0.0	0.1	2.0	0.1	2.3
0.0	20.6	48.3	6.8	1.0	8.2	642.6	1.4	0.0	0.0	0.1	0.2	0.1	2.2	0.1	1.4
0.0	21.6	46.2	20.4	0.8	12.9	1020.0	1.9	0.0	1.4	0.2	0.5	0.2	3.1	0.2	3.4
0.0	18.8	44.2	27.9	1.0	10.9	797.6	1.3	0.0	0.0	0.0	0.1	0.1	1.9	0.1	1.4
1.9	12.3	0.0	42.8	2.5	24.5	603.8	1.0	43.5	0.0	1.4	1.6	0.3	7.6	0.6	17.7
0.0	4.0	8.3	1.6	0.1	1.1	152.5	0.3	0.0	0.0	0.0	0.0	0.0	0.3	0.0	0.6
4.8	22.8	0.0	53.4	3.1	162.8	1.4	2.3	2.3	0.6	23.1	1.1	0.1	2.1	0.4	104.6
3.1	14.1	0.0	19.8	1.1	36.6	0.9	1.5	0.0	0.4	14.3	0.0	0.1	2.0	0.2	67.3
1.9	16.3	0.0	15.9	1.9	36.0	0.9	1.5	1.4	0.4	14.3	0.1	0.1	1.2	0.2	66.3
0.0	5.8	79.9	31.5	3.2	47.6	502.4	0.8	1.7	1.5	0.0	0.2	0.1	1.6	0.1	11.9
0.0	1.7	57.0	78.2	23.8	15.3	95.2	2.3	145.4	18.8	0.0	0.1	0.4	2.9	0.1	24.5
0.0	9.5	51.9	53.6	11.8	11.9	309.4	1.2	76.5	8.5	0.0	0.1	0.2	1.8	0.1	30.6
0.0	0.0	2.6	11.1	0.3	9.4	182.8	0.1	7.7	0.9	0.9	0.0	0.0	0.2	0.0	1.7
0.0	1.7	57.0	78.2	23.8	15.3	95.2	2.3	145.4	18.8	0.9	0.1	0.4	2.9	0.1	24.5
0.0	1.3	45.1	50.2	0.6	53.6	911.2	6.5	7.7	6.5	0.0	0.0	0.0	1.1	0.2	43.4
0.0	1.1	17.0	11.1	0.3	36.6	714.9	0.3	17.0	0.0	0.1	0.0	0.0	0.2	0.0	1.4
0.0	4.5	90.0	63.0	0.6	19.8	198.0	2.5	48.6	1.7	0.0	0.1	0.0	1.7	0.1	31.8
0.0	1.1	64.6	50.2	0.4	49.3	321.3	4.6	26.4	3.1	0.0	0.0	0.2	3.1	0.1	35.7
0.0	0.5	61.2	51.9	0.3	29.8	323.0	2.5	22.1	0.0	0.9	0.0	0.1	0.9	0.1	9.4
0.0	1.6	76.5	53.6	1.2	43.4	193.0	6.2	5.1	1.8	0.0	0.0	0.0	4.2	0.1	0.9
0.0	3.8	47.6	28.1	5.7	31.5	313.7	2.3	77.4	11.6	0.0	0.3	0.4	2.6	0.1	64.3
0.0	10.7	68.9	52.7	5.9	49.3	354.5	74.1	76.5	3.2	0.0	0.1	0.2	1.4	0.1	26.4
0.0	1.3	22.4	33.0	4.6	19.5	96.2	26.6	11.2	3.5	0.0	0.1	0.0	1.1	0.0	14.2
0.0	1.3	21.0	37.0	4.9	27.7	149.5	31.9	6.7	3.9	0.0	0.1	0.1	1.1	0.1	15.1
0.0	3.4	18.9	13.0	0.3	18.3	143.8	0.3	6.8	0.7	0.0	0.0	0.0	0.5	0.0	11.5
0.0	0.3	18.7	6.8	0.3	36.6	675.8	0.3	17.0	0.0	0.0	0.0	0.0	0.3	0.0	1.4
0.0	0.7	0.0	0.0	0.0	0.0	985.0	0.0	0.0	0.0	0.0	0.0	0.0	0.0	0.0	0.0
0.0	2.4	4.0	11.0	0.8	0.0	120.0	0.0	5.0	4.0	0.0	0.1	0.1	0.8	0.0	0.0
0.0	0.1	11.7	2.3	0.2	2.0	13.4	0.1	4.0	0.1	0.0	0.0	0.0	0.2	0.0	0.2
0.0	0.9	12.4	4.7	0.1	2.8	24.1	0.1	3.9	0.1	0.0	0.0	0.0	0.2	0.0	0.6
0.0	2.5	221.4	75.5	3.5	52.5	216.3	1.6	23.0	2.9	1.2	0.0	0.0	3.5	0.1	2.3
0.0	1.2	30.6	16.2	0.5	36.6	599.3	0.3	17.0	0.0	0.0	0.0	0.0	0.1	0.0	1.4
0.0	1.3	4.0	35.6	0.1	5.3	30.4	0.3	9.2	2.0	0.1	0.0	0.1	0.0	0.0	3.3
0.0	205.0	114.8	0.0	0.0	0.0	0.0	0.0	0.0	0.0	2.5	0.0	0.0	0.0	0.0	0.0
0.0	12.0	0.0	0.0	0.0	0.0	0.0	0.0	0.0	0.0	0.0	0.0	0.0	0.0	0.0	0.0
2.2	9.5	0.0	5.1	0.4	21.5	1.7	0.2	2.3	1.8	1.5	0.0	0.0	0.2	0.1	4.0
0.5	7.3	13.6	5.7	1.5	14.5	627.4	2.3	0.0	0.0	0.1	0.0	0.0	0.5	0.1	38.0
0.0	8.0	0.0	2.0	0.2	0.0	290.0	0.0	0.0	0.0	0.0	0.0	0.0	0.3	0.0	0.0
1.6	4.8	0.0	9.8	6.9	17.6	284.8	0.6	3.9	13.3	0.0	0.4	0.1	4.7	0.4	0.0
0.2	0.2	0.0	1.7	0.1	10.3	43.9	0.2	2.2	0.0	0.0	0.0	0.0	0.5	0.0	1.7
1.5	9.3	0.0	37.1	0.4	21.8	216.3	0.3	17.3	0.5	0.0	0.0	0.1	0.5	0.1	11.1
0.8	9.7	0.0	25.0	0.3	21.0	194.0	0.3	7.4	0.0	0.0	0.0	0.0	0.4	0.1	0.0
1.4	9.5	0.0	36.0	0.4	21.5	178.6	0.4	2.6	0.0	0.4	0.0	0.0	0.3	0.1	5.7
0.3	7.6	0.0	0.9	0.7	3.1	289.7	0.1	9.1	0.0	0.0	0.1	0.1	0.4	0.0	0.9
2.4	4.1	0.0	4.8	0.5	30.9	276.7	0.5	9.6	0.1	0.0	0.1	0.0	0.4	0.1	0.0
2.0	4.0	0.0	2.6	0.5	32.0	155.6	0.5	0.0	0.0	0.3	0.0	0.0	0.5	0.1	0.0
0.2	0.6	0.0	2.6	0.1	2.1	44.5	0.1	1.5	0.0	0.0	0.0	0.0	0.2	0.0	1.4
0.8	6.7	0.0	11.6	0.7	15.6	80.2	0.4	0.6	0.1	0.0	0.1	0.0	0.6	0.0	5.1
1.5	5.6	0.0	17.3	0.8	27.5	83.3	0.6	4.3	0.3	0.0	0.1	0.0	0.4	0.0	6.5
1.2	4.6	0.0	21.8	0.9	20.4	97.5	0.5	1.1	0.0	0.0	0.1	0.0	0.2	0.0	3.7
1.1	4.4	0.3	25.2	0.7	20.1	89.6	0.4	1.4	0.0	0.0	0.0	0.0	0.3	0.0	6.0
1.0	7.1	1.4	29.2	0.7	18.7	56.7	0.4	2.0	0.0	0.0	0.0	0.1	0.2	0.0	7.4
1.2	4.5	0.3	25.8	0.6	24.4	116.0	0.5	0.6	0.0	0.0	0.0	0.1	0.9	0.0	9.1
1.3	4.9	0.3	29.8	0.7	21.0	78.8	0.4	0.0	0.0	0.0	0.0	0.1	0.1	0.0	6.8
1.2	5.0	0.3	28.6	0.7	20.4	79.9	0.4	0.0	0.0	0.0	0.1	0.0	0.3	0.0	6.0
1.4	4.7	0.3	26.4	0.7	22.1	77.1	0.4	1.4	0.0	0.0	0.1	0.0	0.3	0.0	6.2

Code	Food Name	Unit Amount	Kilocalories (kcal)	Protein (g)	Carbohydrate (g)
19439	Snack, Kudos Whole-Grain Bars, chocolate chip/M&M Mars	4.0-oz bar	437.0	5.8	67.7
19407	Snack, low-fat granola bar, crunchy almond/brown sugar/Kellogg	4.0-oz bar	390.0	8.0	78.0
19441	Snack, meat-based sticks, smoked	1.0 oz	155.9	6.1	1.5
19031	Snack, Nutri-Grain Cereal Bars, fruit/Kellogg	4.0-oz bar	368.0	4.4	72.9
19034	Snack, popcorn cakes	1 cake	38.4	1.0	8.0
19806	Snack, popcorn, air-popped	1 Tbsp.	1.9	0.1	0.4
19039	Snack, popcorn, caramel-coated w/peanuts	1.0 oz (2/3 cup)	113.4	1.8	22.9
19040	Snack, popcorn, caramel-coated, no peanuts	1.0 oz	122.2	1.1	22.4
19807	Snack, popcorn, cheese flavor	1 Tbsp.	3.7	0.1	0.4
19035	Snack, popcorn, oil-popped, white corn	1.0 oz	141.8	2.6	16.2
19408	Snack, popcorn, prep in microwave	3 cups	210.0	3.0	20.4
19412	Snack, pork skins, plain	1.0 oz	154.5	17.4	0.0
19042	Snack, potato chips w/o salt	1.0 oz	157.9	2.1	14.5
919975	Snack, potato chips, BBQ flavor	1.0 oz	139.2	2.2	15.0
19809	Snack, potato chips, light	1.0 oz	133.5	2.0	19.0
19411	Snack, potato chips, plain, no salt	1.0 oz	152.0	2.0	15.0
19043	Snack, potato chips, plain, salted	1.0 oz	152.0	2.0	15.0
919985	Snack, potato chips, sour cream & onion	1.0 oz	150.5	2.3	14.6
19047	Snack, pretzel, hard, plain, no salt	1.0 oz	108.0	2.6	22.5
19813	Snack, pretzel, hard, plain, salted	1.0 oz	108.0	2.6	22.5
19050	Snack, pretzel, hard, chocolate-coated	1.0 oz	129.8	2.1	20.1
919978	Snack, pretzel, hard, whole-wheat	1.0 oz (2 sm pretzels)	101.4	3.1	22.7
19052	Snack, rice cake	1 cake	21.0	0.5	4.6
19818	Snack, rice cake, brown rice & multigrain	1 cake	34.8	0.8	7.2
19816	Snack, rice cake, brown rice, plain	1 cake	34.8	0.7	7.3
19524	Snack, sesame stick, wheat-based, no salt	1.0 oz	153.4	3.1	13.2
19857	Snack, taro chips	1.0 oz	141.2	0.7	19.3
19424	Snack, tortilla chips, nacho flavor	1.0 oz	141.2	2.2	17.7
19056	Snack, tortilla chips, nacho, light	1.0 oz	126.2	2.5	20.3
19058	Snack, tortilla chips, plain	1.0 oz	142.0	2.0	17.8
19063	Snack, tortilla chips, ranch flavor	1.0 oz	138.9	2.2	18.3
19059	Snack, tortilla chips, taco flavor	1.0 oz	136.1	2.2	17.9
19062	Snack, trail mix, regular	1.0 oz	131.0	3.9	12.7
6201	Soup, asparagus, canned, made w/H$_2$O	1 cup (8 fl oz)	85.4	2.3	10.7
6009	Soup, beans w/ham, chunky, RTE, canned	1 cup (8 fl oz)	230.9	12.6	27.1
6748	Soup, beef noodle, condensed, canned	1 cup (8 fl oz)	168.2	9.7	18.0
6008	Soup, beef broth or bouillon, dry, made w/H$_2$O	1 packet (6 fl oz)	14.6	1.0	1.4
6147	Soup, beef mushroom, canned, made w/H$_2$O	1 cup (8 fl oz)	73.2	5.8	6.3
6743	Soup, beef vegetable, canned, RTE/Progresso Healthy Classics	1 cup	160.0	10.5	25.6
6722	Soup, beef, chunky, RTE, canned	1 cup (8 fl oz)	170.4	11.7	19.6
6724	Soup, beefy mushroom, dry mix/Lipton Recipe Secrets	1 serving	32.8	0.9	6.6
6402	Soup, beefy onion, dry mix/Lipton Recipe Secrets	1 serving	25.1	0.5	4.7
6002	Soup, black bean, canned, made w/H$_2$O	1 cup (8 fl oz)	116.1	5.6	19.8
906161	Soup, broccoli & cheese, dry mix/Lipton Soup Secrets	1 serving	66.9	1.8	8.9
6411	Soup, cauliflower, dry, made w/H$_2$O	1 cup (8 fl oz)	69.1	2.9	10.7
6011	Soup, cheese, canned, made w/milk	1 cup (8 fl oz)	230.9	9.5	16.2
6413	Soup, chicken broth or bouillon, dry, made w/H$_2$O	1 cup (8 fl oz)	22.0	1.3	1.4
6017	Soup, chicken gumbo, canned, made w/H$_2$O	1 cup (8 fl oz)	56.1	2.6	8.4
6727	Soup, chicken noodle, chunky, canned, RTE	1 cup (8 fl oz)	175.2	12.7	17.0
6022	Soup, chicken rice, canned, made w/H$_2$O	1 cup (8 fl oz)	60.3	3.5	7.2
6025	Soup, chicken vegetable, chunky, RTE, canned	1 cup (8 fl oz)	165.6	12.3	18.9
6012	Soup, chicken w/dumplings, canned, made w/H$_2$O	1 cup (8 fl oz)	96.4	5.6	6.0
6034	Soup, consomme w/gelatin, dry, made w/H$_2$O	1 cup (8 fl oz)	17.5	2.2	2.1
6001	Soup, crab, RTE, canned	1 cup (8 fl oz)	75.6	5.5	10.3
6410	Soup, cream of broccoli, canned, RTE/Progresso Healthy Classics	1 cup (8 fl oz)	128.2	3.5	19.4
6210	Soup, cream of celery, canned, made w/H$_2$O	1 cup (8 fl oz)	90.3	1.7	8.8
6216	Soup, cream of chicken, canned, made w/H$_2$O	1 cup (8 fl oz)	115.2	3.4	9.1
6243	Soup, cream of mushroom, canned, made w/H$_2$O	1 cup (8 fl oz)	129.3	2.3	9.3
6246	Soup, cream of onion, canned, made w/H$_2$O	1 cup (8 fl oz)	107.4	2.8	12.7
6253	Soup, cream of potato, canned, made w/H$_2$O	1 cup (8 fl oz)	73.2	1.8	11.5
6256	Soup, cream of shrimp, canned, made w/H$_2$O	1 cup (8 fl oz)	90.3	2.8	8.2
6582	Soup, cream of vegetable, dry, made w/H$_2$O	1 cup (8 fl oz)	106.6	1.9	12.3
6035	Soup, cup noodles, ramen, chicken flavor, dry/Nissin	1 individual container	296.2	5.6	36.8
6283	Soup, gazpacho, RTE, canned	1 cup (8 fl oz)	46.4	7.1	4.4
6249	Soup, green pea, canned, made w/H$_2$O	1 cup (8 fl oz)	165.0	8.6	26.5

Dietary Fiber (g)	Total Fat (g)	Cholesterol (mg)	Calcium (mg)	Iron (mg)	Magnesium (mg)	Sodium (mg)	Zinc (mg)	Vitamin A (μgRE)	Vitamin C (mg)	Vitamin E (mgαT)	Thiamin (mg)	Riboflavin (mg)	Niacin (mg)	Vitamin B$_6$ (mg)	Folate (μg)
3.6	16.4	136.0	783.0	9.2	70.0	280.0	1.4	1253.0	46.6	10.8	0.2	0.2	1.5	0.1	13.0
6.2	7.4	0.0	35.0	8.6	87.0	291.0	2.2	713.0	0.0	0.0	0.7	0.8	9.5	1.0	0.0
0.0	14.1	37.7	19.3	1.0	6.0	419.6	0.7	47.9	1.9	0.0	0.0	0.1	1.3	0.1	0.0
2.1	7.5	0.0	41.0	4.9	27.0	297.0	4.1	614.0	0.0	0.0	1.0	1.1	13.5	1.4	108.0
0.3	0.3	0.0	0.9	0.2	15.9	28.8	0.4	0.7	0.0	0.0	0.0	0.0	0.6	0.0	1.8
0.1	0.0	0.0	0.1	0.0	0.7	0.0	0.0	0.1	0.0	0.0	0.0	0.0	0.0	0.0	0.1
1.1	2.2	0.0	18.7	1.1	22.7	83.6	0.4	1.7	0.0	0.4	0.0	0.0	0.6	0.1	4.5
1.5	3.6	1.4	12.2	0.5	9.9	58.4	0.2	2.8	0.0	0.3	0.0	0.0	0.6	0.1	0.6
0.1	0.2	0.1	0.8	0.0	0.6	6.2	0.0	0.3	0.0	0.0	0.0	0.0	0.0	0.0	0.1
2.8	8.0	0.0	2.8	0.8	30.6	250.6	0.7	0.6	0.1	0.0	0.0	0.0	0.4	0.1	4.8
1.0	13.2	0.0	8.0	0.7	0.0	415.0	0.0	10.8	3.0	0.0	0.1	0.3	0.7	0.0	0.0
0.0	8.9	26.9	8.5	0.2	3.1	521.1	0.2	11.1	0.1	0.2	0.0	0.1	0.4	0.0	0.0
1.0	10.6	0.0	6.1	0.4	19.2	4.1	0.2	1.6	12.1	0.0	0.1	0.0	1.1	0.2	13.2
1.2	9.2	0.0	14.2	0.5	21.3	212.6	0.3	6.2	9.6	1.4	0.1	0.1	1.3	0.2	23.5
1.7	5.9	0.0	6.0	0.4	25.2	139.5	0.0	7.3	0.8		0.1	0.1	2.0	0.2	7.7
1.4	9.8	0.0	6.8	0.5	19.0	2.3	0.3	0.0	8.8	1.4	0.0	0.1	1.1	0.2	12.8
1.3	9.8	0.0	6.8	0.5	19.0	168.4	0.3	0.0	8.8	1.4	0.0	0.1	1.1	0.2	12.8
1.5	9.6	2.0	20.4	0.5	21.0	177.2	0.3	6.0	10.6	0.0	0.1	0.1	1.1	0.2	17.6
0.8	1.0	0.0	10.2	1.2	9.9	81.9	0.2	0.0	0.0	0.1	0.1	0.2	1.5	0.0	23.5
0.9	1.0	0.0	10.2	1.2	9.9	486.2	0.2	0.0	0.0	0.1	0.1	0.2	1.5	0.0	48.5
0.0	4.7	0.0	21.0	0.6	11.6	161.3	0.3	0.6	0.1	0.0	0.0	0.1	0.2	0.0	2.6
2.2	0.7	0.0	7.8	0.8	8.4	56.8	0.2	0.0	0.3	0.0	0.1	0.1	1.8	0.1	15.1
0.4	0.0	0.0	0.0	0.1	0.0	16.0	0.0	2.8	0.0	0.0	0.0	0.0	0.6	0.0	0.0
0.3	0.3	0.0	1.9	0.2	12.3	22.7	0.2	0.0	0.0	0.0	0.0	0.0	0.6	0.0	1.8
0.4	0.3	0.0	1.0	0.1	11.8	29.3	0.3	0.5	0.0	0.1	0.0	0.0	0.7	0.0	1.9
0.0	10.4	0.0	48.2	0.2	12.8	8.2	0.3	2.6	0.0	0.0	0.0	0.0	0.4	0.0	6.2
2.0	7.1	0.0	17.0	0.3	23.8	97.0	0.1	0.0	1.4	1.4	0.0	0.1	0.1	0.1	5.7
1.5	7.3	0.9	41.7	0.4	23.2	200.7	0.3	11.6	0.5	0.0	0.0	0.1	0.4	0.1	4.0
1.4	4.3	0.9	45.1	0.5	27.5	284.4	0.0	11.9	0.1	0.0	0.1	0.1	0.1	0.1	7.4
1.8	7.4	0.0	43.7	0.4	24.9	149.7	0.4	5.7	0.0	0.4	0.0	0.1	0.4	0.1	2.8
1.1	6.7	0.3	40.0	0.4	25.2	173.5	0.4	7.7	0.3	0.0	0.0	0.1	0.4	0.1	4.8
1.5	6.9	1.4	43.9	0.6	24.9	223.1	0.4	25.8	0.3	0.0	0.1	0.1	0.6	0.1	6.0
0.0	8.3	0.0	22.1	0.9	44.8	64.9	0.9	0.6	0.4	0.0	0.1	0.1	1.3	0.1	20.1
0.5	4.1	4.9	29.3	0.8	4.9	980.9	0.9	43.9	2.7	0.7	0.1	0.1	0.8	0.0	22.0
11.2	8.5	21.9	77.8	3.2	46.2	972.0	1.1	396.1	4.4	0.0	0.1	0.1	1.7	0.1	29.2
1.5	6.2	10.0	30.1	2.2	12.6	1905.1	3.1	125.5	0.8	0.0	0.1	0.1	2.1	0.1	37.7
0.0	0.5	0.0	7.3	0.0	5.5	1021.1	0.1	0.0	0.0	0.0	0.0	0.0	0.3	0.0	0.0
0.2	3.0	7.3	4.9	0.0	9.8	941.8	1.5	0.0	4.6	0.0	0.0	0.1	1.0	0.0	9.8
6.0	1.6	15.0	15.0	1.9	32.5	420.0	1.3	215.0	4.8	0.5	0.1	0.1	2.9	0.3	25.0
1.4	5.1	14.4	31.2	2.3	4.8	866.4	2.6	261.6	7.0	0.2	0.1	0.2	2.7	0.1	13.4
0.1	0.4	0.2	10.8	0.1	0.0	645.2	0.0	0.0	0.2	0.0	0.0	0.0	0.1	0.0	0.0
0.4	0.6	0.0	11.2	0.1	0.0	606.6	0.0	0.0	0.7	0.0	0.0	0.0	0.1	0.0	0.0
4.4	1.5	0.0	44.5	2.1	42.0	1198.0	1.4	49.4	0.7	0.1	0.1	0.1	0.5	0.1	24.7
0.7	2.9	2.9	46.4	0.2	0.0	545.3	0.0	0.0	3.0	0.0	0.0	0.0	0.1	0.0	3.7
0.0	1.7	0.0	10.2	0.5	2.6	842.6	0.3	0.0	2.6	0.0	0.1	0.1	0.5	0.0	2.6
1.0	14.6	47.7	288.7	0.8	20.1	1019.1	0.7	148.1	1.3	0.3	0.1	0.3	0.5	0.1	10.0
0.0	1.1	0.0	14.6	0.1	4.9	1483.5	0.0	12.2	0.0	0.0	0.0	0.0	0.2	0.0	2.4
2.0	1.4	4.9	24.4	0.9	4.9	954.0	0.4	14.6	4.9	0.0	0.0	0.0	0.7	0.1	4.9
3.8	6.0	19.2	24.0	1.4	9.6	849.6	1.0	122.4	0.0	0.8	0.1	0.2	4.3	0.0	38.4
0.7	1.9	7.2	16.9	0.7	0.0	814.6	0.3	65.1	0.2	0.1	0.0	0.0	1.1	0.0	1.0
0.0	4.8	16.8	26.4	1.5	9.6	1068.0	2.2	600.0	5.5	0.0	0.0	0.2	3.3	0.1	12.0
0.5	5.5	33.7	14.5	0.6	4.8	860.4	0.4	53.0	0.0	0.1	0.0	0.1	1.8	0.0	2.4
0.0	0.0	0.0	7.5	0.1	7.5	3312.5	0.0	0.0	0.0	0.0	0.0	0.0	0.6	0.0	4.0
0.7	1.5	9.8	65.9	1.2	14.6	1234.6	1.5	51.2	0.0	0.0	0.2	0.1	1.3	0.1	14.6
3.6	4.1	7.1	60.5	1.8	21.4	843.7	0.4	46.3	8.5	0.6	0.0	0.1	0.5	0.1	42.7
0.7	5.6	14.6	39.0	0.6	7.3	949.2	0.2	31.7	0.2	0.9	0.0	0.0	0.3	0.0	2.4
0.2	7.2	9.6	33.6	0.6	2.4	969.6	0.6	55.2	0.2	0.2	0.0	0.1	0.8	0.0	1.7
0.5	9.0	2.4	46.4	0.5	4.9	880.8	0.6	0.0	1.0	1.2	0.0	0.1	0.7	0.0	4.9
1.0	5.3	14.6	34.2	0.6	4.9	927.2	0.1	29.3	1.2	0.0	0.1	0.1	0.5	0.0	6.8
0.5	2.4	4.9	19.5	0.5	2.4	1000.4	0.6	29.3	0.0	0.0	0.0	0.0	0.5	0.0	2.9
0.2	5.2	17.1	17.1	0.5	9.8	976.0	0.8	14.6	0.0	0.8	0.0	0.0	0.4	0.0	3.7
0.5	5.7	0.0	31.2	0.5	10.4	1170.0	0.3	2.6	3.9	1.2	1.2	0.1	0.5	0.0	7.8
0.0	14.1	0.0	0.0	2.2	0.0	1433.6	0.0	0.0	0.0	0.0	0.0	0.0	0.0	0.0	0.0
0.5	0.2	0.0	24.4	1.0	7.3	739.3	0.2	261.1	7.1	0.5	0.0	0.0	0.9	0.1	9.8
2.8	2.9	0.0	27.5	2.0	40.0	917.5	1.7	20.0	1.8	0.1	0.1	0.1	1.2	0.1	1.8

Code	Food Name	Unit Amount	Kilocalories (kcal)	Protein (g)	Carbohydrate (g)
6287	Soup, hearty chicken noodle, dry mix/Lipton Cup-a-Soup	1 envelope	61.4	2.6	10.2
6204	Soup, lentil ham, RTE, canned	1 cup (8 fl oz)	138.9	9.3	20.2
6027	Soup, Manhattan clam chowder, canned, made w/H$_2$O	1 cup (8 fl oz)	78.1	2.2	12.2
6039	Soup, minestrone, canned, RTE/Progresso Healthy Classics	1 cup (8 fl oz)	122.9	4.8	20.3
6430	Soup, nacho cheese	1 cup (8 fl oz)	105.4	3.8	6.4
6230	Soup, New England clam chowder, canned, made w/H$_2$O	1 cup (8 fl oz)	95.2	4.8	12.4
6302	Soup, noodle w/chicken broth, dry mix/Lipton Soup Secrets	1 Tbsp.	62.1	2.1	9.2
6045	Soup, onion, canned, made w/H$_2$O	1 cup (8 fl oz)	57.8	3.8	8.2
6730	Soup, split pea w/ham, canned, made w/H$_2$O	1 cup (8 fl oz)	189.8	10.3	28.0
6192	Soup, split pea w/ham, chunky, RTE, canned	1 cup (8 fl oz)	184.8	11.1	26.8
6099	Soup, tomato rice, made w/H$_2$O	1 cup (8 fl oz)	118.6	2.1	21.9
6559	Soup, tomato vegetable, dry, made w/H$_2$O	1 cup (8 fl oz)	55.7	2.0	10.2
6359	Soup, tomato, canned, made w/H$_2$O	1 cup (8 fl oz)	85.4	2.0	16.6
6159	Soup, tomato, canned, made w/milk	1 cup (8 fl oz)	161.2	6.1	22.3
6065	Soup, turkey noodle, canned, made w/H$_2$O	1 cup (8 fl oz)	70.3	4.0	8.9
6066	Soup, turkey vegetable, canned, made w/H$_2$O	1 cup (8 fl oz)	72.0	3.1	8.6
6471	Soup, turkey, chunky, RTE, canned	1 cup (8 fl oz)	134.5	10.2	14.1
6301	Soup, vegetable, chunky, RTE, canned	1 cup (8 fl oz)	122.4	3.5	19.0
6068	Soup, vegetarian vegetable, canned, made w/H$_2$O	1 cup (8 fl oz)	72.3	2.1	12.0
22693	Stew, beef stew, canned entree	1 cup	218.1	11.5	15.7
924055	Stew, beef & vegetable	1 cup	220.5	16.0	15.0
906162	Stew, chicken vegetable/Bounty	7.5 oz	166.1	10.5	15.1
924190	Stew, ratatouille, homemade	1/2 cup	132.7	1.2	5.9
19337	Stuffing, brownberry sage and onion stuffing mix, dry mix/Best Foods	1/2 cup	255.3	8.9	47.2
924174	Sugar substitute, Equal	1 package	4.0	0.0	1.0
18356	Sweet roll, cheese	1 oz	102.2	2.0	12.4
18357	Sweet roll, cinnamon-raisin, commercially prep	1 large	308.8	5.1	42.2
919959	Sweet, All-Fruit Strawberry Spread/Polaner	1 Tbsp.	41.5	0.1	10.3
919904	Sweet, baking chocolate/Bakers	1 oz	141.1	3.1	9.0
919916	Sweet, chewing gum	1 stick	10.2	0.0	2.9
919902	Sweet, chewing gum, sugarless	1 piece	8.0	0.0	2.0
19166	Sweet, cocoa, dry powder, unsweetened	1 Tbsp.	12.4	1.1	2.9
19172	Sweet, fruit butter, apple	1 Tbsp.	29.4	0.1	7.3
19703	Sweet, gelatin, dry mix, low kcal w/aspartame, prep w/H$_2$O	1 cup	16.4	2.6	1.6
19296	Sweet, gelatin, dry, prep w/H$_2$O	1 cup	159.3	3.2	37.8
19283	Sweet, honey, strained/extracted	1 Tbsp.	63.8	0.1	17.3
19717	Sweet, Ice Popsicle	1 double stick	92.2	0.0	24.2
19280	Sweet, ices/sorbet, pineapple-coconut	1 Tbsp.	14.0	0.0	3.0
918860	Sweet, ices/sorbet/water, fruit, low kcal w/aspartame	1 bar	12.2	0.3	3.2
919905	Sweet, Italian ice, restaurant-prep	1.0 fl oz	15.4	0.0	3.9
19297	Sweet, jam, low kcal	1 Tbsp.	18.0	0.0	5.1
19719	Sweet, jams & preserves	1 Tbsp.	48.4	0.1	12.9
919907	Sweet, jellies	1 Tbsp.	51.5	0.1	13.5
919906	Sweet, jelly, low kcal	1.0 oz	4.2	0.0	1.0
19303	Sweet, maraschino cherry	1.0 oz	96.0	0.1	24.6
19304	Sweet, marmalade, orange	1 Tbsp.	49.2	0.1	13.3
19305	Sweet, molasses	1 Tbsp.	53.2	0.0	13.8
19251	Sweet, pectin, unsweetened, dry mix	1/4 package	39.0	0.0	10.8
19334	Sweet, Solo Poppy Seed Filling/Sokol	1 Tbsp.	59.7	0.9	10.5
19335	Sweet, sugar, brown	1 tsp. packed	17.3	0.0	4.5
19340	Sweet, sugar, granulated, white	1 tsp.	16.3	0.0	4.2
19336	Sweet, sugar, maple	1 piece (1 oz/1.75" x 1.25" x 0.5")	99.1	0.0	25.5
19113	Sweet, sugar, powdered/confectioner's, white	1 tsp.	9.7	0.0	2.5
19349	Sweet, syrup, chocolate, fudge-type	1 Tbsp.	59.5	0.8	10.7
19351	Sweet, syrup, corn, dark	1 Tbsp.	56.4	0.0	15.3
19362	Sweet, syrup, corn, light	1 Tbsp.	56.4	0.0	15.3
19129	Sweet, syrup, maple	1 Tbsp.	52.4	0.0	13.4
19360	Sweet, syrup, pancake	1 Tbsp.	57.4	0.0	15.1
19355	Sweet, syrup, pancake, reduced-kcal	1/4 cup	98.4	0.0	26.6
19365	Sweet, topping, butterscotch or caramel	1 Tbsp.	51.7	0.3	13.5
19367	Sweet, topping, marshmallow cream	1.0 oz	90.2	0.2	22.1
19137	Sweet, topping, pineapple	2 Tbsp.	106.3	0.0	27.9
919984	Sweet, topping, strawberry	1 Tbsp.	53.3	0.0	13.9
924200	Syrups, chocolate, genuine chocolate flavor, lite/Hershey	1 Tbsp.	25.0	0.3	5.8
924201	Taco	6.0 oz	369.4	20.7	26.7

Dietary Fiber (g)	Total Fat (g)	Cholesterol (mg)	Calcium (mg)	Iron (mg)	Magnesium (mg)	Sodium (mg)	Zinc (mg)	Vitamin A (µgRE)	Vitamin C (mg)	Vitamin E (mgαT)	Thiamin (mg)	Riboflavin (mg)	Niacin (mg)	Vitamin B$_6$ (mg)	Folate (µg)
0.3	1.2	14.2	5.9	0.5	0.0	591.4	0.0	0.0	0.1	0.0	0.1	0.1	1.3	0.0	17.0
0.0	2.8	7.4	42.2	2.7	22.3	1319.4	0.7	34.7	4.2	0.0	0.2	0.1	1.4	0.2	49.6
1.5	2.2	2.4	26.8	1.6	12.2	578.3	1.0	97.6	3.9	0.7	0.0	0.0	0.8	0.1	9.8
1.2	2.5	0.0	38.6	1.7	31.3	470.0	0.7	135.0	0.7	0.7	0.1	0.1	1.0	0.1	60.3
0.0	7.2	0.0	78.0	0.6	0.0	754.0	0.0	270.8	5.0	0.0	0.0	0.1	0.3	0.0	0.0
1.5	2.9	4.9	43.9	1.5	7.3	915.0	0.8	0.0	2.0	0.1	0.0	0.0	1.0	0.1	3.7
0.3	1.9	14.4	3.4	0.5		723.8	0.0	0.0	0.1	0.0	0.2	0.1	1.0	0.0	19.8
1.0	1.7	0.0	26.5	0.7	2.4	1053.2	0.6	0.0	1.2	0.3	0.0	0.0	0.6	0.0	15.2
2.3	4.4	7.6	22.8	2.3	48.1	1006.9	1.3	45.5	1.5	0.0	0.1	0.1	1.5	0.1	2.5
4.1	4.0	7.2	33.6	2.1	38.4	964.8	3.1	487.2	7.0	0.1	0.1	0.1	2.5	0.2	4.6
1.5	2.7	2.5	22.2	0.8	4.9	815.1	0.5	76.6	14.8	0.8	0.1	0.0	1.1	0.1	13.6
0.5	0.9	0.0	7.6	0.6	20.2	1146.1	0.2	20.2	6.1	0.8	0.1	0.0	0.8	0.1	10.1
0.5	1.9	0.0	12.2	1.8	7.3	695.4	0.2	68.3	66.4	2.5	0.1	0.1	1.4	0.1	14.6
2.7	6.0	17.4	158.7	1.8	22.3	744.0	0.3	109.1	67.7	2.6	0.1	0.2	1.5	0.2	20.8
0.8	2.1	5.0	12.6	1.0	5.0	838.3	0.6	30.1	0.3	0.1	0.1	0.1	1.4	0.0	20.1
0.5	3.0	2.4	16.8	0.8	4.8	902.4	0.6	242.4	0.0	0.1	0.0	0.0	1.0	0.0	4.8
0.0	4.4	9.4	49.6	1.9	23.6	922.8	2.1	715.1	6.4	0.0	0.0	0.1	3.6	0.3	11.1
1.2	3.7	0.0	55.2	1.6	7.2	1010.4	3.1	588.0	6.0	0.6	0.1	0.1	1.2	0.2	16.6
0.5	1.9	0.0	21.7	1.1	7.2	821.8	0.5	301.3	1.4	0.8	0.1	0.0	0.9	0.1	10.6
3.5	12.5	37.1	27.8	1.6	32.5	946.6	1.9	494.2	10.2	0.2	0.2	0.1	2.9	0.3	25.5
2.0	11.0	71.0	29.0	2.9	0.0	292.0	5.3	1138.0	17.0	0.0	0.1	0.2	4.7	0.3	37.0
0.0	7.0	0.0	29.0	1.2	0.0	1055.0	0.0	1463.4	5.0	0.0	0.0	0.1	3.4	0.0	0.0
0.0	12.3	0.0	27.8	0.6	16.1	164.8	0.2	40.7	20.7	0.0	0.1	0.0	0.6	0.1	17.1
3.6	3.4	0.0	0.0	2.6	0.0	1125.6	0.0	0.0	0.0	0.0	0.0	0.0	0.0	0.0	0.0
0.0	0.0	0.0	0.0	0.0	0.0	0.0	0.0	0.0	0.0	0.0	0.0	0.0	0.0	0.0	0.0
0.3	5.2	21.6	33.5	0.2	5.4	101.4	0.2	21.9	0.1	0.0	0.0	0.0	0.2	0.0	12.2
2.0	13.6	54.8	59.8	1.3	14.1	317.9	0.5	53.1	1.7	3.6	0.3	0.2	2.0	0.1	43.2
0.0	0.0	0.0	0.0	0.0	0.0	3.6	0.0	0.0	0.0	0.0	0.0	0.0	0.0	0.0	0.0
0.5	14.6	0.0	23.0	2.0	86.0	1.0	1.0	3.4	0.0	0.0	0.0	0.1	0.4	0.0	3.0
0.0	0.0	0.0	0.0	0.0	0.0	0.2	0.0	0.0	0.0	0.0	0.0	0.0	0.0	0.0	0.0
0.0	0.0	0.0	5.0	0.0	0.0	0.0	0.0	0.0	0.0	0.0	0.0	0.0	0.0	0.0	0.0
1.8	0.7	0.0	6.9	0.7	26.9	1.1	0.4	0.1	0.0	0.0	0.0	0.0	0.0	0.0	0.0
0.3	0.0	0.0	2.4	0.1	0.9	0.7	0.0	2.0	0.1	0.0	0.0	0.0	0.0	0.0	1.7
0.0	0.0	0.0	4.7	0.0	2.3	112.3	0.1	0.0	0.0	0.0	0.0	0.0	0.0	0.0	0.2
0.0	0.0	0.0	5.4	0.1	2.7	113.4	0.1	0.0	0.0	0.0	0.0	0.0	0.0	0.0	0.0
0.0	0.0	0.0	1.3	0.1	0.4	0.8	0.0	0.0	0.1	0.0	0.0	0.0	0.0	0.0	0.4
0.0	0.0	0.0	0.0	0.0	1.3	15.4	0.0	0.0	0.0	0.0	0.0	0.0	0.0	0.0	0.0
0.1	0.3	0.0	0.0	0.4	0.6	4.3	0.0	0.0	1.6	0.0	0.0	0.0	0.0	0.0	0.1
0.0	0.1	0.0	1.0	0.1	1.0	2.6	0.0	0.0	0.0	0.0	0.0	0.0	0.1	0.0	0.0
0.0	0.0	0.0	0.3	0.0	0.0	1.2	0.0	0.0	0.1	0.0	0.0	0.0	0.2	0.0	1.5
0.5	0.0	0.0	1.0	0.0	0.0	7.0	0.0	0.0	0.0	0.0	0.0	0.0	0.0	0.0	1.0
0.2	0.0	0.0	4.0	0.1	0.8	8.0	0.0	0.2	1.8	0.0	0.0	0.0	0.0	0.0	6.6
0.2	0.0	0.0	1.5	0.0	1.1	6.8	0.0	0.4	0.2	0.0	0.0	0.0	0.0	0.0	0.2
0.5	0.0	0.0	1.0	0.0	0.0	4.0	0.0	0.0	0.0	0.0	0.0	0.0	0.0	0.0	5.0
0.3	0.1	0.0	0.0	0.0	0.0	0.0	0.0	0.0	0.0	0.0	0.0	0.0	0.0	0.0	0.0
0.0	0.0	0.0	7.6	0.0	0.4	11.2	0.0	1.0	1.0	0.0	0.0	0.0	0.0	0.0	7.2
0.0	0.0	0.0	41.0	0.9	48.4	7.4	0.1	0.0	0.0	0.0	0.0	0.0	0.2	0.1	0.0
1.0	0.0	0.0	0.8	0.3	0.1	24.0	0.1	0.0	0.0	0.0	0.0	0.0	0.0	0.0	0.1
0.0	1.6	0.0	58.0	0.0	0.0	13.3	0.0	0.0	0.0	0.0	0.0	0.0	0.0	0.0	0.0
0.0	0.0	0.0	3.9	0.1	1.3	1.8	0.0	0.0	0.0	0.0	0.0	0.0	0.0	0.0	0.0
0.0	0.0	0.0	0.0	0.0	0.0	0.0	0.0	0.0	0.0	0.0	0.0	0.0	0.0	0.0	0.0
0.0	0.1	0.0	25.2	0.5	5.3	3.1	1.7	0.6	0.0	0.0	0.0	0.0	0.0	0.0	0.0
0.0	0.0	0.0	0.0	0.0	0.0	0.0	0.0	0.0	0.0	0.0	0.0	0.0	0.0	0.0	0.0
0.5	1.5	0.3	13.8	0.2	8.7	58.8	0.1	0.7	0.0	0.5	0.0	0.0	0.1	0.0	0.7
0.0	0.0	0.0	3.6	0.1	1.6	31.0	0.0	0.0	0.0	0.0	0.0	0.0	0.0	0.0	0.0
0.0	0.0	0.0	0.6	0.0	0.4	24.2	0.0	0.0	0.0	0.0	0.0	0.0	0.0	0.0	0.0
0.0	0.0	0.0	13.4	0.2	2.8	1.8	0.8	0.0	0.0	0.0	0.0	0.0	0.0	0.0	0.0
0.0	0.0	0.0	0.2	0.0	0.4	16.6	0.0	0.0	0.0	0.0	0.0	0.0	0.0	0.0	0.0
0.0	0.0	0.0	0.6	0.0	0.0	120.0	0.0	0.0	0.0	0.0	0.0	0.0	0.0	0.0	0.0
0.2	0.0	0.2	10.9	0.0	1.4	71.5	0.0	5.5	0.1	0.0	0.0	0.0	0.0	0.0	0.4
0.0	0.1	0.0	0.8	0.1	0.6	13.7	0.0	0.0	0.0	0.0	0.0	0.0	0.0	0.0	0.3
0.4	0.0	0.0	9.2	0.2	0.8	26.5	0.2	0.8	24.6	0.0	0.0	0.0	0.0	0.0	1.3
0.2	0.0	0.0	5.0	0.2	0.8	4.4	0.1	0.4	5.2	0.0	0.0	0.0	0.1	0.0	0.4
0.4	0.1	0.0	1.9	0.0	2.6	24.0	0.0	0.0	0.0	0.0	0.0	0.0	0.0	0.0	0.2
2.0	20.6	57.0	221.0	2.4	71.0	802.0	3.9	147.0	2.0	0.0	0.2	0.1	3.2	0.2	23.0

Code	Food Name	Unit Amount	Kilocalories (kcal)	Protein (g)	Carbohydrate (g)
18386	Toaster muffin, blueberry	1 toaster muffin	103.3	1.5	17.6
918387	Toaster muffin, corn	1 toaster muffin	114.2	1.7	19.1
18493	Toaster pastry, Pop Tart, brown sugar cinnamon/Kellogg	1 pastry	219.0	2.7	32.2
18480	Toaster pastry, Pop Tart, cherry, low-fat/Kellogg	1 pastry	191.9	2.3	39.8
18477	Toaster pastry, Pop Tart, frosted apple cinnamon, low-fat/Kellogg	1 pastry	191.4	2.2	40.0
18479	Toaster pastry, Pop Tart, frosted brown sugar cinnamon, low-fat)/Kellogg	1 pastry	188.0	2.4	39.2
18481	Toaster pastry, Pop Tart, frosted brown sugar cinnamon/Kellogg	1 pastry	211.0	2.5	34.2
18489	Toaster pastry, Pop Tart, frosted strawberry, low-fat/Kellogg	1 pastry	190.8	2.1	40.3
18490	Toaster pastry, Pop Tart, frosted strawberry/Kellogg	1 pastry	202.8	2.3	37.6
11693	Toaster pastry/Pop Tart, fruit (apple/blueberry/cherry/strawberry/Kellogg	1 Pop Tart	204.4	2.4	37.0
18363	Tomato, crushed, canned	1/2 cup	16.0	0.8	3.6
18449	Tortilla, corn, ready-to-cook	1 medium tortilla (6" diam)	57.7	1.5	12.1
18448	Tortilla, toco shell, baked	1 large (6.5" diam)	98.3	1.5	13.1
5600	Tuna Helper	1 serving	301.8	14.4	29.4
924187	Turkey patty, breaded, fried	1 patty	266.0	13.2	14.8
5296	Turkey pot pie, frozen/Swanson	7.0 oz	380.2	10.9	36.1
5295	Turkey roast, light & dark meat, no bone, frozen, seasoned, ckd	3.5 oz	155.0	21.3	3.1
5189	Turkey w/gravy, frozen	1 pkg (5.0 oz)	95.1	8.3	6.5
5293	Turkey, breaded turkey nuggets w/USDA commodity meat, cooked/Pierre product #193	3.5 oz	347.0	18.2	10.2
924210	Turkey, breast w/skin, roasted	3.5 oz	189.0	28.7	0.0
5187	Turkey, dark meat w/skin, roasted	3.5 oz	221.0	27.5	0.0
51619	Turkey, dark meat, no skin, roasted	3.5 oz	187.0	28.6	0.0
5211	Turkey, fryer/roaster, dark meat w/skin, roasted	3.5 oz	182.0	27.7	0.0
5221	Turkey, fryer/roaster, dark meat, no skin, roasted	3.5 oz	162.0	28.8	0.0
5209	Turkey, fryer/roaster, light meat w/skin, roasted	3.5 oz	164.0	28.8	0.0
5201	Turkey, fryer/roaster, light meat, no skin, roasted	3.5 oz	140.0	30.2	0.0
51617	Turkey, fryer/roaster, wing, no skin, roasted	3.5 oz	163.0	30.9	0.0
5305	Turkey, ground, cooked	3.5 oz	235.0	27.4	0.0
5285	Turkey, leg w/skin, roasted	3.5 oz	208.0	27.9	0.0
5181	Turkey, light & dark meat, diced, seasoned	3.5 oz	138.0	18.7	1.0
5185	Turkey, light meat w/skin, roasted	3.5 oz	197.0	28.6	0.0
5165	Turkey, light meat, no skin, roasted	3.5 oz	157.0	29.9	0.0
5294	Turkey, smoked	3.5 oz	118.0	19.6	0.7
5245	Turkey, wing w/skin, roasted	3.5 oz	229.0	27.4	0.0
17089	Veal, breast, whole, boneless, lean, braised	3.5 oz	218.0	30.3	0.0
17138	Veal, sirloin, lean & fat, roasted	6.0 oz	343.4	42.7	0.0
11886	Vege juice, carrot, canned	6.0 oz	73.6	1.7	17.1
11001	Vege juice, tomato, canned w/o salt	6.0 oz	31.3	1.4	7.8
11004	Vege, alfalfa seeds, sprouted, raw	1 cup	9.6	1.3	1.2
11009	Vege, artichokes (globe or French) boiled, drained, no salt	1 medium	150.0	10.4	33.5
11705	Vege, arugula/roquette, raw	1 cup	5.0	0.5	0.7
11015	Vege, asparagus, boiled, drained	1/2 cup	21.6	2.3	3.8
11707	Vege, asparagus, canned, drained	1/2 cup	17.1	1.9	2.2
11011	Vege, asparagus, frozen, boiled, drained, no salt	4 spears	16.8	1.8	2.9
11028	Vege, bamboo shoots, canned, drained	1/2 cup	7.2	0.9	1.2
11045	Vege, bean sprouts, mung, mature seeds, sprouted, stir fried	1/2 cup	3.6	0.4	0.6
11046	Vege, bean sprouts, navy, mature seeds, sprouted, raw	1 cup	93.6	8.5	18.0
11052	Vege, beans, snap, green, raw	1 cup	35.0	1.9	8.1
11722	Vege, beans, snap, yellow, raw	1 cup	37.8	2.0	8.7
11081	Vege, beets, boiled, drained	1/2 cup	37.4	1.4	8.5
11090	Vege, broccoli florets, raw	1 cup	63.4	4.9	10.3
22600	Vege, broccoli in cheese-flavored sauce, frozen/Green Giant	1/2 cup	39.8	4.2	7.4
11095	Vege, broccoli spears, frozen, boiled, drained, no salt	1/2 cup	21.8	2.4	4.2
11093	Vege, broccoli, chopped, frozen, boiled, drained, no salt	1/2 cup	23.5	2.6	4.5
11099	Vege, Brussels sprouts, boiled, drained, no salt	1/2 cup, 4 sprouts	32.0	2.0	6.8
11110	Vege, cabbage, boiled, drained, no salt	1/2 cup	13.2	0.6	2.7
11749	Vege, cabbage, common (Danish/domestic/pointed) fresh harvest, raw	1 cup	15.4	0.7	3.1
11970	Vege, cabbage, Napa, cooked	1/2 cup	8.4	0.4	1.9
11960	Vege, carrots, baby, raw	1 cup or 6 baby carrots	28.0	1.0	6.8
11128	Vege, carrots, canned, drained	1/2 cup	32.9	0.8	7.7
11131	Vege, carrots, frozen, boiled, drained, no salt	1/2 cup	26.3	0.9	6.0
11136	Vege, cauliflower, boiled, drained, no salt	1/2 cup	14.3	1.1	2.5
11138	Vege, cauliflower, frozen, boiled, drained, no salt	1/2 cup	11.8	1.0	2.3
11967	Vege, cauliflower, green, cooked, no salt	1/2 cup	28.8	2.7	5.7
11965	Vege, cauliflower, green, head, raw	1 cup	32.0	3.0	6.3

Dietary Fiber (g)	Total Fat (g)	Cholesterol (mg)	Calcium (mg)	Iron (mg)	Magnesium (mg)	Sodium (mg)	Zinc (mg)	Vitamin A (µgRE)	Vitamin C (mg)	Vitamin E (mg αT)	Thiamin (mg)	Riboflavin (mg)	Niacin (mg)	Vitamin B$_6$ (mg)	Folate (µg)
0.6	3.1	2.0	4.3	0.2	4.0	157.7	0.1	22.1	0.0	0.6	0.1	0.1	0.7	0.0	18.2
0.5	3.7	4.3	6.3	0.5	4.6	141.9	0.1	6.6	0.0	0.0	0.1	0.1	0.8	0.0	18.8
0.8	9.2	0.0	15.5	1.8	8.0	214.0	0.6	0.0	0.0	0.0	0.2	0.2	2.0	0.2	40.0
0.6	2.9	0.0	5.7	1.8	4.7	221.5	0.2	0.0	0.0	0.0	0.2	0.2	2.0	0.2	52.0
0.6	2.9	0.0	5.7	1.8	4.7	205.9	0.2	0.0	0.0	0.0	0.2	0.2	2.0	0.2	52.0
0.6	2.8	0.0	7.0	1.8	5.0	209.5	0.2	0.0	0.0	0.0	0.2	0.2	2.0	0.2	50.0
0.7	7.4	0.0	14.5	1.8	7.5	184.5	1.2	0.0	0.0	0.0	0.2	0.2	2.0	0.2	40.0
0.6	3.0	0.0	5.2	1.8	4.2	201.2	0.2	0.0	0.0	0.0	0.2	0.2	2.0	0.2	52.0
0.5	5.0	0.0	11.4	1.8	5.2	169.0	0.2	0.0	0.0	0.0	0.2	0.2	2.0	0.2	52.0
1.1	5.3	0.0	13.5	1.8	9.4	217.9	0.3	1.6	0.3	1.2	0.2	0.2	2.0	0.2	33.8
1.0	0.1	0.0	17.0	0.7	10.0	66.0	0.1	35.0	4.6	0.3	0.0	0.0	0.6	0.1	6.5
1.4	0.7	0.0	45.5	0.4	16.9	41.9	0.2	0.0	0.0	0.0	0.0	0.0	0.4	0.1	29.6
1.6	4.7	0.0	33.6	0.5	22.1	77.1	0.3	0.0	0.0	0.8	0.0	0.0	0.3	0.1	22.1
0.0	14.0	0.0	0.0	0.0	0.0	916.0	0.0	0.0	0.0	0.0	0.0	0.0	0.0	0.0	0.0
0.5	16.9	58.3	13.2	2.1	14.1	752.0	1.4	10.3	0.0	2.2	0.1	0.2	2.2	0.2	26.3
0.0	21.4	0.0	29.0	2.4	0.0	719.0	0.0	393.4	2.0	0.0	0.3	0.2	3.1	0.0	0.0
0.0	5.8	53.0	5.0	1.6	22.0	680.0	2.5	0.0	0.0	0.4	0.0	0.2	6.3	0.3	5.0
0.0	3.7	25.6	19.9	1.3	11.4	786.7	1.0	18.5	0.0	0.0	0.0	0.2	2.6	0.1	5.7
0.3	25.8	57.0	28.0	1.9	15.0	567.0	1.9	0.0	0.0	2.8	0.2	0.2	4.3	0.2	22.0
0.0	7.4	74.0	21.0	1.4	27.0	63.0	2.0	0.0	0.0	0.0	0.1	0.1	6.4	0.5	6.0
0.0	11.5	89.0	33.0	2.3	23.0	76.0	4.2	0.0	0.0	0.6	0.1	0.2	3.5	0.3	9.0
0.0	7.2	85.0	32.0	2.3	24.0	79.0	4.5	0.0	0.0	0.6	0.1	0.2	3.6	0.4	9.0
0.0	7.1	117.0	27.0	2.3	23.0	76.0	3.8	0.0	0.0	0.0	0.0	0.2	3.4	0.3	9.0
0.0	4.3	112.0	26.0	2.4	24.0	79.0	4.1	0.0	0.0	0.0	0.1	0.2	3.5	0.4	10.0
0.0	4.6	95.0	18.0	1.6	26.0	57.0	2.1	0.0	0.0	0.0	0.0	0.1	6.3	0.5	6.0
0.0	1.2	86.0	15.0	1.6	28.0	56.0	2.1	0.0	0.0	0.0	0.0	0.1	6.9	0.6	6.0
0.0	3.4	102.0	26.0	1.8	22.0	78.0	3.8	0.0	0.0	0.1	0.0	0.2	4.1	0.6	7.0
0.0	13.2	102.0	25.0	1.9	24.0	107.0	2.9	0.0	0.0	0.3	0.1	0.2	4.8	0.4	7.0
0.0	9.8	85.0	32.0	2.3	23.0	77.0	4.3	0.0	0.0	0.6	0.1	0.2	3.6	0.3	9.0
0.0	6.0	55.0	1.0	1.8	17.0	850.0	2.0	0.0	0.0	0.0	0.0	0.1	4.8	0.3	5.0
0.0	8.3	76.0	21.0	1.4	26.0	63.0	2.0	0.0	0.0	0.1	0.1	0.1	6.3	0.5	6.0
0.0	3.2	69.0	19.0	1.4	28.0	64.0	2.0	0.0	0.0	0.1	0.1	0.1	6.8	0.5	6.0
0.0	3.9	42.9	7.1	0.5	92.9	996.4	1.9	0.0	0.0	0.0	0.0	0.1	3.6	0.4	0.0
0.0	12.4	81.0	24.0	1.5	25.0	61.0	2.1	0.0	0.0	0.2	0.1	0.1	5.7	0.4	6.0
0.0	9.8	116.0	9.0	0.8	22.0	68.0	4.2	0.0	0.0	0.4	0.1	0.3	9.0	0.3	15.0
0.0	17.8	173.4	22.1	1.6	44.2	141.1	5.7	0.0	0.0	0.7	0.1	0.6	15.1	0.5	25.5
1.5	0.3	0.0	44.2	0.8	25.8	53.4	0.3	2014.8	15.6	0.0	0.2	0.1	0.7	0.4	7.0
1.5	0.1	0.0	16.6	1.1	20.2	18.4	0.3	103.0	33.7	1.7	0.1	0.1	1.2	0.2	36.6
0.8	0.2	0.0	10.6	0.3	8.9	2.0	0.3	5.3	2.7	0.0	0.0	0.0	0.2	0.0	11.9
16.2	0.5	0.0	135.0	3.9	180.0	285.0	1.5	54.0	30.0	0.6	0.2	0.2	3.0	0.3	153.0
0.3	0.1	0.0	32.0	0.3	9.4	5.4	0.1	47.4	3.0	0.1	0.0	0.0	0.1	0.0	19.4
1.4	0.3	0.0	18.0	0.7	9.0	9.9	0.4	48.6	9.7	0.3	0.1	0.1	1.0	0.1	131.4
1.4	0.6	0.0	14.4	1.6	9.0	258.3	0.4	47.7	16.6	0.4	0.1	0.1	0.9	0.1	86.0
1.0	0.3	0.0	13.8	0.4	7.8	2.4	0.3	49.2	14.6	0.8	0.0	0.1	0.6	0.0	80.8
0.6	0.1	0.0	7.2	0.1	1.8	2.4	0.3	0.0	0.0	0.0	0.0	0.0	0.2	0.1	1.4
0.2	0.0	0.0	4.2	0.1	2.7	42.0	0.1	0.6	0.1	0.0	0.0	0.0	0.1	0.0	2.9
0.0	1.0	0.0	19.2	2.5	133.2	16.8	1.2	0.0	20.8	0.0	0.5	0.3	1.5	0.2	127.6
3.8	0.2	0.0	61.3	1.1	30.0	11.3	0.6	50.0	5.1	0.2	0.0	0.1	0.5	0.1	28.8
4.1	0.2	0.0	66.2	1.2	32.4	12.2	0.6	14.9	5.5	0.2	0.0	0.1	0.5	0.1	31.1
1.7	0.2	0.0	13.6	0.7	19.6	242.3	0.3	3.4	3.1	0.0	0.0	0.0	0.3	0.1	68.0
3.7	0.5	0.0	19.4	1.7	33.4	44.0	0.5	30.8	29.0	0.0	0.1	0.1	1.3	0.0	84.7
0.0	0.5	0.0	68.2	1.2	35.5	38.3	0.6	426.0	132.3	2.4	0.1	0.2	0.9	0.2	100.8
2.3	0.1	0.0	39.8	0.5	15.6	202.8	0.2	147.4	31.3	1.3	0.0	0.1	0.4	0.1	23.4
2.5	0.1	0.0	42.8	0.5	16.8	218.4	0.3	158.3	33.7	1.4	0.0	0.1	0.4	0.1	47.4
2.0	0.4	0.0	28.1	0.9	15.6	200.5	0.3	56.2	48.4	0.0	0.1	0.1	0.5	0.1	46.8
1.7	0.3	0.0	18.6	0.1	4.8	153.0	0.1	7.8	12.1	0.0	0.0	0.0	0.2	0.1	12.0
1.6	0.3	0.0	21.7	0.1	5.6	5.6	0.1	9.1	14.1	0.1	0.0	0.0	0.2	0.1	14.0
0.8	0.1	0.0	16.5	0.2	5.3	6.3	0.1	4.6	14.7	0.0	0.0	0.0	0.1	0.0	19.8
2.2	0.1	0.0	98.0	1.0	58.8	238.0	0.2	16.8	2.8	0.0	0.0	0.0	0.4	0.1	39.6
2.4	0.1	0.0	22.6	0.5	9.5	48.2	0.2	1792.2	1.7	0.3	0.0	0.0	0.4	0.2	10.1
2.6	0.1	0.0	20.4	0.3	7.3	215.4	0.2	1292.1	2.0	0.0	0.0	0.0	0.3	0.1	7.9
1.7	0.3	0.0	9.9	0.2	5.6	150.0	0.1	1.2	27.5	0.0	0.0	0.0	0.3	0.1	27.3
1.7	0.1	0.0	10.5	0.3	5.6	157.5	0.1	1.2	19.4	0.0	0.0	0.0	0.2	0.1	25.4
3.0	0.3	0.0	28.8	0.6	17.1	233.1	0.6	12.6	65.3	0.0	0.1	0.1	0.6	0.2	36.9
3.3	0.3	0.0	32.0	0.7	19.0	23.0	0.6	14.0	72.6	0.0	0.1	0.1	0.7	0.2	41.0

Code	Food Name	Unit Amount	Kilocalories (kcal)	Protein (g)	Carbohydrate (g)
11142	Vege, celeriac, boiled, drained, no salt	1/2 cup	27.0	1.0	5.9
11143	Vege, celery, raw	1/2 cup or 2 stalks	14.4	0.7	3.2
11148	Vege, chard, Swiss, boiled, drained, no salt	1/2 cup	17.6	1.7	3.6
11162	Vege, collards, boiled, drained, no salt	1/2 cup	19.2	1.6	3.6
11656	Vege, corn pudding, homemade	1 cup	232.5	7.8	55.8
11190	Vege, corn salad, raw	2/3 cup (#6 scoop)	182.0	7.3	21.3
11774	Vege, corn, yellow, kernels, frozen, boiled w/salt, drained	1/2 cup	52.5	1.6	12.6
11771	Vege, corn, yellow, sweet, canned, solids & liquid, no added salt	1/2 cup	88.6	2.1	22.3
11174	Vege, corn, yellow, sweet, cream-style, regular pack, canned	1/2 cup	83.0	2.5	20.4
11179	Vege, corn, yellow, sweet, kernels, frozen, boiled, drained, no salt	1/2 cup	73.9	2.5	17.5
11172	Vege, corn, yellow, sweet, whole kernel, canned, drained	1/2 cup	67.2	2.3	16.4
11192	Vege, cowpeas (blackeyes), immature seeds, boiled, drained, no salt	1/2 cup	81.5	2.7	17.1
11205	Vege, cucumber, raw	1 cup	4.8	0.2	1.0
11210	Vege, eggplant (Brinjal) boiled, drained, no salt	1/2 cup, 1" cubes	27.7	0.8	6.6
11213	Vege, endive (escarole) raw	1 Tbsp., 1" pieces	1.3	0.1	0.3
11957	Vege, fennel bulb, raw	1 cup	150.0	4.6	31.7
11950	Vege, fungi, mushroom, enoki, raw	1 cup	79.5	2.6	20.4
11987	Vege, fungi, mushroom, oyster, raw	1 medium: 3.35" long	1.0	0.1	0.2
11269	Vege, fungi, mushroom, shiitake, ckd, no salt	1/2 cup, 4 mushrooms	39.6	1.1	10.3
11261	Vege, fungi, mushrooms, boiled, drained, no salt	1 mushroom	3.2	0.3	0.6
11260	Vege, fungi, mushrooms, slices, raw	10 slices	9.6	0.7	2.0
924135	Vege, green pepper, stuffed, homemade	1 pepper	172.1	10.4	32.0
11961	Vege, hearts of palm, canned	1/2 cup	122.4	9.4	12.1
11971	Vege, herb, cilantro, raw	1 Tbsp., chopped	2.3	0.2	0.4
11234	Vege, kale, boiled, drained, no salt	1/2 cup	18.2	1.2	3.7
11242	Vege, kohlrabi, boiled, drained, no salt	1/2 cup	24.7	1.5	5.7
11245	Vege, lambsquarters, boiled, drained, no salt	1 Tbsp., chopped	3.6	0.4	0.6
11246	Vege, leeks (bulb & lower-leaf portion) raw	1 leek	38.4	1.0	9.4
11250	Vege, lettuce, butterhead (Boston/bibb) leaves, raw	3.5 grams	101.0	8.8	21.3
11251	Vege, lettuce, cos/romaine, raw	1 small leaf	0.7	0.1	0.1
11252	Vege, lettuce, iceberg, head, raw	1 inner leaf	1.4	0.2	0.2
11253	Vege, lettuce, looseleaf, raw	1 small head	38.9	3.3	6.8
11796	Vege, lotus root, boiled w/salt, drained	1 cup, shredded	10.1	0.7	2.0
11974	Vege, mushrooms, sauteed	1 Tbsp., cubes	7.5	0.2	1.8
11805	Vege, onions, boiled w/salt, chopped, drained	1 ring	40.7	0.5	3.8
11282	Vege, onions, chopped, raw	1 Tbsp., chopped	4.2	0.1	1.0
11291	Vege, onions, spring (tops & bulb) chopped, raw	1 Tbsp.	17.5	0.4	4.2
11298	Vege, parsnip, peeled, raw	1 cup, slices	61.6	1.0	14.8
11318	Vege, peas & carrots, canned, regular pack, solids & liquid	1/2 cup	92.2	5.6	17.0
11323	Vege, peas & carrots, frozen, boiled, drained, no salt	1/2 cup	38.4	2.5	8.1
11301	Vege, peas w/edible pod—snow/sugar, boiled, drained, no salt	1/2 cup	33.6	2.6	5.6
11305	Vege, peas, green, boiled, drained, no salt	1/2 cup	67.2	4.3	12.5
11308	Vege, peas, green, canned, regular pack, drained	1/2 cup	58.7	3.8	10.7
11980	Vege, pepper, chili, green, canned	1/2 cup	16.7	1.0	3.3
11670	Vege, pepper, hot chili, raw	1/2 cup	14.7	0.5	3.2
11632	Vege, pepper, jalapeno, canned, solids & liquid	1 pepper	7.8	0.2	1.8
11979	Vege, pepper, jalapeno, raw	1/2 cup chopped	23.0	0.8	4.0
11333	Vege, pepper, sweet, green, chopped/sliced, raw	3.5 oz	18.0	1.0	3.9
11821	Vege, pepper, sweet, red, raw	3.5 oz	18.0	1.0	3.9
11951	Vege, pepper, sweet, yellow, raw	1 Tbsp.	2.5	0.1	0.6
11973	Vege, pickles, bread & butter	10 strips	14.0	0.5	3.3
11937	Vege, pickles, cucumber, dill	2 slices	13.2	1.2	2.6
11941	Vege, pickles, cucumber, sour, slices/spears	1 large (4" long)	14.9	0.4	3.0
11940	Vege, pickles, cucumber, sweet, gherkins	1 large gherkin (3" long)	3.9	0.1	0.8
11970	Vege, pickles, fresh pack	1 medium	41.0	0.1	11.1
11975	Vege, pickles, kosher	2 slices	1.8	0.2	0.3
11976	Vege, pickles, sweet & sour	1.0 oz	6.7	0.6	1.2
11383	Vege, potato, mashed, granules w/milk, prep w/water & margarine	1/2 cup	358.0	10.9	77.7
11672	Vege, potato pancakes, homemade	1/2 cup	83.0	2.1	13.8
11414	Vege, potato salad, homemade	1 cup	284.2	4.3	39.0
11410	Vege, potato wedges, frozen, USDA Commodity	1 cup	357.5	6.7	27.9
11385	Vege, potato, au gratin, mix, prep w/H2O, whole milk & butter	1/6 of 5.5-oz package	81.6	2.3	19.3
11376	Vege, potato, canned, drained	1 potato (2.5" diam)	116.1	2.3	27.0
11675	Vege, potato, flesh & skin, cooked in microwave, no salt	1/2 cup of whole potatoes	66.0	1.8	14.8
11674	Vege, potato, flesh & skin, baked, no salt	1 potato: 2.33" x 4.75"	220.2	4.6	51.0

Dietary Fiber (g)	Total Fat (g)	Cholesterol (mg)	Calcium (mg)	Iron (mg)	Magnesium (mg)	Sodium (mg)	Zinc (mg)	Vitamin A (μgRE)	Vitamin C (mg)	Vitamin E (mgαT)	Thiamin (mg)	Riboflavin (mg)	Niacin (mg)	Vitamin B6 (mg)	Folate (μg)
0.0	0.2	0.0	26.0	0.4	12.0	297.0	0.2	0.0	3.6	0.0	0.0	0.0	0.4	0.1	3.4
1.3	0.1	0.0	33.6	0.3	9.6	72.8	0.1	10.4	4.9	0.3	0.0	0.0	0.3	0.1	17.6
1.8	0.1	0.0	51.0	2.0	75.7	365.2	0.3	276.3	15.8	0.0	0.0	0.1	0.3	0.1	7.6
2.1	0.3	0.0	88.1	0.3	12.6	186.5	0.3	231.6	13.5	0.7	0.0	0.1	0.4	0.1	68.8
7.0	1.9	0.0	7.5	1.5	72.5	10.0	1.6	52.5	12.0	0.0	0.4	0.2	3.8	0.6	76.3
0.0	8.9	167.0	66.8	0.9	25.1	91.9	0.8	60.1	4.7	0.0	0.7	0.2	1.6	0.2	42.3
1.4	0.4	0.0	3.3	0.3	13.1	174.7	0.3	0.0	4.5	0.0	0.0	0.1	0.8	0.1	31.2
1.5	0.5	0.0	3.7	0.5	20.9	3.7	0.7	12.3	5.7	0.1	0.0	0.1	1.2	0.1	55.1
2.1	0.5	0.0	5.3	0.4	24.2	285.6	0.5	25.2	8.5	0.1	0.0	0.1	1.2	0.1	51.8
2.0	0.6	0.0	3.4	0.4	15.1	2.5	0.3	10.9	5.4	0.0	0.1	0.1	1.4	0.1	30.0
2.0	0.4	0.0	3.4	0.3	16.0	4.2	0.3	18.5	2.6	0.1	0.1	0.1	1.1	0.1	26.0
4.2	0.3	0.0	107.5	0.9	43.7	201.6	0.9	66.4	1.8	0.0	0.1	0.1	1.2	0.1	106.7
0.3	0.1	0.0	5.6	0.1	4.8	0.8	0.1	2.8	1.1	0.0	0.0	0.0	0.0	0.0	5.6
2.5	0.2	0.0	5.9	0.3	12.9	236.6	0.1	5.9	1.3	0.0	0.1	0.0	0.6	0.1	14.3
0.1	0.0	0.0	0.4	0.0	0.7	0.2	0.1	0.4	0.1	0.0	0.0	0.0	0.0	0.0	1.0
0.0	1.8	0.0	110.0	1.2	32.0	12.0	1.2	0.0	13.0	0.0	0.1	0.1	0.3	0.2	24.3
19.6	0.2	0.0	44.5	1.6	23.2	9.8	0.4	0.0	0.0	0.0	0.0	0.2	1.8	0.0	10.6
0.1	0.0	0.0	0.0	0.0	0.5	0.1	0.0	0.0	0.4	0.0	0.0	0.0	0.1	0.0	0.9
1.5	0.2	0.0	2.2	0.3	10.1	172.8	1.0	0.0	0.2	0.0	0.0	0.1	1.1	0.1	15.0
0.3	0.1	0.0	0.7	0.2	1.4	28.6	0.1	0.0	0.5	0.0	0.0	0.0	0.5	0.0	2.2
1.0	0.1	0.0	4.4	0.3	6.0	170.0	0.3	0.0	0.0	0.0	0.0	0.0	0.6	0.0	4.9
20.4	3.9	0.0	671.6	4.9	175.8	16.7	1.2	4993.2	20.5	3.7	0.1	0.7	4.4	0.7	153.6
0.4	4.0	0.0	30.4	1.5	0.0	226.1	0.0	40.5	28.8	0.0	0.1	0.3	1.8	0.0	0.0
0.2	0.1	0.0	4.7	0.3	3.1	34.5	0.1	0.0	0.6	0.0	0.0	0.0	0.0	0.0	3.2
1.3	0.3	0.0	46.8	0.6	11.7	168.4	0.2	481.0	26.7	0.0	0.0	0.0	0.3	0.0	8.6
0.9	0.1	0.0	21.3	0.3	16.2	218.5	0.3	3.4	45.9	0.0	0.0	0.0	0.3	0.1	10.3
0.2	0.1	0.0	29.2	0.1	2.6	29.9	0.0	109.6	4.2	0.0	0.0	0.0	0.1	0.0	1.5
1.2	0.2	0.0	37.2	1.4	17.4	12.4	0.1	6.2	5.2	0.0	0.0	0.0	0.2	0.1	30.1
0.0	0.5	0.0	14.0	3.1	35.0	10.0	1.6	4.0	12.6	0.0	0.2	0.1	1.2	0.2	67.0
0.1	0.0	0.0	1.6	0.0	0.7	0.3	0.0	4.9	0.4	0.0	0.0	0.0	0.0	0.0	3.7
0.2	0.0	0.0	3.6	0.1	0.6	0.8	0.0	26.0	2.4	0.0	0.0	0.0	0.1	0.0	13.6
4.5	0.6	0.0	61.6	1.6	29.2	29.2	0.7	106.9	12.6	0.9	0.1	0.1	0.6	0.1	181.4
1.1	0.2	0.0	38.1	0.8	6.2	5.0	0.2	106.4	10.1	0.2	0.0	0.0	0.2	0.0	27.9
0.0	0.0	0.0	0.7	0.0	0.9	1.1	0.0	0.0	0.0	0.0	0.0	0.0	0.0	0.0	1.1
0.1	2.7	0.0	3.1	0.2	1.9	37.5	0.0	2.3	0.1	0.0	0.0	0.0	0.4	0.0	6.6
0.3	0.0	0.0	2.4	0.0	0.9	1.8	0.0	0.5	0.4	0.0	0.0	0.0	0.0	0.0	2.0
0.5	0.0	0.0	12.9	0.1	4.6	1.1	0.1	0.0	3.8	0.1	0.0	0.0	0.0	0.1	8.3
3.0	0.2	0.0	28.1	0.4	22.0	7.6	0.2	0.0	9.9	0.8	0.1	0.0	0.6	0.1	44.2
5.6	0.5	0.0	31.3	1.8	29.6	15.7	1.2	66.1	17.1	0.7	0.2	0.1	1.5	0.1	49.6
2.5	0.3	0.0	18.4	0.8	12.8	243.2	0.4	620.8	6.5	0.0	0.2	0.1	0.9	0.1	20.8
2.2	0.2	0.0	33.6	1.6	20.8	192.0	0.3	10.4	38.3	0.0	0.1	0.1	0.4	0.1	23.3
4.4	0.2	0.0	21.6	1.2	31.2	191.2	1.0	48.0	11.4	0.0	0.2	0.1	1.6	0.2	50.6
3.5	0.3	0.0	17.0	0.8	14.5	1.7	0.6	65.5	8.2	0.3	0.1	0.1	0.6	0.1	37.7
2.1	0.3	0.0	8.7	0.3	10.5	8.1	0.2	21.1	51.3	0.4	0.1	0.0	0.8	0.2	18.0
1.2	0.2	0.0	25.2	0.9	2.8	277.9	0.1	9.1	23.9	0.0	0.0	0.0	0.4	0.1	37.8
0.0	0.1	0.0	3.2	0.1	4.3	0.3	0.1	3.8	25.1	0.0	0.0	0.0	0.3	0.1	14.3
2.2	0.8	0.0	19.6	1.6	12.8	1420.4	0.3	144.5	8.5	0.6	0.0	0.0	0.3	0.2	11.9
0.9	0.2	0.0	8.0	0.5	7.0	4.0	0.1	29.0	41.2	0.0	0.1	0.0	1.1	0.1	9.9
0.0	0.2	0.0	8.0	0.5	7.0	4.0	0.1	334.0	41.2	0.0	0.1	0.0	1.1	0.1	9.9
0.2	0.0	0.0	0.8	0.0	0.9	0.2	0.0	53.0	17.7	0.0	0.0	0.0	0.0	0.0	2.0
0.5	0.1	0.0	5.7	0.2	6.2	1.0	0.1	12.5	95.4	0.0	0.0	0.0	0.5	0.1	13.5
0.0	0.1	0.0	5.6	0.2	5.0	3.8	0.2	5.0	0.6	0.0	0.0	0.0	0.3	0.0	22.2
1.6	0.3	0.0	0.0	0.5	5.4	24.3	0.0	20.3	1.4	0.1	0.0	0.0	0.0	0.0	1.0
0.4	0.1	0.0	0.0	0.1	1.4	422.8	0.0	5.3	0.4	0.1	0.0	0.0	0.0	0.0	0.2
0.4	0.1	0.0	1.4	0.2	1.4	6.3	0.0	4.6	0.4	0.1	0.0	0.0	0.1	0.0	0.4
0.0	0.0	0.0	4.4	0.1	1.2	1.7	0.6	1.4	0.5	0.0	0.0	0.0	0.1	0.0	6.5
0.8	0.1	0.0	18.8	0.5	7.3	15.1	0.0	171.6	9.9	0.6	0.0	0.1	0.4	0.0	17.4
0.0	1.1	2.0	142.0	3.5	74.0	82.0	1.2	9.0	16.0	0.0	0.2	0.3	4.2	0.9	29.9
1.9	2.3	2.1	32.6	0.6	16.8	245.7	0.3	13.7	3.2	0.0	0.0	0.1	0.8	0.2	7.5
4.1	13.7	0.0	38.4	2.0	24.3	954.9	0.4	2.6	8.8	0.1	0.3	0.1	2.8	0.3	21.1
3.3	20.5	170.0	47.5	1.6	37.5	1322.5	0.8	82.5	25.0	0.0	0.2	0.2	2.2	0.4	16.8
1.1	1.0	0.0	80.9	0.4	16.6	544.7	0.2	18.7	4.0	0.0	0.0	0.1	1.1	0.0	10.5
2.7	0.1	0.0	10.8	0.4	27.0	325.4	0.4	0.0	10.0	0.1	0.1	0.0	1.8	0.4	12.0
2.1	0.2	0.0	58.5	1.1	21.0	325.5	0.6	0.0	11.4	0.1	0.1	0.0	1.3	0.2	6.8
4.8	0.2	0.0	20.2	2.7	54.5	492.9	0.6	0.0	26.1	0.0	0.2	0.1	3.3	0.7	22.2

Code	Food Name	Unit Amount	Kilocalories (kcal)	Protein (g)	Carbohydrate (g)
11363	Vege, potato, flesh only, baked, no salt	1 potato: 2.33" x 4.75"	145.1	3.1	33.6
11365	Vege, potato, flesh only, boiled in skin, no salt	1 potato (2.5" diam)	118.3	2.5	27.4
11367	Vege, potato, flesh only, boiled w/o skin, no salt	1 potato (2.5" diam)	118.3	2.5	27.4
911405	Vege, potato, French fries, frozen, fried in oil & lard	10 strips	101.4	1.6	15.8
11403	Vege, potato, French fries, frozen, oven-heated, no salt	10 strips	157.5	2.0	19.8
11391	Vege, potato, hashed brown, plain, frozen, cooked	4.0 oz	94.3	2.4	20.4
11930	Vege, potato, mashed, dried flakes w/o milk, prep w/whole milk & margarine	1/2 cup	118.7	2.0	15.8
11371	Vege, potato, mashed, homemade w/milk & margarine	1/2 cup	113.4	2.2	15.1
11396	Vege, potato, O'Brien, frozen	1/2 cup	111.3	2.0	17.5
11387	Vege, potato, scalloped, mix, prep w/H$_2$O, whole milk & butter	1/6 of 5.5-oz package	93.1	2.0	19.2
11364	Vege, potato, skin only, baked, no salt	skin from 1 potato: 2.33" x 4.75"	114.8	2.5	26.7
11401	Vege, potato, whole, frozen, boiled, drained, no salt	3.5 oz	65.0	2.0	14.5
11426	Vege, pumpkin pie mix, canned	1/2 cup	7.4	1.2	0.9
11424	Vege, pumpkin, canned, no salt	1/2 cup	41.5	1.3	9.9
11952	Vege, radicchio, raw	1 cup	6.9	0.6	1.5
11676	Vege, radish sprouts, raw	1 cup, shredded	9.2	0.6	1.8
11430	Vege, radish, Oriental (Daikon) raw	1 cup	314.4	9.2	73.5
11439	Vege, sauerkraut, canned, solids & liquid	1 cup, slices	109.1	4.4	24.7
11677	Vege, shallots, peeled, raw	1/4 cup	12.5	0.4	2.9
11452	Vege, soybean sprouts, mature seeds, sprouted, raw	3.5 oz	72.0	2.5	16.8
11853	Vege, soybeans, green, boiled w/salt, drained	1/2 cup	38.1	4.0	3.1
11461	Vege, spinach, canned, drained	1/2 cup	13.8	1.8	2.3
11463	Vege, spinach, chopped or leaf, frozen	1/2 cup	22.2	2.5	3.4
11457	Vege, spinach, raw	10-oz package	61.6	6.9	11.7
11484	Vege, squash, acorn, boiled, drained, no salt	1 cup	6.6	0.9	1.1
11486	Vege, squash, butternut, baked, no salt	1 cup	12.0	0.3	3.1
11493	Vege, squash, spaghetti, boiled or baked, drained, no salt	1 cup, cubes	55.4	1.4	13.2
11642	Vege, squash, summer, all varieties, boiled, drained, no salt	1/2 cup	15.4	0.7	3.3
11641	Vege, squash, summer, all varieties, slices, raw	1/2 cup	18.0	0.8	3.9
11644	Vege, squash, winter, all varieties, baked, no salt	1/2 cup	74.1	1.7	16.6
11872	Vege, succotash (corn & lima beans) frozen, boiled w/salt, drained	1 large: 3.12" x 0.6"	18.4	0.8	3.9
11508	Vege, sweet potato, baked in skin, no salt	1/2 cup	98.9	1.7	23.3
11659	Vege, sweet potato, candied, homemade	1/2 cup	172.2	2.7	39.8
11647	Vege, sweet potato, canned w/syrup, drained	1/2 cup	224.7	1.4	45.7
11954	Vege, tomatillos, raw	1 can (No. 3 vacuum/404x307)	280.7	26.5	43.7
11540	Vege, tomato juice, canned, w/salt	1/2 cup, sliced	21.8	0.7	4.0
11887	Vege, tomato paste, canned w/salt	1/2 cup, chopped	11.4	0.5	2.8
11888	Vege, tomato puree, canned w/salt	1/2 cup	395.6	16.9	97.8
11549	Vege, tomato sauce, canned	1/2 cup	39.4	1.6	8.7
11533	Vege, tomato, red, canned, stewed	1 slice or wedge	3.2	0.2	0.6
11531	Vege, tomato, red, canned, whole	1 tomato	31.1	1.1	7.5
11883	Vege, tomato, red, cherry, ripe, raw, Jun-Oct	1/2 cup	23.4	1.1	5.4
11660	Vege, tomato, red, ripe, stewed	1 Tbsp.	4.1	0.2	0.9
11885	Vege, tomato, red, ripe, whole, canned, no added salt	1 medium	97.2	2.4	16.1
11529	Vege, tomato, red, ripe, whole, raw	yield from recipe	114.8	5.6	26.4
11537	Vege, tomato, red, w/green chilies, canned	1/2 cup	25.8	1.0	5.7
11955	Vege, tomato, sun-dried	1/2 cup	32.0	1.0	7.8
11956	Vege, tomato, sun-dried, oil packed, drained	1 cup	673.4	36.8	145.5
11565	Vege, turnip, boiled, drained, no salt	1 piece	0.6	0.0	0.1
11590	Vege, water chestnut, Chinese, canned, solids & liquid	10-oz package, mashed	309.6	13.6	66.9
11578	Vegetable juice cocktail, canned	3.5 oz	48.0	0.6	11.0
11159	Vegetable salad, cole slaw, homemade	1 cup	48.2	1.7	10.2
11581	Vegetables, mixed, canned, drained solids	1/2 cup	41.4	0.8	7.4
924281	Vegetarian manicotti	10-oz package	162.3	7.9	36.0
22246	Vegetarian, beef stew, canned entree/Nestle Chef-Mate	1 serving	190.3	14.0	21.0
22121	Vegetarian, Better'n Burgers/Vegan Burgers, frozen/Worthington, Morningstar	1 patty	28.9	2.3	2.9
22126	Vegetarian, Big Franks, meatless, frozen/Worthingfoods, Loma Linda	1 patty	91.0	13.9	7.5
22122	Vegetarian, Breakfast Patties/Worthington, Morningstar	1 patty	88.2	9.0	1.1
22363	Vegetarian, Breakfast Stuff-Its, egg & cheese pockets, frozen/SunnyFresh	1 patty	79.4	9.9	3.7
22120	Vegetarian, Burger Crumbles/Worthington, Morningstar	1 serving	147.2	6.8	14.7
924269	Vegetarian, Chili Mac/Worthington	1 cup	231.0	22.2	6.6
22215	Vegetarian, chili w/beans, canned entree/Nestle Chef-Mate	1 cup	316.8	11.5	22.9
924060	Vegetarian, chili w/beans/Worthington	1 cup	412.4	17.7	29.0
22216	Vegetarian, chili w/o beans, canned entree/Nestle Chef-Mate	1 cup	323.4	14.1	20.6
22217	Vegetarian, corned beef hash, canned entree/Nestle Chef-Mate	1 cup	430.0	18.6	17.6

Dietary Fiber (g)	Total Fat (g)	Cholesterol (mg)	Calcium (mg)	Iron (mg)	Magnesium (mg)	Sodium (mg)	Zinc (mg)	Vitamin A (μgRE)	Vitamin C (mg)	Vitamin E (mgαT)	Thiamin (mg)	Riboflavin (mg)	Niacin (mg)	Vitamin B$_6$ (mg)	Folate (μg)
2.3	0.2	0.0	7.8	0.5	39.0	376.0	0.5	0.0	20.0	0.0	0.2	0.0	2.2	0.5	14.2
2.7	0.1	0.0	6.8	0.4	29.9	326.4	0.4	0.0	17.7	0.1	0.1	0.0	2.0	0.4	13.6
2.4	0.1	0.0	6.8	0.4	29.9	5.4	0.4	0.0	17.7	0.1	0.1	0.0	2.0	0.4	13.6
2.0	3.8	0.0	3.9	0.6	11.1	15.0	0.2	0.0	6.4	0.1	0.1	0.0	1.1	0.2	7.8
1.6	8.3	6.5	9.5	0.4	17.0	108.0	0.2	0.0	5.2	0.0	0.1	0.0	1.6	0.1	14.5
1.6	0.7	0.0	11.5	1.1	12.7	25.3	0.2	0.0	9.4	0.0	0.1	0.0	1.9	0.1	4.8
2.4	5.9	14.7	51.5	0.2	18.9	348.6	0.2	22.1	10.2	0.7	0.1	0.1	0.7	0.0	7.8
2.3	5.2	3.2	36.8	0.2	20.0	276.2	0.3	21.0	6.3	0.0	0.1	0.1	0.8	0.0	7.4
2.1	4.4	12.6	27.3	0.3	18.9	309.8	0.3	21.0	6.4	0.0	0.1	0.0	1.1	0.2	8.3
2.2	1.2	1.3	16.1	0.5	15.3	410.3	0.2	0.0	4.3	0.1	0.0	0.0	1.2	0.0	8.2
4.6	0.1	0.0	19.7	4.1	24.9	149.1	0.3	0.0	7.8	0.0	0.1	0.1	1.8	0.4	12.5
1.4	0.1	0.0	7.0	0.8	11.0	256.0	0.3	0.0	9.4	0.0	0.1	0.0	1.3	0.2	8.4
0.0	0.2	0.0	15.2	0.9	14.8	4.3	0.1	75.7	4.3	0.0	0.0	0.0	0.4	0.1	14.1
3.5	0.3	0.0	31.7	1.7	28.1	294.0	0.2	2691.3	5.1	0.0	0.0	0.1	0.4	0.1	15.0
0.0	0.0	0.0	28.0	0.9	29.2	19.4	0.1	56.8	9.0	0.0	0.0	0.0	0.2	0.0	4.9
0.4	0.1	0.0	7.6	0.2	5.2	8.8	0.2	1.2	3.2	0.9	0.0	0.0	0.1	0.0	24.0
0.0	0.8	0.0	729.6	7.8	197.2	322.5	2.5	0.0	0.0	0.0	0.3	0.8	3.9	0.7	341.9
4.4	0.3	0.0	79.8	0.9	30.6	26.6	0.5	0.0	10.6	0.0	0.1	0.3	0.7	0.4	35.0
0.0	0.0	0.0	6.6	0.2	3.7	2.1	0.1	202.0	1.4	0.0	0.0	0.0	0.0	0.1	4.2
0.0	0.1	0.0	37.0	1.2	21.0	12.0	0.4	119.0	8.0	0.0	0.1	0.0	0.2	0.3	34.2
0.4	2.1	0.0	27.7	0.6	28.2	4.7	0.5	0.5	3.9	0.0	0.1	0.0	0.5	0.0	37.6
1.4	0.2	0.0	81.6	2.1	52.2	42.0	0.5	491.4	5.9	0.6	0.1	0.1	0.3	0.1	87.5
2.6	0.4	0.0	97.1	1.8	65.5	87.8	0.5	752.3	15.8	1.1	0.1	0.1	0.3	0.1	67.9
6.6	0.5	0.0	321.2	3.3	151.8	708.4	1.5	1711.6	27.1	0.0	0.1	0.4	0.9	0.3	236.5
0.8	0.1	0.0	29.7	0.8	23.7	23.7	0.2	201.6	8.4	0.6	0.0	0.1	0.2	0.1	58.3
0.0	0.0	0.0	12.3	0.2	8.7	72.0	0.0	210.0	4.5	0.0	0.0	0.0	0.3	0.0	5.8
2.9	0.5	0.0	43.1	0.7	22.6	520.7	0.4	22.6	7.2	0.0	0.1	0.0	1.7	0.2	16.4
1.1	0.2	0.0	20.8	0.3	18.5	182.5	0.3	22.3	4.2	0.0	0.0	0.0	0.4	0.1	15.5
1.3	0.3	0.0	24.3	0.3	21.6	0.9	0.4	26.1	5.0	0.1	0.0	0.0	0.5	0.1	18.1
5.3	1.2	0.0	26.6	0.6	15.2	450.3	0.5	676.4	18.2	0.0	0.2	0.0	1.3	0.1	53.2
0.0	0.1	0.0	2.7	0.2	8.5	40.5	0.1	4.6	1.3	0.0	0.0	0.0	0.2	0.0	5.2
2.9	0.1	0.0	26.9	0.4	19.2	236.2	0.3	2094.7	23.6	0.3	0.1	0.1	0.6	0.2	21.7
3.0	0.5	0.0	34.4	0.9	16.4	21.3	0.4	2796.2	28.0	0.5	0.1	0.2	1.0	0.4	18.2
3.9	5.3	13.1	42.6	1.9	18.0	114.8	0.2	687.2	11.0	0.0	0.0	0.1	0.6	0.1	18.7
0.0	4.3	0.0	950.6	10.0	325.4	1850.2	0.6	1122.9	242.4	0.0	0.3	1.3	3.1	0.7	45.9
1.3	0.7	0.0	4.8	0.4	13.6	0.7	0.1	7.5	8.0	0.3	0.0	0.0	1.3	0.0	4.8
0.3	0.0	0.0	6.0	0.4	7.4	241.9	0.1	37.5	12.3	0.6	0.0	0.0	0.5	0.1	13.3
21.6	0.6	0.0	217.5	6.0	233.2	175.5	2.2	2259.8	152.9	0.7	1.2	1.0	12.0	0.6	157.1
1.7	0.5	0.0	12.3	0.8	24.6	18.5	0.2	98.4	26.4	0.0	0.1	0.1	1.5	0.2	11.6
0.2	0.0	0.0	1.0	0.1	1.6	8.4	0.0	30.0	3.2	0.0	0.0	0.0	0.1	0.0	5.8
1.1	0.1	0.0	36.6	0.8	13.3	245.3	0.2	59.9	12.7	0.4	0.1	0.0	0.8	0.0	6.0
1.2	0.2	0.0	36.9	0.7	14.8	182.0	0.2	73.8	17.5	0.4	0.1	0.0	0.9	0.1	9.6
0.2	0.1	0.0	0.9	0.1	2.1	1.7	0.0	11.1	3.4	0.1	0.0	0.0	0.1	0.0	2.0
2.1	3.3	0.0	32.0	1.3	18.5	559.7	0.2	82.4	22.4	1.6	0.1	0.1	1.4	0.1	13.5
6.0	0.8	0.0	181.2	3.3	72.5	60.4	1.0	362.4	85.8	2.3	0.3	0.2	4.4	0.5	47.1
1.4	0.4	0.0	6.2	0.6	13.5	11.1	0.1	76.3	23.5	0.5	0.1	0.1	0.8	0.1	18.5
0.0	0.2	0.0	32.0	0.6	13.5	266.9	0.2	71.3	18.2	0.0	0.1	0.0	0.8	0.1	12.4
32.1	7.8	0.0	287.1	23.7	506.3	5468.0	5.2	227.1	102.3	0.0	1.4	1.3	23.6	0.9	177.5
0.1	0.0	0.0	0.7	0.0	0.2	8.6	0.0	0.0	0.3	0.0	0.0	0.0	0.0	0.0	0.3
21.9	1.8	0.0	363.5	2.9	196.0	48.3	4.6	14.2	119.0	0.0	0.4	0.3	2.1	0.8	51.1
0.2	0.2	0.0	12.0	0.6	22.0	362.0	1.1	22.0	4.1	0.0	0.0	0.0	0.2	0.1	15.9
1.7	0.1	0.0	31.8	1.5	0.0	732.3	0.5	611.2	49.0	0.0	0.1	0.1	1.6	0.5	0.0
0.9	1.6	4.8	27.0	0.4	6.0	13.8	0.1	49.2	19.6	0.0	0.0	0.0	0.2	0.1	15.9
12.1	0.4	0.0	68.8	2.3	60.5	96.3	1.3	1177.0	8.8	1.0	0.2	0.3	2.3	0.2	52.3
0.0	5.3	128.5	39.8	0.7	3.6	283.3	0.3	0.0	0.0	0.2	0.0	0.2	0.1	0.0	0.0
0.5	0.9	4.9	9.5	0.2	5.3	179.0	0.4	46.7	0.4	0.1	0.0	0.0	0.5	0.0	0.0
4.3	0.5	0.0	86.7	2.9	16.2	382.5	0.7	0.0	0.0	0.0	0.3	0.6	4.1	0.2	245.7
1.1	5.3	0.0	7.6	0.7	0.0	166.8	0.9	0.0	0.0	0.0	0.2	0.5	4.3	0.5	0.0
2.0	2.8	0.8	18.2	1.9	1.1	259.2	0.4	0.0	0.0	0.3	5.4	0.1	1.8	0.2	0.0
1.0	7.6	93.4	62.7	0.9	2.6	233.0	0.2	65.3	0.0	0.1	0.1	0.2	1.5	0.0	0.0
5.1	12.9	0.0	79.2	6.4	2.2	476.3	1.6	0.0	0.0	0.7	9.9	0.4	3.0	0.5	0.0
0.0	19.9	0.0	28.0	1.9	28.0	854.0	2.0	490.0	4.0	0.0	0.1	0.5	3.5	0.1	40.0
11.1	25.0	55.7	88.6	4.8	45.5	1171.4	3.9	301.1	0.8	1.2	0.1	0.2	3.5	0.2	0.0
6.0	20.6	0.0	55.0	2.4	53.0	926.0	2.0	738.0	4.0	0.0	0.1	0.8	2.5	0.2	30.0
3.0	31.6	85.0	67.5	4.5	45.0	1587.5	4.5	302.5	1.8	1.6	0.1	0.3	4.8	0.3	0.0

Code	Food Name	Unit Amount	Kilocalories (kcal)	Protein (g)	Carbohydrate (g)
22119	Vegetarian, deli franks/Worthington, Morningstar	1 cup	485.8	24.2	29.1
22118	Vegetarian, Garden Patties, frozen/Worthington, Morningstar	1 patty	166.2	15.5	5.5
22125	Vegetarian, Harvest Burger, original flavor, vege protein patty, original flavor	1 patty	160.2	15.1	13.7
22223	Vegetarian, macaroni and cheese, canned entree/Nestle Chef-Mate	1 patty	137.3	18.0	7.0
22127	Vegetarian, Natural Touch Garden Vege Patty, frozen/Worthington	1 cup	283.4	10.8	35.4
22128	Vegetarian, Natural Touch Vegan Burgers, frozen/Worthington	1 cup	448.6	42.2	38.4
22360	Vegetarian, sandwich, Egg & Cheese Biscuit, pre-ckd, frozen/SunnyFresh	1 patty	91.0	13.9	7.5
22361	Vegetarian, sandwich, Egg, Ham & Cheese Biscuit, pre-ckd, frozen/SunnyFresh	1 serving	223.7	9.9	24.6
22224	Vegetarian, Sausage N' Shells, canned entree/Nestle Chef-Mate	1/2 cup	244.4	12.3	25.3
22123	Vegetarian, Spicy Black Bean Burger/Worthington, Morningstar	1 patty	117.8	4.6	5.8
22218	Vegetarian, Spicy Chili with Beans, canned entree/Nestle Chef-Mate	1 cup	371.9	38.2	49.3
924030	Vegetarian, stew, beef vegetable/Worthington	1 cup	422.5	16.9	32.8
18367	Waffle, plain, homemade	1 lg	217.5	4.6	26.4
18365	Waffle, plain/buttermilk, frozen, ready to heat	1 sm	98.9	2.7	11.2
1072	Whipped dessert topping, nondairy, pressurized can	2 Tbsp.	13.2	0.3	1.2
1073	Whipped dessert topping, nondairy, semi-solid, frozen	1 Tbsp.	10.5	0.0	0.6
901913	Whipped topping, nondairy/Cool Whip	2 Tbsp.	28.6	0.1	2.1
19393	Yogurt, frozen, chocolate, soft serve	1/2 cup	129.6	2.9	14.4
19293	Yogurt, frozen, vanilla, soft serve	1/2 cup	115.2	2.9	17.9
1121	Yogurt, low-fat w/fruit, 10 g protein/8 oz	8.0 oz	360.9	9.1	54.9
1117	Yogurt, low-fat, plain, 12 g protein/8 oz	8.0 oz	225.3	9.0	42.3
1119	Yogurt, low-fat, vanilla, 11 g protein/8 oz	8.0 oz	143.7	11.9	16.0
901906	Yogurt, low-fat, Yoplait	6.0 oz	145.3	8.4	23.5
1116	Yogurt, whole milk, plain, 8 g protein/8 oz	8.0 oz	256.5	9.6	42.6

Dietary Fiber (g)	Total Fat (g)	Cholesterol (mg)	Calcium (mg)	Iron (mg)	Magnesium (mg)	Sodium (mg)	Zinc (mg)	Vitamin A (µgRE)	Vitamin C (mg)	Vitamin E (mgαT)	Thiamin (mg)	Riboflavin (mg)	Niacin (mg)	Vitamin B$_6$ (mg)	Folate (µg)
6.1	30.3	88.6	45.5	3.0	38.0	1593.9	7.5	0.0	1.5	0.3	0.2	0.3	6.3	0.6	0.0
4.1	9.2	0.7	25.5	0.9	5.4	641.2	0.6	0.0	0.0	1.9	0.2	0.0	0.0	0.0	0.0
5.4	5.1	0.9	64.8	1.6	39.6	513.0	0.8	102.6	0.0	1.3	8.7	0.1	0.0	0.0	38.7
5.7	4.1	0.0	101.7	3.9	0.0	411.3	0.0	0.0	0.0	0.0	0.0	0.0	0.0	0.0	0.0
3.3	11.0	27.8	202.4	1.9	32.9	1343.4	1.6	55.7	0.0	0.2	0.3	0.3	2.5	0.1	0.0
15.1	14.2	2.5	181.4	4.6	110.9	1436.4	2.2	287.3	0.0	3.7	24.3	0.4	0.0	0.0	0.0
4.3	0.5	0.0	86.7	2.9	16.2	382.5	0.7	0.0	0.0	0.0	0.3	0.6	4.1	0.2	245.7
0.1	9.8	115.0	106.5	2.5	3.6	728.4	0.3	59.3	0.1	2.4	0.2	0.3	2.0	0.0	0.0
0.3	8.5	16.4	12.5	1.0	16.4	304.2	0.7	42.1	0.0	1.4	0.2	0.1	2.0	0.2	0.0
0.0	8.9	110.9	101.0	2.2	3.0	563.3	0.3	57.4	0.0	2.0	0.2	0.3	2.0	0.0	0.0
15.4	2.5	2.5	182.2	6.0	141.7	1619.2	3.0	45.5	0.0	1.2	26.1	0.5	0.0	0.7	0.0
4.3	24.7	55.7	83.5	5.4	53.1	1485.1	2.8	210.0	1.3	2.1	0.1	0.1	3.0	0.3	0.0
1.1	10.3	2.7	93.0	1.2	15.0	458.3	0.4	19.5	0.2	0.0	0.2	0.2	1.2	0.1	9.0
0.0	4.8	23.5	86.7	0.8	6.5	173.7	0.2	22.1	0.1	0.0	0.1	0.1	0.7	0.0	15.6
0.0	0.9	0.7	6.3	0.0	0.7	4.6	0.0	3.4	0.0	0.0	0.0	0.0	0.0	0.0	0.3
0.0	0.9	0.0	0.2	0.0	0.0	2.5	0.0	1.9	0.0	0.0	0.0	0.0	0.0	0.0	0.0
0.0	2.3	0.0	0.6	0.0	0.2	2.3	0.0	7.7	0.0	0.0	0.0	0.0	0.0	0.0	0.0
0.0	5.8	14.4	72.0	0.0	14.4	57.6	0.3	28.8	0.0	0.0	0.0	0.1	0.0	0.0	0.0
1.6	4.3	3.6	105.8	0.9	19.4	70.6	0.4	31.0	0.2	0.1	0.0	0.2	0.2	0.1	7.9
0.0	12.7	4.5	324.6	0.7	31.8	197.5	1.0	129.4	1.8	0.1	0.1	0.5	0.7	0.2	13.6
0.0	2.6	10.2	313.9	0.1	30.1	120.8	1.5	27.2	1.4	0.1	0.1	0.4	0.2	0.1	19.3
0.0	3.5	13.8	414.5	0.2	39.6	159.4	2.0	36.3	1.8	0.1	0.1	0.5	0.3	0.1	25.4
0.0	2.1	8.3	291.2	0.1	27.9	111.9	1.4	22.1	1.3	0.1	0.1	0.3	0.2	0.1	17.9
2.7	4.3	13.4	0.0	0.0	0.0	121.5	0.0	0.0	0.0	0.0	0.0	0.0	0.0	0.0	0.0
0.0	0.0	5.0	0.0	0.0	0.0	160.0	0.0	0.0	0.0	0.0	0.0	0.0	0.0	0.0	0.0
0.0	7.9	30.9	292.0	0.1	0.0	111.9	1.4	59.5	1.1	0.0	0.1	0.3	0.2	0.1	18.1

APPENDIX L

2001 Behavioral Risk Factor Surveillance System Questionnaire

The Behavioral Risk Factor Surveillance System (BRFSS) Questionnaire is composed of two major sections: the "core section" and the "optional modules." The components of these two sections from the 2001 BRFSS questionnaire are shown below. Every state participating in the BRFSS is expected to administer the questions in the core section. Although participating states are encouraged to ask the questions in the optional modules, they are not required to administer this part of the questionnaire.

Core Sections

Section 1: Health Status

Section 2: Health Care Access

Section 3: Exercise

Section 4: Hypertension Awareness

Section 5: Cholesterol Awareness

Section 6: Asthma

Section 7: Diabetes

Section 8: Arthritis

Section 9: Immunization

Section 10: Tobacco Use

Section 11: Alcohol Consumption

Section 12: Firearms

Section 13: Demographics

Section 14: Disability

Section 15: Physical Activity

Section 16: Prostate Cancer Screening

Section 17: Colorectal Cancer Screening

Section 18: HIV/AIDS

Optional Modules

Module 1: Diabetes

Module 2: Sexual Behavior

Module 3: Quality of Life and Care Giving

Module 4: Health Care Coverage and Utilization

Module 5: Women's Health

Module 6: Oral Health

Module 7: Asthma History

Module 8: Heart Attack and Stroke

Module 9: Cardiovascular Disease

Module 10: Fruits and Vegetables

Module 11: Weight Control

Module 12: Folic Acid

Module 13: Tobacco Indicators

Module 14: Other Tobacco Products

This appendix includes questions from only the following sections and modules:

- Section 4:   Hypertension Awareness
- Section 5:   Cholesterol Awareness
- Section 7:   Diabetes
- Module 1:   Diabetes
- Module 8:   Heart Attack and Stroke
- Module 9:   Cardiovascular Disease
- Module 10:   Fruits and Vegetables
- Module 11:   Weight Control
- Module 12:   Folic Acid

For the complete BRFSS questionnaire and for additional links regarding the BRFSS, visit the *Nutritional Assessment* website at www.mhhe.com/hper/nutrition.

From the National Center for Chronic Disease Prevention and Health Promotion, National Center for Health Statistics, Centers for Disease Control and Prevention, U.S. Department of Health and Human Services.

SECTION 4: HYPERTENSION AWARENESS

4.1. Have you ever been told by a doctor, nurse, or other health professional that you have high blood pressure?   (83)

1   Yes

2   No **Go to Q5.1**

7   Don't know/Not sure **Go to Q5.1**

9   Refused **Go to Q5.1**

4.2. Are you currently taking medicine for your high blood pressure?   (84)

1   Yes

2   No

7   Don't know/Not sure

9   Refused

SECTION 5: CHOLESTEROL AWARENESS

5.1. Blood cholesterol is a fatty substance found in the blood. Have you ever had your blood cholesterol checked?   (85)

1   Yes

2   No **Go to Q6.1**

7   Don't know/Not sure **Go to Q6.1**

9   Refused **Go to Q6.1**

5.2. About how long has it been since you last had your blood cholesterol checked?   (86)

Read Only If Necessary

1   Within the past year (anytime less than 12 months ago)

2   Within the past 2 years (1 year but less than 2 years ago)

3   Within the past 5 years (2 years but less than 5 years ago)

4   5 or more years ago

7   Don't know/Not sure

9   Refused

5.3. Have you ever been told by a doctor, nurse, or other health professional that your blood cholesterol is high?   (87)

1   Yes

2   No

7   Don't know/Not sure

9   Refused

SECTION 7: DIABETES

7.1. Have you ever been told by a doctor that you have diabetes?   (90)

1   Yes   If "Yes" and female, ask "Was this only when you were pregnant?"

2   Yes, but female told only during pregnancy

3   No

7   Don't know/Not sure

9   Refused

MODULE 1: DIABETES

To be asked following core Q7.1 if response is "yes"

1.   How old were you when you were told you have diabetes?   (180–181)

___ ___   Code age in years **[97 = 97 and older]**

9   8   Don't know/Not sure

9   9   Refused

2.   Are you now taking insulin?   (182)

1   Yes

2   No

9   Refused

3. Are you now taking diabetes pills?   (183)

    1   Yes

    2   No

    7   Don't know/Not sure

    9   Refused

4. About how often do you check your blood for glucose or sugar? Include times when checked by a family member or friend, but do not include times when checked by a health professional.   (184–186)

    1 __ __   Times per day

    2 __ __   Times per week

    3 __ __   Times per month

    4 __ __   Times per year

    8 8 8   Never

    7 7 7   Don't know/Not sure

    9 9 9   Refused

5. About how often do you check your feet for any sores or irritations? Include times when checked by a family member or friend, but do not include times when checked by a health professional.   (187–189)

    1 __ __   Times per day

    2 __ __   Times per week

    3 __ __   Times per month

    4 __ __   Times per year

    8 8 8   Never

    5 5 5   No feet

    7 7 7   Don't know/Not sure

    9 9 9   Refused

6. Have you ever had any sores or irritations on your feet that took more than four weeks to heal?   (190)

    1   Yes

    2   No

    7   Don't know/Not sure

    9   Refused

7. About how many times in the past 12 months have you seen a doctor, nurse, or other health professional for your diabetes?   (191–192)

    __ __   Number of times

    8 8   None

    7 7   Don't know/Not sure

    9 9   Refused

8. A test for hemoglobin "A one C" measures the average level of blood sugar over the past three months. About how many times in the past 12 months has a doctor, nurse, or other health professional checked you for hemoglobin "A one C"?   (193–194)

    __ __   Number of times [76 = 76 or more]

    8 8   None

    9 8   Never heard of hemoglobin "A one C" test

    7 7   Don't know/Not sure

    9 9   Refused

If "no feet" to Q5, go to Q10.

---

9. About how many times in the past 12 months has a health professional checked your feet for any sores or irritations?   (195–196)

    __ __   Number of times

    8 8   None

    7 7   Don't know/Not sure

    9 9   Refused

10. When was the last time you had an eye exam in which the pupils were dilated? This would have made you temporarily sensitive to bright light.   (197)

    Read Only If Necessary

    1   Within the past month (anytime less than 1 month ago)

    2   Within the past year (1 month but less than 12 months ago)

    3   Within the past 2 years (1 year but less than 2 years ago)

    4   2 or more years ago

    8   Never

    7   Don't know/Not sure

    9   Refused

11. Has a doctor ever told you that diabetes has affected your eyes or that you had retinopathy?   (198)

    1   Yes

    2   No

    7   Don't know/Not sure

    9   Refused

12. Have you ever taken a course or class in how to manage your diabetes yourself?   (199)

    1   Yes

    2   No

    7   Don't know/Not sure

    9   Refused

Module 8: Heart Attack and Stroke

Now I would like to ask you about your knowledge of the signs and symptoms of a heart attack and stroke.

1. Which of the following do you think is a symptom of a heart attack? For each, tell me yes, no, or you're not sure.

   a. Do you think pain or discomfort in the jaw, neck, or back are symptoms of a heart attack? (282)

      1 Yes

      2 No

      7 Don't know/Not sure

      9 Refused

   b. Do you think feeling weak, lightheaded, or faint are symptoms of a heart attack? (283)

      1 Yes

      2 No

      7 Don't know/Not sure

      9 Refused

   c. (Do you think) chest pain or discomfort (is a symptom of a heart attack?) (284)

      1 Yes

      2 No

      7 Don't know/Not sure

      9 Refused

   d. (Do you think) sudden trouble seeing in one or both eyes (is a symptom of a heart attack?) (285)

      1 Yes

      2 No

      7 Don't know/Not sure

      9 Refused

   e. (Do you think) pain or discomfort in the arms or shoulder (is a symptom of a heart attack?) (286)

      1 Yes

      2 No

      7 Don't know/Not sure

      9 Refused

   f. (Do you think) shortness of breath (is a symptom of a heart attack?) (287)

      1 Yes

      2 No

      7 Don't know/Not sure

      9 Refused

2. Which of the following do you think is a symptom of a stroke? For each, tell me yes, no, or you're not sure. (288)

   a. Do you think sudden confusion or trouble speaking is a symptom of a stroke?

      1 Yes

      2 No

      7 Don't know/Not sure

      9 Refused

   b. Do you think sudden numbness or weakness of face, arm, or leg, especially on one side, is a symptom of a stroke? (289)

      1 Yes

      2 No

      7 Don't know/Not sure

      9 Refused

   c. (Do you think) sudden trouble seeing in one or both eyes (is a symptom of a stroke?) (290)

      1 Yes

      2 No

      7 Don't know/Not sure

      9 Refused

   d. (Do you think) sudden chest pain or discomfort (is a symptom of a stroke?) (291)

      1 Yes

      2 No

      7 Don't know/Not sure

      9 Refused

   e. (Do you think) sudden trouble walking, dizziness, or loss of balance (is a symptom of a stroke?) (292)

      1 Yes

      2 No

      7 Don't know/Not sure

      9 Refused

   f. (Do you think) severe headache with no known cause (is a symptom of a stroke?) (293)

      1 Yes

      2 No

      7 Don't know/Not sure

      9 Refused

3. If you thought someone was having a heart attack or a stroke, what is the first thing you would do? (294)

Please Read

1   Take them to the hospital

2   Tell them to call their doctor

3   Call 911

4   Call their spouse or a family member
     or

5   Do something else

7   Don't know/Not sure   **Do not read these responses.**

9   Refused

MODULE 9: CARDIOVASCULAR DISEASE

1. To lower your risk of developing heart disease or stroke, are you . . .

    a.   Eating fewer high-fat or high-cholesterol foods?   (295)

         1   Yes

         2   No

         7   Don't know/Not sure

         9   Refused

    b.   Eating more fruits and vegetables?   (296)

         1   Yes

         2   No

         7   Don't know/Not sure

         9   Refused

    c.   More physically active?   (297)

    1   Yes

    2   No

    7   Don't know/Not sure

    9   Refused

2. Within the past 12 months, has a doctor, nurse, or other health professional told you to . . .   (298)

    a.   Eat fewer high-fat or high-cholesterol foods?

         1   Yes

         2   No

         7   Don't know/Not sure

         9   Refused

    b.   Eat more fruits and vegetables?   (299)

         1   Yes

         2   No

         7   Don't know/Not sure

         9   Refused

    c.   Be more physically active?   (300)

         1   Yes

         2   No

         7   Don't know/Not sure

         9   Refused

3. Has a doctor, nurse, or other health professional ever told you that you had any of the following?   (301)

    a.   A heart attack, also called a myocardial infarction

         1   Yes

         2   No

         7   Don't know/Not sure

         9   Refused

    b.   Angina or coronary heart disease   (302)

         1   Yes

         2   No

         7   Don't know/Not sure

         9   Refused

    c.   A stroke   (303)

         1   Yes

         2   No

         7   Don't know/Not sure

         9   Refused

If "yes" to Q3a, continue. Otherwise, go to Q5.

4. At what age did you have your first heart attack?   (304–305)

    __ __ Code age in years

    0   7   Don't know/Not sure

    0   9   Refused

If "yes" to Q3c, continue. Otherwise, go to Q6.

5. At what age did you have your first stroke?   (306–307)

    __ __ Code age in years

    0   7   Don't know/Not sure

    0   9   Refused

If "yes" to question 3a or 3c, continue. Otherwise, go to Q7.

6. After you left the hospital following your **[fill in (heart attack) if "yes" to Q3a or to Q3a and Q3c; fill in (stroke) if "yes" to Q3c and "no" to Q3a]**, did you go to any kind of outpatient rehabilitation? This is sometimes called "rehab."   (308)

    1   Yes

    2   No

    7   Don't know/Not sure

    9   Refused

If respondent is aged 35 years or older, continue with Q7. Otherwise, go to next module.

7. Do you take aspirin daily or every other day?   (309)
   1   Yes **Go to Q9**
   2   No
   7   Don't know/Not sure
   9   Refused

8. Do you have a health problem   If "yes," ask "Is this a
   or condition that makes taking   stomach condition?" Code
                                    upset stomachs as
   aspirin unsafe for you?   stomach problems.   (310)
   1   Yes, not stomach-related **Go to Next Module**
   2   Yes, stomach problems **Go to Next Module**
   3   No **Go to Next Module**
   7   Don't know/Not sure **Go to Next Module**
   9   Refused **Go to Next Module**

9. Why do you take aspirin . . .   (311)
   a.   To relieve pain?
        1   Yes
        2   No
        7   Don't know/Not sure
        9   Refused
   b.   To reduce the chance of a heart attack?   (312)
        1   Yes
        2   No
        7   Don't know/Not sure
        9   Refused
   c.   To reduce the chance of a stroke?   (313)
        1   Yes
        2   No
        7   Don't know/Not sure
        9   Refused

MODULE 10: FRUITS AND VEGETABLES

These next questions are about the foods you usually eat or drink. Please tell me how often you eat or drink each one, for example, twice a week, three times a month, and so forth. Remember, I am only interested in the foods you eat. Include all foods you eat, both at home and away from home.

1. How often do you drink fruit juices such as orange, grapefruit, or tomato?   (314–316)
   1   __ __   Per day
   2   __ __   Per week
   3   __ __   Per month
   4   __ __   Per year
   5   5   5   Never
   7   7   7   Don't know/Not sure
   9   9   9   Refused

2. Not counting juice, how often do you eat fruit?   (317–319)
   1   __ __   Per day
   2   __ __   Per week
   3   __ __   Per month
   4   __ __   Per year
   5   5   5   Never
   7   7   7   Don't know/Not sure
   9   9   9   Refused

3. How often do you eat green salad?   (320–322)
   1   __ __   Per day
   2   __ __   Per week
   3   __ __   Per month
   4   __ __   Per year
   5   5   5   Never
   7   7   7   Don't know/Not sure
   9   9   9   Refused

4. How often do you eat potatoes not including French fries, fried potatoes, or potato chips?   (323–325)
   1   __ __   Per day
   2   __ __   Per week
   3   __ __   Per month
   4   __ __   Per year
   5   5   5   Never
   7   7   7   Don't know/Not sure
   9   9   9   Refused

5. How often do you eat carrots?   (326–328)
   1   __ __   Per day
   2   __ __   Per week
   3   __ __   Per month
   4   __ __   Per year
   5   5   5   Never
   7   7   7   Don't know/Not sure
   9   9   9   Refused

6. Not counting carrots, potatoes, or salad, how many servings of vegetables do you usually eat?   (329–331)
   1   __ __   Per day   Example: A serving of vegetables
                         at both lunch and dinner would be
   2   __ __   Per week   two servings.
   3   __ __   Per month
   4   __ __   Per year
   5   5   5   Never

7   7   7   Don't know/Not sure

9   9   9   Refused

MODULE 11: WEIGHT CONTROL

1. Are you now trying to lose weight?   (332)

   1   **Yes Go to Q3**

   2   No

   7   Don't know/Not sure

   9   Refused

2. Are you now trying to maintain your current weight, that is, to keep from gaining weight?   (333)

   1   Yes

   2   No **Go to Q6**

   7   Don't know/Not sure **Go to Q6**

   9   Refused **Go to Q6**

3. Are you eating either fewer calories or less fat to . . .
   lose weight? **[if "Yes" on Q1]**
   keep from gaining weight? **[if "Yes" on Q2]**   (334)

   1   Yes, fewer calories   **Probe for which.**

   2   Yes, less fat

   3   Yes, fewer calories and less fat

   4   No

   7   Don't know/Not sure

   9   Refused

4. Are you using physical activity or exercise to . . .
   lose weight? **[if "Yes" on Q1]**
   keep away from gaining weight?
   [if "Yes" on Q2]   (335)

   1   Yes

   2   No

   7   Don't know/Not sure

   9   Refused

5. How much would you like to weigh?   (336–338)

   __ __ __   Weight

   pounds

   7   7   7   Don't know/Not sure

   9   9   9   Refused

6. In the past 12 months, has a doctor, nurse, or other health professional given you advice about your weight?   (339)

   1   Yes, lose weight   **Probe for which.**

   2   Yes, gain weight

   3   Yes, maintain current weight

   4   No

   7   Don't know/Not sure

   9   Refused

MODULE 12: FOLIC ACID

1. Do you currently take any vitamin pills or supplements?   (340)

   1   Yes   **Include liquid supplements.**

   2   No **Go to Q5**

   7   Don't know/Not sure **Go to Q5**

   9   Refused **Go to Q5**

2. Are any of these a multivitamin?   (341)

   1   **Yes Go to Q4**

   2   No

   7   Don't know/Not sure

   9   Refused

3. Do any of the vitamin pills or supplements you take contain folic acid?   (342)

   1   Yes

   2   No **Go to Q5**

   7   Don't know/Not sure **Go to Q5**

   9   Refused **Go to Q5**

4. How often do you take this vitamin pill or supplement?   (343–345)

   1   __ __   Times per day

   2   __ __   Times per week

   3   __ __   Times per month

   7   7   7   Don't know/Not sure

   9   9   9   Refused

> **If respondent is 45 years old or older, go to next module.**

5. Some health experts recommend that women take 400 micrograms of the B vitamin folic acid, for which one of the following reasons?   (346)

Please Read

   1   To make strong bones

   2   To prevent birth defects

   3   To prevent high blood pressure
      or

   4   Some other reason

   7   Don't know/Not sure   **Do not read these responses.**

   9   Refused

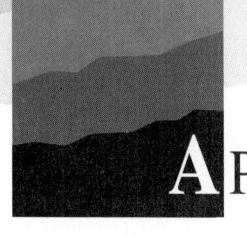

APPENDIX M

SUPPLIERS

The Achievement Center

414 Industrial Lane
Worthington, Minnesota 56187
507-376-3168
507-372-4360 (fax)
www.hickorytech.net/~mrci

American Weights and Measures

16501 Zumaque St.
P.O. Box 227
Rancho Santa Fe, California 92067
800-395-4565
858-204-9699
858-756-0986 (fax)
www.amerweights.com

Beta Technology, Inc.

2841 Mission St.
Santa Cruz, California 95060
800-858-2382
831-457-5709
800-221-8416 (fax)
www.beta-technology.com

Biodynamics Corporation

3511 NE 45th St., #2
Seattle, Washington 98105
800-869-6987
206-526-0205
206-526-0208 (fax)
www.biodyncorp.com

Bodytrends.com

6385 Rose Lane, Suite B
Carpinteria, California 93013
800-549-1667
805-684-8404
www.bodytrends.com

Country Technology, Inc.

P.O. Box 87
Gays Mills, Wisconsin 54631
608-735-4718
608-735-4859 (fax)
www.fitnessmart.com

Creative Health Products, Inc.

5148 Saddle Ridge Rd.
Plymouth, Michigan 48170
800-742-4478
734-996-5900
734-996-4650 (fax)
www.chponline.com

Davco Weight Scales Inc.

P.O. Box 4104
Quesnel, British Columbia, Canada
V2J 3J2
250-747-8371
250-747-8372 (fax)
www.davco.bc.ca

Detecto Scales

366 N. Broadway, Suite 314
Jericho, New York 11753
516-937-0500
516-937-0524 (fax)
www.detectoscale.com

Fat Control, Inc.

19310 Dutton
Stewartstown, Pennsylvania 17363
717-993-3550
www.fatcontrolinc.com

Lafayette Instrument Company

P.O. Box 5729
Lafayette, Indiana 47903
800-428-7545
765-423-1505
765-423-4111 (fax)
www.licmef.com

Life Measurement, Inc.

1850 Bates Ave.
Concord, California 94520
800-426-3763
925-676-6002
925-676-6005 (fax)
www.bodpod.com

Measurement Concepts

43811 SE 143rd St.
North Bend, Washington 98045
888-345-4858
425-831-5963
425-831-6032 (fax)
www.stadiometer.com

Novel Products, Inc.

P.O. Box 408
3266 Yale Bridge Rd.
Rockton, Illinois 61072
800-323-5143
815-624-4888
815-624-4866 (fax)
www.novelproductsinc.com

**Ontario Association of Sport
and Exercise Sciences**

75 Broadway
Orangeville, Ontario
L9W 1K1
519-942-2620
519-942-2285 (fax)
www.oases.on.ca

RJL Systems, Inc.

33955 Harper Ave.
Clinton Twp., Michigan 48035
800-528-4513
810-790-0200
810-790-0205 (fax)
www.rjlsystems.com

Seca Corporation

1352 Charwood Rd., Suite E
Hanover, Maryland 21076
800-542-7322
410-694-9680 (fax)
www.secacorp.com

Seritex, Inc.

1 Madison St.
East Rutherford, New Jersey 07073
973-472-4200   973-472-0222
(fax) www.seritex.com

**Tanita Corporation
of America, Inc.**

2625 South Clearbrook Dr.
Arlington Heights, Illinois 60005
847-640-9241
847-640-9261 (fax)
www.tanita.com

EQUIPMENT

Anthropometric Tapes
Country Technology, Inc.
Creative Health Products, Inc.
Lafayette Instrument Company
Novel Products, Inc.
Ontario Association of Sport and
Exercise Sciences
Seca Corporation
Seritex, Inc.

**Bioelectrical Impedance
Instruments**
American Weights and Measures
Biodynamics Corporation
Bodytrends.com
Country Technology, Inc.
Creative Health Products
Measurement Concepts
RJL Systems, Inc.
Tanita Corporation of America, Inc.

Knee Height & Sliding Calipers
Creative Health Products, Inc.
Lafayette Instrument Company
Seritex, Inc.

**Recumbent Length Measurement
Equipment**
The Achievement Center
Measurement Concepts
Novel Products, Inc.
Seca Corporation
Seritex, Inc.

Skinfold Calipers
Beta Technology, Inc.
Bodytrends.com
Country Technology, Inc.
Creative Health Products, Inc.
Fat Control, Inc.
Lafayette Instrument Company
Novel Products, Inc.
Ontario Association of Sport and
Exercise Sciences
Seca Corporation
Seritex, Inc.

Stadiometers
The Achievement Center
Country Technology, Inc.
Creative Health Products, Inc.
Measurement Concepts

Novel Products, Inc.
Seca Corporation
Seritex, Inc.

Strength Testing
Country Technology, Inc.
Creative Health Products, Inc.
Lafayette Instrument Company
Novel Products, Inc.

Weight Scales
Bodytrends.com
Country Technology, Inc.
Creative Health Products, Inc.
Davco Weight Scales, Inc.
Detecto Scales
Measurement Concepts
Novel Products, Inc.
Ontario Association of Sport and
Exercise Sciences
Seca Corporation
Tanita Corporation of America, Inc.

Whole-Body Plethysmography
Life Measurement, Inc.

2000 CDC Clinical Growth Charts[*]

APPENDIX N

From National Center for Health Statstics, Centers for Disease Control and Prevention, U.S. Department of Health and Human Services.
[*]For additional information relating to the CDC Growth Charts, visit the *Nutritional Assessment* website at www.mhhe.com/hper/nutrition.

Birth to 36 months: Boys
Length-for-age and Weight-for-age percentiles

NAME _____

RECORD # _____

AGE (MONTHS)

Birth 3 6 9 12 15 18 21 24 27 30 33 36

LENGTH

in	cm		cm	in
41				41
40	100	95		40
39		90	100	39
38	95	75		38
37		50	95	37
36	90	25		36
35		10	90	35
34	85	5		

LENGTH (left side)

WEIGHT

Length percentiles: 95, 90, 75, 50, 25, 10, 5

Weight percentiles: 95, 90, 75, 50, 25, 10, 5

AGE (MONTHS)

12 15 18 21 24 27 30 33 36 kg lb

Mother's Stature _____	Gestational	
Father's Stature_____	Age: _____ Weeks	Comment
Date	Age	Weight	Length	Head Circ.	
	Birth				

WEIGHT (lb / kg)

Birth 3 6 9

Revised April 20, 2001.
SOURCE: Developed by the National Center for Health Statistics in collaboration with
the National Center for Chronic Disease Prevention and Health Promotion (2000).
http://www.cdc.gov/growthcharts

Birth to 36 months: Boys
Head circumference-for-age and
Weight-for-length percentiles

NAME _____

RECORD # _____

AGE (MONTHS)

Birth 3 6 9 12 15 18 21 24 27 30 33 36

HEAD CIRCUMFERENCE

in cm ... cm in **HEAD CIRCUMFERENCE**

95
90
75
50
25
10
5

WEIGHT

LENGTH

| cm | 64 66 68 70 72 74 76 78 80 82 84 86 88 90 92 94 96 98 100 | | | | |
| in | 26 27 28 29 30 31 32 33 34 35 36 37 38 39 40 41 | | | | |

Date	Age	Weight	Length	Head Circ.	Comment

cm	46 48 50 52 54 56 58 60 62
in	18 19 20 21 22 23 24

SOURCE: Developed by the National Center for Health Statistics in collaboration with
the National Center for Chronic Disease Prevention and Health Promotion (2000).
http://www.cdc.gov/growthcharts

521

Birth to 36 months: Girls
Length-for-age and Weight-for-age percentiles

NAME _____

RECORD # _____

AGE (MONTHS)

Birth 3 6 9 12 15 18 21 24 27 30 33 36

L E N G T H

W E I G H T

	Mother's Stature _____		Gestational			
	Father's Stature _____		Age: _____ Weeks		Comment	
Date	Age	Weight	Length	Head Circ.		
	Birth					

Revised April 20, 2001.
SOURCE: Developed by the National Center for Health Statistics in collaboration with
the National Center for Chronic Disease Prevention and Health Promotion (2000).
http://www.cdc.gov/growthcharts

Birth to 36 months: Girls
Head circumference-for-age and
Weight-for-length percentiles

NAME _____

RECORD # _____

AGE (MONTHS)

Birth 3 6 9 **12** 15 18 21 **24** 27 30 33 **36**

HEAD CIRCUMFERENCE

in | cm
20 | 52
   | 50
19 | 48
18 | 46
   | 44
17 | 42
16 | 40
15 | 38
14 | 36
   | 34
13 | 32
12 | 30

95
90
75
50
25
10
5

WEIGHT

cm | in
   | 50
22 | 48
21 | 46
20 | 44
19 | 42
18 | 40
17 | 38
16 | 36
   | 34
15 | 32
14 | 30
13 | 28
12 | 26
11 | 24
10 | 22
9 | 20
8 | 18
7 | 16
6 | 14
5 | 12
kg | lb

95
90
75
50
25
10
5

WEIGHT

lb | kg
24 | 11
22 | 10
20 | 9
18 | 8
16 | 7
14 | 6
12 | 5
10 | 4
8 |
6 | 3
   | 2
4 |
2 | 1
lb | kg

LENGTH

cm | 64 66 68 70 72 74 76 78 80 82 84 86 88 90 92 94 96 98 100
in | 26 27 28 29 30 31 32 33 34 35 36 37 38 39 40 41

cm | 46 48 50 52 54 56 58 60 62
in | 18 19 20 21 22 23 24

Date	Age	Weight	Length	Head Circ.	Comment

SOURCE: Developed by the National Center for Health Statistics in collaboration with
the National Center for Chronic Disease Prevention and Health Promotion (2000).
http://www.cdc.gov/growthcharts

523

2 to 20 years: Boys
Stature-for-age and Weight-for-age percentiles

NAME _____

RECORD # _____

Mother's Stature _____ Father's Stature _____				
Date	Age	Weight	Stature	BMI*

*To Calculate BMI: Weight (kg) ÷ Stature (cm) ÷ Stature (cm) x 10,000
or Weight (lb) ÷ Stature (in) ÷ Stature (in) x 703

AGE (YEARS)

12 13 14 15 16 17 18 19 20

STATURE

WEIGHT

AGE (YEARS)

2 3 4 5 6 7 8 9 10 11 12 13 14 15 16 17 18 19 20

Stature percentiles: 95, 90, 75, 50, 25, 10, 5

Weight percentiles: 95, 90, 75, 50, 25, 10, 5

Revised and corrected November 21, 2000.
SOURCE: Developed by the National Center for Health Statistics in collaboration with
the National Center for Chronic Disease Prevention and Health Promotion (2000).
http://www.cdc.gov/growthcharts

524

2 to 20 years: Boys
Bodymass index-for-age percentiles

Date	Age	Weight	Stature	BMI*	Comments

*To Calculate BMI: Weight (kg) ÷ Stature (cm) ÷ Stature (cm) x 10,000
or Weight (lb) ÷ Stature (in) ÷ Stature (in) x 703

BMI

AGE (YEARS)

kg/m²   kg/m²

SOURCE: Developed by the National Center for Health Statistics in collaboration with
the National Center for Chronic Disease Prevention and Health Promotion (2000).
http://www.cdc.gov/growthcharts

525

2 to 20 years: Girls
Stature-for-age and Weight-for-age percentiles

NAME _____

RECORD # _____

Mother's Stature _____	Father's Stature _____			
Date	Age	Weight	Stature	BMI*

*To Calculate BMI: Weight (kg) ÷ Stature (cm) ÷ Stature (cm) x 10,000
or Weight (lb) ÷ Stature (in) ÷ Stature (in) x 703

AGE (YEARS)

12 13 14 15 16 17 18 19 20

STATURE

cm / in
190 — 76
185 — 74
180 — 72
175 — 70
95
90 — 68
75
170 — 66
165 — 64
50
160 — 62
25
10 — 155 — 62
5 — 150 — 60

in / cm
62 — 160
60 — 155
58 — 150
56 — 145
54 — 140
52 — 135
50 — 130
48 — 125
46 — 120
44 — 115
42 — 110
40 — 105
38 — 100
36 — 95
34 — 90
32 — 85
30 — 80

STATURE

WEIGHT

105 — 230
100 — 220
95 — 210
90 — 200
85 — 190
95 — 180
80
90 — 75 — 170
75 — 65 — 160
70 — 150
50 — 60 — 140
55 — 130
25
10 — 50 — 120
5 — 45 — 110

lb / kg
80 — 35
70 — 30
60 — 25
50 — 20
40 — 15
30 — 10

WEIGHT

kg — 35
30
25
20
15
10

AGE (YEARS)

2 3 4 5 6 7 8 9 10 11 12 13 14 15 16 17 18 19 20

Revised and corrected November 21, 2000.
SOURCE: Developed by the National Center for Health Statistics in collaboration with
the National Center for Chronic Disease Prevention and Health Promotion (2000).
http://www.cdc.gov/growthcharts

526

2 to 20 years: Girls
Bodymass index-for-age percentiles

NAME _____

RECORD # _____

Date	Age	Weight	Stature	BMI*	Comments

*To Calculate BMI: Weight (kg) ÷ Stature (cm) ÷ Stature (cm) x 10,000
or Weight (lb) ÷ Stature (in) ÷ Stature (in) x 703

BMI

35
34
33
32
31
30
29
28
27
26
25
24
23
22
21
20
19
18
17
16
15
14
13
12

BMI

27
26
25
24
23
22
21
20
19
18
17
16
15
14
13
12

95
90
85
75
50
25
10
5

kg/m²

AGE (YEARS)

2 3 4 5 6 7 8 9 10 11 12 13 14 15 16 17 18 19 20

SOURCE: Developed by the National Center for Health Statistics in collaboration with
the National Center for Chronic Disease Prevention and Health Promotion (2000).
http://www.cdc.gov/growthcharts

527

Weight-for-stature percentiles: Boys

Date	Age	Weight	Stature	Comments

STATURE

95
90
85
75
50
25
10
5

cm: 80 85 90 95 100 105 110 115 120

in: 31 32 33 34 35 36 37 38 39 40 41 42 43 44 45 46 47

SOURCE: Developed by the National Center for Health Statistics in collaboration with
the National Center for Chronic Disease Prevention and Health Promotion (2000).
http://www.cdc.gov/growthcharts

528

Weight-for-stature percentiles: Girls

Date	Age	Weight	Stature	Comments

STATURE

cm 80 85 90 95 100 105 110 115 120

in 31 32 33 34 35 36 37 38 39 40 41 42 43 44 45 46 47

Percentile lines: 95, 90, 85, 75, 50, 25, 10, 5

SOURCE: Developed by the National Center for Health Statistics in collaboration with
the National Center for Chronic Disease Prevention and Health Promotion (2000).
http://www.cdc.gov/growthcharts

529

APPENDIX O

Triceps Skinfold Norms from NHANES II

From National Center for Health Statistics, Centers for Disease Control and Prevention, U.S. Department of Health and Human Services.

Triceps Skinfold in Millimeters for Persons 6 Months to 19 Years of Age—United States, 1976–1980

Sex and Age	Number of Examined Persons	Mean	Standard Deviation	Percentile								
				5th	10th	15th	25th	50th	75th	85th	90th	95th
Male												
6–11 months	179	10.4	3.1	6.5	7.0	7.0	8.0	10.0	12.0	14.0	15.0	16.0
1 year	370	10.4	2.7	6.5	7.0	7.5	8.5	10.0	12.0	13.0	14.0	15.5
2 years	375	10.2	2.9	6.0	7.0	7.0	8.0	10.0	12.0	13.0	14.5	15.0
3 years	418	10.0	2.6	6.5	7.0	7.5	8.0	9.5	11.5	12.5	13.0	15.0
4 years	404	9.6	3.0	6.0	6.5	7.0	7.5	9.0	11.0	12.0	13.0	15.0
5 years	397	8.9	2.9	5.5	6.0	6.5	7.0	8.0	10.5	11.5	12.5	14.5
6 years	133	9.3	4.4	5.0	5.5	6.0	6.5	8.0	10.5	12.0	13.0	17.5
7 years	148	9.2	4.0	5.0	5.5	6.0	6.5	8.5	11.0	12.0	15.0	17.5
8 years	147	10.5	4.9	5.5	6.0	6.0	7.0	9.0	12.0	16.5	17.0	22.0
9 years	145	10.6	5.7	5.0	5.0	6.0	7.0	9.0	12.5	16.0	19.0	23.0
10 years	157	12.6	6.6	5.0	6.0	6.5	7.5	11.0	16.5	20.0	22.0	26.0
11 years	155	13.3	7.7	4.5	5.5	6.0	7.5	10.5	17.0	22.0	25.0	30.0
12 years	145	12.4	6.4	5.0	6.0	6.0	8.0	11.0	15.0	18.0	21.5	26.5
13 years	173	11.2	7.0	5.0	5.5	6.0	7.0	9.0	12.5	16.5	20.5	22.5
14 years	186	10.4	5.8	4.0	5.0	5.5	6.0	9.0	13.0	15.0	17.0	23.0
15 years	184	10.1	7.2	5.0	5.0	6.0	6.0	7.5	11.0	14.5	18.0	22.0
16 years	178	10.9	6.6	4.5	5.0	5.5	6.5	8.0	13.0	18.5	20.5	25.5
17 years	173	8.5	4.6	4.0	4.5	5.0	5.5	7.0	10.5	12.5	15.0	18.0
18 years	164	11.1	6.6	4.0	5.0	5.0	6.0	9.5	14.5	17.5	19.0	22.5
19 years	148	10.9	6.1	5.0	5.5	6.0	6.5	9.0	13.0	16.0	18.5	23.0
Female												
6–11 months	177	9.9	2.6	6.5	7.0	7.0	8.0	10.0	11.5	12.5	13.0	14.5
1 year	336	10.6	3.3	6.0	7.0	7.5	8.0	10.5	12.0	13.5	15.0	16.5
2 years	336	10.6	3.0	6.0	7.0	7.5	8.0	10.5	12.5	13.5	15.0	16.0
3 years	366	10.3	2.9	6.0	7.0	7.0	8.0	10.0	12.0	12.5	13.5	16.5
4 years	396	10.4	3.1	6.0	6.5	7.5	8.0	10.0	12.0	13.0	14.0	15.5
5 years	364	10.6	3.2	6.0	7.0	7.5	8.5	10.5	12.5	14.0	14.5	16.0
6 years	135	11.0	3.9	6.0	7.0	7.5	8.0	10.0	12.0	14.5	16.0	18.5
7 years	157	11.5	4.5	6.0	7.0	7.5	9.0	10.5	13.0	15.0	18.0	20.0
8 years	123	11.9	5.2	6.0	6.5	7.0	8.5	11.0	14.0	16.0	18.0	21.0

continued

Triceps Skinfold in Millimeters for Persons 6 Months to 19 Years of Age—United States, 1976–1980—*continued*

Sex and Age	Number of Examined Persons	Mean	Standard Deviation	Percentile								
				5th	10th	15th	25th	50th	75th	85th	90th	95th
Female cont'd												
9 years	149	14.3	6.5	7.0	7.5	8.5	10.0	13.0	16.0	20.0	23.0	27.0
10 years	136	14.5	5.9	7.0	8.0	8.0	10.0	13.5	18.0	21.0	22.5	24.5
11 years	140	15.7	6.9	8.0	8.5	9.0	11.0	14.0	19.5	21.5	23.0	29.5
12 years	147	15.1	6.0	7.5	8.0	9.0	11.5	13.5	18.5	21.5	23.0	27.0
13 years	162	15.9	7.9	6.0	7.5	9.0	10.5	15.0	19.0	22.0	25.0	30.0
14 years	178	17.6	7.5	8.0	10.0	10.5	12.0	17.0	21.5	25.0	29.5	32.0
15 years	145	17.1	7.1	8.5	9.5	10.0	11.5	16.5	20.5	24.5	26.0	32.1
16 years	170	19.5	7.2	11.0	11.5	12.0	14.0	18.0	23.0	27.0	30.5	33.1
17 years	134	19.8	7.8	9.5	11.0	11.5	14.0	20.0	24.5	26.5	28.5	34.5
18 years	170	19.9	7.6	11.0	12.0	12.5	14.0	18.0	23.5	27.0	32.5	35.0
19 years	158	20.4	7.6	10.5	11.5	13.0	15.0	19.0	25.0	28.0	30.0	33.5

Triceps Skinfold in Millimeters for Males 18–74 Years of Age—United States, 1976–1980

Race and Age	Number of Examined Persons	Mean	Standard Deviation	Percentile								
				5th	10th	15th	25th	50th	75th	85th	90th	95th
All Races[*]												
18–74 years	5916	12.9	6.7	5.0	6.0	6.5	8.0	12.0	16.0	19.5	22.0	25.5
18–24 years	988	11.6	6.5	4.5	5.0	6.0	6.5	10.0	15.0	17.5	20.0	24.5
25–34 years	1067	12.9	7.0	4.5	5.5	6.5	7.5	11.5	16.5	20.0	23.0	26.0
35–44 years	745	13.8	7.1	5.0	6.0	7.0	9.0	12.5	17.0	20.0	23.0	27.0
45–54 years	690	13.5	6.7	5.5	6.5	7.0	9.0	12.0	16.5	20.0	22.0	25.5
55–64 years	1227	13.2	6.3	5.0	6.0	7.5	9.0	12.0	16.0	19.5	21.5	25.5
65–74 years	1199	12.7	6.1	5.0	6.0	7.0	8.0	11.5	16.0	18.5	21.0	25.0
White												
18–74 years	5148	13.0	6.6	5.0	6.0	7.0	8.0	12.0	16.0	19.5	22.0	25.5
18–24 years	846	11.9	6.5	4.5	5.0	6.0	7.0	10.0	15.0	18.0	20.0	25.0
25–34 years	901	13.1	6.9	5.0	6.0	7.0	8.0	12.0	16.5	20.0	22.5	26.0
35–44 years	653	13.9	7.0	5.5	6.5	7.0	9.0	12.5	17.0	21.0	23.0	27.0
45–54 years	617	13.4	6.5	5.5	6.5	7.5	9.0	12.0	16.5	20.0	21.0	25.0
55–64 years	1086	13.1	5.9	5.5	6.5	7.5	9.0	12.0	16.0	19.0	21.0	24.5
65–74 years	1045	12.9	6.0	5.0	6.5	7.0	8.0	12.0	16.0	19.0	21.0	25.0
Black												
18–74 years	649	12.1	7.8	4.0	4.5	5.0	6.5	10.0	16.0	19.0	23.0	27.0
18–24 years	121	9.7	6.4	4.0	4.0	4.5	5.0	7.5	13.0	15.0	18.5	21.5
25–34 years	139	11.5	7.5	3.5	4.0	5.0	6.0	10.0	15.5	19.0	23.0	24.5
35–44 years	70	13.0	8.1	———	5.0	6.5	9.0	11.0	16.0	18.5	20.0	———
45–54 years	62	15.0	8.7	———	5.5	6.0	9.0	13.0	18.0	25.5	27.5	———
55–64 years	129	12.9	7.8	3.5	4.5	5.5	7.0	10.5	17.5	22.0	25.0	29.0
65–74 years	128	11.6	6.7	4.0	4.5	5.5	7.0	10.0	14.5	16.0	19.5	27.5

[*]Includes all other races not shown as separate categories.

Triceps Skinfold in Millimeters for Females 18–74 Years of Age—United States, 1976–1980

Race and Age	Number of Examined Persons	Mean	Standard Deviation	Percentile								
				5th	10th	15th	25th	50th	75th	85th	90th	95th
*All Races**												
18–74 years	6588	24.9	9.8	11.0	13.0	15.0	17.5	24.0	31.0	35.1	38.0	43.0
18–24 years	1066	20.7	8.6	10.0	11.5	12.5	15.0	19.0	25.0	29.5	32.0	37.0
25–34 years	1170	23.6	9.9	10.0	13.0	14.0	16.5	22.0	29.0	33.5	36.6	43.5
35–44 years	844	26.3	9.8	12.0	14.5	16.5	19.5	25.0	32.6	37.0	40.5	44.5
45–54 years	763	27.5	9.7	12.5	15.0	17.0	20.5	27.0	34.0	38.0	40.5	45.0
55–64 years	1329	27.2	9.5	12.0	15.0	17.5	21.0	26.5	33.0	37.0	40.0	43.6
65–74 years	1416	25.7	9.0	12.0	14.5	16.5	19.0	25.0	31.0	35.0	37.6	42.0
White												
18–74 years	5686	24.7	9.5	11.5	13.5	15.0	17.5	23.5	30.5	35.0	37.5	42.5
18–24 years	892	20.8	8.5	10.5	11.5	13.0	15.0	19.0	25.0	29.0	32.0	37.1
25–34 years	1000	23.3	9.4	10.5	13.0	14.0	16.5	22.0	28.5	33.0	36.0	42.1
35–44 years	726	26.1	9.6	12.0	14.5	16.0	19.0	24.5	32.0	36.5	40.0	44.0
45–54 years	647	27.2	9.4	13.0	15.0	16.5	20.5	27.0	33.0	37.0	40.0	43.1
55–64 years	1176	27.0	9.4	12.5	15.0	17.5	21.0	26.0	32.6	36.5	39.1	43.1
65–74 years	1245	25.5	8.8	12.0	14.5	16.5	19.0	25.0	30.5	34.0	37.0	41.1
Black												
18–74 years	782	26.6	11.6	10.0	12.0	14.0	17.5	25.5	35.0	39.0	42.5	48.0
18–24 years	147	20.6	8.8	8.0	10.0	11.0	14.0	19.0	27.0	31.0	35.0	37.0
25–34 years	145	25.5	12.2	8.0	11.0	13.0	16.0	24.0	32.0	37.0	47.0	49.5
35–44 years	103	28.7	11.4	9.0	14.0	15.5	20.5	29.5	36.6	40.5	45.0	48.0
45–54 years	100	31.6	11.8	10.5	16.0	20.0	23.5	31.5	40.0	43.5	48.5	53.1
55–64 years	135	29.5	10.8	12.0	14.0	18.0	22.0	28.5	38.5	42.0	43.0	46.0
65–74 years	152	29.0	10.5	11.5	14.5	17.0	21.5	29.0	37.0	38.6	44.0	47.5

*Includes all other races not shown as separate categories.

Subscapular Skinfold Norms
from NHANES II

From National Center for Health Statistics, Centers for Disease Control and Prevention, U.S. Department of Health and Human Services.

Subscapular Skinfold in Millimeters for Persons 6 Months–19 Years of Age—United States, 1976–1980

Sex and Age	Number of Examined Persons	Mean	Standard Deviation	Percentile								
				5th	10th	15th	25th	50th	75th	85th	90th	95th
Male												
6–11 months	179	6.5	1.9	4.0	5.0	5.0	5.5	6.0	7.5	8.0	8.5	9.0
1 year	370	6.6	1.9	4.0	4.5	5.0	5.0	6.5	7.5	8.0	9.0	10.5
2 years	375	6.1	2.2	3.5	4.0	4.0	5.0	5.5	7.0	7.5	9.0	10.0
3 years	418	5.7	1.6	4.0	4.0	4.0	4.5	5.5	6.5	7.0	7.5	9.0
4 years	404	5.5	2.2	3.5	3.5	4.0	4.0	5.0	6.0	7.0	7.5	9.0
5 years	397	5.3	2.4	3.0	3.5	4.0	4.0	5.0	6.0	6.5	7.0	8.0
6 years	133	6.0	3.9	3.5	3.5	4.0	4.0	5.0	6.0	8.0	10.0	16.0
7 years	148	5.8	3.1	3.5	4.0	4.0	4.0	5.0	6.0	7.0	7.5	11.5
8 years	147	6.7	4.9	3.5	4.0	4.0	4.5	5.0	6.5	8.0	11.0	21.0
9 years	145	7.0	5.0	3.5	4.0	4.0	4.5	6.0	7.0	10.0	12.0	15.0
10 years	157	8.6	6.6	4.0	4.0	4.5	5.0	6.0	9.5	11.5	17.0	22.0
11 years	155	10.0	8.5	4.0	4.0	4.5	5.0	6.5	10.0	17.5	25.0	31.0
12 years	145	9.2	6.8	4.0	4.5	4.5	5.0	6.5	10.0	15.5	19.0	22.5
13 years	173	9.1	7.3	4.0	4.5	5.0	5.0	7.0	9.0	13.0	15.0	24.0
14 years	186	8.9	5.3	4.5	5.0	5.5	6.0	7.0	9.0	12.0	13.5	20.0
15 years	184	10.0	8.2	5.0	5.5	6.0	6.0	7.5	10.0	12.0	16.0	24.5
16 years	178	10.8	6.4	5.0	6.0	6.5	6.5	9.0	12.5	14.5	21.5	25.0
17 years	173	10.1	5.3	5.5	6.0	6.5	7.0	8.5	11.5	14.0	17.0	20.5
18 years	164	11.9	6.7	6.0	7.0	7.0	8.0	10.0	14.0	16.0	18.0	24.0
19 years	148	12.5	6.9	7.0	7.0	7.5	8.0	10.5	13.5	16.5	22.0	29.0
Female												
6–11 months	177	6.7	1.7	4.5	5.0	5.0	5.5	6.5	7.5	8.0	9.0	10.0
1 year	336	6.7	2.0	4.0	4.0	5.0	5.0	6.5	8.0	8.5	9.5	10.5
2 years	336	6.5	2.2	4.0	4.5	4.5	5.0	6.0	7.5	8.5	9.5	11.0
3 years	366	6.3	2.2	3.5	4.0	4.5	5.0	6.0	7.0	8.0	9.0	11.0
4 years	396	6.2	2.2	3.5	4.0	4.5	5.0	5.5	7.0	8.0	9.0	10.5
5 years	364	6.5	3.5	4.0	4.0	4.5	5.0	5.5	7.0	8.0	10.0	12.0
6 years	135	6.8	3.8	4.0	4.0	4.0	5.0	6.0	7.5	9.0	10.5	14.0
7 years	157	7.0	3.7	3.5	4.0	4.0	4.5	6.0	7.5	9.0	12.0	16.5
8 years	123	7.4	4.9	3.5	4.0	4.5	5.0	6.0	8.0	10.5	12.0	15.0
9 years	149	9.6	7.5	4.0	5.0	5.0	5.5	7.0	9.5	13.0	21.0	29.0
10 years	136	10.4	6.6	4.5	5.0	5.0	6.0	8.0	13.5	18.0	19.5	23.0

continued

Subscapular Skinfold in Millimeters for Persons 6 Months–19 Years of Age—United States, 1976–1980—*continued*

Sex and Age	Number of Examined Persons	Mean	Standard Deviation	Percentile								
				5th	10th	15th	25th	50th	75th	85th	90th	95th
Female cont'd												
11 years	140	11.4	8.1	4.5	5.0	5.5	6.5	8.0	12.0	17.0	22.0	29.0
12 years	147	11.5	7.5	5.0	5.5	6.0	6.5	9.0	13.0	17.0	22.0	29.0
13 years	162	11.9	8.5	4.5	5.5	6.0	7.0	9.5	14.0	17.5	20.0	29.0
14 years	178	13.2	7.7	6.0	6.5	7.0	7.5	10.5	16.0	22.0	26.0	31.0
15 years	145	13.1	6.9	6.0	7.0	7.5	8.5	10.5	16.0	20.5	22.5	27.5
16 years	170	15.2	9.2	6.5	7.5	8.5	9.5	12.0	16.5	23.5	26.0	36.6
17 years	134	15.9	9.2	6.5	7.0	8.0	9.5	13.0	19.5	27.0	29.0	37.0
18 years	170	15.3	8.6	7.0	7.5	8.0	10.0	13.0	18.5	22.0	27.5	34.5
19 years	158	16.0	9.5	7.0	7.5	8.5	9.5	13.0	18.5	23.5	26.5	35.5

Subscapular Skinfold in Millimeters for Males 18–74 Years of Age—United States, 1976–1980

Race and Age	Number of Examined Persons	Mean	Standard Deviation	Percentile								
				5th	10th	15th	25th	50th	75th	85th	90th	95th
All Races[*]												
18–74 years	5916	17.4	8.8	7.0	8.0	9.0	10.5	15.0	22.5	26.0	30.0	34.6
18–24 years	988	13.7	7.5	6.5	7.0	7.5	8.5	11.5	16.0	20.0	23.0	30.0
25–34 years	1067	16.9	8.6	7.0	8.0	9.0	10.0	15.0	22.0	25.5	29.0	34.0
35–44 years	745	18.7	9.2	7.0	8.5	10.0	12.0	17.0	24.0	28.0	30.5	37.0
45–54 years	690	19.4	8.9	7.5	9.0	10.0	12.5	18.0	25.0	29.0	31.0	36.0
55–64 years	1227	18.9	8.4	7.5	9.0	10.0	12.5	18.0	24.0	27.0	30.0	34.5
65–74 years	1199	17.9	8.7	7.0	8.0	9.5	11.0	16.0	23.0	27.5	30.5	35.1
White												
18–74 years	5148	17.3	8.5	7.0	8.0	9.0	11.0	15.5	22.0	26.0	29.5	34.0
18–24 years	846	13.8	7.5	6.5	7.0	7.5	8.5	11.5	16.5	20.5	24.0	30.0
25–34 years	901	16.9	8.3	7.0	8.0	9.0	10.5	15.0	22.0	25.5	29.0	32.5
35–44 years	653	18.5	8.7	7.0	9.0	10.0	12.0	17.0	23.5	27.0	30.0	35.0
45–54 years	617	19.1	8.6	8.0	9.0	10.0	12.5	17.5	24.0	28.5	30.5	35.1
55–64 years	1086	18.9	8.3	7.5	9.5	10.5	12.5	18.0	24.0	27.0	29.5	34.0
65–74 years	1045	18.0	8.5	7.0	8.0	9.5	11.5	16.0	23.0	27.5	30.0	35.0
Black												
18–74 years	649	17.8	10.5	6.5	7.5	8.5	10.0	14.0	24.0	30.0	32.1	38.1
18–24 years	121	12.6	6.6	6.5	7.5	8.0	9.0	10.5	14.5	16.5	19.5	25.0
25–34 years	139	17.2	10.1	7.0	8.0	8.5	9.0	13.0	23.0	27.0	34.0	38.0
35–44 years	70	20.3	12.2	———	8.5	9.5	11.0	17.0	26.0	35.0	40.0	———
45–54 years	62	22.8	11.1	———	8.0	10.0	13.0	21.5	30.0	37.0	37.0	———
55–64 years	129	18.7	9.9	6.0	7.0	8.0	9.5	18.0	26.0	30.0	32.1	37.0
65–74 years	128	18.4	10.4	5.5	7.0	8.0	10.0	15.0	26.5	30.5	33.0	37.0

[*]Includes all other races not shown as separate categories.

Subscapular Skinfold in Millimeters for Females 18–74 Years of Age—United States, 1976–1980

Race and Age	Number of Examined Persons	Mean	Standard Deviation	Percentile								
				5th	10th	15th	25th	50th	75th	85th	90th	95th
*All Races**												
18–74 years	6588	21.2	12.0	7.0	8.0	9.5	11.5	18.0	29.0	35.0	38.5	45.0
18–24 years	1066	16.6	9.9	7.0	7.5	8.0	10.0	13.0	20.5	26.0	31.0	38.0
25–34 years	1170	20.0	12.2	7.0	8.0	8.5	10.5	16.0	27.0	33.5	38.0	45.0
35–44 years	844	22.3	12.4	7.0	8.5	10.0	12.0	19.0	31.0	36.6	40.1	46.5
45–54 years	763	24.1	12.2	7.0	10.0	11.0	14.5	22.0	32.5	37.5	40.5	47.6
55–64 years	1329	23.7	12.3	7.5	9.0	11.0	13.5	22.0	32.0	37.0	41.0	47.0
65–74 years	1416	22.3	11.1	7.0	8.5	10.0	13.0	21.0	30.0	35.0	37.1	43.0
White												
18–74 years	5686	20.5	11.7	7.0	8.0	9.0	11.0	17.0	27.5	34.0	37.5	43.5
18–24 years	892	16.1	9.6	7.0	7.5	8.0	10.0	13.0	19.0	25.0	29.5	37.5
25–34 years	1000	19.1	11.7	7.0	7.5	8.5	10.5	15.0	25.0	32.0	36.0	43.0
35–44 years	726	21.4	12.1	7.0	8.0	9.5	11.5	17.5	30.0	36.0	39.5	46.0
45–54 years	647	23.1	11.8	7.0	9.5	11.0	14.0	20.5	31.0	36.6	40.0	45.0
55–64 years	1176	23.0	12.0	7.0	9.0	11.0	13.0	21.5	31.0	36.0	39.5	45.6
65–74 years	1245	21.8	10.9	6.5	8.5	10.0	13.0	20.5	29.5	34.0	36.1	41.1
Black												
18–74 years	782	26.1	13.3	8.0	9.5	11.0	14.0	25.0	35.5	40.6	45.0	50.0
18–24 years	147	19.1	10.6	7.0	8.0	9.0	11.0	15.0	26.0	31.0	34.0	37.0
25–34 years	145	25.4	13.3	8.5	9.5	11.0	14.0	22.5	35.5	40.6	44.5	48.1
35–44 years	103	27.9	13.0	7.0	10.5	12.0	17.0	28.0	36.5	42.5	46.5	52.0
45–54 years	100	32.0	13.1	11.0	15.0	17.0	22.5	30.5	39.5	45.6	50.5	56.0
55–64 years	135	30.0	13.5	8.0	12.5	13.0	19.5	31.0	40.6	45.0	47.5	50.5
65–74 years	152	27.1	12.1	7.5	9.5	12.0	18.0	27.0	35.5	41.0	44.5	47.0

*Includes all other races not shown as separate categories.

APPENDIX Q

Means, Standard Deviations, and Percentiles of Sum of Skinfold Thickness (mm) by Age for Males and Females of 1 to 74 Years (See Table 7.2 for Interpretation Guidelines)

From Frisancho, AR. 1990. *Anthropometric standards for the assessment of growth and nutritional status.* Ann Arbor: University of Michigan Press. Copyright by the University of Michigan, 1990. Reprinted with permission.

Means, Standard Deviations, and Percentiles of Sum of Skinfold Thickness (mm) by Age for Males and Females of 1 to 74 Years

Age (yrs)	N	Mean	SD	5th	10th	15th	25th	50th	75th	85th	90th	95th
							Males					
1.0–1.9	681	16.8	4.1	11.0	12.0	12.5	14.0	16.5	19.0	21.0	22.0	24.0
2.0–2.9	677	16.0	4.3	10.0	11.0	12.0	13.0	15.5	18.0	20.0	21.5	24.0
3.0–3.9	716	15.4	4.1	10.5	11.0	12.0	13.0	14.5	17.5	19.0	20.5	23.0
4.0–4.9	707	14.5	4.2	9.5	10.5	11.0	12.0	14.0	16.5	18.0	19.0	21.5
5.0–5.9	677	14.2	5.0	9.0	10.0	10.0	11.0	13.0	16.0	18.0	19.0	22.0
6.0–6.9	298	14.3	6.7	8.0	9.0	10.0	10.5	13.0	15.2	18.0	20.0	28.0
7.0–7.9	312	14.8	6.9	8.5	9.0	9.5	10.5	13.0	16.0	19.5	23.0	26.6
8.0–8.9	296	15.6	7.8	8.5	9.0	10.0	11.0	13.5	17.0	20.0	24.5	30.5
9.0–9.9	322	17.0	9.4	8.5	9.5	10.0	11.0	14.0	19.0	24.0	29.0	34.0
10.0–10.9	334	19.1	10.6	9.0	10.0	11.0	12.0	15.5	22.0	27.0	33.5	42.0
11.0–11.9	324	21.4	13.9	9.0	10.0	11.0	12.5	16.5	25.0	33.0	40.0	53.5
12.0–12.9	348	21.0	13.2	9.0	10.0	11.0	12.5	17.0	24.0	34.0	40.5	53.0
13.0–13.9	350	19.8	13.3	8.5	10.5	11.0	12.5	15.0	21.0	29.0	37.0	48.0
14.0–14.9	358	19.4	12.6	9.0	10.0	11.0	12.0	15.0	22.0	27.0	33.0	45.0
15.0–15.9	356	19.3	12.8	10.0	10.5	11.0	12.0	15.0	21.0	27.0	32.5	43.0
16.0–16.9	349	20.0	11.4	10.0	11.5	12.0	13.0	16.0	22.5	27.5	33.5	44.0
17.0–17.9	337	19.1	10.8	10.0	11.0	12.0	13.0	16.0	22.0	27.0	31.5	41.0
18.0–24.9	1748	24.6	13.1	11.0	12.0	13.5	15.0	21.0	30.0	37.0	41.5	50.5
25.0–29.9	1246	27.6	13.9	11.5	13.0	14.0	17.0	24.5	35.0	41.0	46.0	54.5
30.0–34.9	938	30.4	14.1	12.0	14.5	16.5	20.0	28.0	38.0	44.0	49.0	58.0
35.0–39.9	829	30.3	13.3	12.0	14.5	16.5	21.0	29.0	37.0	42.4	47.0	54.5
40.0–44.9	816	30.1	13.3	13.0	15.0	16.5	20.5	28.5	37.0	42.5	47.5	55.0
45.0–49.9	856	30.9	13.6	12.5	15.0	17.5	20.5	29.0	39.0	44.0	48.0	55.0
50.0–54.9	872	30.1	13.1	13.0	15.0	17.0	20.5	28.0	37.5	43.0	48.0	55.5
55.0–59.9	802	29.9	12.7	12.0	15.0	17.0	21.0	28.5	37.0	43.0	47.0	53.5
60.0–64.9	1250	30.5	13.1	13.0	15.5	17.5	21.0	29.0	37.5	43.0	47.0	55.5
65.0–69.9	1770	28.9	13.1	11.0	13.5	16.0	19.5	27.0	36.0	42.0	46.5	53.5
70.0–74.9	1247	28.2	12.4	11.5	14.0	16.0	19.0	26.0	35.0	41.0	45.0	51.0

Means, Standard Deviations, and Percentiles of Sum of Skinfold Thickness (mm) by Age for Males and Females of 1 to 74 Years

Age (yrs)	N	Mean	SD	Percentile								
				5th	10th	15th	25th	50th	75th	85th	90th	95th
				Females								
1.0–1.9	622	16.9	4.5	10.5	12.0	12.0	13.5	16.5	19.5	21.0	23.0	25.0
2.0–2.9	614	16.9	4.5	11.0	12.0	12.5	14.0	16.0	19.0	21.5	23.5	25.5
3.0–3.9	652	16.5	4.5	10.5	11.5	12.0	13.5	16.0	18.5	20.5	21.5	25.0
4.0–4.9	681	16.3	4.7	10.0	11.0	12.0	13.0	15.5	18.5	20.5	22.5	24.5
5.0–5.9	672	16.5	5.9	10.0	11.0	11.5	12.5	15.0	18.5	21.0	24.0	28.5
6.0–6.9	296	16.7	6.5	10.0	10.5	11.0	12.5	15.5	18.5	21.0	23.5	28.0
7.0–7.9	330	17.8	7.1	10.0	11.0	12.0	13.5	16.0	20.0	23.0	26.0	32.5
8.0–8.9	276	20.0	10.7	10.5	11.0	12.0	13.0	17.0	22.5	28.5	31.0	41.5
9.0–9.9	322	22.4	11.8	11.0	12.0	12.5	14.5	19.0	25.5	30.0	39.0	48.9
10.0–10.9	329	23.6	12.1	12.0	12.5	13.0	15.0	20.0	28.5	34.5	40.5	51.0
11.0–11.9	300	25.5	13.6	12.0	13.5	14.5	16.0	22.0	30.0	37.0	42.0	55.0
12.0–12.9	323	26.6	13.3	13.0	14.0	15.0	18.0	23.0	31.0	37.0	44.0	57.0
13.0–13.9	360	28.7	14.6	12.5	14.0	15.5	18.5	24.5	35.5	43.0	47.5	56.5
14.0–14.9	370	30.1	14.3	14.5	16.0	17.5	20.0	26.0	37.0	44.5	48.5	62.0
15.0–15.9	308	30.1	14.1	15.0	17.0	18.0	20.5	26.5	34.5	42.5	48.5	62.5
16.0–16.9	343	33.9	14.9	17.5	20.0	21.5	24.0	30.0	39.5	47.0	53.5	69.5
17.0–17.9	291	34.5	16.2	16.5	18.5	20.0	23.0	31.0	42.0	49.0	55.5	67.4
18.0–24.9	2586	36.1	16.6	16.7	19.0	21.0	24.0	32.0	44.0	52.0	58.5	70.0
25.0–29.9	1907	39.0	18.0	17.5	20.0	22.0	25.5	35.0	48.5	58.0	64.5	73.9
30.0–34.9	1613	43.3	19.8	18.0	22.0	24.5	28.5	39.0	55.0	64.0	71.0	83.0
35.0–39.9	1443	45.2	19.5	19.0	22.5	25.5	30.0	42.0	57.5	66.0	72.2	82.5
40.0–44.9	1378	45.8	18.9	20.0	23.5	27.0	31.0	43.0	58.0	67.0	73.0	80.0
45.0–49.9	953	47.7	19.2	21.0	24.0	27.5	33.5	45.0	59.5	69.0	74.5	81.0
50.0–54.9	992	49.3	18.9	21.0	26.0	30.0	35.5	47.0	61.0	70.0	75.3	83.5
55.0–59.9	868	49.5	19.5	21.0	26.0	29.0	35.0	47.5	62.0	69.5	75.0	85.0
60.0–64.9	1374	49.2	18.6	22.0	27.0	30.0	35.5	48.0	61.0	68.0	74.0	83.5
65.0–69.9	1930	46.3	17.6	21.0	25.0	28.5	34.0	44.0	57.0	64.0	70.0	78.0
70.0–74.9	1458	44.5	17.1	19.0	23.5	27.0	32.0	43.0	56.0	62.0	67.0	75.5

N = number of persons in each age/sex category.
SD = standard deviation.

APPENDIX R

Means, Standard Deviations, and Percentiles of Upper-Arm Muscle Area (cm^2) by Age for Males and Females of 1 to 74 Years (See Table 7.6 for Interpretation Guidelines)

From Frisancho, AR. 1990. *Anthropometric standards for the assessment of growth and nutritional status.* Ann Arbor: University of Michigan Press. Copyright by the University of Michigan 1990. Reprinted with permission.

Means, Standard Deviations, and Percentiles of Upper-Arm Muscle Area (cm^2) by Age for Males and Females of 1 to 74 Years

Age (yrs)	N	Mean	SD	5th	10th	15th	25th	50th	75th	85th	90th	95th
							Percentile					
							Males					
1.0–1.9	681	13.2	2.3	9.7	10.4	10.8	11.6	13.0	14.6	15.4	16.3	17.2
2.0–2.9	672	14.1	3.2	10.1	10.9	11.3	12.4	13.9	15.6	16.4	16.9	18.4
3.0–3.9	715	15.2	3.1	11.2	12.0	12.6	13.5	15.0	16.4	17.4	18.3	19.5
4.0–4.9	707	16.3	2.7	12.0	12.9	13.5	14.5	16.2	17.9	18.8	19.8	20.9
5.0–5.9	676	17.8	3.7	13.2	14.2	14.7	15.7	17.6	19.5	20.7	21.7	23.2
6.0–6.9	298	19.3	4.0	14.4	15.3	15.8	16.8	18.7	21.3	22.9	23.8	25.7
7.0–7.9	312	21.0	4.5	15.1	16.2	17.0	18.5	20.6	22.6	24.5	25.2	28.6
8.0–8.9	296	22.1	4.2	16.3	17.8	18.5	19.5	21.6	24.0	25.5	26.6	29.0
9.0–9.9	322	24.5	5.1	18.2	19.3	20.3	21.7	23.5	26.7	28.7	30.4	32.9
10.0–10.9	333	26.7	5.9	19.6	20.7	21.6	23.0	25.7	29.0	32.2	34.0	37.1
11.0–11.9	324	28.8	6.7	21.0	22.0	23.0	24.8	27.7	31.6	33.6	36.1	40.3
12.0–12.9	348	31.9	7.4	22.6	24.1	25.3	26.9	30.4	35.9	39.3	40.9	44.9
13.0–13.9	350	36.8	9.0	24.5	26.7	28.1	30.4	35.7	41.3	45.3	48.1	52.5
14.0–14.9	358	42.4	9.1	28.3	31.3	33.1	36.1	41.9	47.4	51.3	54.0	57.5
15.0–15.9	356	46.8	9.6	31.9	34.9	36.9	40.3	46.3	53.1	56.3	57.7	63.0
16.0–16.9	350	52.6	10.0	37.0	40.9	42.4	45.9	51.9	57.8	63.6	66.2	70.5
17.0–17.9	337	54.7	10.5	39.6	42.6	44.8	48.0	53.4	60.4	64.3	67.9	73.1
18.0–24.9	1752	50.5	11.6	34.2	37.3	39.6	42.7	49.4	57.1	61.8	65.0	72.0
25.0–29.9	1250	54.1	11.9	36.6	39.9	42.4	46.0	53.0	61.4	66.1	68.9	74.5
30.0–34.9	940	55.6	12.1	37.9	40.9	43.4	47.3	54.4	63.2	67.6	70.8	76.1
35.0–39.9	832	56.5	12.4	38.5	42.6	44.6	47.9	55.3	64.0	69.1	72.7	77.6
40.0–44.9	828	56.6	11.7	38.4	42.1	45.1	48.7	56.0	64.0	68.5	71.6	77.0
45.0–49.9	867	55.9	12.3	37.7	41.3	43.7	47.9	55.2	63.3	68.4	72.2	76.2
50.0–54.9	879	55.0	12.5	36.0	40.0	42.7	46.6	54.0	62.7	67.0	70.4	77.4
55.0–59.9	807	54.7	11.8	36.5	40.8	42.7	46.7	54.3	61.9	66.4	69.6	75.1
60.0–64.9	1259	52.8	11.7	34.5	38.7	41.2	44.9	52.1	60.0	64.8	67.5	71.6
65.0–69.9	1773	49.8	11.6	31.4	35.8	38.4	42.3	49.1	57.3	61.2	64.3	69.4
70.0–74.9	1250	47.8	11.5	29.7	33.8	36.1	40.2	47.0	54.6	59.1	62.1	67.3

Means, Standard Deviations, and Percentiles of Upper-Arm Muscle Area (cm²) by Age for Males and Females of 1 to 74 Years

Age (yrs)	N	Mean	SD	5th	10th	15th	25th	50th	75th	85th	90th	95th
											Percentile	
Females												
1.0–1.9	622	12.3	2.3	8.9	9.7	10.1	10.8	12.3	13.8	14.6	15.3	16.2
2.0–2.9	614	13.3	2.3	10.1	10.6	10.9	11.8	13.2	14.7	15.6	16.4	17.3
3.0–3.9	651	14.3	2.4	10.8	11.4	11.8	12.6	14.3	15.8	16.7	17.4	18.8
4.0–4.9	680	15.4	2.8	11.2	12.2	12.7	13.6	15.3	17.0	18.0	18.6	19.8
5.0–5.9	672	16.7	3.1	12.4	13.2	13.9	14.8	16.4	18.3	19.4	20.6	22.1
6.0–6.9	296	18.0	3.9	13.5	14.1	14.6	15.6	17.4	19.5	21.0	22.0	24.2
7.0–7.9	329	19.3	4.0	14.4	15.2	15.8	16.7	18.9	21.2	22.6	23.9	25.3
8.0–8.9	275	21.1	4.7	15.2	16.0	16.8	18.2	20.8	23.2	24.6	26.5	28.0
9.0–9.9	321	22.9	4.6	17.0	17.9	18.7	19.8	21.9	25.4	27.2	28.3	31.1
10.0–10.9	329	24.3	5.5	17.6	18.5	19.3	20.9	23.8	27.0	29.1	31.0	33.1
11.0–11.9	302	27.6	6.7	19.5	21.0	21.7	23.2	26.4	30.7	33.5	35.7	39.2
12.0–12.9	323	29.7	6.5	20.4	21.8	23.1	25.5	29.0	33.2	36.3	37.8	40.5
13.0–13.9	360	31.9	7.4	22.8	24.5	25.4	27.1	30.8	35.3	38.1	39.6	43.7
14.0–14.9	370	33.9	7.7	24.0	26.2	27.1	29.0	32.8	36.9	39.8	42.3	47.5
15.0–15.9	309	33.8	7.0	24.4	25.8	27.5	29.2	33.0	37.3	40.2	41.7	45.9
16.0–16.9	343	34.8	8.0	25.2	26.8	28.2	30.0	33.6	38.0	40.2	43.7	48.3
17.0–17.9	291	36.1	8.8	25.9	27.5	28.9	30.7	34.3	39.6	43.4	46.2	50.8
18.0–24.9	2588	29.8	8.4	19.5	21.5	22.8	24.5	28.3	33.1	36.4	39.0	44.2
25.0–29.9	1921	31.1	9.1	20.5	21.9	23.1	25.2	29.4	34.9	38.5	41.9	47.8
30.0–34.9	1619	32.8	10.4	21.1	23.0	24.2	26.3	30.9	36.8	41.2	44.7	51.3
35.0–39.9	1453	34.2	11.5	21.1	23.4	24.7	27.3	31.8	38.7	43.1	46.1	54.2
40.0–44.9	1390	35.2	13.3	21.3	23.4	25.5	27.5	32.3	39.8	45.8	49.5	55.8
45.0–49.9	961	34.9	11.8	21.6	23.1	24.8	27.4	32.5	39.5	44.7	48.4	56.1
50.0–54.9	1004	35.6	11.0	22.2	24.6	25.7	28.3	33.4	40.4	46.1	49.6	55.6
55.0–59.9	879	37.1	13.3	22.8	24.8	26.5	28.7	34.7	42.3	47.3	52.1	58.8
60.0–64.9	1389	36.3	11.3	22.4	24.5	26.3	29.2	34.5	41.1	45.6	49.1	55.1
65.0–69.9	1946	36.3	11.3	21.9	24.5	26.2	28.9	34.6	41.6	46.3	49.6	56.5
70.0–74.9	1463	36.0	10.8	22.2	24.4	26.0	28.8	34.3	41.8	46.4	49.2	54.6

N = number of persons in each age/sex category.

SD = standard deviation.

Note: Values for males and females ages 18 years and older have been adjusted for bone area by subtracting 10.0 cm² and 6.5 cm², respectively, from the calculated midupper-arm muscle area.

APPENDIX S

Reference Values for Serum Total Cholesterol and Serum High-Density Lipoprotein, by Sex, Age, Race/Ethnicity, 1988–1994

Data from the National Center for Health Statistics, Centers for Disease Control and Prevention, U.S. Department of Health and Human Services.

Serum Total Cholesterol of Males 4 Years of Age and Older by Age: Mean and Selected Percentiles, United States, 1988–94

Age in Years	Number of Examined Persons	Mean	Standard Deviation	Standard Error of the Mean	Selected Percentiles								
					5th	10th	15th	25th	50th	75th	85th	90th	95th
4 years and older, crude	11,200	192	41.9	0.63	131	142	149	162	189	220	237	248	266
4 years and older, age adjusted		191											
4–5 years	846	161	24.3	1.33	123	133	136	144	159	175	185	192	203
6–8 years	695	166	26.4	1.59	127	135	140	147	165	183	191	203	212
9–11 years	757	172	28.4	1.64	135	140	145	153	171	189	196	209	227
12–15 years	703	158	27.5	1.65	117	124	130	140	158	174	184	192	203
16–19 years	668	158	29.7	1.82	117	123	127	138	156	175	190	200	214
20 years and older, crude	7531	202	41.0	0.75	139	151	160	173	200	228	244	255	273
20 years and older, age adjusted		202											
20–74 years	6587	202	41.0	0.80	139	151	160	173	200	228	244	255	273
20–74 years, age adjusted		201											
20–29 years	1551	180	36.2	1.46	127	137	145	155	177	200	216	225	242
30–39 years	1389	201	39.3	1.68	139	153	162	171	199	228	244	253	267
40–49 years	1169	211	39.2	1.82	147	164	173	186	209	236	249	261	275
50–59 years	829	216	40.8	2.25	154	166	177	191	214	240	257	270	286
60–69 years	1137	217	39.2	1.85	152	169	177	190	215	241	256	270	285
70–79 years	812	208	39.2	2.18	148	159	169	180	205	233	248	256	275
80+ years	644	201	41.0	2.56	140	152	158	170	198	226	244	253	270

Serum Total Cholesterol of Males 4 Years of Age and Older by Race/Ethnicity and Age: Mean and Selected Percentiles, United States, 1988–94

Non-Hispanic White, Age in Years	Number of Examined Persons	Mean	Standard Deviation	Standard Error of the Mean	Selected Percentiles								
					5th	10th	15th	25th	50th	75th	85th	90th	95th
4 years and older, crude	4097	194	41.7	0.8	132	143	150	164	191	222	238	248	267
4 years and older, age adjusted		190											
4–5 years	210	160	22.4	1.8	130	134	140	144	159	174	181	186	197
6–11 years	387	169	26.0	1.5	128	139	144	151	167	184	193	200	216
12–19 years	339	157	28.3	1.8	116	120	126	137	155	173	184	195	205
20 years and older, crude	3161	203	40.4	0.8	141	153	162	174	201	229	244	256	272
20 years and older, age adjusted		201											
20–74 years	2449	203	40.5	1.0	141	153	162	174	201	229	244	256	272
20–74 years, age adjusted		201											
20–29 years	381	179	35.9	2.2	125	137	144	154	175	198	215	224	239
30–39 years	434	201	38.5	2.2	142	156	163	171	199	228	244	253	267
40–49 years	421	212	38.5	2.2	152	166	175	187	209	237	249	261	275
50–59 years	411	216	39.8	2.3	155	166	176	193	213	238	259	272	286
60–69 years	499	217	37.6	2.0	157	171	178	192	215	241	253	267	283
70+ years	1015	206	39.3	1.4	146	155	165	177	203	230	246	255	273

Serum Total Cholesterol of Males 4 Years of Age and Older by Race/Ethnicity and Age: Mean and Selected Percentiles, United States, 1988–94

Non-Hispanic Black, Age in Years	Number of Examined Persons	Mean	Standard Deviation	Standard Error of the Mean	Selected Percentiles								
					5th	10th	15th	25th	50th	75th	85th	90th	95th
4 years and older, crude	3154	188	41.5	0.8	131	140	148	159	184	212	228	240	264
4 years and older, age adjusted		191											
4–5 years	275	164	26.9	1.8	122	127	135	148	164	181	192	200	211
6–11 years	480	172	30.0	1.5	128	137	143	153	169	190	200	207	224
12–19 years	476	166	30.6	1.6	119	131	136	147	163	185	193	201	220
20 years and older, crude	1923	198	42.8	1.1	136	147	155	169	195	222	239	251	275
20 years and older, age adjusted		200											
20–74 years	1813	198	42.7	1.1	136	147	155	169	195	222	238	251	274
20–74 years, age adjusted	1813	200											
20–29 years	456	185	35.6	1.8	133	141	149	161	181	207	221	232	249
30–39 years	451	193	40.1	2.1	134	142	153	162	191	216	227	236	262
40–49 years	333	206	43.2	2.6	143	152	165	178	202	228	249	265	285
50–59 years	203	213	48.4	3.8	136	154	165	180	211	239	255	277	309
60–69 years	268	215	47.8	3.2	148	166	173	181	211	244	263	274	294
70+ years	212	207	42.3	3.2	141	155	159	178	206	233	249	257	289

Serum Total Cholesterol of Males 4 Years of Age and Older by Race/Ethnicity and Age: Mean and Selected Percentiles, United States, 1988–94

Mexican Americans, Age in Years	Number of Examined Persons	Mean	Standard Deviation	Standard Error of the Mean	Selected Percentiles								
					5th	10th	15th	25th	50th	75th	85th	90th	95th
4 years and older, crude	3499	187	42.5	0.9	129	139	146	157	182	212	228	242	260
4 years and older, age adjusted		192											
4–5 years	316	158	26.3	1.9	119	127	133	140	156	172	185	195	204
6–11 years	515	168	26.8	1.5	128	136	139	149	166	185	196	205	215
12–19 years	493	161	30.3	1.8	119	126	132	141	157	177	191	200	213
20 years and older, crude		199	43.1	1.2	137	150	157	171	197	224	241	253	272
20 years and older, age adjusted		203											
20–74 years	2073	200	43.2	1.2	138	150	158	171	197	224	241	253	273
20–74 years, age adjusted	2073	204											
20–29 years	644	184	38.3	1.9	130	142	149	157	177	205	219	232	250
30–39 years	449	205	41.6	2.5	141	157	168	179	200	227	247	257	274
40–49 years	370	212	42.2	2.8	150	163	172	186	210	233	249	266	290
50–59 years	176	215	50.3	4.9	146*	167	179	189	218	235	256	269	279*
60–69 years	337	219	40.6	2.9	160	175	181	188	219	245	258	267	285
70+ years	199	203	41.1	3.7	144*	153	158	173	202	232	241	254	273*

*Value based on a limited number of observations.

Serum Total Cholesterol of Females 4 Years of Age and Older by Age: Mean and Selected Percentiles, United States, 1988–94

Age in Years	Number of Examined Persons	Mean	Standard Deviation	Standard Error of the Mean	Selected Percentiles								
					5th	10th	15th	25th	50th	75th	85th	90th	95th
4 years and older, crude	12,361	197	45.1	0.61	135	145	153	165	191	224	244	257	278
4 years and older, age adjusted		195											
4–5 years	861	164	25.9	1.32	126	134	140	146	163	179	190	197	206
6–8 years	672	166	26.5	1.53	127	136	143	150	165	181	190	196	203
9–11 years	731	169	26.7	1.48	131	137	143	149	167	185	196	205	219
12–15 years	799	164	29.8	1.58	123	130	135	143	160	182	192	201	218
16–19 years	767	171	39.8	2.16	118	128	136	145	164	189	203	217	238
20 years and older, crude	8531	206	44.7	0.73	143	153	161	175	201	233	251	265	284
20 years and older, age adjusted		206											
20–74 years	7429	204	44.2	0.77	142	152	160	173	199	231	249	262	282
20–74 years, age adjusted		204											
20–29 years	1760	183	37.2	1.33	131	141	147	157	179	205	217	229	244
30–39 years	1750	189	34.7	1.24	138	147	153	166	186	209	226	234	250
40–49 years	1300	204	38.2	1.59	150	158	164	177	201	225	245	254	277
50–59 years	962	228	43.8	2.12	166	177	184	199	224	255	273	284	304
60–69 years	1109	235	45.5	2.05	170	183	193	205	230	258	278	290	309
70–79 years	934	233	44.8	2.20	164	177	188	200	233	262	277	287	309
80+ years	716	228	43.3	2.43	165	177	183	196	224	254	270	285	305

Serum Total Cholesterol of Females 4 Years of Age and Older by Race/Ethnicity and Age: Mean and Selected Percentiles, United States, 1988–94

Non-Hispanic White, Age in Years	Number of Examined Persons	Mean	Standard Deviation	Standard Error of the Mean	Selected Percentiles								
					5th	10th	15th	25th	50th	75th	85th	90th	95th
4 years and older, crude	4661	200	45.4	0.8	137	147	154	167	194	227	246	259	280
4 years and older, age adjusted		195											
4–5 years	226	163	23.9	1.8	128	137	140	146	162	177	184	195	208
6–11 years	366	167	25.6	1.6	128	135	143	150	167	183	194	198	212
12–19 years	424	166	36.8	2.1	118	128	134	142	160	185	196	203	227
20 years and older, crude	3645	208	44.6	0.9	144	155	163	177	203	235	252	267	284
20 years and older, age adjusted		206											
20–74 years	2818	206	44.1	1.0	143	153	162	175	201	233	250	263	282
20–74 years, age adjusted		205											
20–29 years	480	183	37.0	2.0	133	141	148	156	182	206	217	229	243
30–39 years	570	188	33.7	1.6	139	147	154	166	185	209	225	233	249
40–49 years	464	205	37.3	2.0	150	158	167	178	202	226	245	253	274
50–59 years	466	230	43.5	2.3	171	179	187	200	226	256	275	285	304
60–69 years	477	234	44.9	2.4	173	184	193	205	229	257	276	288	309
70+ years	1188	232	43.9	1.5	166	178	187	199	232	259	274	285	308

Serum Total Cholesterol of Females 4 Years of Age and Older by Race/Ethnicity and Age: Mean and Selected Percentiles, United States, 1988–94

Non-Hispanic Black, Age in Years	Number of Examined Persons	Mean	Standard Deviation	Standard Error of the Mean	Selected Percentiles								
					5th	10th	15th	25th	50th	75th	85th	90th	95th
4 years and older, crude	3638	193	44.2	0.9	131	142	150	162	187	217	236	251	273
4 years and older, age adjusted		195											
4–5 years	270	167	30.1	2.2	121	131	141	148	165	184	191	201	220
6–11 years	461	173	31.4	1.7	131	141	144	150	169	192	206	213	227
12–19 years	547	170	33.4	1.7	120	130	137	148	167	190	208	216	229
20 years and older, crude	2360	201	45.3	1.1	136	148	157	170	196	226	246	261	284
20 years and older, age adjusted		205											
20–74 years	2209	200	44.7	1.1	136	147	157	169	195	224	244	259	281
20–74 years, age adjusted	2209	203											
20–29 years	577	184	38.2	1.9	129	139	148	158	181	204	216	227	253
30–39 years	596	187	35.4	1.7	132	142	151	164	184	209	221	230	248
40–49 years	420	203	39.5	2.3	141	155	165	177	201	225	241	251	269
50–59 years	255	224	47.2	3.5	152	167	175	193	218	257	272	281	302
60–69 years	270	238	50.2	3.6	170	180	192	207	234	262	284	295	322
70+ years	242	227	48.1	3.7	156	171	178	195	224	257	275	291	304

Serum Total Cholesterol of Females 4 Years of Age and Older by Race/Ethnicity and Age: Mean and Selected Percentiles, United States, 1988–94

Mexican Americans, Age in Years	Number of Examined Persons	Mean	Standard Deviation	Standard Error of the Mean	Selected Percentiles								
					5th	10th	15th	25th	50th	75th	85th	90th	95th
4 years and older, crude	3517	186	42.6	0.9	129	140	145	156	182	210	228	239	261
4 years and older, age adjusted		193											
4–5 years	321	163	28.3	2.0	121	129	138	147	163	183	191	198	206
6–11 years	522	165	30.6	1.7	126	135	141	146	162	180	188	199	209
12–19 years	509	166	33.6	1.9	120	126	133	143	160	185	199	209	224
20 years and older, crude		198	43.3	1.2	139	148	156	167	193	223	238	249	274
20 years and older, age adjusted		204											
20–74 years	2070	197	43.1	1.2	138	147	155	166	192	222	237	249	274
20–74 years, age adjusted	2070	202											
20–29 years	631	183	40.2	2.0	132	140	144	156	177	203	220	232	245
30–39 years	506	191	39.1	2.2	136	146	153	164	187	213	231	238	266
40–49 years	352	205	41.6	2.8	149	158	163	177	202	225	242	254	282
50–59 years	186	222	40.7	3.7	158[*]	182	186	196	218	240	255	268	294[*]
60–69 years	318	229	39.9	2.8	165	180	188	203	230	256	267	282	297
70+ years	172	221	43.1	4.1	153[*]	167	184	198	219	241	262	283	295[*]

[*]Value based on a limited number of observations.

Serum High-Density Lipoprotein (HDL) Cholesterol of Males 4 Years of Age and Older by Age: Mean and Selected Percentiles, United States, 1988–94

Age in Years	Number of Examined Persons	Mean	Standard Deviation	Standard Error of the Mean	Selected Percentiles								
					5th	10th	15th	25th	50th	75th	85th	90th	95th
4 years and older, crude	11,123	47	13.4	0.21	28	32	34	38	45	54	60	64	72
4 years and older, age adjusted		47											
4–5 years	845	50	11.9	0.69	31	36	38	42	49	56	63	66	72
6–8 years	692	53	12.3	0.78	33	38	40	44	52	61	65	68	74
9–11 years	752	54	12.7	0.77	37	39	42	44	53	62	67	71	76
12–15 years	697	48	11.3	0.71	33	36	37	40	47	55	60	63	68
16–19 years	664	46	11.1	0.72	30	33	36	38	45	52	57	61	67
20 years and older, crude	7473	46	13.7	0.26	28	31	34	37	44	53	58	63	72
20 years and older, age adjusted		46											
20–74 years	6535	46	13.6	0.28	28	30	33	37	44	53	58	62	72
20–74 years, age adjusted		46											
20–29 years	1541	47	12.5	0.53	29	33	35	39	45	54	60	63	69
30–39 years	1379	46	13.3	0.60	27	32	34	37	44	52	58	61	70
40–49 years	1152	45	14.8	0.73	26	30	32	36	43	51	58	64	74
50–59 years	823	44	13.9	0.81	27	30	32	36	42	51	56	61	75
60–69 years	1130	46	13.7	0.68	28	31	32	36	43	53	58	63	72
70–79 years	808	46	14.9	0.87	28	31	33	36	44	53	59	63	74
80+ years	640	47	14.2	0.94	29	31	34	38	44	55	63	66	74

Serum High-Density Lipoprotein (HDL) Cholesterol of Males 4 Years of Age and Older by Race/Ethnicity and Age: Mean and Selected Percentiles, United States, 1988–94

Non-Hispanic White, Age in Years	Number of Examined Persons	Mean	Standard Deviation	Standard Error of the Mean	Selected Percentiles								
					5th	10th	15th	25th	50th	75th	85th	90th	95th
4 years and older, crude	4069	46	12.9	0.3	28	31	34	37	44	53	58	62	69
4 years and older, age adjusted		46											
4–5 years	210	49	11.8	1.0	30	35	36	41	48	54	62	64	66
6–11 years	386	52	12.0	0.8	34	38	40	44	51	61	65	68	73
12–19 years	335	45	10.1	0.7	31	34	36	38	44	52	55	59	63
20 years and older, crude	3138	45	13.2	0.3	27	30	33	36	43	52	57	61	71
20 years and older, age adjusted		45											
20–74 years	2431	45	13.1	0.3	27	30	33	36	43	51	57	61	70
20–74 years, age adjusted		45											
20–29 years	378	46	12.1	0.8	28	31	34	38	44	53	59	62	69
30–39 years	431	45	12.7	0.8	26	31	34	37	43	51	55	61	68
40–49 years	416	44	14.1	0.9	26	29	31	35	42	50	54	61	72
50–59 years	409	44	13.6	0.9	26	30	31	35	42	50	55	61	74
60–69 years	495	45	13.3	0.8	28	30	32	36	42	53	58	62	71
70+ years	1009	46	13.6	0.6	28	31	33	36	43	53	59	63	72

Serum High-Density Lipoprotein (HDL) Cholesterol of Males 4 Years of Age and Older by Race/Ethnicity and Age: Mean and Selected Percentiles, United States, 1988–94

Non-Hispanic Black, Age in Years	Number of Examined Persons	Mean	Standard Deviation	Standard Error of the Mean	Selected Percentiles								
					5th	10th	15th	25th	50th	75th	85th	90th	95th
4 years and older, crude	3137	53	15.7	0.3	33	36	38	42	51	61	69	73	83
4 years and older, age adjusted		53											
4–5 years	274	53	11.6	0.8	36	39	42	46	52	59	65	69	75
6–11 years	475	59	14.0	0.7	40	42	44	50	58	68	74	77	86
12–19 years	472	53	12.0	0.6	36	38	42	45	52	60	66	68	73
20 years and older, crude	1916	52	16.7	0.4	32	35	37	41	50	60	68	74	85
20 years and older, age adjusted		52											
20–74 years	1807	52	16.6	0.4	32	35	37	41	49	60	68	74	85
20–74 years, age adjusted	1807	52											
20–29 years	455	53	14.7	0.8	35	37	38	42	51	59	68	73	82
30–39 years	450	52	16.2	0.9	32	35	37	41	49	61	68	73	83
40–49 years	330	53	18.7	1.2	30	34	36	40	48	62	70	80	91
50–59 years	202	51	17.6	1.4	29	33	36	39	47	56	67	77	86
60–69 years	268	51	17.1	1.2	30	34	36	38	48	61	70	74	80
70+ years	211	54	18.4	1.4	33	38	40	43	51	60	67	74	95

Serum High-Density Lipoprotein (HDL) Cholesterol of Males 4 Years of Age and Older by Race/Ethnicity and Age: Mean and Selected Percentiles, United States, 1988–94

Mexican Americans, Age in Years	Number of Examined Persons	Mean	Standard Deviation	Standard Error of the Mean	Selected Percentiles								
					5th	10th	15th	25th	50th	75th	85th	90th	95th
4 years and older, crude	3471	47	12.7	0.3	30	33	35	38	46	54	60	64	70
4 years and older, age adjusted		47											
4–5 years	316	50	12.9	0.9	29	34	38	41	49	58	63	65	72
6–11 years	513	54	12.9	0.7	35	38	41	44	53	63	67	70	75
12–19 years	491	48	11.4	0.6	31	34	37	40	47	54	60	63	67
20 years and older, crude		46	12.5	0.3	28	32	34	37	44	52	58	61	67
20 years and older, age adjusted		45											
20–74 years	2049	46	12.5	0.3	28	32	34	37	44	53	58	61	67
20–74 years, age adjusted	2049	46											
20–29 years	640	46	11.0	0.5	30	33	36	39	45	53	57	61	66
30–39 years	444	46	13.9	0.8	27	31	34	37	44	52	58	64	74
40–49 years	361	44	12.3	0.8	28	30	32	35	41	50	57	60	66
50–59 years	173	46	14.1	1.3	28*	30	33	36	43	54	60	63	80*
60–69 years	335	45	12.8	0.9	30	32	34	37	43	51	57	61	66
70+ years	198	44	12.9	1.1	28*	30	33	37	41	50	57	63	67*

*Value vased on a limited number of observations.

Serum High-Density Lipoprotein (HDL) Cholesterol of Females 4 Years of Age and Older by Age: Mean and Selected Percentiles, United States, 1988–94

Age in Years	Number of Examined Persons	Mean	Standard Deviation	Standard Error of the Mean	Selected Percentiles								
					5th	10th	15th	25th	50th	75th	85th	90th	95th
4 years and older, crude	12,286	54	14.8	0.20	34	38	40	44	53	63	68	73	80
4 years and older, age adjusted		54											
4–5 years	852	48	11.3	0.58	30	35	37	40	47	55	59	62	68
6–8 years	670	50	11.2	0.65	33	38	40	43	49	58	61	65	70
9–11 years	727	51	11.3	0.63	33	38	40	42	50	58	61	66	70
12–15 years	797	51	11.6	0.61	34	37	40	43	50	59	63	66	70
16–19 years	762	52	12.0	0.66	34	38	40	44	52	60	63	67	73
20 years and older, crude	8478	55	15.5	0.25	34	38	41	44	54	64	70	75	83
20 years and older, age adjusted		55											
20–74 years	7382	55	15.4	0.27	34	38	41	45	53	64	70	75	83
20–74 years, age adjusted		55											
20–29 years	1751	55	14.8	0.53	35	38	41	45	53	64	70	75	84
30–39 years	1744	54	15.0	0.54	33	37	40	44	53	64	69	74	81
40–49 years	1282	55	14.0	0.59	36	38	41	45	53	64	68	72	79
50–59 years	955	57	17.2	0.83	34	38	41	45	54	65	73	78	87
60–69 years	1104	56	17.2	0.78	32	37	40	44	53	65	72	78	87
70–79 years	929	56	16.4	0.81	32	36	40	45	55	64	71	75	84
80+ years	713	56	15.9	0.89	33	37	40	44	54	65	71	76	85

Serum High-Density Lipoprotein (HDL) Cholesterol of Females 4 Years of Age and Older by Race/Ethnicity and Age: Mean and Selected Percentiles, United States, 1988–94

Non-Hispanic White, Age in Years	Number of Examined Persons	Mean	Standard Deviation	Standard Error of the Mean	Selected Percentiles								
					5th	10th	15th	25th	50th	75th	85th	90th	95th
4 years and older, crude	4625	54	15.0	0.3	34	38	40	44	53	63	69	73	81
4 years and older, age adjusted		54											
4–5 years	224	46	11.0	0.8	30	34	36	39	46	52	57	61	68
6–11 years	363	49	10.5	0.6	32	38	39	42	48	55	60	62	68
12–19 years	423	51	11.1	0.6	32	37	39	42	51	58	61	64	70
20 years and older, crude	3615	56	15.6	0.3	34	38	41	45	54	64	70	76	84
20 years and older, age adjusted		56											
20–74 years	2793	56	15.6	0.3	34	38	41	45	54	64	70	76	84
20–74 years, age adjusted		56											
20–29 years	475	55	15.2	0.8	36	38	41	44	53	64	71	76	86
30–39 years	566	55	15.1	0.7	33	37	40	44	54	64	69	74	82
40–49 years	456	56	13.7	0.7	37	39	42	46	54	65	69	72	79
50–59 years	464	57	17.7	1.0	34	38	41	45	54	66	75	79	87
60–69 years	473	56	17.1	0.9	31	37	40	44	53	65	72	78	86
70+ years	1181	55	16.0	0.5	32	36	40	44	54	64	71	75	83

Serum High-Density Lipoprotein (HDL) Cholesterol of Females 4 Years of Age and Older by Race/Ethnicity and Age: Mean and Selected Percentiles, United States, 1988–94

Non-Hispanic Black, Age in Years	Number of Examined Persons	Mean	Standard Deviation	Standard Error of the Mean	Selected Percentiles								
					5th	10th	15th	25th	50th	75th	85th	90th	95th
4 years and older, crude	3614	57	15.6	0.3	36	39	42	46	55	65	72	77	85
4 years and older, age adjusted		57											
4–5 years	263	53	11.7	0.9	35	38	42	45	52	59	64	69	76
6–11 years	460	56	12.9	0.7	36	41	44	47	56	65	70	72	78
12–19 years	543	56	13.5	0.7	36	40	43	46	54	62	70	73	80
20 years and older, crude	2348	57	16.4	0.4	35	39	42	46	55	66	73	79	86
20 years and older, age adjusted		58											
20–74 years	2198	57	16.2	0.4	35	39	42	46	55	66	73	78	85
20–74 years, age adjusted	2198	57											
20–29 years	576	58	14.6	0.7	37	41	44	48	57	66	72	77	84
30–39 years	595	57	15.7	0.8	36	39	42	46	54	66	72	78	85
40–49 years	415	55	17.3	1.0	34	37	40	43	52	63	71	77	86
50–59 years	252	57	15.5	1.2	35	39	41	46	55	67	73	77	85
60–69 years	269	60	19.2	1.4	34	39	42	47	57	70	77	82	89
70+ years	241	61	18.9	1.4	35	40	42	47	58	72	80	86	92

Serum High-Density Lipoprotein (HDL) Cholesterol of Females 4 Years of Age and Older by Race/Ethnicity and Age: Mean and Selected Percentiles, United States, 1988–94

Mexican Americans, Age in Years	Number of Examined Persons	Mean	Standard Deviation	Standard Error of the Mean	Selected Percentiles								
					5th	10th	15th	25th	50th	75th	85th	90th	95th
4 years and older, crude	3504	52	13.2	0.3	33	37	39	43	51	59	65	69	77
4 years and older, age adjusted		52											
4–5 years	321	49	11.0	0.8	32	36	38	41	49	56	60	62	65
6–11 years	520	51	11.7	0.6	34	38	40	43	50	58	63	67	73
12–19 years	507	53	12.4	0.7	35	38	40	44	52	59	64	69	76
20 years and older, crude		52	13.8	0.4	33	36	38	42	51	60	66	71	77
20 years and older, age adjusted		53											
20–74 years	2061	52	13.8	0.4	33	36	38	42	50	59	66	71	77
20–74 years, age adjusted	2061	52											
20–29 years	628	53	13.4	0.7	34	37	39	44	51	59	66	71	77
30–39 years	506	51	13.7	0.8	31	36	38	42	50	59	65	70	77
40–49 years	348	50	12.7	0.8	32	35	37	41	49	57	62	65	70
50–59 years	184	55	15.4	1.4	34[*]	38	42	45	52	63	71	77	87[*]
60–69 years	318	54	14.7	1.0	32	36	40	44	52	63	69	73	81
70+ years	172	55	16.1	1.5	34[*]	36	39	44	54	65	71	76	80[*]

*Value based on a limited number of observations.

*Example of a Form That Can
Be Used for Self-Monitoring
Eating Behavior*

Food Record

Name _____ Day of week _____ Date _____

Time	Time Spent	Food Eaten—How Prepared	Amount	Place, Person(s) with Whom Food Was Eaten, Other Activities, Mood/Feelings

Remember: Do not alter your normal diet while keeping this record. For the requested information, provide responses that are as accurate as possible.

APPENDIX U

Compentency Checklist for Nutrition Counselors

This can be used by counselors to identify the competencies they already possess and those they want to develop.

From Raab C, and Tillotson JL. 1985. *Heart to heart: A manual on nutrition counseling for the reduction of cardiovascular disease risk factors.* Bethesda, MD: U.S. Department of Health and Human Services: Public Health Service; National Institutes of Health.

Nutrition Information for Particular Patient	Performance Objectives	Needs More Work	Not Attempted Yet	Good
1. Counselor knows the essential elements and rationale behind patient's prescribed diet (e.g., low-fat, low-sodium, etc.)	1a. Is familiar with all the food categories of the diet	_____	_____	_____
	1b. Is comfortable with substitutions and rationale for selection of food	_____	_____	_____
	1c. Is prepared to help patient adapt diet to his or her needs	_____	_____	_____
2. Counselor has knowledge of local eating patterns.	2a. Has some grasp of regional customs and of what foods are available in area	_____	_____	_____
	2b. Is familiar with frequently patronized restaurants and food chains and will ask patient his or her favorites	_____	_____	_____
3. At the outset, counselor makes reasonably sure that patient's knowledge of prescribed diet is adequate.	3a. Takes a history to find out patient's dietary background	_____	_____	_____
	3b. At first session, discusses long-term goals and explains diet thoroughly, making sure patient understands	_____	_____	_____
	3c. Eliminates patient's knowledge gaps (by discussing diet further, giving examples, using visuals, etc.) so following sessions can concentrate on goal setting	_____	_____	_____
	3d. Initially, asks patient for food diary; analyzes with patient to assess current diet and eating behavior	_____	_____	_____
Communication Skills				
4. Counselor sets appropriate tone for counseling sessions through preparation, manner, and physical setting.	4a. Makes appointment with patient, allowing enough time for comfortable, thorough discussion	_____	_____	_____
	4b. Arranges for private, quiet setting	_____	_____	_____

continued

Nutrition Information for Particular Patient	Performance Objectives	Needs More Work	Not Attempted Yet	Good
Communication Skills—(cont'd)				
	4c. Establishes patient's ability to see and to read and speak English; adapts counseling if necessary	_____	_____	_____
	4d. Shows interest in patient as an individual, looks for his or her particular needs and preferences	_____	_____	_____
	4e. Maintains relaxed, comfortable manner; makes patient feel at ease	_____	_____	_____
	4f. Indicates intentions to talk and to listen	_____	_____	_____
5. Counselor prepares self and patient for continuing relationship over a specified period.	5a. Explains initially the necessity of follow-up over time	_____	_____	_____
	5b. Outlines plans for working with patient—a certain number of sessions over a certain period of time with occasional contact by phone and mail	_____	_____	_____
6. Counselor uses principles of good communication.	6a. Uses primarily open-ended questions (rather than those answered by yes or no)	_____	_____	_____
	6b. Guards against doing most of the talking; shows ability to listen	_____	_____	_____
	6c. Is able to tolerate periods of silence	_____	_____	_____
	6d. Shows nonjudgmental, noncritical attitude toward patient's eating pattern and chosen lifestyle	_____	_____	_____
	6e. Uses words patient can understand			
7. Counselor communicates interest and confidence both nonverbally and verbally.	7a. Shows poise and interest through posture and "body language"	_____	_____	_____
	7b. Has frequent eye contact with patient	_____	_____	_____
	7c. Uses gestures and words to encourage patient to communicate freely, without putting words in patient's mouth	_____	_____	_____
Counseling Approaches				
8. Counselor is aware that the change process is the responsibility of the patient.	8a. Does not assume responsibility for changes or consequences	_____	_____	_____
	8b. Does not become too ego-involved in patient's eventual success or failure	_____	_____	_____
9. Counselor is aware of need for patient to recognize manageable goals.	9a. Helps patient choose an initial goal that is easily achieved	_____	_____	_____
	9b. Helps patient set specific and short-term goals that are progressively more challenging	_____	_____	_____
	9c. Is able to help patient evaluate goals	_____	_____	_____
	9d. Helps patient avoid failure through too large or too many goals	_____	_____	_____
10. Counselor is able to help patient set up recordkeeping and/or tally systems.	10a. Can help patient verbalize a method appropriate to the task	_____	_____	_____
	10b. Can suggest alternate methods for patient's consideration without dictating choice	_____	_____	_____
	10c. Emphasizes need for accurate records	_____	_____	_____

Nutrition Information for Particular Patient	Performance Objectives	Needs More Work	Not Attempted Yet	Good
Counseling Approaches—cont'd				
	10d. Is able to help patient review food records patient can understand	_____	_____	_____
11. Counselor is aware of the need to examine and anticipate obstacles that will interfere with progress.	11a. Can review with patient potential obstacles in social, personal, and physical environments	_____	_____	_____
	11b. Can help patient identify actual or potential problems and deal with these by encouraging patient to restructure environment and by role playing problem situations with him or her	_____	_____	_____
	11c. Discusses how patient will deal with possible failure	_____	_____	_____
12. Counselor is able to define own role in giving support and feedback.	12a. Can avoid taking the major responsibility	_____	_____	_____
	12b. Can place the responsibility for change on patient	_____	_____	_____
	12c. Is aware of own biases and belief systems and is able to ignore them	_____	_____	_____
13. Counselor is able to evaluate progress toward the stated goal.	13a. Is able to give patient feedback about progress	_____	_____	_____
	13b. Keeps notes in sufficient detail to depict patient's responsibilities and progress	_____	_____	_____
	13c. Measures progress by a combination of biological measures, food intake evaluation, and subjective judgments, with an emphasis on changing *behavior*	_____	_____	_____
14. Counselor encourages patient to get family and friends involved.	14a. Helps patient recognize their strong influence on him or her, suggests that patient ask openly for their support	_____	_____	_____
	14b. Suggests that patient ask them to participate in some way: sharing new tastes and habits, helping with food selection, limiting inappropriate foods	_____	_____	_____
	14c. Can help patient cope with negative feedback through anticipating and rehearsing problem situations	_____	_____	_____
	14d. Can evaluate whether they are potentially supportive or destructive	_____	_____	_____
	14e. Can utilize them as a support without losing sight of the primary responsibility resting with patient	_____	_____	_____
15. Counselor is able to understand that his or her role is not simply that of information-giver or instructor.	15a. Acts as facilitator for patient	_____	_____	_____
	15b. Is appropriately assertive	_____	_____	_____
	15c. Is able to resist "lecturing"	_____	_____	_____
16. Counselor is aware of the need to keep patient task-oriented.	16a. Recognizes delaying tactics and distractions	_____	_____	_____
	16b. Is able to redirect the session toward specifics	_____	_____	_____
	16c. Responds pleasantly but professionally to patient's attempts at humor	_____	_____	_____

GLOSSARY

A

absorptiometry The measurement based on the uptake of energy from radiation (e.g., photons or X rays) by the tissue or medium being measured (e.g., bone mineral content).

accuracy The degree to which a measured value represents the real, or true, value.

acromion process The spine of the scapula (shoulder blade) extending toward the outside of the body. The acromion process, or tip, is used as an anatomic landmark in arm anthropometric measurements (e.g., midarm circumference and triceps skinfold measurement).

actuarial data Statistical information relating to life expectancy, collected by the insurance industry and used, for example, to develop height-weight charts.

Adequate Intake The recommended daily dietary intake level assumed to be adequate and based on experimentally determined approximations of nutrient intake by a group of healthy people. It is an observational standard used when there are insufficient data available to determine a Recommended Dietary Allowance. One of four nutrient reference intakes included in the Dietary Reference Intakes.

age-adjusted death rate The number of deaths in a specific age group for a given calendar year, divided by the population of the same age group as of July 1 of that year. (The quotient being multiplied by 1000.) Also known as "age-specific" death rate.

air displacement plethysmography An approach to measuring body volume that is based on the difference between the volume of air within an empty chamber of known volume and the volume of air when a subject is inside the chamber. The volume of air the subject displaces when inside the chamber is equivalent to the subject's volume, from which body density and percent body fat can then be calculated.

albumin A serum protein, produced by the liver, used as an indicator of nutritional status.

anabolism The process by which body cells convert simple biological substances into more complex compounds.

android obesity Excess body fat that is predominantly within the abdomen and upper body, as opposed to the hips and thighs. This is the typical pattern of male obesity.

anemia A hemoglobin level below the normal reference range for individuals of the same sex and age.

anergy A less than expected or absent immune reaction in response to the injection of antigens within the skin.

angina pectoris Chest pain caused by lack of oxygen supply (known as ischemia) within the heart muscle or myocardium.

anorexia nervosa A condition of disturbed or disordered eating behavior characterized by a refusal to maintain a minimally normal body weight, an intense fear of gaining weight (not alleviated by losing weight), and a distorted perception of body shape or size in which a person feels overweight (either globally or in certain body areas), despite being markedly underweight.

antecedent A preceding event, condition, or cause. Behaviorists regard an action as being preceded by an antecedent. Behavior modification theory holds that, when antecedents to behaviors are recognized, the antecedents can be modified or controlled to decrease the occurrence of negative behaviors and increase the occurrence of positive behaviors. This is referred to as stimulus control.

anthropometry Measurement of the body (stature, weight, circumferences, and skinfold thickness).

apoproteins Special proteins, found in lipoproteins, that control the interaction and metabolic fate of lipoproteins. Apoproteins activate enzymes that modify the composition and structure of lipoproteins, are involved in the binding and ingestion of lipoproteins by cells, and participate in the exchange of lipids between lipoproteins of different classes.

appendicular skeleton The portion of the skeleton that contains the bones of the limbs, pelvis, clavicles, and scapulae.

Archimedes' principle The fact that an object's volume, when submerged in water, equals the volume of water the object displaces. Thus, if the mass and the volume of a body are known, the density of that body can be calculated. This principle is used to determine whole-body density in hydrostatic weighing.

arm muscle area An indicator of total body muscle calculated from the triceps skinfold thickness and midarm circumference.

arteriography A radiographic study of an artery or arterial system in which contrast medium is injected into an artery to determine the condition of the artery (e.g., narrowing due to atherosclerosis).

atherogenic Atherosclerosis-producing.

atherosclerosis A progressive disorder beginning in childhood with the appearance of lesions in the form of fatty streaks in the lining of the coronary arteries or aorta. These may eventually progress to fatty and fibrous plaques or even larger, more complicated lesions. As the lesions develop, the progressive narrowing of the vessels reduces blood flow to the tissues supplied by the affected vessels.

attenuated Becoming weakened or thinned. For example, X-ray beams are attenuated by passing through body tissue.

auscultation The act of listening for sounds arising from organs (e.g., heart and lungs), typically using a stethoscope.

axial skeleton The part of the skeleton composed of the skull, vertebral column, sternum, and ribs.

B

balance sheet approach The most common method of estimating per capita food availability at the national level. Food exports, nonfood use (e.g., livestock feed, seed, and industrial use), and year-end inventories are subtracted from data on beginning-year inventories, total food production, and imports to arrive at an estimate of per capita food availability.

balloon angioplasty A surgical procedure in which a balloon catheter is inserted through the skin into a narrowed blood vessel and inflated to enlarge its interior opening, or lumen, in order to increase blood flow through the affected vessel.

basal metabolic rate (BMR) An individual's energy expenditure measured in the postabsorptive state (no food consumed during the previous 12 hours) after resting quietly for 30 minutes in a thermally neutral environment. (Room temperature is perceived as neither hot nor cold.)

behavior modification A behavioral change theory that attempts to alter previously learned behavior or to encourage the learning of new behavior through a variety of action-oriented methods, as opposed to changing feelings or thoughts.

Behavior Risk Factor Surveillance System An ongoing data-collection program administered by the U.S. Centers for Disease Control and Prevention to monitor state-level prevalence of the major behavioral risks associated with the leading causes of premature morbidity and mortality. It provides state-specific data on personal health behavior and disease risk factors, which allow states to better target their resources for disease risk factor intervention and health promotion activities.

beriberi A disease resulting from thiamin deficiency and characterized by nervous tingling throughout the body, poor arm-leg coordination, deep calf muscle pain, heart enlargement, and occasional edema.

bias A measure of inaccuracy or departure from accuracy.

binge eating The practice of eating an unusually large amount of food in a discrete period of time.

bioelectrical impedance The measure of resistance to an alternating current in an organism. Used to estimate total body water from which percent body fat and lean body mass can be calculated using various equations.

biological marker A nutrient, food component, or metabolite that can be objectively measured and used to represent dietary or nutrient intake.

biopsy The removal and examination of tissue samples to determine the presence or concentration of certain nutrients (or the presence or absence of disease).

BMI Body mass index.

body cell mass The metabolically active, energy-requiring mass of the body.

body composition The proportions of various tissues (fat, muscle, and bone) or elements (e.g., hydrogen, potassium, carbon, calcium, nitrogen) making up the body, usually expressed as percent body fat and percent lean body mass.

body density The mass of the body per unit volume, generally measured by hydrostatic weighing. Percent body fat can then be estimated from body density using the Siri or Brozek equations.

body mass index *See* Quetelet's index.

bulimia nervosa An eating disorder characterized by episodes of binge eating followed by some behavior to prevent weight gain, such as purging, fasting, or exercising excessively.

bypass surgery A surgical procedure creating an auxiliary flow, a shunt, or a pathway around a diseased or malfunctioning body area to restore normal or nearly normal body function (e.g., coronary bypass, intestinal bypass).

C

cachexia Profound physical wasting and malnutrition usually associated with chronic disease, advanced acquired immune deficiency syndrome, alcoholism, or drug abuse.

cadaver A dead body used for anatomic, anthropometric, or other study. Only by analyzing cadavers can direct measurement of human body composition be made.

calorie count Calculation of the energy and nutrient value of foods eaten by a subject, such as a hospitalized patient.

calorimetry Measurement of a subject's energy expenditure.

cancer A group of diseases characterized by abnormal growth of cells that, when uncontrolled, invade other tissues or organs, interfering with their normal function and nutrition.

cardiovascular disease A variety of pathologic processes pertaining to the heart and blood vessels (coronary artery disease and hypertension).

case-control study Comparison of current disease status with the level of past exposure to some factor of interest (e.g., some nutrient or dietary component) in two groups of subjects (cases and controls), in an attempt to determine how past exposure to the factor relates to currently existing disease.

catabolism The breaking down of more complex compounds into simple biological substances, generally resulting in energy release.

cerebrovascular disease A group of disorders, characterized by decreased blood supply to the brain, resulting from hemorrhage of or atherosclerosis within the cerebral arteries.

CHD Coronary heart disease.

CHI Creatinine-height index.

cholesterol A fatlike sterol found in animal products and normally produced by the body. It serves as a precursor for bile acids and steroid hormones and is an essential component of the plasma membrane and the myelin sheaths of nerves. Serum cholesterol levels are causally related to risk for coronary artery disease.

chronic disease A disease progressing over a long period of time, such as coronary heart disease, certain cancers, stroke, diabetes mellitus, and atherosclerosis.

chylomicrons Lipoproteins synthesized in the small intestine that transport dietary triglycerides from the small intestine to adipose tissue, muscle, and the liver. They are 90% triglyceride by weight and are naturally found in serum shortly after meals, but they are not normally present in fasting serum.

cirrhosis Inflammation of the interstitial tissue of an organ, especially the liver.

closed questions Questions that are restrictive and allow an interviewer to control answers and ask for specific information. They are often answered by a simple yes or no response.

coding Assigning a number to each food item recorded in a 24-hour recall or food record that identifies the food for purposes of computerized nutrient analysis.

coefficient of variation (CV) A measure of precision calculated by dividing the standard deviation by the mean and multiplying by 100 (CV = SD ÷ mean × 100).

cognitive restructuring Elimination of negative, irrational thoughts through increasing awareness of one's self-talk, disputing and changing negative self-talk, and using cognitive rehearsal and thought stopping.

cohort study *See* longitudinal study.

computed tomography (CT) An imaging technique producing highly detailed cross-sectional body images from computerized processing of X-ray beam transmission through body tissues of differing density.

computer hardware The physical components of a computer (e.g., the monitor, disc drives, central processing unit, and keyboard).

conjunctival impression cytology Microscopic examination of the conjunctival epithelial cells used to detect early morphologic changes indicative of vitamin A deficiency.

consequences Events that follow and are causally linked to certain behaviors. Consequences reinforce, or reward, the behavior they follow, and they may be positive, negative, or neutral. When consequences are positive, behavior is more likely to be repeated. Behavior followed by negative consequences is less likely to be repeated.

Continuing Survey of Food Intakes by Individuals (CSFII) A national survey of individual dietary intake intended to be conducted annually by the USDA (except when the Nationwide Food Consumption Survey is in progress).

coronary heart disease (CHD) A disease of the heart resulting from inadequate circulation of blood to local areas of the heart muscle. The disease is almost always a consequence of focal narrowing of the coronary arteries by atherosclerosis and is known as ischemic heart disease or coronary artery disease.

correlational study A research design in which the occupance of one variable is compared with the occupance of another variable within the same population. The study is useful for generating hypotheses regarding the associations between suspected risk factors and disease risk.

creatine A nitrogen-containing compound, 98% of which is found in muscle in the form of creatine phosphate. Creatine spontaneously dehydrates to form creatinine, which is then excreted unaltered in the urine.

creatinine The end product of creatine metabolism. Twenty-four-hour urinary creatinine excretion is used as an index of body muscle mass.

creatinine-height index (CHI) An index or a ratio sometimes used to assess body protein status. CHI = 24-hour urinary creatinine excretion ÷ expected creatinine excretion of a reference adult of the same sex and stature × 100.

cross-sectional survey A study design in which disease and various factors of interest are simultaneously examined in groups at a specific period of time.

CSFII Continuing Survey of Food Intakes by Individuals.

CT Computed tomography.

CV Coefficient of variation.

D

Daily Reference Value (DRV) A dietary reference value serving as a basis for the Daily Values. DRVs are for nutrients (e.g., total fat, cholesterol, total carbohydrate, and dietary fiber) for which no set of standards existed before passage of the Nutrition Labeling and Education Act of 1990.

Daily Value (DV) A dietary reference value appearing on the nutrition labels of foods regulated by the FDA and the USDA as part of the Nutrition Labeling and Education Act of 1990. It is derived from the Daily Reference Values (DRVs) and the Reference Daily Intakes (RDIs). The daily value on food labels shows the percent of the DRVs or RDIs that a serving of food provides.

deciliter (dL) A unit of volume in the metric system. One deciliter equals 10^{-1} liter, 1/10 of a liter, or 100 milliliters.

deficiency diseases Diseases caused by a lack of adequate dietary nutrients, vitamins, or minerals (e.g., rickets, pellagra, beriberi, xerophthalmia, and goiter).

densitometry Measurement of body density.

density *See* body density.

deuterium A radioactive hydrogen isotope having twice the mass of common light hydrogen atoms. Known as "heavy hydrogen."

deuterium oxide "Heavy water" composed of oxygen and deuterium (D_2O or ^2H_2O). Used in the determination of total body water.

DHHS United States Department of Health and Human Services.

diabetes mellitus A metabolic disorder characterized by inadequate insulin secretion by the pancreas or the inability of certain cells to use insulin and resulting in abnormally high serum glucose levels. Diabetes mellitus can be classified as type 1 diabetes, type 2 diabetes, or gestational diabetes mellitus (GDM).

Dietary Goals for the United States Seven dietary goals established by the U.S. Senate Select Committee on Nutrition and Human Needs in 1977 for improving the quality of the American diet.

Dietary Reference Intakes Reference values that are quantitative estimates of nutrient intakes to be used for planning and assessing diets for apparently healthy people in various life-stage and gender groups in the United States and Canada. The Dietary Reference Intakes include the Estimated Average Requirement, the Recommended Dietary Allowance, the Adequate Intake, and the Tolerable Upper Intake Level.

diet history An approach to assessing an individual's usual dietary intake over an extended period of time (e.g., past month or year). This typically involves Burke's four assessment steps: collecting general information about the subject's health habits, questioning the subject about his or her usual eating pattern, performing a "cross check" on the data given in step 2, and having the subject complete a 3-day food record.

Diet Quality Index An instrument developed by researchers at the Department of Nutrition at the University of North Carolina, Chapel Hill, to assess the overall diet quality of groups and to evaluate risk for chronic disease related to dietary pattern.

dilution techniques An approach to indirectly measure total body water (TBW). A known concentration and volume of a tracer is given to a subject orally or parenterally, time is allowed for the tracer to equilibrate with the subject's body water, and the concentration of the tracer is analyzed in a sample of the subject's blood, urine, or saliva.

direct calorimetry Measurement of the body's heat output using an airtight, thermally insulated living chamber.

distal Away from the center of the body.

diurnal variations Cyclical changes occurring throughout the day.

dL Deciliter.

DPA Dual-photon absorptiometry.

DRV Daily Reference Value.

dual-energy X-ray absorptiometry (DXA) An approach for measuring bone mineral content in the appendicular skeleton, axial skeleton, or whole body using an X-ray source operating at two energy levels.

dual-photon absorptiometry (DPA) An approach for measuring bone mineral content using photons at two different energy levels derived from a radioisotopic source (gadolinium-153).

duplicate food collections A direct method of calculating nutrient intake in which subjects place an identical portion of all foods and beverages consumed during a specified period in collection containers. This is then chemically analyzed at a laboratory for nutrient content, which provides a potentially more accurate determination of actual nutrient intake; it is compared with calculations based on food composition data.

DV Daily Value.

DXA Dual-energy X-ray absorptiometry.

E

electrolyte An electrically charged particle (anion or cation), present in solution within the body, that is capable of conducting an electrical charge. Sodium, chloride, potassium, and bicarbonate are electrolytes commonly found in the body.

enrichment The replacement of certain nutrients lost in food during processing according to some standard stipulated by law.

enteral nutrition The delivery of food or nutrients into the esophagus, stomach, or small intestine through tubes to improve nutritional status.

epidemiology The study of the distribution and determinants of disease and health outcomes in human populations in order to generate evidence that contributes to the prevention of disease and adverse health outcomes and the promotion of health.

erythrocyte Red blood cell, or RBC.

essential lipid The small amount of lipid (constituting about 1.5% to 3% of lean body weight), serving as a structural component of cell membranes and the nervous system, that is necessary for life.

Estimated Average Requirement The daily dietary intake level estimated to meet the nutrient requirement of 50% of healthy individuals in a particular life stage and gender group. One of four nutrient reference intakes included in the Dietary Reference Intakes.

estimated food record A method of recording individual food intake in which the amounts and types of all food and beverages are recorded for a specific period of time, usually ranging from 1 to 7 days. Portion sizes are estimated using household measures (e.g., cups, tablespoons, teaspoons), a ruler, or containers (e.g., coffee cups, bowls, glasses). Certain items (e.g., eggs, apples, 12-ounce cans of soda) are counted as units.

etiology The cause of a disease or an abnormal condition.

F

false negative Nutrient intake misclassified as adequate when it is actually inadequate.

false positive Nutrient intake misclassified as inadequate when it is actually adequate.

fatty streak The initial step of atherosclerosis, usually beginning in childhood, in which lipids (primarily cholesterol and its esters) become deposited in macrophages and smooth muscle cells within the inner lining of large elastic and muscular arteries.

FDA Food and Drug Administration.

femtoliter (fL) A unit of volume in the metric system. One femtoliter equals 10^{-15} liter.

ferritin The combination of the protein apoferritin and iron that functions as the primary storage form for body iron. It is primarily found in the liver, spleen, and bone marrow.

ferritin model A model for assessing the prevalence of iron deficiency, requiring abnormal values for at least two of the following measurements: serum ferritin level, transferrin saturation, and erythrocyte protoporphyrin level.

fibrous plaque A collection of lipids within the arterial walls during adolescence and early adulthood, creating a projection into the channel, or lumen, of the artery, resulting in impaired blood flow and oxygen delivery to a tissue or an organ.

fL Femoliter.

food balance sheet *See* balance sheet approach.

food exchange system A meal planning method, originally developed for the diabetic diet, that simplifies control of energy consumption, helps ensure adequate nutrient intake, and allows considerable variety in food selection.

food frequency questionnaire A questionnaire listing foods on which individuals indicate how often they consume each listed item during certain time intervals (daily, weekly, or monthly). Standard portion sizes are used and an estimate of nutrient intake is provided on the questionnaire. Sometimes referred to as the semi-quantitative food frequency or list-based diet history approach.

food inventory record An approach to household food consumption measurement in which total household food use is calculated by subtracting food on hand at the end of the survey period (ending inventory) from the sum of food on hand at the start of the survey period (beginning inventory) and food brought into the household during the survey.

food list-recall approach A method of measuring household food consumption in which an interviewer, using a detailed listing of foods, asks the respondent to recall the amount of food used by the household during the preceding week and the amount paid for purchased items. This approach has been used in the Nationwide Food Consumption Survey (NFCS).

fortification The addition of nutrients to food at a nutrient concentration greater than originally present and/or the addition of nutrients not initially existing in food.

four-compartment model A body composition model viewing the body as being composed of four chemical groups: water, protein, mineral, and fat.

Frankfort horizontal plane An imaginary plane intersecting the lowest point on the margin of the orbit (the bony socket of the eye) and the tragion (the notch above the tragus, the cartilaginous projection just anterior to the external opening of the ear). This plane should be horizontal with the head and in line with the spine.

G

g Gram.

generalized equations Regression equations for estimating body density or percent body fat from anthropometric measures that are applicable to population groups varying widely in adiposity and age.

glycosylated hemoglobin Hemoglobin bound to glucose. Under conditions of healthy blood glucose control, a certain percentage of hemoglobin can be expected to be glycated, or bound to glucose. Under conditions of elevated blood glucose levels (e.g., poorly controlled diabetes), the percent of glycosylated hemoglobin is increased.

goiter Thyroid gland enlargement caused by dietary iodine deficiency.

gram A unit of mass in the metric system. One gram equals 10^{-3} kilogram, 1 pound equals 453.5924 grams, and 1 ounce equals 28.350 grams.

gynoid obesity Excess body fat that is predominantly within the hips and thighs, as opposed to within the abdomen and upper body. This is the usual pattern of female obesity.

H

HANES Health and Nutrition Examination Survey.

HDL High-density lipoprotein.

Healthy Eating Index An instrument developed by the U.S. Department of Agriculture to provide a single summary measure of overall dietary quality.

height-weight indices Various ratios or indices expressing body weight in terms of height. Among these are Quetelet's index and Benn's index.

hemoglobin The iron-containing protein pigment of red blood cells that carries oxygen to body cells. Blood hemoglobin levels can reflect iron status (e.g., abnormally low hemoglobin may mean anemia).

HHANES Hispanic Health and Nutrition Examination Survey.

high-density lipoprotein (HDL) A serum lipoprotein synthesized by the liver and intestine that transports cholesterol within the bloodstream. As the serum level of HDL increases, risk of coronary artery disease decreases.

hydrostatic weighing Underwater weighing. The most widely used technique of determining whole-body density, based on Archimedes' principle.

hydroxyapatite Calcium and phosphate crystals providing rigidity to teeth and bones.

hyperlipidemia Excessively high levels of lipids in the blood.

hypermetabolism An increased rate of energy and protein metabolism accompanying trauma, infection, burns, or surgery.

hypertension Persistently elevated arterial blood pressure.

hypervitaminosis A An excessive consumption of vitamin A.

I

IDL Intermediate-density lipoproteins.

iliac crest   The crest, or top, of the ilium (the largest of three bones making up the outer half of the pelvis). The crest is the bony spine located just below the waist. Used as an anatomic landmark in skinfold measurement sites.

impedance   The opposition to an alternating current, composed of two elements: resistance and reactance.

imputed data   Data used by compilers of food composition tables when certain nutrient data are unavailable. These data are obtained from similar foods or ingredients for which data are more complete.

incidence   The number of new events or cases of a disease in a defined population, within a specified time period.

index of nutritional quality (INQ)   A concept related to nutrient density that allows the quantity of a nutrient per 1000 kcal in a food, meal, or diet to be compared with a nutrient standard.

indirect colorimetry   The determination of energy expenditure by measuring the body's oxygen consumption and carbon dioxide production.

infarct   The death of local tissues fed by an obstructed artery or occluded venous drainage because of insufficient blood supply.

infectious disease   Any disease caused by the invasion and multiplication of microorganisms, such as bacteria, fungi, or viruses.

infrared interactance   When infrared light is projected through the skin, some of the energy is reflected from the skin and underlying tissues. Estimates of body composition are made by analyzing certain characteristics of this reflected energy.

INQ   Index of nutritional quality.

intermediate-density lipoproteins (IDL)   Lipoprotein particles created by the removal of triglycerides from VLDL. IDL is a midway product in the conversion of VLDL to LDL.

International Unit (IU)   An amount defined by the International Conference for Unification of Formulae and used to express the quantity of certain substances.

intraindividual variability   Change in an individual's nutrient intake from day to day.

in vivo neutron activation analysis   *See* neutron activation analysis.

iron deficiency   The depletion of body iron stores, corresponding to the second and third stages in the development of iron deficiency.

iron-deficiency anemia   A low hemoglobin value found in association with iron deficiency. Theoretically, anemia corresponds to the third stage of iron deficiency.

iron overload   An excessive accumulation of iron storage in tissues.

ischemia   Impaired blood flow, causing oxygen-nutrition deprivation to associated tissues, resulting in pain (e.g., angina pectoris) or, if severe enough, tissue death, as in heart attack.

IU   International Unit.

J

joule   A unit of work or energy in the metric system. The amount of work done by a force of 1 newton acting over the distance of 1 meter. *See also* kilojoule.

K

kat/L   The SI unit of enzyme activity. One katal per liter is the amount of enzyme necessary to catalyze a reaction at the rate of 1 mole of substrate per second per liter (mol $\cdot$ s^{-1} $\cdot$ L^{-1}).

kcal   Kilocalorie.

kg   Kilogram.

kilocalorie (kcal)   The amount of energy required to raise the temperature of 1 liter of water 1° C. A unit of heat equal to 1000 calories. Also known as a large calorie. One kcal equals 0.239 kilojoule.

kilogram (kg)   A unit of mass in the metric system. One kilogram equals 1000 grams, or 2.2046 pounds.

kilojoule (kj)   A unit of work or energy in the metric system. A kilojoule equals 1000 joules. A kilojoule is equivalent to 4.18 kcal. *See also* joule.

kj   Kilojoule.

kwashiorkor   A protein deficiency, generally seen in children, characterized by edema, growth failure, and muscle wasting.

L

lapse   A single or temporary recurrence of an unwanted habit or behavior that one has overcome or has turned from for a period of time.

LDL   Low-density lipoprotein.

LDL receptors   Molecules on the surface of plasma membranes of hepatic and peripheral cells that recognize and remove low-density lipoprotein from the blood.

leading question   A question that contains an implicit or explicit suggestion about the expected desired answer.

lipoproteins   Spherical macromolecular complexes of lipids (triglycerides, cholesterol, cholesterol esters, and phospholipids) and special proteins known as apoproteins that transport lipids from sites of absorption or synthesis to sites of storage or metabolism via the blood. They include chylomicrons, LDL, IDL, VLDL, and HDL.

list-based diet history   *See* food frequency questionnaire.

longitudinal study   Cohort study. A study design comparing future exposure to various factors in a group (cohort) of subjects in an attempt to determine how exposure with the factors relates to diseases that may develop.

low-density lipoprotein (LDL)   A serum lipoprotein whose primary role is transporting cholesterol to the various cells of the body. LDL contains approximately 70% of the serum's total cholesterol, is considered the most atherogenic (atherosclerosis-producing) lipoprotein, and is the prime target of attempts to lower serum cholesterol. Low serum levels of LDL cholesterol are desirable.

M

μ The Greek letter mu, used as a prefix in such instances as μg (microgram) and μL (microliter), where it indicates 10^{-6}, or one-millionth.

m Meter.

magnetic resonance imaging (MRI) A technology allowing both imaging of the body and *in vivo* chemical analysis without radiation hazard to the subject.

malnutrition This can mean any nutrition disorder but usually refers to failing health caused by long-term nutritional inadequacies.

marasmic kwashiorkor A combination of chronic energy deficiency and chronic or acute protein deficiency.

marasmus Predominantly an energy (kilocalorie) deficiency presenting with significant loss of body weight, skeletal muscle, and adipose tissue mass, but with serum protein concentrations relatively intact.

MCV Mean corpuscular (red blood cell) volume.

MCV model A model for assessing the prevalence of iron deficiency that requires abnormal values for at least two of the following measurements: mean corpuscular volume, transferrin saturation, or erythrocyte protoporphyrin level.

mean A value calculated by summing all the observations in a sample and dividing the sum by the number of observations. Also referred to as the arithmetic mean or, simply, average. One of three measures of central tendency, along with median and mode.

median The observation that divides the distribution into equal halves, with 50% of the observations above and 50% of the observations below this point. Also known as the 50th percentile. One of the three measures of central tendency, along with mean and mode.

menopause The cessation of monthly menses.

meter (m) A unit of distance in the metric system. One meter equals 100 centimeters, 1000 millimeters, and 39.37 inches.

Metropolitan relative weight An individual's actual body weight divided by the midpoint value of weight range for a given height (obtained from a Metropolitan Life Insurance Company height-weight table) and then multiplied by 100. *See also* relative weight.

mg Milligram.

MI Myocardial infarction.

midaxillary line An imaginary line running vertically through the middle of the axilla, used as an anatomic landmark in skinfold measurements.

milligram (mg) A unit of mass in the metric system. 10^{-3} gram, or one-thousandth of a gram.

millimeter (mm) A unit of distance in the metric system. 10^{-3} meter, or 1/1000 of a meter.

millimole (mmol) 10^{-3} mole, or 1/1000 of a gram.

missing foods Foods eaten but not reported by participants of nutritional surveys.

mm Millimeter.

mmol Millimole.

mode The observation that occurs most frequently. One of the three measures of central tendency, along with mean and median.

modeling Observational learning, or imitation. A learning process in behavior modification in which observers learn new behaviors by watching the actions of a model.

morbidity Illness or sickness.

morphology The study of the shape and structure of organisms, organs, or parts.

mortality Death.

myocardial infarction (MI) Heart attack. The death of an area of heart tissue caused by blockage of the coronary artery feeding that area.

myocardium Heart muscle.

N

National Health and Nutrition Examination Survey (NHANES) A continuous, annual cross-sectional survey, conducted by the U.S. Department of Health and Human Services, that assesses food intake, height, weight, blood pressure, vitamin and mineral levels, and a number of other health parameters in a statistically selected group of Americans.

National Nutrition Monitoring System (NNMS) A congressionally mandated system in which the USDA and USDHHS are to work cooperatively in collecting data relating to health and nutritional status measurements, food composition measurements, dietary knowledge, attitude assessment, and surveillance of the food supply.

Nationwide Food Consumption Survey (NFCS) A survey of food consumption at the household and individual levels, conducted by the USDA.

NCEP National Cholesterol Education Program.

NCHS National Center for Health Statistics.

negative nitrogen balance A condition in which nitrogen loss from the body exceeds nitrogen intake. Negative nitrogen balance is often seen in the case of illness, trauma, burns, or recovery from major surgery.

negative reinforcer An unpleasant consequence of a behavior that maintains and strengthens the behavior by the negative reinforcer's being removed from the situation.

neutral questions Questions that allow a client to respond without pressure or direction from the interviewer.

neutron activation analysis A technology allowing in vivo measurement of the body's content of calcium, iodine, hydrogen, sodium, chloride, phosphorus, carbon, and other elements. A neutron beam is directed to the subject, and the response of various elements within the body allows estimation of the quantities of these elements.

NFCS Nationwide Food Consumption Survey.

NHANES National Health and Nutrition Examination Survey.

NHANES I The first National Health and Nutrition Examination Survey.

NHANES II The second National Health and Nutrition Examination Survey.

NHANES III The third National Health and Nutrition Examination Survey.

NHES National Health Examination Survey.

nitrogen balance A condition in which nitrogen losses from the body are equal to nitrogen intake. Nitrogen balance is the expected state of the healthy adult.

NLEA Nutrition Labeling and Education Act.

NMR Nuclear magnetic resonance.

nomogram A graphic device with several vertical scales allowing calculation of certain values when a straightedge is connected between two scales and the desired value is read from a third scale.

nonambulatory Unable to walk (ambulate).

nonquantitative food frequency questionnaire A food frequency questionnaire assessing frequency of food consumption but not the size of food servings.

nuclear magnetic resonance (NMR) Earlier name for magnetic resonance imaging (MRI).

nutrient database A compilation of data on the nutrient content of various foods. The database may exist in book form or as an electronic file accessible by computer.

nutrient density The nutritional composition of foods expressed in terms of nutrient quantity per 1000 kcal. If the quantity of nutrients per 1000 kcal is great enough, then the nutrient needs of a person will be met when his or her energy needs are met.

nutritional assessment The measurement of indicators of dietary status and nutrition-related health status of individuals or populations to identify the possible occurrence, nature, and extent of impaired nutritional status (ranging from deficiency to toxicity).

nutritional epidemiology The application of epidemiologic principles to the study of how diet and nutrition influence the occurrence of disease.

nutritional monitoring The assessment of dietary or nutritional status at intermittent times with the aim of detecting changes in the dietary or nutritional status of a population.

nutritional screening The process of identifying characteristics known to be associated with nutrition problems in order to pinpoint individuals who are malnourished or at risk for malnutrition.

nutritional surveillance Continuous assessment of nutritional status for the purpose of detecting changes in trend or distribution in order to initiate corrective measures.

Nutrition Labeling and Education Act (NLEA) A law passed by the U.S. Congress in 1990, mandating nutrition labeling for virtually all processed foods regulated by the U.S. Food and Drug Administration, authorizing appropriate health claims on food labels, and calling for activities to educate consumers about food labels.

O

obesity An excessive accumulation of body fat.

observational standards A dietary standard based on clinical observation, as opposed to scientific measurement of actual need.

olecranon process The bony projection of the distal ulna at the elbow. Used as an anatomic landmark in upper-arm anthropometric measurements.

open questions Questions providing individuals with considerable freedom in deciding the amount and type of information to give in answering an interviewer's questions.

osteoporosis A condition in which bone mineral content is decreased, resulting in greater susceptibility to bone fracture, deformity, and pain.

overnutrition The condition resulting from the excessive intake of foods in general or particular food components.

overweight Body weight in excess of a particular standard and sometimes used as an index of obesity.

P

parallax The apparent difference in the reading of a measurement scale (e.g., a skinfold caliper's needle) when viewed from various points not in a straight line with the eye.

parenteral nutrition The process of administering nutrients directly into veins to improve nutritional status.

pellagra A niacin deficiency syndrome characterized by inflamed mucous membranes, mental deterioration, diarrhea, and eruptions in skin areas exposed to light or injury.

PEM Protein-energy malnutrition.

percentiles Divisions of a distribution into equal, ordered subgroups of hundredths. The 50th percentile is the median. The 90th percentile, for example, is an observation whose value exceeds 90% of the set of observations and is exceeded by only 10%.

peripheral vascular disease Atherosclerotic changes within the aorta, iliac, and femoral arteries, affecting blood flow in the body's periphery.

pg Picograms.

phantom foods Foods not eaten but reported as having been eaten by participants of nutrition surveys.

picograms (pg) A unit of mass in the metric system. One picogram equals 10^{-12} gram, or one-trillionth of a gram.

plethysmography *See* air displacement plethysmography.

population-specific equations Regression equations for estimating body density or percent body fat from anthropometric measures that can be applied only to population groups sharing certain features, such as sex, age, and adiposity.

positive nitrogen balance Nitrogen intake exceeds nitrogen loss from the body. This is commonly seen during growth, pregnancy, and recovery from trauma, surgery, or illness.

positive reinforcer Any consequence (reward) that maintains and strengthens behavior by its presence. (The positive reinforcer makes the behavior more likely to recur.)

postprandial After a meal.

power-type indices Indices such as Quetelet's index and Benn's index.

precision The difference in results when the same measurement is repeatedly performed on the same sample.

prevalence The existing cases of a disease or another condition in a given population at a designated time.

protein-energy malnutrition (PEM) An inadequate consumption of protein and energy, resulting in a gradual body wasting and increased susceptibility to infection.

provisional tables Provisional data supplied by the United States Department of Agriculture for special nutrients or foods, such as dietary fiber, bakery foods, vitamin K, fatty acids, and sugar, that are often released years before more complete data are available.

proximal Toward the center of the body.

Q

QCT Quantitative computed tomography.

quantitative computed tomography (QCT) An imaging technique consisting of an array of X-ray sources and radiation detectors aligned opposite each other. As the X-ray beams pass through the subject, they are weakened, or attenuated, by the body's tissues and eventually picked up by the detectors. Data from the detectors are then transmitted to a computer, which reconstructs the subject's cross-sectional anatomy, using mathematic equations adapted for computer processing.

quantitative food frequency questionnaire *See* semi-quantitative food frequency questionnaire.

quantitative ultrasound The transmission of high-frequency sound waves through bone to determine its fracture risk.

Quetelet's index Weight in kilograms divided by height in meters squared (kg/m^2). The most widely used weight-height or power-type index.

R

rational-emotive therapy (RET) A counseling approach based on the premise that emotional disturbances are a product of irrational thinking. RET holds that emotions are primarily the result of our beliefs, evaluations, interpretations, and reactions to life situations, which in turn determine our behavior. Behavior is altered by correcting the thought process using methods such as cognitive restructuring, language changing, cognitive rehearsal, and thought stopping.

RDA Recommended Dietary Allowance.

RDIs Reference Daily Intakes.

reality therapy A therapy based primarily on the work of psychiatrist William Glasser and his premise that every person's behavior is an attempt to fulfill his or her basic human needs (behavior driven completely from within). Emphasis is placed on individual responsibility for actions and client participation in decision making.

Recommended Dietary Allowance The average daily dietary intake level sufficient to meet the nutrient requirement of nearly all (97% to 98%) healthy individuals in a particular life stage or gender group. One of four nutrient reference intakes included in the Dietary Reference Intakes.

recumbent The position of lying down. Recumbent length, for example, is obtained with the subject lying down and is generally reserved for children younger than 24 months of age or for children between 24 and 36 months who cannot stand erect without assistance.

REE Resting energy expenditure.

Reference Daily Intakes (RDIs) A set of dietary references that serves as the basis for the Daily Values and are based on the Recommended Dietary Allowances (RDAs) for essential vitamins and minerals and, in selected groups, protein. The RDIs replace the U.S. Recommended Daily Allowances (U.S. RDAs).

regression equations Equations developed by comparing a variety of anthropometric measures with measurements of body density (usually by hydrostatic weighing) to see which anthropometric measures are best at predicting body density. A statistical process called multiple-regression analysis is used to develop the equations.

relapse The resumption of an unwanted habit or behavior that one has, for a period of time, overcome or turned from.

relative weight A subject's actual body weight divided by the midpoint value of weight range for a given height and then multiplied by 100. *See also* Metropolitan relative weight.

reliability *See* reproducibility.

remodeling The dynamic process of skeletal change in which bones are constantly undergoing resorption and reformation.

reproducibility Also known as reliability. The ability of a method to yield the same measurement value on two or more different occasions, assuming that nothing has changed in the interim.

resting energy expenditure (REE) Also known as resting metabolic rate. This term is used for metabolic rate or energy expenditure in the awake, resting, and postabsorptive individual.

RET Rational-emotive therapy.

rickets A condition, especially found in infants and children, characterized by malformed bones, delayed fontanel closure, and muscle pain, due to a deficiency of vitamin D.

S

scurvy An ascorbic acid (vitamin C) deficiency disease characterized by anemia, spongy and bleeding gums, and capillary hemorrhages.

self-contract An agreement an individual makes with himself or herself to help build commitment to behaviorial change.

semi-quantitative food frequency questionnaire A food frequency questionnaire that assesses both frequency and portion size of food consumption. *See also* food frequency questionnaire.

sensitivity A test's ability to indicate an abnormality where there is one.

serum proteins Proteins present in serum (the liquid portion of clotted blood) that are often regarded as indicators of the body's visceral protein status (e.g., albumin).

shortfall nutrients Nutrients whose intakes are below recommended levels among a significant part of the population.

SI Système International.

signs Observations made by a qualified examiner during a physical examination.

single-photon absorptiometry (SPA) An approach for measuring bone mineral content using photons at a single energy level derived from a radioisotopic source (iodine-125).

skinfold thickness A double fold of skin that is measured with skinfold calipers at various body sites.

software program The entire set of programs, procedures, and related documentation associated with computer programs. The list of program commands that operate a particular program on the computer.

somatic protein Protein contained in the body's skeletal muscles.

SPA Single-photon absorptiometry.

specificity A test's ability to indicate normalcy where there is no abnormality.

stadiometer A device capable of measuring stature in children over 2 years of age and in adults. This measure is taken in a standing position.

standard deviation A measure of how much a frequency distribution varies from the mean.

stature Standing height.

stimulus control A behavior modification technique in which behavioral antecedents are recognized and modified or controlled to decrease the occurrence of negative behaviors and to increase the occurrence of positive behaviors.

stroke A blockage or rupture of a blood vessel supplying the brain, with resulting loss of consciousness, paralysis, or other symptoms.

Subjective Global Assessment A clinical approach to assessing the nutritional status of a patient using information gained from the patient's history and physical examination.

supine The position in which one is lying on his or her back.

surrogate source A source of information about a subject's behavior (e.g., dietary practices) from a source other than the subject. Typical surrogate sources include a spouse, child, close relative, and friend of the subject.

symptoms Disease manifestations that the patient is usually aware of and often complains of.

Système International (SI) An international system of measurement units allowing the interchangeability of information between nations and disciplines.

T

TEF Thermal effect of food.

thermic effect of exercise Energy expenditure resulting from physical activity.

thermic effect of food (TEF) Also known as diet-induced thermogenesis or the specific dynamic action of food. TEF is the increased energy expenditure following food consumption or administration of parenteral or enteral nutrition caused by absorption and metabolism of food and nutrients.

TOBEC Total body electrical conductivity.

Tolerable Upper Intake Level The highest level of daily nutrient intake likely to pose no risk for adverse health effects for almost all apparently healthy individuals in the general population. As intake increases above this level, risk for adverse (toxic) effects increases. One of four nutrient reference intakes included in the Dietary Reference Intakes.

total body electrical conductivity (TOBEC) A method of assessing body composition in which a subject is placed in an electromagnetic field (EMF). Since electrolytes within the fat-free mass are capable of conducting electricity, the degree to which the EMF is disrupted is related to the amount of fat-free mass within the subject's body.

transferrin The form in which iron is transported within the blood.

tritium An isotope of hydrogen having three times the mass of ordinary hydrogen. It is commonly used as a tracer in the determination of total body water.

24-hour recall A method of dietary recall in which a trained interviewer asks the subject to remember in detail all foods and beverages consumed during the past 24 hours. This information is recorded by the interviewer for later coding and analysis.

two-compartment model A body composition model that views the body as being composed of two compartments: fat mass and fat-free mass, or, according to an alternative approach, adipose tissue and lean body mass.

U

ulna The larger, inner bone of the forearm. Used as an anatomic landmark in arm anthropometry.

ultrasound A diagnostic method used for imaging internal organs and estimating the thickness of subcutaneous adipose tissue. High-frequency sound waves are transmitted into the body from a transducer (sound transmitter) applied to the skin surface. As ultrasound strikes the interface between two tissues differing in density (e.g., adipose tissue and muscle), some of it is reflected back and received by the transducer. Alterations between the signal as it is transmitted and received are used to image internal organs and to determine subcutaneous tissue thickness.

undernutrition A condition resulting from the inadequate intake of food in general or particular food components.

underwater weighing *See* hydrostatic weighting.

USDA United States Department of Agriculture.

USRDA U.S. Recommended Daily Allowances.

U.S. Recommended Daily Allowances (USRDA) A set of nutrition standards developed by the FDA for use in regulating the nutrition labeling of food. They were replaced by the Reference Daily Intakes.

V

validity The ability of an instrument to measure what it is intended to measure. Validating a method of measuring dietary intake, for example, involves comparing measurements of intake obtained by that method with intake measurements obtained by some other accepted approach.

very low-density lipoprotein (VLDL) A lipoprotein, present in blood, that is synthesized by the liver and primarily carries triglyceride to cells for storage and metabolism.

viscera Organs of the body (such as liver, kidneys, heart).

visceral protein Protein found in the body's organs or viscera, as well as that in the serum and in blood cells.

VLDL Very low-density lipoprotein.

W

waist circumference The distance around the horizontal plane through the abdomen at the level of the iliac crest of a standing subject. This measurement is used as an index of abdominal fat content.

weighed-food record A method of recording individual food intake in which the amounts and types of all food and beverages are recorded for a specific period of time, usually ranging from 1 to 7 days. Portion sizes are determined by accurate weighing.

weight-height indices *See* height-weight indices.

WIC Special Supplemental Nutrition Program for Women, Infants, and Children.

X

xerophthalmia An eye disease caused by vitamin A deficiency in which the conjunctiva and cornea dry and thicken, in part because of decreased mucus production. If not treated in earlier stages with vitamin A supplements, permanent damage may ensue, with softening of the cornea and subsequent blindness.

INDEX